Pathways to Pregnancy and Parturition

Pathways to Pregnancy and Parturition

P.L. Senger, Ph.D.
Professor of Animal Sciences
Department of Animal Sciences
Washington State University
Pullman, Washington 99164-6332 USA

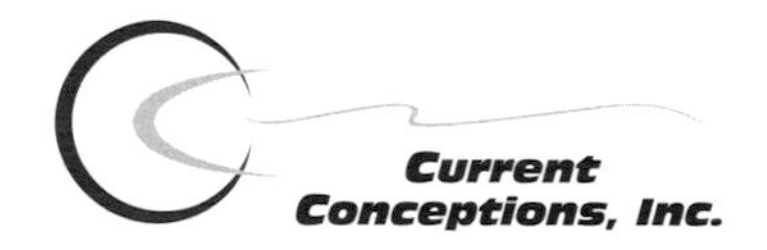

Current Conceptions, Inc.
Washington State University Research & Technology Park
1615 NE Eastgate Blvd.
Pullman, WA 99163-5607

ISBN 0-9657648-0-X

1st Revised Edition
Phillip L. Senger, Author

Printing: The Mack Printing Group-Science Press, Ephrata, PA.

Additional Copies may be ordered from:

Current Conceptions, Inc.
c/o Hayden, Ross, and Co.
Attn: Tracey Hostetler
P.O. Box 9043
315 S. Almon
Moscow, ID 83843

Phone: 208 882 5547
FAX: 208-882-3724

Cover designed by Sonja Oei
Cover photograph credits - Radiography: Vickie L. Mitzimburg and Sonja R. Fenimore
Photography: Henry Moore, Jr.
Pre-press layout by J. Richard Scott

Dedication

To paraphrase Hodding Carter, there are two lasting benefits we can give our students, children and other people we associate with. "**One is roots and the other is wings.**"

This book is dedicated to Dr. R.G. (Dick) Saacke and his wife, Ann, a couple who have been models for countless students, fellow educators/professionals, friends and their own children in emphasizing the importance of uncompromising commitment to high standards and values (**roots**). At the same time, they have always encouraged others to fly and to enjoy their journey (**wings**).

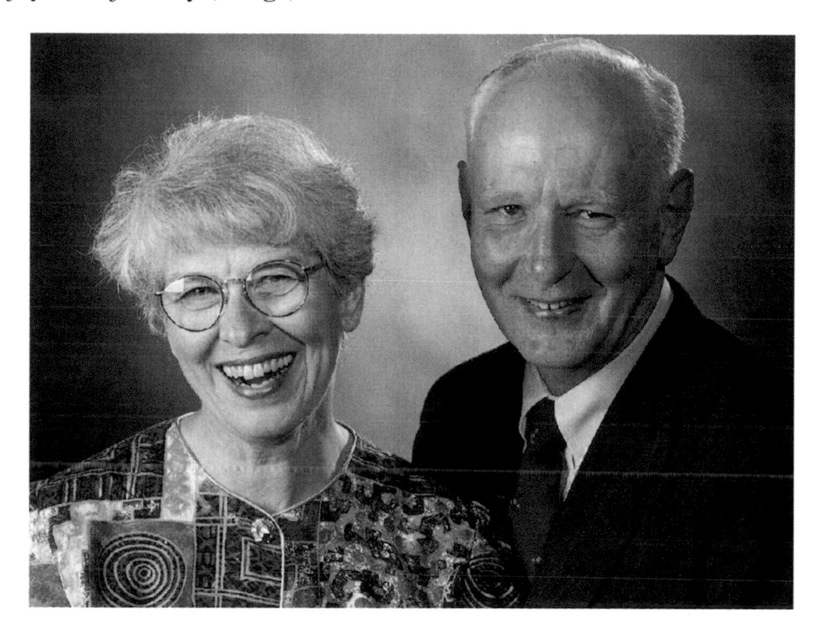

Note: Dedicating an educational instrument in reproductive physiology to Dr. Saacke (my graduate mentor and friend) is something like dedicating a set of blueprints to Frank Lloyd Wright. One is inevitably nervous that the blueprints will not measure up. Regardless, I hope the spirit of trying to enlighten students shows through in this work.

The Author

P.L. (Phil) Senger grew up in Cary, North Carolina and received his B.S. in Zoology from North Carolina State University. He was awarded the M.S. and Ph.D. in reproductive physiology from the Department of Dairy Science at Virginia Polytechnic Institute and State University. He is Professor of Animal Sciences at Washington State University, where his primary teaching responsibilities have included systemic physiology, reproductive physiology and artificial insemination/pregnancy detection. He has authored over 200 scientific, educational and popular press papers. Dr. Senger has received four teaching awards including the American Society of Animal Science Distinguished Teaching Award in 1998, and two awards for research in reproductive physiology. He is married and has three daughters. He enjoys racquetball, skiing, fishing and gardening.

Preface

This book is written for students, not my colleagues. In general, college textbooks are too lofty. They often target the instructor and assume that the students have a higher level of knowledge than they really do. I have tried to strike the proper balance by presenting the main physiologic concepts without unessential detail. At the same time, I have tried to provide a format from which instructors can incorporate additional information according to their own specific priorities and expertise.

I am a firm believer that learning should be stimulating, interesting and fun, not a task. In this light, I have broken textbook tradition and included some humor and amazing notes in "**Further Phenomena for Fertility.**"

Acknowledgements

Inspiration

During preparation of this book, I have received encouragement beyond belief from colleagues all over the world. This has come about because of their strong commitment to educating students in the field of reproductive physiology. The following individuals have provided special encouragement and support throughout the course of this project:

J.R. Carlson
Associate Dean and Associate Director of the Agriculture Research Center
Washington State University
Pullman, WA 99164-6240

E. K. Inskeep, Professor of Animal Sciences
Division of Animal and Veterinary Science
West Virginia University
Morgantown, WV 26506-6108

R.G. Saacke, Professor of Dairy Science
Department of Dairy Science
Virginia Polytechnic Institute and State University
Blacksburg, VA 24061

Martha A. Senger (my wife of 30 years who has supported most everything I wanted to do!)

Blood, Sweat & Tears

This has been, at times, an exhausting process. People with huge work ethics who don't get tired easily have made immense contributions. Students have played an important role in the development of this text. The following are acknowledged for contributions ranging from tireless typing to critical reviews to specimen preparation:

Cheryl A. Dudley (G^3) typed the first drafts of this book entirely from dictation. Her tireless efforts helped this work germinate and develop roots.

Coordinators of Student Reviews (Spring 1995): **Wayne H. Wilson; Jacinda L. Pickett; Sarah N. Hagerty; Joel A. Edmonds**.

This textbook was used and critiqued in draft form by over 300 students at four universities. The following are acknowledged for their contributions and for their patience with the early drafts of this book:

The students in ANPH 225 at West Virginia University (Spring semester, 1996) under the professorships of **Drs. R.A. Dailey**, **E.K. Inskeep**, **R.L. Cochrane**, and **P.E. Lewis**.

The students in AN 310 at Colorado State University (Spring semester, 1996) under the professorship of **Dr. Thomas W. Geary**.

The students in AN 220 at North Carolina State University (Spring semester, 1996) under the professorship of **Dr. Allison M. Benoit**.

The students in AS 350 at Washington State University under the professorships of **Dr. P.L Senger (G^3)** (Spring semester, 1995) and **Dr. J.J. Reeves** (Spring semester, 1996 and 1997).

The following undergraduate students played a direct role in preparing and providing materials for the final product:

Melinda N. Dawson (typing), **Monica E. Axtell (G^3)** (color layout and specimen preparation), **Joel M. Abbott** (specimen preparation), **Amy E. Sroufe (G^3)** (typing), **Jolene L. Schmidt** (specimen acquisition), **Amy E. Senger** (typing and promotion), and **Juan Martín Rivas Poletti** (exchange student, Asuncion, Paraguay).

Know-How and Knowledge

These professionals provided scientific and technical expertise. Without their help, self-publishing this book would have been impossible.

Carolyn C. Abbott - relief graphics.

Jeanne C. Andersen (G^3) - editing/proofing.

Pascal Derde (DVM) - equine specimen removal and preparation, Cavel West, Inc., Redmond, OR.

Vickie L. Mitzimberg and **Sonja R. Fenimore** - radiograph preparation, Veterinary Teaching Hospital, College of Veterinary Medicine, Washington State University.

Henry Moore, Jr. (G^3) and **Charles E. Royce** - all color photography, Biomedical Communications Unit, College of Veterinary Medicine, Washington State University.

Sonja L. Oei (G^3) - graphic illustrations and art.

J. Richard Scott (G^3) - pre-press layout of text and illustrations.

D.L. Snyder - assistance in specimen removal and preparation, Washington State University Meats Laboratory.

Bryan A. Toms - final layout and printing coordination, Science Press, Ephrata, PA.

The following reproductive physiologists made valuable contributions to the scientific content of one or more chapters in this book:

R.P. Amann (Emeritus, Colorado State University)
J.H. Britt (North Carolina State University)
R.A. Dailey (West Virginia University)
D.R. Deaver (Pennsylvania State University)
M.A. Diekman (Purdue University)
M.J. Fields (University of Florida)
S.P. Ford (Iowa State University)
D.W. Forrest (Texas A&M University)
D.L. Foster (University of Michigan)
G.R. Gallagher (Berry College)
T.W. Geary (Colorado State University)
R.D. Geisert (Oklahoma State University)
E.K. Inskeep (West Virginia University)
L. Johnson (Texas A&M University)
J.E. Kinder (University of Nebraska)
J.W. Knight (Virginia Polytechnic Institute and State University)
A.R. Menino, Jr. (Oregon State University)
M.A. Mirando (Washington State University)
M.L. O'Connor (Pennsylvania State University)
J.E. Parks (Cornell University)
J.J. Reeves (Washington State University)
R.G. Sasser (University of Idaho)
R.W. Silcox (Brigham Young University)
C.M. Ulibarri (Washington State University)
C.J.G. Wensing (Institute of Animal Science and Health, Lelystad, The Netherlands)
G.L. Williams (Texas A&M University, Beeville)

During the development of this book a group of eight people made the majority of the day-to-day contributions. As this project evolved, this group became known as "Senger's Gonadal Gossip Gang." The "gang" is pictured on the inside of the back cover, and individuals are identified in the above acknowledgements with "G^3" after their names.

Table of Contents

Pathways to Pregnancy and Parturition

1 Introduction to Reproduction

Take-Home Message

Reproduction is a sequence of events beginning with development of the reproductive system in the embryo. After the animal is born, it must grow and achieve puberty by acquiring the ability to produce fertile gametes. This ability must be accompanied by reproductive behavior and copulation. After copulation, the sperm and egg meet, fertilization occurs, and it is followed by development of the preattachment embryo. The conceptus attaches to the uterus by a specialized organ called the placenta. It allows the conceptus to grow and develop to term. The fully developed fetus is born and the female giving birth to it must reestablish cyclicity before she can become pregnant again.

Reproductive physiology is a relatively new science and most of our knowledge of the subject has been generated during the past 75 years. Both poor reproductive efficiency and high reproductive efficiency are costly. Poor reproductive efficiency results in suboptimal production of animal products. High reproductive efficiency in humans and vermin results in excessive population growth. Knowledge and understanding of the reproductive process will become increasingly important as the human population continues to grow and resources become increasingly scarce.

Welcome to the exciting and fascinating subject of reproductive physiology. Among the many scientific subjects in the natural sciences, knowledge about reproductive physiology commands interest even among those who have no scientific inclination at all. In its broadest sense, the subject of reproductive physiology carries with it interest, imagination, expectation, emotion and an intrinsic desire to know more. The average person on the street couldn't care less about Boyle's Law, Beer's Law, the periodic table or the phylogenetic organization of the plant and animal kingdoms. But, mention copulation, ejaculation, spermatozoa, pregnancy, the uterus, fertilization, embryo development or any of the myriad terms associated with reproduction and most people will be interested. Almost without exception, everyone wants to know more about the reproductive process, whether it relates to humans, food producing animals, their pet or just acquiring more basic knowledge.

Pathways to Pregnancy and Parturition is intended to help you develop a solid scientific understanding of the principles of reproduction in food producing animals. Further, it is intended to help you become fluent in the language of the subject matter. If you develop this fluency, you will enjoy a lifetime of understanding that will enable you to adapt successfully to new knowledge and technology that will affect reproduction in animals as well as humans.

PATHWAYS TO PREGNANCY AND PARTURITION includes the following aids to learning:

- ***sequence maps***
- ***take-home messages***
- ***fact boxes***
- ***bold type words***

As you read the chapters in this book you will encounter several features that are intended to make learning and understanding easy. The text of each chapter begins with a "**Take-Home Message**." This feature provides you with the main points of the chapter before you engage the details. Presenting the "Take-Home Message" first should establish some questions in your mind that will then be answered later in the chapter. The "Take-Home Message" is also intended as a study guide, highlighting the main points of each chapter.

Fact boxes are included throughout each chapter to give you a "quick read" and to highlight important points, terms and/or sequences.

Many words and terms in this textbook are in bold print. Those are important key words. You should understand them, know how to pronounce them, know how to spell them and be able to use them correctly in a discussion or in writing. In addition to the explanations appearing in the text, these terms are also defined in the glossary at the end of the book.

At the end of each chapter is a short section called "**Additional Reading**." Several important sources containing additional in-depth information about the subject of the chapter are listed. In general, these are scientific review papers that will provide detail beyond what is presented in the chapter.

There are some remarkable reproductive phenomena throughout the animal kingdom. The section entitled "**Further Phenomena for Fertility**" is intended to present some of the interesting facts, observations and even myths relating to the topics of each chapter. This section will give species other than food producing animals a place to shine.

Successful reproduction requires an orderly sequence of events. As you use ***Pathways to Pregnancy and Parturition***, you will encounter a "**sequence map**" at the beginning of each chapter (Figure 1-1). In the "sequence map," each major event is represented by a black dot with a white border around it. A sign, reading "**You are here**" lets you know exactly where the chapter you are reading fits in the sequence of reproductive events. Each event in the "sequence map" has one or more chapters dedicated to it. These events are described briefly below.

"Prenatal Development" (Chapter 4)

Sex of the embryo is determined at the time of fertilization. However, the development of a male or a female reproductive tract and the anterior and posterior pituitary occurs during development of the embryo.

"Acquisition of Puberty" (Chapter 6)

After the animal is born, it enters a period of growth and development which precedes the development of reproductive function. After a critical body size is reached, the hypothalamus and pituitary begin to produce hormones and the reproductive system gains full function.

"Tract Function" (Chapters 2 and 3)

Complete anatomical structure and function of the male and female reproductive tract are required before successful reproduction can take place. Knowledge of the function and structure of the reproductive organs is essential for complete understanding.

"Regulation of Reproduction" (Chapter 5)

After the animal reaches puberty, the reproductive system is regulated precisely by an intricate interplay of hormones produced by the anterior pituitary and the gonads. This interplay of hormones results in cyclicity in the female and spermatogenesis in the male.

"Cyclicity" (Chapters 7, 8 and 9)

The female must exhibit estrous cycles. An estrous cycle is characterized as a repeated sequence of events, usually beginning with behavioral estrus (heat) and ending with a subsequent behavioral estrus several weeks later. The estrous cycle consists of the follicular phase and the luteal phase.

"Spermatogenesis" (Chapter 10)

After puberty, the male acquires the ability to produce large quantities of spermatozoa. These spermatozoa are produced on a continual basis in most males. Control of spermatogenesis is under the influence of pituitary hormones. Males are capable of producing between 1 and 25 billion spermatozoa per day.

"Reproductive Behavior and Copulation" (Chapter 11)

One of the characteristics associated with the acquisition of full reproductive potential is the display of reproductive behavior culminating in copulation and deposition of sperm into the female reproductive tract. The physiologic regulation of reproductive behavior is one

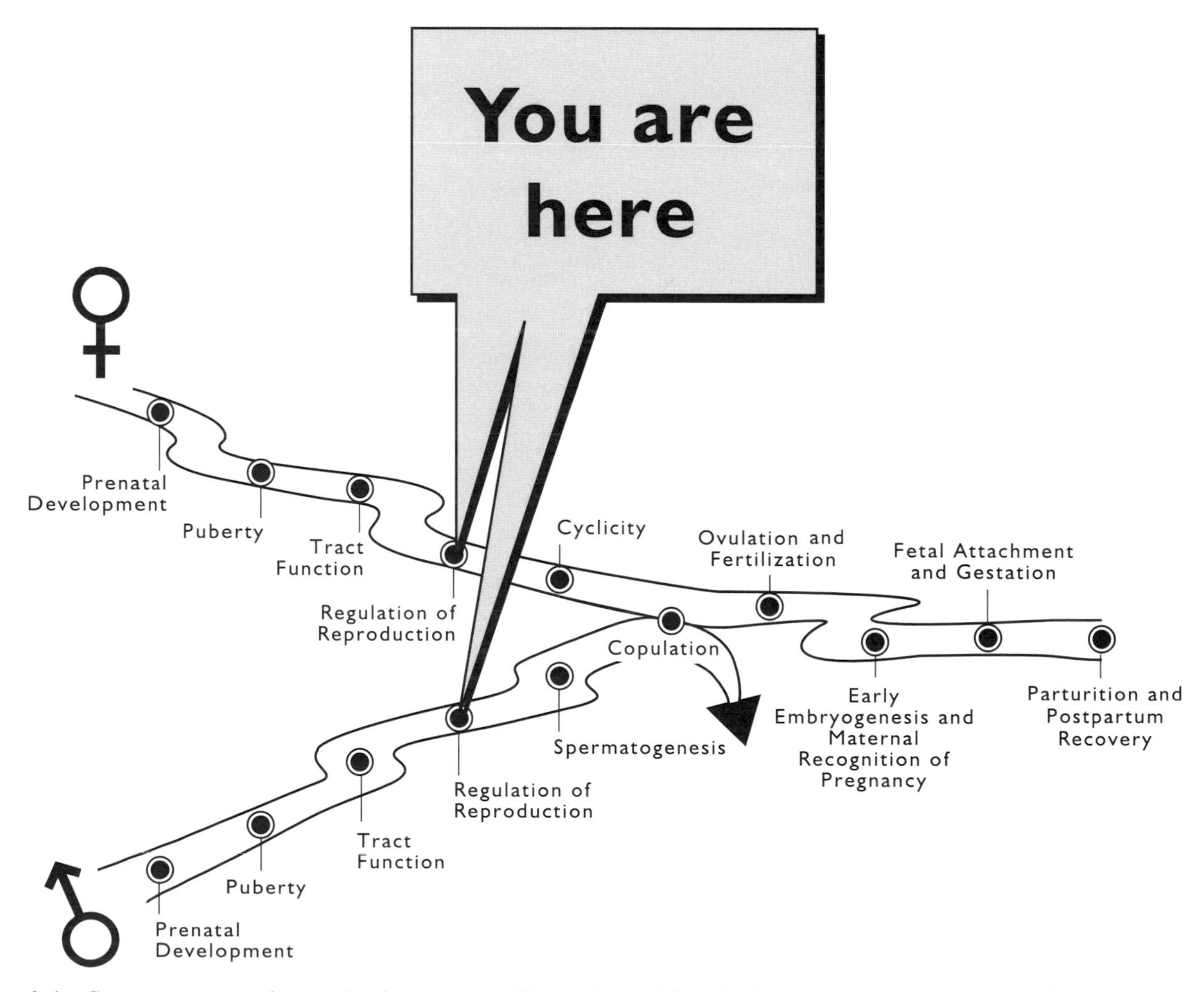

Figure 1-1. Sequence map of reproductive events. The male and female have a common sequence of developmental events until after copulation. After copulation the female bears the responsibility for gestation and parturition. The arrow on the male pathway indicates his departure from the sequence after copulation. The sign "You are here" indicates where the chapter you are reading fits into the sequence of reproductive events.

of the most interesting, yet poorly understood components of reproductive physiology.

"Ovulation and Fertilization" (Chapter 12)

In most species, ovulation occurs after copulation. Fertilization then occurs and is the result of a series of cellular changes in the sperm and the oocyte within the female reproductive tract.

"Early Embryogenesis and Maternal Recognition of Pregnancy" (Chapter 13)

After fertilization, the embryo begins to develop and sends biochemical signals to the dam, physiologically "notifying" her that she is pregnant. Failure of these signals to be sent or recognized results in the termination of pregnancy.

"Placentation and the Endocrinology of Gestation and Parturition" (Chapter 14)

If successful maternal recognition of pregnancy occurs, then the fetus will attach to the uterus, forming a placenta which controls the exchange of nutrients and gases between the fetus and the dam. This transient organ (the placenta) also produces hormones important for successful gestation. Successful birth (parturition) concludes the series of reproductive events. Parturition is a carefully orchestrated interplay of endocrine and muscular events.

The study of reproductive physiology started with Aristotle around 350 B.C. But, most of our knowledge has been generated during the past century.

Now that you know the features of ***Pathways to Pregnancy and Parturition***, you should have some knowledge of the historical development of reproductive physiology and why reproduction is important.

Aristotle provided the first recorded information on how he thought the reproductive system functioned in his book entitled ***Generation of Animals***. He believed that the fetus arose from menstrual blood. He had no way of observing spermatozoa in the ejaculate or the beginnings of embryo development. Therefore, he concluded, based on the observation that menstruation did not occur during pregnancy, that the fetus was derived from menstrual blood. He also proposed that the conversion of menstrual blood to a fetus was initiated by seminal fluid deposited in the female during copulation. Aristotle also thought that semen was derived from all parts of the body and that the testes were simply pendular weights which kept the transport ducts (the ductus deferens) from becoming kinked or plugged with seminal fluid. Considering that Aristotle had no research tools whatsoever, his speculations were not totally unreasonable.

The next major observation in reproductive physiology, occurring almost 2,000 years later, was made by Fallopius, who described the oviducts. The name **Fallopian tube** reflects his discovery. A student of Fallopius, Coiter, discovered the **corpus luteum** in 1573. It wasn't until almost 100 years later that a scientist named Regnier de Graaf described the antral follicle, which has been named the **Graafian follicle** in honor of his discovery. De Graaf killed female rabbits at half-hour intervals after they had copulated. He discovered that the number of "scar-like" wounds on the surface of the ovaries (we now know these to be ovulation sites) usually corresponded with the number of embryos in the uterus of the rabbit. However, de Graaf thought that the entire follicle was the egg.

A major technological breakthrough in the study of reproductive physiology was made by a Dutch scientist named van Leeuwenhoek, who developed a simple microscope. A medical student suggested to van Leeuwenhoek that semen might contain living cells. Using his microscope, van Leeuwenhoek observed semen and discovered that it contained small particles that moved about. He referred to these particles as "animalcules."

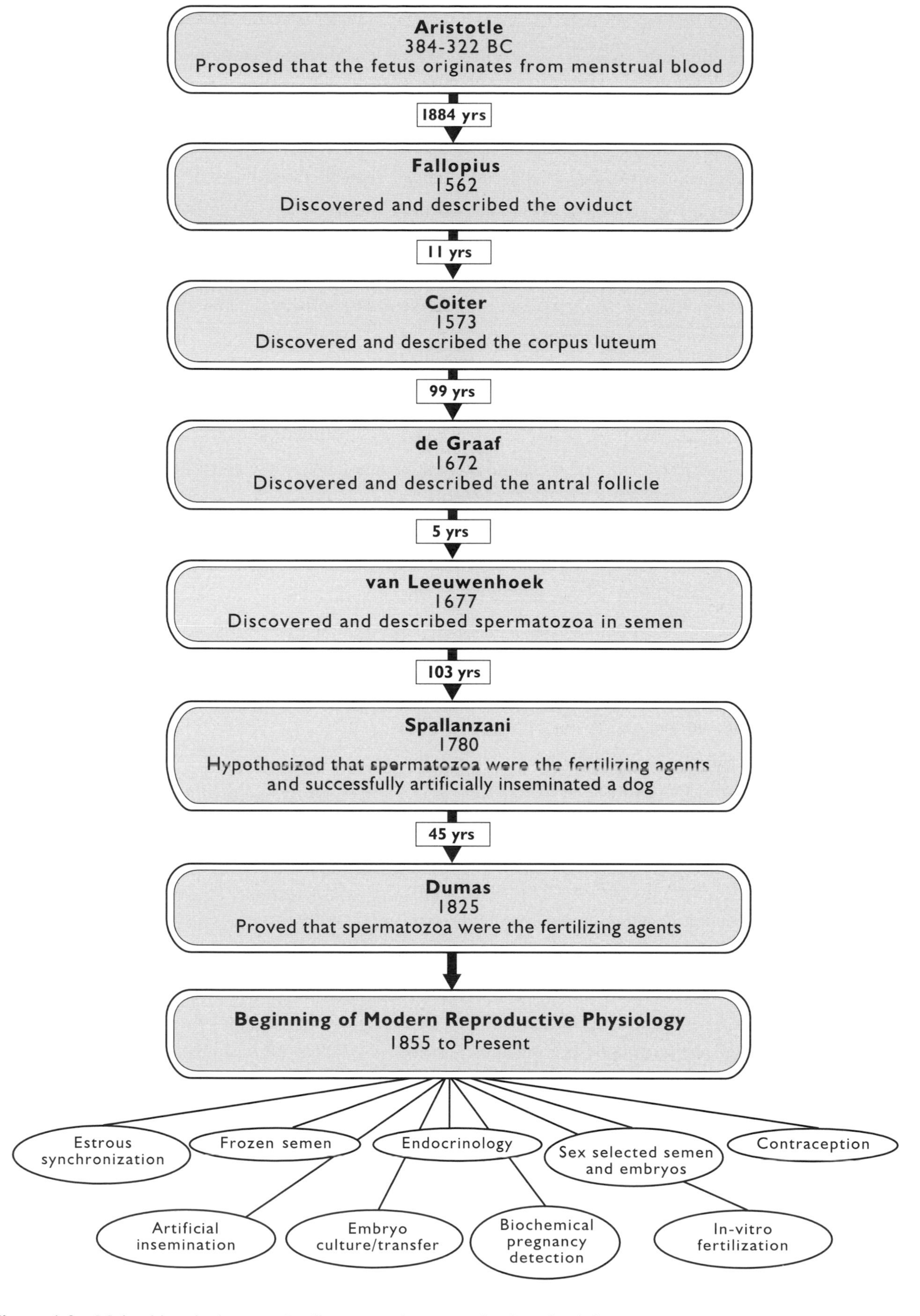

Figure 1-2. Major historical events leading to modern reproductive physiology.

While the first "animalcules" were observed in semen from a man afflicted with a venereal disease, van Leeuwenhoek found that similar "animalcules" were present in semen from males of many species and published a paper on his observations in 1677. The discovery that semen contained "animalcules" (spermatozoa) led to an outburst of speculation regarding their function. The most widely accepted speculation of the day was that the "animalcules" contained fully formed individuals within their cellular confines. In other words, the sperm head was thought to contain a microscopic, yet fully formed individual.

The father of modern artificial insemination was an Italian priest named Spallanzani. He showed that one drop of dog semen diluted with 25 pounds of fluid retained its ability to fertilize. Using the dog, he performed the first artificial insemination.

The fertilization process was not described until it was discovered that follicles contained ova and were precursors to the early embryo. A scientist named Dumas collected bodies about 1 mm in diameter from rabbit follicles. This discovery led Dumas to conclude that the "animalcules," now called spermatozoa, were responsible for uniting with the ovum and producing an embryo. Using rabbits, he demonstrated in 1825 that spermatozoa were the fertilizing agents. This early description of fertilization marked the beginning of modern reproductive physiology. Over 2,000 years elapsed from the original conjectures of Aristotle until it was understood that spermatozoa from the male were required to fertilize ova from the female. The major historical events leading to development of the modern discipline of reproductive physiology are presented in Figure 1-2.

The era of modern reproduction physiology that followed can be characterized as an "explosion of knowledge." Recognition that the gonads produce steroid hormones that alter the function of the reproductive tissues and that the anterior pituitary controls the function of the gonads were major milestones. The understanding that females experience reproductive cyclicity and that they ovulate with predictable frequency continued the explosion of knowledge. Development of the radioimmunoassay for the measurement of hormones enabled the precise description of hormonal profiles in both the male and female. These discoveries opened the door for the development of methods for artificial manipulation of reproductive processes. Understanding spermatozoal physiology and how these cells function in test-tube environments led to successful artificial insemination in several species. In fact, worldwide success of artificial insemination can be traced to the understanding of basic spermatozoal physiology in the 1940s and 1950s. It wasn't until the 1960s that it was understood that prostaglandin $F_{2\alpha}$ regulated the length of the estrous cycle in most mammalian females. The discovery that prostaglandin $F_{2\alpha}$ was the luteolysin made it possible to manipulate and alter estrous cycles and to control the time of ovulation.

Techniques such as separation of the X and Y bearing spermatozoa ("sexed semen"), embryo transfer, embryo freezing, electronic estrous detection and time-released spermatozoa lead the forefronts of reproductive physiology research.

A 3% improvement in birth rate results in an additional:

- ***1 million beef calves/year***
- ***3.2 million pigs/year***
- ***3.7 million gallons of milk/year***

Once a certain fundamental level of understanding had been achieved, scientists began to develop ways to perturb or to manipulate reproductive events. Such manipulations are a major goal in reproductive physiology research today. Development of basic techniques for the generation of fundamental understanding of reproductive processes has resulted in significant breakthroughs in technology for both enhancing and limiting reproduction. Techniques for enhancing reproduction are important when one considers that animal-derived food products are based on the ability of the species to reproduce. Small improvements in reproduction have profound positive effects on overall efficiency of production. For example, litter size in swine is an important characteristic that is a function of ovulation rate, fertilization rate and number of live pigs born. In dairy cows, failure to produce one calf per year results in compromised milk production. Thus, the efficiency of milk production is reduced. In beef cattle, the reproducing cow is the fundamental production unit. Production of less than one calf per year reduces the efficiency of the beef herd. In sheep, the ability to give birth to twins and to nurse these individuals to weaning significantly improves production.

Any factor that improves reproductive performance even slightly has the potential of having a large impact on the efficiency of food animal production. For example, there are approximately 35 million beef cows in the national beef herd. If the overall reproductive rate could be improved by only 3%, an additional 1.05 million beef calves would be born in one year. In swine, a 3% increase in pigs weaned would translate into an increase of 3.2 million pigs per year in the national swine herd. In the national dairy herd, a 3% increase in pregnancy rate would translate into an additional 3.7 million gallons of milk per year. As production traits (rate of gain, milk production per cow, feed efficiency, etc.) continue to improve, increasing physiologic/metabolic demands will be imposed on the breeding female. Therefore, it is likely that a high level of reproductive efficiency will be more and more difficult to maintain in the future. Furthermore, there will always be a need for managers of food animal enterprises, their veterinarians and related agribusiness service personnel to have a strong understanding of reproductive physiology, because proper application of new technology will require this knowledge.

There will be an increasing demand in the future for the development of new techniques to limit rather than enhance reproductive function. The human population must be controlled so that overpopulation does not erode worldwide resources and quality of life. Elimination of costly wastes associated with overpopulation of pets must be accomplished. In addition, methods to control the population growth of vermin and insects through reproductive manipulation will be needed as environmental concerns preclude the use of chemical control. As the above needs become more pressing, there will be an increasing need for understanding the reproductive processes in more and more species. In addition to basic scientific understanding, better educational techniques must be developed to disseminate knowledge regarding reproductive processes so that individuals without specialized training can appreciate and apply techniques that will ultimately improve the quality of life for all species. Basic knowledge and understanding are the prerequisites for the solution to any problem. It is the intent of this book to provide the tools for basic understanding and knowledge of reproductive physiology, primarily in food producing animals. However, the principles described herein will undoubtedly have value and application to reproductive issues in other species, including the human.

2 The Organization and Function of the Female Reproductive Tract

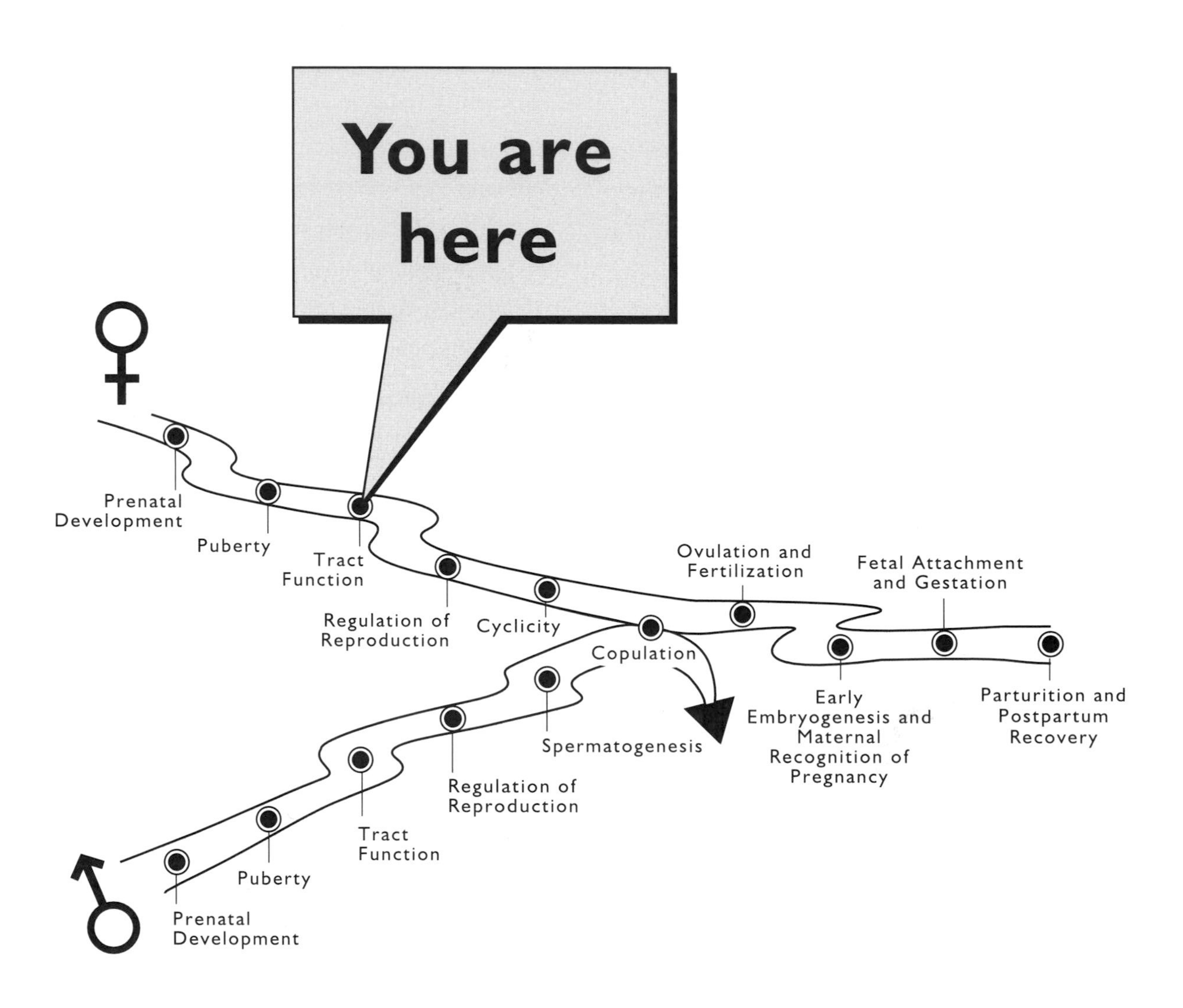

Take-Home Message

The female reproductive tract includes the ovaries, oviducts, uterus, cervix, vagina and the external genitalia. The ovaries produce gametes and a variety of hormones which act upon other parts of the reproductive tract. The oviducts provide the optimal environment for fertilization and preattachment development of the embryo. The uterus provides the environment for sperm transport, early embryogenesis and the site for attachment of the conceptus. The cervix is a barrier which secretes mucus during estrus and produces a cervical seal during pregnancy. The vagina is the copulatory organ and produces lubricating mucus during the time of estrus. Each tubular part of the tract has an outer serosal layer which is continuous with the peritoneum, a muscularis consisting of a longitudinal and circular layer of smooth muscle, a submucosal layer and a mucosal layer lining the lumen of each organ.

Structures of the female reproductive tract include the **ovaries** (the female gonads), **oviducts**, **uterus**, **cervix, vagina** and **external genitalia**. In all food producing species, the reproductive tract lies directly beneath the rectum and is separated by the **rectogenital pouch** (Figure 2-1). In the cow and mare, this fortuitous anatomical relationship provides the opportunity for manual palpation (manipulation per rectum) and/or ultrasonic examination of the female reproductive tract to: 1) diagnose the ovarian status of the female; 2) diagnose pregnancy by determining the presence or absence of a fetus or of fetal membranes located within the uterus; 3) manipulate the tract for insertion of an artificial insemination syringe or 4) identify reproductive tract abnormalities. The rectum of the sow and ewe is too small for the human arm to be inserted and thus palpation per rectum cannot be performed in these females.

The female tract is a series of tubes; each tube is organized in concentric layers called the:

- ***serosa (outer)***
- ***muscularis***
- ***submucosa***
- ***mucosa (inner)***

In its simplest form, the female reproductive tract can be considered as a series of interconnected tubes. Each of these tubes has distinct anatomical features. Thus, each tubular component can be easily identified. The tubular components of the female tract are the oviducts, uterus, cervix and vagina. Each component of the reproductive tract is characterized by having four distinct concentric layers. If you were to observe a cross-section of any one of the tubular components of the female reproductive tract you would see that the cross-section is composed of similar layers across all regions of the tract. These components are the **serosa, muscularis, submucosa** and **mucosa** (Figure 2-5). The outer **serosal** coating is a single-cell layer of squamous (flattened) cells which simply cover the surface of the reproductive tract. The **muscularis** is usually a double layer of smooth muscle consisting of an outer longitudinal layer and an inner circular layer. The purpose of the muscularis is to provide the tubular components with the ability to contract. Such contractions are important for the transport of secretory products, gametes (spermatozoa and ova) and early embryos to the appropriate location within the tract. The muscularis of the uterus is also important in expulsion of the fetus and fetal membranes during parturition.

Immediately beneath the muscularis is the **submucosa**. The submucosa is a layer of varying thick-

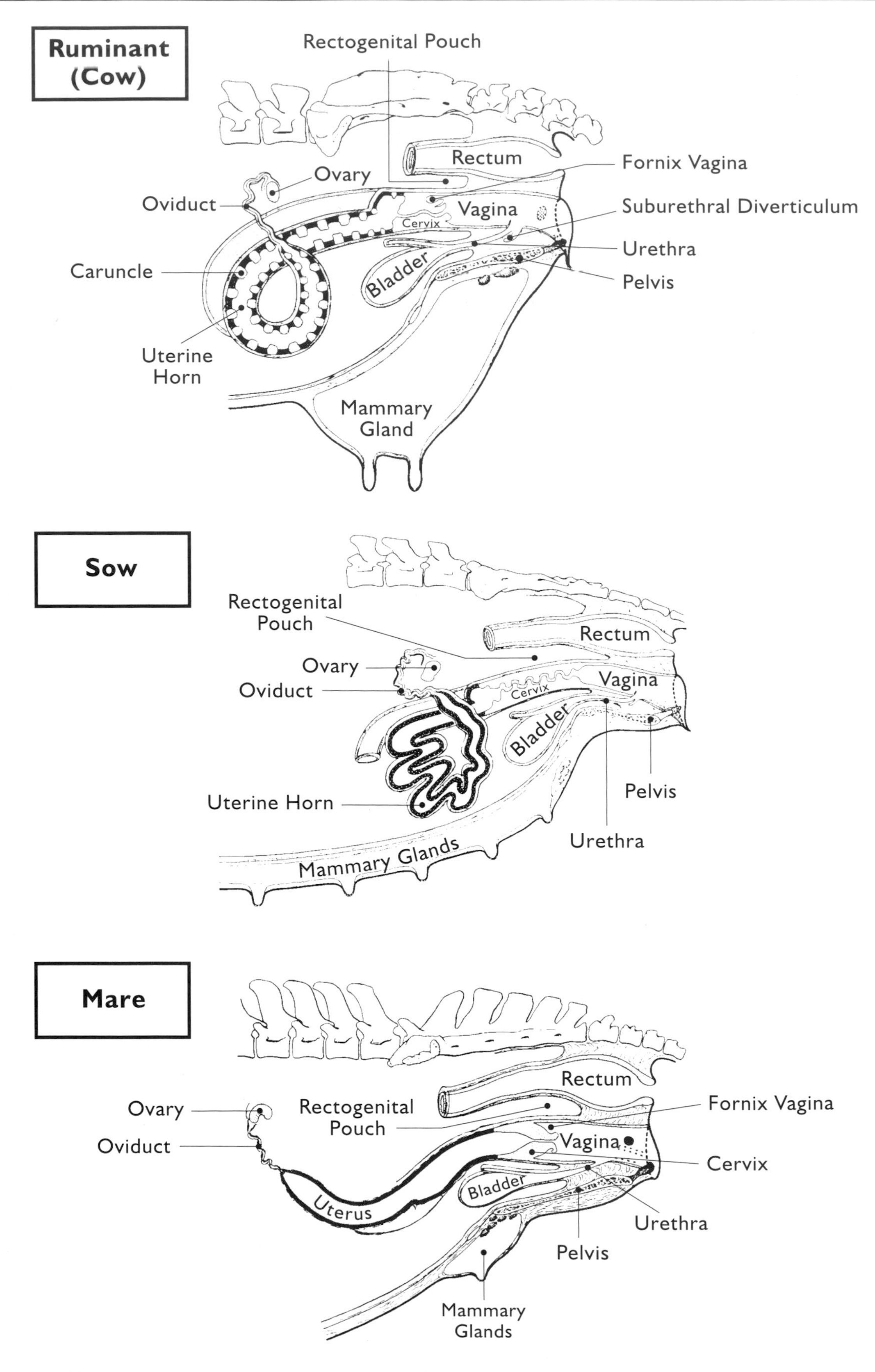

Figure 2-1. The reproductive organs in the ruminant (cow as an example), sow and mare as seen from midsagittal views. Note the relationship of the tract to the rectum. Modified from Ellenberger and Baum (1943), *Handbuch der vergleichenden Anatomie der Haustiere*, 18th Edition, Zietzschmann, Ackerknecht and Grau, eds. Permission from Springer-Verlag, New York.

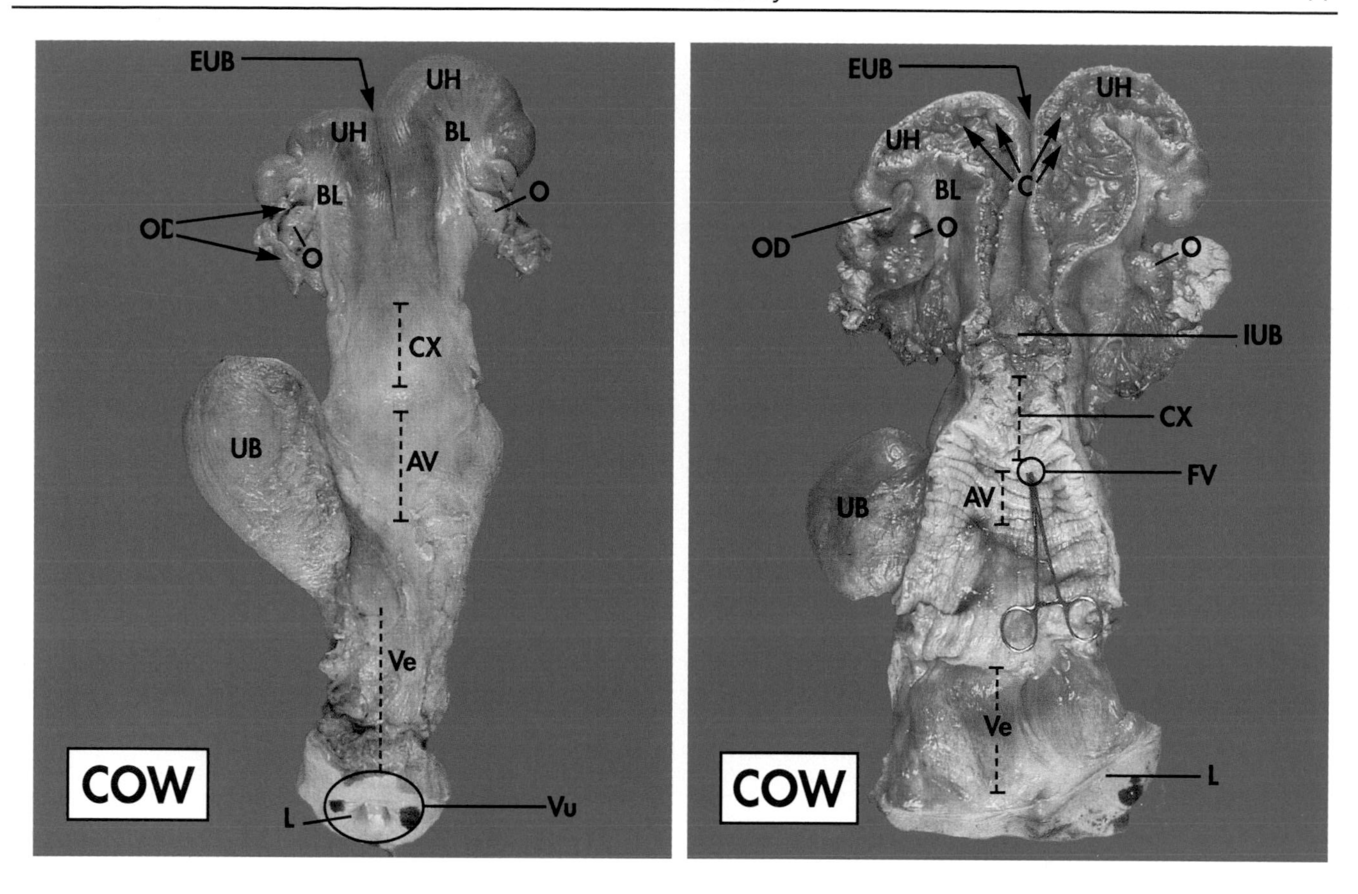

Figure 2-2. Dorsal view of excised reproductive tracts from the cow and ewe. Left panels are intact. Specimens in the right panels have been opened to expose the interior of the tract. AV = Anterior Vagina; BL = Broad Ligament (mesometrial portion); C = Caruncle; CX = Cervix; EUB = External Uterine Bifurcation; IUB = Internal Uterine Bifurcation; L = Labia; O = Ovary; OD = Oviduct; UB = Urinary Bladder; UH = Uterine Horn; Ve = Vestibule; Vu = Vulva. Tip of forceps is in fornix vagina.

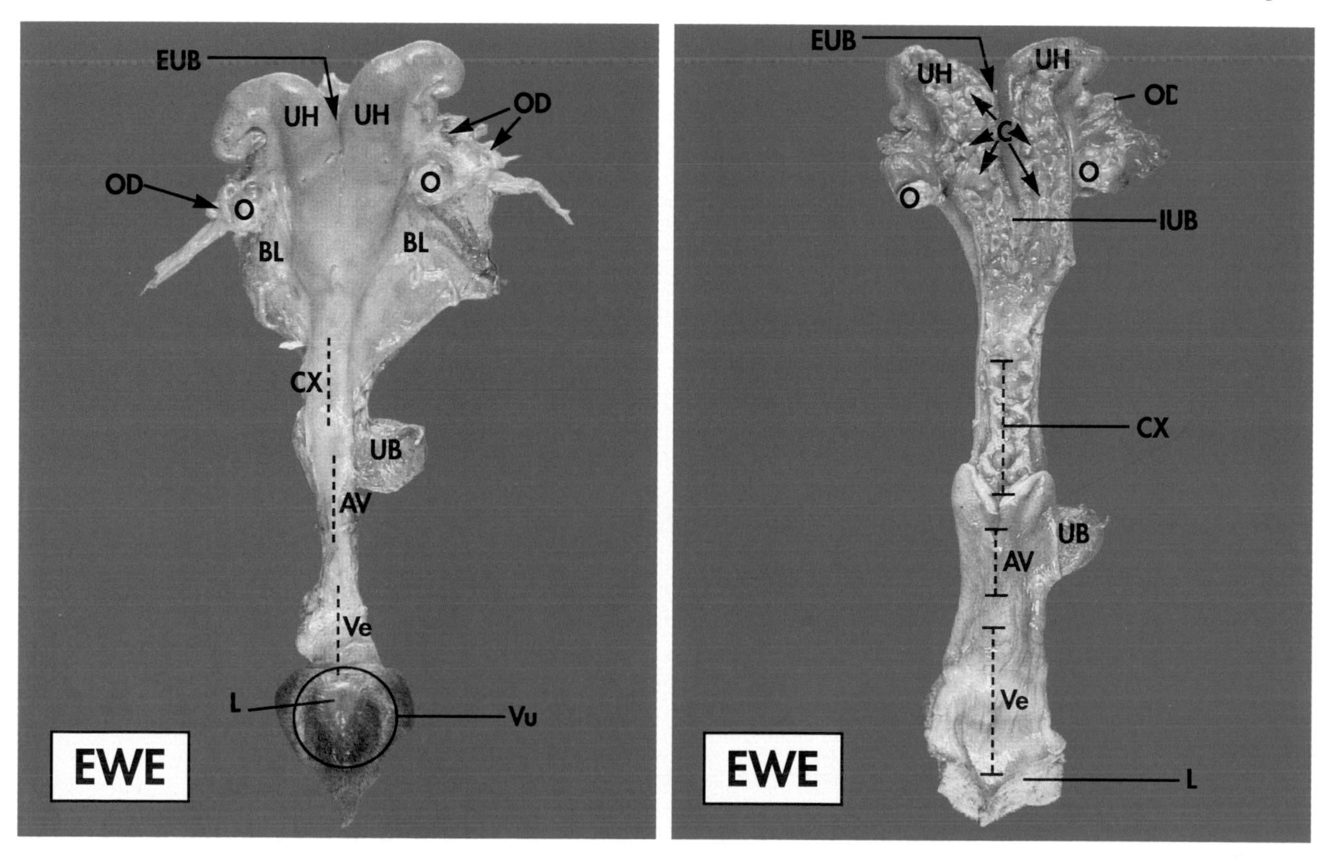

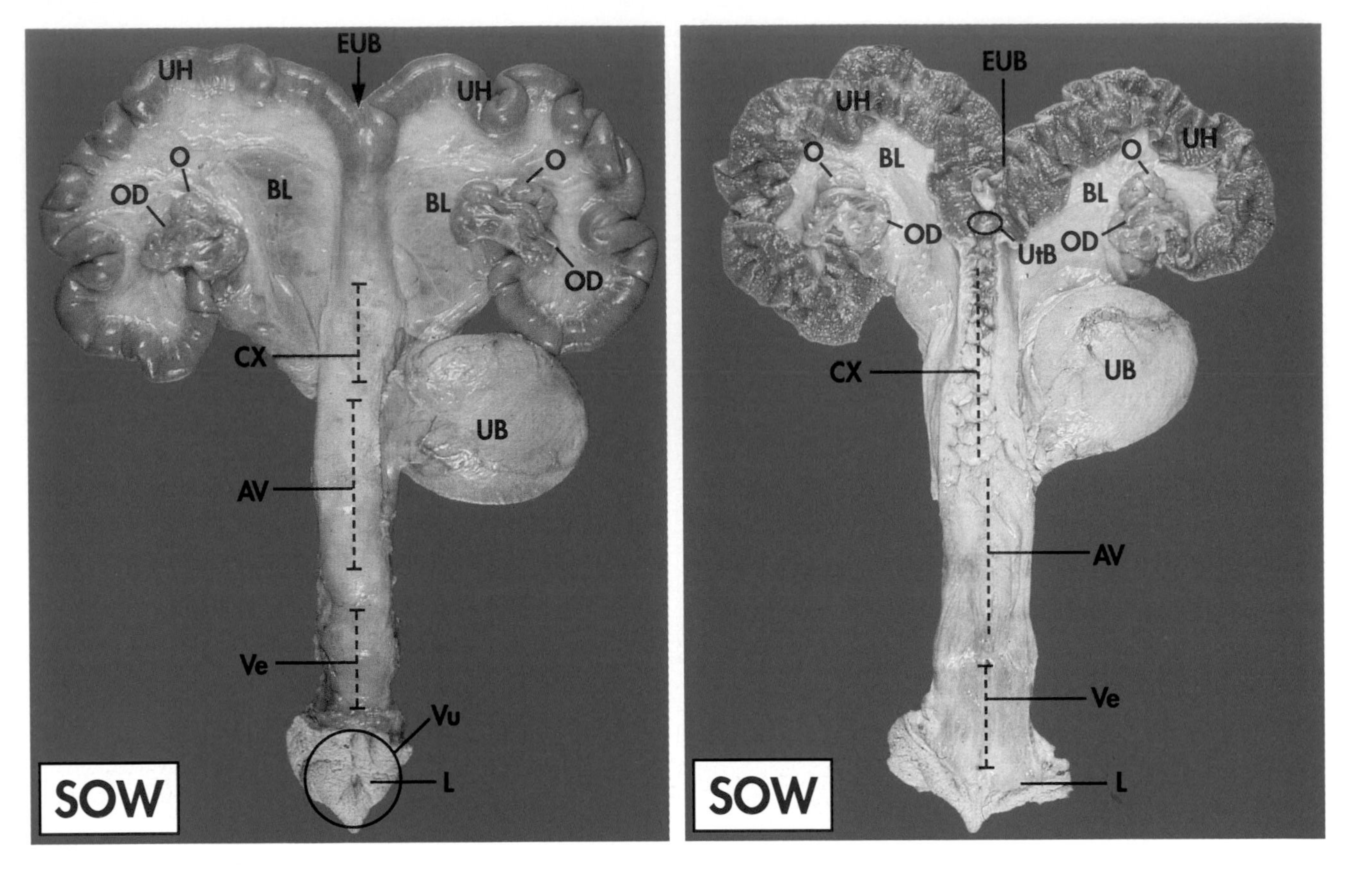

Figure 2-3. Dorsal view of excised reproductive tracts from the sow and mare. Left panels are intact specimens. Specimens in the right panels have been opened to expose the interior of the tract. AV = Anterior Vagina; BL = Broad Ligament (mesometrial portion); CX = Cervix; EUB = External Uterine Bifurcation; L = Labia; O = Ovary; OD = Oviduct; TF = Transverse Fold; UB = Urinary Bladder; UtB = Uterine Body; UH = Uterine Horn; Ve = Vestibule; Vu = Vulva.

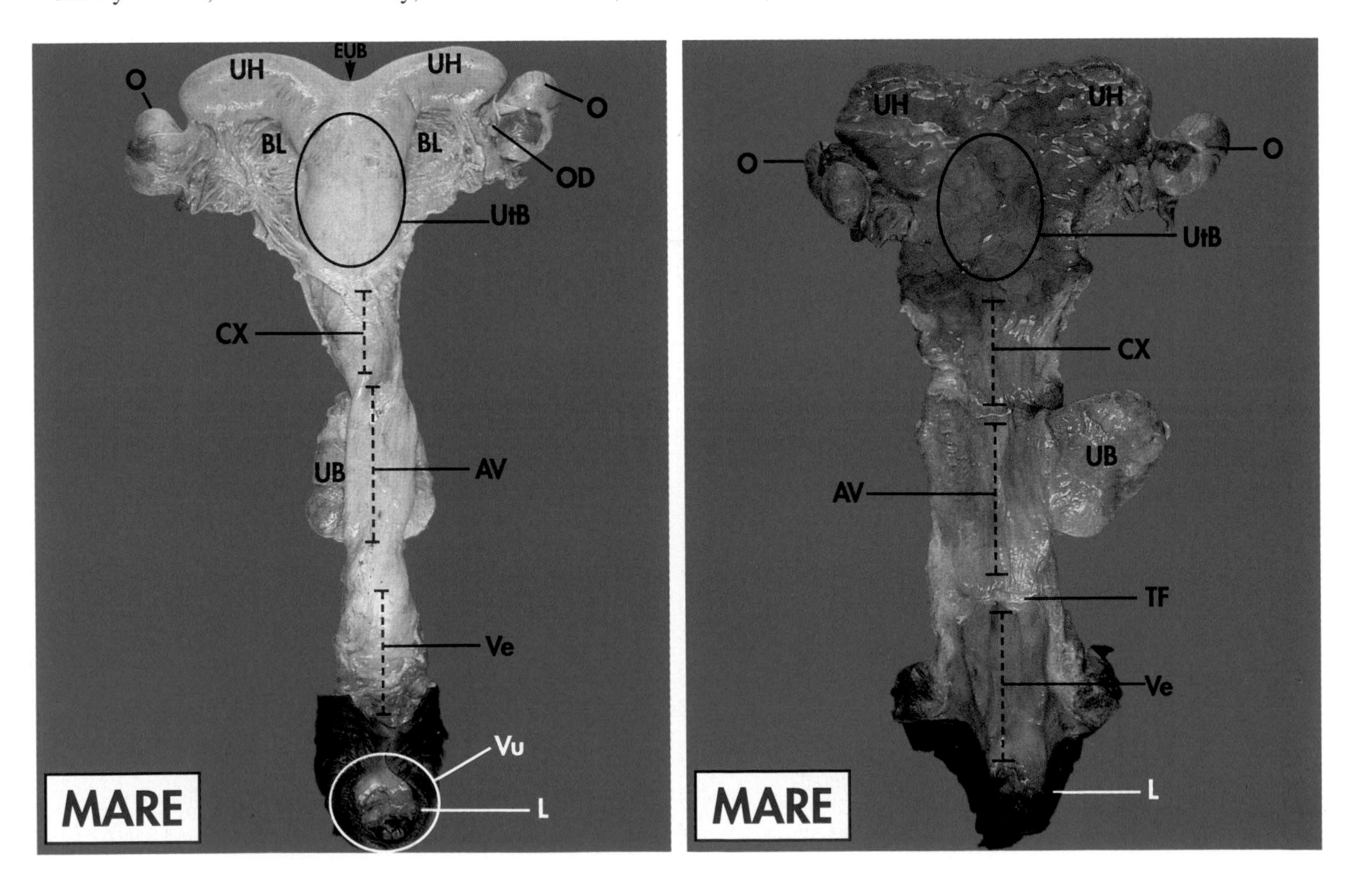

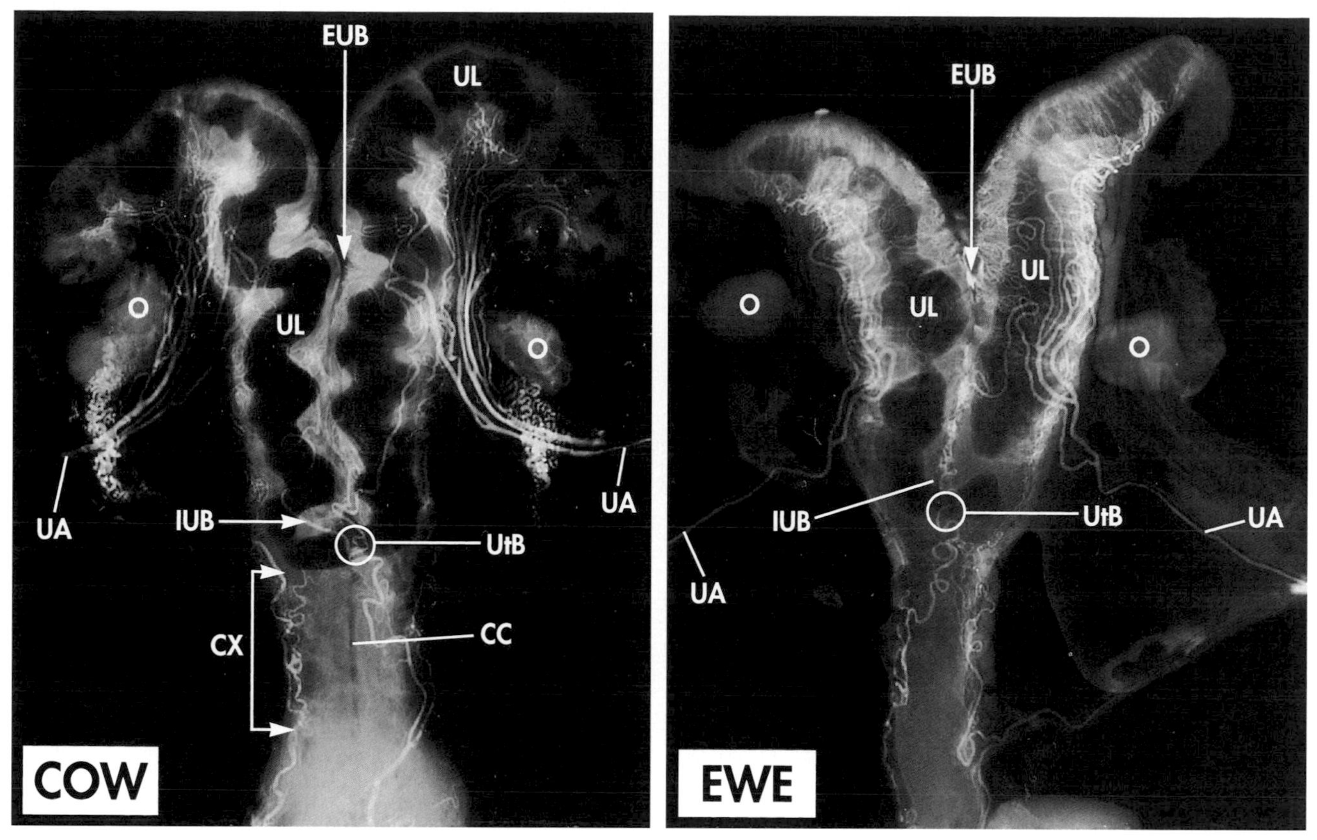

Figure 2-4. Radiographs of excised reproductive tracts of the cow, sow, ewe and mare. The uterine artery was infused with radiopaque contrast medium so that the blood supply to the uterus can be visualized. The lumen of the tract can be visualized because air was infused. Circled area = Uterine Body (UtB); AV = Anterior Vagina; CC = Cervical Canal; CX = Cervix; EUB = External Uterine Bifurcation; IP = Interdigitating Prominences; IUB = Internal Uterine Bifurcation; O = Ovary; UA = Uterine Artery; UL = Uterine Lumen; UB = Urinary Bladder.

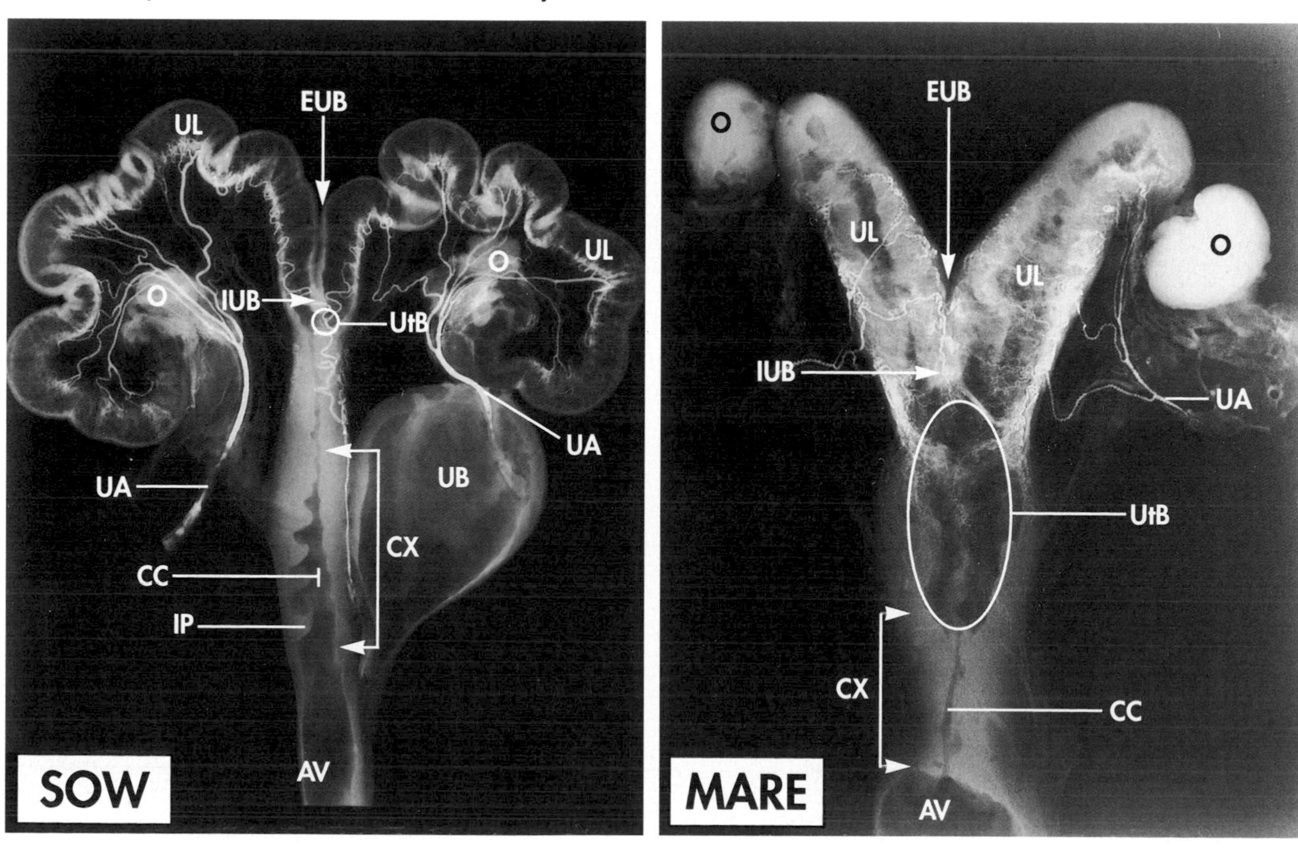

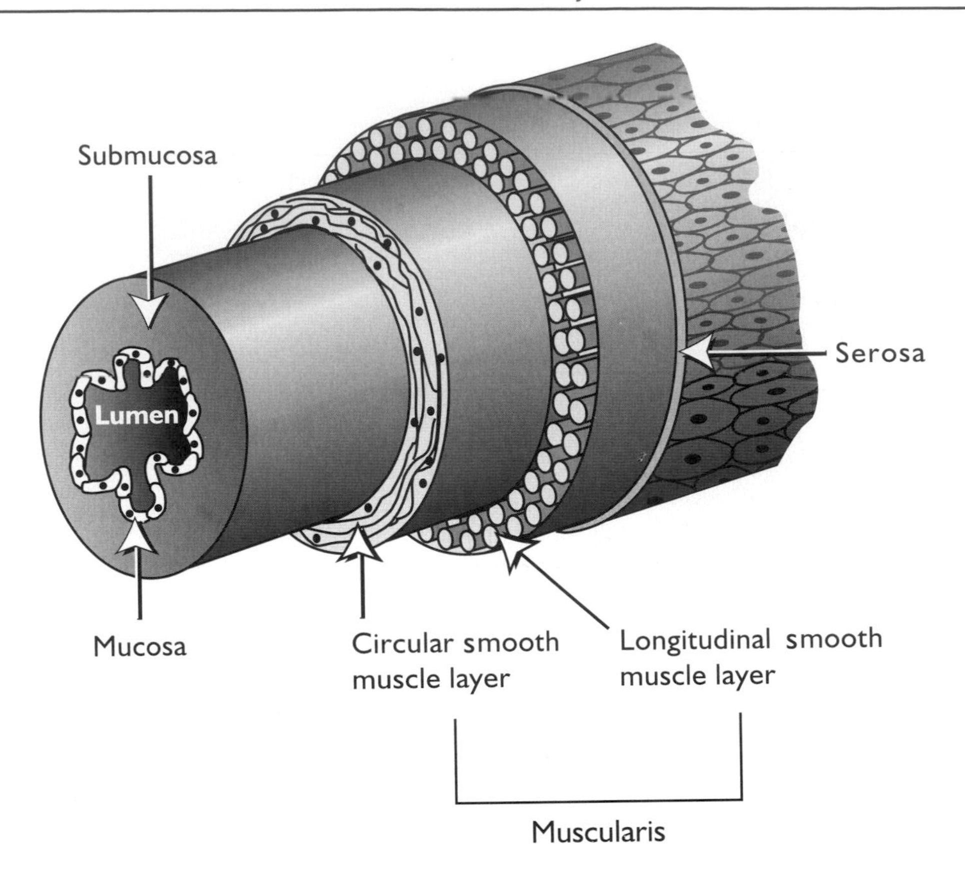

Figure 2-5. Schematic of the typical tubular composition in a cross section of the tubular portions of the female reproductive tract. The lumen is lined with epithelium called the mucosa, which is supported by the submucosa. Typically, the muscularis is composed of an inner layer of circular smooth muscle and an outer longitudinal layer of smooth muscle. The serosa is the connective tissue covering the tract. (Graphic by Sonja Oei.)

ness (depending on the specific anatomical region of the tract) that houses blood vessels, nerves and lymphatics. It also serves as a supporting tissue for the mucosal layer. The lumen in all the parts of the reproductive tract is lined with a secretory layer of epithelium known as the **mucosa**. Each part of the female reproductive tract is lined by a different type of mucosal epithelium. Each type of mucosal epithelium performs a different function depending on the region of the tract in which it is located. For example, the oviduct is lined with a mixture of ciliated and simple columnar epithelium. The cells produce fluids and also move materials along the oviduct because of ciliary action (Figure 2-9). The posterior vagina is lined with stratified squamous epithelium (Figure 2-16) which provides the organ with protection during copulation.

The reproductive tract is surrounded by the peritoneum, which forms the broad ligament.

The reproductive tract develops in a retroperitoneal position behind the peritoneum (see Chapter 4). The peritoneum is the connective tissue lining of the abdominal cavity and completely surrounds or covers the reproductive tract. During embryonic development the tract grows and begins to push against the peritoneum (Figure 2-6). As the tract continues to grow it becomes completely surrounded by the peritoneum. A portion of the peritoneum eventually fuses to form a double layered connective tissue sheet which supports and suspends the ovaries, oviduct, uterus, cervix and the anterior vagina. This suspensory tissue is called the **broad ligament** and can be seen *in situ* (in its normal

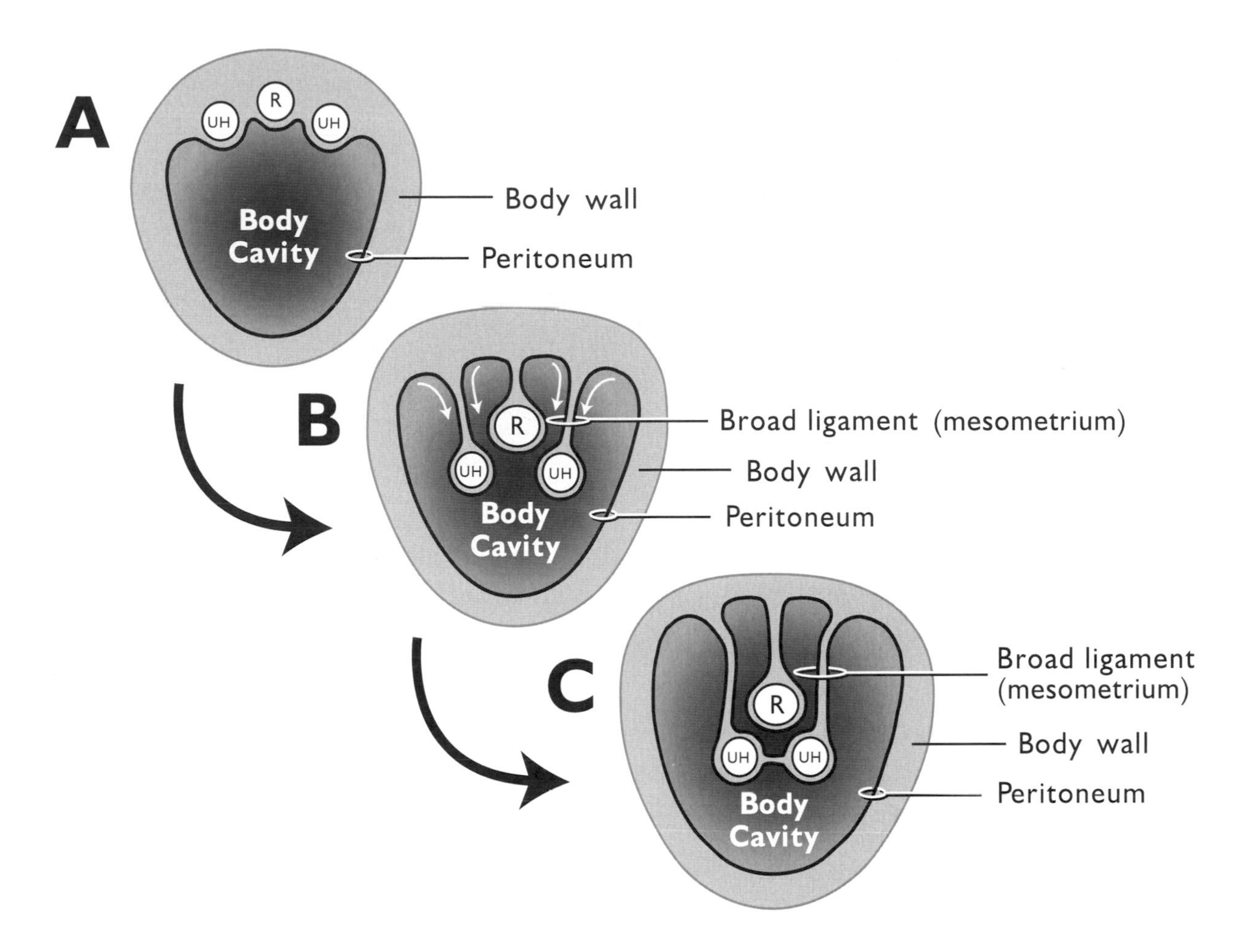

Figure 2-6. Embryonic development of the broad ligament. Initially, the uterine horns develop dorsal to the peritoneum (A). As the development continues, (UH = Uterine Horn; R = Rectum), it pushes into the body cavity (arrows in B) and eventually becomes completely surrounded by a layer of peritoneum (C). The broad ligament consists of two layers of peritoneum which "sandwiches" the tract between them (B and C). Each layer of peritoneum is continuous with the peritoneal lining of the body cavity. (Graphic by Sonja Oei.)

place or place of origin) in Figure 2-7. The broad ligament houses the vascular supply, the lymphatic drainage and nerves. It consists of several anatomical components which support the various organs of the female tract.

Components of the broad ligament are the:

- ***mesovarium***
- ***mesosalpinx***
- ***mesometrium***

The anterior (cranial) portion of the broad ligament attaches to and supports the ovary. This component is called the **mesovarium** and can be observed in Figure 2-7. The mesovarium houses the blood and lymphatic vessels and nerves which supply the ovary and forms the **hilus** (Figure 2-8) of the ovary. An additional supportive ligament for the ovary is also present in most species. This ligament is the **utero-ovarian ligament** (Figure 2-10) and, as the name implies, it attaches the ovary to the uterus.

The **oviduct (salpinx)** is surrounded and supported by a thin, serous part of the broad ligament known as the **mesosalpinx**. This delicate subdivision of the

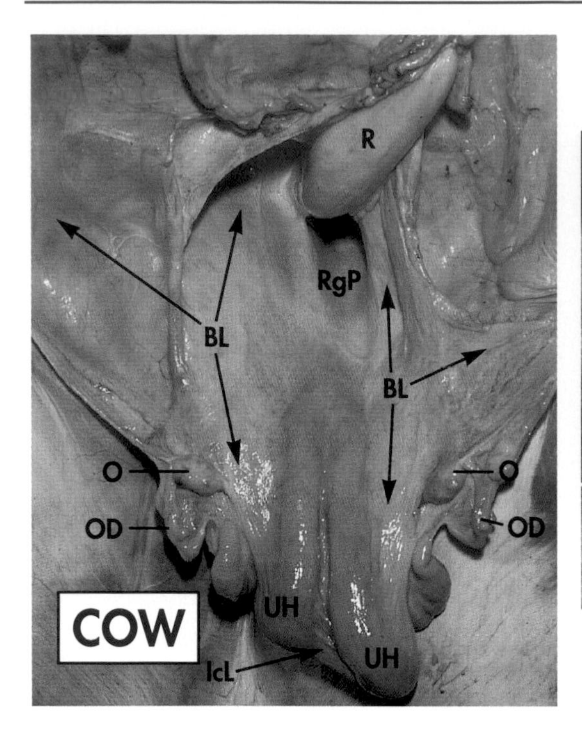

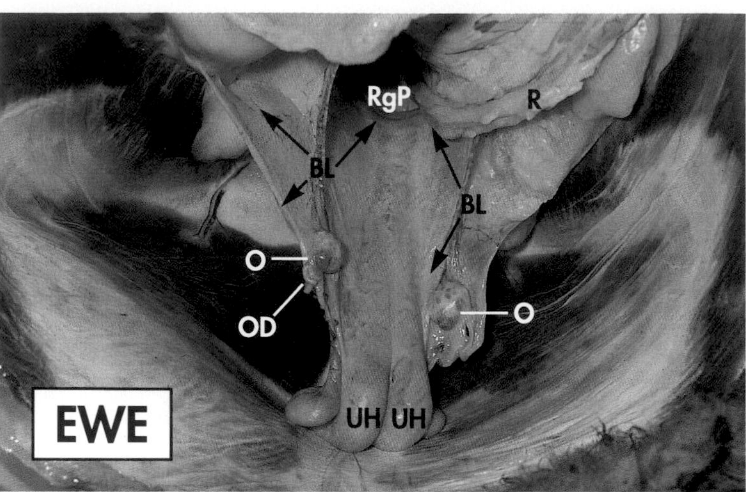

Figure 2-7. Caudal view of the cow, ewe, sow and mare (mare with permission from Ginther, O. J.; see additional reading) reproductive tracts *in situ*. Intestines have been removed so that the reproductive tract is in full view. The tract is suspended by the broad ligament (BL) which is attached dorsally and is continuous with the peritoneum. BL = Broad Ligament; IcL = Intercornual Ligament; O = Ovary; OD = Oviduct; R = Rectum; RgP = Rectogenital Pouch; UH = Uterine Horn.

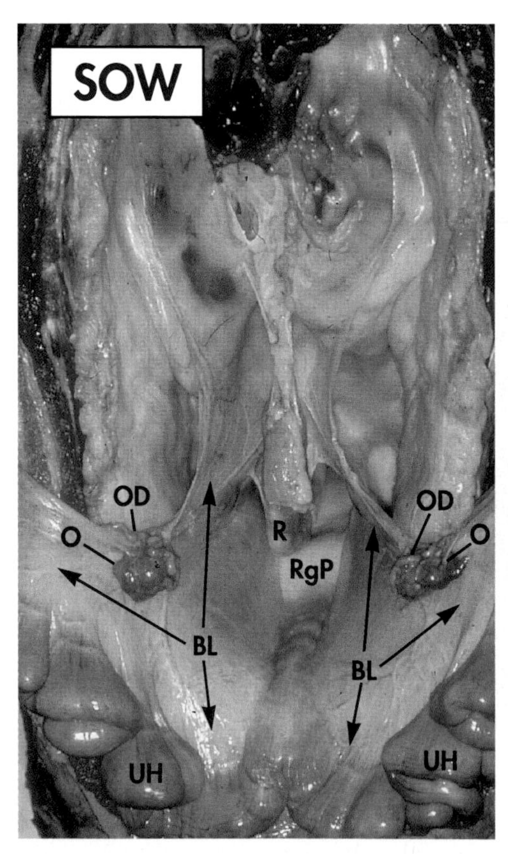

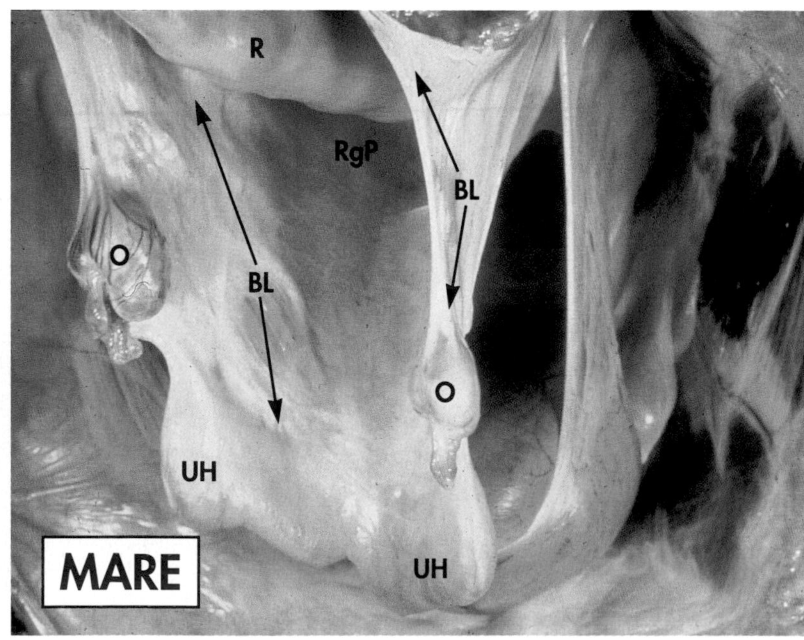

broad ligament not only supports the oviducts but serves as a bursa-like pouch that surrounds the ovary. The mesosalpinx helps to orient the infundibulum so that ova released at ovulation have a high probability of being directed into the oviduct. The nature and orientation of the mesosalpinx in the cow, ewe, mare and sow can be observed in Figure 2-10.

The **mesometrium** is the largest and most conspicuous part of the broad ligament. It supports the **uterine horns (cornua)** and the body of the uterus. The dorsal portion of the mesometrium is continuous with the dorsal peritoneum and thus the uterus literally "hangs" from the dorsal body wall (Figures 2-6 and 2-7).

The Ovary Is an Organ of Constant Change

No other organ in the female body undergoes such a predictable and dramatic series of changes in such a short period of time as the ovary. For example, within about a three week period of time in the cow, pig and mare, ovulation occurs and the **follicles** are completely transformed into a functional **corpus luteum** producing progesterone. The corpus luteum is then destroyed, new follicles develop and produce large quantities of estrogen, ovulation occurs again and a

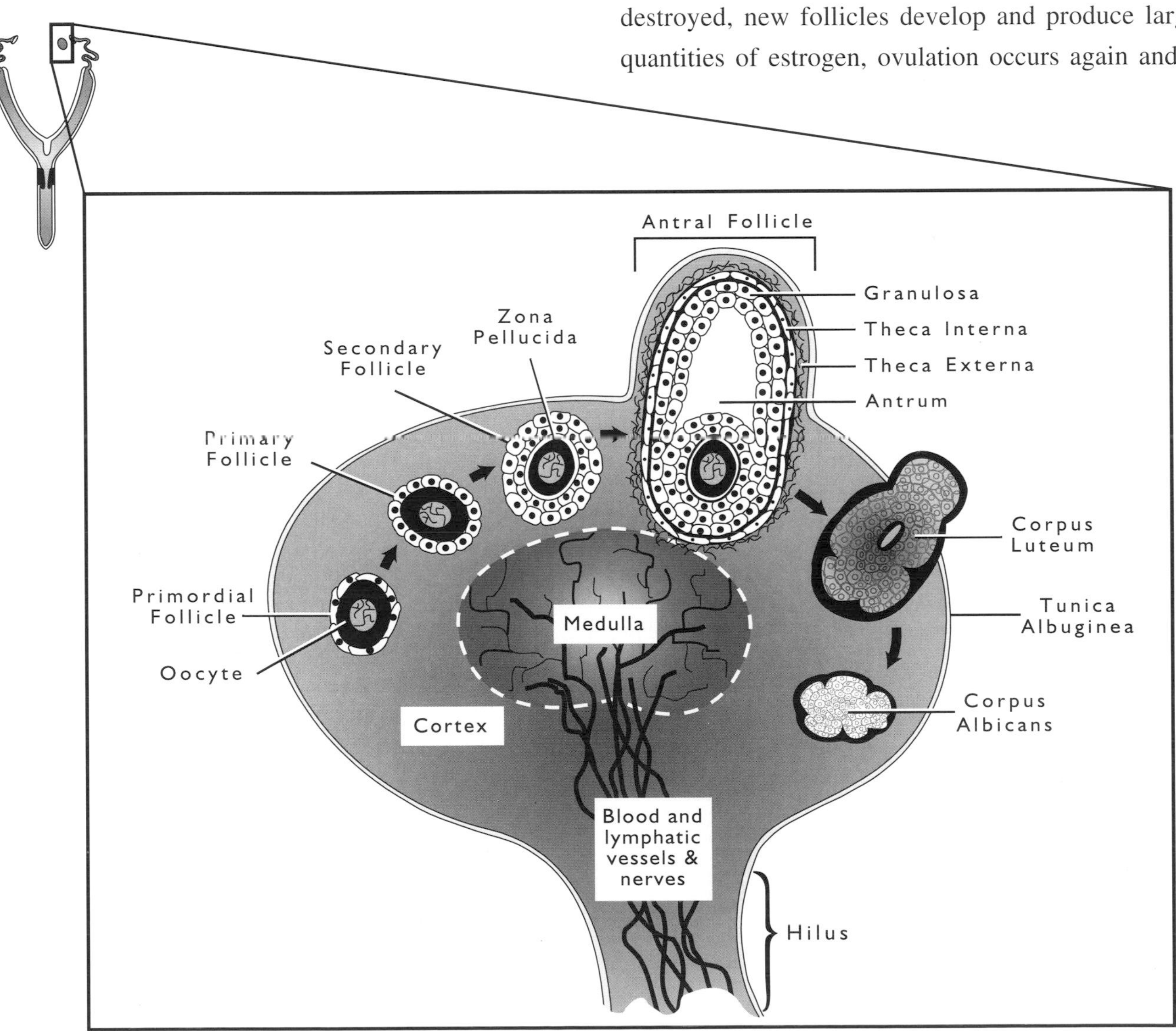

Figure 2-8. Schematic illustration of the ovary showing the primary structures and their sequence of development. It should be noted that, in general, all types of follicles are present within the ovary at any point in time. However, developing and functional corpora lutea may or may not be present depending on the stage of the estrous cycle. With the exception of the mare, development (and regression) of all ovarian structures occurs at random locations within the ovary. (Graphic by Sonja Oei.)

complete estrous cycle has occurred. This not only causes profound physiologic and behavioral changes in the female, but also causes profound morphologic changes in the ovary itself. These changes will be described in detail in Chapters 7, 8, 9 and 11.

The **ovary** is a round knot-like structure, the primary functions of which are to produce female gametes (the ova) and the hormones **estrogen** and **progesterone**. The ovary also produces **oxytocin**, **relaxin**, **inhibin** and **activin**. Details about these hormones will be presented in subsequent chapters. The ovary is composed of an outer connective tissue surface called the **tunica albuginea.** The tunica albuginea is covered by a single layer of cuboidal cells called the germinal epithelium. This layer has no function relating to production of the germinal cells and is thus erroneously named. Beneath the tunica albuginea is a zone referred to as the **ovarian cortex**. Generally (the mare is the exception), the ovarian cortex houses the population of oocytes which will develop into mature follicles and eventually ovulate. The ovarian cortex also houses the functional corpus luteum, abbreviated **CL** (plural = **corpora lutea**), and the degenerating corpora lutea known as **corpora albicantia** (singular = corpus albicans). Corpora lutea ("yellow bodies") are relatively large, conspicuous structures that produce progesterone. Corpora albicantia can readily be observed on ovaries of most species. The word "albicans" is derived from the word "albino," which implies a white color. Corpora albicantia appear as white, scar-like structures and represent corpora lutea in various stages of degeneration from previous estrous cycles. A good example of a corpus albicans can be seen in Figure 2-10 (sow).

The central part of the ovary is called the **ovarian medulla**. The medulla houses the vasculature, nerves and the lymphatics and is composed of dense connective tissue.

Morphologically, the ovaries of the mare present several important exceptions to the information presented above. First, the ovarian medulla and cortex are reversed (cortex inside, medulla outside) when compared to the cow, ewe and sow. Second, ovulation occurs at only one location in the mare's ovary, while it occurs at random locations in the ovaries of the cow, ewe and sow. Ovulation in the mare occurs in the **ovulation fossa**. Third, follicles can be palpated per rectum in the mare, but corpora lutea cannot. This is because corpora lutea do not protrude from the ovarian surface but penetrate into the ovarian tissue.

The ovaries of most females are relatively dense, turgid structures that can be distinguished tactilely from other tissues in the immediate anatomical vicinity using palpation per rectum. By inserting the arm into the rectum, the ovaries can be palpated by carefully manipulating the cranial portion of the tract. Determination of ovarian functional status can be made by identifying various structures (CL or follicles) on the ovaries. Utilization of an ultrasound probe inserted into the rectum allows detailed characteristics of ovarian structures in the cow and the mare. Recent use of this technology (see Chapter 8) has enabled a greater understanding of follicular growth patterns.

The primary ovarian structures are:

- ***primary follicles***
- ***secondary follicles***
- ***antral follicles***
- ***corpora lutea***
- ***corpora albicantia***

Within any region of the ovarian cortex, one can encounter several different types of **ovarian follicles** (Figure 2-8). The various types of ovarian follicles represent different stages of follicular development and maturity. The process whereby immature follicles develop into more advanced follicles and become candidates for ovulation is referred to as **folliculogenesis** (see Chapter 8 for details).

There are four types of follicles present within the ovary. **Primordial follicles**, which are microscopic, are the most immature and are the smallest encountered in the ovarian cortex. The oocyte (egg) within the primordial follicle is surrounded by a single layer of flattened (squamous) cells (Figure 2-8). The primordial follicle will develop into a slightly more advanced follicle called the **primary follicle**. The primary follicle is characterized by having an oocyte which is surrounded by a single layer of cuboidal (cube-like) epithelium or follicular cells (Figure 2-8). Females are born with a lifetime supply of primordial and primary follicles. Primary follicles do not divide into other primary follicles. Instead, they either develop into a more advanced secondary follicle or they degenerate. A **secondary follicle**, also microscopic, is characterized as having two or more layers of follicle cells, but without an **antrum** or cavity (Figure 2-8). In general, the oocyte within a secondary follicle is characterized as being surrounded by a relatively thick translucent layer called the **zona pellucida**. An **antral follicle** is characterized by a fluid-filled cavity called the antrum. The fluid within the antrum is called **follicular fluid**. Sometimes the antral follicle is referred to as a **tertiary follicle**. When the tertiary follicle becomes a dominant preovulatory follicle, it is sometimes called a **Graafian follicle**. Some antral follicles can be observed with the naked eye on the surface of the ovaries. They appear as blister-like structures that vary in size from less than 1 mm to several centimeters (Figure 2-10). The sizes of these follicles vary depending on their stage of development or regression and upon species.

Antral follicles consist of three distinct layers. These layers are the **theca externa,** the **theca interna** and the **granulosal cell layer** (Figure 2-8). The theca externa is composed primarily of loose connective tissue that completely surrounds and supports the follicle. The layer just beneath the theca externa is the theca interna. Cells of the theca interna are responsible for the production of androgens under the influence of LH (see Chapters 5 and 8). Beneath the theca interna is the granulosal cell layer (sometimes called the **membrana granulosa**). It is separated from the theca interna by a thin basement membrane. The granulosal cells produce a variety of materials and possess receptors to FSH. The most important products of these cells are estrogen, inhibin and follicular fluid. Granulosal cells are also believed to govern the maturation of the oocyte.

When dominant antral follicles ovulate, small blood vessels rupture, causing local hemorrhage. This small amount of bloody tissue can be observed with the naked eye. In addition to the rupture of these small blood vessels, the loss of fluid from the antrum of the follicle causes the follicle to collapse into many folds. Because of this in-folding (a type of implosion), a small portion of the granulosal and thecal layers are pushed to the apex of the follicle. This small protrusion of tissue, coupled with the rupture of blood vessels, yields a structure called the **corpus hemorrhagicum**. After the formation of the corpus hemorrhagicum ("bloody body"), the cells of the theca interna and the granulosal cells differentiate into luteal cells to form a corpus luteum. A detailed, full-color photographic presentation of corpora lutea formation as it relates to progesterone production during the estrous cycle is presented in Chapter 9 (Figures 9-3 through 9-6). The corpus luteum produces progesterone and is essential for the maintenance of pregnancy.

The oviducts consist of the:

- ***infundibulum***
- ***ampulla***
- ***isthmus***

A schematic illustration of the oviduct is presented in Figure 2-9. The **infundibulum** is the terminal end (cranial or ovarian end) of the oviduct and consists of a funnel-shaped opening. This funnel-like opening forms a pocket that "captures" the newly ovulated oocyte. The surface of the infundibulum is covered with many velvety, finger-like projections called **fimbriae**. The fimbriae greatly increase the surface area of the infundibulum and cause it to glide or slip over the entire surface of the ovary near the time of ovulation.

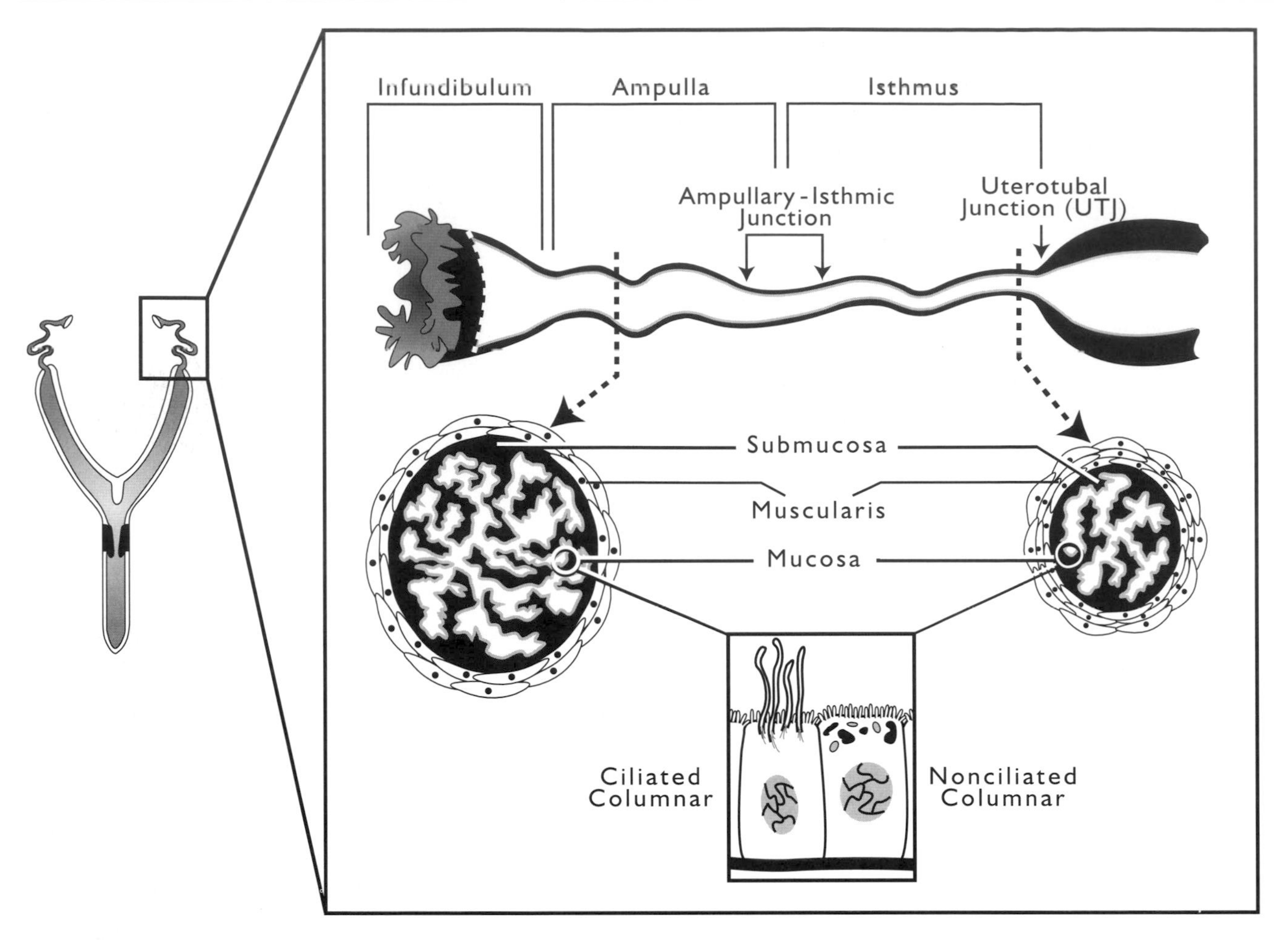

Figure 2-9. Schematic illustration of the oviduct and its components. (Graphic by Sonja Oei.)

Such an action maximizes the chance that the oocyte will be "captured" after ovulation and transported through an opening called the **ostium** into the ampulla of the oviduct. The relationship of the infundibulum to the ovary is presented in Figure 2-10. The surface area of the infundibulum ranges from 6 to 10 cm^2 in sheep to 20 to 30 cm^2 in cattle. The infundibulum leads directly into a thick portion of oviduct called the **ampulla**. The ampulla occupies one-half or more of the oviductal length and merges with the isthmus of the oviduct. The ampulla has a relatively large diameter, with the internal portions being characterized as having many fern-like mucosal folds with ciliated epithelium (Figure 2-9). The junction between the ampulla and the isthmus (**ampullary-isthmic junction**) is generally ill-defined. In the mare, the ampullary-isthmic junction serves as a control point that allows only fertilized oocytes to pass into the isthmus and eventually into the uterus.

The **isthmus** is smaller in diameter than the ampulla. It is connected directly to the uterus and the point of juncture is called the **uterotubal junction**. The isthmus has a thicker muscular wall than the ampulla and has fewer mucosal folds.

The primary function of the smooth muscle layer (muscularis) of the oviduct is to transport newly ovulated oocytes and spermatozoa to the site of fertilization (the ampulla). Gamete transport by the oviduct requires that spermatozoa and ova move in opposite directions so that they encounter each other in the ampulla. The mechanisms controlling gamete transport by the oviduct are not well understood.

The mucosa of the oviduct secretes substances that provide the optimum environment for the free-floating, unfertilized oocyte. It also sustains spermatozoal function until the oocyte arrives after ovulation. There is increasing evidence that the epithelium of the oviduct

Figure 2-10. Relationship of the mesosalpinx to the oviduct in the cow, ewe, sow and mare. The infundibulum is a delicate membrane-like component of the oviduct, which is in close apposition to the ovary. Arrows indicate the direction of oocyte /embryo transport within the oviduct toward the uterus.
AF = Antral Follicle
CA = Corpus Albicans
If = Infundibulum
Ms = Mesosalpinx
O = Ovary
OD = Oviduct
UH = Uterine Horn
UOL = Utero-Ovarian Ligament
UL =Uterine Lumen

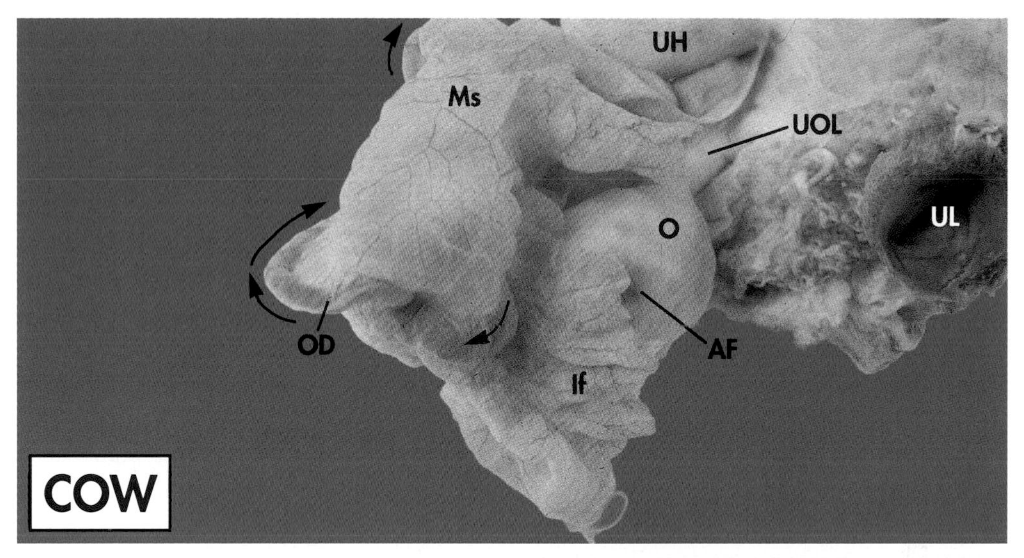

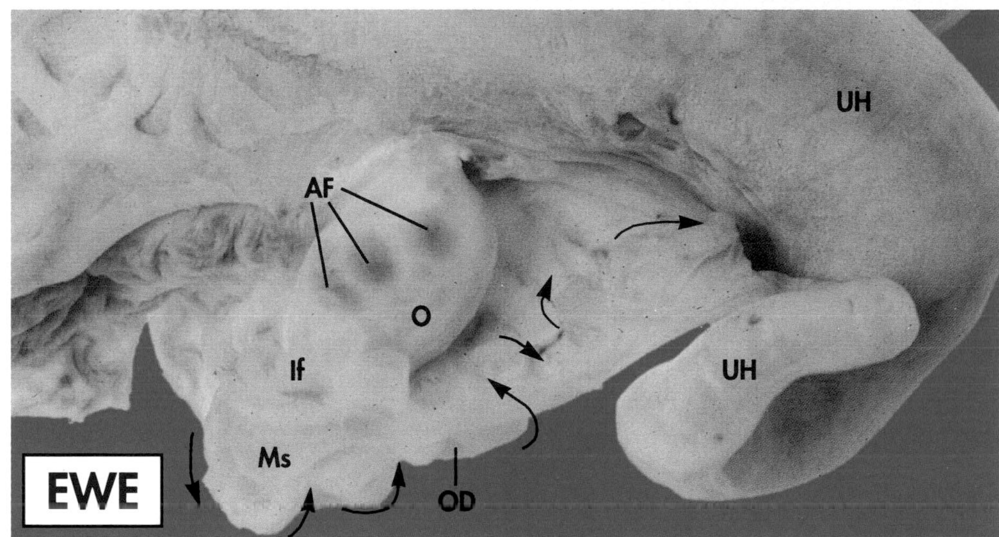

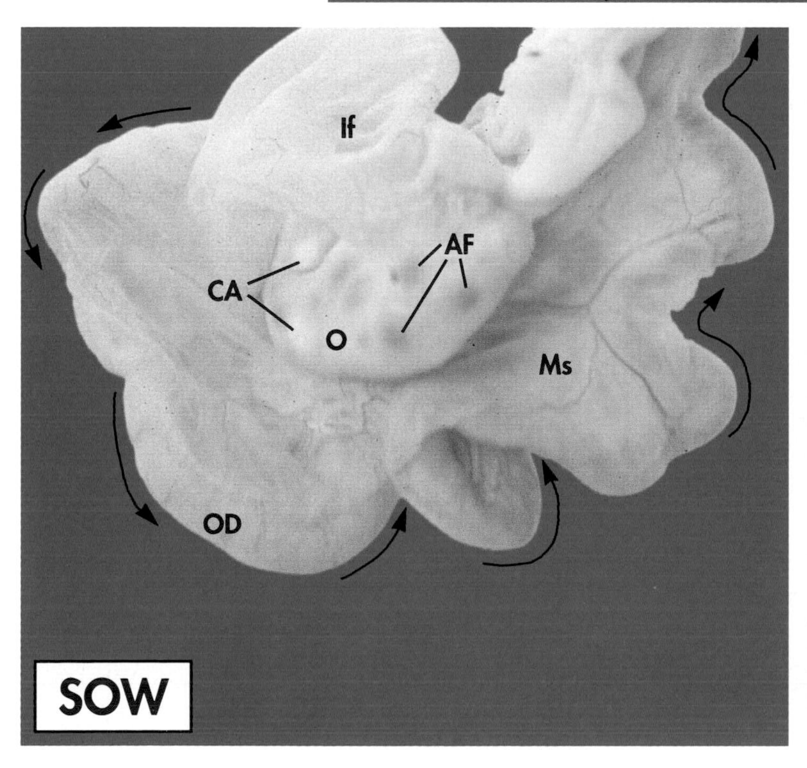

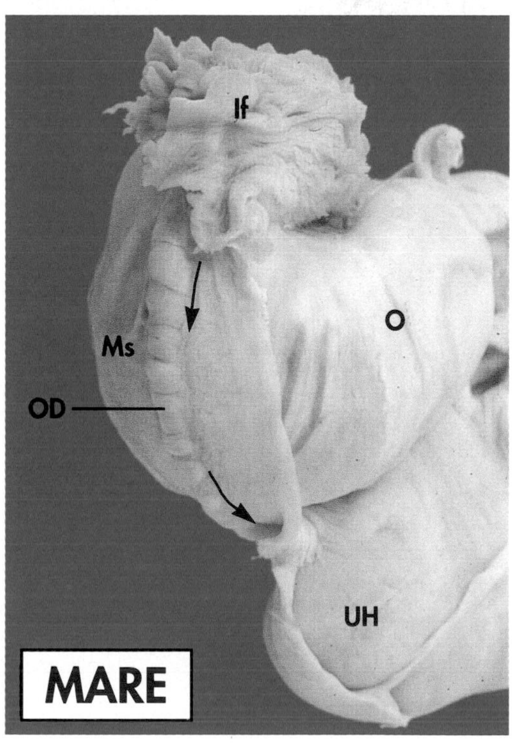

produces substances that facilitate the fertilizing capability of spermatozoa. After fertilization, the newly formed zygote must reside in the oviduct for a few days before it enters the uterus. Thus, the composition of the fluid secreted by the cells lining the oviduct is important for providing a suitable environment for the development of the early embryo.

In the cow, the **uterotubal junction** (UTJ) is believed to regulate the movement of the embryo into the uterus. Under conditions of high estradiol, the uterotubal junction forms a "kink" (like a kink in a hose), thus blocking movement of embryos. As estradiol levels decrease, this kink straightens out; the lumen of the isthmus is no longer blocked by the kink and embryos can enter the uterine lumen with relative ease. In other species, the oviduct attaches to the uterus without an obvious kink-like anatomical constriction. In swine, constriction of the uterotubal junction serves as a major barrier to sperm transport and prevents excessive numbers of spermatozoa from reaching the ampulla. Such blockage is believed to be important in the prevention of polyspermy in swine.

The Uterus Is the Organ of Pregnancy

The uterus connects the oviducts to the cervix. In most mammals, the uterus consists of two **uterine horns** or **cornua**. The degree to which the uterine horns are developed constitutes the basis for classification of mammalian uteri.

Among mammals there are three distinct anatomical types of uteri (Figure 2-11). The first of these is a **duplex uterus,** characterized as having two cervical canals which separate each uterine horn into distinct compartments. There are two types of duplex uteri. The first is characterized by having a single vaginal

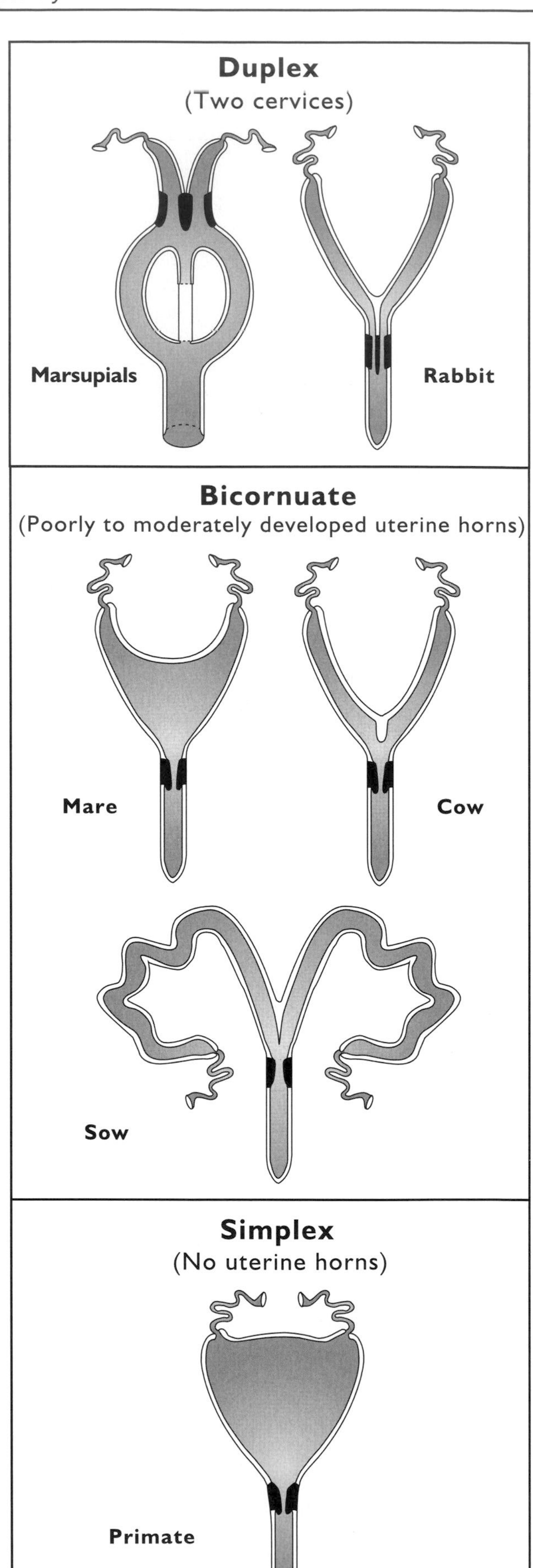

Figure 2-11. Types of uteri found in mammals. The solid black area in each example represents the cervix. (Graphic by Sonja Oei.)

canal opening to the exterior. On the interior it bifurcates (splits) into two vaginas and two cervices. Marsupials have this type of uterus. In the opossum, this interesting female anatomical configuration is accommodated by the male, which possesses a forked penis. It is believed that after intromission, the male opossum deposits semen in each of the two sides of the reproductive tract simultaneously. The second, less complex type of duplex uterus is found in the rabbit. In this type of duplex uterus, there are two uterine horns and two distinct cervical canals connecting with a single vaginal canal. Therefore, in species like the rabbit it is possible to artificially inseminate the female into one horn with sperm from one male and to artificially inseminate the contralateral (opposite) horn with semen from another male; the offspring will represent two genetic types. The rabbit is an excellent animal to use for the study of various experimental seminal or embryo treatments, because transuterine migration of the gametes or embryos is not likely to occur.

The **bicornuate uterus** is characterized as having two uterine horns and a small uterine body. The length of the uterine horns is dependent on the degree of fusion between the paramesonephric ducts in the developing female fetus (see Chapter 4 for details). In species where there is a high degree of fusion (mare) there are short uterine horns and a relatively large uterine body. When a moderate degree of fusion occurs, uterine horns of intermediate length result (cow, ewe and goat). And, when little fusion takes place between adjacent paramesonephric ducts, long uterine horns result (sow). In all types of bicornuate uteri the uterus opens into the vagina through a single cervical canal. In your readings outside of this book you will encounter the term "bipartite uterus." The term "bipartite" was once used to describe bicornuate uteri with short (mare) to moderate length (cow) uterine horns. In an attempt to simplify the classification of mammalian uteri, the suggestion has been made that the term "bipartite" be dropped from the uterine classification nomenclature. This suggestion has been followed here. An **internal** and **external uterine bifurcation** of the horns can be distinguished in the bicornuate uterus (Figure 2-4).

The **simplex uterus** is characterized as having a single uterine body. Only small rudiments of a structure resembling a uterine horn may be apparent. Fusion of the paramesonephric ducts is almost complete, resulting in a single-chambered uterus without horns. The simplex uterus is found in primates, including humans.

The unique names of the components of the uterus are:

- ***serosa = perimetrium***
- ***muscularis = myometrium***
- ***mucosa + submucosa = endometrium***

The uterus consists of a serosal layer called the **perimetrium,** which is part of the peritoneum. It is continuous with the serosal layer covering the mesosalpinx. The perimetrium is quite thin and almost transparent. Beneath the serosal layer is a longitudinal layer of smooth muscle. The longitudinal layer of smooth muscle is easy to recognize because of the creases, or small ridges, that run in an anterior-posterior direction. Beneath the longitudinal smooth muscle layer is a circular layer. The smooth muscle cells wrap around the uterine horn in a circular fashion. Collectively, the outer longitudinal layer and the inner circular muscle layer are referred to as the **myometrium**. The myometrium has several physiologic responsibilities. One of the most important is to provide motility (a form of contraction) for the uterus. In species other than the mare, the myometrium has a high degree of tone (a partial state of contraction) when estrogen is the predominant steroidal hormone. Muscular tone (in this case myometrial tone) is a condition where a partial state of contraction exists. A high degree of tone can be palpated (felt) as turgidity or hardness and is distinguished easily from a soft or flaccid uterus, found when estrogen is low and progesterone is high. Uterine tone is presumably related to transport mechanisms for sperm and mucus-like material produced by the uterus. The transport mechanisms for spermatozoa will be addressed in more detail in Chapter 12. Under the influence of progesterone, the myometrium has a low degree of tone. This lack of tone is appropriate, since it is during this time that the embryo will enter the uterus for eventual attachment. A high degree of motility would undoubtedly minimize the possibility of successful attachment of the conceptus. A third important function of the myometrium includes its role during **parturition**. During parturition, the myometrium becomes a major driving force for expulsion of the fetus and fetal membranes.

The inner portion of the uterus is composed of the **mucosa** and **submucosa.** The mucosa and the submucosa of the uterus comprise the **endometrium**. The mucosal epithelium is responsible for secreting materials into the lumen of the uterus which enhance embryo development and sperm survival. The uterine glands develop from the mucosal layer of the uterus. They penetrate into the submucosa and begin to coil under the influence of estrogen (Figure 2-12). However, they reach full secretory capacity under the influence of progesterone. Uterine glands produce materials which are believed to be important to the survival and function of the preimplantation embryo. The submucosa is predominantly connective and supporting tissue and houses the uterine glands. A distinct difference between lower mammals and primates, particularly humans, is that the endometrium of the uterus in the human is sloughed to the exterior. The endometrial glands in domestic mammals are not sloughed. The functionality of the uterine glands changes during the estrous cycle in a type of secretory "waxing and waning." In other words, secretory activity of the uterine glands changes as a function of the stage of the estrous cycle. The mechanisms

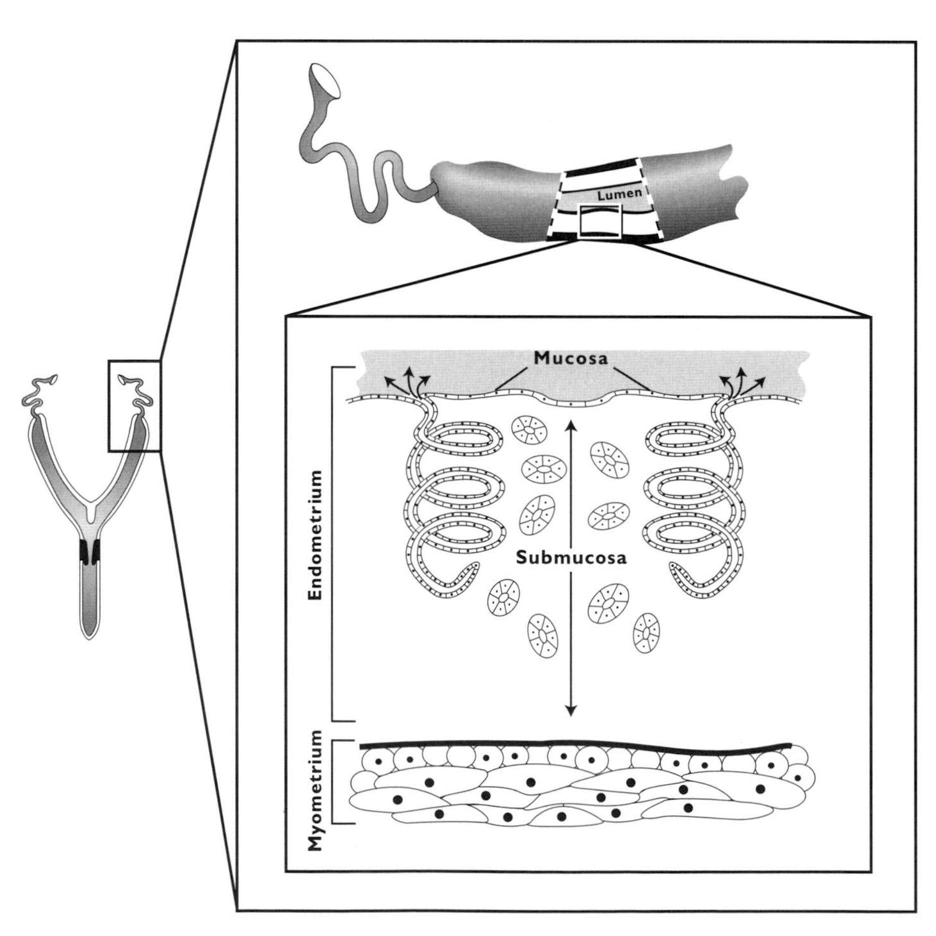

Figure 2-12. Schematic illustration of uterine tissue. Uterine glands develop from the endometrial mucosa, penetrate into the submucosa and become coiled. They secrete material into the lumen of the uterus (arrows). (Graphic by Sonja Oei.)

Figure 2-13. Excised uterine tissue from the cow, ewe, sow and mare. The uterus has been opened so that the endometrial surface can be visualized. In the cow and the ewe, caruncles (C) can be observed as protrusions from the endometrial surface. Blood vessels (V) are white, cord-like structures located beneath the surface of each caruncle. The endometrium of the sow and mare is characterized as having many endometrial folds (EF). Both the caruncles and the endometrial folds contribute to the maternal placenta if pregnancy occurs.
C = Caruncles
EF = Endometrial Folds
M = Myometrium
O = Ovary
UOL = Utero-Ovarian Ligament
V = Blood Vessels

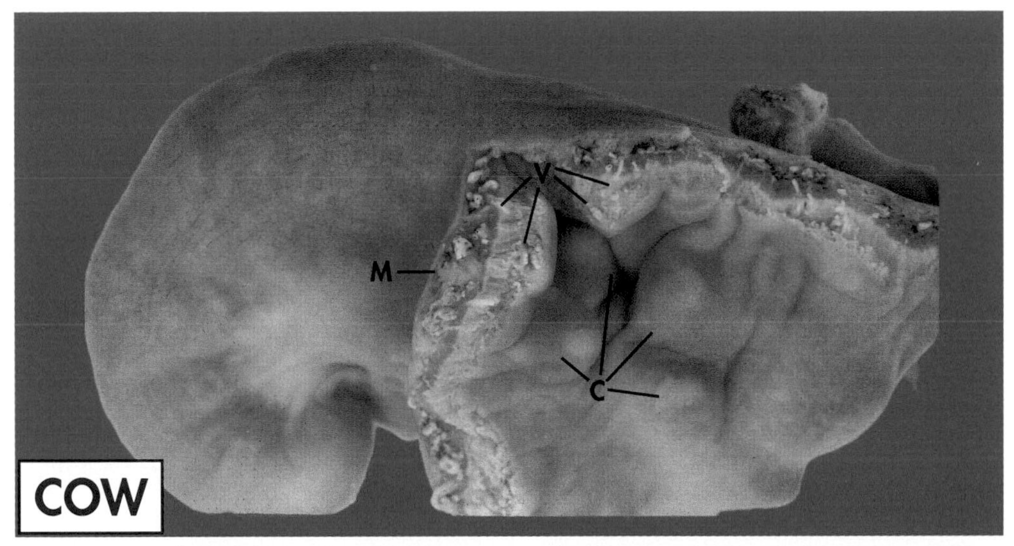

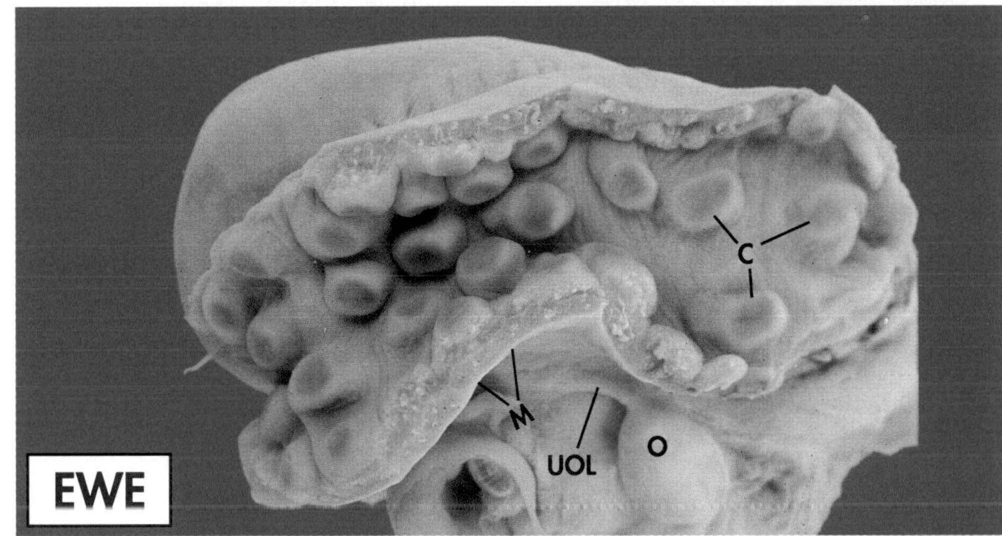

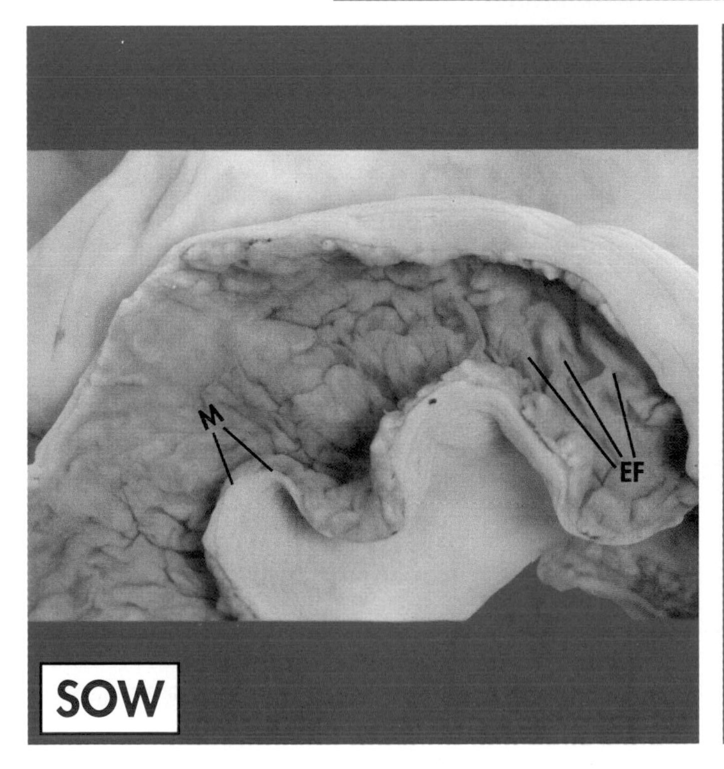

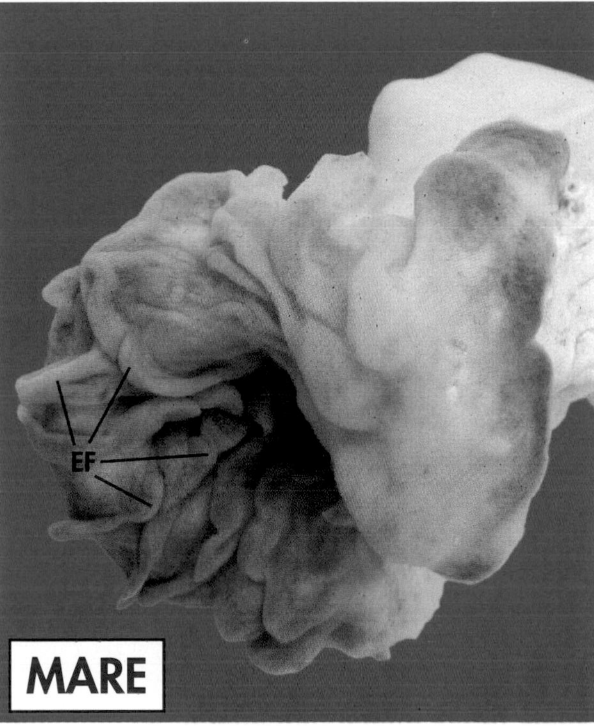

whereby uterine glands may be lost (or replenished) in domestic animals remains undefined.

The primary functions of the uterus are:
- ***sperm transport***
- ***luteolysis and control of cyclicity***
- ***environment for preattachment embryo***
- ***maternal contribution to the placenta***
- ***expulsion of the fetus and fetal placenta***

At a critical time during the estrous cycle the cells of the uterine endometrium produce **prostaglandin $F_{2\alpha}$**. Prostaglandin $F_{2\alpha}$ causes luteolysis or regression of the corpus luteum if the animal is not pregnant. Details of these important mechanisms are presented in Chapter 9.

In ruminants, the surface of the endometrium is characterized as having small, nonglandular areas that protrude from the surface of the endometrium. These small protruberances are referred to as **caruncles** and can be observed with a high degree of detail in Figure 2-13. These caruncular regions are highly vascularized and will give rise to the maternal portion of the placenta if attachment of the embryo occurs. In contrast to the cow and ewe, the endometrium of the sow and mare have no caruncles. Their endometrium is characterized by having many endometrial folds (Figure 2-13). The folds will provide the uterine surface for the development of the placenta.

The cervix provides lubrication, a flushing system and a barrier during pregnancy.

The cervix is a thick-walled, noncompliant organ that serves as a barrier to sperm transport in the ewe and cow, but not in the sow and mare. The cervix also isolates the uterus from the external environment during pregnancy by forming a barrier consisting of highly viscous mucus. Cervical anatomy differs significantly among species (Figure 2-15). In general, however, it can be characterized as having a cervical canal (lumen) which is surrounded by folds or rings protruding into the cervical canal (Figure 2-14). In the cow and the ewe, there are several of these rings that form interlocking finger-like projections (Figure 2-15). In the sow, the rings interdigitate in a very intimate fashion (Figure 2-15). These interdigitations require a special penile adaptation in the boar. The boar has a corkscrew or spiral twist in the glans penis so that during copulation the boar's penis becomes "locked" into the cervix. Thus, in the pig, initial deposition of the semen occurs in the cervix. Because of the large volume (200-500 ml), most of the ejaculate quickly enters the uterus. The distinguishing feature of the mare's cervix is the presence of conspicuous, loose folds of mucosa that protrude into the vagina. The cervix of the mare is soft during estrus. During copulation the penis of the stallion presses against the soft cervix. Semen is ejaculated under high pressure and enters the uterus during ejaculation.

A primary role of the cervix in the cow and ewe is to produce mucus during estrus. In the sow and mare, a much smaller quantity of mucus is produced. This mucus flows from the cervix toward the exterior and lubricates the vagina during copulation. Foreign material introduced during copulation (including sperm) is flushed out of the tract by cervical mucus. This flushing action brought about by outflow of mucus probably minimizes introduction of microorganisms into the uterus. The biochemical and physical properties of the mucus change as the stage of the estrous cycle changes. Details regarding the role of the cervix in transport of spermatozoa will be presented in Chapter 12.

During pregnancy the cervix is responsible for isolation of the conceptus within the uterus from the external environment. Under the influence of progest-

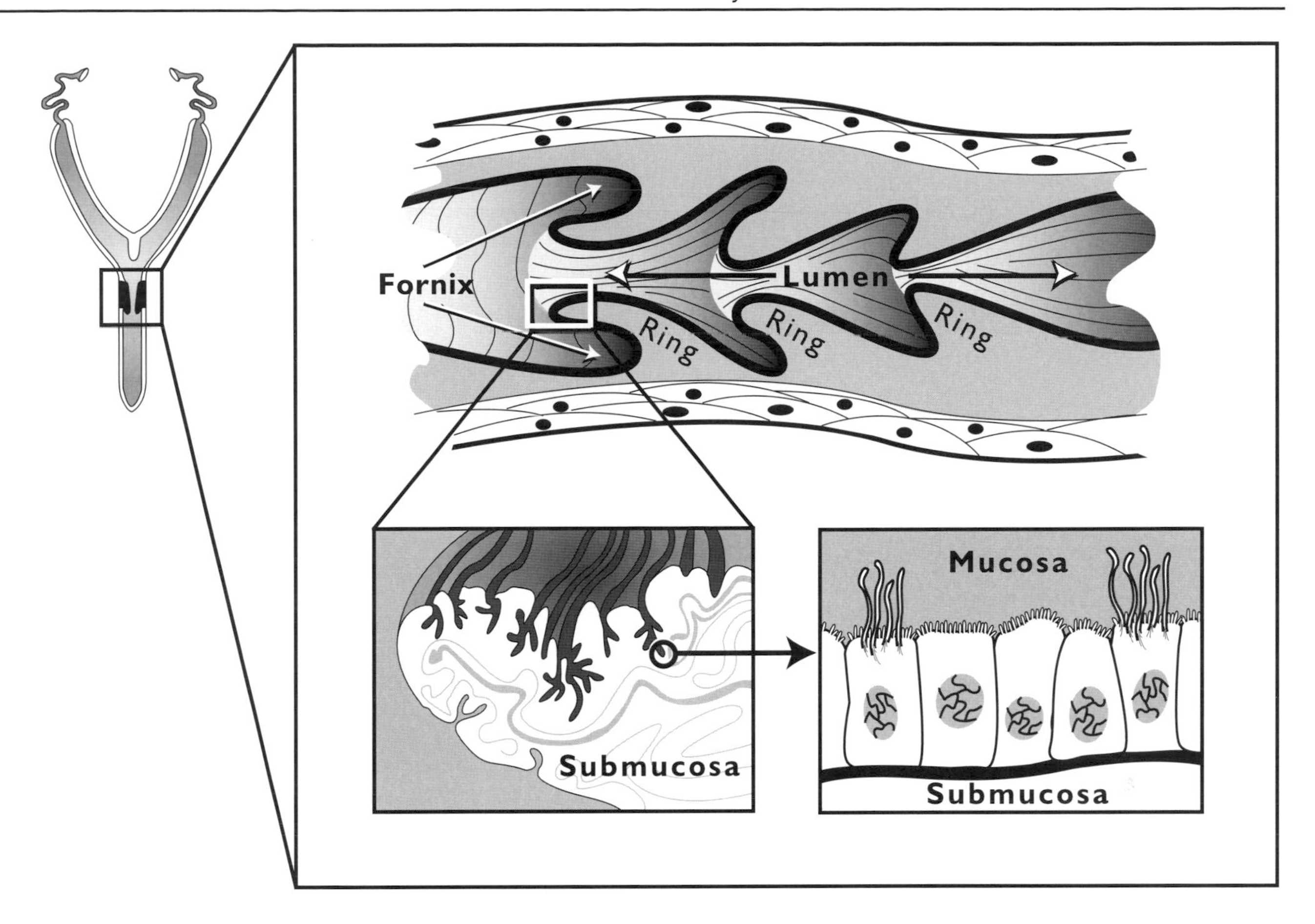

Figure 2-14. A schematic illustration of the cervix. In the cow, ewe and sow the cervix has distinct rings which protrude into the lumen. The surface of the cervix has many crypts and folds which are covered with columnar epithelium. Some cells are ciliated. In the cow, a distinct fornix is present. To observe actual specimens see Figure 2-15. (Graphic by Sonja Oei.)

erone, the mucus becomes quite viscous. In fact, the viscous mucus temporarily "glues" the folds of the cervix together so that foreign material cannot enter the uterus during gestation. This barrier is referred to as the **cervical seal of pregnancy**. Disruption of the cervical seal of pregnancy will generally cause abortion, because microorganisms can gain access to the interior of the uterus, causing infection and subsequent embryonic death.

The Vagina Is the Copulatory Organ

The primary function of the vagina is to serve as a copulatory organ, as well as the site for expulsion of urine during micturition. The vagina has a poorly organized and ill-defined muscular layer and a well developed, highly adapted mucosal epithelium.

The mucosal epithelium varies depending on the specific region of the vagina. The luminal epithelium region of the vagina near the cervix (anterior vagina) is generally columnar and highly secretory in nature. In the cow and mare the cervix protrudes into the anterior vagina, forming a large crypt, or pocket, around the cervix. This crypt is referred to as the **fornix vaginae** (Figures 2-14, 2-15 and 2-16). Spermatozoa are deposited in the fornix vaginae by the bull during natural service. The fornix vaginae is composed of columnar epithelial cells which, as in the cervix, secrete copious quantities of mucus during estrus. The sow does not have a fornix vaginae. Towards the posterior, the vagina begins to change its cellular composition. As you will see in Chapter 4, this organ is formed embryologically from two distinct anatomical regions. The

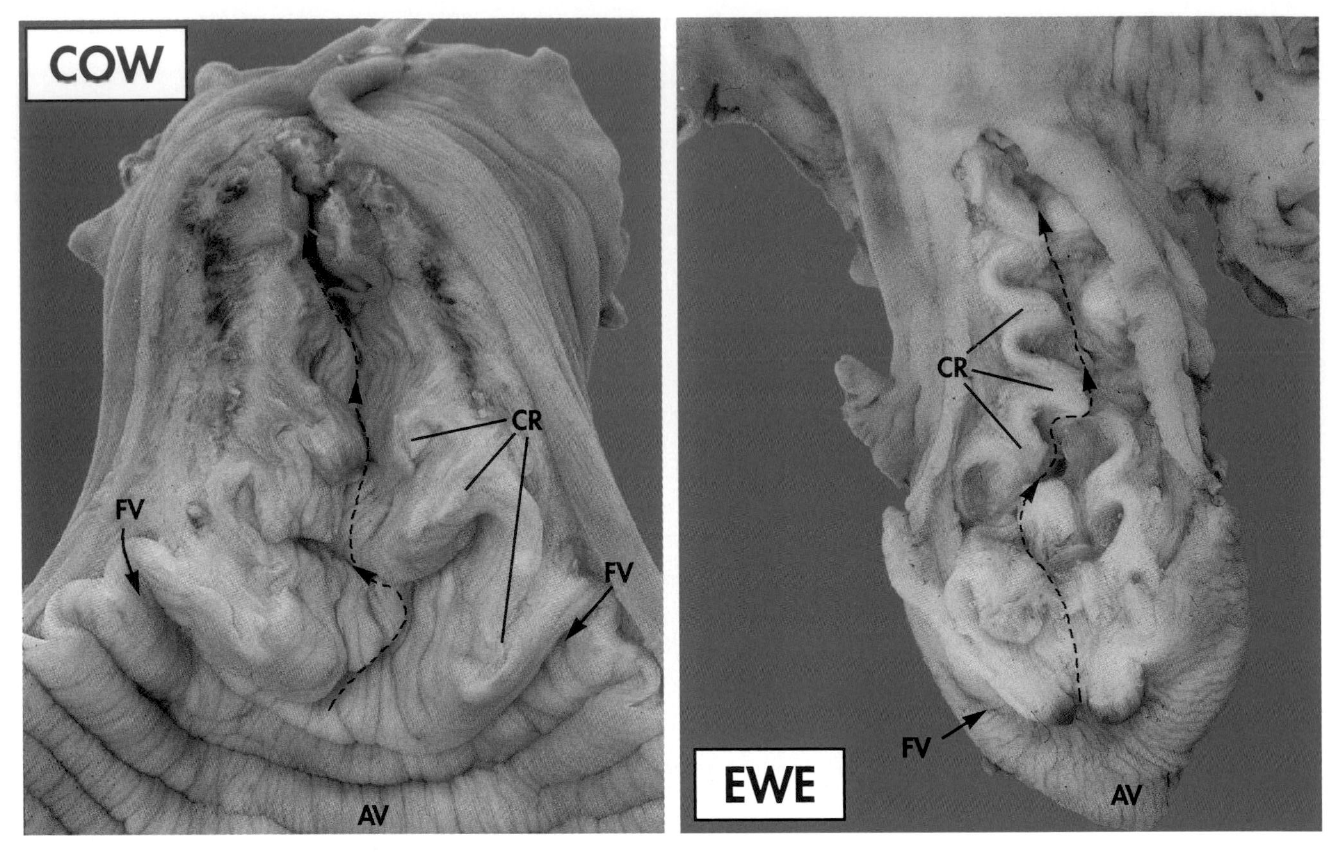

Figure 2-15. Excised cervical tissue from the cow, ewe, sow and mare. The cervix of the cow and ewe have distinct, well developed protrusions called cervical rings (CR). The sow has interdigitating prominences (IP). The mare has no cervical rings but has many longitudinal cervical folds (CF) which are continuous with the endometrial folds of the uterus. Arrows indicate the pathway of the cervical canal from the anterior vagina (AV) toward the uterus. AV = Anterior Vagina; CF = Cervical Folds; CR = Cervical Rings; FV = Fornix Vagina; IP = Interdigitating Prominences; Ut = Uterus.

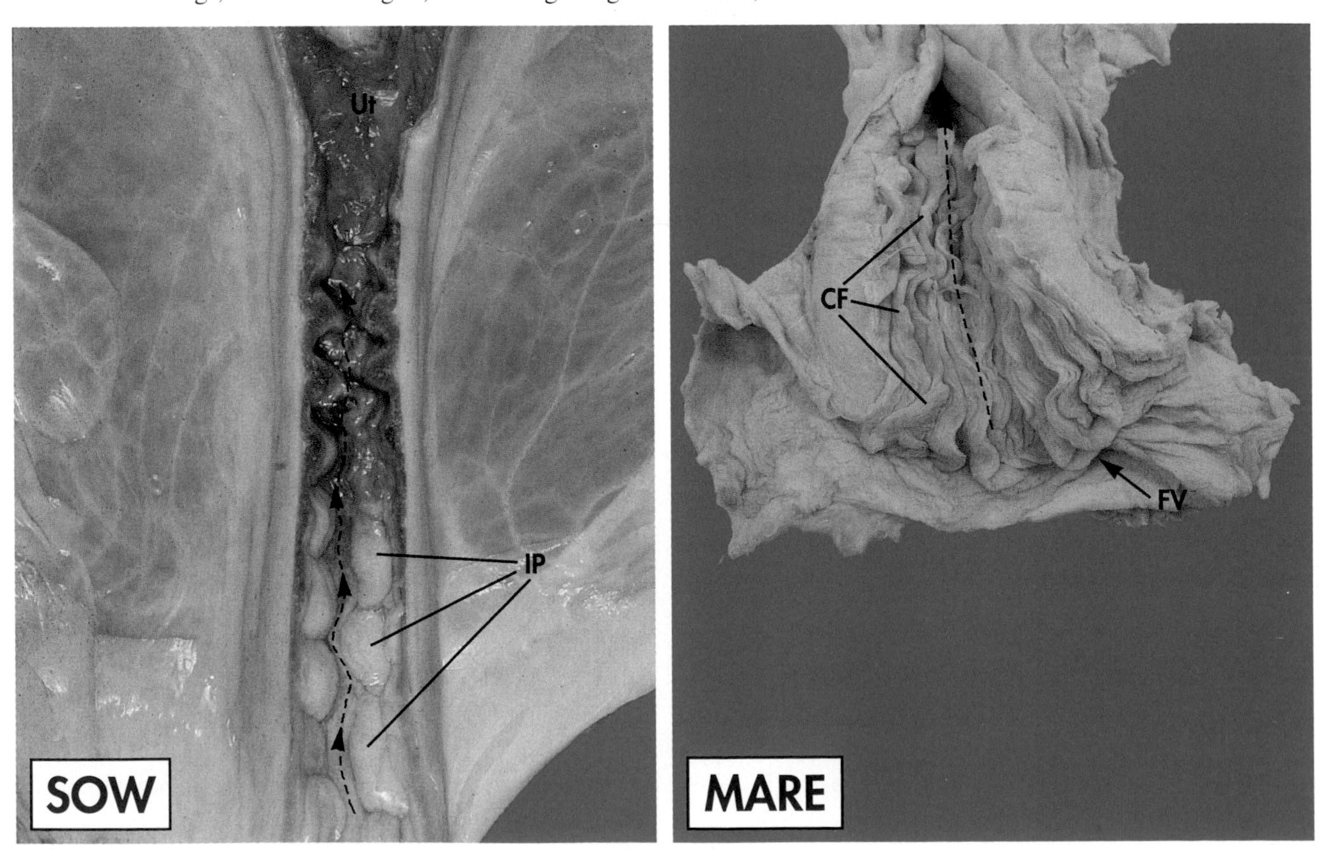

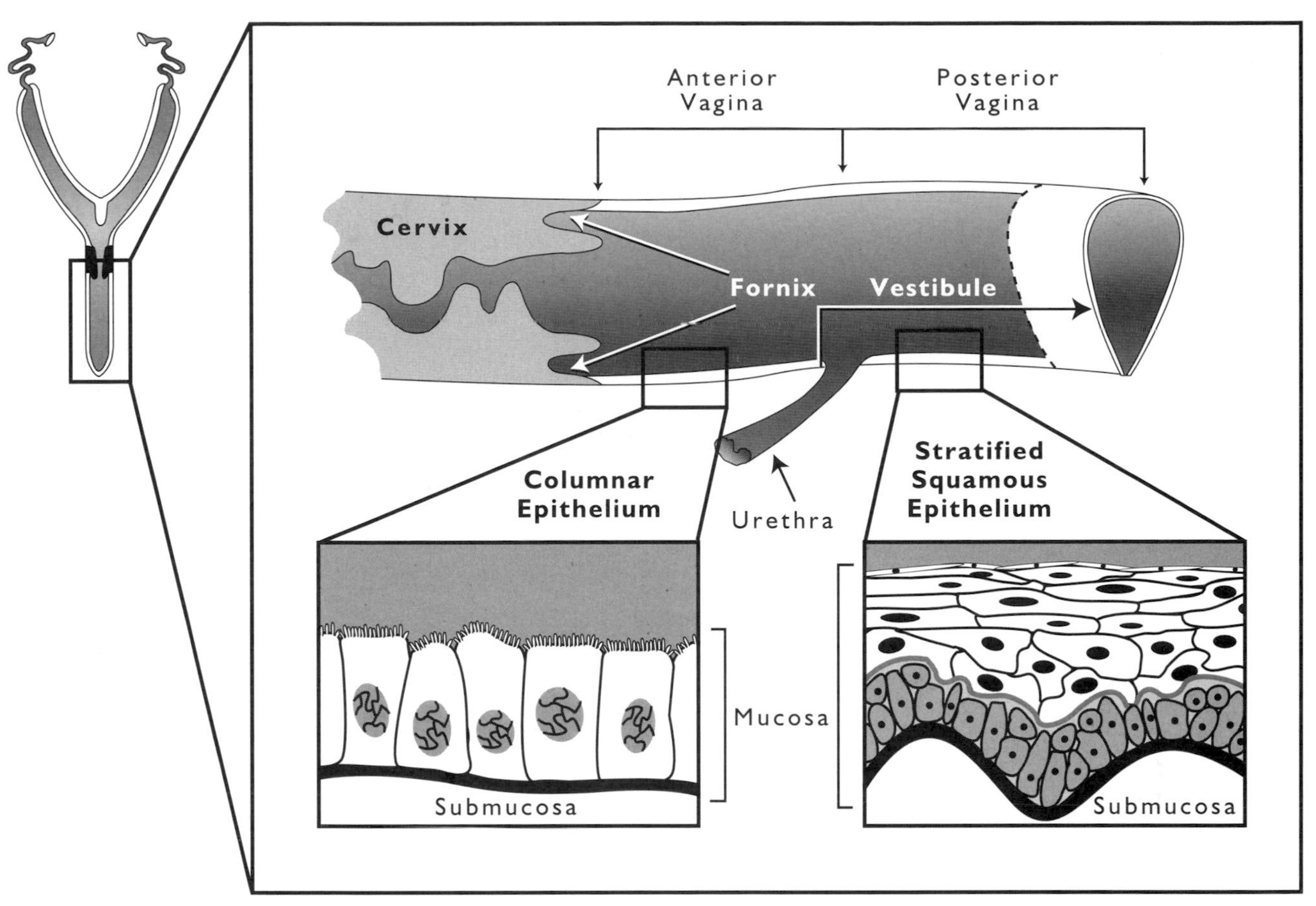

Figure 2-16. A schematic illustration of the vagina illustrating the differences in the mucosal surfaces between the anterior and posterior vagina. (Graphic by Sonja Oei.)

anterior vagina originates from the Müllerian ducts and fuses with the posterior vagina which originated from an invagination of the urogenital sinus. Thus, it is not surprising to see two distinct types of cells lining the anterior and posterior vagina. The anterior vagina is characterized as having a high degree of secretory activity as evidenced by **columnar epithelium**, and some ciliated columnar epithelium. The posterior vagina is characterized as having **stratified squamous epithelium** (the same type of epithelium that comprises the skin) (Figure 2-16). The degree of secretory activity and the thickness of the stratified squamous epithelium in the posterior vagina change with the endocrine status of the female. During the time of estrogen dominance, during estrus, the stratified squamous epithelium thickens dramatically.

Since the posterior vagina, or the **vestibule,** develops from the ventral part of the cloaca, it belongs to both the urinary and the genital systems (see Chapter 4). The vestibule is the portion of the vagina that is common to the urinary system and the reproductive system (Figure 2-16). It extends from the level of the external urethral orifice to the labia of the vulva. In most species, if the floor of the vagina is carefully dissected, one can encounter **Gartner's ducts**. These often open directly into the vestibule and are blind sacs which represent the remnants of the **Wolffian duct**. These have no apparent function and simply represent an embryonic remnant of the male reproductive system of the embryo.

In the floor of the vestibule of the sow and the cow is a small, blind pouch which lies immediately ventral to the urethral opening. This blind pouch is referred to as the **suburethral diverticulum** (Figure 2-1). A **diverticulum** is a tube which diverts its pathway from a main tube. The function of the suburethral diverticulum is unknown, but sometimes inexperienced inseminators can position the insemination rod or pipette into this blind pouch. Also, this blind pouch can be used as a landmark for the installation of a catheter to collect urine directly from the cow's bladder.

The **vulva** is the external part of the female reproductive tract. It consists of two **labia** (major and minor) which meet in the medial portion of the tract to form a **commissure** (site of union). Under most conditions, the labia form a closure which minimizes the entrance of foreign material into the vagina.

The skin of the labia is part of the integument and has numerous sebaceous and sweat glands and hair follicles. The labia consist mainly of adipose tissue into which are imbedded small bundles of smooth muscle which are known as **constrictor vulvae** muscles. The purpose of these muscles is to insure that the commissure remains intact.

The region in the female that surrounds the anus and the vulva and covers the pelvic outlet is referred to as the **perineum**. Between the dorsal commissure and the anus is a bridge of skin which is sometimes torn during parturition, generally resulting from an oversized or malpositioned fetus.

The ventral commissure of the vestibule houses the **clitoris**, the female homologue of the glans penis. It is composed of erectile tissue and is covered with stratified squamous epithelium. It is well supplied with sensory nerve endings. The onset of estrus, accompanied by high estrogen levels, generally results in a continuous state of erection of the clitoris. The functional significance of this highly sensitized area has not been well established in domestic animals. However, clitoral stimulation at the time of insemination has been shown to increase conception rates by artificial insemination by up to 6% in beef cows, but not in heifers. The submucosa of the vestibule also houses the **vestibular glands** (also called Bartholin's glands). These glands are located in the posterior portion of the vestibule and actively secrete a mucous-like material during estrus.

Further Phenomena for Fertility

Early myths and folklore referred to "vagina dentata" which described a vagina with teeth. Vagina dentata is said to symbolize fear of castration, the dangers of sexual intercourse, of birth, etc.

The female bedbug has no vagina (and apparently does not display estrus). The male "drills" into the abdomen with his pointed penis and deposits semen directly into the body cavity.

The Italian anatomist Gabriello Fallopius (1532-1562) is perhaps most widely recognized for his description of the oviducts which bear his name. Fallopius, a recognized early authority on syphilis, has also been credited with the invention of the condom. His Gallico Liber Absoltismus (published posthumously in 1564) contains a description of a "linen sheath" that is credited with decreasing the spread of syphilis that was very prevalent in Europe during his lifetime.

The word "hysterectomy" means surgical removal of the uterus. The word is derived from a notion espoused by Plato (347-266 BC). He thought that the uterus was a multichambered organ that could wander about the body causing hysteria in the host woman. He thought that if a woman went too long without becoming pregnant her uterus would become indignant and would wander around the body causing extreme anxiety, hysteria, respiratory insufficiency and all sorts of diseases. The cure was removal of the uterus, which removed the possibility of hysteria and disease. In spite of its ancient and erroneous origin the term hysterectomy is still used today in the highest level of medical and scientific practice. A more descriptive term for removal of uterus would be "uterectomy." Author's Theory: This myth probably was originated by Greek males who recognized that pregnancy required copulation. The anxiety / disease causing fable "legitimized" their desire for frequent copulation.

Most birds have only a left ovary and oviduct which are functional. Some birds have two functional ovaries, but only the left oviduct is functional. Thus, when the right ovary ovulates there is nowhere for the oocyte to go except into the body cavity, where it is reabsorbed (the truest form of recycling). The oocyte cannot enter the left oviduct because a mesentery separates the right ovary from the left oviduct.

In the female hyena, the clitoris is very well developed. In fact, it is so well developed that it is almost impossible to distinguish the male hyena from the female hyena. The female also has a false scrotum. Of further note is the fact that the female is the dominant sex and produces as much or more testosterone than the typical male.

Additional Reading

Dyce, K.M., W.O. Sack and C.J.G. Wensing. 1996. *Textbook of Veterinary Anatomy.* 2nd Edition, W.B. Saunders Co., Philadelphia.

Ginther, O.J. 1992. *Reproductive Biology of the Mare.* 2nd Edition, Equiservices Publishing, Cross Plains, WI (608-798-4910).

Schummer, A., R. Nickel and W.O. Sack. 1979. *The Viscera of the Domestic Mammals.* 2nd Revised Edition, Springer-Verlag, New York.

3 The Organization and Function of the Male Reproductive System

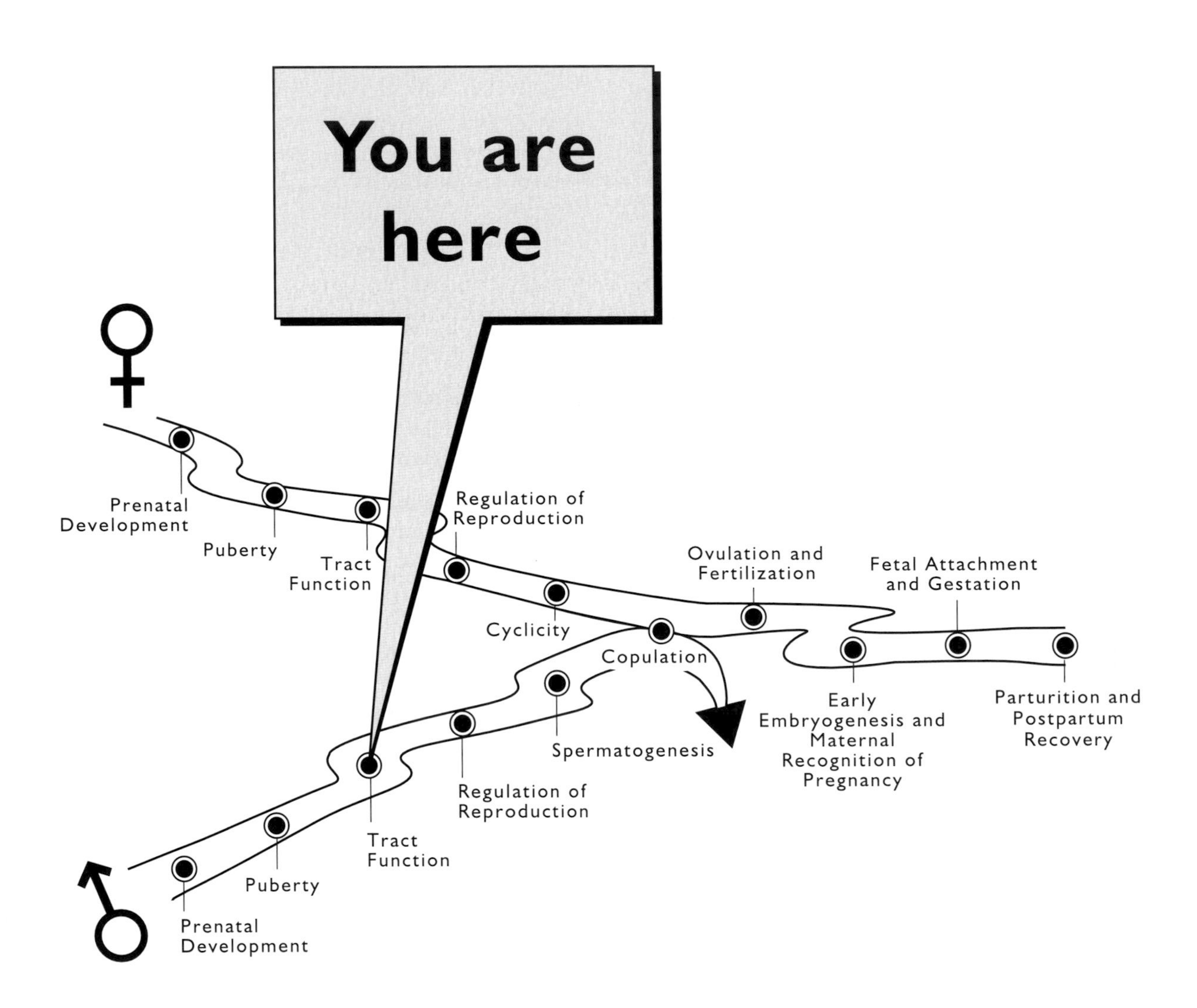

Take Home Message

The male reproductive system consists of the spermatic cord, testis, epididymis, accessory sex glands and the penis. The testis produces spermatozoa and testosterone, as well as other substances such as inhibin, estrogen and several proteins. The epididymis provides the environment for final maturation of spermatozoa and serves as a storage organ for these cells. The accessory sex glands produce seminal plasma and the penis is the copulatory organ.

The male reproductive system is analogous to a manufacturing complex (Figure 3-1). The primary products of the "manufacturing" process are fertile spermatozoa. Hormones (such as testosterone) and other secretory products (epididymal fluid and seminal plasma) of the male system contribute to the efficiency of the overall manufacturing and delivery process.

The **testes** serve as the manufacturing and assembly plant for spermatozoa and have an immense potential output. In fact, spermatozoal production in mammals ranges from < 1 to 25 billion spermatozoa per day for both testes in normal males. This computes to an amazing production rate of around 35,000 to 290,000 spermatozoa per second. Once produced, spermatozoa pass through the rete tubules and the efferent ducts, and enter the **head** (caput) and **body** (corpus) of the **epididymis** (the "finishing shops"). In the head and body of the epididymis, spermatozoa undergo changes which allow them to become fertile. After gradual transport through the body and head over several days, spermatozoa enter the **tail** (cauda) of the epididymis. The tail of the epididymis is equivalent to a warehouse and shipping center. Spermatozoa in the tail of the epididymis are capable of fertilization and are motile if diluted into an appropriate buffer solution. The tail of the epididymis serves as a storage organ for spermatozoa prior to ejaculation and, in the sexually inactive male, may contain 4 to 8 days production of sperm. In males who are ejaculating with regular frequency, fewer sperm may be found. Upon sexual excitation, the spermatozoa in the tail of the epididymis are "shipped" via contractions of the epididymal duct and the **ductus deferens** to a new location in the reproductive tract, the **pelvic urethra.** Final alterations and packaging take place during emission when spermatozoa are mixed with fluids produced by the **accessory sex glands.** Collectively this mixture of fluids (from the epididymal tail and the accessory sex glands) is known as **seminal plasma**. Mixing of seminal plasma with spermatozoa causes dilution and undoubtedly some biochemical and surface changes which facilitate spermatozoal function. Once sperm are mixed with seminal plasma, they are available for delivery by ejaculation. The delivery system is the **penis** and specific muscles responsible for **erection**, **protrusion of the penis** and **ejaculation** of semen.

The basic components of the male reproductive system are the:
- ***spermatic cord***
- ***scrotum***
- ***testis***
- ***excurrent duct system***
- ***accessory sex glands***
- ***penis and muscles for protrusion, erection and ejaculation***

The remainder of the chapter will assist you in developing knowledge about the anatomy and function of the specific components of the male reproductive system.

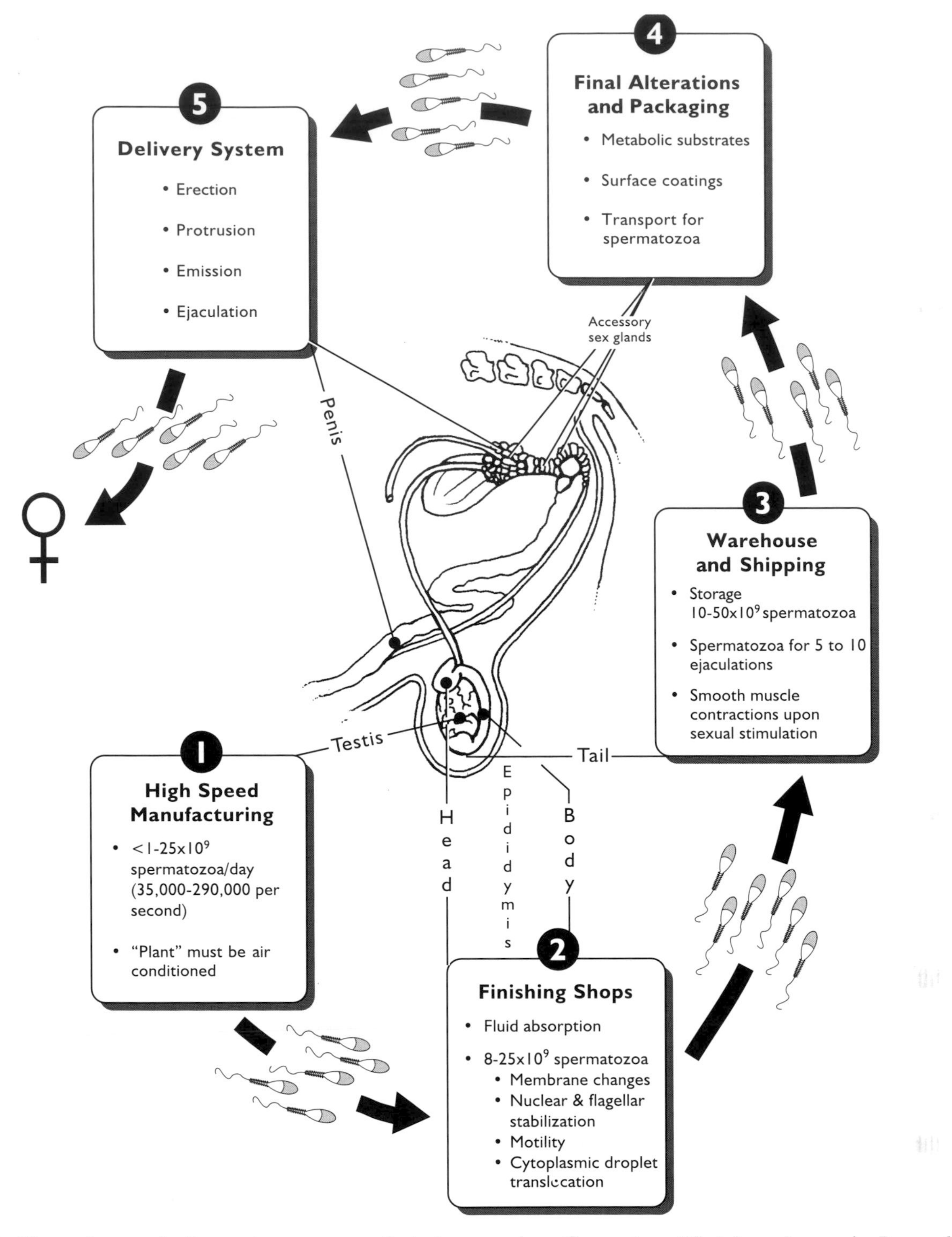

Figure 3-1. The male reproductive system as a manufacturing complex. Concept modified from Amann in *Proceedings of the 14th NAAB Technical Conference*, 1986. (Graphic by Sonja Oei.)

The Spermatic Cord Suspends the Testis

The **spermatic cord** extends from the inguinal ring (the passageway from the body cavity into the scrotum) to its attachment on the dorsal pole of the testis. It suspends the testis in the scrotum (Figures 3-2 through 3-5). It is most highly developed in males like the ram and bull which have a pendulous scrotum. The spermatic cord provides the pathway to and from the body for the testicular vasculature, lymphatics and nerves. The spermatic cord also houses the ductus deferens, the **cremaster muscle** and a specialized vascular network called the **pampiniform plexus**.

Bull

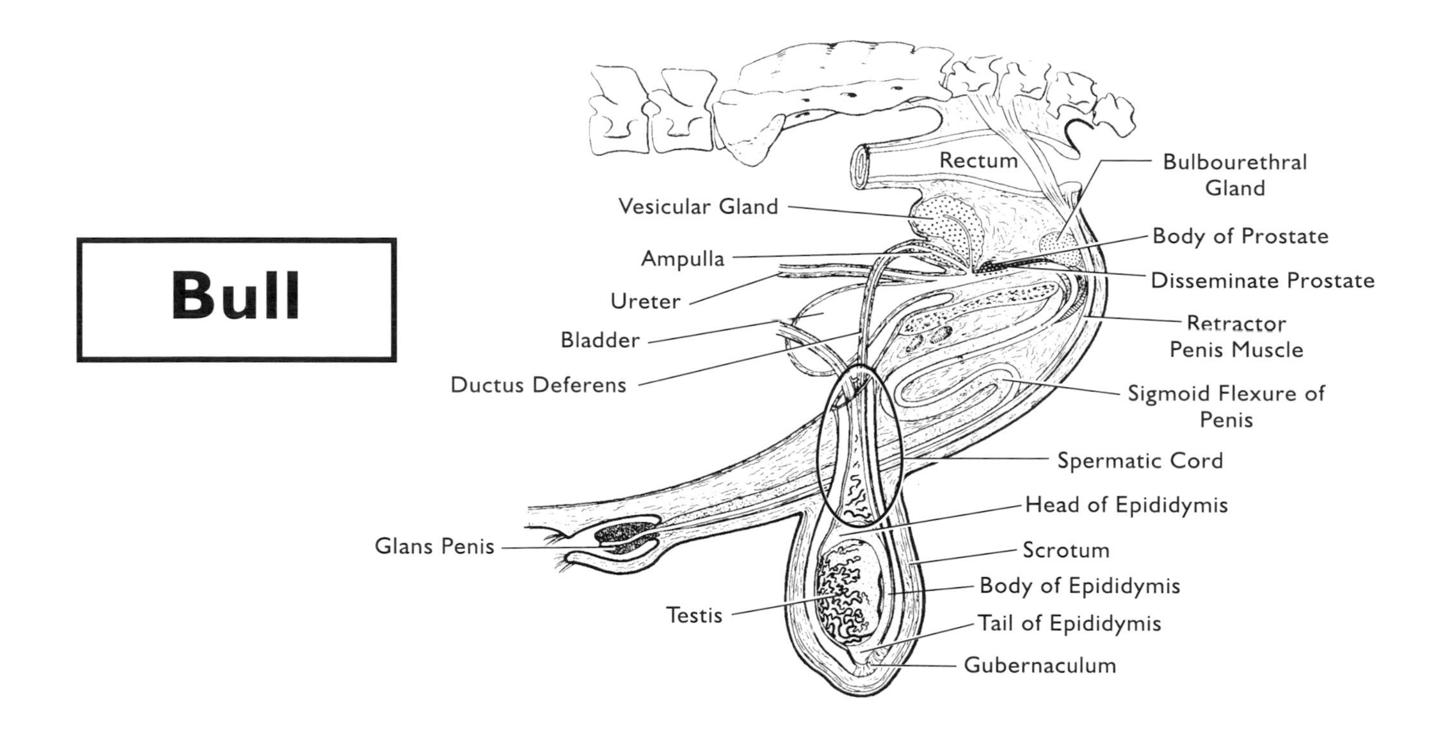

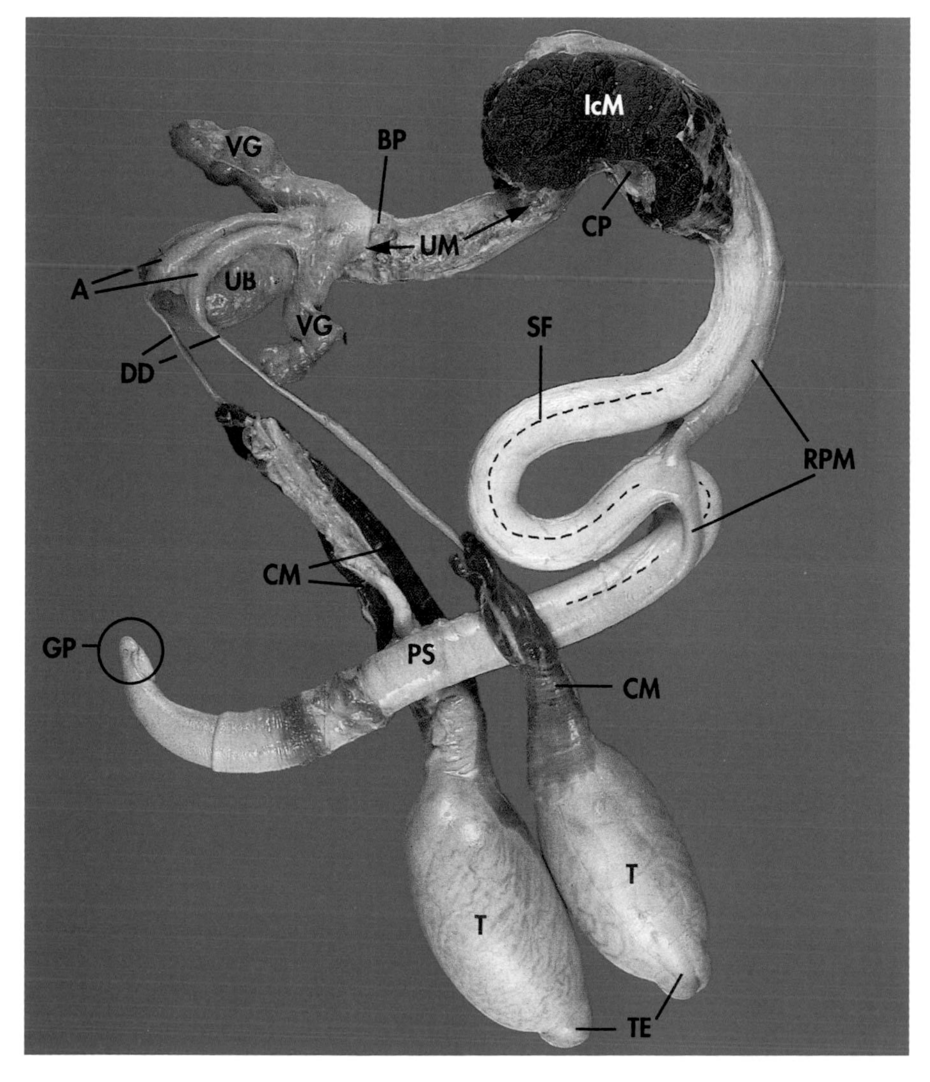

Figure 3-2.

Top Panel

Schematic illustration of a sagittal view of the bull reproductive tract (modified from Ellenberger and Baum, 1943, Handbuch der vergleichenden Anatomie der Haustiere, 18th Edition. Zietzschmann, Ackerknecht and Grau, eds. Permission from Springer-Verlag, New York).

Bottom Panel

Sagittal view of an excised reproductive tract from the bull.

A = Ampulla; BP = Body of Prostate; CM = Cremaster Muscle; CP = Crus Penis; DD = Ductus Deferens; GP = Glans Penis; IcM = Ischiocavernosus Muscle; PS = Penile Shaft; RPM = Retractor Penis Muscle; SF = Sigmoid Flexure; TE = Tail of Epididymis; T = Testis; UM = Urethralis Muscle; UB = Urinary Bladder; VG = Vesicular Gland.

Stallion

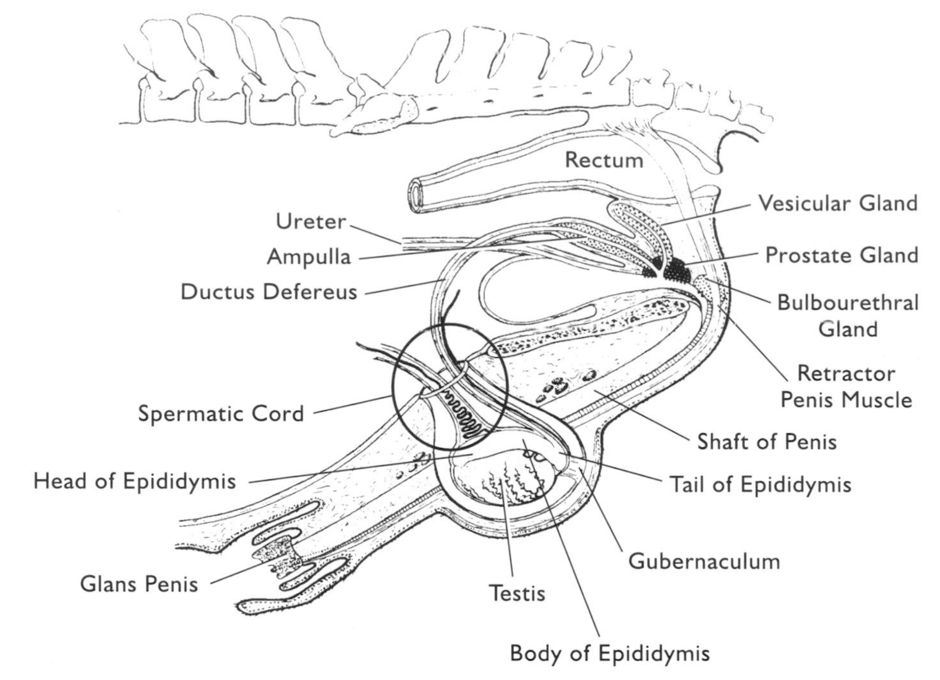

Figure 3-3.
Top Panel
Schematic illustration of a sagittal view of the stallion reproductive tract (modified from Ellenberger and Baum, 1943, Handbuch der vergleichenden Anatomie der Haustiere, 18th Edition. Zietzschmann, Ackerknecht and Grau, eds. Permission from Springer-Verlag, New York).

Bottom Panel
Sagittal view of an excised reproductive tract from the stallion. A = Ampulla; BsM = Bulbospongiosus Muscle; BuG = Bulbourethral Glands; CM = Cremaster Muscle; CP = Crus Penis; DD = Ductus Deferens; GP = Glans Penis; IcM = Ischiocavernosus Muscle; P = Prostate; PS = Penile Shaft; RPM = Retractor Penis Muscle; T = Testis; TE = Tail of Epididymis; U = Ureters; UB = Urinary Bladder; VG = Vesicular Gland.

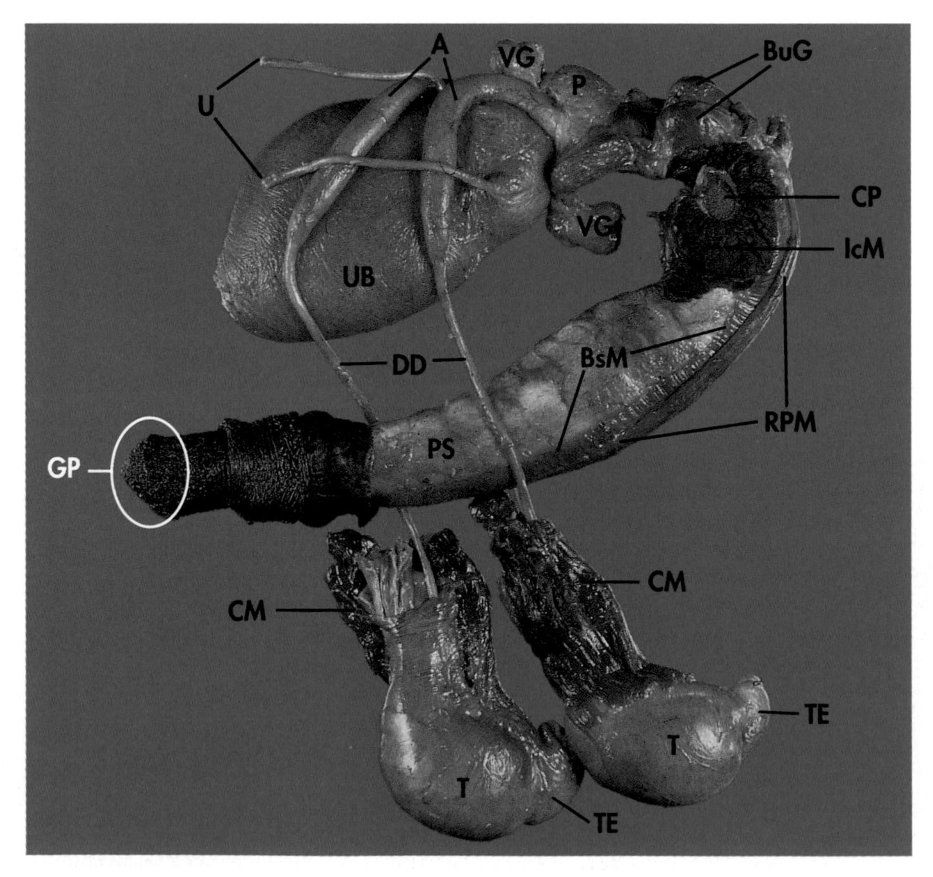

Boar

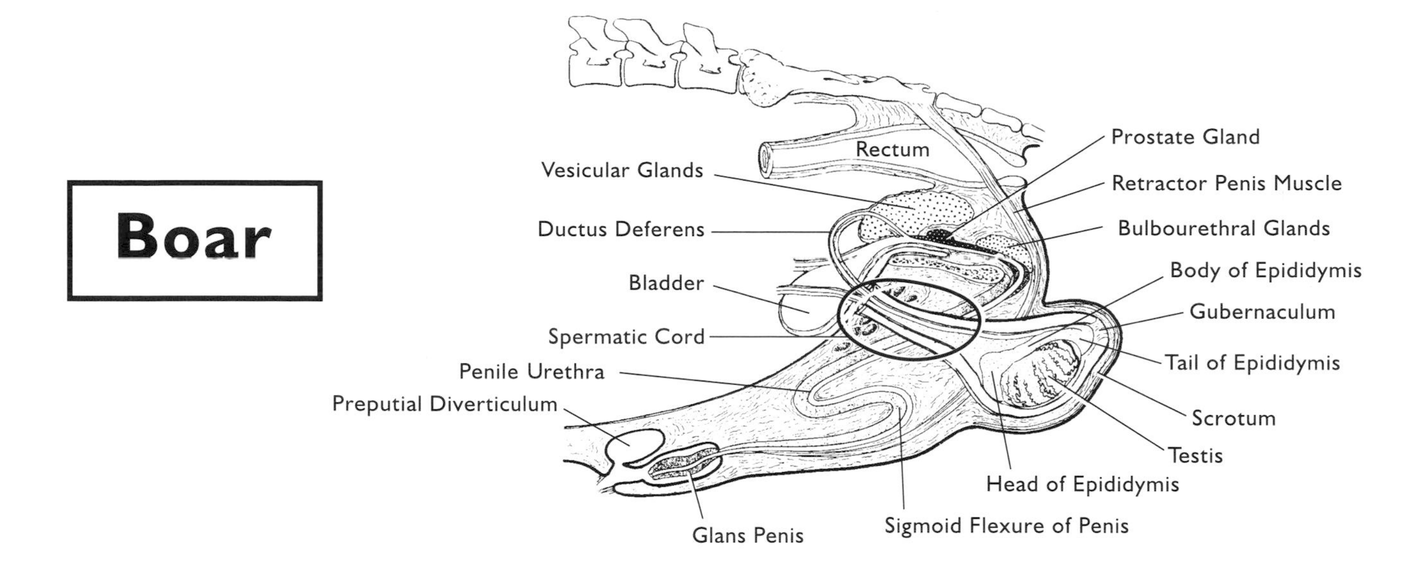

Figure 3-4.
Top Panel
Schematic illustration of a sagittal view of the boar reproductive tract (modified from Ellenberger and Baum, 1943, Handbuch der vergleichenden Anatomie der Haustiere, 18th Edition. Zietzschmann, Ackerknecht and Grau, eds. Permission from Springer-Verlag, New York).

Bottom Panel
Sagittal view of an excised reproductive tract from the boar. BE = Body of Epididymis; BsM = Bulbo-spongiosus Muscle; BuG = Bulbourethral Glands; CP = Crus Penis; DD = Ductus Deferens; GP = Glans Penis; HE = Head of Epididymis; IcM = Ischiocavernosus Muscle; PS = Penile Shaft; PG = Prostate Gland; RPM = Retractor Penis Muscle; TE = Tail of Epididymis; T = Testis (left - t. vaginalis intact; right - t. vaginalis removed); UM = Urethralis Muscle; UB = Urinary Bladder; VG = Vesicular Glands.

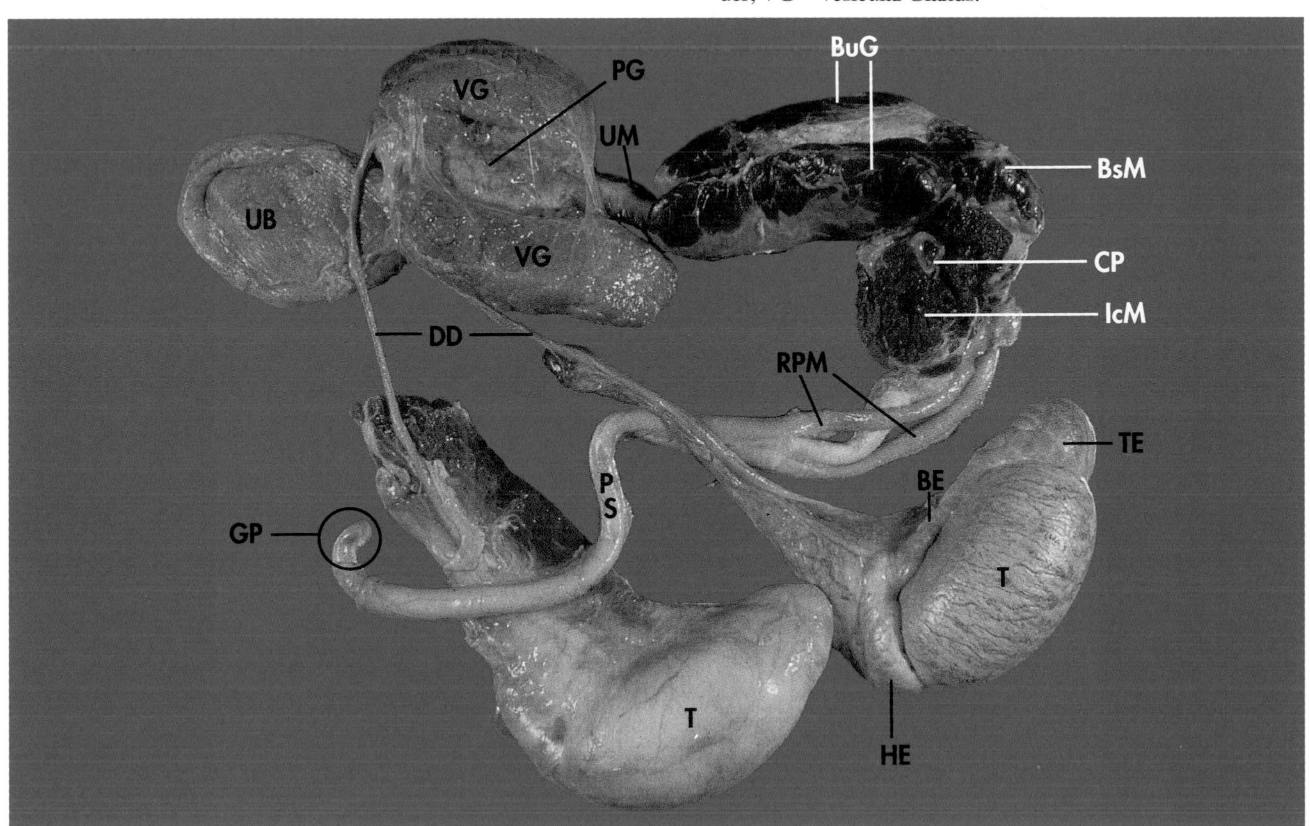

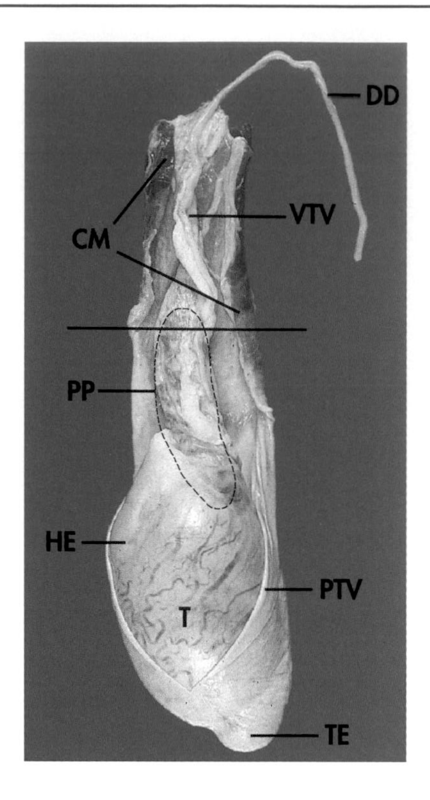

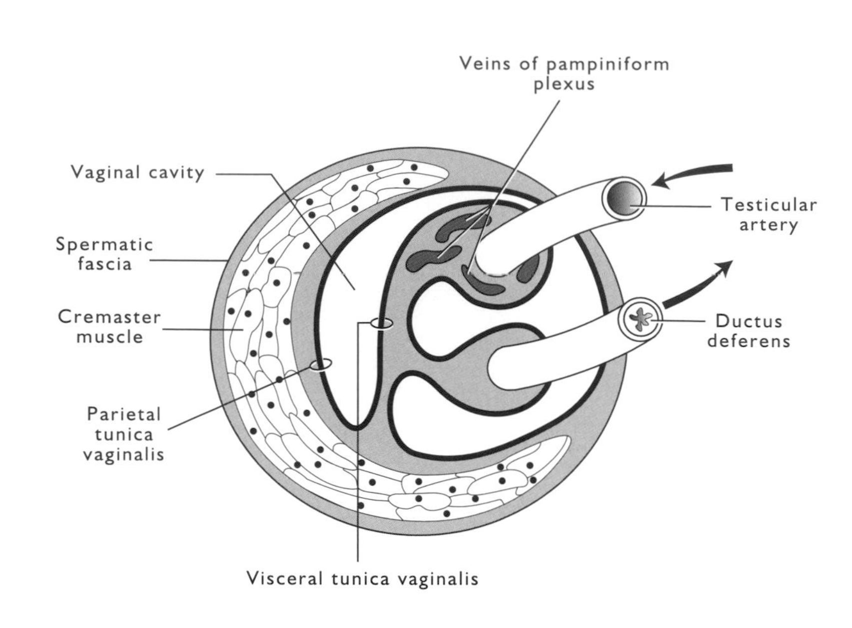

Figure 3-5. Excised spermatic cord and testis of the bull (left panel) and a schematic illustration of a cross section of the spermatic cord (right panel). Arrows indicate direction of fluid flow. The line across the excised spermatic cord indicates the approximate plane of the cross-sectional schematic. The excised spermatic cord has been incised to expose the interior. CM = Cremaster Muscle; DD = Ductus Deferens; HE = Head of Epididymis; PP = Pampiniform Plexus; PTV = Parietal Tunica Vaginalis; T = Testis; TE = Tail of Epididymis; VTV = Visceral Tunica Vaginalis. (Schematic modified from Dyce, Sack and Wensing, *Textbook of Veterinary Anatomy. 2nd Edition.)*

The functions of the spermatic cords are to:

- ***provide vascular, lymphatic and neural connection to the body***
- ***provide a heat exchanger (pampiniform plexus)***
- ***house the cremaster muscle***

The pampiniform plexus is a vascular structure consisting of an intimately intertwined artery and vein (Figures 3-6 and 3-7). This highly specialized structure is important for proper temperature control of the testis. In most mammals the testes must be 4 to 6°C cooler than the body in order for spermatogenesis (manufacture of spermatozoa) to occur. The spermatic artery leaves the body and enters the spermatic cord as an uncoiled vessel (Figures 3-6 and 3-7). As it approaches the testis, the spermatic artery becomes highly coiled and is intimately intermingled with a network of veins. The complex, intimate network of the spermatic artery and the spermatic veins forms a **countercurrent heat exchanger** (Figure 3-6). Heat from the warm (39°C) blood from the body is transferred to the cooler (33°C) venous blood leaving the surface of the testes (Figure 3-6). This venous blood has been cooled by direct heat loss from the testicular veins through the skin of the scrotum. Maintenance of low testicular temperature is obligatory for spermatogenesis in food producing mammals and man. Disruption or modification of this cooling mechanism will severely compromise, if not completely suppress spermatogenesis.

In addition to serving as a heat exchanger, the pampiniform plexus also serves as a **pulse pressure eliminator**. Pulse pressure exists in all arteries throughout the body. Pulse pressure is what you feel when you palpate the radial artery in your wrist or the carotid artery in your neck. It is the difference between **systolic pressure** (heart contraction) and **diastolic pressure** (heart relaxation). For example, if systolic pressure is 120 mm Hg and diastolic pressure is 80 mm Hg, the pulse pressure is 40 mm Hg. In the case of the **spermatic artery**, this pulse pressure is almost eliminated between the inguinal ring and the surface of the testis (Figure 3-7). Thus, blood entering the testis is almost "pulseless." However, the mean arterial pressure (the average of systolic and diastolic pressure) is only slightly reduced. The mechanism whereby the arterial pulse pressure is eliminated is not known. It has been proposed that the spermatic artery has a higher compliance (elasticity) than other arteries of comparable size. The functional significance of this pulse elimination is not understood clearly.

The close relationship between the venous and the arterial blood supply in the pampiniform plexus results in some opportunity for exchange of testosterone between the two vessels (Figure 3-6). Because testosterone is at high concentrations in the venous drainage from the testicle, and levels are low in the arterial blood from the body supplying the testicle, testosterone moves from the vein to the artery (Figure 3-6). This concentration gradient allows some testosterone to be recirculated back into the testicle. In this context, the pampiniform plexus is fundamentally quite similar to the vascular countercurrent exchange system between the uterine vein and ovarian artery in the female, where $PGF_{2\alpha}$ is transferred to the ovary (see Chapter 9).

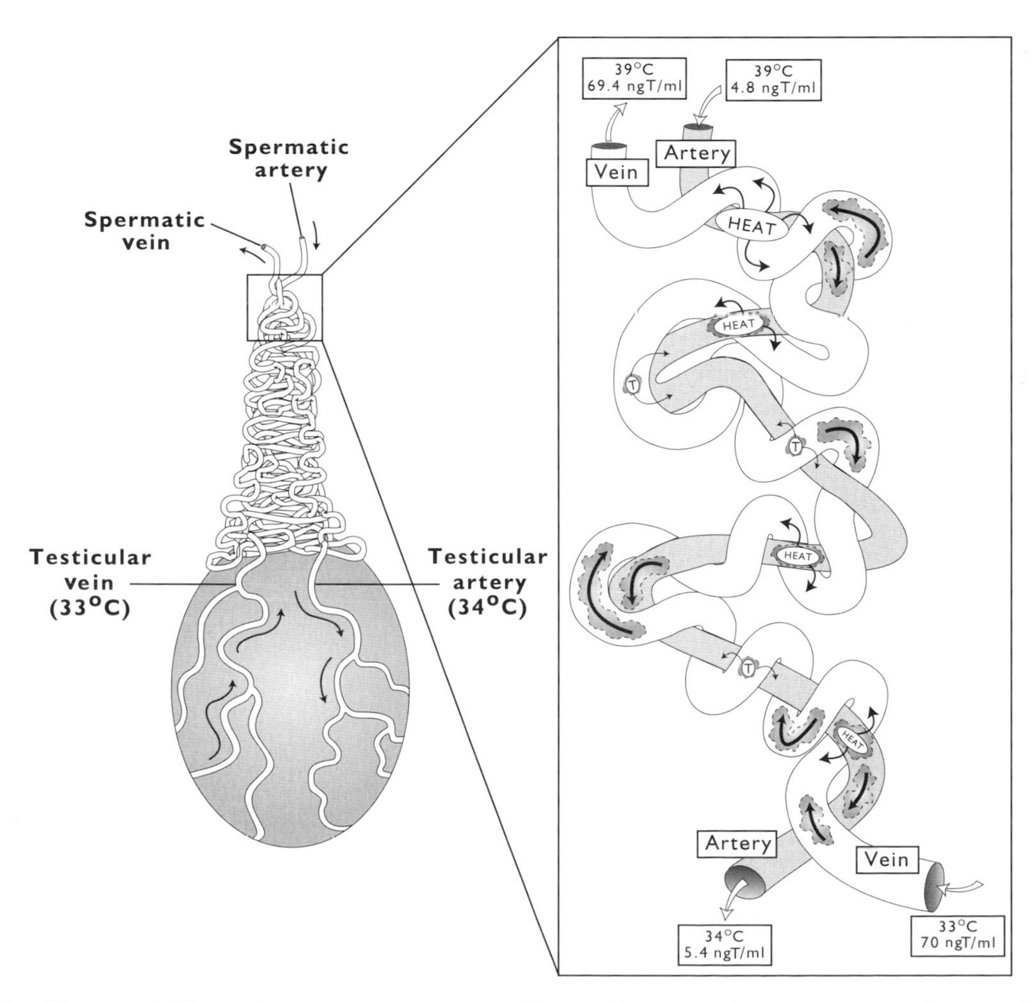

Figure 3-6. The pampiniform plexus as a countercurrent heat exchanger and testosterone exchanger. Warm (39°C) arterial blood is cooled on its way to the testis because the artery lies in close apposition to the veins returning cooler blood (33°C) to the body and a large (6°C) temperature gradient exists. (Graphic by Sonja Oei.)

The Testes Are Supported by the Cremaster Muscle

The primary muscle supporting the testis and coursing the length of the spermatic cord is the cremaster muscle (Figures 3-2 through 3-5). The cremaster is a striated muscle which is continuous with the internal abdominal oblique muscle. It helps support the testis and aids in control of testicular temperature. Its temperature control function is probably related to the fact that when the cremaster muscle contracts and relaxes, it creates a "pumping action" on the pampiniform plexus, thus facilitating blood flow and enhancing cooling efficiency. In some species (the ram and, to some degree, the bull) sexual excitation promotes a high degree of intermittent contractile activity of the cremaster muscle. During sexual excitation the testes move up and down in a rapid manner. Unlike the smooth muscle in the scrotum (**tunica dartos**), the cremaster muscle is not capable of sustained contractions. Therefore, it is reasonable to assume that the function of the cremaster muscle is more related to facilitating blood movement in the pampiniform plexus than providing sustained contractions for elevating the testes close to the body wall during exposure to cold temperatures. The cremaster muscle may be important in short-term elevation of the testicles during fear or high planes of excitement. Such a function would tend to protect the pendular testes during periods of physical confrontation or flight from danger.

Not all animals possess pendular testes and thus do not have a scrotum. Birds, elephants, sloths, armadillos and some marine mammals (whales and dolphins) have testes located inside the body in a **retroperitoneal position**. Thus, mechanisms associated with temperature regulation are not important in these species, except where loss of control of deep body temperature occurs. The testes of some mammals (rat and rabbit) move into and out of the body cavity throughout their lives through a patent inguinal canal. The evolutionary basis for the descent of the testes and the need for testicular cooling is not clear.

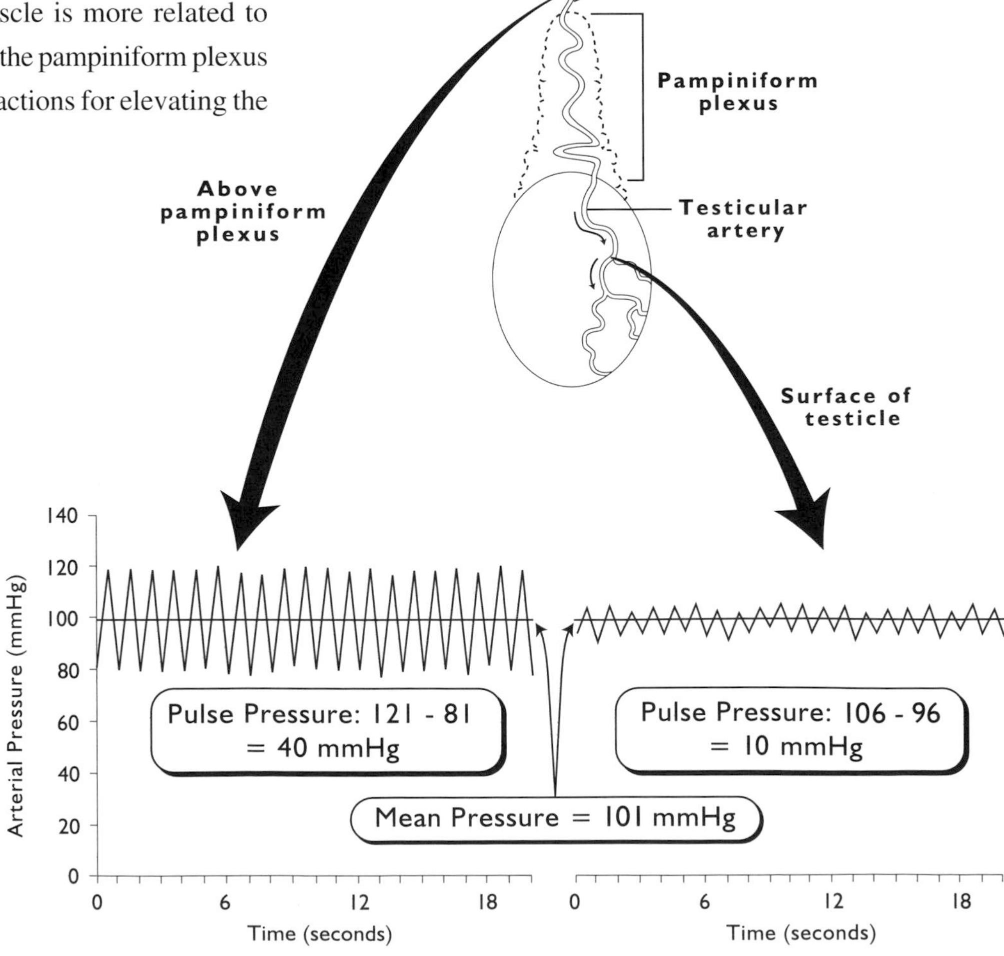

Figure 3-7. Pulse pressure in the spermatic artery (above the pampiniform plexus) and the testicular artery (below the pampiniform plexus) in the ram. (Graphic by Sonja Oei.)

The Scrotal Skin Serves as a Temperature Sensor and a Cooling System

The **scrotum** is a two lobed sack. It protects and supports the testes and is required for proper temperature regulation. The scrotum consists of four major layers. They are: 1) the **skin**; 2) the **tunica dartos**; 3) the **scrotal fascia**; and 4) the **parietal tunica vaginalis** (Figure 3-11).

The scrotal skin is heavily populated with sweat glands. These sweat glands are required for maintenance of proper testicular temperature. The scrotal sweat glands are innervated by sympathetic nerves (Figure 3-8). When the male experiences either elevated body temperature or elevated scrotal temperature, the hypothalamus detects this change and sends nerve impulses to the sweat glands. Sweating allows the scrotum (and thus the testes) to be cooled by evaporative heat transfer.

The scrotal skin is endowed with large numbers of thermosensitive nerves. These sensory nerves govern both the degree of scrotal sweating and respiratory rate of the animal. In fact, in the ram changes in scrotal temperature can bring about dramatic changes in respiratory rate. For example, the rate of respiration of fully fleeced Merino rams begins to increase gradually when the skin temperature of the scrotum rises above 36°C. If the temperature of the scrotal skin continues to increase (40-42°C), the respiratory rate will increase suddenly and the ram will begin to pant (polypnea). Respiratory frequencies as high as 200 breaths per minute can occur under these conditions (Figure 3-9). Warming an equivalent area of the flank or other parts of the body results in only small increases in respiratory rate. This response clearly shows that there is a highly developed neural pathway originating in the scrotum and terminating in the respiratory center of the brain (Figure 3- 8).

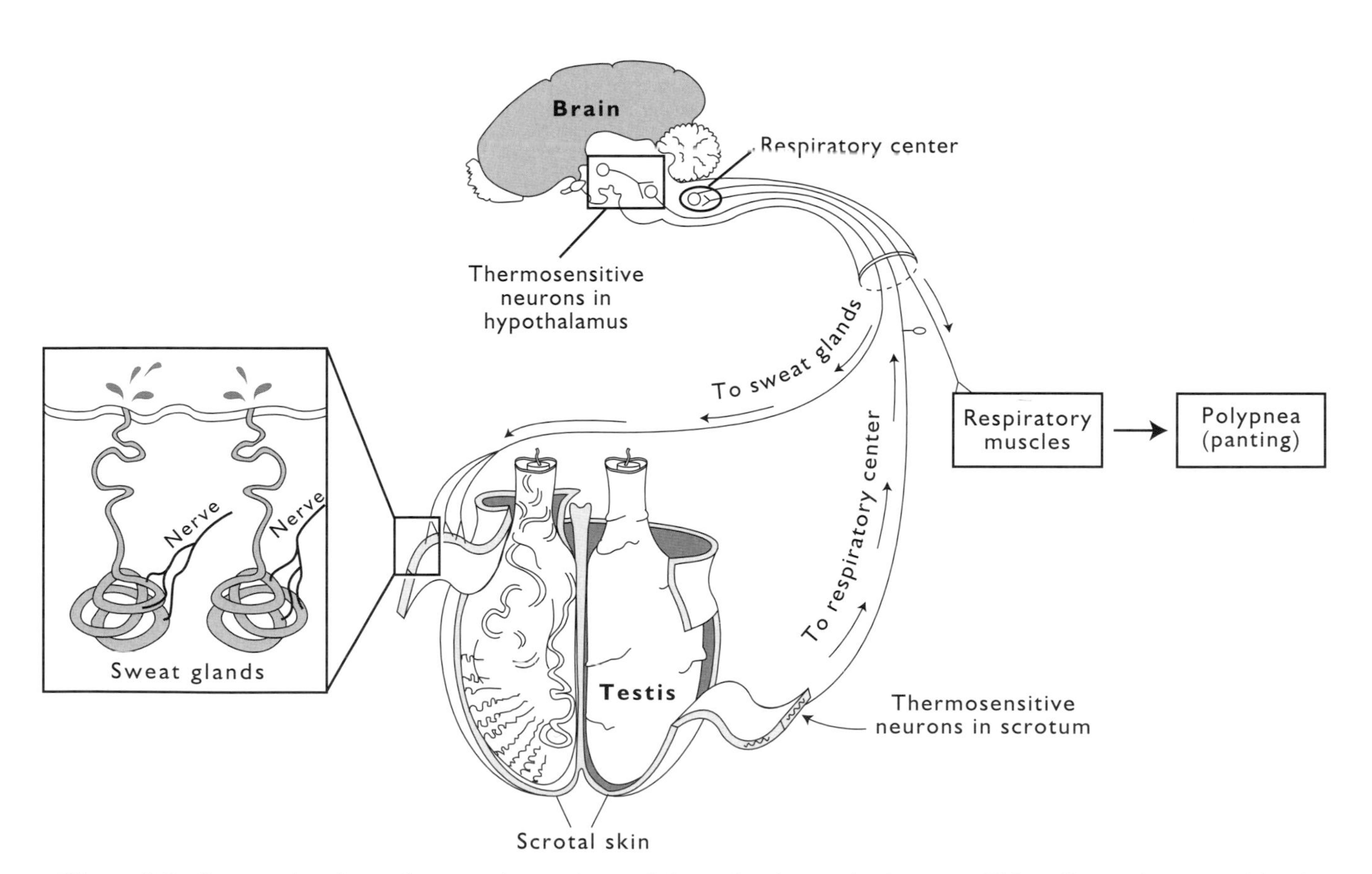

Figure 3-8. Proposed pathway for scrotal sweating and thermal polypnea in the ram. This reflex pathway resulting in polypnea is not activated until scrotal temperature reaches about 36°C. (Graphic by Sonja Oei.)

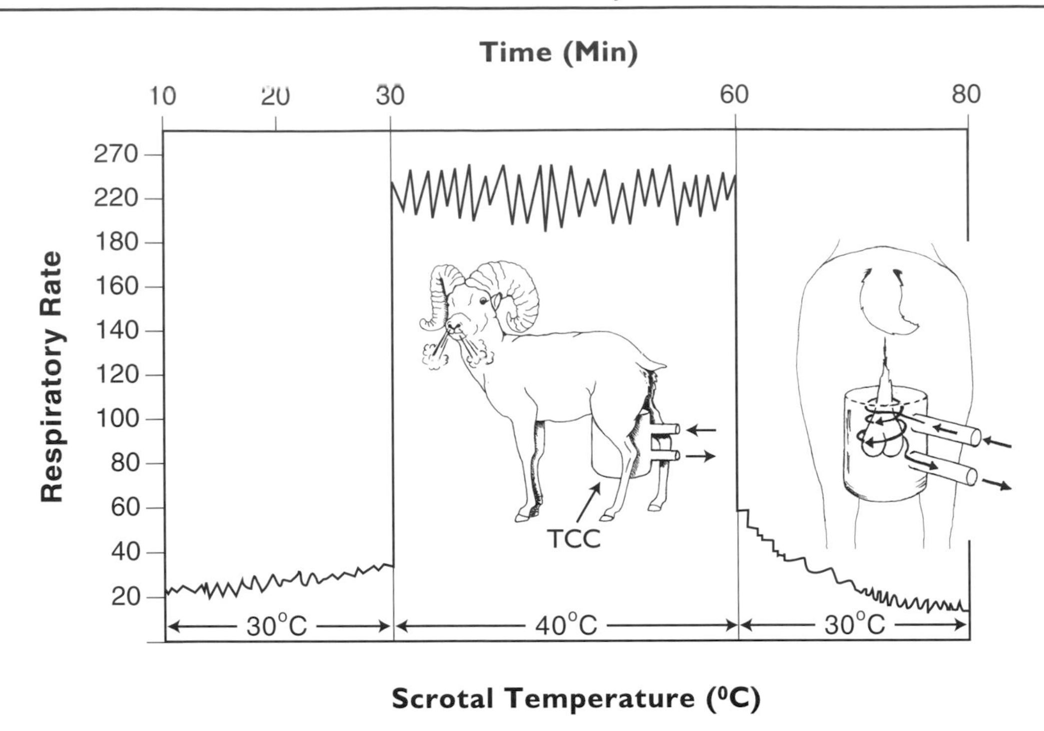

Figure 3-9. Warming of the scrotum using a temperature controlled chamber (TCC-arrow) in a fully fleeced ram causes little change in respiratory rate until the scrotal temperature reaches 40°C. When a scrotal temperature of 40°C is reached, marked polypnea occurs with respiratory rates often exceeding 200 cycles/min. When scrotal temperature returns to about 30°C, respiratory rates suddenly return to normal. (Adapted from Waites, *The Testis* Vol. 1. Johnson, Gomes and Vandemark.)

> ***The scrotum is a:***
> - ***thermosensor***
> - ***radiator***
> - ***protective sac***

While cooling of the testes is obligatory to normal spermatogenesis, constant cooling does not appear to be necessary. For example, Australian researchers found that exposure of the scrotum to hot temperatures for periods of 16 hours per day did not influence spermatozoal numbers. But a reduction in **motility** and percentage of live spermatozoa occurred when the testes were heated for only 8 hours per day. An additional important finding was that when 16 hours per day of heat was applied to the scrotum, reduced survival of embryos produced by normal females was observed. There appears to be significant variability with regard to the effect of scrotal heating upon spermatozoal production and viability. Further research is needed in this important area since the ambient temperature can often be managed/manipulated in the environment of the sexually active male, especially males used for artificial insemination.

The ability to measure the cooling capacity of the testes is difficult. Historically, the cooling capacity and thermal regulatory function of the testes was measured by small temperature sensors which were installed surgically in the vasculature and/or in the testicular tissue. A noninvasive technology called **infrared thermography**, is currently being utilized by Canadian researchers to assess the cooling capacity of the testes. Infrared thermography measures the infrared emissions from a heat producing body. Thus, this technique quantitates the heat released from the surface of the testes. Theoretically, males with faulty testicular cooling capacity can be identified and eliminated as breeding males. While this technique has not reached the stage where it can be applied to everyday livestock management activities, it has promise for evaluating testicular cooling capacity in bulls.

In general, the scrotal skin (and spermatic cord) in mammals contains little fat. However, under certain management conditions, accumulation of scrotal fat may be a problem. For example, beef bulls being fed for maximum rate of gain in bull test stations are evaluated for their efficiency of growth. Under conditions of maximum nutrient intake, fat may accumulate in the scrotum as well as the spermatic cord. Such accumulation of fat would decrease the cooling effectiveness of the scrotum and pampiniform plexus and thus may reduce spermatogenic efficiency, spermatozoal viability and fertility.

The Tunica Dartos Has the Ability to Elevate the Testes for a Sustained Period of Time

The **tunica dartos** (also called the **dartos muscle**) is an open mesh-like smooth muscle layer which lies just beneath the scrotal skin (Figure 3-11). The degree of contraction of this smooth muscle is constantly being adjusted in response to changes in scrotal skin temperature. The sensory nerves initiating the changes in the tone (degree of contraction) of the tunica dartos are located in the scrotal skin. Unlike the striated muscle (cremaster muscle), the smooth muscle of the tunica dartos can maintain sustained contractions. This characteristic allows the testes to be held close to the body for sustained periods during cold temperatures. On the contrary, during the hot summer months, the tunica dartos relaxes and thus the surface area of the scrotum increases substantially to facilitate cooling. This increase in surface area of the scrotum is closely linked to scrotal perspiration. As the scrotum perspires, the increased surface area allows for a greater rate of evaporative heat loss and more rapid and efficient cooling.

Development and maintenance of the contractile characteristics of the tunica dartos are under androgen control. For example, the ability of the tunica dartos to contract in response to cold temperatures is lost in castrated males because testosterone is absent.

Artificial manipulation of the scrotum has been used to sterilize beef bulls. The scrotum may be artificially shortened to hold the testes next to the body, resulting in elevated testicular temperature and causing significantly reduced spermatogenesis. A bull subjected to this procedure is referred to as a "**short scrotumed**" bull, which physiologically is an artificial cryptorchid (see Chapter 4). The testes are artificially forced into the dorsal region of the scrotum by placing a large rubber band around the lower portion of the scrotum. In 3 to 4 weeks the lower scrotum sloughs at the juncture of the rubber band because of restricted circulation. As you might expect, the weight of the testes in these bulls is less than in unaltered bulls. In fact, they are about one-half the weight of an unaltered bull. "Short scrotumed" males, while sterile, maintain normal testosterone levels, and thus maintain a high rate of growth. Research has shown that "short scrotumed" bulls have increased efficiency of growth and have leaner carcasses compared to steers. Although this technique is not in widespread use, it illustrates the importance of an intact scrotum for testicular cooling. Furthermore, it illustrates the importance of androgens for growth and leanness.

The testes are the primary reproductive organs in the male. Their functions are to produce:

- ***spermatozoa***
- ***hormones and proteins***
- ***fluids***

The testes are paired organs which vary considerably in size and shape among species. They are considered the primary reproductive organs in the male because they produce both **spermatozoa** and the androgen **testosterone**. In addition, they produce inhibin, estrogens and a variety of proteins believed to be important to spermatozoal function. They also produce fluid which originates primarily from the seminiferous tubules. This fluid serves as a vehicle in which spermatozoa are suspended and facilitates their removal from the testes. The fluid produced by the testes

Figure 3-10. Excised testicles from the bull, boar and stallion. The parietal tunica vaginalis (PTV) has been incised and reflected away from the testis. The lower right panel illustrates the intimate relationship between the tunica albuginea (TA) and the visceral tunica vaginalis (VTV). CM = Cremaster Muscle; DD = Ductus Deferens; EB = Epididymal Body; EH = Epididymal Head; ET = Epididymal Tail; PP = Pampiniform Plexus; PTV = Parietal Tunica Vaginalis; T = Testis; TA = Tunica Albuginea; VTV = Visceral Tunica Vaginalis.

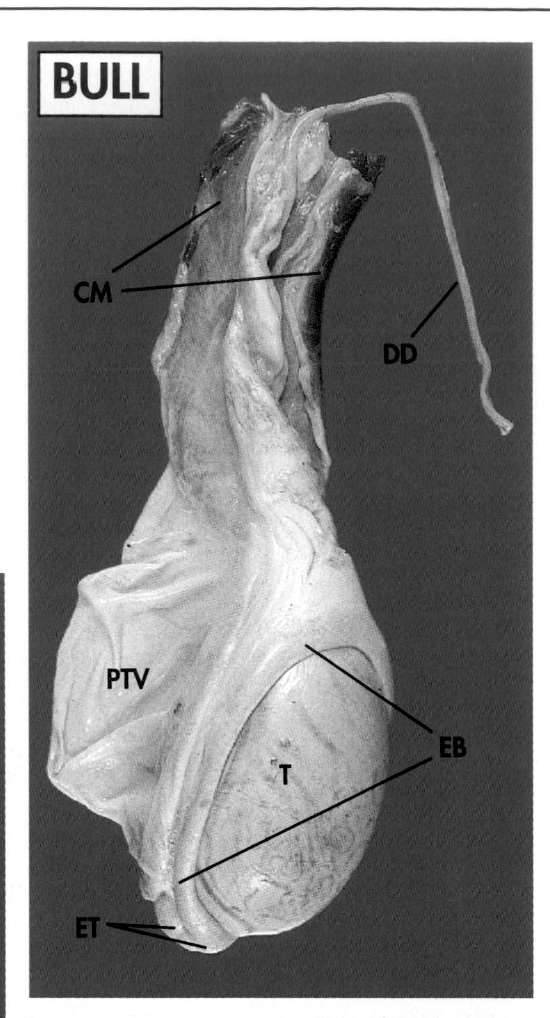

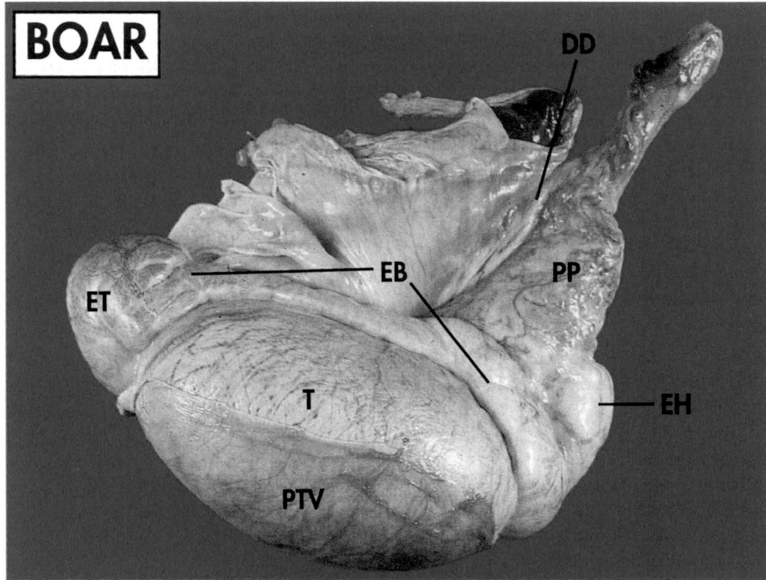

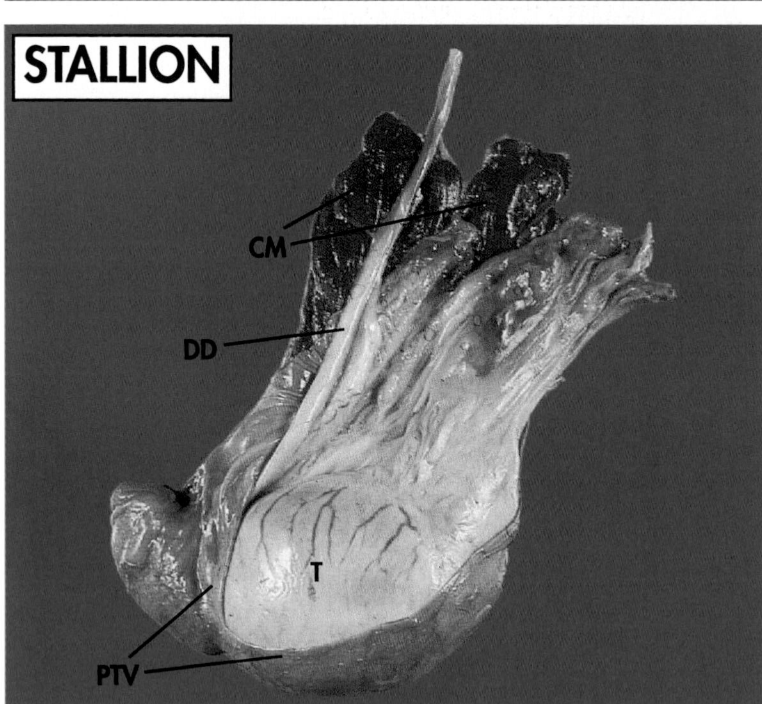

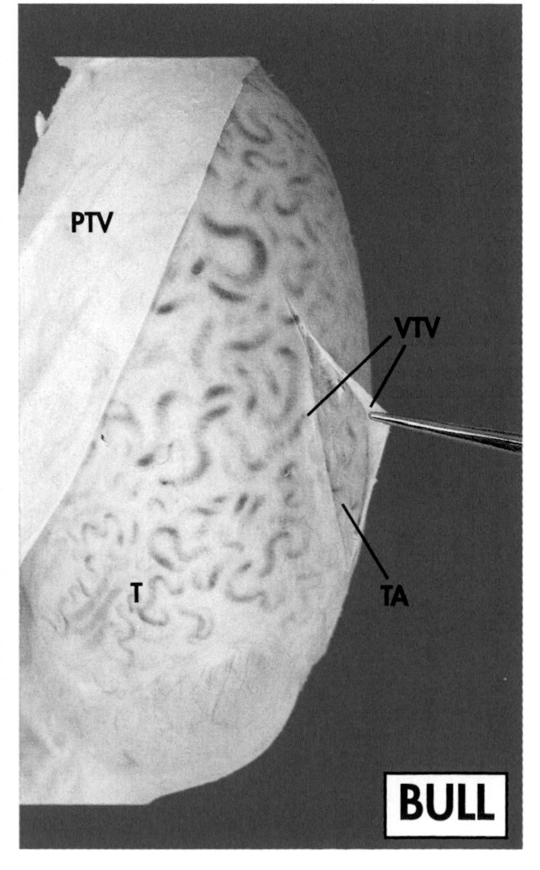

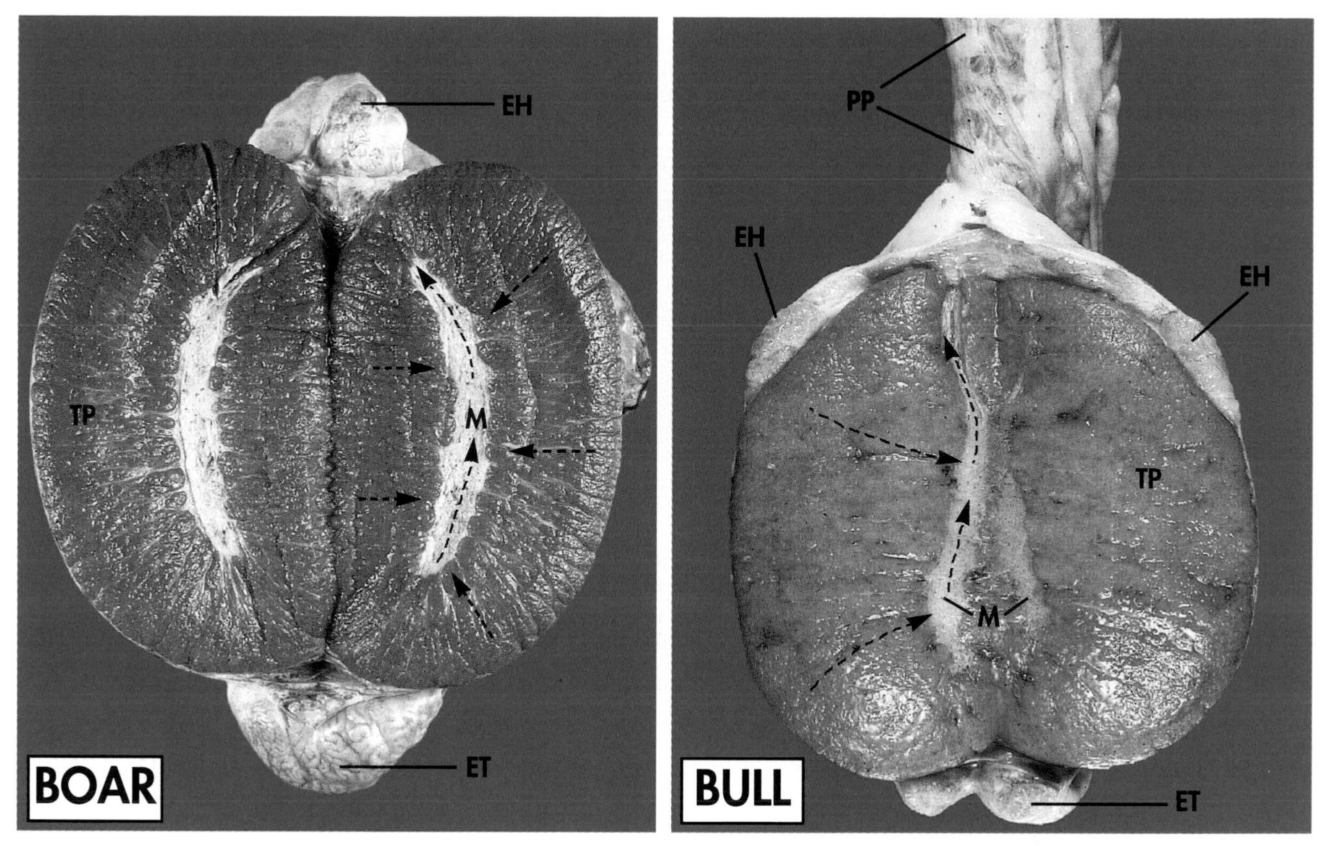

Figure 3-11. The top two panels show a testis from a boar and a bull which have been incised longitudinally to expose the testicular parenchyma (TP) and the mediastinum (M). Arrows denote direction of flow of spermatozoa and fluids toward the efferent ducts and the head of the epididymis. The efferent ducts are not visible in these photographs. EH = Epididymal Head; ET = Epididymal Tail; M = Mediastinum; PP = Pampiniform Plexus; TP = Testicular Parenchyma.
The bottom panel is a schematic illustration of the scrotum, the connective tissue supporting structures and the tubular pathway of the typical mammalian testis. (Graphic by Sonja Oei; modified from Davis, Langford and Kirby; *The Testis* Vol. 1 Johnson, Gomes and Vandemark).

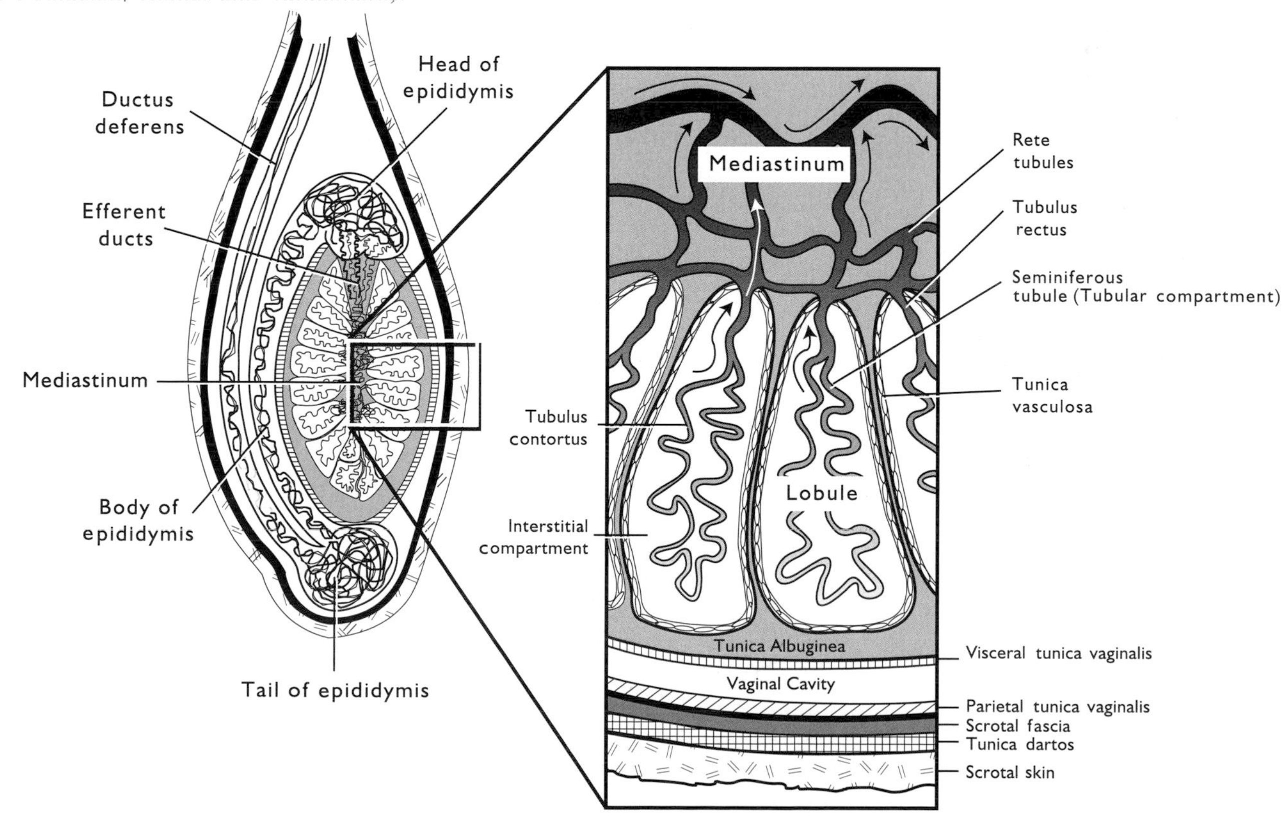

(sometimes called rete fluid) also contains synthetic products of the Sertoli cells.

> *The testis consists of the:*
> - *testicular capsule*
> - *parenchyma*
> - *mediastinum*
> - *rete tubules*

The Testicular Capsule Is a Dynamic "Suborgan" Covering the Testes

The covering of the testis, or **testicular capsule** is composed of two layers. They are the **visceral tunica vaginalis** and the connective tissue capsule known as the **tunica albuginea**. The visceral tunica vaginalis is closely associated with the tunica albuginea and these two layers can be separated using careful dissection (Figure 3-10). The tunica albuginea sends many finger-like projections into the parenchyma of the testicle. These septal projections join with the **mediastinum** (Figure 3-11). The interior surface of the tunica albuginea and the septal divisions forming the lobules is quite vascular and this surface is thus called the **tunica vasculosa** (Figure 3-11).

The testicular capsule was once considered to be an inert covering whose sole function was to form the outer boundary of the testes. It is now apparent that the testicular capsule is not an inert connective tissue boundary but a dynamic "suborgan" capable of undergoing changes in direct response to hormones and neurotransmitters. The tunica albuginea is not only composed of connective tissue, but contains smooth muscle fibers. Contractions of capsular smooth muscle can be induced by both acetylcholine and norepinephrine. These two important compounds cause contraction and relaxation of smooth muscle in the blood vessels and visceral organs throughout the body. Rhythmic cycles of contractions and relaxation of the testicular capsule serve to provide a pumping action thought to facilitate movement of spermatozoa into the rete tubules and efferent ducts.

> *The testicular parenchyma consists of:*
> - *seminiferous tubules*
> - *interstitial cells of Leydig*
> - *capillaries*
> - *lymphatic vessels*
> - *connective tissue*

The word **parenchyma** refers to the specific cellular mass of a gland or organ that is supported by a network of connective tissue. The major cellular mass of the testis is therefore referred to as the parenchyma. It is a soft, tan (sometimes brown or gray) mass made up of seminiferous tubules and interstitial tissue (blood vessels, nerves, lymphatics, connective tissue and Leydig cells) (Figure 3-11). The parenchyma can be divided into the **tubular compartment** and the **interstitial compartment** (Figure 3-11). The tubular compartment consists of **seminiferous tubules** and all of the cells and material inside them. The interstitial compartment consists of all cells and materials outside the seminiferous tubules, such as blood vessels, connective tissue, lymphatics, nerves and the **interstitial cells of Leydig,** which produce testosterone.

The mediastinum is the central connective tissue core of the testis (Figure 3-11) which houses ducts called rete tubules. The rete tubules (or rete testis) are tiny channels through which spermatozoa are transported out of the testis (Figure 3-11). The dense connective tissue of the mediastinum helps prevent compression or collapse of the rete tubules so spermatozoa and fluid originating in the seminiferous tubules can move freely out of the testis.

The seminiferous tubules (comprising the tubular compartment of the parenchyma) are microscopic.

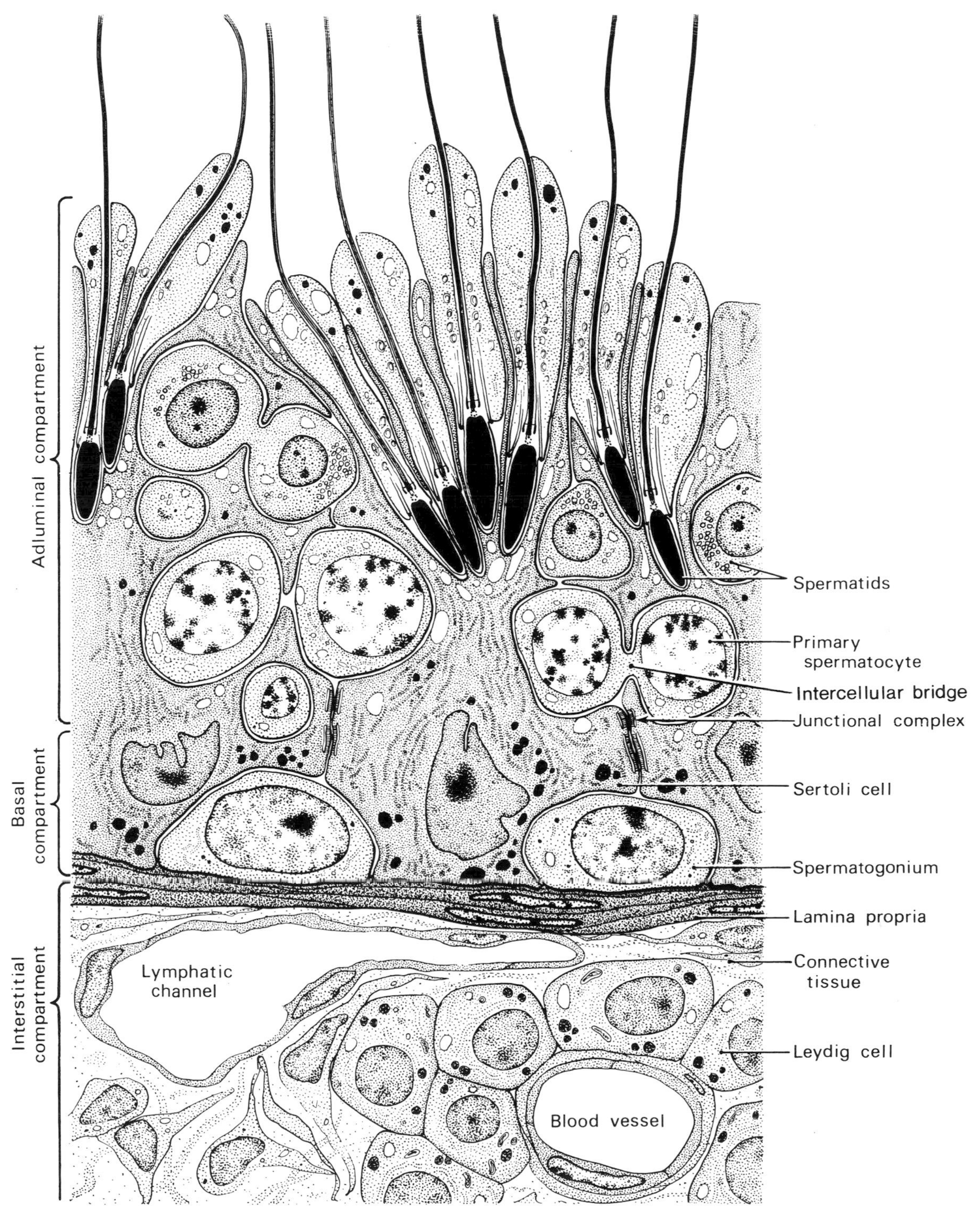

Figure 3-12. A portion of a seminiferous tubule showing the relationship of the germ cells to the adjacent Sertoli cells. Formation of spermatozoa in the seminiferous epithelium starts near the basement membrane. Here a spermatogonium divides to form other spermatogonia and, ultimately, primary spermatocytes. The primary spermatocytes are moved from the basal compartment through the junctional complexes between adjacent Sertoli cells into the adluminal compartment where they eventually divide to form secondary spermatocytes (not shown) and spherical spermatids. The spermatogonia, primary spermatocytes, secondary spermatocytes and spherical spermatids all develop in the space between two or more Sertoli cells and are in contact with them. During elongation of the spermatid nucleus, the spermatids are repositioned by the Sertoli cells to become imbedded within long pockets in the cytoplasm of an individual Sertoli cell. When released as a spermatozoon, a major portion of the cytoplasm of each spermatid remains as a residual body (cytoplasmic droplet) within a pocket of the Sertoli cell cytoplasm. Note the intracellular bridges between adjacent germ cells in the same cohort or generation. (From Amann, *Journal of Dairy Science* Vol. 66, No. 12, 1983.)

They form highly convoluted loops, the ends of which join with the **rete tubules**. Each loop of a seminiferous tubule is composed of a convoluted portion (**tubulus contortus**) and a straight portion (**rectus**) which join the rete tubule (Figure 3-11). Spermatogenesis takes place predominantly in the convoluted portion of the tubule.

> ***The tubular compartment consists of:***
> - ***seminiferous epithelium***
> - ***Sertoli cells***
> - ***developing germ cells***
> - ***peritubular cells***

The seminiferous tubule is composed of a basement membrane and a layer of **seminiferous epithelium** (also called the **germinal epithelium**) (Figure 3-12). The tubule is surrounded by peritubular cells which are contractile. Their contraction and the flow of fluid secreted by **Sertoli cells** allows newly formed spermatozoa to move into the rete tubules.

The seminiferous epithelium consists of two major regions known as the **basal compartment** and the **adluminal compartment.** Sertoli cells are anchored to the basement membrane and surround the developing population of germ cells. The relationship between the Sertoli cells and the germinal elements is shown in Figure 3-12.

Sertoli cells are the only somatic cells in the seminiferous epithelium. Once believed to be simply a supportive component for the germinal elements, they are now considered to be the cellular "governors" of spermatogenesis. Each Sertoli cell "hosts" a maximum number of developing germ cells, characteristic for a given species. Hence, testes with high numbers of Sertoli cells are capable of producing large numbers of spermatozoa. Conversely, testes with small numbers of Sertoli cells can only produce small numbers of spermatozoa. Sertoli cells are analogous to the granulosal cells of the ovarian follicle. However, unlike granulosal cells, the Sertoli cell contains receptors for both FSH and testosterone. Because Sertoli cells possess receptors to different hormones (protein and steroid), they have the capability of producing a variety of substances. A few examples are: 1) **androgen binding protein (ABP)**, a testosterone transport protein; 2) **sulfated glycoproteins (SGP) 1 and 2,** which are believed to be related to fertility acquisition (SGP-1) and to provide a detergent effect to allow cells and fluids to move through the tubular network of the testis (SGP-2); 3) **transferrin**, an iron transport protein believed to be required for successful spermatogenesis; and 4) **inhibin**, as in the female, a suppressor of FSH.

Adjacent Sertoli cells are tightly attached to each other on their lower lateral surfaces by a band of specialized junctions called **junctional complexes (tight junctions**). The Sertoli cell junctional complexes separate the germinal epithelium into a basal compartment (Figure 3-12) which houses spermatogonia and early primary spermatocytes, and an adluminal compartment which houses all other germ cells. The name basal compartment reflects its position just above the basement membrane of the seminiferous tubule. The adluminal compartment implies a region adjacent to the lumen of the seminiferous tubule. The cell types found in the adluminal compartment are **primary** and **secondary spermatocytes** and **spermatids**. The junctional complexes between Sertoli cells form a specialized permeability barrier that prevents large molecular weight materials and immune cells from gaining access to the adluminal compartment.

> ***The blood-testis barrier prevents immunologic destruction of developing germ cells.***

The peritubular cells surrounding the seminiferous tubule and the Sertoli cell junctional complexes form the **blood-testis barrier**. The primary purpose of the blood-testis barrier is to prevent autoimmune reactions from destroying the developing germ cells. Materials in the interstitial compartment are first screened by the peritubular layer surrounding the seminiferous epithelium. The peritubular layer thus acts as the first barrier against large molecular weight materials (mainly immunoglobulins).

The junctional complexes between Sertoli cells serve as the second barrier against immune cells and immunoglobulins. The most important feature of the blood-testis barrier is the exclusion of immune cells (macrophages and lymphocytes) and immunoglobulins (antibodies) from the adluminal compartment. This exclusion is important since these materials would recognize the developing germinal elements as being foreign because they are undergoing meiosis. Therefore, they are immunologically different from other cells within the body and thus generate an immune response. In addition to forming the blood-testis barrier, the Sertoli cell junctional complexes provide a type of control for materials entering and, at least in part, leaving the adluminal compartment.

The Excurrent Duct System Allows for Final Maturation, Storage and Delivery of Spermatozoa to the Pelvic Urethra

The efferent ducts converge to a single duct, **the epididymal duct**. The function of the efferent ducts is to convey newly formed spermatozoa and tubular fluid (rete fluid) into the epididymal duct. The head of the epididymis contains the point of connection between the efferent ducts and the initial segment of the epididymal duct (see Chapter 4 for embryologic origin). The function of the epididymis is to provide the environment for final maturation of spermatozoa, resulting in acquisition of motility and potential fertility. The epididymis also serves as a storage reservoir for spermatozoa. Epididymal function is androgen dependent.

The excurrent duct system consists of:

- ***efferent ducts***
- ***the epididymal duct***
- ***the ductus deferens***

The epididymis is organized into three distinct regions known as the head (caput), the body (corpus) and the tail (cauda) (Figures 3-2, 3-3, 3-4, 3-10, 3-11 and 3-14).

The epididymal duct is a single, highly convoluted duct ranging in length from 30 to 60 meters depending on species. It is surrounded by smooth muscle. This muscular layer is responsible for rhythmic contractions of the duct, forcing spermatozoa to travel along its course to the tail. The time required to transport spermatozoa from the proximal head of the epididymis to the distal tail is referred to as **epididymal transit time**.

Table 3-1. Time required (days) for passage of spermatozoa through the various parts of the epididymal duct.

Species	Head	Body	Tail	Total
Boar	3	2	4-9	9-14
Bull	2	2	10	14
Ram	1	3	8	12
Stallion	1	2	6	9

Adapted from Fournier-Delpech and Thibault in *Reproduction in Mammals and Man*. Thibault, Levasseur and Hunter, Eds. Ellipses Press, Paris. 1993.

Epididymal transit time through the head and body is remarkably constant among species (Table 3-1). Smooth muscle in the tail of the epididymis tends to be quiescent except during periods of sexual excitation. When sexual stimulation occurs, the smooth muscle of the distal tail begins to contract vigorously, thus moving spermatozoa into the ductus deferens. Epididymal transit time through the head and body is not altered by sexual excitation. However, the number of sperm in the distal tail can be altered dramatically by the frequency of ejaculation. In sexually rested males, the sperm content of the tail is maximal, while males experiencing a high ejaculation frequency have 25% to 45% fewer sperm in the epididymal tail. Spermatozoa spending an unusually long time in the tail (such as after long periods of sexual rest) may be of poor quality when compared to sperm from animals ejaculated routinely (once or twice weekly). Some males tend to accumulate sperm in the epididymis rather than void them periodically, which probably constitutes a loss of viability.

The epididymal duct provides the environment for acquisition of fertility by spermatozoa.

It is important to recognize that the epididymis is a dynamic organ which not only controls the maturation and fertility acquisition of spermatozoa but also controls their exit from the male reproductive system. With sperm production rates of several billion per day, it is easy to imagine that if the epididymis did not provide continual movement of sperm out of the male reproductive tract, there would be a buildup of immense pressure. Spermatozoal removal from the epididymis is caused by periodic contractions of the epididymis and ductus deferens, resulting in a gradual trickle of spermatozoa out of the tail, through the ductus deferens, into the pelvic urethra where they are flushed out of the tract during urination. This trickle allows removal of sperm from the epididymis on a continual basis. There is no reabsorption of sperm in the epididymal duct.

Factors that control epididymal transit are poorly understood but it is almost certain to be under the control of the nervous and the endocrine systems. Materials such as oxytocin, acetylcholine, prostaglandins and angiotensin II (a powerful vasoconstrictor produced by the kidney) have been shown to alter epididymal motility *in vitro*.

The changes in spermatozoal function and the epididymal contents are summarized in Figure 3-14. As spermatozoa enter the efferent ducts and epididymal duct, their concentration is low because they are diluted in **rete fluid.** Most of this fluid is absorbed by the epithelium of the efferent ducts and the proximal head of the epididymis. Spermatozoa are concentrated immensely in the epididymis. For example, spermatozoal concentrations in the head of the epididymis may be 25 to 50 million, while in the tail concentration may exceed 2 billion. Changes in spermatozoal concentrations are the result of fluid reabsorption and secretion along the course of the epididymis. Not only is fluid absorbed, but the spectrum of proteins and other molecules in the fluid bathing the sperm is changed along the course of the epididymal duct.

The total spermatozoal content of the epididymal duct, the ductus deferens and the ampulla is referred to as the **extragonadal reserves** (**EGR**). Only the distal tail reserves are eligible for ejaculation. On a per ejaculate basis, the number of sperm removed from the tail reserves can be increased dramatically when the male is subjected to a series of sexual preparation maneuvers such as false mounting or restraint from mounting. Sexual preparation likely stimulates release of oxytocin from the posterior pituitary. This causes contractions of the smooth muscle surrounding the tail of the epididymis which move spermatozoa into the ductus deferens. Oxytocin also causes contractions of the smooth muscle in the ductus deferens which transports spermatozoa to the pelvic urethra where they are positioned for

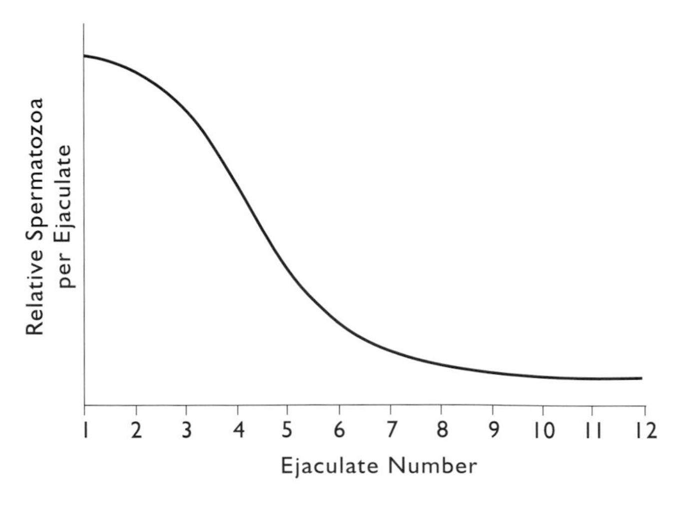

Figure 3-13. Influence of sequential ejaculation upon relative spermatozoa per ejaculate. This graph illustrates depletion of spermatozoal reserves in the distal tail of the epididymis.

ejaculation. These mechanisms will be detailed in Chapter 11.

It is important to recognize that even though a male might have adequate spermatozoal production by the testes, depletion of the reserves in the tail of the epididymis can occur rapidly if repeated ejaculations take place (Figure 3-13). For example, in mature bulls sperm in the ejaculate can be reduced to near zero after eight to ten successive ejaculations during a relatively short time period (several hours). Therefore, the number of fertile breedings a male can achieve will be limited by the size of his sperm reserves in the epididymal tail. From a practical viewpoint, the number of females a male can service in a 1-2 day period is dependent on his epididymal tail reserves, not the spermatozoal producing capability of the testes. It should be emphasized that when males are exposed to several females in estrus at the same time there is a strong likelihood that the male will select one of the females and inseminate her repeatedly. Such repeated insemination of a single female can deplete the reserves in the tail of the epididymis and thus compromise the chances of successful

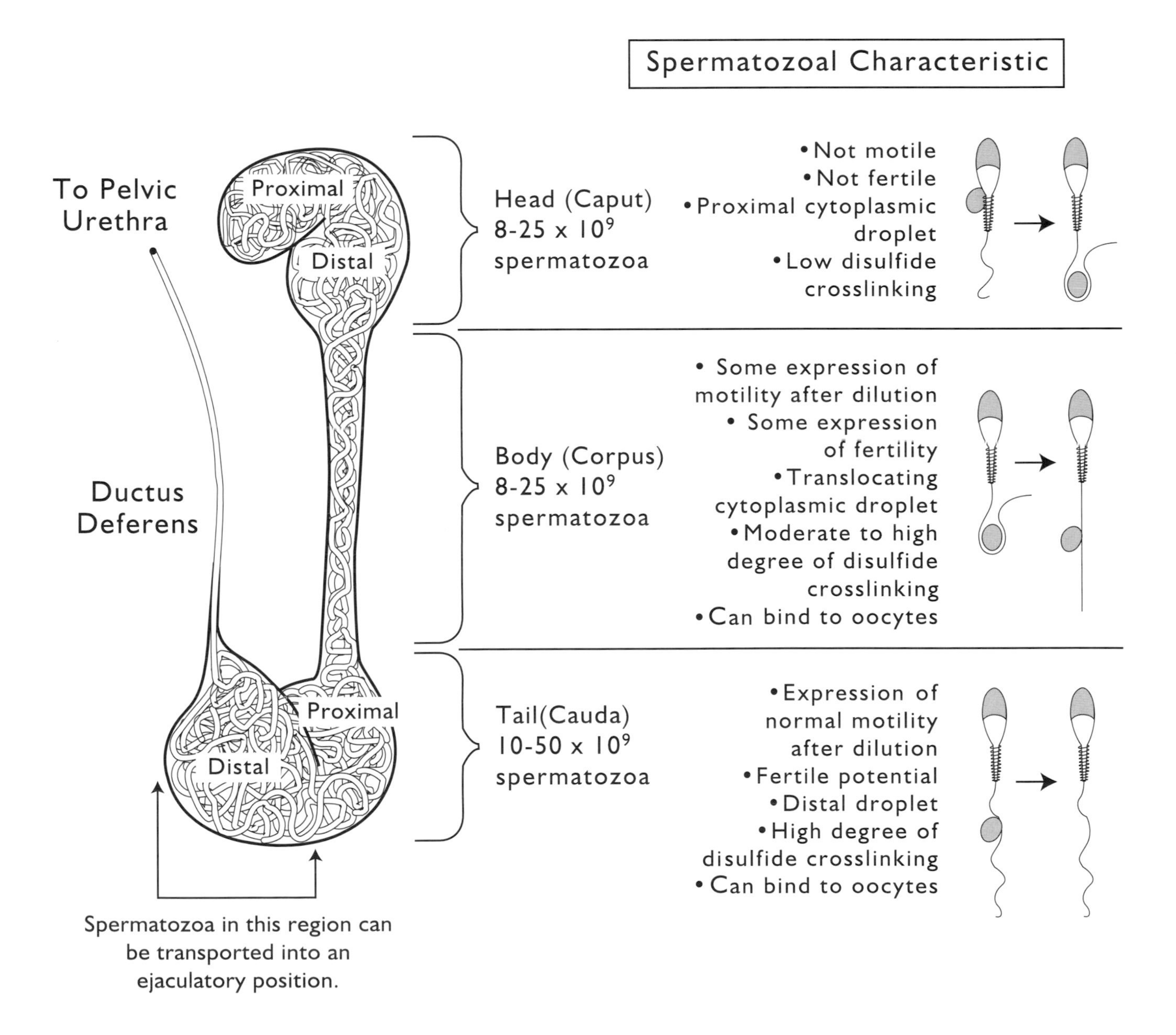

Figure 3-14. The epididymis of a typical mammal. (Graphic by Sonja Oei.)

pregnancies in other females that are in estrus the same day.

Spermatozoa entering the head of the epididymis possess a cytoplasmic droplet located near the base of the head of the spermatozoa. This droplet is referred to as the **proximal cytoplasmic droplet.** As spermatozoa move through the epididymis, the droplet moves down their tails and is called a **translocating cytoplasmic droplet**. Spermatozoa in the tail of the epididymis possess a **distal cytoplasmic droplet** (Figure 3-14). Normally, the distal droplet is lost in the distal tail or during ejaculation. A high proportion of ejaculated spermatozoa retaining a cytoplasmic droplet indicates faulty epididymal maturation.

Seminal Plasma Is a Non-Cellular Fluid Vehicle for Spermatozoal Delivery to the Female

The epididymis and accessory sex glands are responsible for production of secretions which contribute to the liquid, noncellular portion of semen known as the seminal plasma. **Seminal plasma** is not required for fertility, but is important in natural insemination where a fluid vehicle for delivery of the sperm is needed. Spermatozoa that are removed from the tail of the epididymis are equally as fertile as those that are ejaculated. In fact, when dairy bulls of genetic superiority die, spermatozoa can be flushed from the epididymal tail, processed and frozen. Artificial removal of these reserves can result in the generation of 600 to 1000 additional units of frozen semen.

In some species (the boar and stallion), the seminal plasma possesses special coagulation properties that plug the female reproductive tract and minimize loss of spermatozoa following copulation and ejaculation. The accessory sex glands secrete their products into the lumen of the pelvic urethra.

Seminal plasma is produced by the:

- ***epididymis***
- ***ampulla***
- ***vesicular glands (seminal vesicles)***
- ***prostate gland***
- ***bulbourethral glands (Cowper's glands)***

The **ampullae** are enlargements of the ductus deferens that open directly into the pelvic urethra. The enlargement is the result of a dramatic increase in the mucosal portion within the ampulla. The mucosa of the ampulla forms numerous pockets. The boar does not have conspicuous ampullae.

The **vesicular glands** are paired glands which are dorsocranial to the pelvic urethra. The secretions of the vesicular glands empty directly into the pelvic urethra. These glands were originally named the seminal vesicle. Early anatomists erroneously imagined that these glands were reservoirs for spermatozoa because there was a visual similarity between the secretion of these glands and ejaculated semen. While the vesicular glands do serve as a reservoir for their own secretions, they do not serve as a reservoir for spermatozoa. The vesicular glands have openings within the pelvic urethra which are separate from those of the ampullae. In bulls and boars the vesicular gland contributes to a large proportion of the ejaculate volume. The gross anatomical configurations of the vesicular glands vary significantly among species. These are illustrated in Figure 3-15. In the bull and ram the vesicular glands are lobulated. In the boar they are also well developed and contribute to a viscous, milky component of the seminal plasma. In the stallion the vesicular glands are elongated, hollow pouches.

The **prostate gland** lies in close proximity to the junction between the bladder and pelvic urethra. There is great species variation with regard to shape

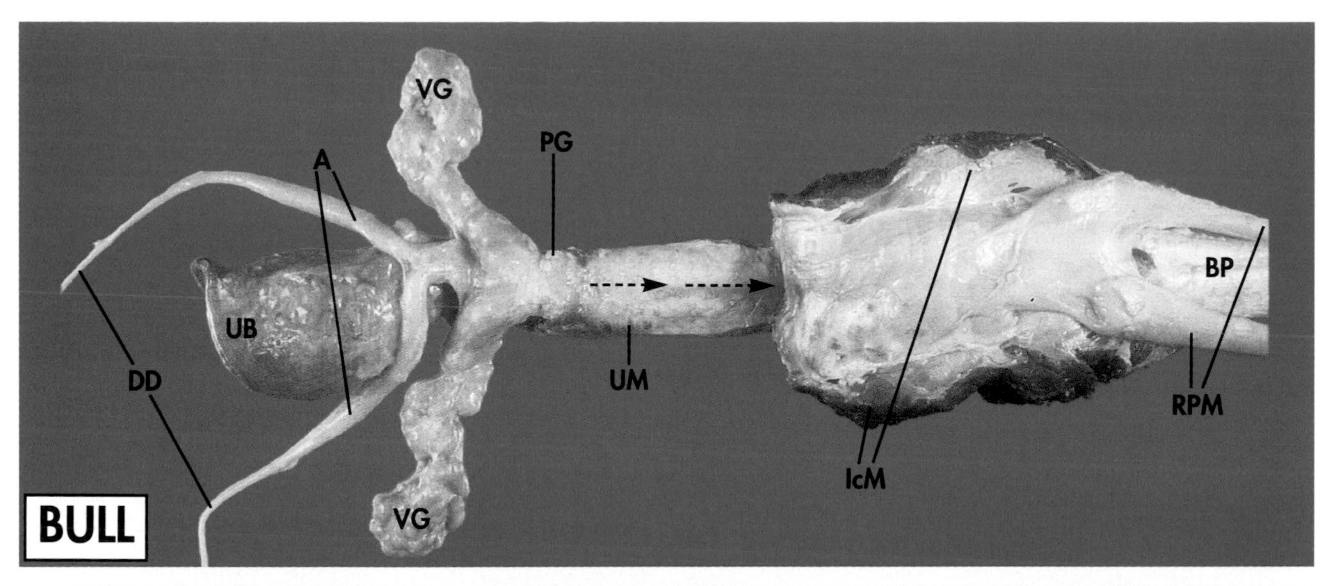

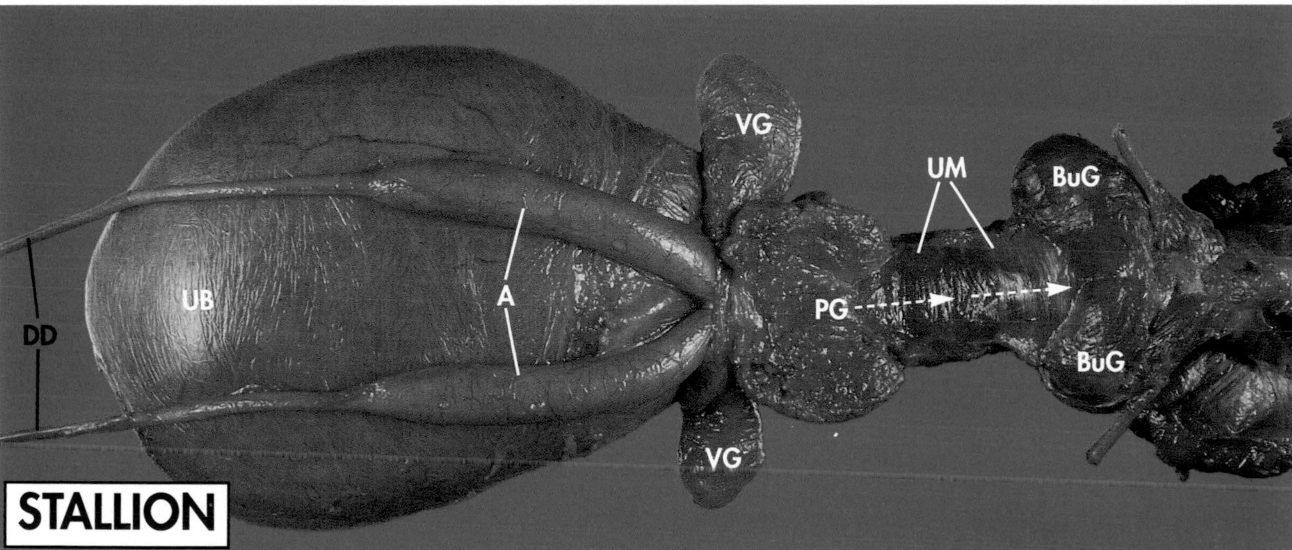

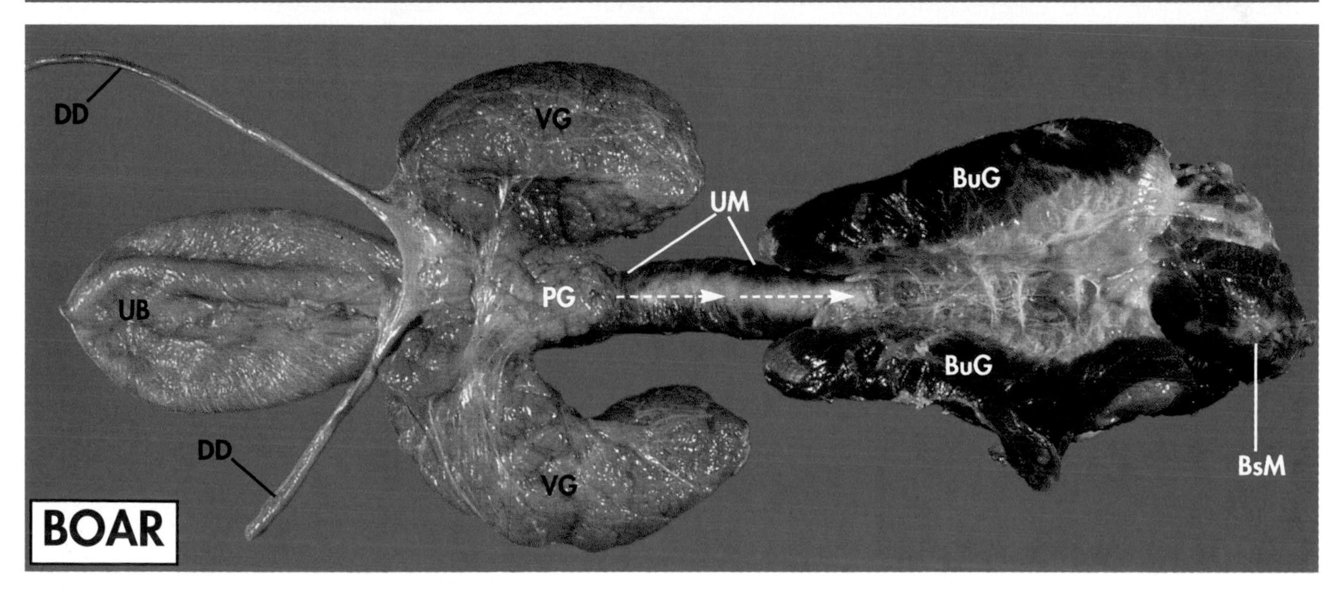

Figure 3-15. Dorsal view of the pelvic urethral region of the bull, boar and stallion*. A = Ampulla; BP = Base of Penis; BuG = Bulbourethral Glands; BsM = Bulbospongiosus Muscle; DD = Ductus Deferens; IcM = Ischiocavernosus Muscle; PG = Prostate Gland (Body); RPM = Retractor Penis Muscle; VG = Vesicular Glands; UB = Urinary Bladder; UM = Urethralis. *(arrows indicate the direction of fluid flow during emission and ejaculation)

and location. The prostate may have two structural forms. The first involves a **corpus prostate** in which the prostate is outside of the urethralis muscle and is visible as a heart-shaped (boar), or an H-shaped (stallion) structure. The second type is a **disseminate prostate** in which glandular tissue is distributed along the dorsal and lateral walls of the pelvic urethra. The disseminate prostate is sometimes referred to as the **urethral gland**. To observe the disseminate prostate one must make an incision in the pelvic urethra and expose the prostatic tissue. In the bull the prostate has two distinct forms and the corpus prostate is located near the neck of the bladder. In the boar the disseminate prostate is the major portion of the gland and the body of the prostate is often partially concealed by the vesicular glands. The ram does not have a prostatic body and its prostate is entirely disseminate. In contrast, the stallion has no disseminate prostate and the glands are characterized by two lateral lobes.

The **bulbourethral glands** are paired glands located on either side of the pelvic urethra near the ischial arch. These glands are usually small and ovoid and are characterized by being quite dense due to the high degree of fibrous connective tissue within the gland. In the ram, bull and stallion these glands are small and buried under the bulbospongiosus muscle. The boar is the notable exception with regard to the size of the bulbourethral glands. They are very large and dense and lie on the surface of the caudal two thirds of the pelvic urethra. These glands produce a viscous secretion which is important because it provides the gel fraction of the ejaculate and causes the seminal plasma to coagulate following ejaculation.

Secretions of the accessory sex glands contain an immense variety of components and ions, most of which have not been assigned a function. In general, most substances found in blood, including hormones and enzymes, can be found in seminal plasma. It is beyond the scope of this book to detail all of the secretory products of the accessory sex glands. However, among the most unique are fructose, which serves as an energy source for spermatozoa, citric acid, inositol, ergothioneine and prostaglandins.

The presence of these materials with regard to specific accessory sex glands varies among species. It should be emphasized that with the exception of fructose as an energy source, the precise role of the other materials is not known.

The accessory sex glands are dependent on testosterone for full development and maintenance of their structure and function. In fact, the weights of accessory sex glands can be used as a bioassay for androgens. In the absence of androgens, the weights of the accessory sex glands will be quite low. In contrast, when androgens are present the weights of the accessory sex glands are normal and their secretory activities are normal.

The Penis Is the Copulatory Organ

The penis consists of:
- ***a base***
- ***a shaft***
- ***the glans penis***
- ***crus penis***

The **penis** is composed of three parts. These are the **base (root) of the penis** where it is attached to the ischial arch, **the shaft** (the main portion of the penis) and **the glans penis,** which is the specialized distal end.

The glans penis is heavily populated with sensory nerves and is the homologue of the clitoris in the female. Stimulation of the glans penis is the primary factor initiating the mechanisms of ejaculation. Bulls, boars and rams have a fibroelastic penis with limited erectile tissue encased in a non-expandable, dense connective tissue structure. In species with a fibroelastic penis, there is a **sigmoid flexure** (Figures 3-2 through 3-4). This is an S-shaped configuration along the shaft of the penis. The sigmoid flexure allows the penis to be

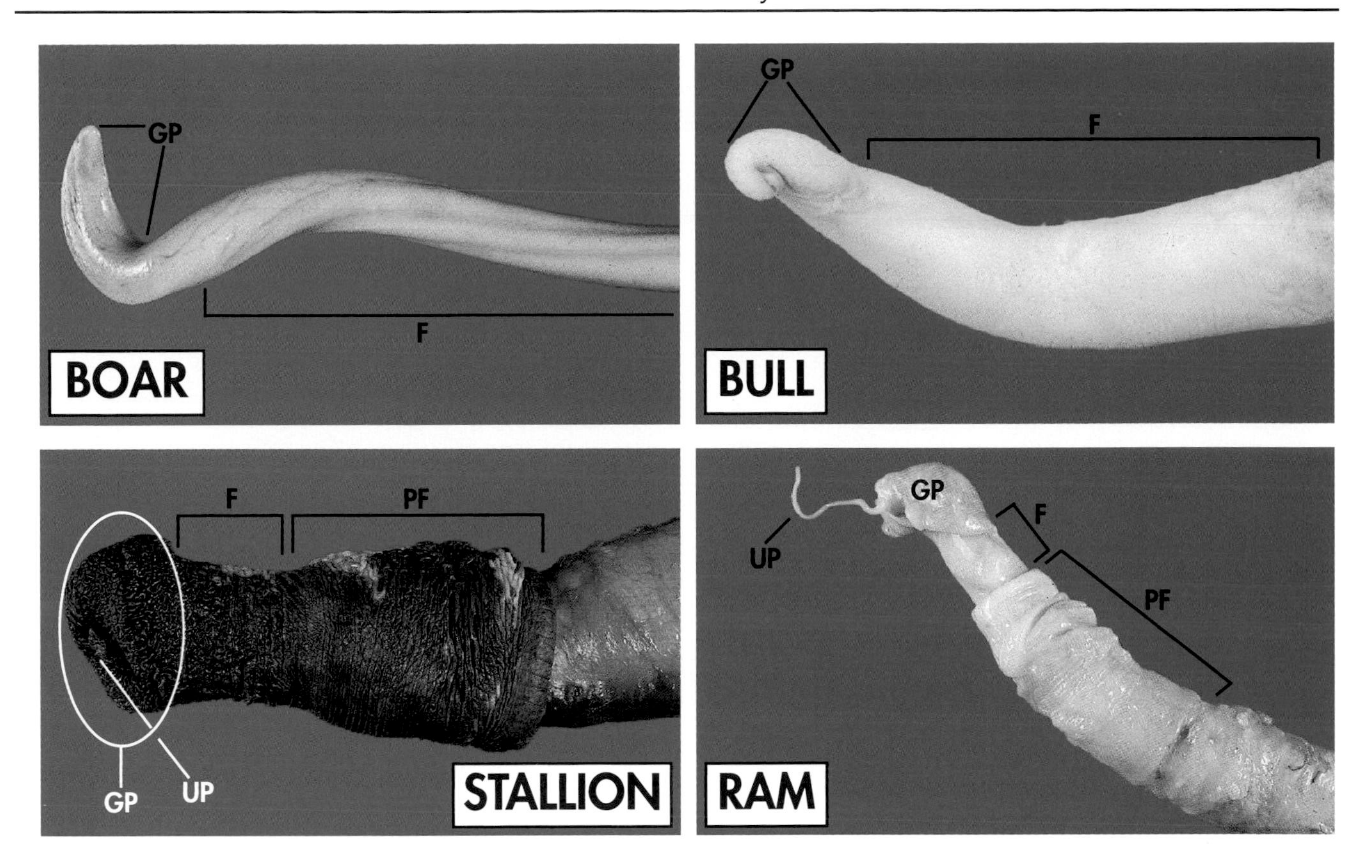

Figure 3-16. Top panels are photographs of distal ends of penises. Bottom panels are cross-sections of the penile shaft. Bull cross-section is near the caudal end. Stallion is cranial to the scrotum. BsM = Bulbospongiosus; CC = Corpus Cavernosum; CS = Corpus Spongiosum; DEC = Dorsal Erection Canals; F = Free end of penis; GP = Glans Penis; PF = Preputial Fold; RPM = Retractor Penis Muscle; TA = Tunica Albuginea; T = Trabeculae (from tunica albuginea); U = Urethra; UP = Urethral Process.

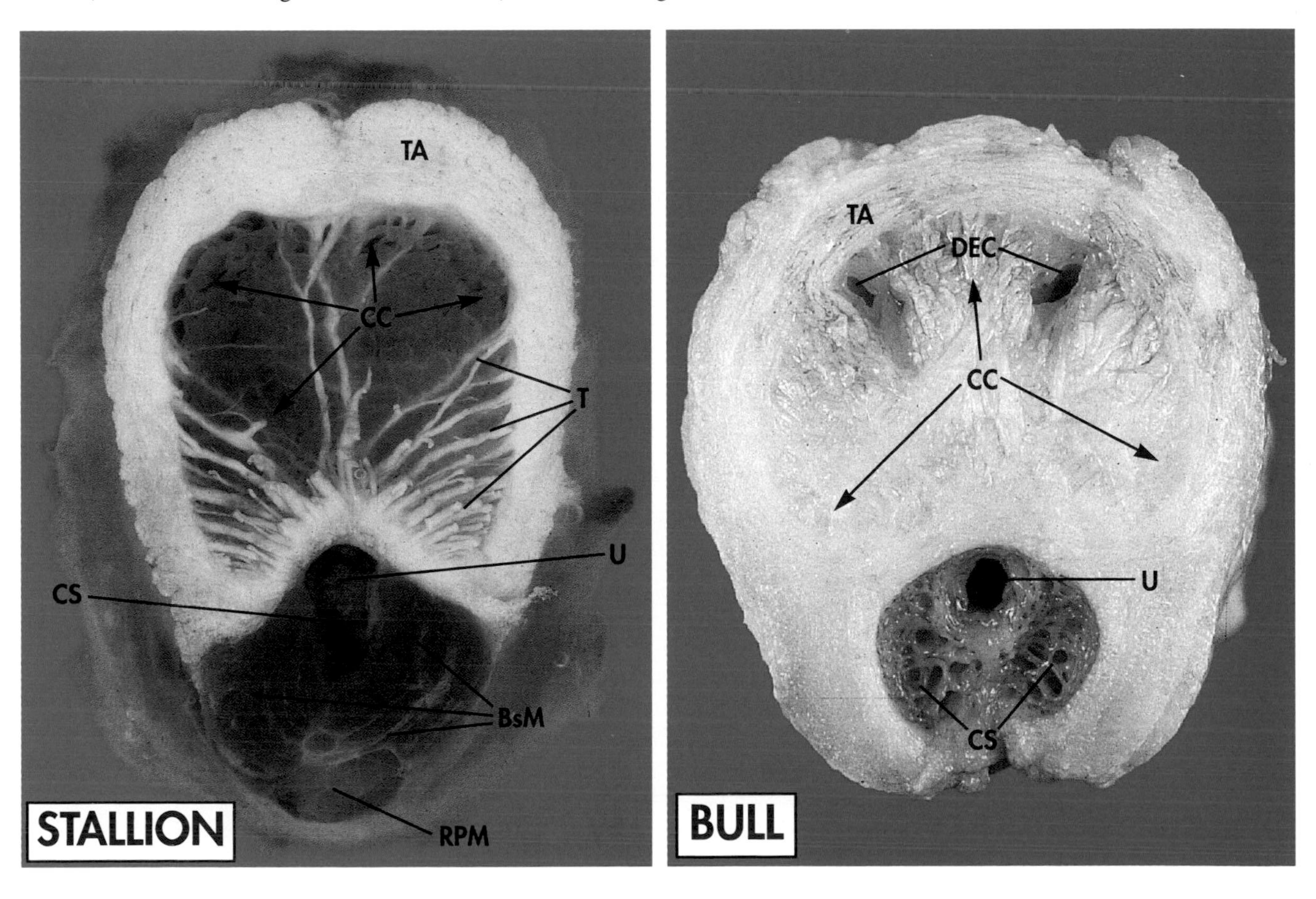

retracted inside the body until erection occurs. Erection is a simple stiffening without a change in diameter. The sigmoid flexure is maintained by a pair of smooth muscles known as the **retractor penis muscles** (Figures 3-2 through 3-4). These are attached dorsally to the coccygeal vertebrae and attached ventrally to the ventrolateral sides of the penis. When contracted, the retractor penis muscle holds the penis inside the sheath. When relaxed, the penis protrudes.

The shaft of the penis has an area of spongy, erectile tissue known as the **corpus cavernosum,** which makes up the majority of the penile interior. In the ventral portion of the penis immediately surrounding the **penile urethra** is another area of spongy erectile tissue called the **corpus spongiosum**. Erection in the bull, boar and ram is brought about by a combination of relaxation of the retractor penis muscles and the rushing of blood into the corpus cavernosum and the corpus spongiosum (Figure 3-16). The mechanism of erection and ejaculation will be presented in Chapter 11. In the stallion the penis contains much larger quantities of erectile tissue (cavernous tissue) compared to the bull, ram and boar (Figure 3-16).

Erection, Protrusion of the Penis and Ejaculation Are Under Muscular Control

The paired **ischiocavernosus muscles**, the muscles associated with the pelvic urethra and the penis, vary in size and form depending on the species. The ischiocavernosus muscles are relatively short paired muscles in the area of the root of the penis. These are strong muscles enclosing the crura which insert broadly on the lateral surface of the penis above the sigmoid flexure. They also connect the penis to the ischial arch.

Muscles associated with the pelvic urethra and the penis are the:

- ***urethralis***
- ***bulbospongiosus***
- ***ischiocavernosus***
- ***retractor penis***

The **urethralis** is a striated muscle that surrounds the pelvic urethra in a circular manner. The urethralis muscle is a thick, powerful muscle responsible for movement of seminal plasma and spermatozoa into the penile urethra. The urethralis muscle is shown in Figure 3-15. The **bulbospongiosus muscle** overlaps the root of the penis and extends down the caudal and ventral surfaces. In the boar, ram and bull it extends only part way down the penis. This muscle also covers the bulbourethral glands. The function of the bulbospongiosus muscles is to empty the extrapelvic part of the urethra.

Further Phenomena for Fertility

In many mammalian species (bats, rodents, carnivores, shrews, moles and many primates--but not humans) there is a penile bone called the os penis or baculum. The baculum of the raccoon has a gentle sigmoid shape and makes an attractive, unique cocktail stirring device when cleaned, sterilized and polished.

The fully engorged penis of the bull elephant weighs over 25 kilograms (about 55 lbs).

The penis of lizards and snakes is paired and is called a hemipenis. It is an extension of the cloaca and is everted into the cloaca of the female during copulation. It contains spines and/ or ridges which help sustain intromission.

In Brazil there is a species of monkey that has huge testicles relative to his body size. Unlike most mammals, this species of monkey has no competition amongst males for the right to breed

the female. Instead, the female will copulate with many males in sequence. Therefore, the male with the largest testicles (which produce the most sperm) has the greatest probability of fathering the new baby monkey.

The word "testis" is derived from Latin and meant "witness" or "spectator." English words "testify" and "testament" were derived from testis. The reason for this derivation is not known. However, it has been proposed that the testes were witnesses to virility. Romans required that a witness be an adult intact male. Prepubertal boys, women or eunuchs could not serve as witnesses. Placing the hand on the testicle (or someone else's testicles) was a requirement while testifying in some cultures.

The prepuce of the male dromedary (one-humped camel) is pendulous and contains three groups of muscles which change the direction of the preputial orifice from caudal during urination to cranial during erection.

Additional Reading

Nickel, R., A. Schummer and E. Seiferle. 1979. *The Viscera of Domestic Mammals*. 2nd Revised Edition. Springer-Verlag, New York.

Dyce, K.M., W.O. Sack and C.J.G. Wensing. 1996. *Textbook of Veterinary Anatomy*. 2nd Edition, W.B. Saunders Co., Philadelphia.

Johnson, A.D., W.R. Gomes and N.L. Vandemark, eds. 1970. *The Testis*. Vol. I. Academic Press, New York.

4 Embryogenesis of the Pituitary Gland and the Male or Female Reproductive System

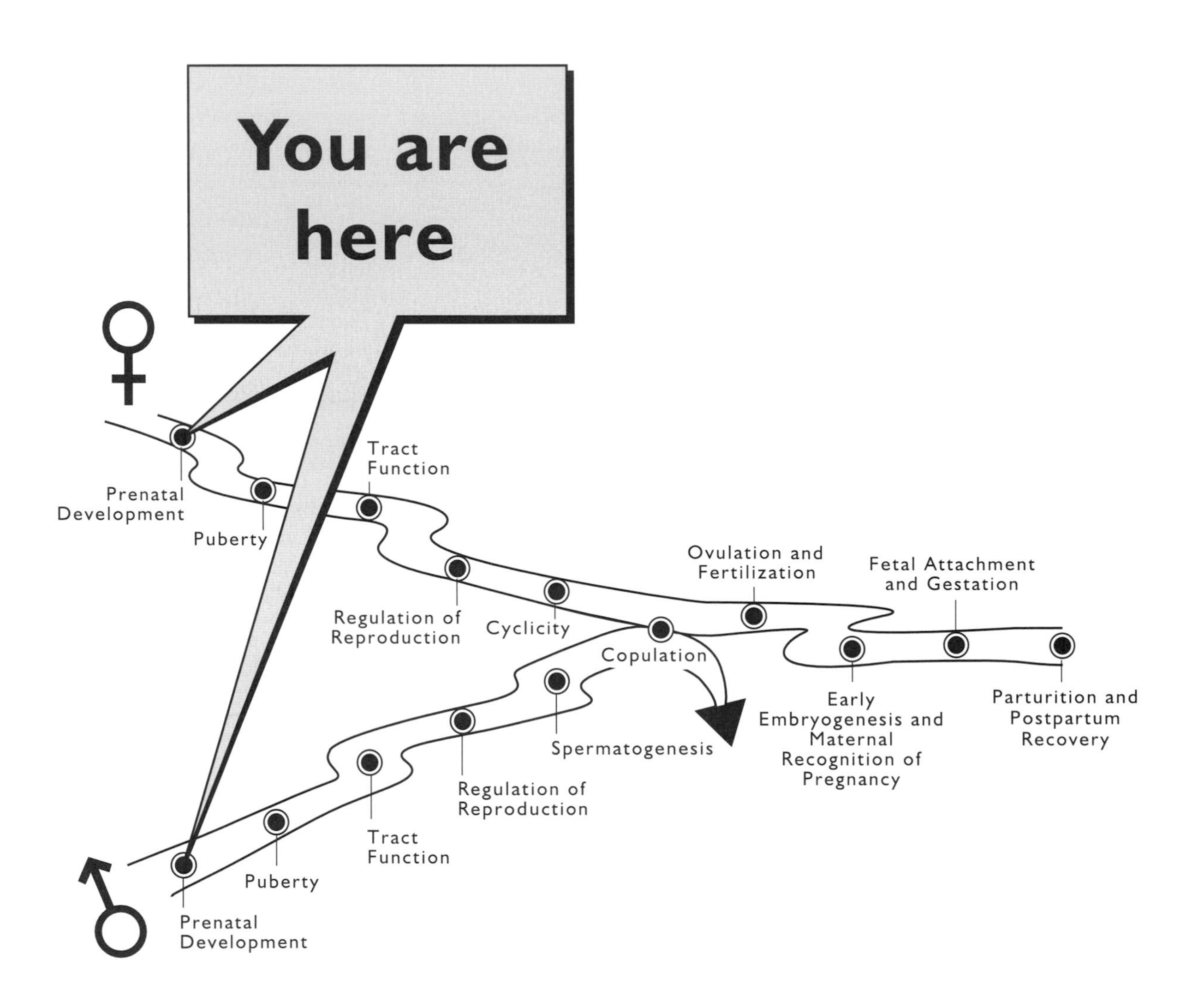

Take-Home Message

The anterior and posterior pituitary originate from two distinctly different tissues (neural and epithelial) and two distinctly different anatomical regions in the developing embryo. The anterior pituitary originates from the roof of the mouth and the posterior pituitary originates from the brain. The embryonic gonad develops into a testis or an ovary, depending upon the chromosomal makeup of the cells of the genital ridge. The development of the male reproductive tract requires the presence of testis determining factor (TDF), and the development of the female tract requires its absence. Both the male and the female reproductive tract originate from a series of tubes. In the male, the mesonephric tubules and ducts are utilized to form the excurrent duct system. In the female, the paramesonephric duct forms the oviducts and the uterus.

The embryogenesis (development of the embryo) of the pituitary and the male and female reproductive tracts is a remarkably coordinated series of events involving the merging of several types of tissue that will ultimately form complete glands and organs. The normal development of the urogenital system in mammals is among the most complex of all organ systems and requires critical timing for complete development. Embryogenesis of the reproductive system must be understood from a practical viewpoint, because it represents a possible limitation to reproductive performance in food producing animals. For example, faulty embryogenesis often results in sterility of either the male or the female. The information presented in this chapter will not contain strict timelines because these vary significantly among species. However, the sequence of events presented is similar among most mammalian species.

During embryogenesis various cells form organs that **differentiate** from discrete **germ layers** that make up the embryo. **Differentiation** is the process whereby a primitive group of unspecialized cells develops into a functional, recognizable group of cells that have a common function. The germ layers, which

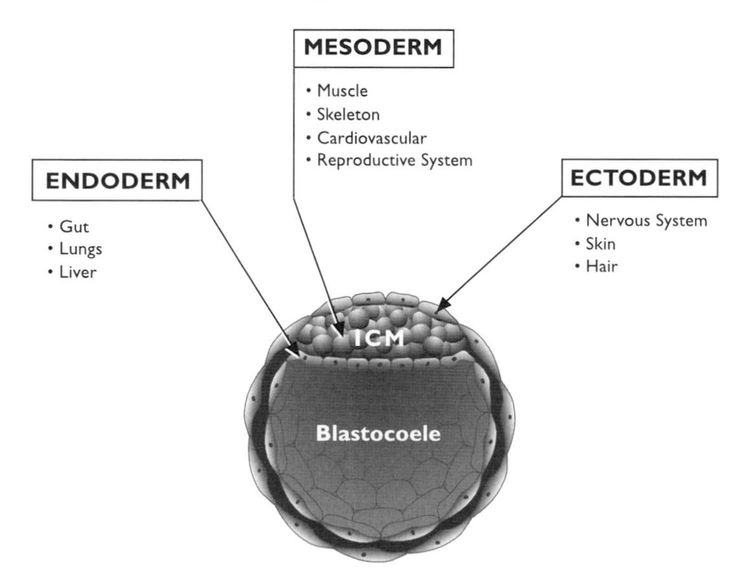

Figure 4-1. Derivation of the primary embryonic germ layers from the blastocyst. The inner cell mass (ICM) gives rise to the embryo and the three germ layers (endoderm, mesoderm and ectoderm) will develop into various organs.

Table 4-1. The origin of various organs and organ systems from the embryonic germ layers. (**Bold words** indicate organs of reproductive importance.)

Ectoderm	Mesoderm	Endoderm
Nervous system	Muscle	Digestive system
- hypothalamus	Blood vessels	(including liver and pancreas)
- posterior pituitary	Reproductive system	Pulmonary system
- anterior pituitary	**- gonads (male and female)**	Most glands
- skin, hair, nails, sweat glands (including mammary glands)	**- uterus, cervix, part of vagina**	
Oral cavity	**- epididymis, vas deferens**	
Nasal cavity (including anterior pituitary)	**- accessory sex glands**	
Reproductive tract	Renal system	
- portions of the vagina and vestibule	Skeletal system	
- penis, clitoris		

appear prior to attachment of the embryo to the uterus, are called the **endoderm, mesoderm** and **ectoderm**. The endoderm (endo=inside, derm=skin) is the innermost cellular layer of the embryo and will eventually give rise to the gut, liver, lungs, pancreas and other endocrine organs. The ectoderm (ecto=outer, derm=skin) develops from the outer cells of the inner cell mass. As you will see in Chapter 13, the inner cell mass is a clump of cells which will become the embryo. The ectoderm will give rise to the central nervous system, sense organs, mammary glands, sweat glands, skin, hair, claws and hooves. The middle layer of the embryo is referred to as the mesoderm (meso=middle, derm=skin). The mesoderm develops between the ectoderm and the endoderm. This germ layer gives rise to the circulatory, skeletal, muscular and renal systems. Most of the reproductive system is derived from the mesoderm. A more complete listing of tissue derivations is presented in Table 4-1.

The Pituitary Gland Originates from the Brain and from Tissue in the Roof of the Mouth

The **posterior pituitary** originates from neural tissue of the brain, while the **anterior pituitary** originates from the tissue in the roof of the embryo's mouth. Tissue in the roof of the mouth, called **stomodeal ectoderm**, will give rise to the glandular tissue of the anterior pituitary. Early in embryo development a **diverticulum** (a sac or pouch diverting from a main tube, channel or cavity) develops from the floor of the brain and grows ventrally toward the roof of the **stomodeum** (the embryonic mouth) (Figure 4-2A, B and C). The specific region of the brain from which this diverticulum develops is called the **infundibulum**. At the same time that the infundibulum is developing, another diverticulum originates from the roof of the stomodeum and grows dorsally. This diverticulum is called **Rathke's pouch,** or sometimes **Rathke's pocket** (Figure 4-2A, B and C). As Rathke's pouch continues to develop, it loses its continuity with the stomodeum and forms a discrete body of cells that become closely associated with the developing infundibulum (Figure 4-2). The cells of Rathke's pouch differentiate to form the **adenohypophysis** (the anterior pituitary). The prefix **adeno** refers to tissues that are glandular in nature. While the cells of the adenohypophysis are differentiating into various specialized cells capable of producing a variety of hormones, the infundibulum differentiates to form the **neurohypophysis** (posterior pituitary).

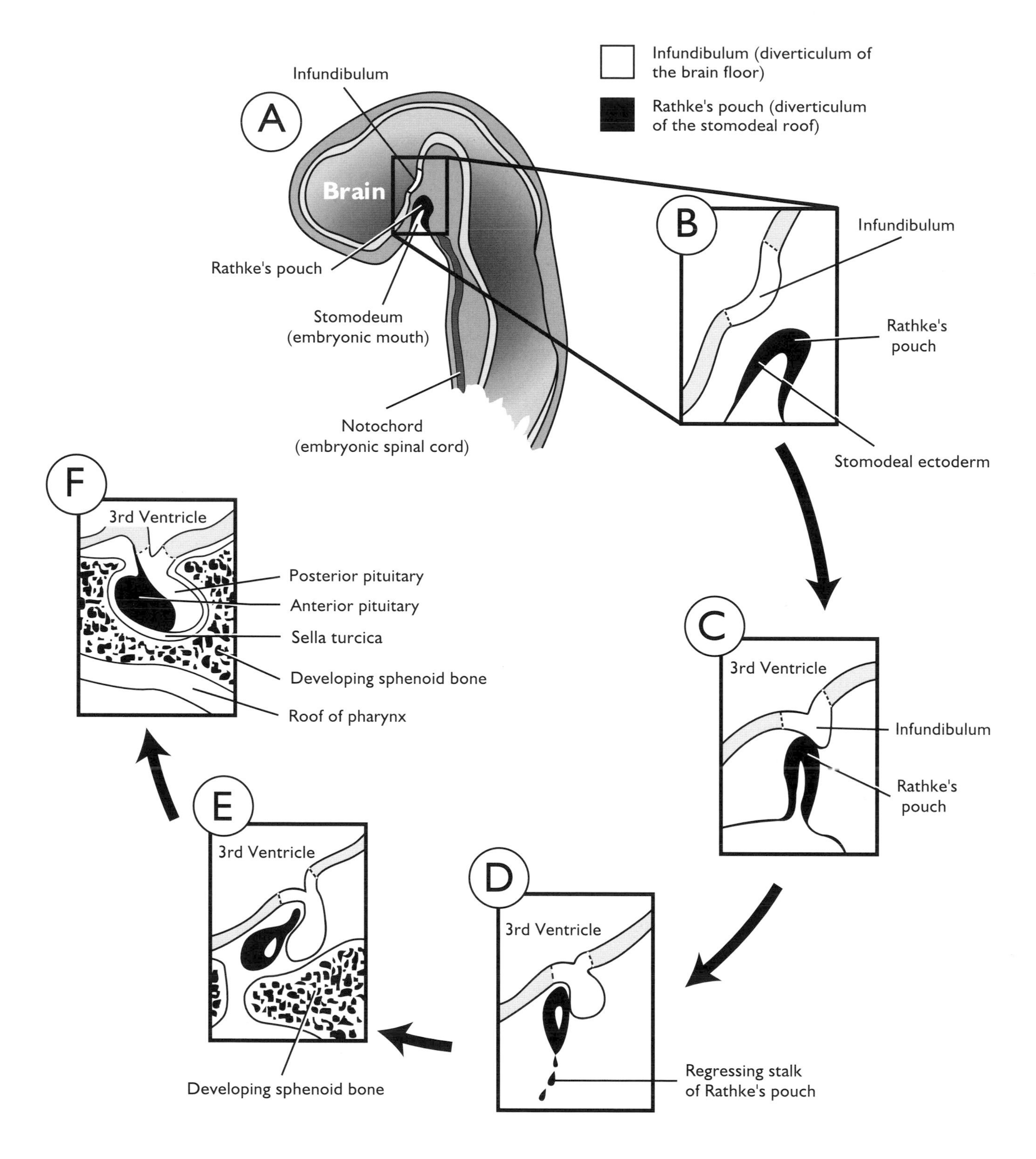

Figure 4-2. Development of the anterior and posterior pituitary. The posterior lobe of the pituitary is formed from a diverticulum (outpocketing) from the floor of the brain. The third ventricle is a cavity within the brain which will be described more completely in Chapter 5. Once this outpocketing begins to form, it is referred to as the infundibulum (A,B). The anterior lobe forms as an evagination from the stomodeal ectoderm. This stomodeal ectoderm is referred to as Rathke's pouch (A,B,C,D). Eventually, Rathke's pouch completely separates from the stomodeal ectoderm and becomes intimately associated with the posterior pituitary. Both the anterior and posterior pituitary eventually become surrounded by the bony vault known as the sella turcica. Modified with permission from Churchill Livingstone from *Human Embryology,* William J. Larson.

Hypophysis = pituitary
Adenohypophysis = anterior pituitary
Neurohypophysis = posterior pituitary

The posterior pituitary contains the axons and nerve terminals (telodendria) of neurons whose cell bodies are located in the hypothalamus (see Chapter 5). As development of the pituitary nears its completion, a bone of the cranium known as the **sphenoid bone** (Figure 4-2F) begins to form around both the anterior and posterior pituitary. This highly protective cavity is known as the **sella turcica**. This bony cavity is so named because it resembles the side view of a Turkish saddle.

It is important to understand that the dual embryonic origin allows the anterior and posterior pituitary to perform entirely different functions. For example, the nerves of the posterior pituitary cause a direct and rapid release of oxytocin which causes milk ejection by the mammary gland. In contrast, the adjacent anterior pituitary gland consists of specialized glandular epithelial cells that produce glycoprotein hormones like follicle stimulating hormone and luteinizing hormone, which cannot be produced by the nerve cells.

Sexual Differentiation of the Reproductive Tract Involves Specific Substances

The initial step in sex determination is at fertilization when a sperm delivers either an X (female) or Y (male) chromosome to the oocyte. Thus, the sex of the individual is determined at fertilization and the genetic control of sex differentiation has been established. In the early embryo (first 15% of gestation), when the yolk sac is still present, primordial (primitive) germ cells develop. These cells originate from the inner lining of the yolk sac (Figure 4-3A and B). The primordial germ cells migrate by amoeboid movement from the yolk sac into the hindgut and finally reside in the undifferentiated gonad (Figure 4-3B and C). The sex of the embryo cannot be determined in the undifferentiated gonad. The undifferentiated gonad is located on the inner surface of the dorsal body wall and is known at this time in development as the **genital ridge** (Figure 4-3B and C). It will form the gonads in the male or the female. The genital ridge forms medial to the embryonic renal systems which will be described below. Most of the primordial germ cells populate the genital ridge in the region of the tenth thoracic vertebra. Primordial germ cells that do not reside in this area will degenerate. During the time primordial germ cells are colonizing the genital ridges, they are undergoing mitosis and their numbers increase significantly.

When the primitive germ cells arrive in the genital ridge they stimulate cells in this region to proliferate. This results in the formation of compact strands of tissue called **primitive sex cords** (Figure 4-3). These proliferating sex cords cause the genital ridges to enlarge and push toward the developing kidney (mesonephros).

The reproductive system develops in close proximity to and at the same time as the renal system.

During its development the embryo utilizes three morphologically distinct renal systems. The first, called the **pronephros (pronephric kidney)**, is a nonfunctional remnant of a primitive form of kidney found in lower animals. Early in embryogenesis, the pronephros regresses and is replaced by a functional, bilateral pair of intermediate kidneys known as the **mesonephros (mesonephric kidney)** (Figure 4-4). The mesonephros produces urine which is drained by a bilateral pair of ducts called the **mesonephric ducts**. These ducts may also be called **Wolffian ducts**. The mesonephric ducts extend caudally and empty into the **urogenital sinus** (Figure 4-4). By the first 10% to 15% of gestation the final form of kidney begins to appear. This final renal form is known as the **metanephros (metanephric kidney)**. It will develop functional nephrons and will serve as the functional form of kidney in adult mammals. The metanephros becomes functional by the first 30% to 35% of gestation.

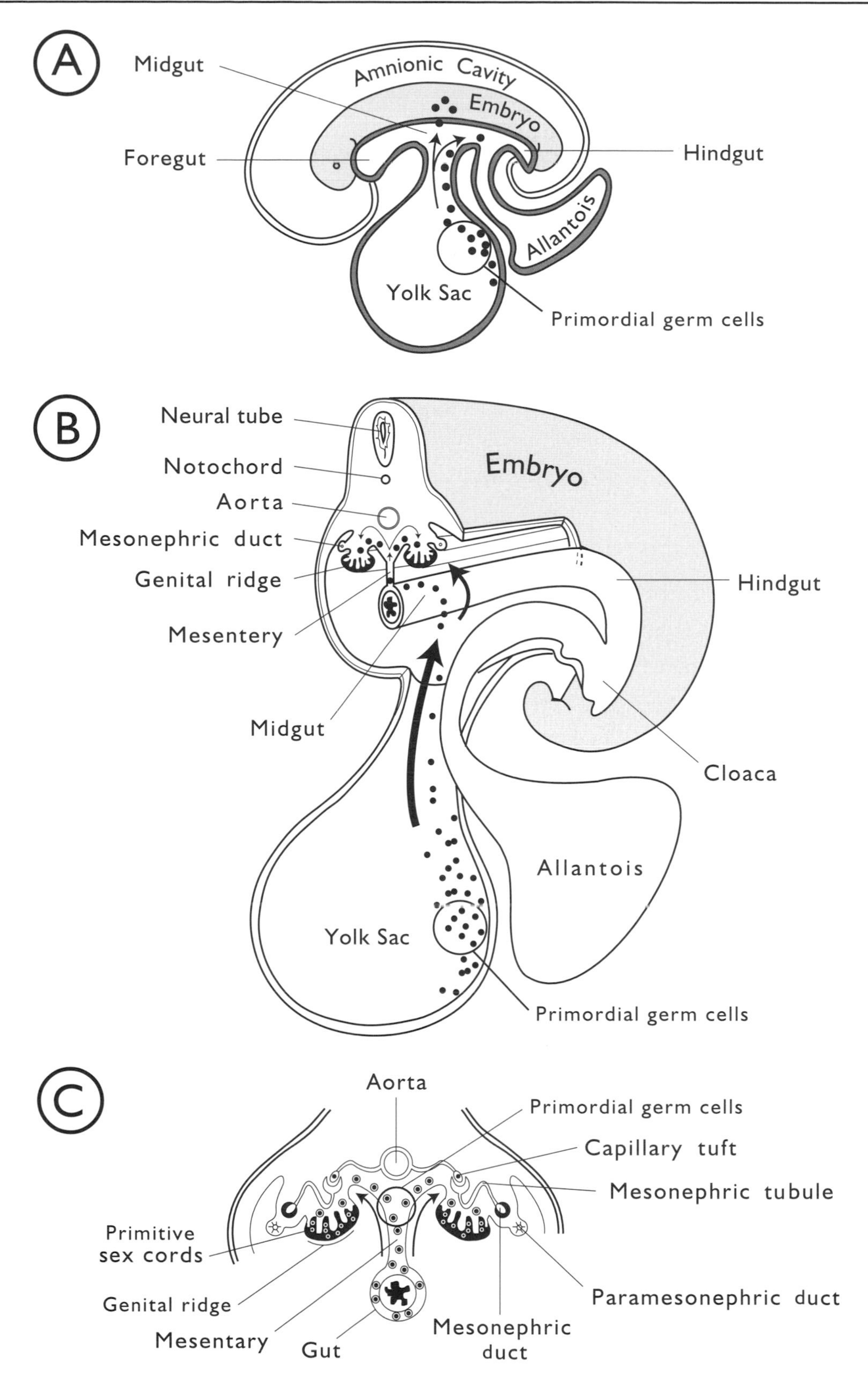

Figure 4-3. Migration of primordial germ cells from the yolk sac into the genital ridge (the indifferent gonad). **A**. Migration of primordial germ cells from the yolk sac into the midgut region of the embryo as seen from a lateral view. **B**. Primordial germ cells migrate by ameboid motion around the midgut, enter the mesentery and take up residence in the genital ridge. **C**. A transverse section showing migration of primordial germ cells being incorporated into the sex cords of the indifferent gonad. Notice the close relationship between the paramesonephric duct, the mesonephric duct and tubule and the genital ridge. Modified from Dyce, Sack and Wensing, *Textbook of Veterinary Anatomy*, 2nd Edition, with permission from W.B. Saunders Co.

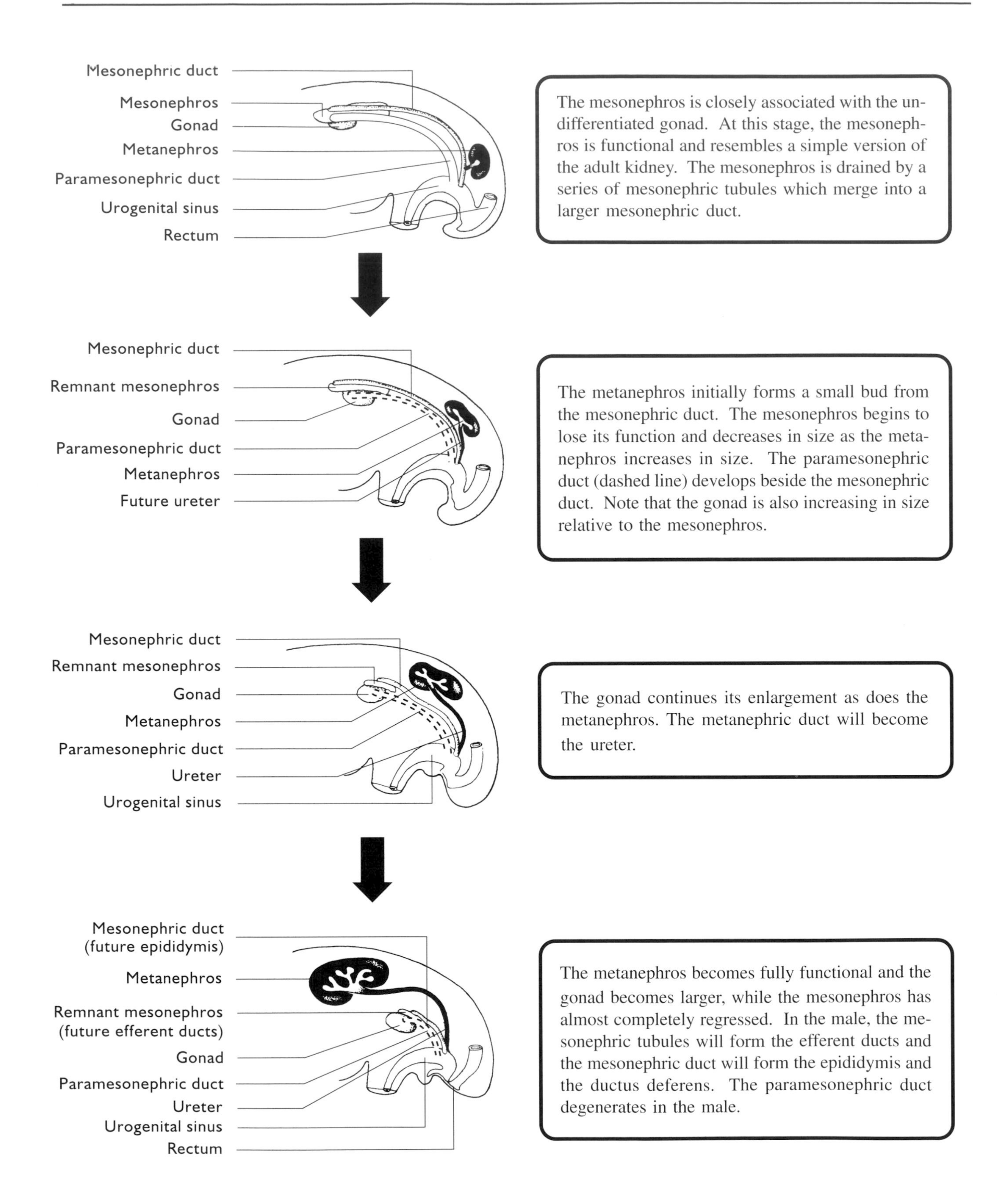
Mesonephric duct
Mesonephros
Gonad
Metanephros
Paramesonephric duct
Urogenital sinus
Rectum
The mesonephros is closely associated with the undifferentiated gonad. At this stage, the mesonephros is functional and resembles a simple version of the adult kidney. The mesonephros is drained by a series of mesonephric tubules which merge into a larger mesonephric duct.
Mesonephric duct
Remnant mesonephros
Gonad
Paramesonephric duct
Metanephros
Future ureter
The metanephros initially forms a small bud from the mesonephric duct. The mesonephros begins to lose its function and decreases in size as the metanephros increases in size. The paramesonephric duct (dashed line) develops beside the mesonephric duct. Note that the gonad is also increasing in size relative to the mesonephros.
Mesonephric duct
Remnant mesonephros
Gonad
Metanephros
Paramesonephric duct
Ureter
Urogenital sinus
The gonad continues its enlargement as does the metanephros. The metanephric duct will become the ureter.
Mesonephric duct (future epididymis)
Metanephros
Remnant mesonephros (future efferent ducts)
Gonad
Paramesonephric duct
Ureter
Urogenital sinus
Rectum
The metanephros becomes fully functional and the gonad becomes larger, while the mesonephros has almost completely regressed. In the male, the mesonephric tubules will form the efferent ducts and the mesonephric duct will form the epididymis and the ductus deferens. The paramesonephric duct degenerates in the male.

Figure 4-4. Development of the metanephros and regression of the mesonephros with associated development of the gonad. Modified from Dyce, Sack and Wensing *Textbook of Veterinary Anatomy*, 2nd Edition, with permission from W.B. Saunders Co.

At the same time the mesonephros is developing, a new pair of ducts beside the mesonephric ducts begin to develop. These ducts are called the **paramesonephric ducts** or **Müllerian ducts.** They form on either side of the mesonephric duct, thus paramesonephric (Figures 4-4, 4-6, 4-9 and 4-10). Even though the mesonephric and the paramesonephric ducts are both present, the embryo is still "uncommitted" with regard to its sex at this time. Sexual differentiation of the organs *per se* still has not occurred. This stage is referred to as the **sexually indifferent stage** because morphologic discrimination between the male and female embryo cannot be made by simple observation.

Sexual Differentiation Is Controlled by a Single Substance Directed by a Gene on the Y Chromosome

Females possess two X chromosomes, whereas males have one X and one Y sex chromosome. These sex chromosomes determine whether the embryo will become a male and develop testes or will become a female and develop ovaries. The substance that controls the pathway toward either male or female development is called **testis determining factor (TDF)** and is controlled by a gene on the Y chromosome. The X chromosome does not have such a gene. When testis determining factor is synthesized by the sex cords (Figure 4-5) within the primitive gonad, the development of the male reproductive system is stimulated. The absence of TDF results in the development of a female reproductive system. The pathway of events controlled by TDF is presented in Figure 4-5.

> ***Part of the male tract is derived from the mesonephros***
> - ***mesonephric tubules → efferent ducts***
> - ***mesonephric ducts → epididymis and ductus deferens***

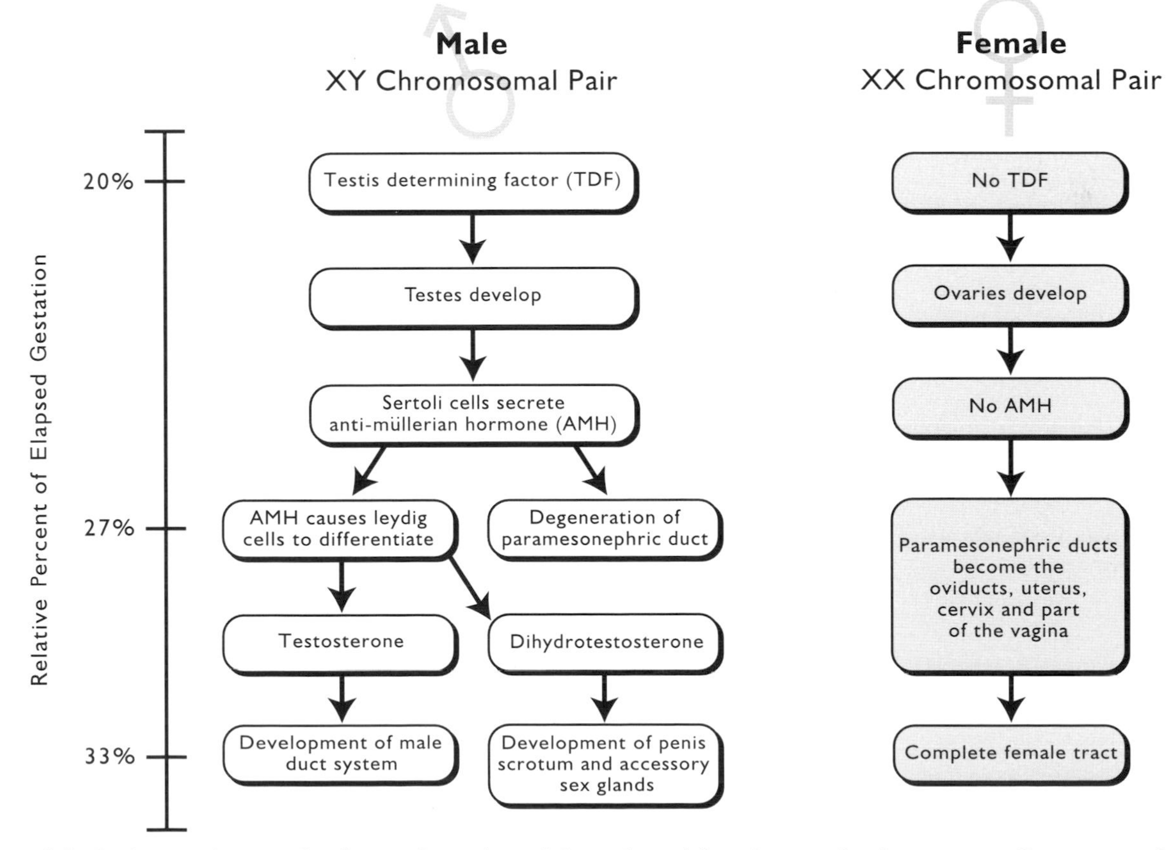

Figure 4-5. Pathway of events leading to formation of the male and female reproductive system. Percentage of gestation based on a human timeline.

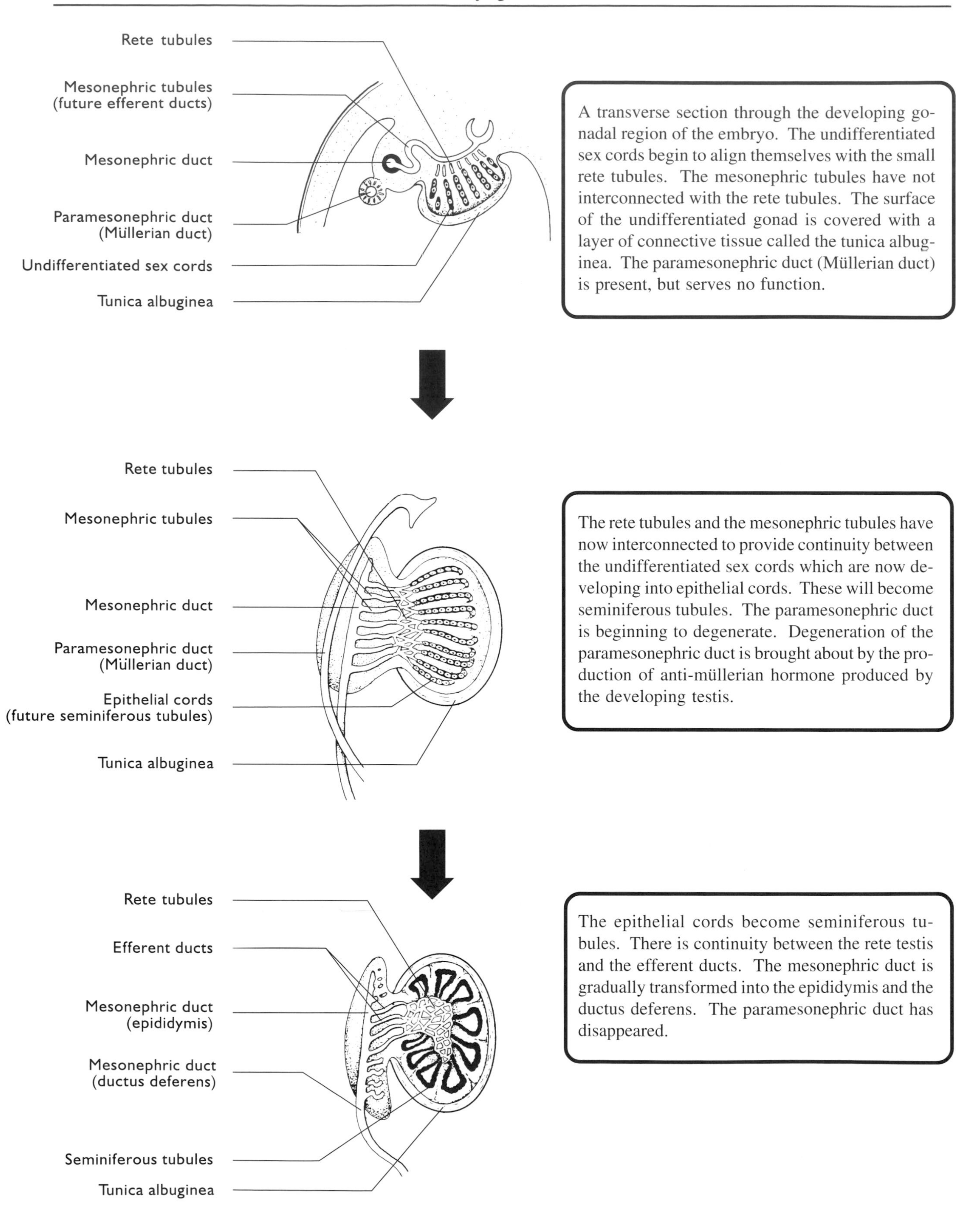
Rete tubules
Mesonephric tubules
(future efferent ducts)
Mesonephric duct
Paramesonephric duct
(Müllerian duct)
Undifferentiated sex cords
Tunica albuginea
A transverse section through the developing gonadal region of the embryo. The undifferentiated sex cords begin to align themselves with the small rete tubules. The mesonephric tubules have not interconnected with the rete tubules. The surface of the undifferentiated gonad is covered with a layer of connective tissue called the tunica albuginea. The paramesonephric duct (Müllerian duct) is present, but serves no function.
Rete tubules
Mesonephric tubules
Mesonephric duct
Paramesonephric duct
(Müllerian duct)
Epithelial cords
(future seminiferous tubules)
Tunica albuginea
The rete tubules and the mesonephric tubules have now interconnected to provide continuity between the undifferentiated sex cords which are now developing into epithelial cords. These will become seminiferous tubules. The paramesonephric duct is beginning to degenerate. Degeneration of the paramesonephric duct is brought about by the production of anti-müllerian hormone produced by the developing testis.
Rete tubules
Efferent ducts
Mesonephric duct
(epididymis)
Mesonephric duct
(ductus deferens)
Seminiferous tubules
Tunica albuginea
The epithelial cords become seminiferous tubules. There is continuity between the rete testis and the efferent ducts. The mesonephric duct is gradually transformed into the epididymis and the ductus deferens. The paramesonephric duct has disappeared.

Figure 4-6. Developmental sequence of the testis. Modified from Dyce, Sack and Wensing, *Textbook of Veterinary Anatomy*, 2nd Edition, with permission from W.B. Saunders Co.

In the male embryo, portions of the mesonephric kidney are appropriated for use in the reproductive tract at about the same time that the paramesonephric ducts begin to degenerate. Between 5 and 15 **mesonephric tubules** penetrate into the primitive gonad and make connections with the primitive sex cords via the **rete testis**. The rete testis is a network of tiny ducts that connect the seminiferous tubules to the **efferent ducts**. The efferent ducts are derived from the mesonephric tubules (Figure 4-6). The mesonephric duct will give rise to the epididymis and vas deferens. Together, the **efferent ducts**, the **epididymis** and the **ductus deferens** are appropriated to become the **excurrent extragonadal duct system** of the male reproductive tract.

The Testes Are Formed at the Level of the Ribs. They Descend into the Scrotum Late in Gestation

In most mammals, the testes descend into the **scrotum**. The descent of the testes is a series of complex events, the mechanisms of which are not completely understood. Regardless of the details, we know that the descent of the testes depends on the proper growth and regression of a ligamentous cord known as the **gubernaculum** (Figure 4-7). The gubernaculum (also called the **gubernaculum testis**) is a connective tissue organ that attaches to the ventral pole of the testis and extends to the inguinal region of the developing fetus (Figure 4-7). Changes in the regional growth of the gubernaculum cause the testes to descend into the scrotum by mechanical means.

> ***The descent of the testes has three phases:***
> - ***growth and elongation of the body away from the testes***
> - ***rapid growth of the distal gubernaculum***
> - ***regression of the gubernaculum***

The testes lie in a retroperitoneal position (Figure 4-7) and are attached caudally to the ligamentous gubernaculum. The gubernaculum extends caudally and resides in the area of the future scrotum. As the testes and gubernaculum begin to grow, they push out into the peritoneum. This "pushing-out" causes the peritoneum to wrap around the gubernaculum as well as the testes.

Overall, the descent of the testes can be divided into three phases. The first phase involves growth and elongation of the body away from the stationary testis. The second phase involves the rapid growth of the distal gubernaculum. The distal portion of the gubernaculum is that portion which has passed through the inguinal ring (Figure 4-7) and forms an outgrowth into the future scrotum. This phase of rapid gubernacular growth results in the testes being pulled from the region of the tenth thoracic vertebra to the inguinal ring. The third phase involves the shrinkage of the gubernaculum within the scrotum to pull the testes through the inguinal ring. Continued shrinkage of the gubernaculum results in the vaginal process being attached to the ventral pole of the testis and to the inner ventral surface of the scrotum (Figure 4-7).

After complete descent of the testes, you can see that the **vaginal process** (processus vaginalis) is continuous with the peritoneal cavity, and the testis is surrounded by a double layer of peritoneum (Figure 4-7). The layer of peritoneum immediately adjacent to the testis is the **visceral tunica vaginalis**, and the layer away from the testis is referred to as the **parietal tunica vaginalis** (see Chapter 3 for actual example). The space between the visceral and parietal tunica vaginalis is continuous with the body cavity that houses the viscera. These tunicae are slippery and allow the testis to move freely within the scrotum during physical activity and during contraction of the external cremaster and the tunica dartos muscles.

Now that you are able to visualize the mechanics of testicular descent, it is important to understand the factors that control this important event. The most

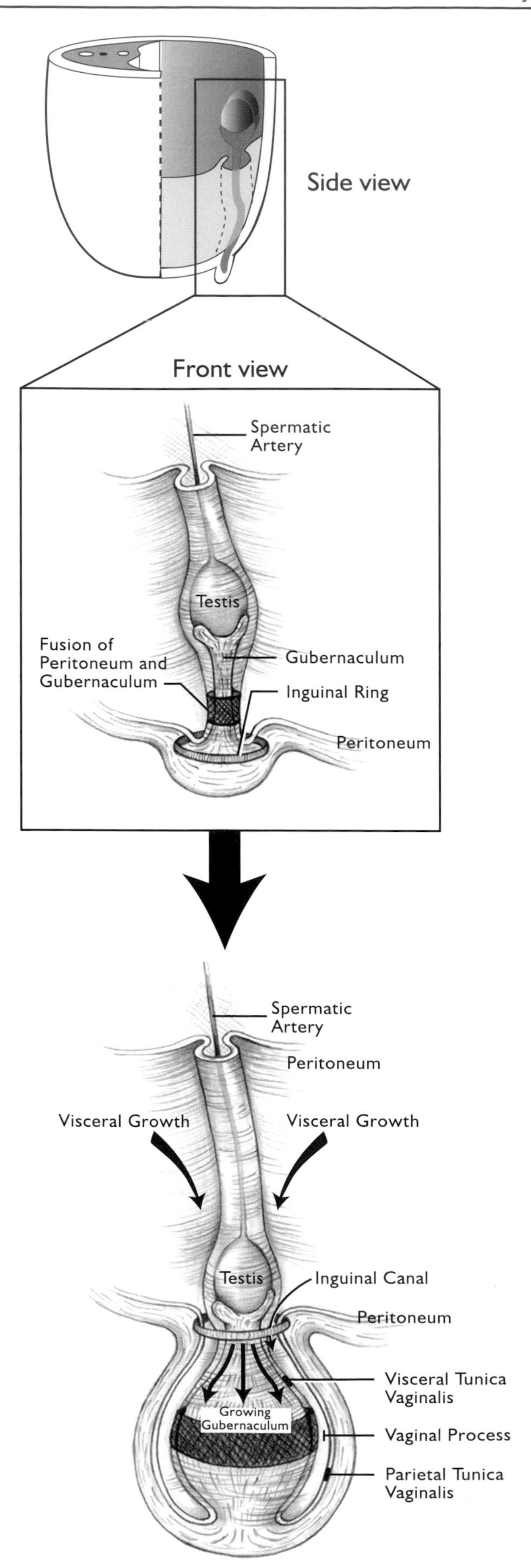

Before actual descent occurs, the testes lie in a retroperitoneal position and are attached caudally to the ligamentous gubernaculum. Cells of the peritoneum infiltrate the gubernaculum in the inguinal region and form a junction with it. This fusion is important because it binds the peritoneum to the gubernaculum and will allow the vaginal process to form as the distal gubernaculum grows toward and into the scrotal region.

After the gubernaculum penetrates the inguinal ring, there is rapid growth of the distal gubernaculum which results in pulling of both the testes and the peritoneum (vaginal process) into the scrotum. This rapid growth of the gubernaculum in the scrotal region is the "force" responsible for mechanically moving the testes into the inguinal canal.

Figure 4-7. Major steps in the descent of the testes. Growth and subsequent retraction of the gubernaculum causes the testes to descend from the level of the tenth thoracic vertebra into the scrotum. (Graphics by Sonja Oei.)

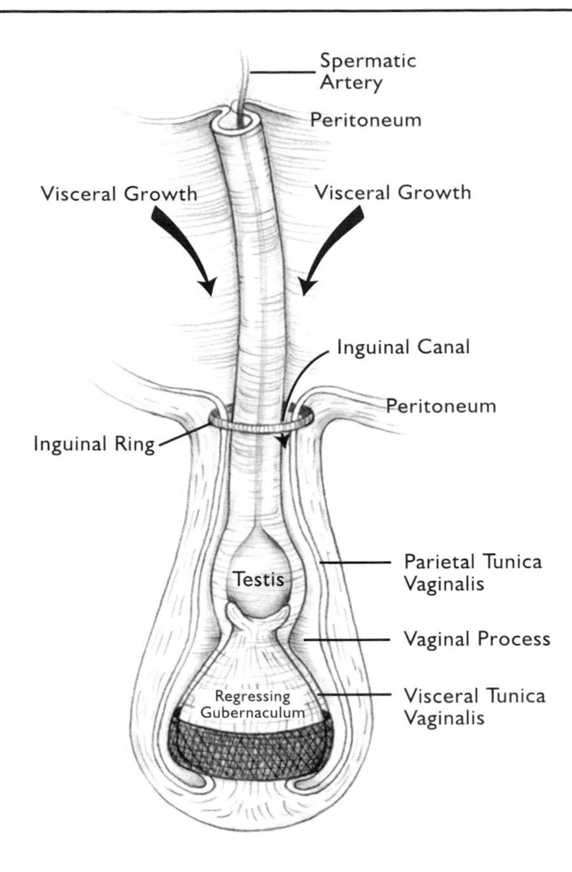

Once the testis is in the inguinal region, it is pulled through the inguinal canal because of regression ("contraction") of the gubernaculum. Also, it is possible that the pressure associated with visceral growth helps "push" the testis or at least hold it near the inguinal ring.

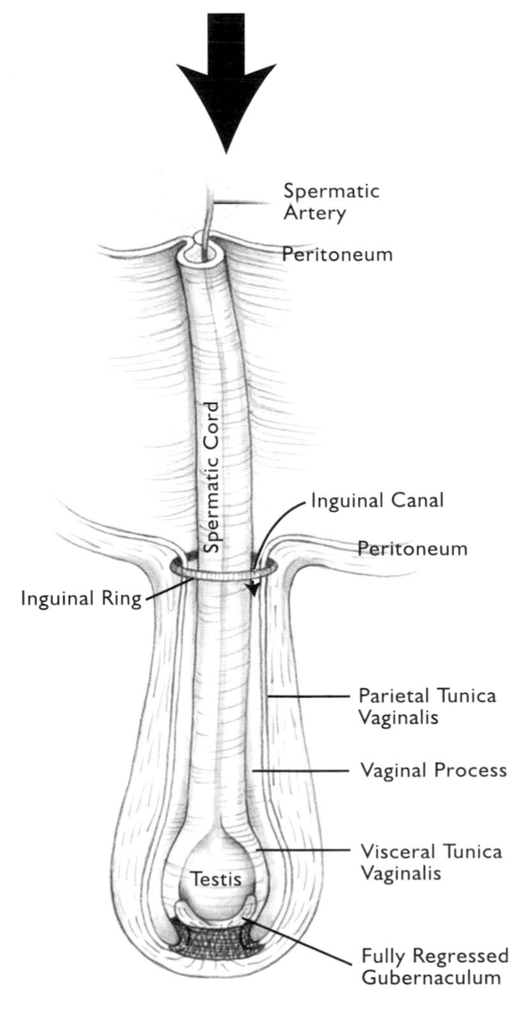

The gubernaculum continues to regress. As this regression occurs, it continues to move the testis deeper into the scrotum and cause a complete encapsulation of the testis by the inner layer of the peritoneum known as the Visceral tunica vaginalis. The outer layer of the peritoneum is the parietal layer of the tunica vaginalis. When the testis has fully descended, the gubernaculum has regressed to a small knot which attaches the testis to the distal scrotum. The vaginal process contributes to the two tunicae of the testis. The inner (visceral) layer covers the testis, epididymis and spermatic cord and the outer (parietal) layer forms a continuous fold which lies directly adjacent to (but is not attached to) the visceral tunica vaginalis.

important components of testicular descent are growth (initial phase) and regression (second phase) of the gubernaculum. An important question is, "What controls this growth and regression?" You must remember that the single most important event in testicular descent is rapid and dramatic growth of the gubernaculum during the initial phase. The presence of the testes is required for this growth to occur. It is now clear, however, that this growth is not dependent on the presence of Leydig cells, testosterone, testosterone receptors or gonadotropins. Castration experiments (Figure 4-8) indicate that the testis is essential for normal gubernacular growth. However, supplementation with gonadotropins and testosterone in castrated fetal pigs cannot promote gubernacular growth (Figure 4-8). Therefore, it appears that there is a testicular component other than testosterone which causes the dramatic gubernacular growth associated with the first phase of testicular descent. Recently, Dutch scientists have discovered a low molecular weight material (less than 3,500 daltons) which was extracted from fetal pig testes. This factor induced gubernacular growth *in vitro* (Figure 4-8). The Dutch researchers proposed that the testis produces a factor during embryogenesis which causes specific growth of the gubernaculum. They suggested that the factor(s) be called "**descendin.**" Precise biochemical identification and characterization of the factor(s) has yet to be completed.

Regression of the gubernaculum results in the final passage through the inguinal canal and orientation of the peritoneum around the testis in the scrotum. While there appears to be a specific substance which governs gubernacular growth ("descendin"), factors that cause gubernacular regression have not been identified.

Cryptorchidism is a condition in which the testes do not descend into the scrotum.

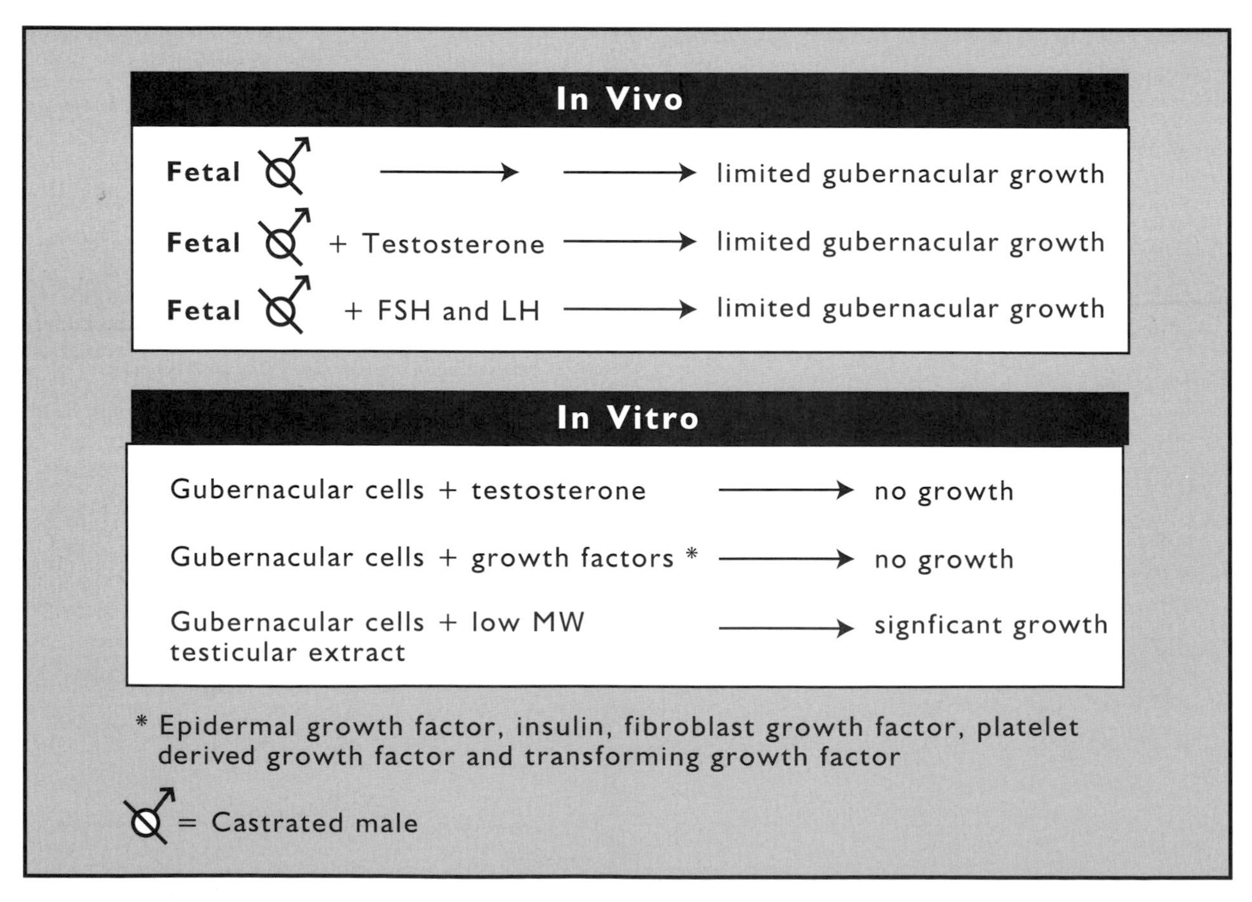

Figure 4-8. Effects of various *in vivo* and *in vitro* treatments upon growth of the gubernaculum.

Descent of the testes from the body cavity into the scrotum occurs by mid-gestation in the bull and the ram and during the last quarter of gestation in the boar. In the stallion, the testes enter the scrotum either just before or just after birth. Failure of the testes to descend into the scrotum is called **cryptorchidism**. The prefix "crypt" means hidden, concealed or not visible to the naked eye. "Orchid" is a Latinized-Greek word referring to the testis. Thus, the word cryptorchid literally means "a testis which is hidden from view." Bilateral cryptorchidism results in sterility. However, cryptorchid testes are capable of producing testosterone. Thus, the cryptorchid male possesses secondary sex characteristics that are normal and has normal reproductive behavior.

Because of the continuity between the vaginal process and the body cavity, it is possible for portions of intestine to pass into the vaginal process and enter the scrotum. Such a condition exists when the inguinal canal does not close completely. When a portion of the intestine passes through the inguinal canal into the vaginal process a condition known as an **inguinal hernia** exists. In humans, diagnosis of the presence of an inguinal hernia can easily be made by applying pressure to the lateral inguinal regions and asking the patient to cough. Such a maneuver allows the physician to feel the intestine rebound (or bounce) during the cough, inside the tunica vaginalis.

Development of the Female Reproductive Tract Requires the Absence of Testis Determining Factor

In the absence of TDF, certain cells of the sex cords differentiate into primitive follicle cells and the bulk of the genital ridge becomes the ovary (Figure 4-9).

Genetic females contain the X chromosome, which lacks the gene that governs the production of TDF (Figure 4-5). As a result, cells in the primitive gonad of the female do not differentiate into Sertoli cells. Since there are no Sertoli cells, anti-müllerian hormone cannot be produced. Therefore, the Leydig cells cannot produce testosterone and the male reproductive tract cannot develop. The development of the female reproductive tract takes place because of the absence of TDF which drives the male chain of events shown in Figure 4-5.

In the absence of TDF, the epithelial cords, or sex cords, fragment into cellular clusters, each enclosing a primitive germ cell. These clusters of germ cells penetrate less deeply into the interior of the future ovary than in the male. Thus, primordial follicles are formed along the outer surface of the ovary, and will eventually become the cortex of the ovary. Rete formation in the ovary is not pronounced (Figure 4-9), and a direct connection between the rete tubules and the mesonephric tubules does not occur. Therefore, there is no tubular outlet for the gametes. The development of the follicles (Figure 4-9) occurs throughout prenatal life and eventually the number of gametes (follicles) will become maximum and the female embryo will be born with a pool of oocytes from which folliculogenesis will occur for her reproductive lifetime. Figure 4-9 summarizes the major steps culminating in the formation of the ovary.

The ducts of the female reproductive tract are provided by the paramesonephric ducts. The anterior part of each paramesonephric duct runs parallel to the mesonephric duct (Figures 4-3 and 4-4). The anterior part of the mesonephric duct remains open to the peritoneal cavity, but the caudal end butts against the dorsal wall of the urogenital sinus (Figures 4-4 and 4-10).

The uterus and vagina result from a fusion of the paramesonephric ducts.

The oviducts, uterus, cervix and anterior vagina develop from the paramesonephric ducts. The paramesonephric ducts fuse together near their attachment to the posterior wall of the primitive urogenital sinus. The degree to which these ducts fuse determines the type of uterus the animal will have in adult life (see Chapter 2).

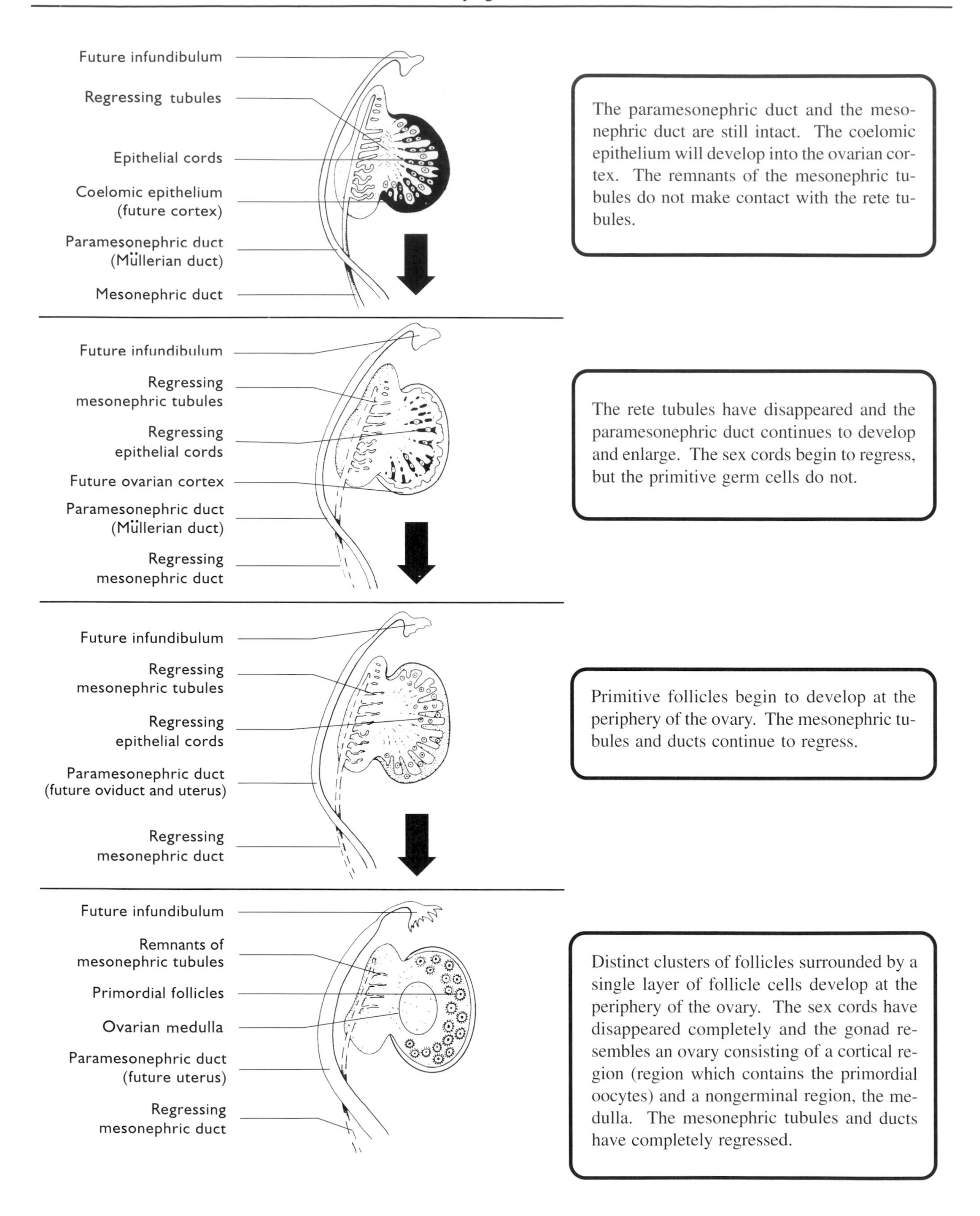

Future infundibulum
Regressing tubules
Epithelial cords
Coelomic epithelium
(future cortex)
Paramesonephric duct
(Müllerian duct)
Mesonephric duct
The paramesonephric duct and the mesonephric duct are still intact. The coelomic epithelium will develop into the ovarian cortex. The remnants of the mesonephric tubules do not make contact with the rete tubules.
Future infundibulum
Regressing
mesonephric tubules
Regressing
epithelial cords
Future ovarian cortex
Paramesonephric duct
(Müllerian duct)
Regressing
mesonephric duct
The rete tubules have disappeared and the paramesonephric duct continues to develop and enlarge. The sex cords begin to regress, but the primitive germ cells do not.
Future infundibulum
Regressing
mesonephric tubules
Regressing
epithelial cords
Paramesonephric duct
(future oviduct and uterus)
Regressing
mesonephric duct
Primitive follicles begin to develop at the periphery of the ovary. The mesonephric tubules and ducts continue to regress.
Future infundibulum
Remnants of
mesonephric tubules
Primordial follicles
Ovarian medulla
Paramesonephric duct
(future uterus)
Regressing
mesonephric duct
Distinct clusters of follicles surrounded by a single layer of follicle cells develop at the periphery of the ovary. The sex cords have disappeared completely and the gonad resembles an ovary consisting of a cortical region (region which contains the primordial oocytes) and a nongerminal region, the medulla. The mesonephric tubules and ducts have completely regressed.

Figure 4-9. Development of the ovary, the paramesonephric ducts and regression of the mesonephros. Modified from Dyce, Sack and Wensing, *Textbook of Veterinary Anatomy*, 2nd Edition, with permission from W.B. Saunders Co.

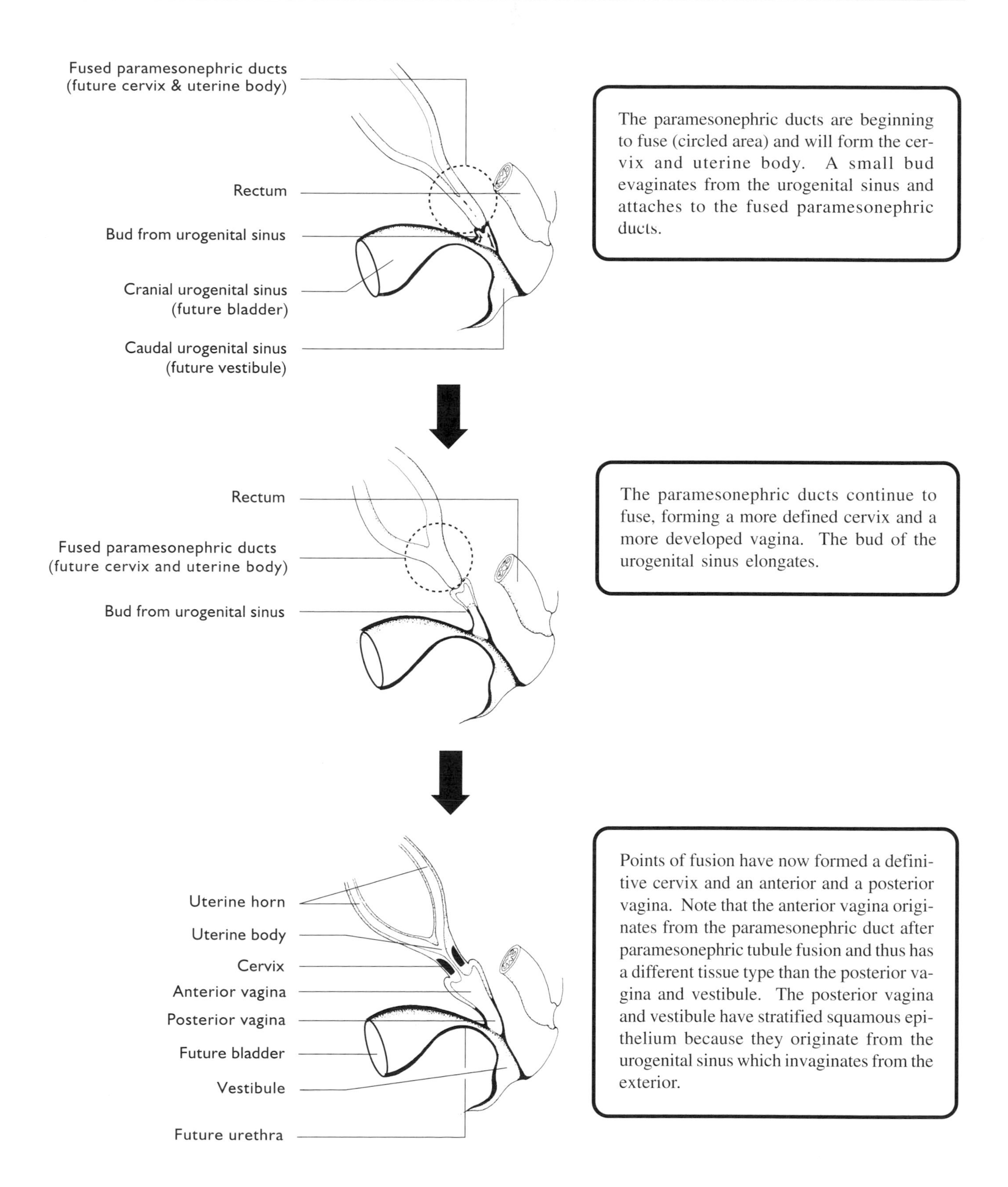

Figure 4-10. Fusion of paramesonephric ducts with the urogenital sinus to form the vagina. The purpose of this figure is to illustrate how the paramesonephric ducts fuse with a bud of the urogenital sinus. This results in the anterior vagina, cervix and uterus being of one tissue origin (mesoderm) and the posterior vagina and vestibule from another (ectoderm). Modified from Dyce, Sack and Wensing, *Textbook of Veterinary Anatomy*, 2nd Edition, with permission from W.B Saunders Co.

Anterior

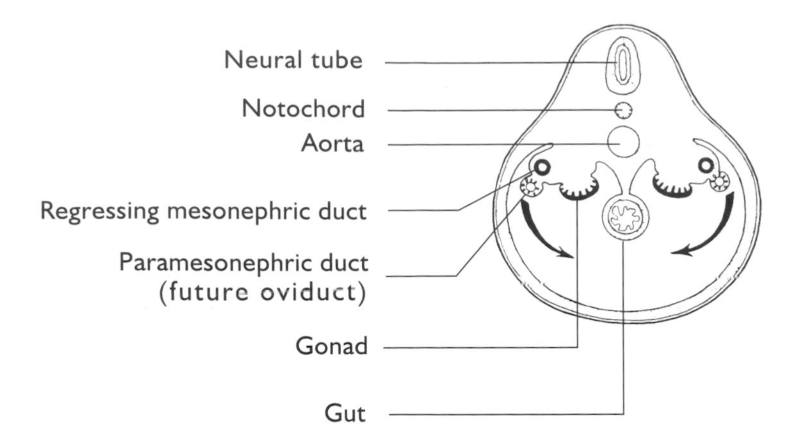

In the more anterior region of the embryo the gonad and paramesonephric duct are quite separated. They may move ventrally (arrows) but never entirely fuse. Thus, the ovary and the more anterior portions of the future uterus and oviducts (paramesonephric ducts) never fuse.

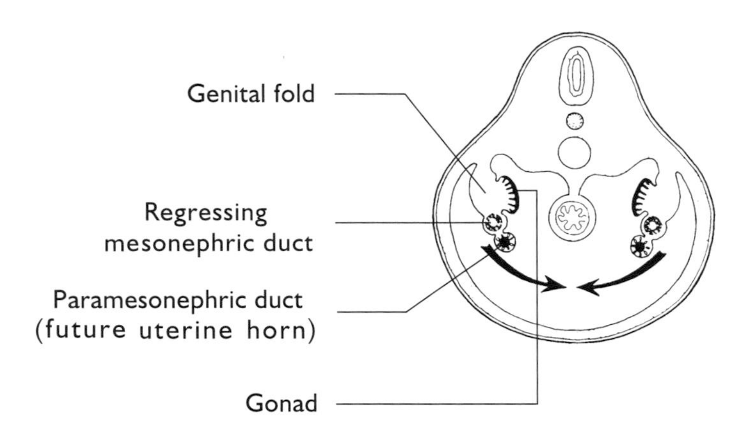

As the section becomes more posterior, the gonadal ridges as well as the paramesonephric ducts become more closely associated during their ventral movement. However, they still do not completely fuse.

Posterior

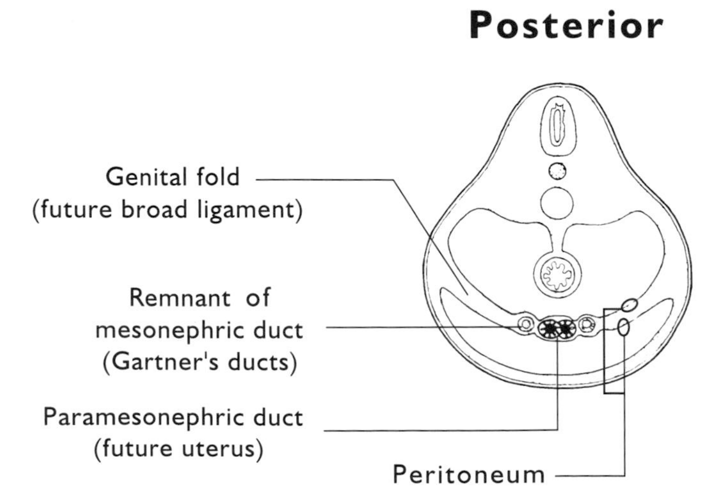

In the more posterior regions, the paramesonephric ducts have completely fused, thus creating either the body of the uterus or the cervix. The remnants of the mesonephric ducts sometimes embed themselves in the wall of the vagina; these remnants can be seen in the adult animal and are called Gartner's ducts. It should be noted that the reproductive tract is sandwiched between two layers of peritoneum referred to as the genital fold. This connective tissue layer from the peritoneum forms the broad ligament which supports the female reproductive tract in the abdominal cavity.

Figure 4-11. Transverse sections from anterior (top) to posterior (bottom) illustrating the formation of the supportive structures of the female tract from the genital fold. Modified from Dyce, Sack and Wensing, *Textbook of Veterinary Anatomy*, 2nd Edition, with permission from W.B. Saunders Co.

You can see in Figure 4-10 that the caudal tip of the fused paramesonephric ducts fuses with a small bud protruding from the urogenital sinus. This fusion results in a duct system that is continuous from the exterior to the interior. Note that the anterior vagina, cervix and uterus originate from the paramesonephric ducts (and thus mesoderm). The posterior vagina and vestibule originate from the ectoderm, which is a portion of the urogenital sinus.

It is important to note that both the male and female gonad and duct system originate behind the peritoneum **(retroperitoneal)**. Even though it appears that the reproductive tract, particularly that of the female, is inside the body cavity, it is indeed located outside the peritoneum. This supportive tissue is known as the broad ligament and surrounds the uterus, supporting it from a dorsal and lateral aspect. Figure 4-11 shows that the entire reproductive tract originates behind the peritoneum. In fact, the female tract is "sandwiched" between the genital fold. The genital fold will become the broad ligament consisting of the mesometrium, the mesosalpinx and the mesovarium. Recall from Chapter 2 that the female tract is suspended by the broad ligament that is continuous with the dorsal peritoneum.

A freemartin is a heifer born twin to a bull. The heifer calf is sterile.

In cattle, a condition exists that results in abnormal embryogenesis of the female reproductive tract. This condition is referred to as "**freemartinism**." A freemartin results because of a unique condition during the formation of the placenta in the cow. In the bovine, the extra embryonic membranes fuse to form a common chorion. These membranes occupy the same cotyledon. Thus, there is a common blood supply between the male fetus and the female fetus. Because of this shared blood supply, both embryos will be exposed to the same hormonal milieu (i.e., the female will be exposed to testosterone and anti-müllerian hormone from the male fetus). This common blood supply is established by about day 39 of gestation. In the bovine, the development of the testes occurs before the development of the ovaries. In fact, the testes are recognizable by day 40, whereas the ovaries require several weeks longer to develop. As you now know, the testes produce a substance called anti-müllerian hormone. This hormone inhibits the growth of the paramesonephric ducts (Müllerian ducts). Since the female twin is exposed to anti-müllerian hormone as the female reproductive tract is developing, the paramesonephric ducts do not develop completely. This incomplete development results in reproductive tracts which are "blind" and **canalization** (formation of a canal or lumen) is not complete. In addition, the potential ovaries cease to grow and do not develop the appropriate complement of germ cells. Therefore, the ovaries are incapable of producing estrogen and often produce substantial amounts of testosterone as well as androstenedione. This atypical form of steroidogenesis not only causes abnormal female reproductive tract development, but also "programs" the central nervous system so that the genetic female behaves similarly to a male. The response of the freemartin to this elevated level of testosterone and androstenedione may range from lack of noticeable physical and behavioral characteristics to significant "bullish" behavior. From a practical perspective, the freemartin can be used quite effectively as an animal to detect estrus. Since these animals' central nervous system has been programmed to be male-like, they are generally more aggressive in seeking out other females in estrus. By supplementing freemartin heifers with exogenous androgens, maleness can be further accentuated.

Further Phenomena for Fertility

All species do not develop a distinct sex (separate testes and ovaries) like this chapter explains. Some individuals possess both an ovary and a testis and are called hermaphrodites. Sea basses are synchronous hermaphrodites, meaning that fertile spermatozoa and oocytes in an ovotestes are present at the same time within a single fish. Self-fertilization is possible, but these fish have group-spawning events to insure genetic heterogeneity. Self-fertilization is advantageous if a sea bass is not present at the spawning event.

Testicles sometimes stray from the normal path of descent. In humans, they have been found under the skin of the root of the penis and in front of the anus.

In some species the guardian of embryogenesis is the male. The female bell toad lays her eggs in strings 3 to 4 feet long. The male wraps the egg string around his body. For about one month he serves as the "uterus," making sure that he and the eggs are exposed to the appropriate environment. He hides during the day (because he doesn't want his buddies to see him) and seeks water at night to moisten the eggs. Apparently, at "parturition" (hatching), the male sits in the water and the tadpoles swim away. We do not know the endocrine basis for this phenomenon.

In 1975, there were approximately 125 million babies born in the world. Of these, 6 million had chromosomal disorders, biochemical disorders or major congenital birth defects that required extensive medical resources. The most frequent type of disorder was a major congenital defect (4 million) because of faulty embryogenesis.

In chickens (and some ducks and doves) "sex" can be reversed after birth. Removal of the functional left ovary results in the development of the nonfunctional right gonad into a testis or ovotestis (a gonad containing follicles of ovulatory size and tubules with spermatozoa). The younger the bird at ovariectomy, the greater the probability that the right gonad will develop into a testis. The older the bird, the greater the probability that an ovotestis will develop.

Additional Reading

Dubois, Paul. 1993. "The Hypothalamic-Pituitary Axis: Embryological, Morphological and Functional Aspects" in *Reproduction in Mammals and Man.* Thibault, C., M.C. Levasseur and R.H.F. Hunter, eds., Ellipses, Paris.

Fentener van Vlissingen, J.M.F., E.J.J. von Zoelen, P.J.F. Ursem and C.J.G. Wensing. 1988. "*In vitro* model of the first phase of testicular descent: Identification of a low molecular weight factor from fetal testes involved in proliferation of gubernaculum testis cells and distinct from polypeptide growth factors and fetal gonadal hormones." *Endo.* 123:2868-2877. *(Author's note: This paper is the first suggesting the existence of "descendin.")*

George, F.W. and J.D. Wilson. 1994. "Sex Determination and Differentiation" in *Physiology of Reprod.* 2nd Edition Vol. 2., E. Knobil and J.D., Neill, eds., Raven Press, New York.

Larsen, William J. 1993. *Human Embryology.* Churchill Livingstone, New York.

5 Regulation of Reproduction - Nerves, Hormones and Target Tissues

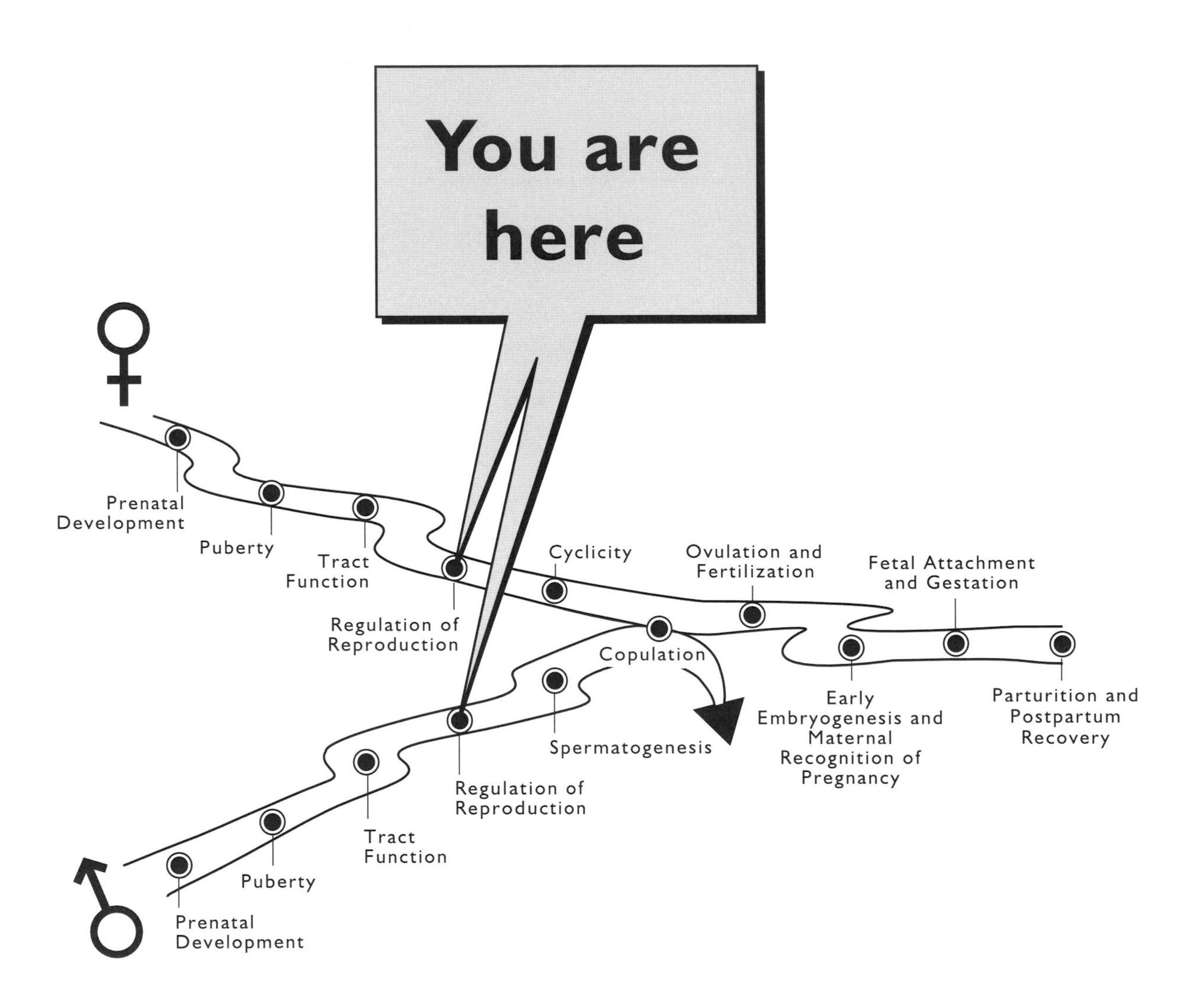

Take Home Message

Hormones originate from endocrine glands or nerves. They enter the blood and cause cells in target tissues containing specific receptors to produce new products or new hormones. The original hormones and the products of their action are necessary for successful reproduction. Protein hormones act via plasma membrane receptors and exert effects in the cytoplasm of the cell. Steroid hormones act through nuclear receptors and cause transcription and translation that results in the production of new proteins. Both types of hormones cause changes in the function of the target cells.

Reproduction is regulated by a remarkable interplay between the **nervous system** and the **endocrine system**. These two systems interact in a consistent display of teamwork to initiate, coordinate and regulate all reproductive functions. In order to understand and appreciate the role of these two systems, you must first focus on the control that each system exerts independently.

Neural control is exerted by:
- ***simple neural reflexes***
- ***neuroendocrine reflexes***

The fundamental responsibility of the nervous system is to translate or **transduce** external stimuli into neural signals which bring about a change in the reproductive organs and tissues. The fundamental pathways of nervous involvement are a **simple neural reflex** and a **neuroendocrine reflex.** The functional components of these two pathways are sensory neurons, the spinal cord, efferent neurons (nerves leaving the spinal cord and traveling to the target tissue) and **target tissues.** Target tissues are those organs which respond to a specific set of stimuli.

The basic difference between the simple neural reflex and the neuroendocrine reflex is the type of delivery system each employs. For example, a simple neural reflex employs nerves which release their neurotransmitters (messengers) directly onto the target tissues. In other words, the target tissue is directly innervated by a neuron. In contrast, a neuroendocrine reflex requires that a **neurohormone** (a substance released by a neuron) enter the blood and act on a remote target tissue. Neurons releasing neurotransmitters may also be referred to as **neurosecretory cells**. Direct innervation of the target tissue does not exist in the neuroendocrine reflex. Instead, the neurohormone in the blood is the messenger between the neurosecretory cell and the target tissue.

Neural Reflexes and Neuroendocrine Reflexes Cause Rapid Changes in Target Tissues

In a simple neural reflex, sensory neurons (also afferent sensory neurons) synapse directly with **interneurons** in the spinal cord (Figure 5-1). These interneurons synapse with efferent neurons which travel directly to the target tissue. The target tissue responds to the neurotransmitter released by the efferent neuron. A **neurotransmitter** is a substance of small molecular weight which is released from the terminals of nerves that causes other nerves to fire or causes contraction of smooth muscle that surrounds portions of the reproductive tract (Figure 5-1). An example of a simple neural reflex in reproduction is ejaculation. A stimulus originating in the glans penis is recognized by sensory neurons. Signals are then transmitted to the spinal cord where they synapse with efferent neurons that cause a series of highly coordinated muscular contractions re-

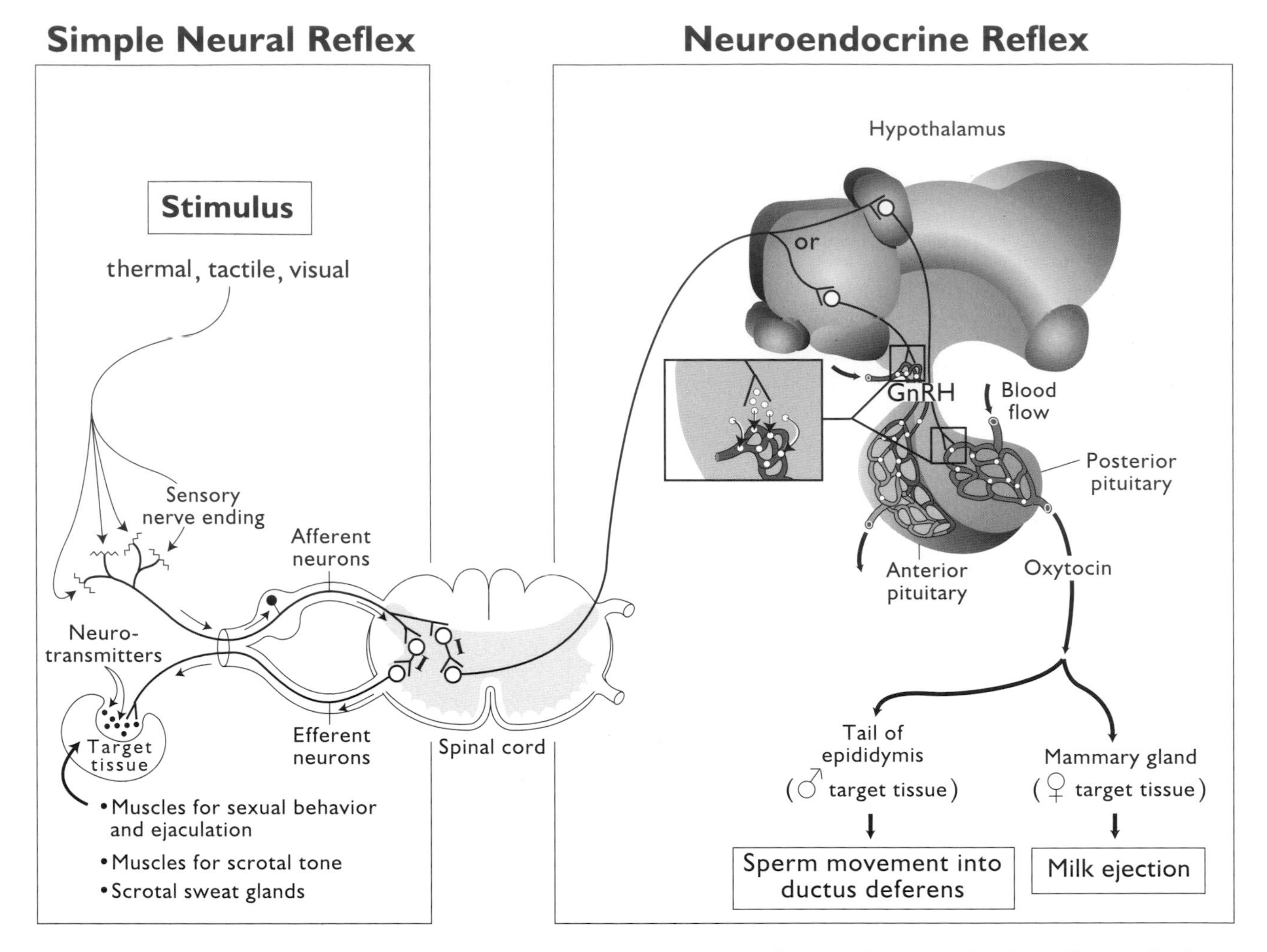

Figure 5-1. Reproductive processes are controlled by simple neural reflexes and neuroendocrine reflexes. Both reflexes are initiated by sensory nerves which travel to the spinal cord. Here, the sensory nerves synapse with interneurons (I). Efferent neurons either travel directly to the target tissue (simple neural reflex) or to the hypothalamus (neuroendocrine reflex). Hypothalamic neurons release neurohormones which enter the blood and then activate the target tissue, which can be the anterior pituitary or other tissues such as the mammary gland or the epididymis. (Graphic by Sonja Oei.)

sulting in expulsion of semen. Another example of a simple neural reflex that impacts the reproductive system (described in Chapter 3) involves temperature sensitive neurons located in the scrotum. When scrotal temperature decreases, sensory neurons in the scrotum recognize this decrease and send sensory signals to the spinal cord. Efferent nerves travel to the tunica dartos in the scrotum and release neurotransmitters which initiate contraction that elevates the testicles to bring them closer to the body, thus warming them.

The **neuroendocrine reflex** (Figure 5-1) is quite similar to a simple neural reflex. This type of reflex is also initiated with sensory input to synaptic junctions at interneurons in the spinal cord. Efferent neurons traveling from the spinal cord **synapse** with other neurons in the hypothalamus. The hypothalamic neurons release small molecular weight materials from their terminals. These materials are referred to as neurohormones because they are released into the blood rather than directly onto the target tissue. Neurohormones released into capillaries travel to a target tissue elsewhere in the body. The classic example of a neuroendocrine reflex is the suckling reflex. When suckling occurs, sensory nerves in the teat of the lactating female recognize the tactile stimulus. These sensory signals travel to the spinal cord and then to the hypothalamus where they synapse with other nerves. The hypothalamic neurons then depolarize ("fire"), causing release of **oxytocin** directly from nerve terminals located in the posterior pituitary. Oxytocin is stored as a neurosecretory material in the nerve terminals of the posterior pituitary. When these neurosecretory cells "fire," oxytocin is released, enters the blood, travels to the target tissue (in this case, myoepithelial cells of the mammary gland) and causes these cells to contract, resulting in milk let-down (milk ejection from the mammary alveoli). In addition, other forms of stimuli, such as visual or auditory, can cause milk let-down if the animal is preconditioned to respond to these stimuli. For example, the sight or sound of the newborn may elicit a similar response without direct mammary stimulation. Also, many dairy cows entering the milking parlor receive visual or auditory stimuli prior to actual mammary stimulation by either the sight or sounds of the equipment and begin to experience milk let-down prior to entering the parlor.

Inhibitory neurons block or stop the action of other excitatory neurons.

The neural pathways illustrated in Figures 5-1 and 5-2 deal exclusively with excitatory neurons (neurons which cause other neurons or tissues to be excited or activated). However, another type of neuron is widespread throughout the central nervous system. This type of neuron is known as an **inhibitory neuron** and rather than excite, it inhibits other neurons. In order to understand fully the possible action of inhibitory neurons, you must first understand the functional difference between inhibitory and excitatory neurons. The distinguishing feature between the inhibitory and excitatory neurons is

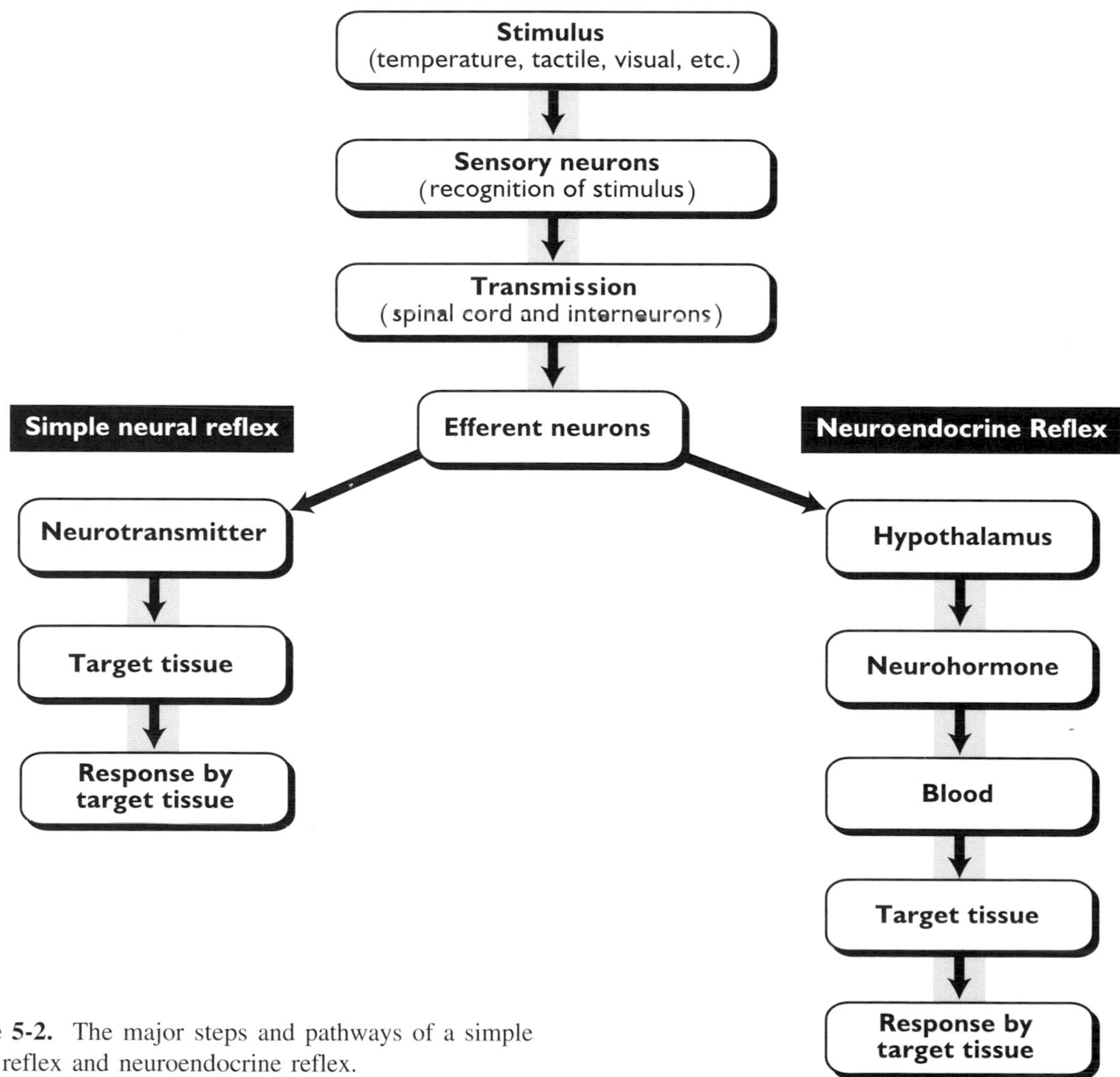

Figure 5-2. The major steps and pathways of a simple neural reflex and neuroendocrine reflex.

the type of neurotransmitter that is released from each. An **excitatory neurotransmitter** will increase the probability of a postsynaptic action potential (firing of the nerve). An **inhibitory neurotransmitter** will decrease the chance of a postsynaptic action potential. Thus, the probability that the postsynaptic neuron will fire is controlled by the ratio of presynaptic excitation and presynaptic inhibition.

The hypothalamus is the neural control center for reproductive hormones.

The hypothalamus is a complex portion of the brain consisting of clusters of nerve cell bodies. The clusters, or groups of nerve cell bodies are called **hypothalamic nuclei,** each of which has a specific name. For example, groups of hypothalamic nuclei which influence reproduction are named the surge center and the tonic center (Figure 5-3). Neurons in these regions produce **gonadotropin releasing hormone** (GnRH). Neurons in the paraventricular nucleus (PVN) produce oxytocin. The hypothalamic nuclei surround a small cavity known as the third ventricle, found in the center of the brain (Figure 5-3). It should be understood that various hypothalamic nuclei have different functions and are stimulated by different sets of conditions.

Neurons in the hypothalamus communicate with the anterior pituitary utilizing a special circulatory modification known as the hypothalamo-hypophyseal portal system.

Axons from the cell bodies of the surge and tonic centers extend into the pituitary stalk region where the nerve endings (terminal boutons) terminate on a sophisticated and highly specialized capillary network. This capillary network is referred to as the **hypothalamo-hypophyseal portal system** (Figure 5-4). The terminal boutons of the hypothalamic neurons release neuropeptides, which enter the specialized capillary system at the stalk of the pituitary. Blood enters the capillary system from the **superior hypophyseal artery,** which divides into small arterial capillaries at the level of the pituitary stalk. This portal system enables extremely small quantities (picograms) of releasing hormones to be deposited in the capillary plexus (**primary portal plexus**) of the pituitary stalk. Releasing hormones are then transferred immediately to a second capillary plexus in the anterior pituitary where the releasing hormone causes pituitary cells to release other hormones. The hypothalamo-hypophyseal portal system is important because it allows minute quantities of releasing hormones to act directly on the cells of the anterior pituitary before dilution by the systemic circulation.

The posterior pituitary does not contain a portal system. Neurohormones are deposited directly into capillaries in the posterior pituitary.

The posterior pituitary is organized quite differently from the anterior pituitary (Figure 5-5). Neurons from certain hypothalamic nuclei extend directly into the posterior pituitary where the neurohormone is released into a simple arteriovenous capillary plexus. For example, cell bodies in the paraventricular nucleus synthesize oxytocin which is transported down the axon to the posterior pituitary where it is released into the blood.

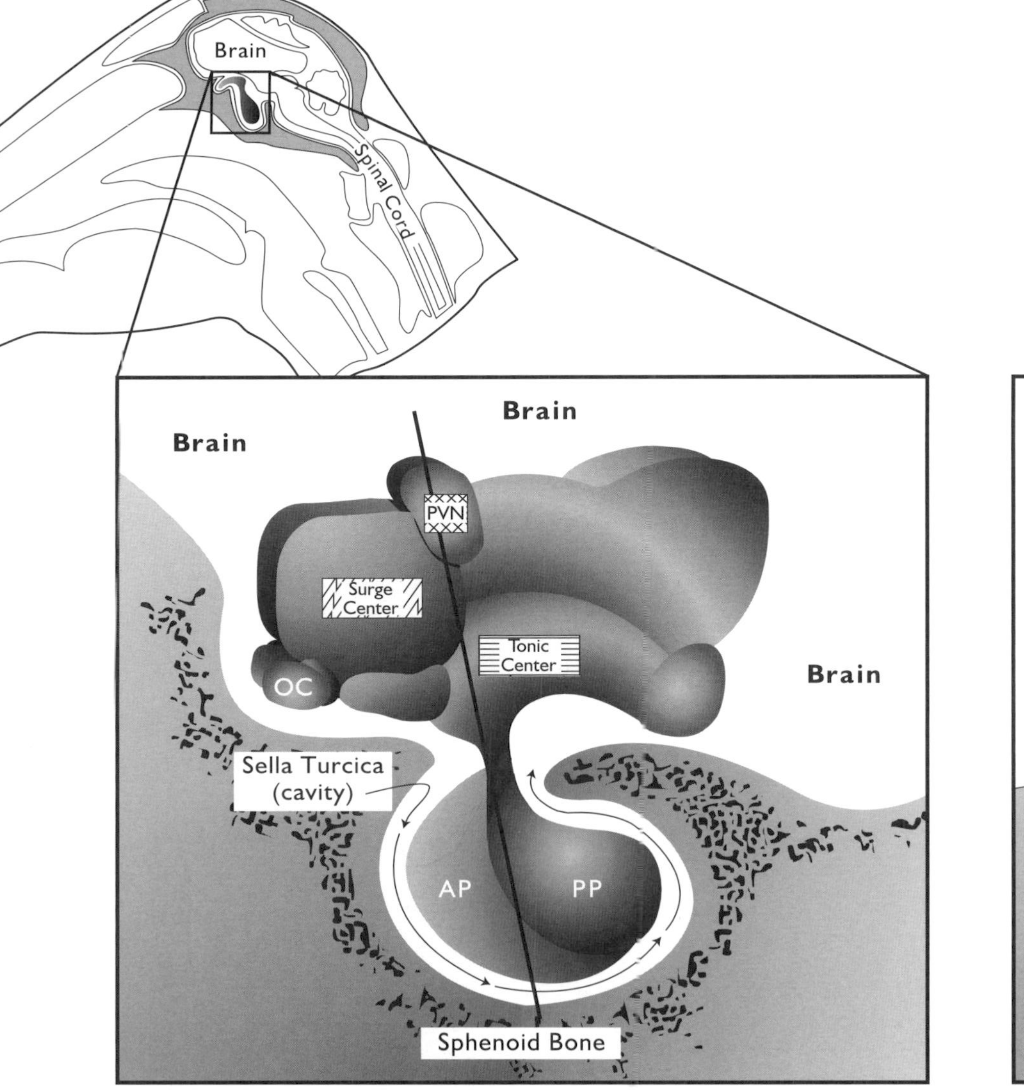

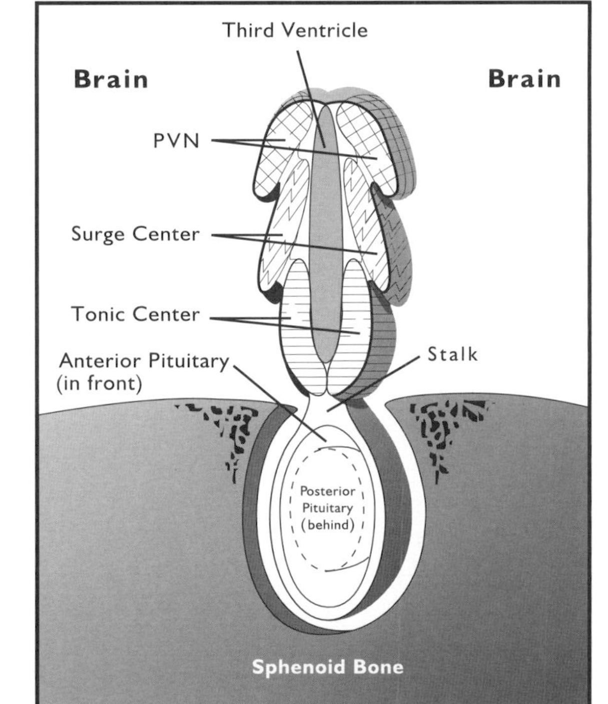

Figure 5-3. The anatomy of the typical mammalian hypothalamus and pituitary. The hypothalamus is a specialized ventral portion of the brain consisting of groups of nerve cell bodies called hypothalamic nuclei, which appear as lobules in the figure. The surge center, the tonic center and the paraventricular nucleus (PVN) have direct influence on reproduction. The anterior and posterior pituitary are positioned in a depression of the sphenoid bone called the sella turcica. The right panel (frontal view) illustrates the relationship of the paraventricular nucleus (PVN), the surge center and the tonic center to the third ventricle and pituitary. The vertical line in the left panel (sagittal view) represents the plane of section shown in the right panel. Notice that the third ventricle, a brain cavity, separates the lateral portions of the hypothalamus. AP = Anterior Pituitary, PP = Posterior Pituitary, OC = Optic Chiasm. (Graphic by Sonja Oei.)

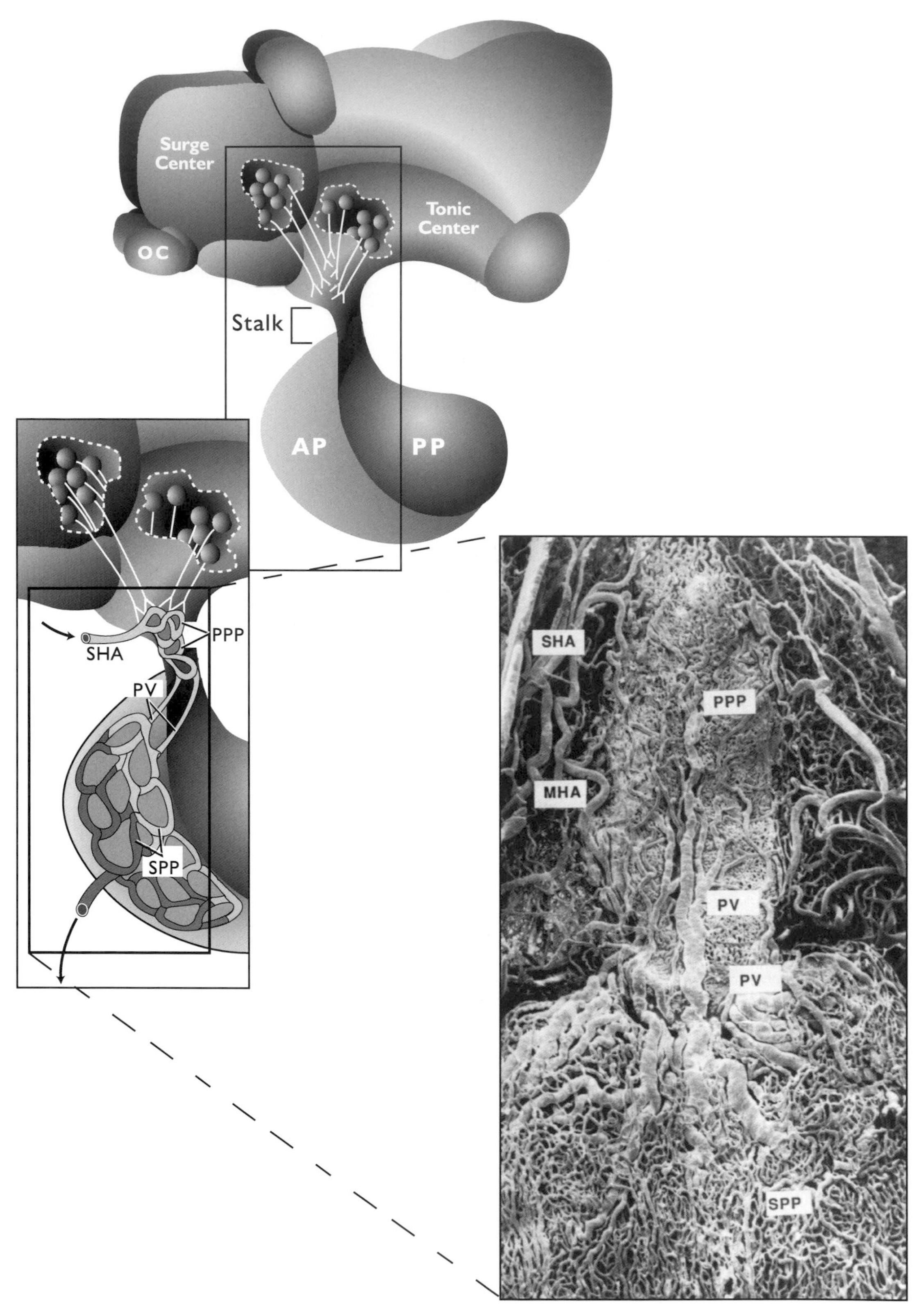

Figure 5-4. Axons from neurons in the surge center and the tonic center extend to the stalk region where their endings terminate upon blood vessels of the hypothalamo-hypophyseal portal system. This portal system consists of: the superior hypophyseal artery (SHA); the primary portal plexus (PPP), where the surge center and tonic center neurons terminate; the medial hypophyseal artery (MHA) which supplies part of the anterior pituitary; the portal vessels (PV) which transport blood containing releasing hormones; and the secondary portal plexus (SPP) which delivers blood (and releasing hormones) to the cells of the anterior pituitary. The photograph at the right is a scanning electron micrograph of the hypothalamo-hypophyseal portal system after vascular injection with latex (Mercox). It was provided with permission by Dr. H. Duvernoy, Faculte de medecine et de Pharmacie de Besancon, Laboratoire d'Anatomie, Place St. Jacques, 25030 Besancon, France. (Graphic by Sonja Oei.)

Endocrine Control is Generally Slower, but Longer Lasting Than Neural Control

In contrast to neural regulation, the endocrine system relies on **hormones** to cause responses. A hormone is a substance produced by a gland that acts on a remote tissue (**target tissue**) to bring about a change in the target tissue. These changes may involve alterations in metabolism, synthetic activity and secretory activity.

Extremely small quantities of a hormone can cause dramatic physiologic responses. Hormones act at blood levels ranging from nanograms (10^{-9}) to picograms (10^{-12}) per ml of blood (Table 5-1).

Exponent		Name
1.0		**gram**
10^{-1}	.1	
10^{-2}	.01	
10^{-3}	**.001**	**milligram**
10^{-4}	.000,1	
10^{-5}	.000,01	
10^{-6}	**.000,001**	**microgram**
10^{-7}	.000,000,1	
10^{-8}	.000,000,01	
10^{-9}	**.000,000,001**	**nanogram**
10^{-10}	.000,000,000,1	
10^{-11}	.000,000,000,01	
10^{-12}	**.000,000,000,001**	**picogram**

Table 5-1. Illustration of exponents, decimal places and common weight designations used in describing quantities of substances. The shaded area indicates range of hormone weights per milliliter of blood that cause physiologic responses.

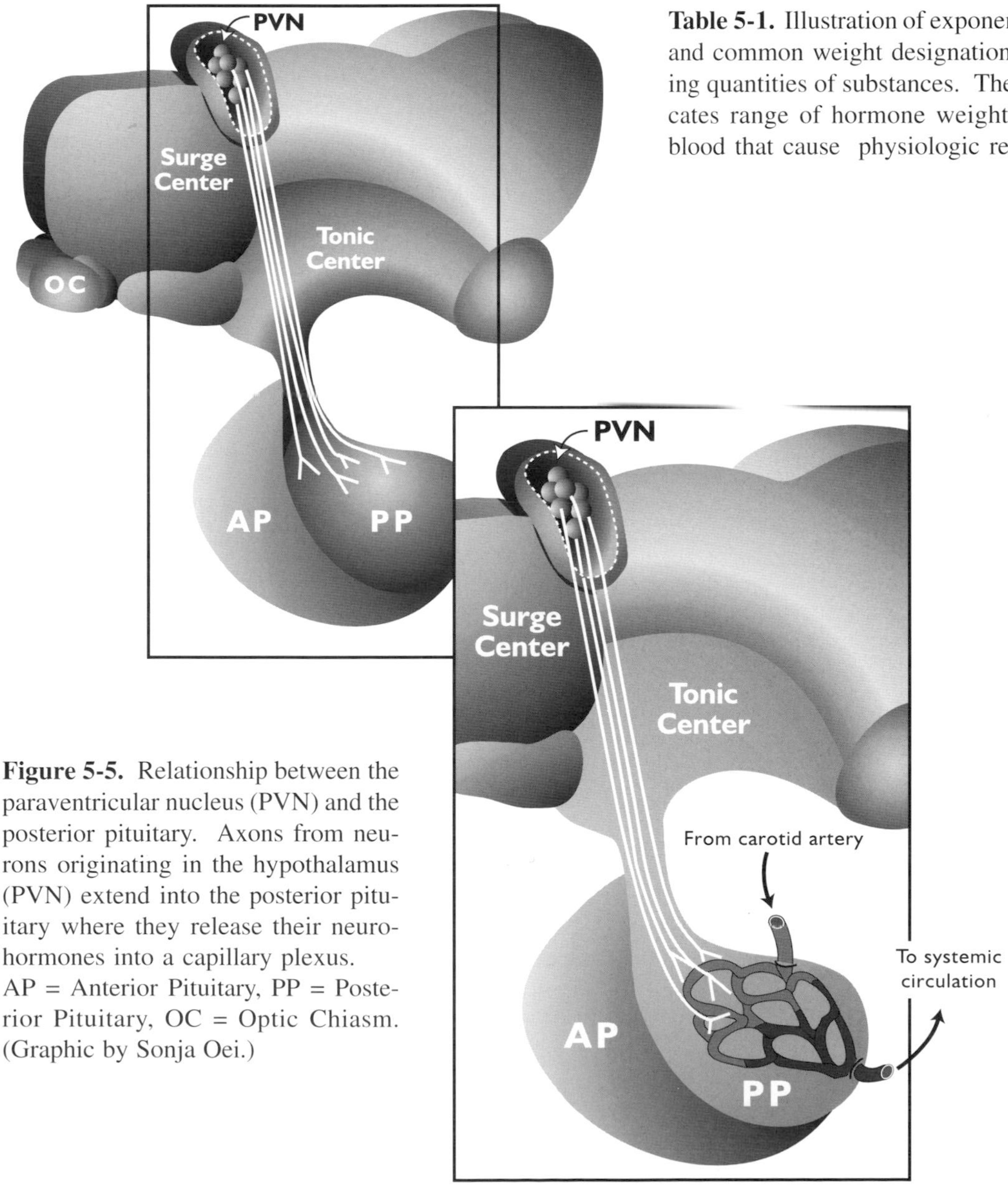

Figure 5-5. Relationship between the paraventricular nucleus (PVN) and the posterior pituitary. Axons from neurons originating in the hypothalamus (PVN) extend into the posterior pituitary where they release their neurohormones into a capillary plexus. AP = Anterior Pituitary, PP = Posterior Pituitary, OC = Optic Chiasm. (Graphic by Sonja Oei.)

The ability to measure extremely small quantities of hormones has brought about an explosion of knowledge regarding the quantities, patterns of secretions and roles of hormones as they relate to reproductive processes. Much of this exciting information will be presented in chapters which follow.

Hormones are characterized as having relatively short half-lives. Hormonal **half-life** is defined as the time required for one-half of a quantity of a hormone to disappear from the blood or from the body. Short half-lives are important because once the hormone is secreted and released into the blood and causes a response, it is degraded so that further or unnecessary responses do not occur. It should be emphasized, however, when hormones are continually produced (such as progesterone during pregnancy), the action brought about by the hormone continues for as long as the hormone is present. Compared to nervous control, hormonal control is slower and has durations of minutes, hours or even days.

> ***Reproductive hormones:***
> - ***act in minute quantities***
> - ***have short half-lives***
> - ***bind to specific receptors***
> - ***regulate intracellular biochemical reactions***

In order for a hormone to cause a response, it must first interact specifically with the target tissue. For this interaction to occur, the cells of the target tissue must have receptors that bind the hormone. Binding of the hormone with its specific receptor initiates a series of intracellular biochemical reactions which will be discussed later in this chapter.

Hormonal regulation of a biochemical reaction is generally tied to secretory activity of the target cell. When exposed to a hormone, the target cell synthesizes substances which are not produced unless the hormone is present. For example, estradiol (produced by the ovary), causes the cells of the cervix to secrete mucus. This change is caused by a series of biochemical or synthetic pathways within the cells of the cervix. These will be detailed later in this chapter.

Reproductive hormones can be classified according to their source of origin, their primary mode of action and their biochemical classification. Table 5-2 summarizes hormonal classification by source, by target tissue and by their primary actions. Details about these hormones will be presented in subsequent chapters where their function will be specifically described in the female (Chapters 6, 7, 8, 9,11, 13 and 14) and in the male (Chapters 6, 10 and 11).

Glandular Origin Constitutes One Method of Hormonal Classification

Hypothalamic hormones are produced by neurons in the hypothalamus. Their role is to cause the release of other hormones from the anterior pituitary. The primary releasing hormone of reproduction is **gonadotropin releasing hormone (GnRH)** (Figure 5-6). **Neuropeptides** of hypothalamic origin are very small molecules generally consisting of less than twenty amino acids. These small peptides are synthesized and released from neurons in the hypothalamus. The most important neuropeptide governing reproduction is GnRH. The amino acid sequence for GnRH, a decapeptide, is shown in Figure 5-6. The molecular weight of GnRH is only 1,183 daltons.

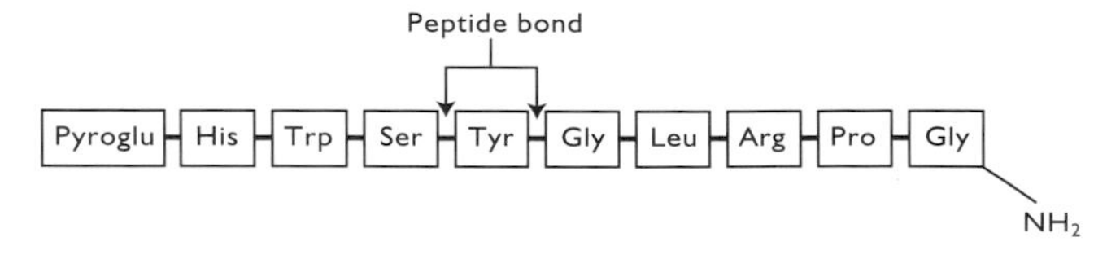

Figure 5-6. Amino acid sequence of GnRH.

Pituitary hormones are released into the blood from the anterior and posterior pituitary. The primary reproductive hormones from the anterior pituitary are **follicle stimulating hormone (FSH)**, **luteinizing hormone (LH)** and **prolactin.** **Oxytocin** is the primary reproductive hormone released from the posterior pituitary.

Gonadal hormones originate from the gonads and affect the function of the hypothalamus, anterior pituitary and tissues of the reproductive tract. Gonadal hormones also initiate the development of secondary sex characteristics which cause "maleness" or "femaleness." In the female, the ovary produces estrogens, progestogens, inhibin, some testosterone, oxytocin and relaxin. In the male, the testes produce testosterone and other androgens, inhibin and some estrogens.

Reproductive hormones originate from the:
- ***hypothalamus***
- ***pituitary***
- ***gonads***
- ***uterus***
- ***placenta***

Hormones are also produced by the uterus and the placenta. These are responsible for governing cyclicity and maintenance of pregnancy. An example of a uterine hormone is **prostaglandin $F_{2\alpha}$ ($PGF_{2\alpha}$)**. Placental hormones include **progesterone**, **estrogen**, **equine chorionic gonadotropin (eCG)** and **human chorionic gonadotropin (hGC)** during gestation.

Mode of Action Is Another Method of Hormonal Classification

Neurohormones are synthesized by neurons and are released directly into the blood so that they can cause a response in target tissues elsewhere in the body. A neurohormone can act on any number of tissues provided that the tissue has cellular receptors for the neurohormone. An example is oxytocin of posterior pituitary origin.

Releasing hormones are also synthesized by neurons in the hypothalamus and cause release of other hormones from the anterior pituitary. They can also be classified as neurohormones because they are synthesized and released by neurons. An example is gonadotropin releasing hormone (GnRH) which controls the release of FSH and LH from the anterior pituitary.

Gonadotropins are hormones released by the **gonadotroph cells** of the anterior pituitary and they stimulate the gonads. The suffix "**tropin**" means having an affinity for. Thus, these hormones have an affinity for the gonads (the ovary and the testis). Gonadotropins are **follicle stimulating hormone (FSH)** and **luteinizing hormone (LH).** Luteinizing hormone is responsible for causing ovulation and stimulating the corpus luteum (CL) to produce progesterone. Luteinizing hormone causes testosterone production in the male. Follicle stimulating hormone causes follicular growth in the ovary of the female. It stimulates Sertoli cells in the male and is probably a "key player" in governing spermatogenesis.

Reproductive hormones function as:
- ***releasing factors for other hormones***
- ***gonadotropins***
- ***sexual promoters (steroids)***
- ***pregnancy maintenance hormones***
- ***luteolytic hormones***

Sexual promoters (estrogen, progesterone, testosterone) are produced by the gonads of both the male and the female to stimulate the reproductive tract, to regulate the function of the hypothalamus and the anterior pituitary and to regulate reproductive behavior. These hormones also cause the development of secondary sex characteristics. The sexual promoters are the driving force for all reproductive function.

Human chorionic gonadotropin (hCG) and **equine chorionic gonadotropin** (eCG) are produced by the early embryo (conceptus). These placental hormones cause stimulation of the maternal ovary.

Pregnancy maintenance hormones are in high concentrations during times of pregnancy. They are responsible for maintenance of pregnancy (e.g., progesterone) and, in some cases, assisting the female in her lactation ability. **Placental lactogen** promotes development of the mammary gland of the dam and is therefore **lactogenic**.

General metabolic hormones promote metabolic well-being. Such hormones are **thyroxin** from the thyroid gland, **the adrenal corticoids** from the adrenal cortex and **growth hormone (somatotropin)** from the anterior pituitary. Thyroxin regulates metabolic rate of the animal. The adrenal corticoids perform a host of functions ranging from mineral metabolism to regulation of inflammatory responses. Growth hormone helps regulate growth, lactation and protein metabolism. These general metabolic hormones are all necessary for optimum reproduction. However, they are considered to exert an indirect rather than a direct effect on reproductive function.

Luteolytic hormones cause destruction of the corpus luteum. The suffix "**lytic**" is a derivative of the word lysis. Lysis means decomposition, disintegration or dissolution. Luteolytic hormones, therefore, cause disintegration of the corpus luteum. The major luteolytic hormone is **prostaglandin $F_{2\alpha}$** ($PGF_{2\alpha}$). As you shall see in Chapter 9, $PGF_{2\alpha}$ causes a decrease in secretion of progesterone by the corpus luteum.

Biochemical classifications include:
- ***peptides***
- ***glycoproteins***
- ***steroids***
- ***prostaglandins***

Glycoproteins are polypeptide hormones which contain carbohydrate moieties and range in molecular weight from several hundred to 70,000 daltons. Some glycoprotein hormones are composed of two side-by-side polypeptide chains which have carbohydrates attached to each chain. These polypeptide chains have

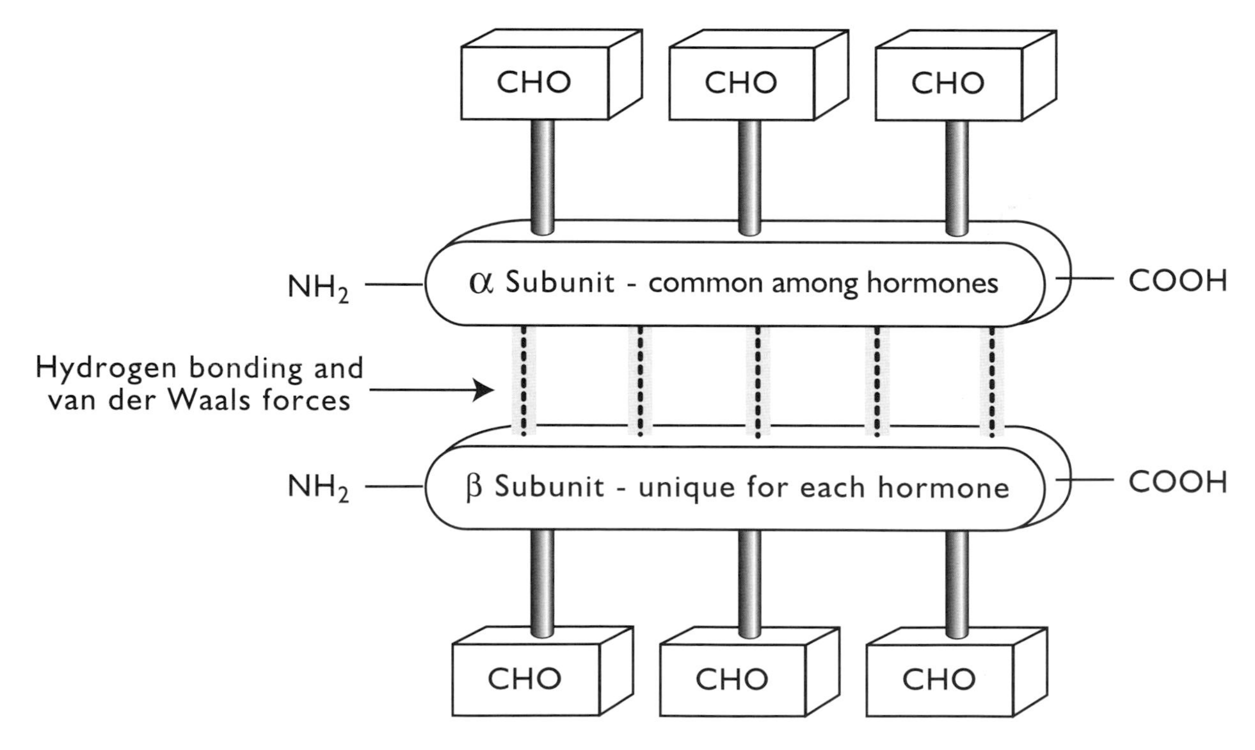

Figure 5-7. Schematic diagram of an anterior pituitary glycoprotein hormone. The α and β subunits are held together non-covalently by hydrogen bonding and van der Waals forces (dotted lines). Carbohydrate (CHO) moieties are shown in boxes and are covalently bonded to the α or β subunit.

been designated by biochemists as the **alpha (α) and beta (β) subunits** (Figure 5-7). The anterior pituitary produces glycoprotein hormones which all have the same α subunit but different β subunits. The α subunit for FSH, LH and thyroid stimulating hormone (TSH) are identical within species. However, the β subunit is unique to each individual hormone and gives each of these glycoprotein hormones a high degree of specificity and function. Individual α and β subunits of these molecules have no biological activity. If an α subunit of one hormone is combined with the β subunit of another hormone, the activity will be determined by the hormone which contributed the β subunit. The α and β subunits are held together with hydrogen bonds and van der Waals forces and thus <u>are</u> <u>not</u> covalently attached (Figure 5-7).

Inhibin is another glycoprotein hormone that contains an α and one of two possible β subunits (designated β_A or β_B). This hormone appears to have the same physiologic activity regardless of which β subunit is present.

Researchers have identified a protein from follicular fluid that consists of two β subunits. They have termed this material "**activin**." "Activin" has been shown to cause release of FSH in pituitary cells in culture. It therefore causes the opposite of inhibin in-vitro. This function has not been demonstrated in the intact animal and thus, it is not as yet considered a hormone.

Prolactin is an example of a protein that consists of a single polypeptide chain rather than containing an α and β subunit.

Dispersed along each subunit of the hormone are carbohydrate moieties that are believed to protect the molecule from short-term degradation, which might occur during transport in the blood and interstitial compartments to target tissues. The quantity of carbohydrate moieties on the surface of the protein is believed to determine the duration of the hormone's half-life. In other words, the higher the degree of glycosylation (number of carbohydrate moieties), the longer the half-life of the hormone. Recent research findings indicate that a single glycoprotein hormone may have as many as 6 to 8 subtypes in which the degree of glycosylation varies significantly among them. Control of the genetic expression of these subtypes is not understood. Glycoprotein hormones can be degraded easily by proteolytic enzymes in the digestive tract. Therefore, they are not effective when given orally.

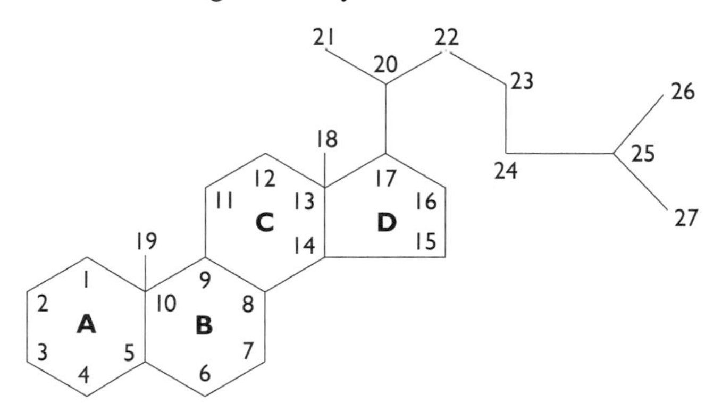

Figure 5-8. The standardized labeling of the steroid molecule. A, B, C and D designate specific rings. Numbers designate specific carbons.

Steroid hormones have a common molecular nucleus called the **cyclopentanoperhydrophenanthrene nucleus**. The molecule is composed of four rings designated A, B, C and D. Each carbon in the ring has a number, as shown in Figure 5-8.

Steroids are synthesized from cholesterol through a series of complex pathways involving many enzymatic conversions. Figure 5-9 illustrates the major biochemical transformations that occur in the gonadal steroid synthetic pathway. Notice the high degree of structural similarity between estradiol and testosterone. Steroid molecules are sexual promoters and cause profound changes in both the male and female reproductive tract and these will be discussed in later chapters.

Prostaglandins were first discovered in seminal plasma of mammalian semen and were believed to originate from the prostate gland. Thus, these compounds were named prostaglandins. The seminal vesicles are now known to produce more prostaglandin than the prostate, at least in the ram. Prostaglandins are among the most ubiquitous and physiologically active substances in the body. They are lipids consisting of 20-carbon unsaturated hydroxy fatty acids that are derived from arachidonic acid. There are at least six biochemical pros-

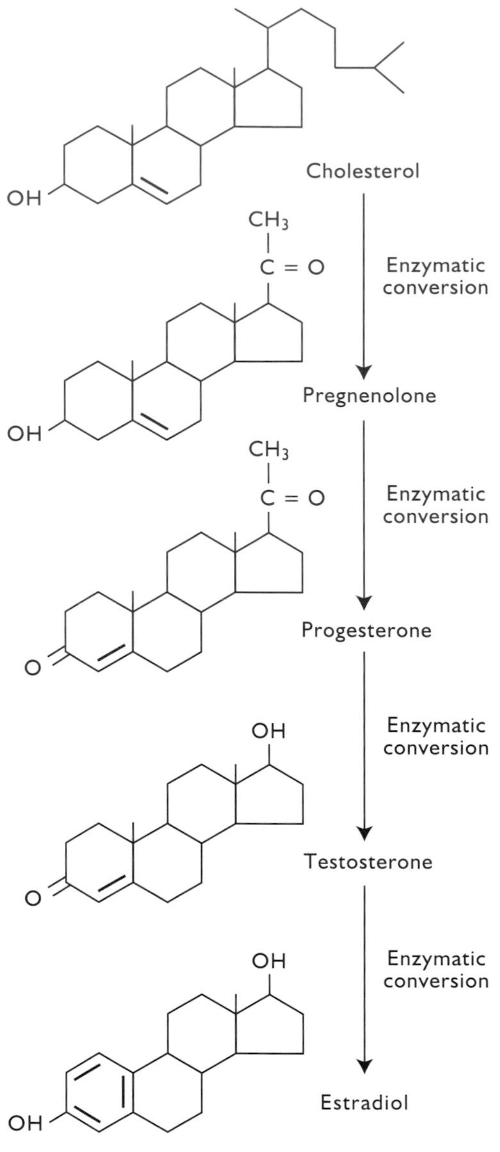
OH
Cholesterol
CH3
C = O
Enzymatic conversion
OH
Pregnenolone
CH3
C = O
Enzymatic conversion
O
Progesterone
OH
Enzymatic conversion
O
Testosterone
OH
Enzymatic conversion
OH
Estradiol

Figure 5-9. Condensed version of reproductive steroid synthetic pathway.

taglandins and numerous metabolites with an extremely wide range of physiologic activity. For example, prostaglandin E_2 (PGE_2) lowers blood pressure, while prostaglandin $F_{2\alpha}$ ($PGF_{2\alpha}$) increases blood pressure. Prostaglandins also stimulate uterine smooth muscle, influence lipid metabolism and mediate inflammation. As far as the reproductive system is concerned, the two most important prostaglandins are $PGF_{2\alpha}$ and PGE_2 (Figure 5-10). Ovulation is controlled, at least in part, by $PGF_{2\alpha}$ and PGE_2.

The discovery that $PGF_{2\alpha}$ caused luteolysis (destruction of the corpus luteum) in the female opened a new world of application for the control of the estrous cycle. Use of prostaglandins as a tool for reproductive management is now routine. Prostaglandins are rapidly degraded in the blood. In fact, almost all of $PGF_{2\alpha}$ is removed from the blood during one pass through the pulmonary circulation. Thus, $PGF_{2\alpha}$ has an extremely short half-life (seconds).

Hormone action requires the presence of specific receptors on target cells.

Endocrine glands are composed of many cells which synthesize and secrete specific hormone molecules. These hormone molecules enter the blood and are transported to every cell in the body. In spite of the fact that every cell in the body is exposed to the hormone, only certain cells are capable of responding to the hormone. Tissues containing these cells are called **target tissues**.

Prostaglandin $F_{2\alpha}$ ($PGF_{2\alpha}$)

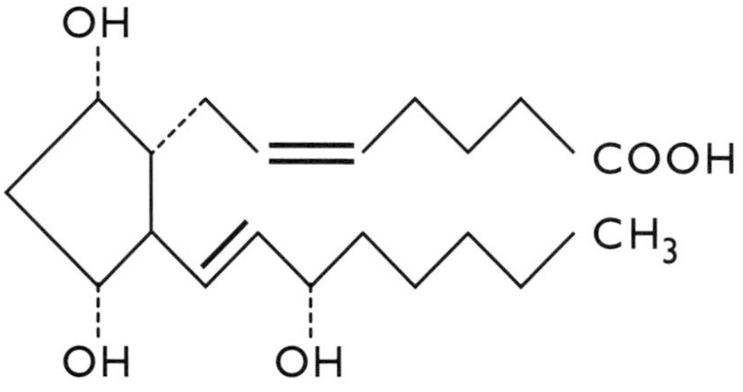
OH
COOH
CH3
OH
OH

Prostaglandin E_2 (PGE_2)

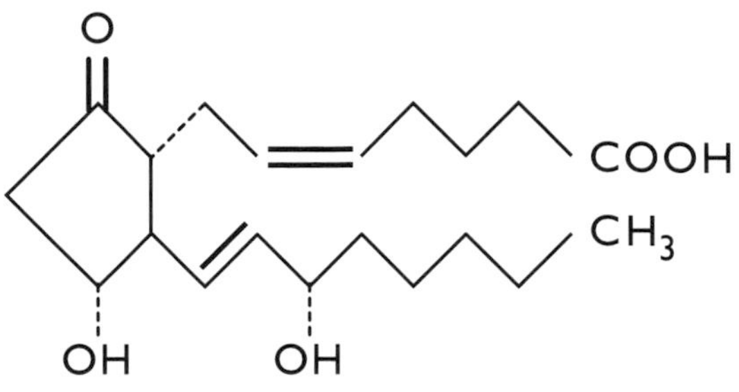
O
COOH
CH3
OH
OH

Figure 5-10. Structure of $PGF_{2\alpha}$ and PGE_2. The dashed lines represent bonds which extend into the plane of the page.

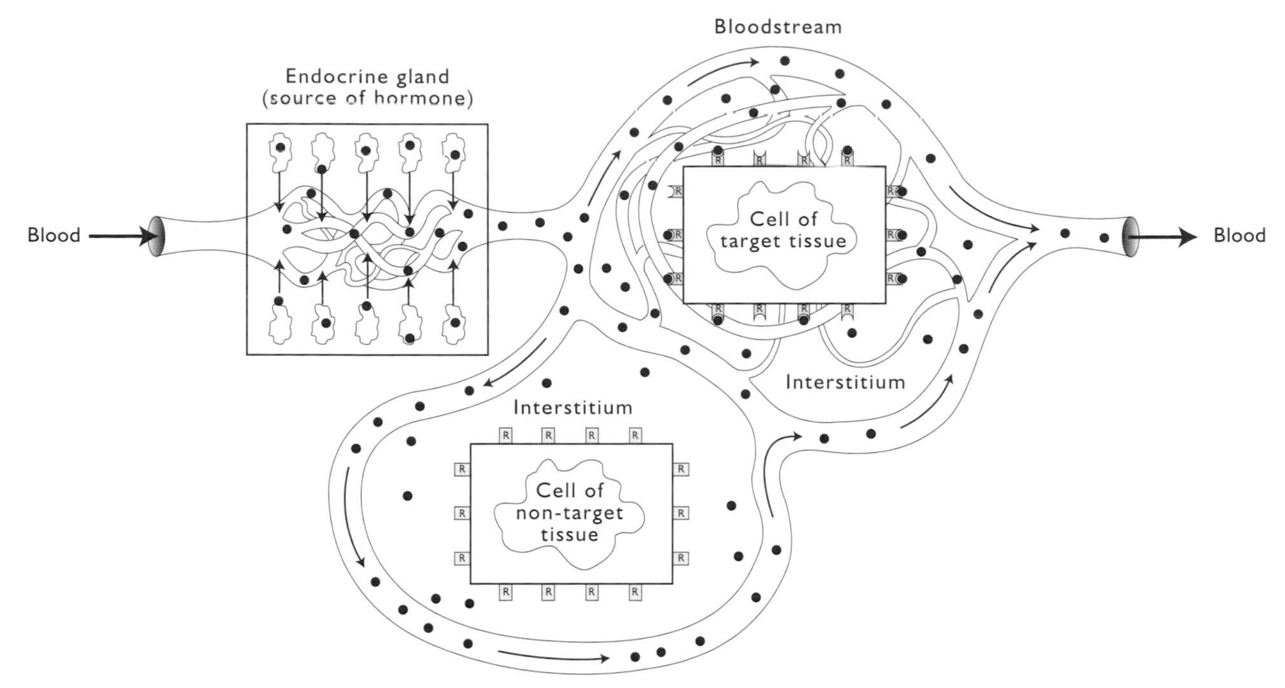

Figure 5-11. Schematic representation of target versus non-target tissues. Hormones (black spheres) are produced by the endocrine gland and are released into the blood. The blood delivers the hormone to the target tissues. Target tissues contain receptors (R) which specifically bind the hormone. Nontarget tissues also have receptors (R) but for other hormones. The specific hormone shown here will not bind to these receptors. Therefore, the non-target tissue will not respond. (Graphic by Sonja Oei.)

For example, if a hormone's responsibility is to cause the cervix to synthesize mucus, other organs such as the liver, the kidney or the pancreas will not produce mucus.

Target tissues are distinguished from other tissues because their cells contain specific molecules which bind a specific hormone. These specific molecules located in the cells of target tissues are known as **hormone receptors** (Figure 5-11). Receptors have a specific affinity or degree of attraction for a specific hormone and thus bind it. Once the receptor of the cells making up the target tissue has bound the hormone, the target tissue begins to perform a new function. Often, the target tissue produces another hormone which acts upon another tissue elsewhere in the body.

> ***Protein hormones utilize plasma membrane bound receptors. Steroid hormones diffuse into the cell and attach to a specific nuclear receptor.***

Receptors for protein hormones are an integral part of the plasma membrane of the target cell. They contain three distinct regions. These regions are re-

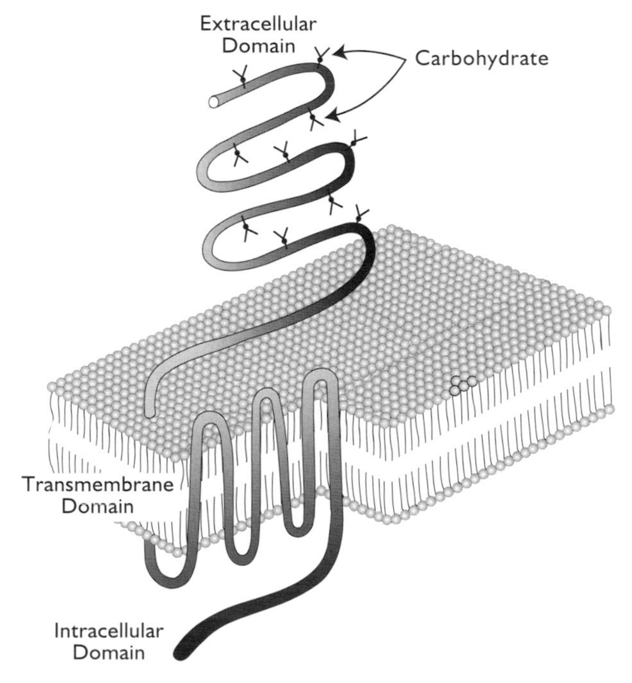

Figure 5-12. Schematic illustration of the LH receptor showing the extracellular, transmembrane and intracellular domains.(Graphic by Sonja Oei.)

Table 5-2. Summary of Reproductive Hormones

Name of Hormone (Abbrev.)	Biochemical Classification	Source	Male Target Tissue
Gonadotropin Releasing Hormone (GnRH)	Neuropeptide (decapeptide)	Hypothalamic surge and tonic centers	Anterior pituitary (gonadotroph cells)
Luteinizing Hormone (LH)	Glycoprotein	Anterior pituitary (gonadotroph cells)	Testis (interstitial cells of Leydig)
Follicle Stimulating Hormone (FSH)	Glycoprotein	Anterior pituitary (gonadotroph cells)	Testis (Sertoli cells)
Prolactin	Protein	Anterior pituitary (lactotroph cells)	Testis and brain
Oxytocin (OT)	Neuropeptide (octapeptide)	Synthesized in the hypothalamus, stored in the posterior pituitary; synthesized by corpus luteum.	Smooth muscle of epididymal tail, ductus deferens and ampulla
Estradiol (E_2)	Steroid	Granulosal cells of follicle, placenta, Sertoli cells of testis	Brain
Progesterone (P_4)	Steroid	Corpus luteum and placenta	
Testosterone (T)	Steroid	Interstitial cells of Leydig, cells of theca interna in female	Accessory sex glands, tunica dartos of scrotum, seminiferous epithelium, skeletal muscle
Inhibin	Glycoprotein	Granulosal cells (female) Sertoli cells (male)	Gonadotrophs of anterior pituitary
Prostaglandin $F_{2\alpha}$($PGF_{2\alpha}$)	Prostaglandin (C-20 fatty acid)	Uterine endometrium, vesicular glands	Epididymis
Prostaglandin E_2 (PGE_2)	Prostaglandin (C-20 fatty acid)	Ovary, uterus, embryonic membranes	
Human chorionic gonadotropin (hCG)	Glycoprotein	Trophoblast of blastocyst (chorion)	
Equine chorionic gonadotropin (eCG)	Glycoprotein	Chorionic girdle cells	
Placental lactogen	Protein	Placenta	

Table 5-2. Summary of Reproductive Hormones

Female Target Tissue	Male Primary Action	Female Primary Action
Anterior pituitary (gonadotroph cells)	Release of FSH and LH from anterior pituitary	Release of FSH and LH from anterior pituitary
Ovary (cells of theca interna and luteal cells)	Stimulates testosterone production	Stimulates ovulation, formation of corpora lutea and progesterone secretion
Ovary (granulosal cells)	Sertoli cell function	Follicular development and estradiol synthesis
Mammary cells, corpus luteum in some species (rat and mouse)	Can induce maternal behavior in females and males	Lactation, maternal behavior and corpora lutea function (some species)
Myometrium and endometrium of uterus, myoepithelial cells of mammary gland	$PGF_{2\alpha}$ synthesis and pre-ejaculatory movement of spermatozoa	Uterine motility, promotes uterine $PGF_{2\alpha}$ synthesis, milk ejection
Hypothalamus, entire reproductive tract and mammary gland	Sexual behavior	Sexual behavior, GnRH, elevated secretory activity of the entire tract, enhanced uterine motility
Uterine endometrium, mammary gland, myometrium, hypothalamus		Endometrial secretion, inhibits GnRH release, inhibits reproductive behavior, promotes maintenance of pregnancy
Brain, skeletal muscle, granulosal cells	Anabolic growth, promotes spermatogenesis, promotes secretion of accessory sex glands	Substrate for E_2 synthesis, abnormal masculinization (hair patterns, voice, behavior, etc.)
Gonadotrophs of anterior pituitary	Inhibits FSH secretion	Inhibits FSH secretion
Corpus luteum, uterine myometrium, ovulatory follicles	Affects metabolic activity of spermatozoa, causes epididymal contractions	Luteolysis, promotes uterine tone and contraction, ovulation
Early corpus luteum, oviduct (mare)		Ovulation, assists in maternal recognition of pregnancy (mare)
Ovary	Increase growth of fetal testis	Facilitate production of progesterone by ovary
Ovary		Causes formation of accessory corpora lutea
Mammary gland of dam		Mammary stimulation of dam

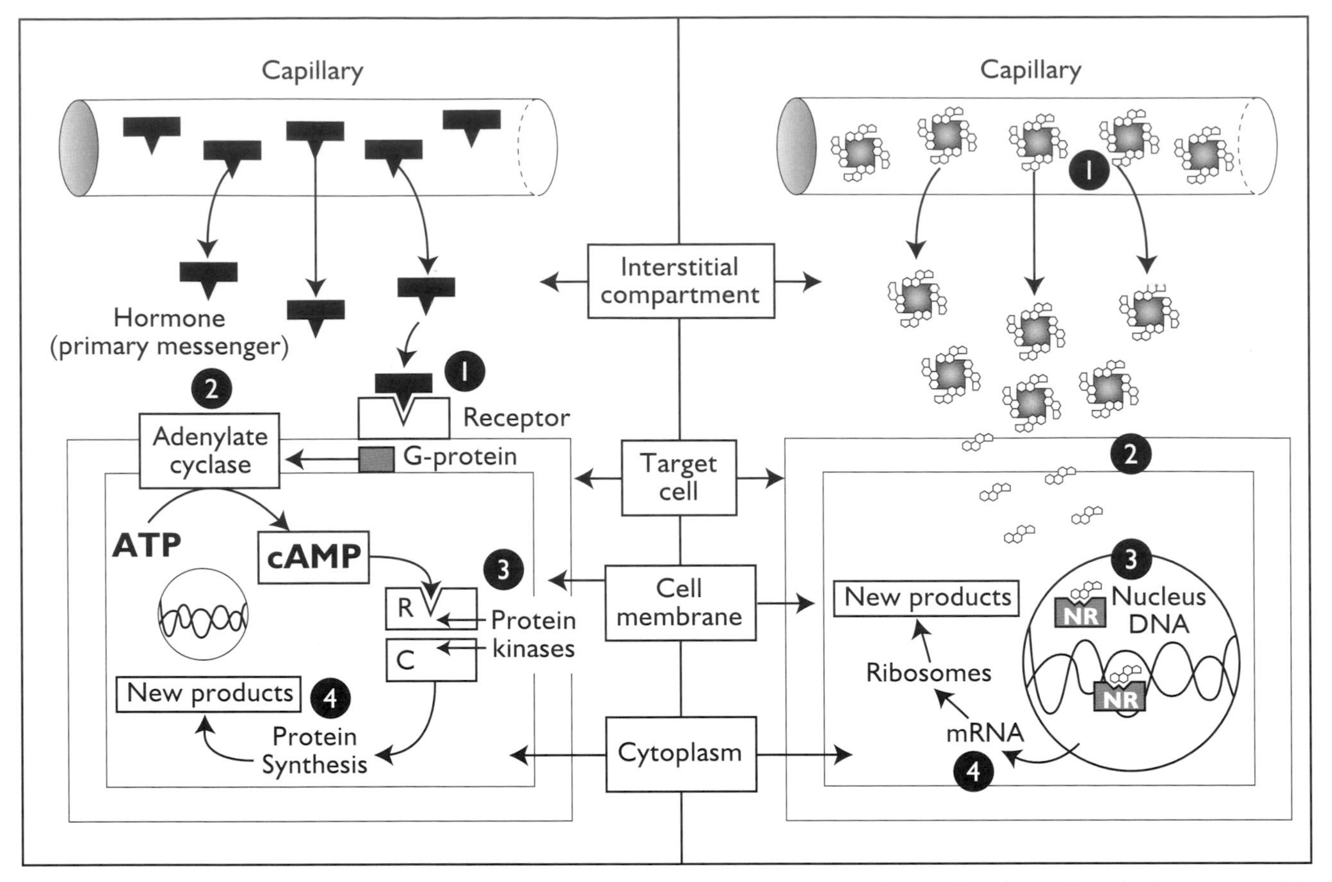

Figure 5-13. Schematic illustrations of protein and steroid hormone mechanisms of action. Protein hormones ultimately activate protein kinases via cAMP. Cyclic AMP activates the regulatory subunit (R) which, in turn, activates the catalytic subunit (C) of the enzyme resulting in activation of other enzymes by phosphorylation. This allows the construction of new products for reproduction. Steroids diffuse through the plasma membrane, cytoplasm and nuclear membrane of the target cell. They bind to nuclear receptors which (NR) trigger mRNA production and eventually protein synthesis. (Circled numbers in the figure are steps of action described in the text.) (Graphic by Sonja Oei.)

ferred to as **receptor domains**. The configuration of the LH receptor consists of an **extracellular domain**, a **transmembrane domain** and an **intracellular domain** (Figure 5-12).

The extracellular domain has a specific site which binds the specific hormone. When this site is occupied, the transmembrane domain changes its configuration and thus activates other membrane proteins known as G-proteins. The function of the intracellular domain of the receptor is not clear.

In contrast to the action of protein hormones, steroid action requires nuclear receptors. Steroid hormones are passively transported through the cell membrane of all target cells because of their lipid solubility, but they bind to specific receptors within the nucleus of only target cells.

Steps of protein hormone action are:

- ***hormone-receptor binding***
- ***adenylate cyclase activation***
- ***protein kinase activation***
- ***synthesis of new products***

Protein Hormones: Steps of Action

Step 1- <u>Hormone-Receptor Binding</u>. The hormone diffuses from the blood into the interstitial compartment and binds to a membrane receptor which is specific for the hormone. The binding occurs on the surface of the membrane of the target tissue cells (Figures 5-11 and 5-13). In general, receptors to the gonadotropins are sparsely distributed on the surface of the target cells. In fact, only 2,000 to 20,000 LH or FSH receptors are present per follicle cell. Hormone-receptor binding is believed to be brought about by a specific geometric configuration of the receptor which "fits" the geometric configuration of the hormone. The hormone receptor binding is much like fitting two adjacent pieces of a puzzle together. The affinity of the hormone-receptor binding varies among hormones.

Step 2-<u>Adenylate Cyclase Activation</u>. The hormone-receptor complex activates a membrane bound enzyme known as **adenylate cyclase**. Adenylate cyclase activity is mediated by a membrane bound protein called a **G-protein.** When the hormone receptor complex is formed, the G-protein is transformed in a way that activates adenylate cyclase (Figure 5-13). The activation of this enzyme causes the conversion of **ATP** to **cyclic AMP** (cAMP) within the cytoplasm of the cell. This cyclic AMP has been termed the "**second messenger**" in the pathway because cAMP must be present before further "downstream" events can occur. The primary messenger is the hormone itself.

Step 3-<u>Protein Kinase Activation</u>. Cyclic AMP causes the activation of a family of control enzymes located in the cytoplasm called **protein kinases**. These protein kinases are responsible for activating enzymes in the cytoplasm which convert substrates into products. Protein kinases consist of a regulatory and a catalytic subunit. The regulatory subunit binds cAMP, and this binding causes activation of the catalytic subunit which initiates the conversion of existing substrates to new products.

Step 4-<u>Synthesis of New Products</u>. The products made by the cell are generally secreted and these secretory products have specific functions towards enhancing reproductive processes. For example, the gonadotropins (FSH and LH) bind to follicle cells in the ovary which results in the synthesis of a new product, estradiol. When steroids are synthesized, they are not actively secreted, but simply diffuse through the plasma membrane into the interstitial spaces and into the blood.

Steps of steroid hormone action are:
- ***steroid transport***
- ***movement through the cell membrane and cytoplasm***
- ***binding of steroid to nuclear receptor***
- ***mRNA synthesis and protein synthesis***

Steroid Hormones: Steps of Action

Step 1-<u>Steroid Transport</u>. Steroid hormones are transported in the blood by a complex system. Steroids are not water soluble and therefore cannot be transported as free molecules. Therefore, they must attach to molecules that are water soluble. Steroids bind to a variety of plasma proteins in a nonspecific manner. Some steroids have specific carrier proteins. These transport proteins carry steroids in the blood and interstitial fluid to the cell membranes of all cells.

Step 2-<u>Movement through the Cell Membrane and Cytoplasm</u>. When the steroid-carrier protein complex travels into the interstitial compartment and comes in contact with target cells, the steroids disassociate from the carrier protein and diffuse through the plasma membrane because of their lipid solubility (Figure 5-13). After the steroid molecule enters the cell, it diffuses through the cytoplasm and into the nucleus.

Step 3-<u>Binding of Steroid to Nuclear Receptor</u>. If the cell is a target cell, the steroid binds to a specific nuclear receptor. The steroid-receptor binding

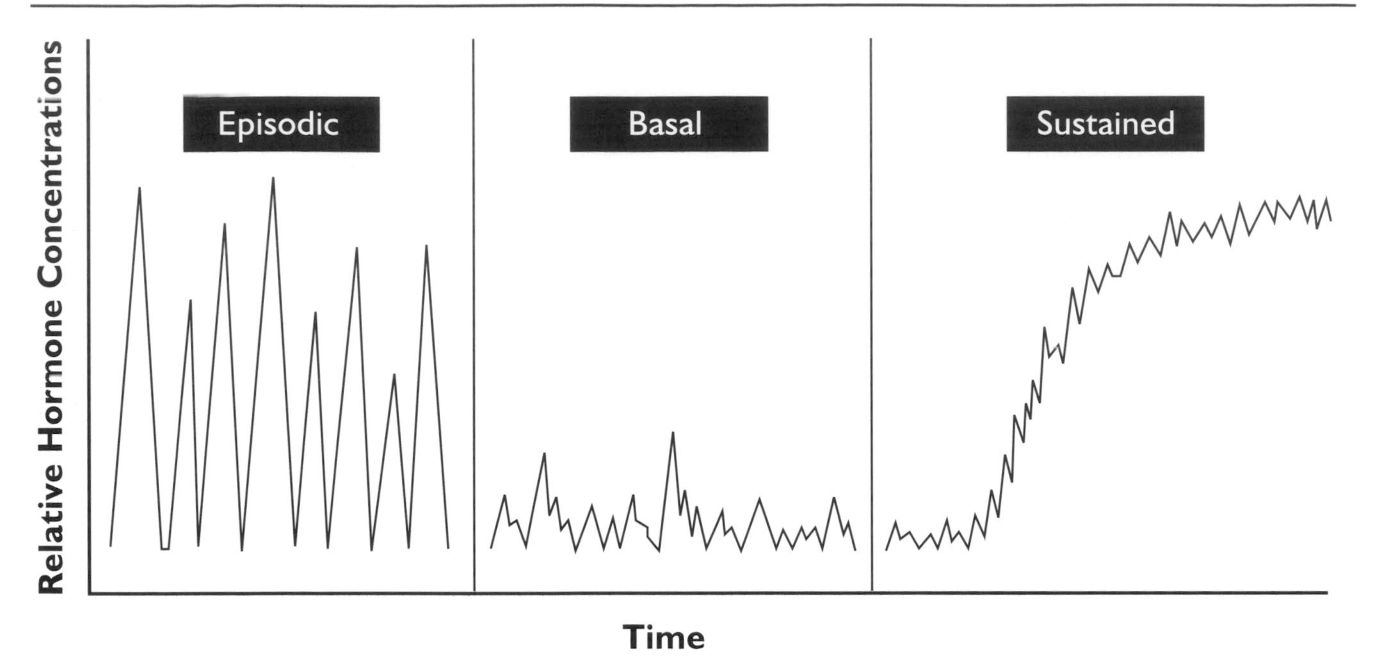

Figure 5-14. Typical patterns of hormonal secretion by the reproductive system. The patterns illustrated may occur independently or in combination.

is similar to protein-receptor binding in that the steroid must "fit" the receptor. The steroid-receptor complex initiates DNA-directed messenger RNA synthesis (transcription).

Step 4-<u>mRNA Synthesis and Protein Synthesis</u>. The newly synthesized mRNA leaves the nucleus and attaches to ribosomes where it directs the synthesis of specific proteins which will enhance the reproductive process. A few examples of steroid-directed synthesis are: 1) mucus from the cervix during estrus; 2) "uterine milk" from the uterine glands; and 3) seminal plasma components from the accessory sex glands in the male.

> ***"Strength" of hormone action depends on:***
> - ***pattern and duration of secretion***
> - ***half-life***
> - ***receptor density***
> - ***receptor-hormone affinity***

The physiologic activity of a hormone depends on several factors including pattern and duration of hormone secretion, half-life of the hormone, receptor density and receptor-hormone affinity. These factors determine the magnitude and the duration of action of hormones.

In general, hormones are secreted in three types of patterns (Figure 5-14). One type is episodic secretion, which generally is associated with hormones under nervous control. When nerves in the hypothalamus "fire," neuropeptides are released in a sudden burst (episode), and thus hormones from the anterior pituitary tend to be released in an episodic manner as well. A typical pattern of episodic release is shown in Figure 5-14. A second type of secretion is a basal (tonic) pattern. Here, the hormone stays low, but fluctuates with low amplitude pulses. Sustained hormone release is a third type of hormonal pattern or profile. In this type, the hormone remains elevated, but in a relatively steady, stable fashion for a long period of time (days to weeks). Steroids tend to be secreted in a more stable fashion because the glands producing the steroids are generally producing them continuously rather than as a function of neural activity (which causes a pulsatile release). High progesterone during diestrus or pregnancy is an example of a sustained pattern of hormone secretion.

In general, hormones that are controlled by nervous activity have a short duration of secretion which is the result of bursts of neural activity. Hormones not directly linked to nervous activity, such as gonadal steroids, generally have a longer, more sustained release profile.

Half-Life of a Hormone Determines How Long It Will Act

Different hormones have different durations (different life expectancies) within the systemic circulation. The rate at which the hormone is cleared from the circulation determines its half-life. The longer the half-life, the greater the potential biological activity. Some hormones have exceptionally short half-lives ($PGF_{2\alpha}$), while other hormones have quite long half-lives (eCG).

The density of target tissue receptors varies as a function of the cell type as well as the degree to which hormones promote (**up-regulate**), or inhibit (**down-regulate**) synthesis of hormone receptors. Factors such as animal condition and nutrition may play a role in influencing receptor numbers. As you will see later on, different hormones promote synthesis of receptors to either themselves or other hormones. For example, FSH promotes the synthesis of LH receptors by the follicular cells. The higher the degree to which a cell is populated with receptors, the higher the degree of potential response by the target cell.

Hormonal potency is influenced by:
- ***receptor density***
- ***hormone receptor affinity***

Receptors vary with regard to their affinity for various hormones. In general, the greater the affinity of the hormone for the receptor, the greater the biologic response.

Hormone **agonists** are **analogs** (having a similar molecular structure) which bind to the specific receptor and initially cause the same biologic effect as the native hormone. Some agonists promote greater physiological activity because they have greater affinity for the hormone receptor. Other analogs, called **antagonists**, have greater affinity for the hormone receptor, but promote weaker biologic activity than the native hormone. Antagonists decrease the response of target cells by having a weaker biological activity than the native hormone or by occupying hormone receptors and thus preventing the native hormone from binding. In either case, the antagonist interferes with native hormone action.

Pheromones are Another Class of Substances Which Cause Remote Effects

In addition to molecules that are transported by blood, an additional class of materials exists which directly influences reproductive processes. These materials are called **pheromones**. Pheromones are substances secreted to the outside of the body. They are generally volatile and are detected by the olfactory system (and perhaps the vomeronasal organ) by members of the same species. Pheromones cause specific behavioral or physiologic responses by the percipient. Pheromones are known to influence the onset of puberty, the identification of females in estrus by the males and other behavioral traits. More details regarding the impact of pheromones will be presented in Chapters 6 and 11.

<u>Further Phenomena for Fertility</u>

The word pituitary is derived from the Latin word "pituita" which means mucus. The existence of the pituitary gland was recognized as early as 200 AD. It was thought to be a mucus-secreting organ for lubrication of the throat. Mucus from the pituitary was thought to be transported into the nose and then into the nasopharynx where it could lubricate the throat.

The dramatic effects of male castration have been recognized for over 2,000 years. The testis was known to control virility and sterility. Castration was always (and still is) regarded as a catastrophic event. However, castration in humans was deemed useful under certain sets of conditions such as generating guardians for harems.

The scientific discipline of endocrinology originated from a belief in "organ magic." Consumption of human or animal organs was thought to increase powers or cure ailments. For example, warriors thought that eating the hearts of their enemy increased their courage. Eating the thyroids of sheep was thought to improve the intelligence of the mentally retarded; liver from wolves cured liver ailments; brain from rabbits cured nervousness and fox lungs cured respiratory disorders. Throughout recorded history sex gland consumption was believed to increase sexual prowess. As early as 1400 BC, Hindus prescribed testicular tissue for male impotence. The "birthday" of modern endocrinology was stimulated by the famous report of Brown-Séquard who injected himself with testicular extracts. The aging Brown-Séquard reported in 1889 that these extracts reversed the effects of age, made him feel significantly more vigorous and corrected his failing memory. His report, even though erroneous, prompted a rush of "gland treatments" by the medical profession of the day. Brown-Séquard's error stimulated careful scrutiny by scientists and physicians. This scientific scrutiny led to the development of modern endocrinology.

In the 19th century, French doctors reported that the eating of frog legs by French soldiers in North Africa caused two outbreaks of priapism (painful and prolonged penile erection). The attending physicians noted that the symptoms amongst the soldiers resembled those seen in men who had overindulged in a drug called cantharidin (popularly known as "Spanish Fly"). This material is extracted from a beetle for its purported value as an aphrodisiac. One of the attending French physicians dissected a local frog and discovered that its gut was full of beetles which produced cantharidin. Recently, researchers have shown that frogs eating this beetle have levels of cantharidin in their thigh muscles that are sufficiently high enough to cause human priapism.

Additional Reading

Bear, M.F., B.W. Connors and M.A. Paradiso. 1996. *Neuroscience: Exploring the Brain.* Williams & Wilkins, Baltimore.

Cupps, P.T., ed. 1991. *Reproduction in Domestic Animals*, 4th Edition. Academic Press, New York.

Thibault, C., M.C. Levasseur and R.H.F. Hunter, eds. 1993. *Reproduction in Mammals and Man.* Ellipses, Paris.

6 The Onset of Puberty

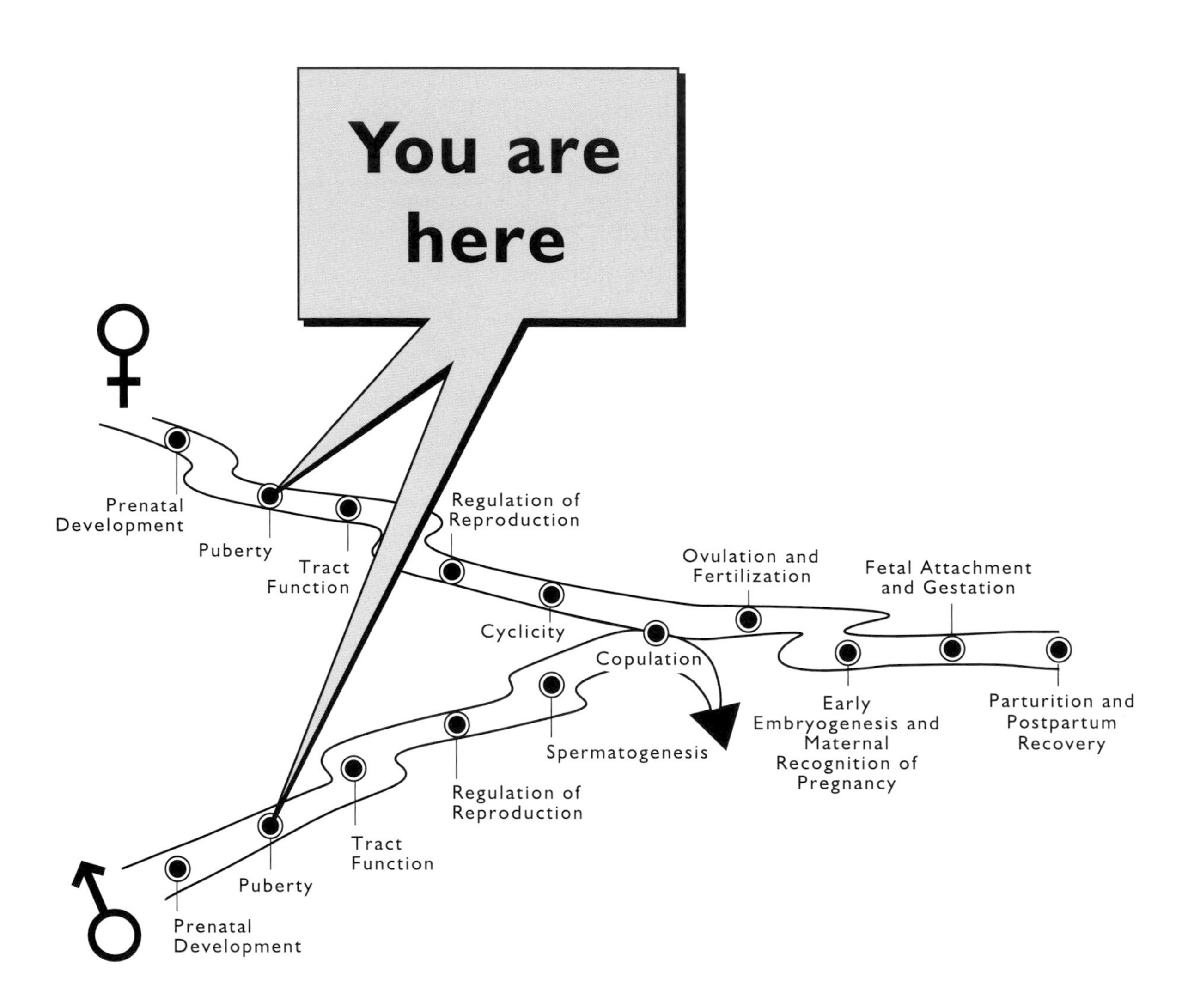

Take Home Message

Puberty is the process of acquiring reproductive competence. The onset of puberty depends upon the ability of specific hypothalamic neurons to produce GnRH in sufficient quantities to promote and support gametogenesis. In the female, hypothalamic GnRH neurons must develop the ability to respond to estradiol positive feedback before they can produce sufficient quantities of GnRH to cause ovulation. Development of hypothalamic GnRH neurons is influenced by: 1) development of threshold body size; 2) exposure to a variety of environmental and social cues; and 3) the genetics of the animal. Puberty in the male appears to be less dependent on body size and social factors than in the female.

Puberty can be defined generally in both the male and female as the ability to accomplish reproduction successfully. Puberty should be considered as a process, not a single event. The word puberty originated from the Latin word *pubscere*, which means "to be covered with hair." This definition applies to the development of hair in the pubic area, armpits and legs in women and men. Also, the development of the beard in men is an indicator of pubescence. While the original definition of the word puberty was fashioned after observable traits in humans, it obviously does not apply to other animals. The obligatory physiologic requirement for pubertal onset in mammals is the development of specific hypothalamic neurons so that there is release (from the neurons) of adequate quantities of gonadotropin releasing hormone (GnRH) at appropriate frequencies. Thus, GnRH can stimulate release of gonadotropic hormones which promote gametogenesis, steroidogenesis and development of reproductive tissues. Development of these specific hypothalamic GnRH neurons is influenced by 1) acquisition of threshold body size, 2) exposure to certain environmental or social cues and 3) the genetics of the animal.

The Onset of Puberty Has Many Definitions in Females

Several criteria can be used to define puberty in the female. Some examples are presented below.

Age at first estrus (heat). This is the age at which the female displays her first estrus. The age at first estrus is relatively easy to determine because females display outward behavioral signs of sexual receptivity, especially in the presence of the male. The first estrus generally is not accompanied by ovulation. Thus, the age at first estrus may not reflect acquisition of full reproductive capability.

Age at first ovulation. This is the age at which the first ovulation occurs. To determine critically when ovulation occurs, manual or visual validation is required. This can be accomplished using palpation of the ovary per rectum in animals which are large enough to permit insertion of the hand and arm into the rectum (cow and mare). Also, ultrasonographic imaging can be used to determine ovarian status. When ovulation has occurred, a soft depression on the surface of the ovary can be palpated. In smaller animals (sow and ewe) surgical procedures allowing the ovary to be visualized enable direct determination of ovulation. In addition, laparoscopic diagnosis can be used to determine when ovulation occurs. All of the above techniques require frequent observations of the ovary to determine precisely when ovulation occurred. Thus, although age at ovulation is a good criterion for puberty, it is difficult to determine.

Age at which a female can support pregnancy without deleterious effects. This definition is most applicable from a management standpoint in food producing animals. The goal for food producing species is to generate the highest possible number of offspring in the shortest time interval without compromising the well-being of the dam or the neonate. Acquisition of a threshold body size is important in controlling the onset of puberty. The energy requirements for follicular development, ovulation and ova/embryo transport are quite small. However, the "metabolic costs" of pregnancy and lactation are high. Thus, it makes biologic sense that the female cross a "metabolic threshold" before puberty occurs.

The Onset of Puberty Has Many Definitions in Males

As in the female, the onset of puberty in the male can be defined in several ways.

Age when behavioral traits are expressed. Generally, males of most species acquire reproductive behavioral traits (mounting and erection) before they acquire the ability to ejaculate and produce spermatozoa. These behavioral traits are relatively easy to determine since mounting behavior and erection of the penis can be observed readily.

Age at first ejaculation. The process of ejaculation is quite complex and requires closely coordinated development of nerves, specific muscles and expulsion of seminal fluids from the accessory sex glands. When development of all these components occurs, ejaculation can take place. Generally, the ability to ejaculate substantially precedes the ability to produce sufficient spermatozoa to achieve pregnancy.

Age when spermatozoa first appear in the ejaculate. The male acquires the ability to produce seminal fluid and to ejaculate before spermatozoa are available in the tail of the epididymis. To determine precisely when the first spermatozoa are available, one must collect ejaculates at least once per week. This is relatively easy to do, since ejaculates can be collected by artificial means from the boar, bull, ram or stallion. After behavioral characteristics have developed and the male is willing to mount a receptive female (or surrogate female), frequent seminal collections can be made. This enables determination of the age at which spermatozoa appear in the ejaculate.

Age when spermatozoa first appear in the urine. As you have read in Chapter 3, most of the spermatozoa produced by the testes are lost in the urine during periods of sexual rest (sexual abstinence). The presence of spermatozoa in the urine clearly indicates that spermatogenesis is occurring. Frequent collection of urine is difficult in large animals and requires special equipment.

Age when the ejaculate contains a threshold number of spermatozoa. Even though an ejaculate may contain spermatozoa, there may be insufficient numbers to accomplish optimum fertilization. Therefore, the presence of a threshold (minimum number) of spermatozoa is required. These thresholds vary among species. In general, they reflect minimum seminal characteristics required to achieve pregnancy following copulation. From a practical viewpoint, this is the most valid criterion for puberty since it defines the ability of the male to provide enough spermatozoa for successful fertilization.

The age at which puberty is acquired varies among and within species. This variation is summarized in Table 6-1. The factors contributing to the variation in pubertal onset constitute the discussion in the remainder of this chapter.

Table 6-1. Average ages (Range) of Puberty in the Male and Female of Various Species

Species	Male	Female
Bovine	11 mo (7-18)	11 mo (9-24)
Ovine	7 mo (6-9)	7 mo (4-14)*
Porcine	7 mo (5-8)	6 mo (5-7)
Equine	14 mo (10-24)	18 mo (12-19)

*Because of seasonal effects in the ewe, the range is quite large. (See Figure 6-8).

Release of GnRH in High Frequency Pulses From Specific Hypothalamic Neurons Is Required for the Onset of Puberty

In order for the male and the female to experience puberty, the hypothalamic GnRH neurons must be capable of releasing high frequency and high amplitude pulses of GnRH. Before puberty, neurons in the hypothalamus cannot release GnRH in a pattern of high pulse frequency or high amplitude. Therefore, in the prepubertal animal, gonadotropin (FSH and LH) secretion is minimal and neither folliculogenesis nor spermatogenesis can occur.

Genetics (breed) influence age at puberty.

The breed of the animal has an important influence on the age at which puberty is attained in both the male and the female. For example, dairy heifers reach puberty at around 7 to 9 months of age, while British beef breeds reach puberty between 12 and 13 months. *Bos indicus* breeds may not reach puberty until 24 months of age. Table 6-2 summarizes the influence of breed upon age of puberty in cattle, swine and sheep.

Table 6-2. Influence of Breed on Age at Puberty in Various Classes of Food Producing Animals.

Species	Average Age at Puberty (Months)	
	Female	Male
Cattle		
Holstein	8.5	9.0
Brown Swiss	11.6	8.8
Angus	12.4	9.8
Hereford	13.0	10.8
Brahman	19.0	17.0
Swine		
Meishan	3.1	3.0
Large White	6.3	5.8
Yorkshire	7.0	6.5
Sheep		
Rambouillet	9.2	
Finnish Landrace	8.6	

In addition to genetic factors, at least two additional factors impact the development of the hypothalamic GnRH neurons in the female. They are 1) development of a threshold body size and/or composition and 2) exposure to certain environmental or social cues.

The female must reach a threshold body size before puberty can be achieved.

In virtually all female mammals, a certain body size is required before the onset of puberty can be initiated. A current hypothesis contends that the female must develop a certain degree of "fatness" before reproductive cycles can be initiated. The relationship between metabolic status and development of GnRH neurons has not been completely described, but there is good evidence that metabolic signals effect the development of the hypothalamic neurons and thus their production of GnRH.

Certain external or social factors influence the onset of puberty in the female.

There are a number of external factors which modulate the onset of puberty and these vary significantly among species. These factors include 1) season during which the animal is born (sheep), 2) the photoperiod which the animal is experiencing during the onset of puberty (sheep), 3) the presence or absence of the opposite sex during the peripubertal period (swine and cattle) and 4) the density of the groups (within the same sex) in which the animals are housed (swine).

How Do the Hypothalamic GnRH Neurons Acquire the Ability to Release GnRH in High Frequency Pulses?

It has been well established that the onset of puberty is not limited by the potential performance of the gonads or the anterior pituitary. For example, the anterior pituitary of the prepubertal animal will produce FSH and LH if stimulated by exogenous GnRH. Also, the ovaries of prepubertal females will respond by producing follicles and estradiol when stimulated with FSH and LH. Therefore, the onset of puberty is not limited by the gonadotropin producing ability of the anterior pituitary or the ability of the ovary to respond to gonadotropins. The failure of the hypothalamus to produce sufficient quantities of GnRH to cause gonadotropin release is known to be the major factor limiting pubertal onset.

The developing hypothalamus can be compared to a rheostatically controlled switch for a lighting system. As the rheostatically controlled switch is gradually turned up, the lights in the room gradually become brighter and brighter until they reach full intensity. Likewise, the development of the hypothalamus occurs in a gradual fashion during growth of the animal, rather than suddenly, like an on-off switch. The factors that cause the rheostatically controlled switch (hypothalamus) to turn-up will be described in subsequent sections of this chapter.

As you have read previously (Chapter 5), the hypothalamus contains a **tonic GnRH center** and a **preovulatory GnRH center (surge center)**. Before ovulation can occur, full neural activity of the surge center must be achieved (Figure 6-1). Such an activity results in sudden bursts of GnRH known as the **preo-**

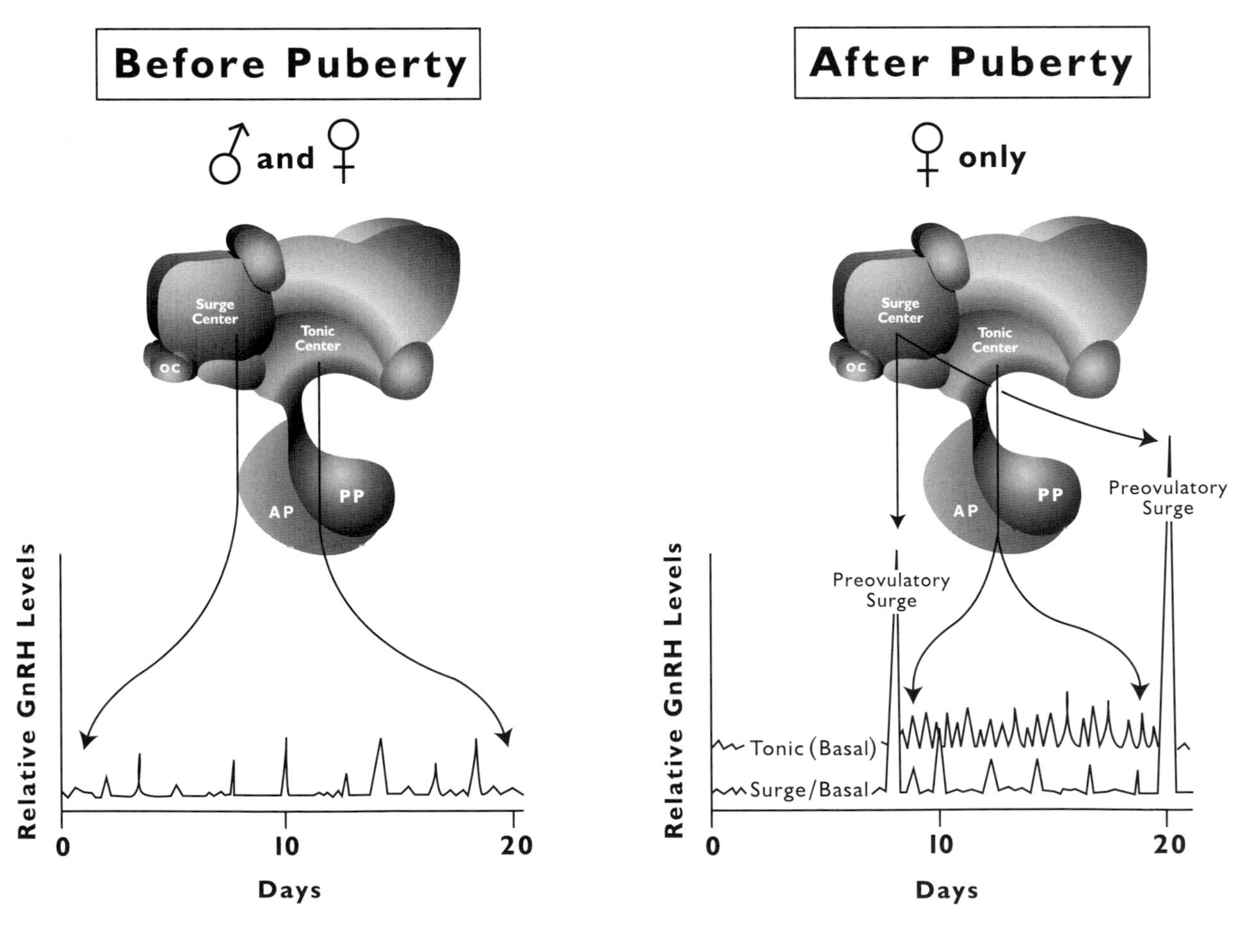

Figure 6-1. Before puberty in the female and male, GnRH neurons in both the tonic and surge center of the hypothalamus release low amplitude and low frequency pulses of GnRH (left panel). After puberty in the female, the tonic center controls basal levels of GnRH but they are higher than in the prepubertal female. The surge center controls basal levels and the preovulatory surge of GnRH. The male does not develop a surge center. (Graphic by Sonja Oei.)

vulatory GnRH surge. In other words, the GnRH neurons must fire frequently and release large quantities of GnRH to cause the preovulatory LH surge (Figure 6-2). Inability of the surge center to function results in ovulation failure. In addition to the need to have a functional surge center in the female, the tonic center must also reach a certain functional state. The tonic GnRH center regulates the tonic frequency of LH pulses. The frequency of GnRH pulses is thought to be controlled by a "pulse generator" in the hypothalamus. This "pulse generator" is believed to read internal signals (nutrients, metabolites and blood estradiol) and external signals such as day length and the presence of the male or female. Such recognition influences the release of GnRH and ultimately the time of puberty. Specific details of the control of the preovulatory surge during the estrous cycle are presented in Chapter 8.

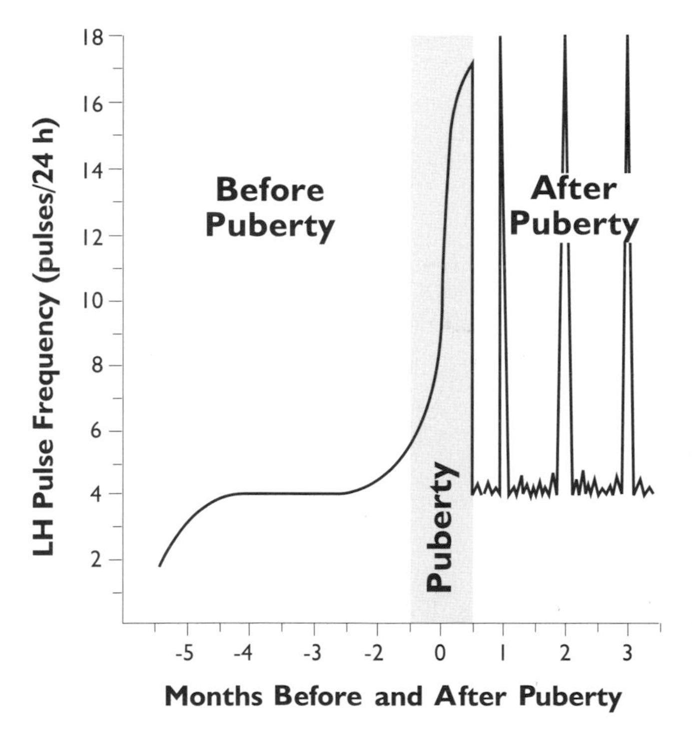

Figure 6-2. Frequency of LH pulses (as a reflection of GnRH pulses) in heifers prior to the onset of puberty. Note the substantial time required (approximately 2 months) for the pulse frequency to become high enough for puberty to be achieved. The variation in LH pulse frequency after puberty reflects the changes occurring during the estrous cycle. The LH pulse frequency during midcycle is similar to frequencies of the prepubertal female. (Modified from Kinder *et al.* 1994.)

Before puberty, females have low ovarian estradiol and low hypothalamic sensitivity to estradiol, resulting in low frequency GnRH pulses.

It appears that the prepubertal female is characterized by having 1) a lack of gonadal estradiol to stimulate the surge center and 2) a lack of sensitivity to estradiol in the surge center. The surge center is capable of functioning at a very early age when experimentally stimulated. However, under normal conditions it remains relatively dormant until puberty. For example, in the prepubertal female, the tonic GnRH center stimulates LH pulses from the anterior pituitary. The amplitude of these LH pulses can be as great as those of the postpubertal female. However, the frequency of the GnRH pulses in the prepubertal female is much lower than the frequency of GnRH pulses in the postpubertal female (Figures 6-1 and 6-2). Prior to puberty, low-frequency GnRH pulses provide an insufficient stimulus to cause the anterior pituitary to release FSH and LH. Therefore, follicular development (even though it does occur before puberty), cannot result in high circulating estradiol concentrations. Estradiol therefore remains below the minimum threshold that is necessary to trigger firing of GnRH neurons in the surge center.

As the prepubertal female matures, her hypothalamus becomes more and more sensitive to estradiol.

Figure 6-3 illustrates the influence of exogenous estradiol upon LH release as a function of age in prepubertal ewes. Remember that LH increases in direct response to the GnRH released by hypothalamic neurons. Therefore, blood LH is a direct indicator of hypothalamic GnRH release. Notice in Figure 6-3 that as the age of the ewe lamb increases, the amplitude of the LH surge increases when estradiol is administered. Clearly, the hypothalamus has the ability to exhibit some response to estradiol at a very early age (7 weeks). But, the hypothalamus doesn't reach its maximum capacity for GnRH production until about 27 weeks, the normal age of puberty in the ewe.

The hypothalamus is inherently female. Testosterone defeminizes the hypothalamus during embryogenesis and "eliminates" the GnRH surge center in the male.

During prenatal development in the male, testosterone from the fetal testis "defeminizes" the brain. In contrast, the female fetus has no testis to produce testosterone and she therefore develops a GnRH surge center in the hypothalamus. In order for testosterone to "defeminize" the hypothalamus, it must first be converted to estradiol. Since the fetal ovaries produce estradiol, a logical question is, "Why doesn't the female hypothalamus become "defeminized"? The answer to this question lies in the inability of fetal estradiol in the female to cross the blood-brain barrier and gain access to the hypothalamus. A protein called **alpha-fetoprotein** binds estradiol and prevents it from crossing the blood-brain barrier. Therefore, estradiol cannot affect the hypothalamus. Testosterone, on the other hand, crosses the blood-brain barrier, is converted to estradiol in the brain and "defeminizes" the hypothalamus, thus minimizing surge center function. Figure 6-4 summarizes the effect of alpha-fetoprotein on the hypothalamus.

The female hypothalamus contains a surge center and a tonic center. The male hypothalamus does not appear to have a surge center.

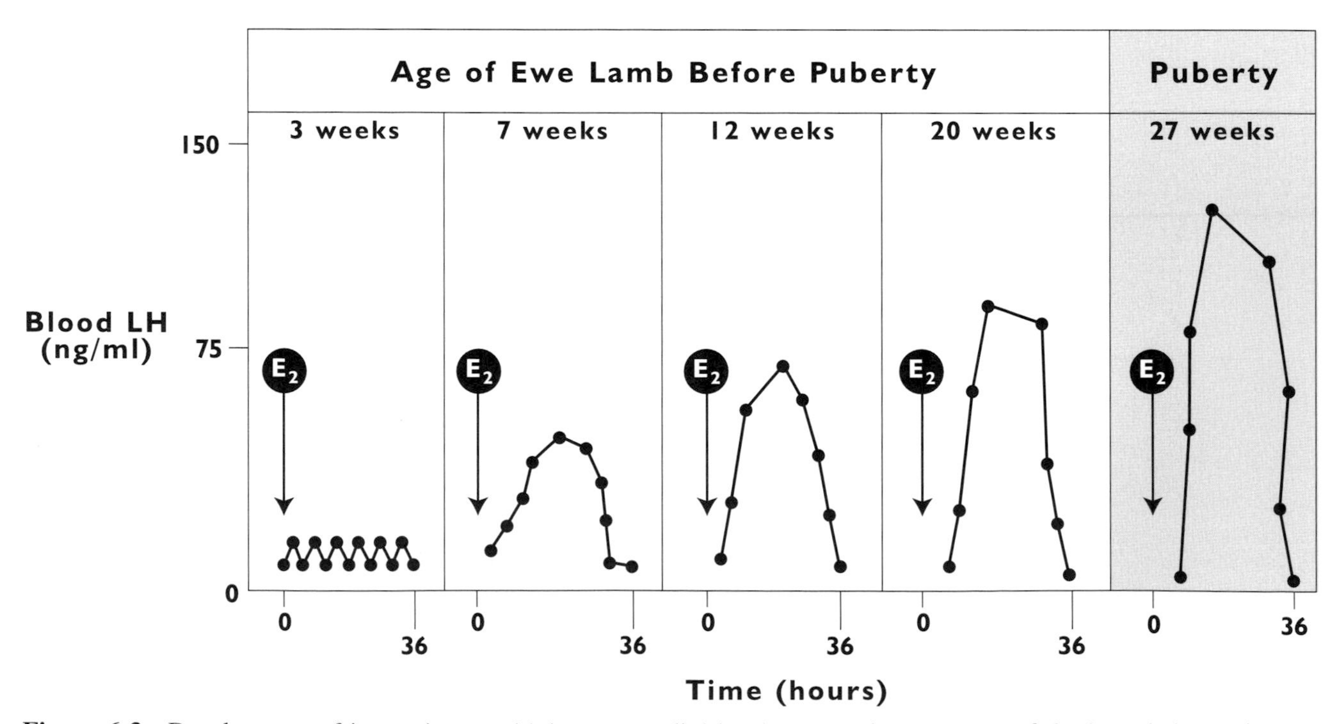

Figure 6-3. Development of increasing sensitivity to estradiol by the preovulatory center of the hypothalamus in ewe lambs. Secretion of LH is a reflection of GnRH release from the preovulatory center in the hypothalamus. Estradiol was administered for 36 hours (arrows) by subcutaneously implanting silastic capsules containing estradiol. (Modified from Foster, 1994.)

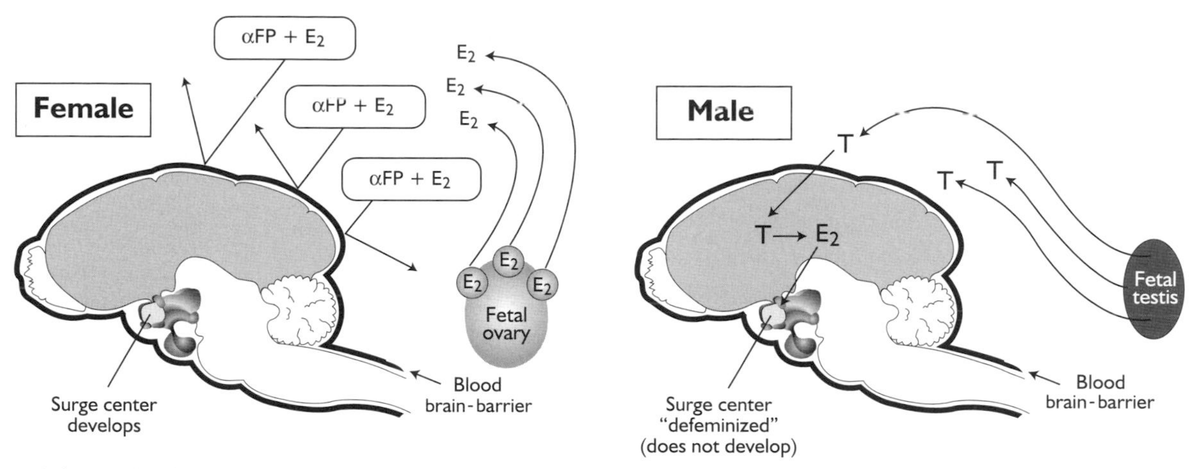

Figure 6-4. Alpha fetoprotein (αFP) combines with estradiol (E_2) from the fetal ovary. The αFP-E_2 complex cannot cross the blood brain barrier and thus E_2 cannot enter the brain to affect the hypothalamus. Testosterone (T) from the fetal testis readily enters the brain where it is converted to E_2 which defeminizes the surge center. (Graphic by Sonja Oei.)

The fundamental difference in the endocrine profiles of the postpubertal male and female is that LH does not surge in the male, but maintains a relatively consistent episodic release in a day-in day-out fashion. These episodes occur every 2 to 6 hours in the postpubertal male. This steady GnRH episodic rhythm also results in steady episodes of LH and, in turn, an episodic release of testosterone. In contrast, you can readily see in Figure 6-5 that LH and estradiol surge about every 20 days in the female. During the time between the surges, low amplitude repeated pulses are present.

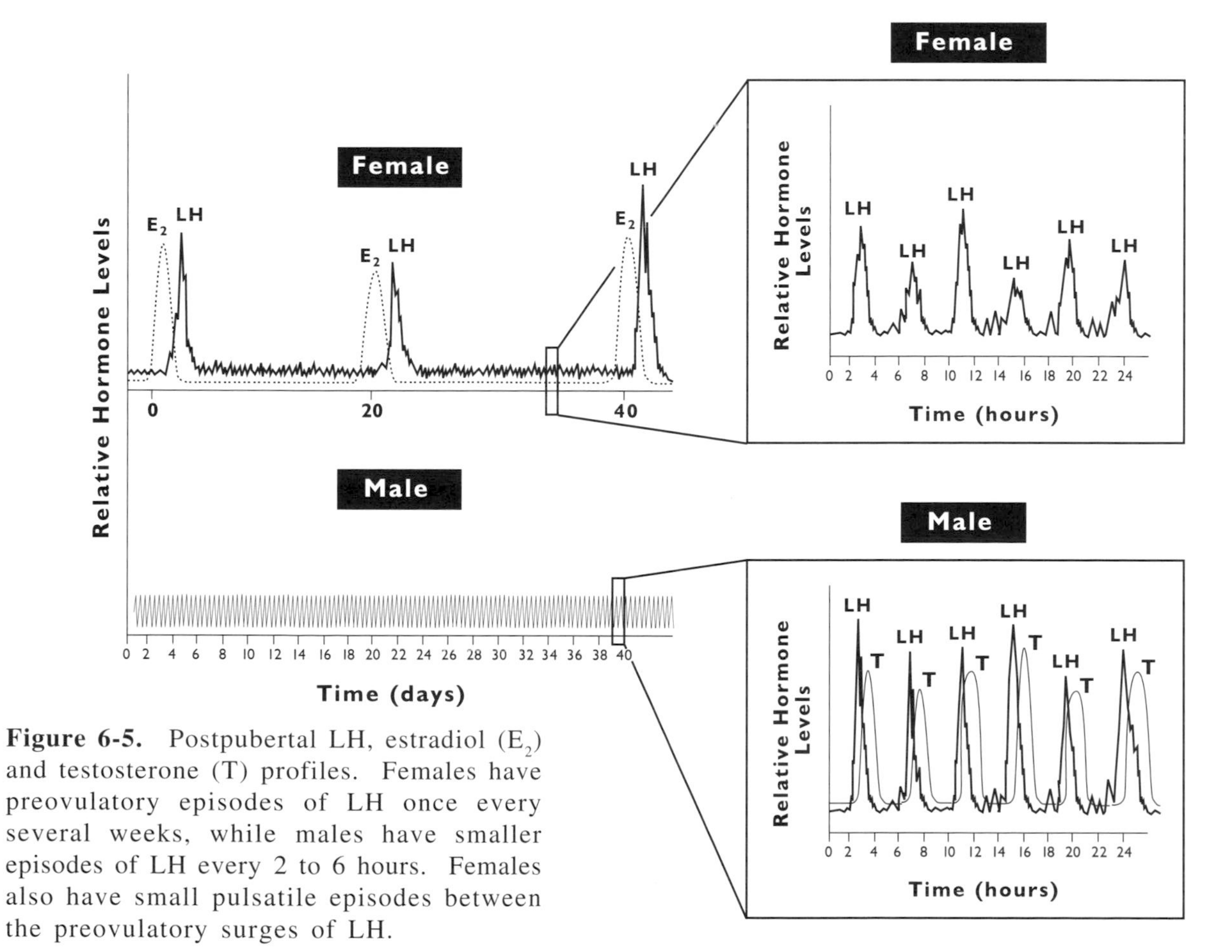

Figure 6-5. Postpubertal LH, estradiol (E_2) and testosterone (T) profiles. Females have preovulatory episodes of LH once every several weeks, while males have smaller episodes of LH every 2 to 6 hours. Females also have small pulsatile episodes between the preovulatory surges of LH.

A Certain Degree of "Fatness" Is Required for the Onset of Puberty in the Female

Nutritional intake in the newborn is directed almost exclusively towards body maintenance. The priority for the neonate is to use its energy towards maintenance of vital physiologic functions. Therefore, nonessential processes such as reproduction are of low priority. As the neonate begins to grow, energy consumption increases, body mass becomes larger and the relative surface area of the body decreases. This allows a shift in the metabolic expenditure so that nonvital physiological functions begin to develop. As this shift occurs, the overall metabolic rate decreases and more internal energy becomes available for nonvital body functions. This excess internal energy can be converted into fat stores and the young animal begins to place priority on reproduction and the onset of puberty begins. The threshold level of fat accumulation required for the onset of puberty has not been determined.

It should be emphasized that "fatness" alone does not promote the onset of puberty. Females can be extremely fat at a very young age and not be pubertal. Both age and amount of body fat are important in regulating the age of pubertal onset.

> ***GnRH neurons detect "moment-to-moment" changes in blood glucose and fatty acids.***

The central question regarding how metabolic status triggers puberty is, "what metabolic factors effect GnRH neurons and how are these factors recognized?" There is evidence to indicate that initiation of high frequency GnRH pulses is under the influence of glucose and free fatty acid levels in the blood. For example, when female hamsters were treated concurrently with inhibitors of fatty acid (methylpalmoxorate) and glucose oxidation (2-deoxyglucose, 2DG) their estrous cycles were disrupted. The rationale for using inhibitors of glucose and fatty acid oxidation was that these inhibitors reduce available internal energy. Thus, effects on reproduction could be studied while normal energy balance was maintained versus when it was disrupted. When these metabolic inhibitors were injected into ovariectomized prepubertal ewes, pulsatile LH secretion was suppressed almost immediately (Figure 6-6). The rationale for using ovariectomized ewe lambs was to remove all possible effects of ovarian steroids on the hypothala-

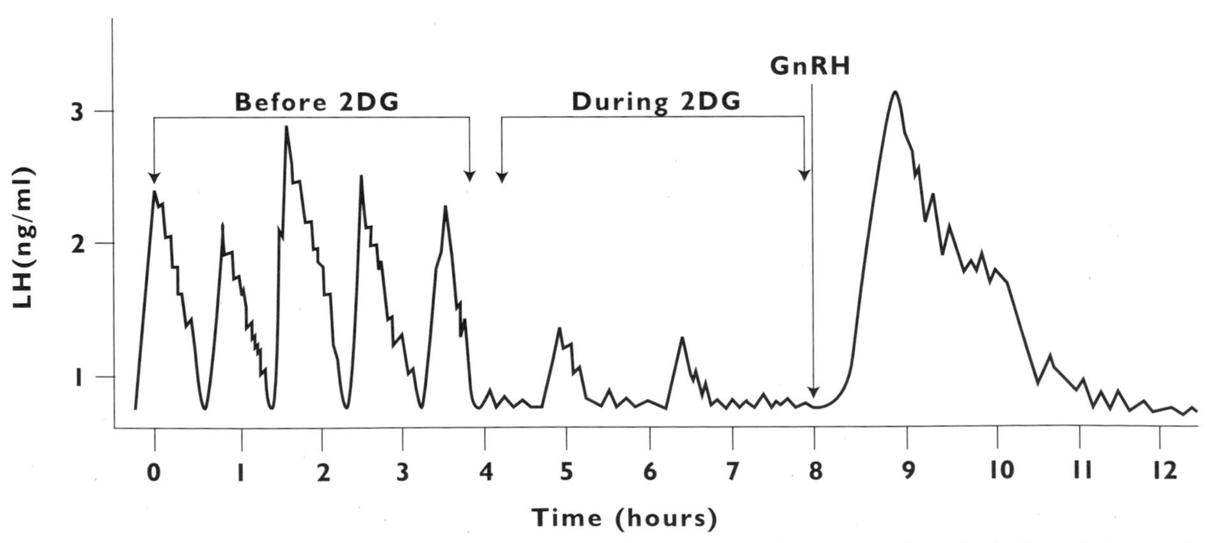

Figure 6-6. In an ovariectomized ewe lamb, low amplitude LH pulses occur hourly before 2-deoxyglucose (Before 2DG) was given to each animal. When the ewe lambs were treated with 2DG, the frequency and amplitude of the LH pulses were reduced significantly (During 2DG). When the same animal receiving 2DG was treated with exogenous GnRH, a small surge of LH resulted. These data suggest that moment-to-moment regulation of GnRH occurs only when glucose is available for metabolism. (Modified from Foster, 1994.)

mus. Thus, the researchers were able to interpret the results based solely on the action of the metabolic inhibitors without confounding effects associated with ovarian steroids. In addition to reduced frequency, the amplitude of the LH pulses also decreased in some sheep. These data strongly suggest that the hypothalamic GnRH neurons (or the "pulse generator neurons") are sensitive to concentrations of glucose in the circulating blood.

A practical illustration of the impact of nutrition on the age of pubertal onset in dairy heifers is shown in Figure 6-7. A major goal in the management of the dairy heifer is to achieve a successful, uncomplicated birth by 24 months. In order for this to occur, appropriate nutrition and adequate body size must be achieved. Figure 6-7 describes the relationship between age and weight of heifers as it relates to the onset of puberty and nutritional level. Curve A illustrates the growth rate and age at onset of puberty (first estrus) when heifers were fed to gain 2.0 pounds per day for the first 12 months. Heifers fed this diet reached puberty between 6 and 8 months. If continued into the second year, this feeding regimen can result in over-conditioned heifers. The second nutritional level (curve B) allows the heifer to reach the same target weight (1200 pounds at 24 months), but heifers grow at a uniform weight of 1.5 pounds per day

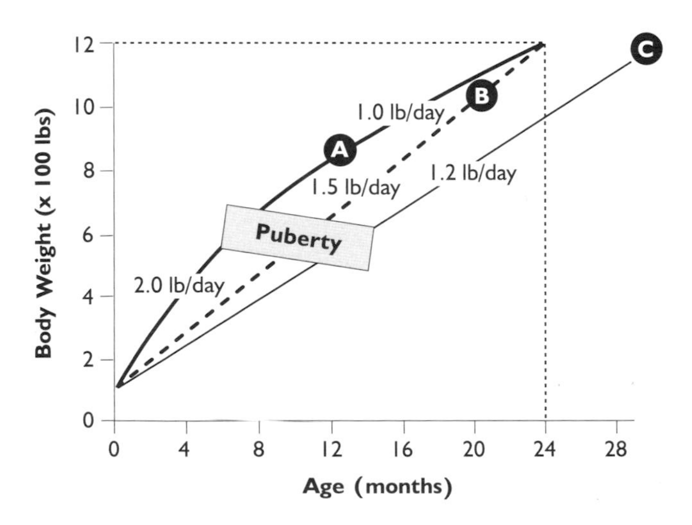

Figure 6-7. Relationship between plane of nutrition, growth and average daily gains upon the onset of puberty in Holstein heifers. (Modified from Head in *Large Herd Dairy Management*, Van Horn and Wilcox, eds. American Dairy Science Association.)

for the entire 24 month period. All heifers in this group will be in estrus for the first time between 9 and 11 months of age. Growth illustrated in curve C is slower (1.2 pounds per day), resulting from restricted feeding or lower quality feeds. Most of these heifers will reach puberty by 12 months, but they will be too small for successful pregnancy and parturition even though they are capable of becoming pregnant.

The mechanism whereby energy metabolism is detected and converted to hypothalamic neural activity has not been described. It is believed, however, that a so-called "pulse generator" (a group of neurons in the hypothalamus) detects the metabolic status of the animal and regulates the rate of GnRH release.

"Fatness" for puberty in the male is not understood.

Little research has been conducted on the influence of metabolic status on the onset of puberty in the male. Restriction of energy intake to 70% of recommended amounts delays the onset of puberty in the male. However, it is not clear whether the "degree of fatness" theory is appropriate. The energy expenditure associated with spermatogenesis and copulation is "microscopic" in comparison to the energy expenditure associated with gestation, parturition and lactation. Therefore, it is reasonable to hypothesize that the impact of metabolic status on the onset of puberty in the male is not nearly as critical as it is in the female.

Environmental and Social Conditions Impact the Onset of Puberty in the Female

External factors have a significant influence upon the onset of puberty. These factors include season of birth (with resultant photoperiod differences) and social cues such as the presence of the male or size of the social group in which females are housed. In general, environmental information is perceived by sensory neurons of the optic and olfactory systems. Stimuli are processed by the central nervous system and delivered as neural inputs to the GnRH neurons of the hypothalamus. The net effect is that the hypothalamus gains the ability to produce high frequency and high amplitude pulses of GnRH at an earlier age (provided that optimum size and energy balance requirements are met).

Season of Birth and Photoperiod Are Important Modulators of Pubertal Onset

The month of birth will influence the age of puberty, particularly in seasonal breeders, provided no artificial illumination alters natural photoperiod cues. Sheep are seasonal breeders that begin their estrous cycles in response to short day lengths. In natural photoperiods, spring-born lambs receiving adequate nutrition attain puberty during the subsequent fall. The age at puberty is about 5 to 6 months after birth. In contrast, fall-born lambs do not reach puberty until about 10 to 12 months after birth. As seen in Figure 6-8, both sets of lambs (fall-born and spring-born) reach puberty only after the day length decreases significantly in the months of September and October. It should be noted in Figure 6-8 that those animals which were fall-born reached puberty faster as a group than did the spring-born lambs. For example, all (100%) of the fall-born lambs displayed estrus within 17 days of each other, while only about 25% of the spring-born lambs displayed estrus within 30 days. The length of time from the

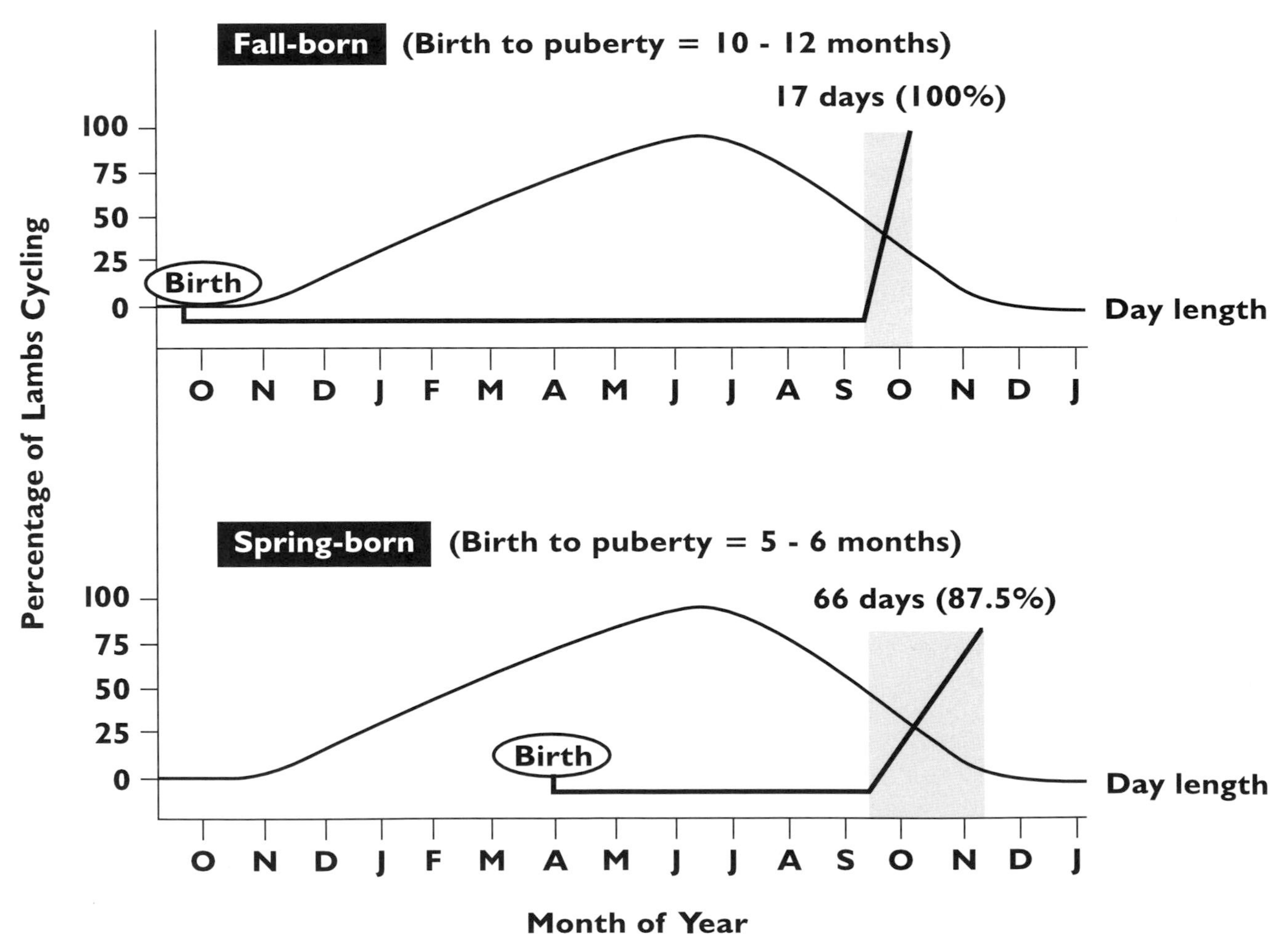

Figure 6-8. Influence of season of birth (fall-born vs. spring-born) upon onset of puberty as judged by the percentage of lambs displaying estrous cycles (shaded area). Notice that all of the fall-born lambs began cycles within 17 days of one another. However, they were 48 to 50 weeks of age when the cyclicity began. In contrast, spring-born lambs reached puberty at a much younger age and less synchronously. There were 65 days between the first and last lambs cycling. (Modified from Foster, 1994.)

onset of the breeding season until the spring-born lambs began to display estrus was about 66 days, almost 4 times as long as the fall-born lambs. The strong influence of season of birth may be related to the larger body size of fall-born lambs than the spring-born lambs. Fall-born lambs reached the proper size/fatness when short days commenced, compared to spring-born lambs. Spring-born lambs have less time to reach the appropriate body size/composition for pubertal onset during their first reduced photoperiod (fall). Therefore, puberty occurs over a longer time and is delayed by up to 2 months when compared to fall-born lambs.

In heifers there is good evidence that age at puberty is influenced by the season of birth. For example, heifers born in autumn tend to reach puberty earlier than those born in spring. Exposure during the second six months of their life to long photoperiods and spring/summer-like temperatures hastens the onset of puberty. It appears that the sequence of exposure to photoperiod is important because exposure to short days during the first six months of life (fall-born calves) followed by increasing day lengths during the second six months (spring and summer) has been associated with the earliest age of puberty in heifers.

There are significant sex differences in the timing of puberty. For example, spring-born ram lambs begin reproductive development at about 10 weeks of age during midsummer, as judged by the onset of spermatogenesis. Spring-born ewe lambs, however, do not reach puberty until 25 to 35 weeks after birth (see Figure 6-8). Season of birth does not affect the age of puberty in bull calves.

Social Cues Alter the Onset of Puberty

Social cues significantly impact the onset of puberty in many mammalian species. Such mediation is caused by olfactory recognition of **pheromonal** substances present in the urine. While the original work demonstrating this phenomenon was conducted in rodents, enhancement of the onset of puberty by the presence of the male has been demonstrated in the ewe, sow and cow. The evolutionary advantage of such a stimulus is obvious. Females reaching puberty in the presence of the male have a greater opportunity to become pregnant. One should be reminded that pubertal onset cannot be accelerated in animals which have not achieved the appropriate metabolic body size to trigger hypothalamic responsiveness to estradiol.

Small groups of gilts housed together have delayed onset of puberty.

Certain social cues inhibit the onset of puberty. Gilts housed in small groups have delayed puberty when compared to gilts housed in larger groups. If prepubertal gilts are housed in groups of 10 or more, these females will enter puberty at the expected time. However, if the group size is decreased to only two or three gilts, they will enter puberty at a later time than their counterparts housed in larger groups (Figure 6-9).

Presence of the male hastens the onset of puberty.

If gilts are housed in small groups and exposed to a boar, these females will enter puberty at an earlier age than either of their large or small grouped counterparts which are not exposed to a boar. An important point to recognize is that the presence of the male, either in visual contact with the females or in direct physical contact with them, will hasten the onset of puberty in gilts (Figure 6-9). Such observations are valuable for

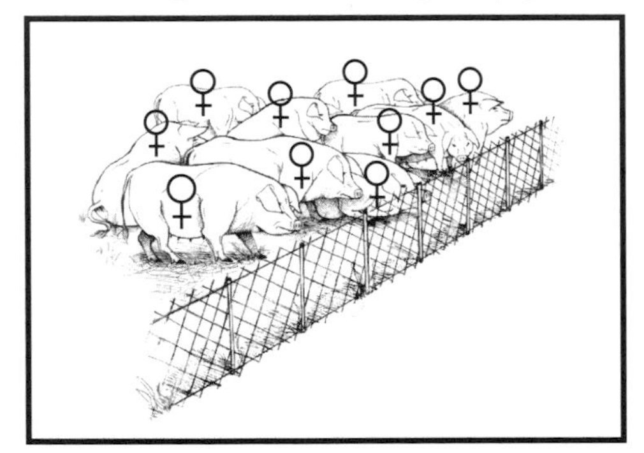

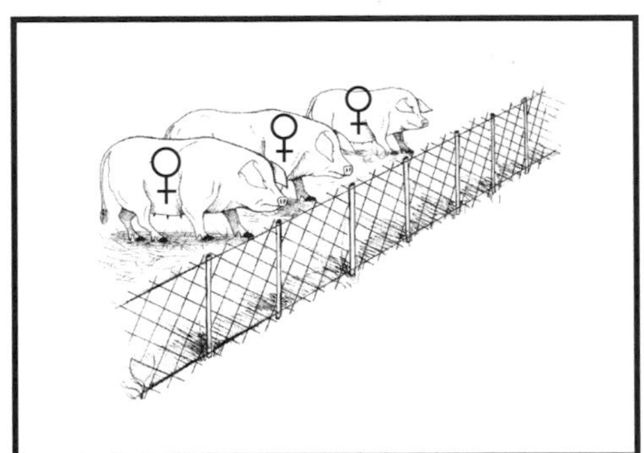

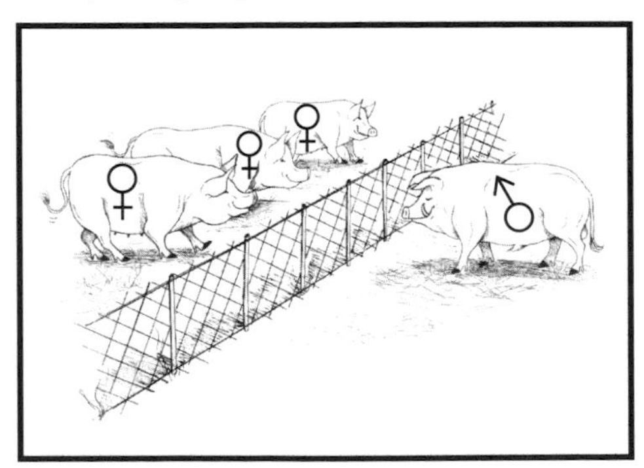
Small female group and boar
(no physical contact)
Accelerated puberty (24 weeks)

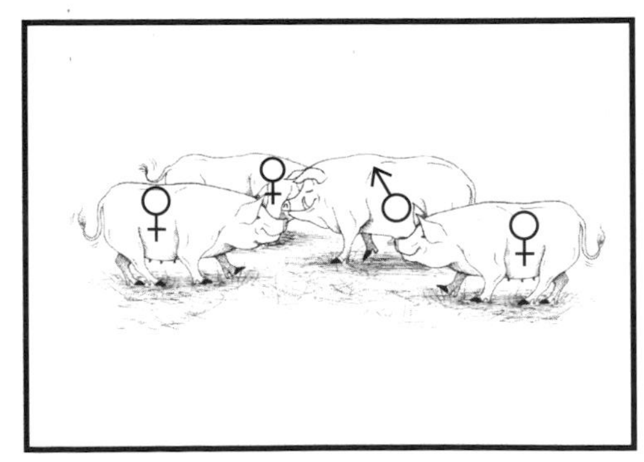
Small female group and boar
(physical contact)
Accelerated puberty (24 weeks)

Figure 6-9. Gilts housed in large groups (10 or more) reach puberty at the normal time (28 weeks). Those housed in small groups have delayed puberty (32 weeks). Gilts exposed to a boar, either within sight of or with direct physical contact, experience accelerated puberty. (Graphic by Sonja Oei.)

swine management because the age of puberty can be reduced by properly managing the social environment.

Nebraska researchers have shown conclusively that bulls accelerate the onset of puberty in beef heifers. However, there was an interaction between growth rate and exposure to the bull. For example, heifers with a high growth rate (1.75 lb/day) and exposure to a bull for about 6 months reached puberty at about 375 days. Those with a moderate growth rate (1.4 lb/day) coupled with bull exposure (6 months) reached puberty at about 422 days. Figure 6-10 summarizes the influence of growth rate and exposure to a bull upon the age at puberty in beef heifers. Heifers with a high growth rate which were exposed to the bull attained puberty 74 days earlier than heifers with a moderate growth rate and no exposure to a bull. Heifers with moderate growth rate and exposure to bulls reached puberty 53 days earlier than moderately growing heifers without bulls. Clearly, presence of the bull hastens the onset of puberty in the beef heifer.

Unfortunately, little research has been conducted describing the effect of female-on-male or male-on-male social influences and their impact on the onset of puberty. Virtually all of the research has been conducted describing the influence of the male on the onset of puberty in the female rather than the opposite.

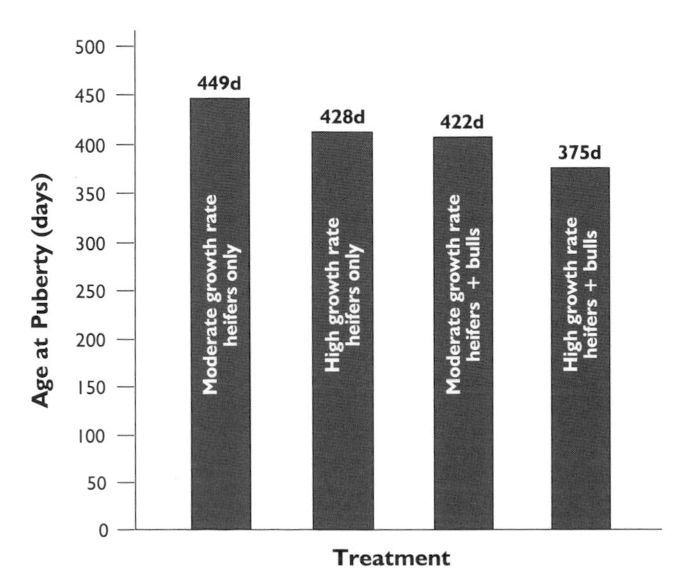

Figure 6-10. Influence of growth rate and bull exposure upon the age of puberty in beef heifers.

The Story on the Onset of Puberty Is Not Complete

As you now know, the onset of puberty involves the capability of the hypothalamic neurons to produce high frequency and high amplitude GnRH pulses. This capability is influenced by genetics, by achieving the appropriate energy metabolism/body size and appropriate exposure to external modulators such as photoperiod, size of social groups and the presence of the male.

The exact mechanisms that enable estradiol to control GnRH from the hypothalamus during the peripubertal period are unknown. A major challenge is to understand the impact of metabolism on the development of the hypothalamus. Currently, there is little basic understanding of how the brain recognizes growth so that the proper signals are sent to the hypothalamus and reproduction can commence. As increasing metabolic demands are placed on food producing animals, a better understanding of the impact of metabolism upon hypothalamic function will be imperative.

With regard to social cues, the presence of certain pheromones produced by the same or opposite sex alter the onset of puberty. The pathway whereby these pheromones send their message to the hypothalamus is, as yet, not well defined. We know that the pathway is mediated through the olfactory and the vomeronasal organs (see Chapter 11), but neither specific agents nor a clear pathway have been described. Further, the visual pathway may be quite important in mediating pubertal onset, but this sensory avenue has received little attention.

Minimizing the age at puberty in the male is more advantageous than in the female.

From a genetic improvement/reproductive management standpoint, it would be beneficial if the onset of puberty could be shortened, particularly in the male.

If one could develop techniques to perturb the system in the male so that spermatogenesis would occur 4 to 6 months earlier (particularly in animals where artificial insemination is employed), the generation interval could be reduced and genetic improvement could be accelerated. For example, spermatogenesis is initiated in Holstein bulls at between 9 and 11 months. If puberty could be initiated several months earlier, this would mean that semen from genetically superior bulls could be used earlier in the male's life, and thus expensive bull maintenance and wasteful accumulation of excessive males could be reduced. This same principle could hold true in swine and poultry where considerable reproductive "down-time" is spent waiting for the onset of puberty in the male. Since the female must maintain a successful pregnancy and deliver live offspring, there is clearly a physiologic limit to hastened pubertal onset. Such a limit is not imposed on the male since artificial insemination requires spermatozoa only and does not require that the male reach a threshold body size to support pregnancy and lactation.

Further Phenomena for Fertility

An anomaly of the captive environment for the endangered clouded leopard is that males and females must be paired before they reach puberty. If they are housed together after puberty the male becomes very aggressive and frequently injures or even kills the female. This happens even after long introduction efforts with animals kept in adjacent pens, and making sure that animals are placed together only when the female is in estrus. This behavior does not happen in the wild.

The famous boys' choirs in Europe consisted entirely of prepubertal boys. It was recognized that their high pitched clear voices were "ruined" during and after puberty. Many of these boys were castrated so that their boyhood voices could be retained. Castrato choirs were composed of adult male singers castrated in boyhood so as to retain soprano or alto voices.

In naked mole rats, the dominant female (called the queen) suppresses puberty in the subordinates (i.e. there is no vaginal opening which occurs at puberty). Once thought to be due to the suppressive effects of pheromones, a more recent theory is that the queen actuully uses tactile stimulation to suppress puberty by regularly having physical contact with each female.

There are examples of males being forced to leave their family group when they reach puberty to avoid inbreeding. Some of these encounters can be rather brutal, with the maternal faction ganging up on the newly pubertal males to "kick them out." Examples of this behavior are found in lions and elephants.

In Papua New Guinea, a small group of people (about 2,000) called Sambia practice extensive rituals which they believe promote the onset of puberty in the male. Rituals in the female are not practiced because they believe the female attains reproductive competence through natural means. Up to six intermittent "manhood" initiation rituals are performed. One taboo contends that the reproductive development of the male is compromised by sustained presence with the mother. Boys are traumatically separated from their mothers (and wiped clean of female contaminants) so that puberty can develop. They further believe the young male can produce semen only after long series (years) of homosexual fellatio inseminations following removal of the mother. They think this "injection of semen" is obligatory for the formation of male reproductive capacity.

Additional Reading

Foster, D.L. 1994. "Puberty in the Sheep." In *The Physiology of Reproduction.* 2nd Edition., E. Knobil and J.D. Neil, eds. Raven Press, Ltd., New York.

Kinder, J.E., M.S. Roberson, M.W. Wolfe and T.T. Stampf. 1994. "Management factors affecting puberty in the heifer." In *Factors Affecting Calf Crop* M.J. Fields and R. Sands, eds. CRC Press, Inc.

Plant, T.M. 1994. "Puberty in primates." In *The Physiology of Reproduction,* 2nd Edition. E. Knobil and J.D. Neil, eds. Raven Press, Ltd., New York.

7 The Estrous Cycle-Terminology and Basic Concepts

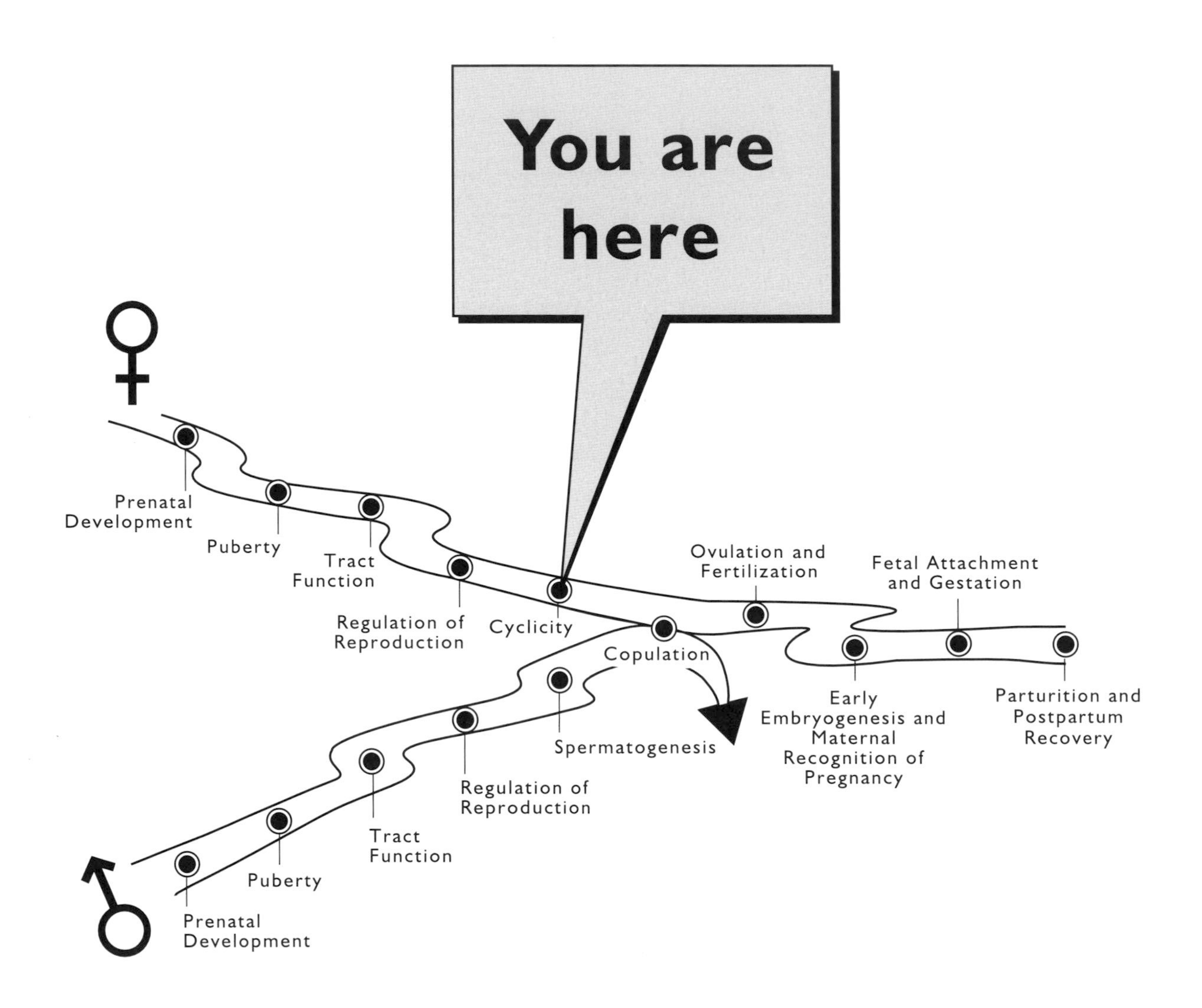

Take Home Message

Estrous cycles provide females with repeated opportunities to become pregnant. Each estrous cycle consists of a relatively short follicular phase and a longer luteal phase. The follicular phase is dominated by the hormone estradiol from ovarian follicles, which causes marked changes in the female tract and initiates sexual receptivity. The luteal phase is dominated by the hormone progesterone from the corpus luteum, which prepares the reproductive tract for pregnancy and inhibits sexual receptivity. Periods when estrous cycles cease are called anestrus. Anestrus is caused by pregnancy, season, lactation, certain forms of stress and pathology.

After puberty the female enters a period of reproductive **cyclicity** which continues throughout most of her productive life. **Estrous cycles** consist of a series of predictable reproductive events beginning at **estrus** (heat) and ending at the subsequent estrus. They continue throughout the adult female's life and are interrupted by pregnancy, nursing and by season of the year in some species. Cyclicity may also cease if nutrition is inadequate or environmental conditions are unusually stressful. Pathologic conditions of the reproductive tract, such as uterine infection, persistent corpora lutea or a mummified fetus may also cause anestrus. **Estrous cycles** provide females with repeated opportunities to copulate and become pregnant. Sexual receptivity and copulation are the primary behavioral events that occur during estrus. Copulation generally occurs during the first half of the estrous cycle and takes place prior to ovulation, providing the opportunity for conception (pregnancy). If conception does not occur, another estrous cycle begins, providing the female with another opportunity to mate and conceive. When conception does occur, the female enters a period of **anestrus** during pregnancy which ends after parturition (giving birth) and uterine involution (repair and returning to normal size).

ESTRUS is a noun.
"The cow is displaying estrus."

ESTROUS is an adjective.
"The length of the estrous cycle in the pig is 21 days."

Terminology Describing Reproductive Cyclicity Can Be Confusing

The words used to describe the estrous cycle are spelled similarly, but have subtly different meanings. The proper use of the words **estrus** and **estrous** must be understood to prevent confusion. The word estrus is a noun, while estrous is an adjective. **Oestrus** and **oestrous** are the preferred spellings in British and European literature. **Estrual** is also an adjective and is used to identify a condition related to estrus. For example, an estrual female is a female in estrus. An estrous cycle is the period between one estrus and the next. Estrus is the period of sexual receptivity. Estrus is commonly referred to as **heat**. The term estrus (oestrus) originated from a Greek word meaning "gadfly, sting or frenzy." This word (oestrus) was used to describe a family of parasitic biting insects (*oestridae*). These insects caused cattle to stampede with their tails flailing in the air as the insect buzzed around them. The behavior occurring in females in estrus was deemed similar to that observed during these insects attacks. Thus, the term oestrus or estrus was applied to the period of sexual receptivity in mammalian females. Another common term used to describe reproductive cycles is **season**. This refers to several estrous cycles that may occur during a certain season of the year. For example, a mare "coming into season" begins to show cyclicity and visible signs of estrus. She will cycle several times during her season.

Examples of other words which can lead to confusion in spelling and usage are: **anestrous** vs. **anestrus** and **polyestrous** vs. **polyestrus**. If the word is used as an adjective, it is spelled -ous. For example, "polyestrous females have repeated estrous cycles." If the word is used as a noun, it is spelled -us. For example, "the female is experiencing anestrus."

Estrous cycles are categorized according to the frequency of occurrence throughout the year. These classifications are **polyestrus, seasonally polyestrus** and **monoestrus.** Polyestrous females, such as cattle, swine and rodents, are characterized as having a uniform distribution of estrous cycles which occur regularly throughout the entire year. Polyestrous females can become pregnant throughout the year without regard to season. Seasonally polyestrous females (sheep, goats, mares, deer and elk) display "clusters" of estrous cycles that occur only during a certain season of the year. For example, sheep and goats are **short-day breeders** because they begin to cycle as day length decreases (autumn). In contrast, the mare is a **long-day breeder** because she initiates cyclicity as day length increases in the spring.

Monoestrous females are characterized as having only one cycle per year. Dogs, wolves, foxes and bears are animals which are characterized as having a single estrous cycle per year. In general, monoestrous females are characterized as having periods of estrus which last for several days. Such a prolonged period of estrus increases the probability that mating and pregnancy can occur.

The Estrous Cycle Consists of Two Major Phases

The estrous cycle can be divided into two distinct phases which are named after the dominant structure present on the ovary during each phase of the cycle. These divisions of the estrous cycle are **the follicular phase** and the **luteal phase**. The follicular phase is the period from the regression of corpora lutea to ovulation. In most mammals, the follicular phase is relatively short, encompassing no more than 20% of the estrous cycle (Figure 7-1). During the follicular phase, the primary ovarian structures are preovulatory follicles which produce the dominant reproductive hormone, **estradiol.**

***Follicles* are the dominant ovarian structure during the follicular phase.**

***Estrogen* (produced by the follicles) is the dominant hormone during the follicular phase.**

The **luteal phase** is the period from ovulation until corpora lutea regression. The luteal phase is much longer than the follicular phase and, in most mammals, occupies about 80% of the estrous cycle (Figure 7-1). During this phase, the dominant ovarian structures are the corpora lutea (CL) and the primary reproductive hormone is **progesterone**. Even though the luteal phase is dominated by progesterone from the CL, follicles continue to grow and regress during this phase. Details of this follicular growth are presented in Chapter 8.

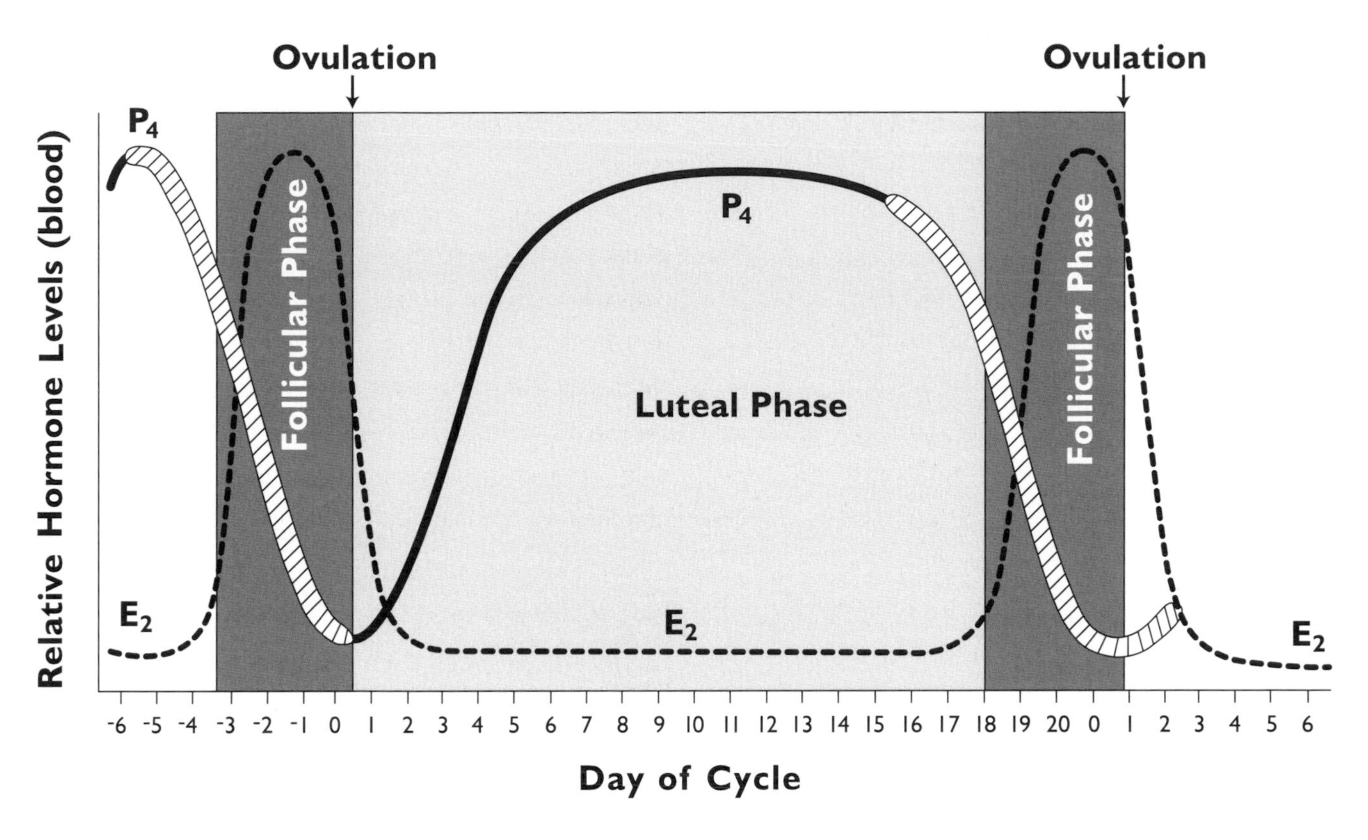

Figure 7-1. Phases of the estrous cycle. The follicular phase begins because luteolysis causes the decline of progesterone (P_4 hatched portion of the curve). Therefore gonadotropins (FSH and LH) are produced. The follicular phase is dominated by estrogen (E_2) produced by ovarian follicles. The follicular phase ends at ovulation. The luteal phase begins after ovulation and includes the development and maximum function of corpora lutea.

Corpora lutea ***are the dominant ovarian structures during the luteal phase.***

Progesterone ***(produced by corpora lutea) is the dominant hormone during the luteal phase.***

The Estrous Cycle Can Be Divided into Four Stages

The four stages of an estrous cycle are **proestrus, estrus, metestrus** and **diestrus**. Each of these stages is a subdivision of the follicular and luteal phases of the cycle. For example, the follicular phase includes proestrus and estrus. The luteal phase includes metestrus and diestrus.

Follicular phase = Proestrus + Estrus

Luteal phase = Metestrus + Diestrus

Proestrus Is the Period Immediately Preceding Estrus

Proestrus begins when progesterone declines as a result of luteolysis (destruction of the corpus luteum) and terminates at the onset of estrus. Proestrus lasts from 2 to 5 days depending on species and is characterized by a major endocrine transition, from a period of progesterone dominance to a period of estrogen dominance (Figure 7-2). The gonadotropins FSH and LH are the primary hormones responsible for this transition. It is during proestrus that follicles are recruited for ovulation and the female reproductive system prepares for the onset of estrus and mating.

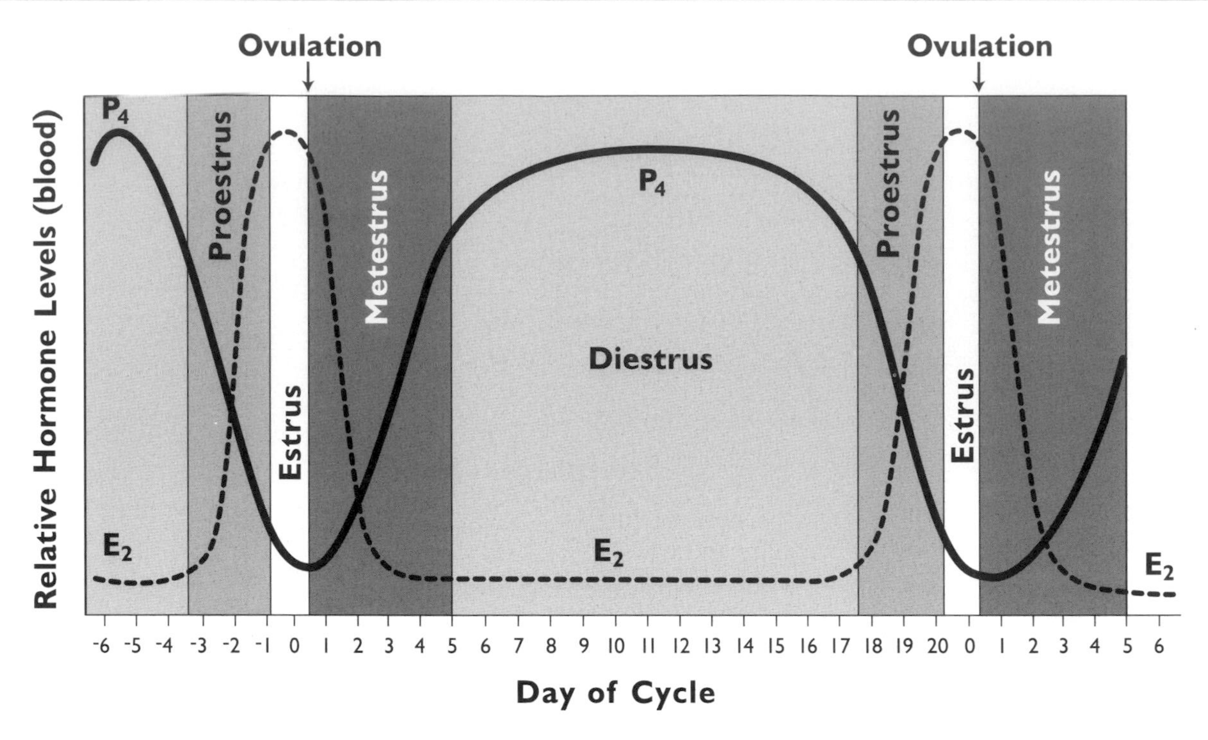

Figure 7-2. Stages of the estrous cycle. Proestrus is characterized by a significant rise in estradiol (E_2). When estradiol reaches a certain level, the female enters estrus. Following ovulation, cells of the follicle are transformed into a corpus luteum during metestrus. Diestrus is characterized by a fully functional CL and high progesterone (P_4).

Estrus Is the Period During Which the Female Allows Copulation

Estrus is the most recognizable stage of the estrous cycle because it is characterized by visible behavioral symptoms such as sexual receptivity and mating. Estradiol is the dominant hormone during this stage of the estrous cycle. It not only induces profound behavioral alterations, but causes major physiologic changes in the reproductive tract.

When a female enters estrus, she does so gradually and is not sexually receptive at first. She may display behavioral characteristics which are indicative of her approaching sexual receptivity. These include increased locomotion, phonation (vocal expression), nervousness and attempts to mount other animals. However, during this early period she will not accept the male for mating. As the period of estrus progresses, so does the female's willingness to accept the male for mating. This willingness is referred to as **standing estrus**. It is during the time of estrus that the female displays a characteristic mating posture known as **lordosis,** so named because of a characteristic arching of the back in preparation for mating. Standing behavior (lordosis) can be observed by humans and used as a diagnostic tool to identify the appropriate time to inseminate the female artificially or to expose her to the breeding male. The average duration of estrus is characteristic for each species. However, the range in the duration of estrus can be quite large even within species (Table 7-1). Understanding and appreciating the magnitude of these ranges is important because it allows one to anticipate the variation and thus for more precise detection of estrus.

Proestrus ***= Formation of ovulatory follicles +*** E_2 ***secretion***
Estrus ***= Sexual receptivity + peak*** E_2 ***secretion + ovulation***
Metestrus ***= CL formation + beginning of*** P_4 ***secretion***
Diestrus ***= Sustained luteal secretion of*** P_4

Table 7-1. Characteristics of Estrous Cycles in Food Producing Animals.

Species	Length of Estrous Cycle		Duration of Estrus		Time from Onset of Estrus to Ovulation	Time from LH Surge to Ovulation
	Mean	Range	Mean	Range		
Cattle	21d	17 - 24d	15h	6 - 24h	24 - 32h	28h
Pig	21d	17 - 25d	50h	12 - 96h	36 - 44h	40h
Sheep	17d	13 - 19d	30h	18 - 48h	24 - 30h	26h
Horse	21d	15 - 26d	7d	2 - 12d	5d	2d

h=hours d=days

Metestrus Is the Transition from Estrogen Dominance to Progesterone Secretion

Metestrus is the period between ovulation and the formation of functional corpora lutea. During early metestrus both estrogen and progesterone are relatively low (Figure 7-2). The newly ovulated follicle undergoes cellular and structural remodeling resulting in the formation of an intraovarian endocrine gland called the corpus luteum (see Chapter 9). This cellular transformation is called **luteinization**. During metestrus, progesterone secretion is detectable soon after ovulation. However, two to five days are usually required after ovulation before the newly formed corpora lutea produce significant quantities of progesterone.

Diestrus Is the Period of Maximum Luteal Function

Diestrus is the longest stage of the estrous cycle and encompasses the period of time when the corpus luteum is fully functional and progesterone production is high. It ends when the corpus luteum is destroyed (luteolysis). High progesterone prompts the uterus to prepare a suitable environment for early embryo development and eventual attachment of the conceptus to the endometrium. Diestrus usually lasts about 10 to 14 days. The duration of diestrus is directly related to the length of time that the corpus luteum remains functional (i.e. produces progesterone). Females in diestrus do not display sexual receptivity.

Anestrus Means "Without Cyclicity"

Anestrus is a condition when the female does not exhibit regular estrous cycles. During anestrus the ovaries are relatively inactive and neither ovulatory follicles nor functional corpora lutea are present. Anestrus is the result of insufficient GnRH release from the hypothalamus to stimulate and maintain gonadotropin secretion.

Anestrus can be caused by:

- ***pregnancy***
- ***presence of offspring***
- ***season***
- ***stress***
- ***pathology***

It is important to distinguish between **true anestrus** caused by insufficient hormonal stimuli and **apparent anestrus** caused by failure to detect estrus or failure to recognize that a female is pregnant. To eliminate true anestrus, one must normally improve the female's nutrition, remove offspring or eliminate stress or pathologic factors. To eliminate apparent anestrus, one must improve detection of estrus, detection of pregnancy, or both.

Gestational Anestrus Is a Normal Condition Brought about by Inhibition of GnRH by Progesterone

From a practical perspective, lack of cyclicity is a major clue that a female is pregnant. Estrous cycles do not occur during pregnancy because elevated progesterone from either the CL and/or the placenta exert a negative feedback on GnRH neurons. This prevents sufficient secretion of FSH and LH from the pituitary to allow follicular development and ovulation. Thus, expression of estrus and potential preovulatory surges of LH are nonexistent. Occasionally however, cows and ewes will display behavioral estrus during pregnancy, but the incidence is low (3% to 5%). The reason for display of estrus in pregnant cows and ewes is not understood. In certain breeds of pregnant sheep (Rambouillet) estrous behavior is seen frequently. Ovulation can be induced during pregnancy by giving exogenous gonadotropins, but pregnant females induced to ovulate generally do not show estrus.

Progesterone declines rapidly just before parturition. Even though progesterone drops rapidly and estradiol increases in the periparturient female, she will remain anestrus for a period of time after parturition. This relatively short period of postpartum anestrus provides time for uterine repair (involution) before an ensuing estrus. It would not be advantageous for a female to display estrus and thus engage in copulation when the uterus is not fully recovered from a previous pregnancy. In addition to the inability to support a new embryo, copulation could introduce microorganisms into the reproductive tract, which could promote postpartum uterine infection.

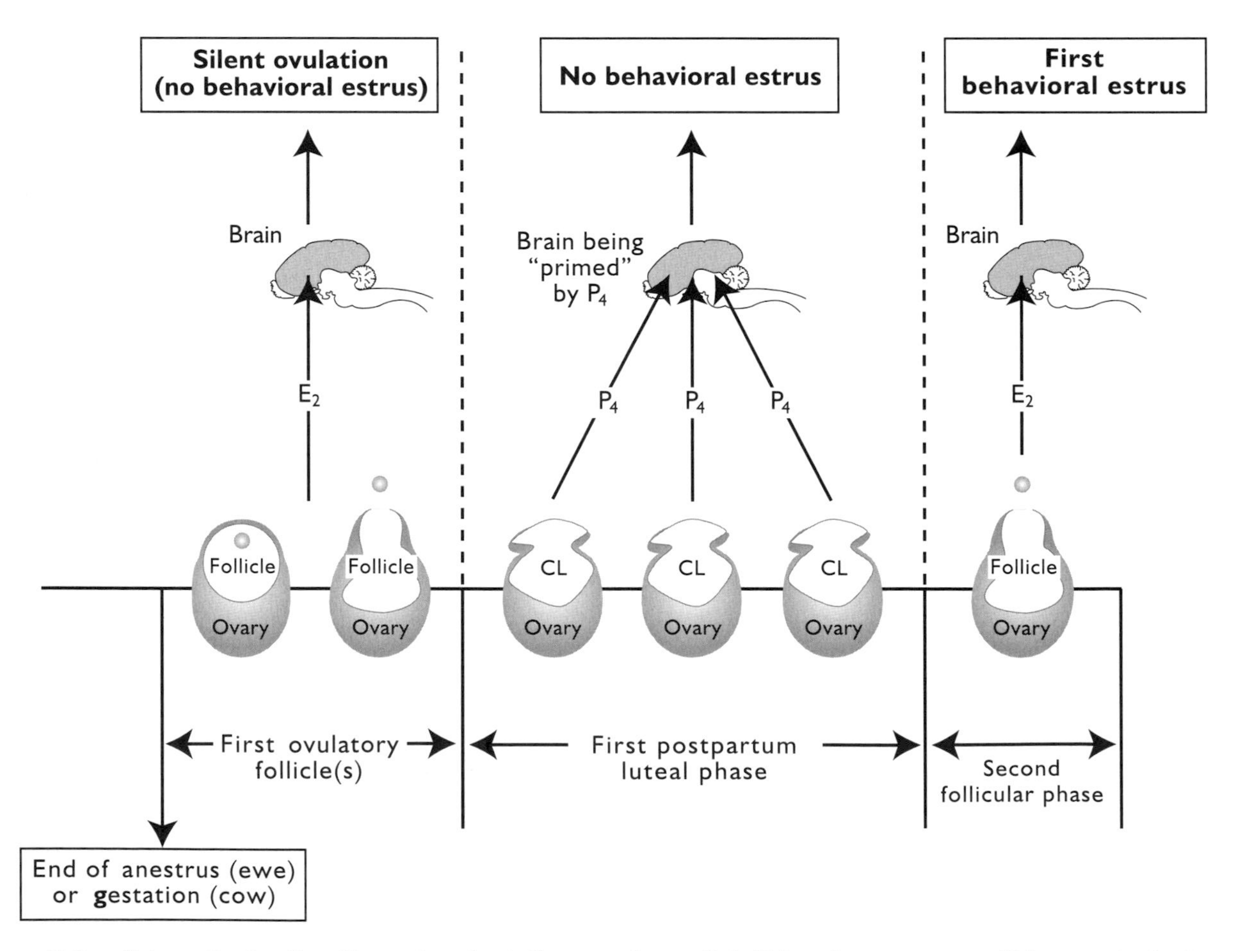

Figure 7-3. Schematic timeline illustrating the influence of estradiol (E_2) and progesterone (P_4) upon the brain, and subsequent behavioral estrus in the cow and ewe. Following seasonal anestrus in the ewe or pregnancy in the cow, the ovary develops a follicle(s) which will often ovulate without an accompanying behavioral estrus (silent ovulation). The corpus luteum produced from the ovulatory follicle produces progesterone (P_4) which "primes" the brain and enables estradiol (E_2) produced by the next ovulatory follicle to elicit behavioral estrus. (Graphic by Sonja Oei.)

Seasonal Anestrus Is a Normal Condition

Seasonal anestrus probably evolved as a way of preventing females from conceiving during periods of the year when survival of the developing embryo and the neonate would be low. For example, preattachment embryo survival is known to be reduced significantly when ambient temperatures and humidity are high during the summer months. High temperatures coupled with high humidity cause elevated body temperature of the pregnant female and can result in death of the preattachment embryo. Females which cycle in the fall (sheep, deer and elk) conceive during times of moderate ambient temperature. Most seasonal breeders give birth during the spring when nutritional conditions favor lactation and neonatal growth following weaning. Females return to cyclicity in the fall when temperatures moderate. Seasonal breeders normally make the transition from the cyclic state to the anestrus state and back again on an annual basis. This transition is controlled by **photoperiod**.

The mare begins to cycle in the spring and generally conceives before the hot summer months. The developing embryo is well established within the uterus before the onset of hot weather. Also, the relatively long length of pregnancy (11 months) enables the foal to be born the following spring, again providing optimum timing for conception and birth as it relates to environmental conditions.

In the ewe, the first ovulation occurring after seasonal anestrus is not accompanied by a behavioral estrus. This situation, whereby an ovulation is not preceded or accompanied by behavioral estrus, is referred to as a **silent ovulation**. For maximal expression of behavioral estrus, progesterone must be present for a certain period of time prior to exposure to estrogen. In other words, progesterone from the first CL formed after the first ovulation and after seasonal anestrus "primes" the brain so that its sensitivity to estrogen is optimized (Figure7-3). When estrogen from the second group of follicles after anestrus appears, the female displays behavioral estrus because her brain has been primed by progesterone thus allowing it to be "turned on" by estrogen. A similar priming effect probably is necessary in cattle, since the first ovulation after parturition (calving) is generally a silent one. The corpus luteum from the first postpartum ovulation provides the cow with a "priming" of progesterone prior to the initiation of postpartum cyclicity (Figure 7-3).

Onset of Seasonal Cyclicity Is Similar to the Onset of Puberty

Seasonal anestrus is characterized by hypothalamic dormancy with regard to GnRH secretion (as in the prepubertal female). Before the breeding season commences, the hypothalamus must be able to release GnRH in sufficient quantities to elicit a response by the anterior pituitary. The release of FSH and LH at levels capable of maintaining follicular development and causing ovulation is required.

Seasonal breeders can be categorized as either **long-day breeders** or **short-day breeders**. The mare is characterized as a long-day breeder because as the day length increases in the spring the mare also begins to cycle. During the short days of the winter months, the mare is in anestrus. Short-day breeders are animals that begin to cycle during the short days of the fall. Animals such as sheep, deer, elk and goats are categorized as short-day breeders. The duration of the breeding season varies among and within species. For example, in sheep, the Merino breed has a period of cyclicity which ranges from 200 to 260 days, while blackface breeds have shorter periods of cyclicity ranging from 100 to 140 days.

The two primary factors which influence the onset of the breeding season are photoperiod and temperature. Photoperiod is by far the most important. It is well known that artificial manipulation of the photoperiod can alter the cyclicity of the seasonal breeder.

A major question that must be answered in order to understand the influence of day length on the onset of reproductive activity is, "How is photoperiod

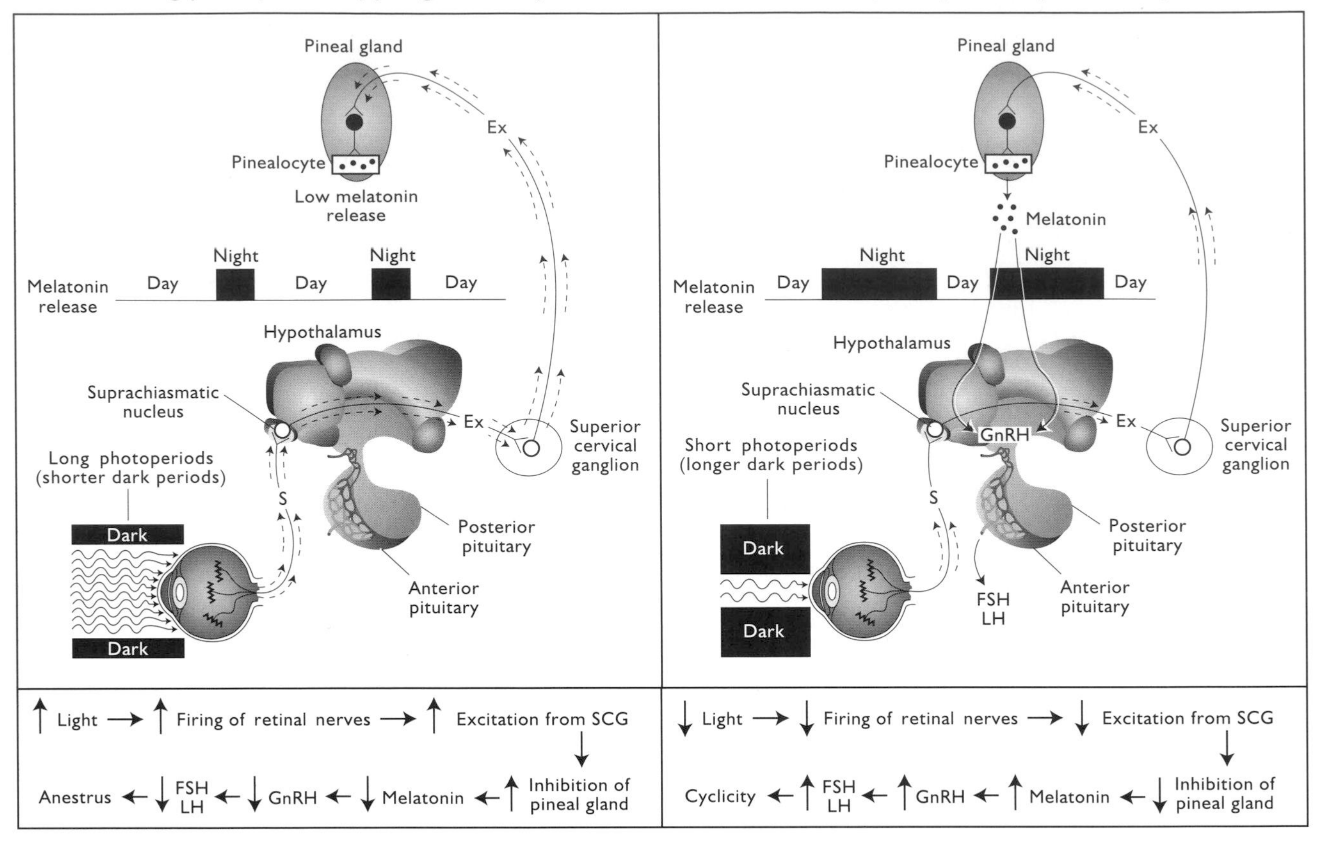

Figure 7-4. Model for the effect of photoperiod on short-day breeders. During long periods of light (left panel), the excitatory neurons (Ex) fire with a high degree of frequency and for a sustained period of time because sensory neurons (S) in the retina of the eye are stimulated. Therefore, the inhibitory neurons (shaded black) in the pineal gland also fire at high frequency and for sustained periods. Sustained release of inhibitory neurotransmitters prevents pinealocytes from synthesizing and releasing large quantities of melatonin. During short photoperiods (right panel), the excitatory pathways are less active and the inhibition on the pinealocytes is decreased. Melatonin is synthesized and released during the night. Therefore, during the longer dark periods the inhibition on the pinealocyte has been reduced. Melatonin stimulates release of GnRH and thus initiates cyclicity. Relative melatonin secretion is illustrated by the black boxes on the melatonin release time-line. Equations at the bottom of each panel summarize the main events of this model. (Graphic by Sonja Oei.)

translated into a physiologic signal?" The basic pathway for induction of cyclicity by short day length is presented in Figure 7-4.

The retina of the eye is stimulated by light. This photoreception is transferred by a nerve tract to a specific area of the hypothalamus known as the **suprachiasmatic nucleus**. From the suprachiasmatic nucleus a second nerve tract travels to the **superior cervical ganglion.** These presynaptic neurons cause the postganglionic neurons to fire. These postganglionic neurons synapse with inhibitory neurons which make contact with cells in the **pineal gland (pinealocytes)**. These cells secrete a material called **melatonin**. During the daylight hours, the light sensed by the retinal cells of the eye activates an excitatory neural pathway at the level of the pineal gland where inhibitory neurons continue to fire, thus inhibiting the release of melatonin from the pinealocytes. In contrast, during the dark hours this inhibitory pathway is shut down because the firing of nerves in the light-sensitive areas in the retina is diminished. Thus, the pathway of inhibition has been disrupted and melatonin can be released from the pinealocytes. Melatonin is synthesized and released only during the night hours. Melatonin stimulates GnRH secretion and thus promotes cyclicity.

> ***Lactational anestrus prevents a new pregnancy before young are weaned.***

Females (cows and swine) nursing their young experience **lactational anestrus** which lasts for variable periods of time. Cyclicity is completely suppressed during lactation in the sow. When weaning takes place, the sow will display estrus and ovulate within 4 to 8 days. In the suckled cow, cyclicity is delayed by as much as 60 days after parturition. The duration of lactational anestrus is influenced by the degree of suckling in the cow. However, suckling in itself does not appear to be important when the frequency is greater than two suckling sessions per day. Suckling sessions of two or less per day promote return to cyclicity, while sessions of greater than two per day tend to cause postpartum anestrus (Figure 7-5). There appears to be a threshold of about two sessions per day above which anestrus will be maintained and below which the cow will return to cyclicity; it does not seem to matter whether there are 3 or 20 suckling sessions per day. In other words, the effect of suckling does not operate in a continuum but rather in a threshold manner.

> ***Mammary stimulation is not totally responsible for lactational anestrus.***

It has been almost universally accepted that repeated sensory stimulation of the teat during suckling causes inhibition of gonadotropin release from the anterior pituitary in the postpartum female. However, recent research findings from Texas A&M University indicate that this long-standing concept is probably incorrect. In fact, data now show that direct neural stimulation of the mammary gland does not inhibit gonadotropin release in the cow. Figure 7-6 illustrates the typical pattern of LH release during *ad libitum* suckling in the beef cow. During the time of intense suckling, LH in the blood is quite low. When the suckling is suddenly terminated (acute weaning), increased episodes of LH

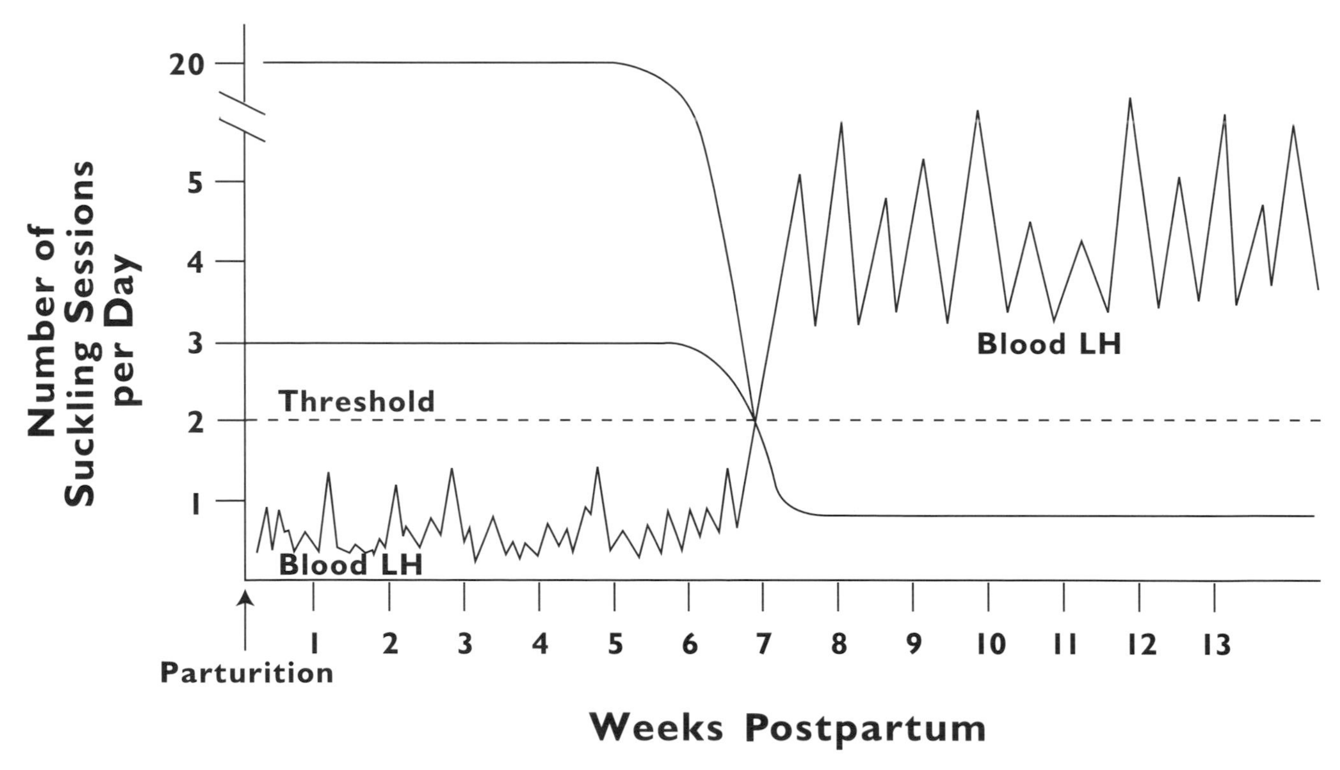

Figure 7-5. Influence of suckling frequency upon blood LH (a direct indication of GnRH release) in postpartum beef cows. Suckling frequency of less than 2 suckling sessions per day promotes return to cyclicity as judged by elevated LH. Greater than 2 suckling sessions per day promotes anestrus. Suckling sessions of 3 or 20 per day do not alter LH secretions. (Derived from the data of Dr. G.L. Williams, Texas A&M University, Beeville.)

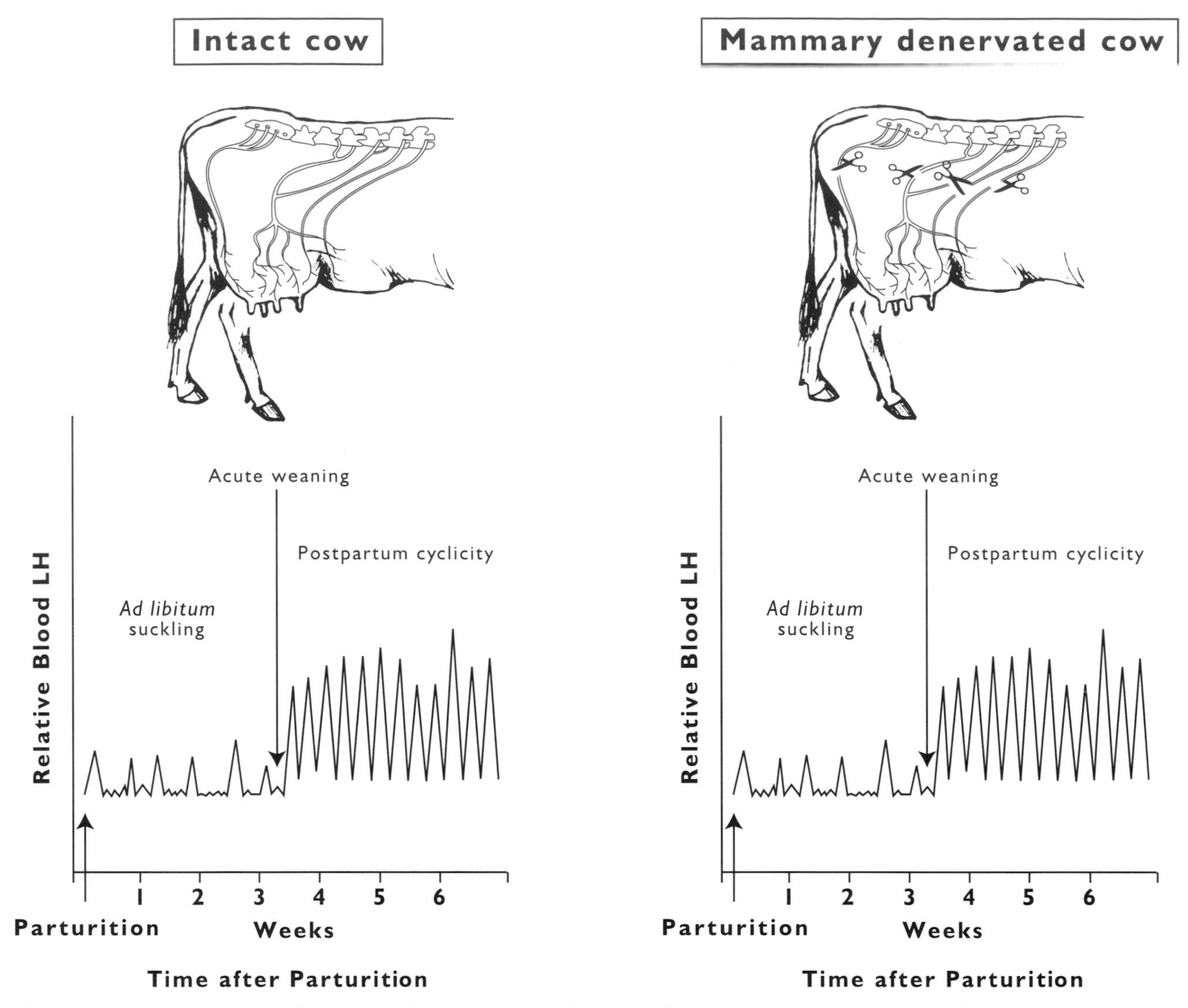

Figure 7-6. *Ad libitum* suckling results in suppression of LH amplitude and pulse frequency. When removal of the calf occurs suddenly (acute weaning), LH pulse frequency and amplitude increases. This phenomenon occurs in both intact and mammary denervated cows. Since cows in both treatments responded the same, suckling cannot be responsible for suppression of LH in the postpartum female. (Graphic by Sonja Oei.)

occur within 2 to 3 days after the calves are removed and the postpartum female resumes cyclicity. The response for the intact cow shown in Figure 7-6 implies that mammary stimulation is the cause of inhibition of GnRH, resulting in basal LH levels during the suckling period. However, when cows were subjected to complete mammary denervation (abolition of the nerve tracts supplying the mammary gland), the response in blood LH was identical to that of the intact cow. Destroying all of the nerves to the mammary gland would be expected to remove immediately any inhibition on the hypothalamus brought about by mammary stimulation. However, as you can see by comparing the right and left panels of Figure 7-6, there was no difference between suckled females with intact neural pathways to the mammary gland when compared to suckled females with the neural pathways to the mammary gland destroyed. Clearly, if suckling alone prevented the hypothalamus from producing GnRH, then females with denervated mammary glands would have hastened elevations of LH following parturition. Since this did not occur, the interpretation is that factors other than teat stimulation are responsible for inhibition of GnRH during the postpartum period. These factors may be 1) visual encounter with the offspring, 2) olfactory encounter with the offspring, 3) auditory encounter with the offspring or all of the above.

It is also now known that the cow's own calf is important to maintenance of postpartum anestrus. If a cow's own calf is replaced with an alien (unrelated calf) the LH secretion increases dramatically and ovarian activity soon follows, even though the alien calf is permitted to suckle. The precise role of calf identity on central nervous system control of gonadotropin release has yet to be fully explained. Regardless, it appears that maintenance of the postpartum anestrus condition is a combination of sensory inputs to the dam apparently involving sight, sound and smell.

In dairy cows, calves are removed from the dam very soon (hours to a few days) after parturition. The fact that dairy cows do not experience lactational anestrus suggests that presence of the calf contributes to lactational anestrus in beef cows.

Anestrus can result from negative energy balance.

Females consuming low quantities of energy or protein often have sustained periods of anestrus. Nutritional anestrus is characterized by an absence of GnRH pulses from the hypothalamus, inadequate secretion of gonadotropins and inactive ovaries. In nursing females, inadequate nutrition will prolong the duration of lactational anestrus. This is particularly true in **primiparous** females (those that have given birth for the first time) where restricted dietary intake is compounded with the energy requirements of lactation and growth. The primiparous female represents one of the most difficult to manage from a reproductive standpoint since growth and lactation impose two strong energy demands. Providing first-calf lactating heifers with optimum nutrition cannot be overemphasized. During early lactation in dairy cows, the metabolic demands for milk production are often so great that the female cannot consume enough dietary energy to meet her metabolic needs. This negative energy balance is often related to delayed postpartum cyclicity (nutritional anestrus). In non-lactating cycling females, prolonged periods of inadequate nutrition will also cause anestrus. However, undernutrition must be severe and must occur for a prolonged period for cyclicity to cease entirely. Nutritionally anestrous females respond to adequate nutrition by resuming their estrous cycles.

Further Phenomena for Fertility

The word "menstrual" (as in menstrual cycle) is derived from the Latin word meaning month. In historical latin folklore the moon was believed to regulate not only the tides of the sea, but also the monthly "emotional tides" of women.

Some female bats are very aggressive and prey on the males of their species, thus minimizing the opportunity for successful copulation and pregnancy. To offset this problem, males hibernate after the females. Thus, males can then safely breed the "sleeping" females. This is not a "silent estrus"!!! Ovulation does not occur until after hibernation. The sperm are stored in the female tract until ovulation when they fertilize the oocytes.

In primitive societies, menstruating women were isolated from the tribe and forced to occupy a small "menstrual hut" located away from the village. Menstruation was believed to be responsible for assorted ills such as crop failures, bad luck in hunting and fishing, death of livestock, failure of food to be preserved and failure of beer to ferment. Reproductive processes were blamed because of ignorance about them.

Dairy cows are afflicted by a condition called cystic ovarian disease, often called "cystic ovaries." One type of cystic ovarian disease results in nymphomania (excessive or uncontrollable sexual desire). Follicles fail to ovulate and produce estradiol, which causes the cow to be in constant estrus.

Women were not employed in the opium industry during the 19th century because it was believed that menstruating women would make the opium bitter.

Hysterectomy does not affect the length of the menstrual cycle in rhesus monkeys or humans. Prostaglandins in low doses seem to stimulate progesterone in the rhesus monkey.

Unlike humans, other animals do not have menopause. For example, chimpanzees live to be forty years old but show no signs of menopause. The female African elephant remains reproductively competent until she is in her nineties.

Additional Reading

Asdell, S.A. 1964. *Patterns in Mammalian Reproduction.* Comstock Publishing Co., Ithaca, N.Y.

Draincourt, M.A., D. Royere, B. Hedou and M.C. Levasseur. 1993. "Oestrus and menstrual cycles." In *Reproduction in Mammals and Man*. C. Thibault, M.C. Levasseur and R.H.F. Hunter, eds. Ellipses, Paris.

Williams, G.L., O.S. Gazai, G.A. Guzman Vega and R.L. Stanko. 1996. Mechanisms regulating suckling mediated anovulation in the cow. *Animal Reproduction Science*. 42: 289-297.

8 The Follicular Phase of the Estrous Cycle

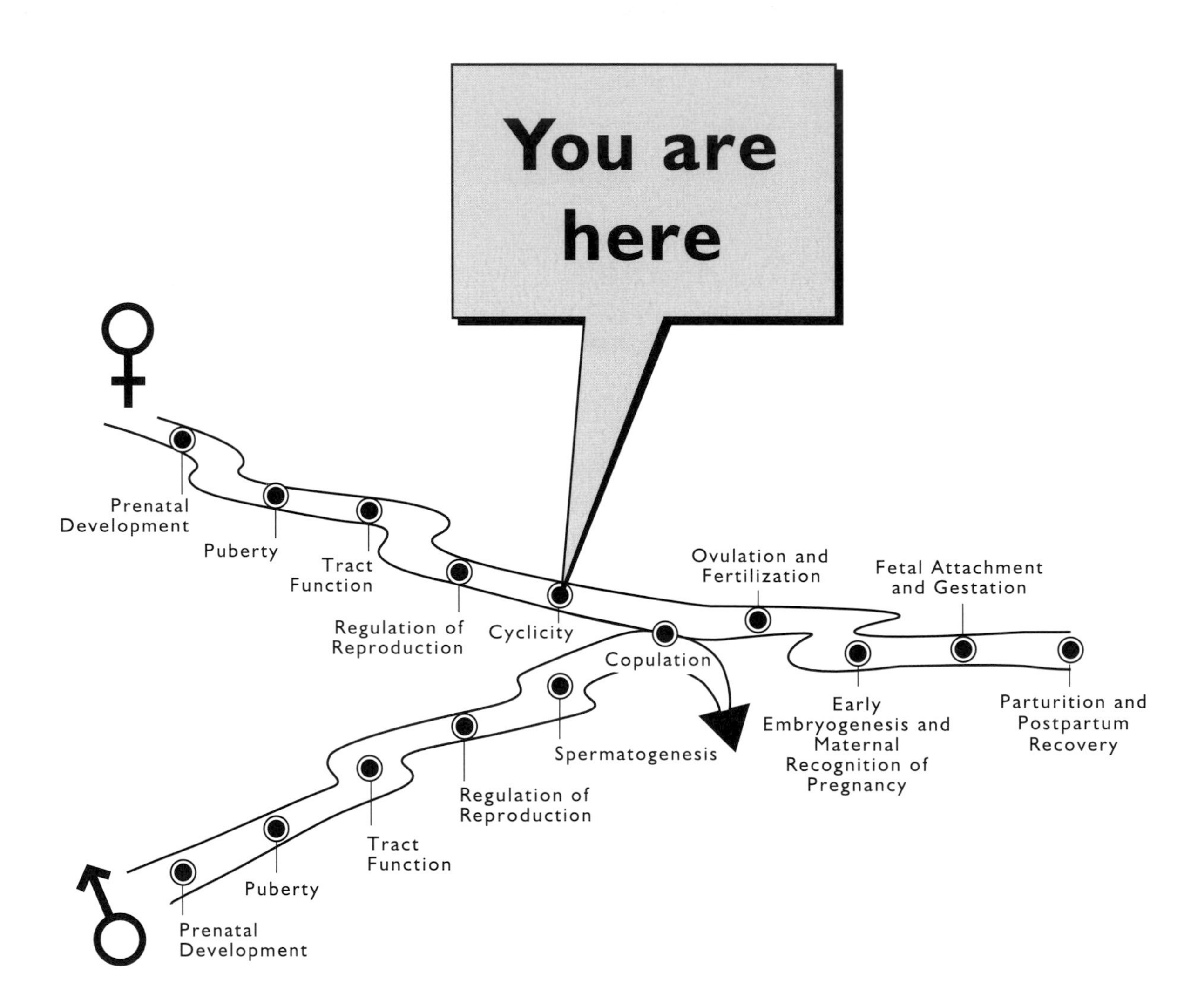

Take Home Message

The follicular phase consists of four major events. They are: 1) gonadotropin release from the anterior pituitary; 2) follicular preparation for ovulation; 3) sexual receptivity; and 4) ovulation. Estrogen produced by developing follicles causes profound changes in the reproductive tract and induces reproductive behavior in preparation for copulation. Estrogen also controls the onset of the preovulatory LH surge which causes ovulation. Ovulation is a cascade of physiological and biochemical changes which culminate in rupture of dominant follicles and release of the oocyte.

It is important to recognize that the follicular phase is initiated after luteolysis which results in a marked reduction in progesterone. Therefore, the negative feedback by progesterone on the hypothalamus is removed and GnRH is released at higher amplitudes and frequencies than during the luteal phase. This causes FSH and LH to be released at higher levels, thus promoting follicular development and the production of estrogen. The main steps in this process are presented in Figure 8-1.

Recall from Chapter 7 that the follicular phase of the estrous cycle consists of **proestrus** and **estrus.** During the follicular phase four significant events take place. They are 1) gonadotropin release from the anterior pituitary, 2) follicular preparation for ovulation, 3) sexual receptivity and 4) ovulation. These components will be described in the remainder of this chapter and in Chapter 11 (Reproductive Behavior).

↓ P_4 from CL
→ ↑ GnRH
→ ↑ FSH and LH
→ Proestrual follicular development
→ ↑ Inhibin → ↓ FSH
→ ↑ Estradiol to threshold → Preovulatory LH surge

Figure 8-1. Primary steps leading to the preovulatory LH surge.

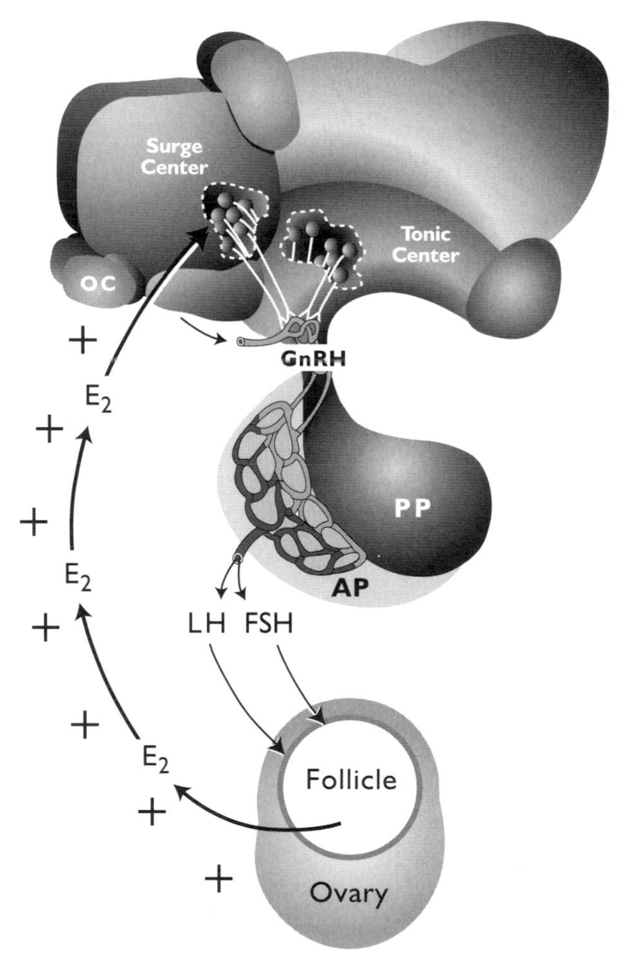

Figure 8-2. Early in the follicular phase, GnRH pulse frequency begins to increase, thus causing FSH and LH to be secreted from the anterior pituitary (AP). These gonadotropins stimulate the ovary to secrete estradiol (E_2) which exerts a positive feedback on the neurons of the hypothalamic surge center. PP= Posterior Pituitary, OC= Optic Chiasm. (Graphic by Sonja Oei.)

Gonadotropin Release Is Controlled by Ovarian Estrogen and Hypothalamic GnRH

The follicular phase is governed by the hypothalamus, the anterior pituitary and the ovary through the production of estradiol and the absence of progesterone. The relationship between these components is illustrated in Figure 8-2.

The hypothalamus plays an obligatory role in regulating estrous cycles because it produces **gonadotropin releasing hormone (GnRH)**, which is responsible for stimulating the release of the gonadotropins FSH and LH.

The tonic and surge centers in the hypothalamus control GnRH release. The surge center responds dramatically to high estradiol.

As you should remember from Chapter 5, secretion of GnRH in the female is controlled by two separate areas in the hypothalamus. These areas are composed of clusters of nerve cell bodies which represent anatomically discrete regions known as **hypothalamic nuclei**. At least two hypothalamic nuclei (the ventromedial nucleus and the arcuate nucleus) comprise the tonic GnRH center. The tonic center is responsible for basal secretion of GnRH. The neurons in this center release small pulses of GnRH over a substantial period of time (days to weeks). The profile of tonic GnRH release is characterized by having many small pulses or episodes (Figure 8-3). These pulses have various frequencies and amplitudes depending on the degree of nervous activity (rate of firing) in the tonic center. Thus, as with many neurally controlled hormonal profiles, this pattern is referred to as an **episodic profile** (see Chapter 5). In contrast, another hypothalamic center known as the **surge center** (also called the preovulatory center) is responsible for the preovulatory release of GnRH that stimulates a surge of LH, causing ovulation. Anatomically, the preovulatory center consists of the preoptic nucleus, the anterior hypothalamic area and the suprachiasmatic nucleus. This center releases basal levels of GnRH until it receives the appropriate stimulus. This stimulus is known to be a threshold level of estrogen in the absence of progesterone. When the estrogen concentration in the blood reaches a certain level, a large quantity of GnRH is released from the terminals of neurons, the cell bodies of which are located in the surge center. Release of GnRH is caused by depolarization (action potentials) originating in the cell bodies of neurosecretory cells. The preovulatory surge of GnRH occurs only once during the estrous cycle. However, tonic release of GnRH occurs during the entire estrous cycle.

The release of GnRH by the tonic and preovulatory centers in the hypothalamus may be compared to water faucets. Tonic (basal) release is analogous to a leaky faucet (Figure 8-3) in which small quantities of water drip from the faucet over a long period of time. In contrast, release of GnRH from the preovulatory center is analogous to opening a faucet fully for a short period of time and then suddenly turning it off. Water gushes forth and then stops. A threshold level of estrogen (without progesterone) is necessary to open the faucet fully.

GnRH release from the tonic center appears to be spontaneous.

As described above, release of GnRH from nerve terminals in the tonic GnRH center of the hypothalamus occurs in periodic pulses. Controls for the pattern of tonic pulsatile GnRH secretion are poorly understood and not easy to study because such small, short-lived pulses are difficult to quantitate. Each GnRH pulse occurs because of simultaneous depolarizations of several GnRH neurons. Each GnRH neuron releases a small quantity of GnRH, and summation of these small quantities causes a pulse or episode to occur. The release of GnRH from the tonic center neurons occurs spontaneously in a rhythmic fashion (see Figure 8-3).

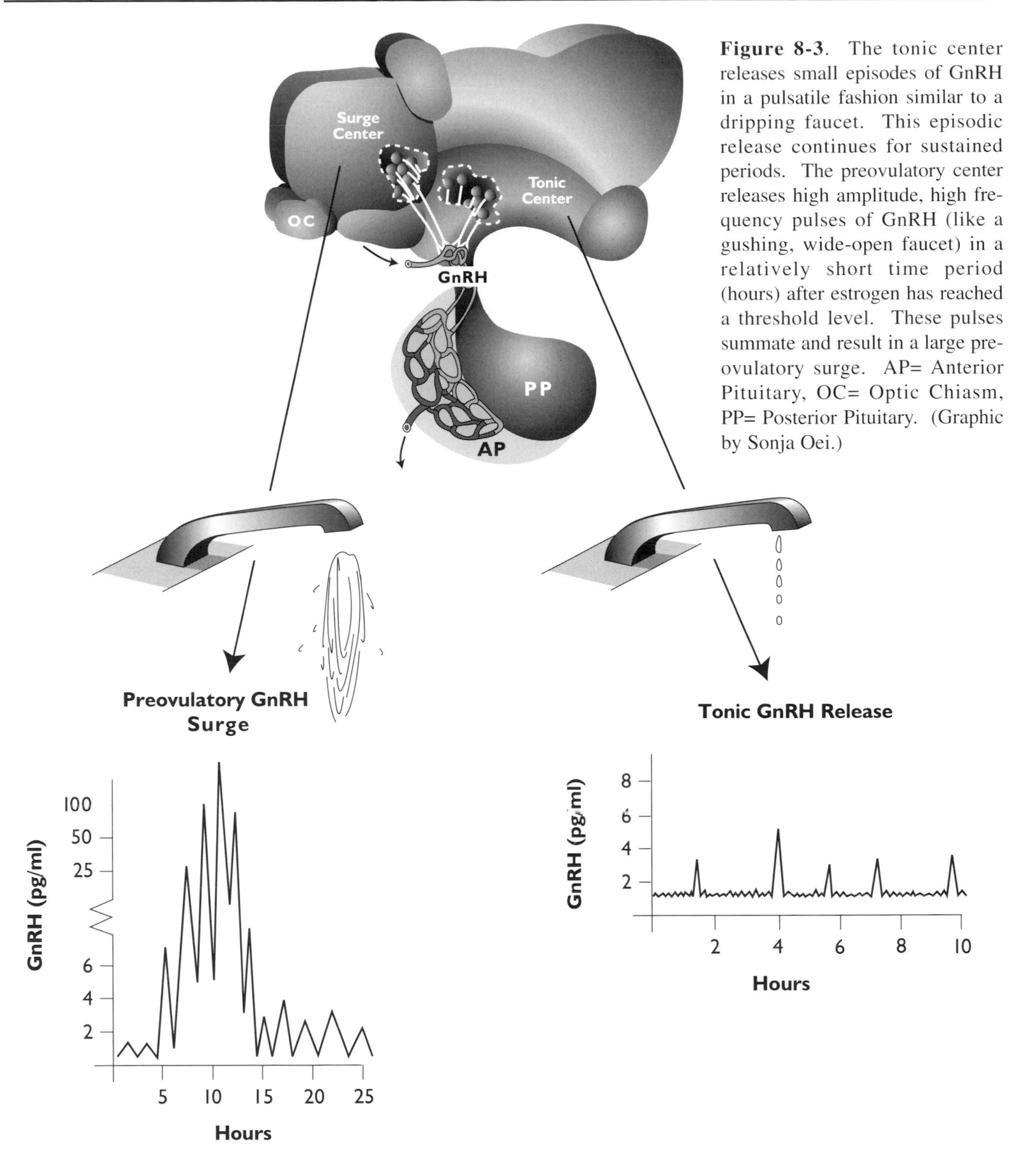

Figure 8-3. The tonic center releases small episodes of GnRH in a pulsatile fashion similar to a dripping faucet. This episodic release continues for sustained periods. The preovulatory center releases high amplitude, high frequency pulses of GnRH (like a gushing, wide-open faucet) in a relatively short time period (hours) after estrogen has reached a threshold level. These pulses summate and result in a large preovulatory surge. AP= Anterior Pituitary, OC= Optic Chiasm, PP= Posterior Pituitary. (Graphic by Sonja Oei.)

In fact, small GnRH episodes occur every 1.5 to 2.0 hours. The GnRH from the tonic center results in LH release which is generally less than 5ng/ml blood serum.

> ***GnRH release from the surge center is controlled by estrogen.***

The preovulatory surge of GnRH is controlled by the combination of high estrogen and low progesterone. In mammals, estrogen in the presence of low progesterone exerts a differential effect on GnRH. For example, estrogen in low levels causes a negative feedback (suppression) on the preovulatory center. That is, low estrogen reduces the level of firing GnRH neurons in the preovulatory center. However, when estradiol levels are high, as they would be during the mid to late follicular phase (Figure 8-4), the preovulatory center responds dramatically by releasing large quantities of GnRH. This stimulation in response to rising concentrations of estradiol is referred to as **positive feedback.** You should recognize that during the middle part of the cycle, when estradiol levels are low and progesterone is high, there is **negative feedback** on the preovulatory center, thus preventing high amplitude pulses of GnRH. During the follicular phase, the follicles begin to produce more and more estrogen (Figure 8-4). Once estradiol reaches a threshold level (or peak), the preovulatory center is "turned on" and releases large quantities of LH in response to GnRH. In fact, the LH surge is at least 10 times greater than a tonic LH pulse.

In summary, elevated GnRH is essential for initiating the follicular phase of the estrous cycle. The tonic center releases small amplitude episodes (pulses) of GnRH which stimulate release of FSH and LH from the anterior pituitary, causing growth and development of ovarian follicles. The surge center is responsible for release of large quantities of GnRH, thus causing a surge of LH that causes ovulation.

Growth of the Antral Follicles Is Stimulated by FSH and LH and Involves Both Growth and Death of These Follicles

Even though the **follicular phase** comprises only about 20% of the estrous cycle, the process of follicular growth and degeneration (known as **follicular dynamics**) occurs continuously throughout the entire estrous cycle. Antral follicles of various sizes develop

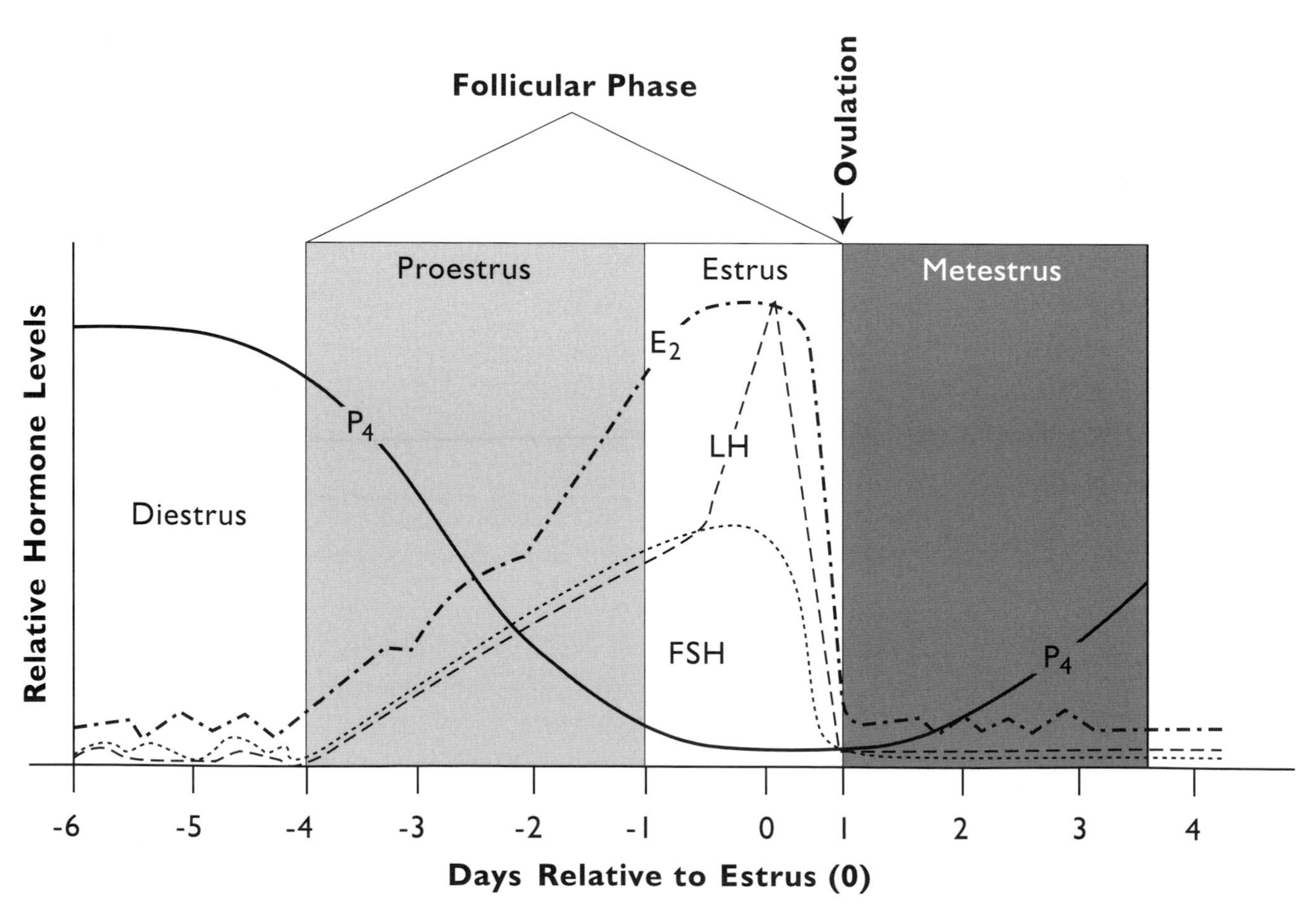

Figure 8-4. Changes in hormones during the follicular phase. As progesterone (P_4) drops, FSH and LH increase together in response to GnRH. FSH and LH cause the production of estradiol (E_2) by ovarian follicles (Figure 8-2). When the follicle reaches a certain maturational stage, it produces inhibin, which suppresses FSH secretion from the anterior pituitary. Thus, FSH does not surge with the same magnitude as LH. When estrogen reaches a threshold level (peak), the preovulatory surge of LH occurs, inducing ovulation.

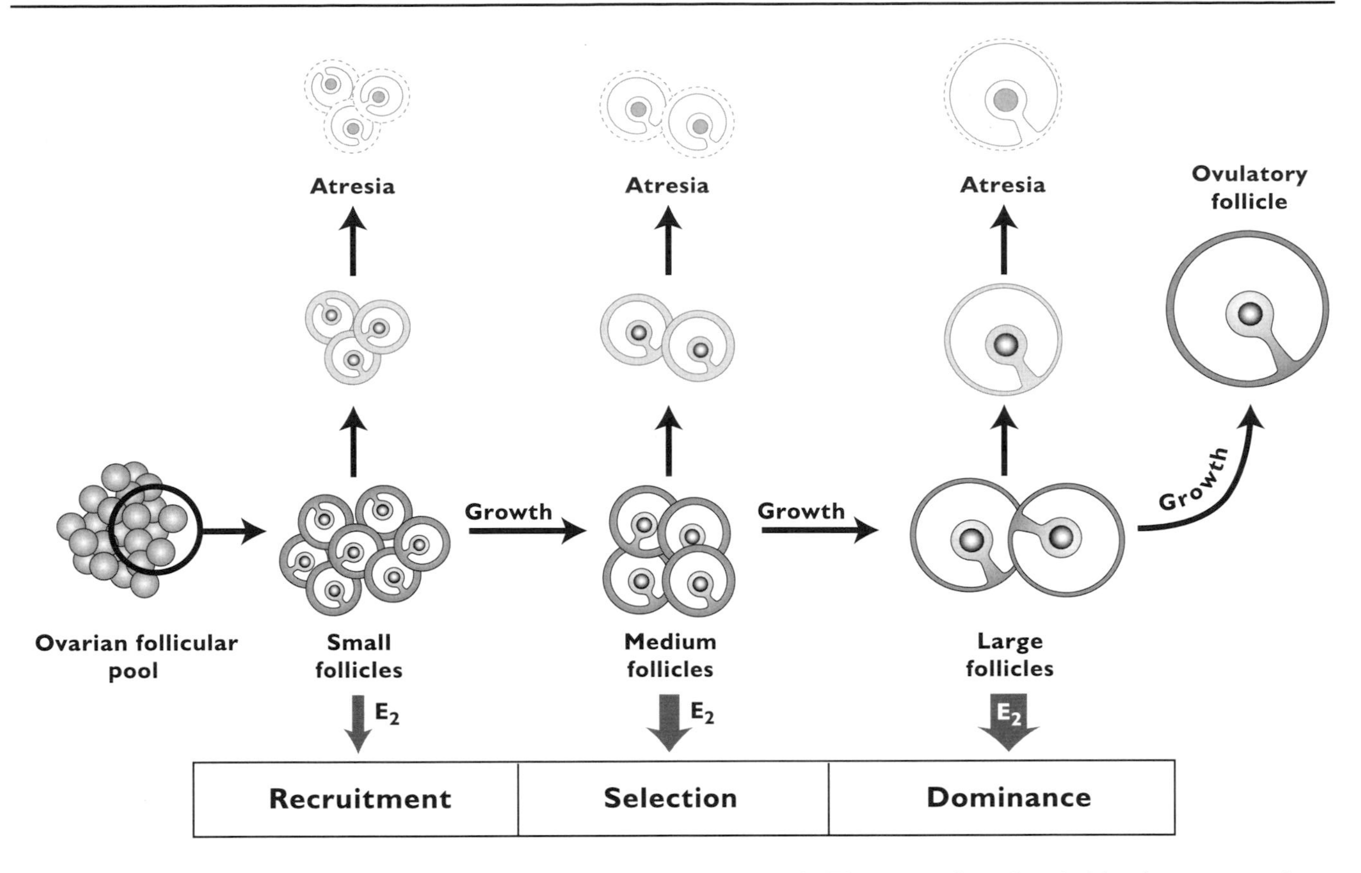

Figure 8-5. Small antral follicles are **recruited** from the ovarian pool. They are **selected** and either become atretic or develop into **dominant** follicles that ovulate. (Graphic by Sonja Oei.)

in response to tonic levels of FSH and LH and these antral follicles are always present. If you were to examine the ovaries at any point during the estrous cycle, you would see a significant number of antral follicles of various sizes. These antral follicles have been classified by scientists studying follicular dynamics as small, medium or large depending on their diameter. For example, in the pig the small, medium and large classifications consist of follicles measuring less than 3mm, 4 to 6mm and greater than 6mm in diameter, respectively. However, in the mare, the sizes of these same classifications are less than 10mm, 10 to 20mm and greater than 20 mm. The number of small antral follicles may exceed 100 for a pair of ovaries in the pig. Large follicles nearly always can be seen on the ovaries in species where only a single follicle ovulates, like the cow and the mare. These large follicles represent those that have reached the greatest size possible under the existing endocrine conditions.

Dynamics of antral follicles consist of:

- ***recruitment***
- ***selection***
- ***dominance***
- ***atresia***

The dynamics of antral follicles involve three major events. These events are **recruitment**, **selection** and **dominance** (Figure 8-5). Recruitment is the phase of follicular development in which a group (cohort) of small antral follicles begins to grow and produce estradiol. Some of the recruited follicles undergo atresia. Following recruitment, a group of growing follicles which have not undergone atresia are selected. Selection involves the emergence of dominant follicles (potentially ovulatory) from the cohort of previously recruited antral follicles. Selected follicles may become dominant or they may undergo atresia. As the selected follicles proceed toward dominance, they continue to produce increasing amounts of estrogen as well as the hormone inhibin. Recall, that inhibin is a protein hormone produced by the follicle that selectively inhibits the release of FSH from the anterior pituitary.

In the cow and the mare, **monotocous** species (giving birth to a single offspring), there are several selected follicles, but only one will develop into the dominant follicle. However, in **polytocous** species (litter bearers) there are multiple dominant follicles. The condition of dominance is characterized by one or more large preovulatory follicles exerting a major inhibitory effect on other antral follicles from the recruited and selected cohort. This inhibitory influence is thought to be caused by a combination of the production of inhibin by the dominant follicle and reduced blood supply to some follicles. Suppressed FSH concentrations in the blood, coupled with reduced blood supply to some follicles results in atresia. Only those follicles receiving a large blood supply (and thus higher levels of gonadotropin) continue to grow.

Atresia occurs continuously throughout folliculogenesis.

The process of **atresia** involves far more follicles than does the process of dominance. In fact, over 90% of ovarian follicles undergo a degenerative process called atresia. Atresia is a Greek word (a = not; tresia = perforated). The word atresia in the follicular context refers to the closure or disappearance of the antrum, which accompanies the degenerative changes of an antral follicle. At any one point in time during the postpubertal reproductive period, the proportion of atretic antral follicles is quite high. For example, if you were to examine the ovaries of a rat, about 70% of antral follicles would be in some stage of atresia. In the mouse 50% are atretic, in the rabbit 60% and in the human 50 to 75%.

As seen in Figure 8-6, during metestrus (days 3 to 5 in cattle), a group of follicles is recruited. However, these follicles do not encounter the appropriate endocrine conditions for continued development and undergo atresia within the ovary. During diestrus, a second follicular wave occurs, but these follicles also undergo atresia. Note that the first two follicular waves begin and terminate during times in the cycle when progesterone is increasing or is at its highest level. Ovulation cannot occur under progesterone dominance. During progesterone dominance, GnRH is released in low quantities and thus FSH and LH are low. It should be

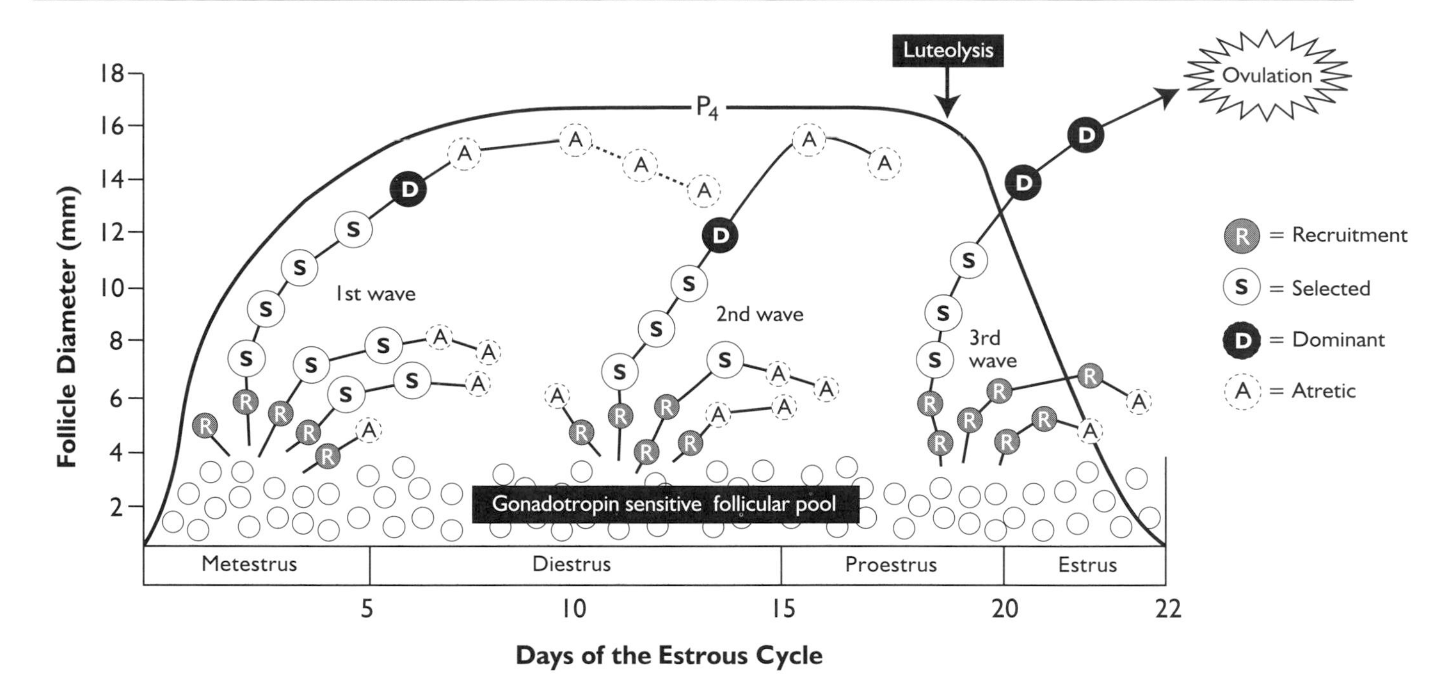

Figure 8-6. Several follicular waves occur during one estrous cycle. The third follicular wave (occurring after luteolysis) results in a dominant follicle which will ovulate. Note in the figure that the first two follicular waves occur either during progesterone elevation (metestrus) or during peak progesterone production (diestrus). Follicles recruited during these phases of the cycle will become atretic. Only those follicles recruited during or after luteolysis will become eligible for ovulation. (Modified from Lucy *et al.*, 1992.)

emphasized that even though follicles in the first two follicular waves become atretic they still produce some estradiol. In fact, midcycle estradiol increases and declines with each follicular wave but blood concentrations are not high. After luteolysis (corpus luteum regression), a third wave of follicles develops. One or more of these follicles will develop into the dominant and the preovulatory follicle. It must be emphasized that the endocrine condition for final follicular development will exist only after luteolysis and subsequent decline in progesterone. Also, the number of follicular waves within a given cycle varies among and within species.

Follicular waves of antral follicles are not unique to the estrous cycle. They occur before puberty, during pregnancy, during anestrus and during the postpartum recovery period. However, follicular waves occurring during these times do not yield dominant follicles which produce threshold levels of estradiol.

The above discussion has focused almost entirely on growth and atresia of antral follicles. You should recognize that the majority of a follicle's lifetime is spent in preantral stages. Recruitment, selection and dominance are relatively short-term processes when compared to the preantral stages.

***Recruitment* = high FSH + low LH + no inhibin**

***Selection* = moderate FSH + moderate LH + low inhibin**

***Dominance* = low FSH + high LH + high inhibin**

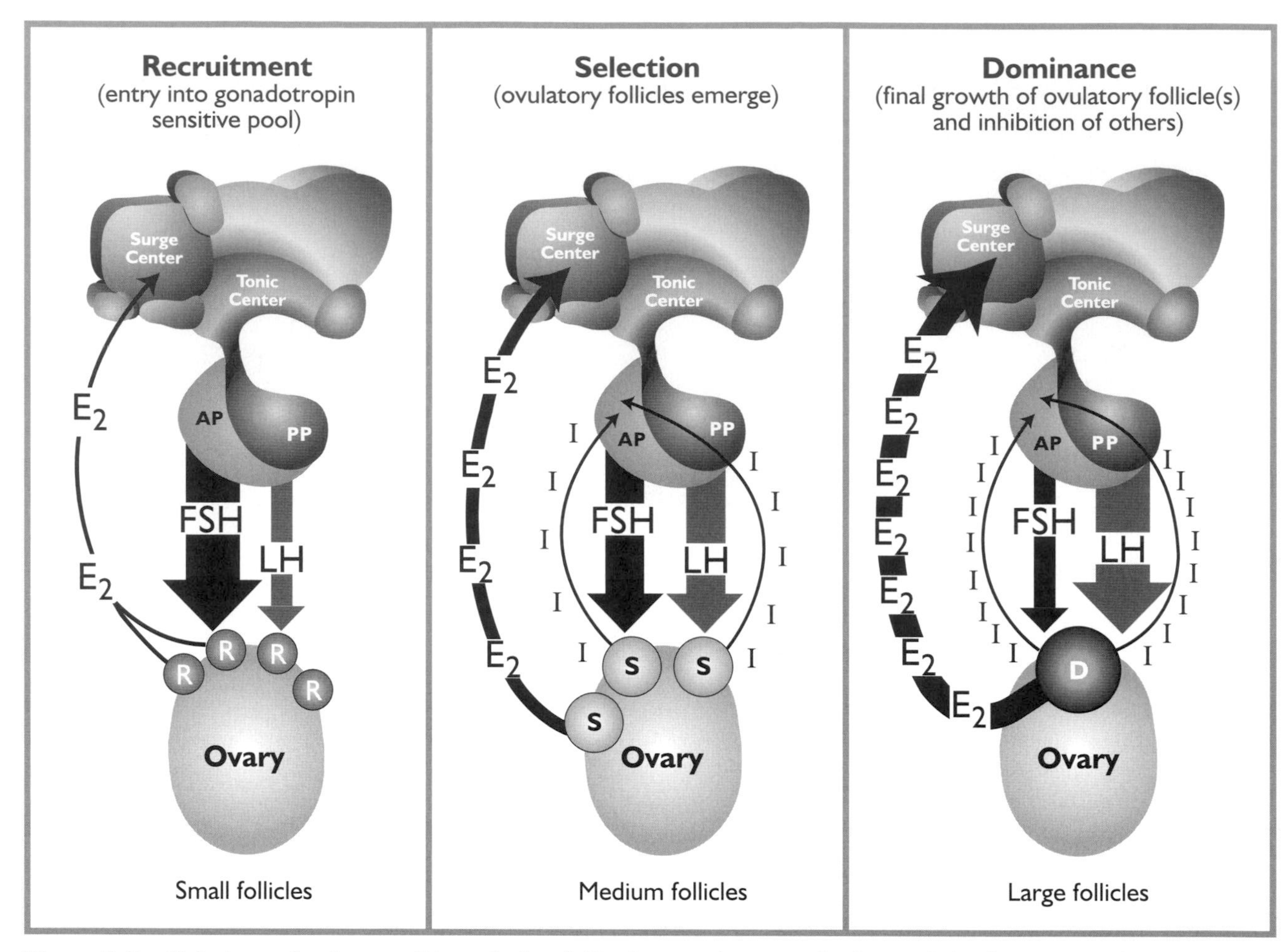

Figure 8-7. Relative endocrine conditions during follicular recruitment, selection and dominance. During recruitment FSH and LH begin to increase, thus promoting follicular development. As the follicles enter the selection phase, inhibin is produced by the follicle and begins to inhibit FSH release by the anterior pituitary. Thus, the relative roles of LH and FSH begin to change and the role of FSH declines and LH increases. As the follicular dominance phase is entered, the large follicle produces more and more estrogen and this prompts the preovulatory center to release a surge of LH. In addition, FSH concentrations are reduced because inhibin has suppressed FSH release from the anterior pituitary almost entirely. This probably causes other antral follicles to undergo atresia. (Modified from Driancourt, *et al.* (1993) in *Reproduction in Mammals and Man.*) (Graphic by Sonja Oei.)

Follicle preparation for ovulation occurs under a set of endocrine conditions that is different from the first two waves. The fundamental difference is that FSH and LH are at higher concentrations than during the time of previous waves because the inhibition of GnRH by progesterone has been removed. Figure 8-7 illustrates the relative roles of FSH and LH during the preovulatory wave of follicle development. Preovulatory follicles are recruited and selected during proestrus and eventually dominate during estrus. Elevated levels of FSH induce recruitment of follicles from the gonadotropin sensitive pool within the ovary. Once the follicles are recruited, they begin to produce estradiol and small quantities of inhibin. As the inhibin levels increase (during selection), the degree of negative feedback on the anterior pituitary increases. Thus, FSH begins to decline and LH begins to become more important than FSH in follicular development. As soon as FSH concentrations decline to a certain point, recruitment of other follicles stops. In addition, excess follicles in the cohort (those originally recruited) become atretic. The stage of dominance is characterized by continued decreasing FSH levels and increasing LH levels. The dominant follicle continues to grow, even though FSH levels are reduced, because apparently the dominant follicle's requirement for FSH is reduced. Estradiol levels from the dominant follicle are now approaching threshold, and the dominant follicle is now reaching its maximum size. When estradiol levels reach threshold, the preovulatory LH surge occurs, which dramatically alters the function of the follicle. The estrogen secretion by the dominant follicle declines abruptly once the preovulatory surge of LH occurs (Figure 8-4).

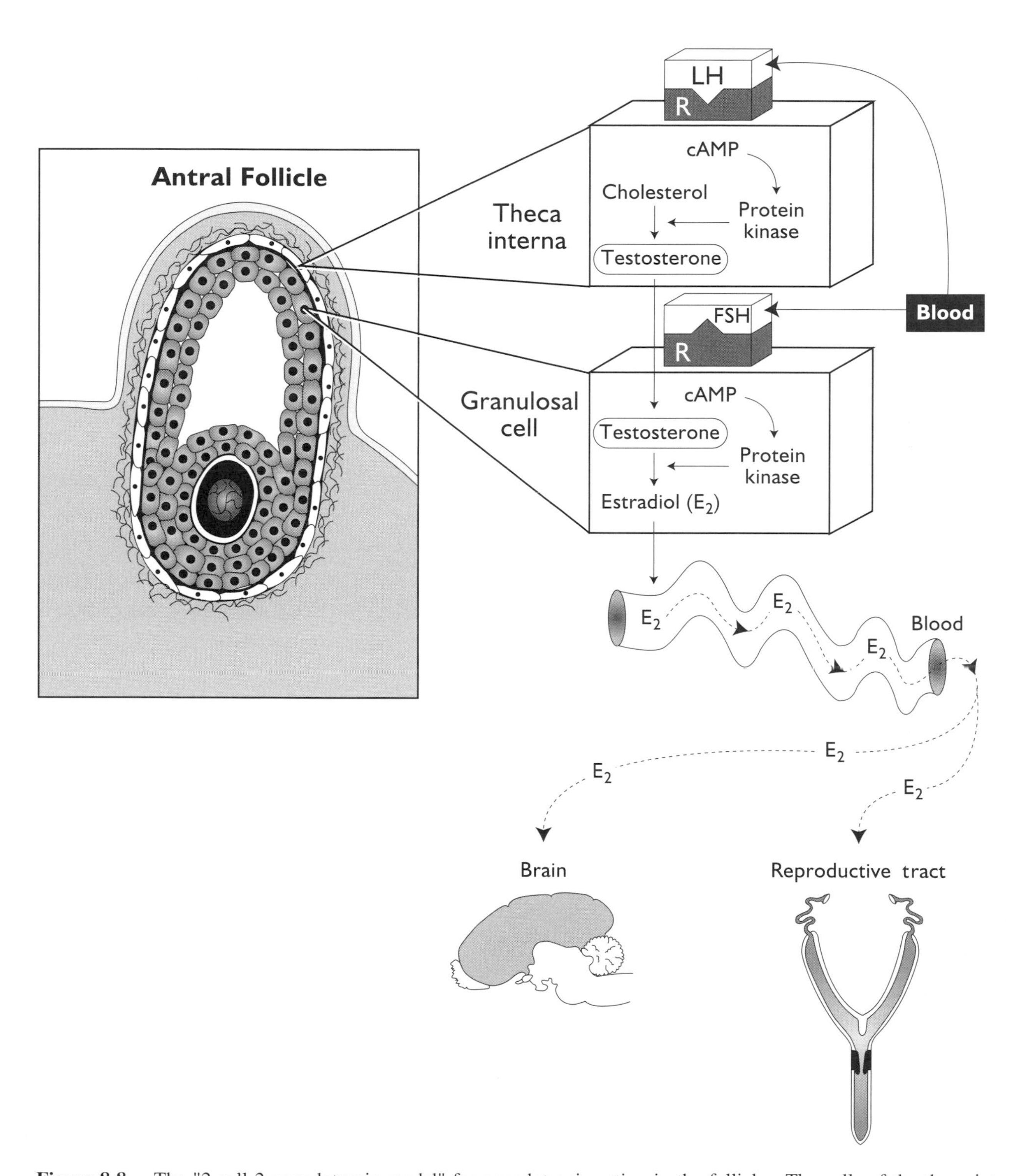

Figure 8-8. The "2-cell 2-gonadotropin model" for gonadotropin action in the follicle. The cells of the theca interna contain receptors to LH. Thecal cells produce testosterone that diffuses into the granulosal cells which contain FSH receptors. Binding of FSH to its receptors causes the synthesis of enzymes which are responsible for the conversion of testosterone to estradiol. (Graphic by Sonja Oei.)

"The 2-Cell, 2-Gonadotropin Model" Describes Estrogen Synthesis

During follicular development, LH binds to LH-specific receptors located on the cells of the theca interna of the developing follicle (Figure 8-8). The binding of LH to its receptors activates a cascade of intracellular events, described in Chapter 5. The net effect is conversion of cholesterol to testosterone. Testosterone then diffuses out of the cells of the theca interna and enters the granulosal cells. The granulosal cells contain receptors for FSH. When FSH binds to its receptor, it causes the conversion of testosterone to estradiol. This 2-cell, 2-gonadotropin pathway continues to function until levels of estrogen increase to a threshold that induces the preovulatory LH surge. An important step in the preparation of the follicle for ovulation is the acquisition of LH receptors by granulosal cells. When the LH receptors are present, the preovulatory LH surge can exert its full effect on the follicle to cause ovulation.

Estrogen Induces Reproductive Behavior

Elevated estradiol coupled with low progesterone induces profound behavioral changes in the female. During the follicular phase, the female becomes sexually receptive and copulation can take place. It is important to recognize that the period of estrus is closely associated with, but precedes ovulation. Estrous behavior culminates with the female standing to be mounted by the male. The physiology of reproductive behavior will be discussed in detail in Chapter 11.

Ovulation results from a cascade of events starting with the LH surge.

The preovulatory surge of LH is critically important because it sets in motion a series of biochemical events that lead to ovulation. Ovulation is a complicated process that involves purposeful destruction of follicular tissue. The main events of the ovulatory cascade resulting from the LH surge are shown in Figure 8-9.

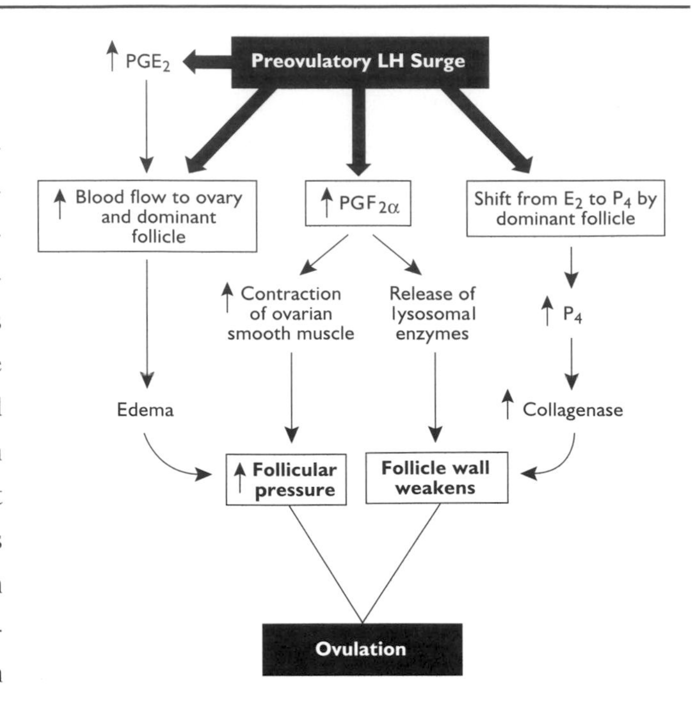

Figure 8-9. Summary of ovarian events caused by the preovulatory LH surge which leads to ovulation.

Ovulation is brought about by:
- ***elevated blood flow***
- ***breakdown of connective tissue***
- ***ovarian contractions***

Hyperemia (local elevated blood flow) is believed to be controlled at the tissue level by histamine and prostaglandin E_2 (PGE_2). Blood flow to the ovary has been shown to increase 7-fold after an injection of human chorionic gonadotropin (hCG), an LH-like hormone. In addition, there is elevated local blood flow to dominant follicles. Accompanying this local hyperemia, the theca interna becomes edematous because of increased vascular permeability brought about by histamine. This edematous condition causes elevated hydrostatic pressure around the follicle which may facilitate its eventual rupture. In addition to increased blood flow brought about by histamine and PGE_2, dominant follicles are thought to produce **angiogenic factors** (substances which promote the growth of new blood vessels). Angiogenic factors have been found in follicular fluid. Thus, the dominant follicle can potentially control its own blood flow during final development. The net effect of elevated blood flow is to ensure that the dominant preovulatory follicle is provided with the necessary hormonal and metabolic ingredients for final maturation.

The Dominant Follicle Begins to Produce Progesterone Before Ovulation

Following the LH surge, the cells of the theca interna begin to produce progesterone instead of testosterone. At first, this transition involves only a small quantity of progesterone which is produced locally (at the follicular level). This local elevation of progesterone is essential for ovulation because progesterone causes an enzyme called **collagenase** to be synthesized by the theca interna cells. Collagenase causes the breakdown of collagen, which is a major component of connective tissue. Connective tissue makes up the tunica albuginea, the outer connective tissue covering the ovary. At the same time that collagenase is "digesting" the collagen of the tunica albuginea, the granulosal cells increase their secretion of follicular fluid, which increases the fluid volume inside the follicle. Thus, follicular enlargement is closely coordinated with the enzymatic degradation of the tunica albuginea. As these two processes advance, the apex of the follicle called the **stigma** begins to push outward and weaken.

Prostaglandins Cause Ovarian Contraction and Aid in Follicular Remodeling

After the LH surge, both prostaglandin $F_{2\alpha}$ and prostaglandin E_2 are synthesized and released locally by the ovary. Prostaglandin $F_{2\alpha}$ causes contractions of the myoid (smooth muscle) components of the ovary. Thus, intermittent contractions may increase pressure locally and force the stigma to protrude even more dramatically from the surface of the ovary. Prostaglandin $F_{2\alpha}$ also causes lysosomes within the granulosal cells to rupture, releasing their enzymatic content. These lysosomal enzymes cause further connective tissue deterioration at the apex of the follicle.

The role of prostaglandin E_2 is to help the follicle remodel itself into a corpus luteum after ovulation. The follicle receives its direction for this reorganization from prostaglandin E_2. Prostaglandin E_2 is believed to activate a tissue reorganization factor called plasminogen. Plasminogen is a material which causes dissolution of blood clots. It is not unique to the ovary and is found throughout the body. Plasminogen helps dissolve the coagulum of the corpus hemorrhagicum.

Some Species Require Copulation Before Ovulation Can Occur

Among mammals there are two types of ovulators. These are known as **spontaneous ovulators** and **reflex (induced) ovulators**. Spontaneous ovulators ovulate with a regular frequency and do not require copulation. Ovulation is brought about totally in response to hormonal changes. Examples of spontaneous ovulators are the cow, sow, ewe, mare and human.

The **reflex (induced) ovulator** requires stimulation of the vagina and/or cervix for ovulation to occur. Examples of reflex ovulators are the rabbit, members of the cat family, the ferret and the mink. Also, camelids (camels, llamas and alpacas) are induced ovulators. With the exception of the rabbit, induced ovulators are sustained copulators. The pathway for induced ovulation is illustrated in Figure 8-10.

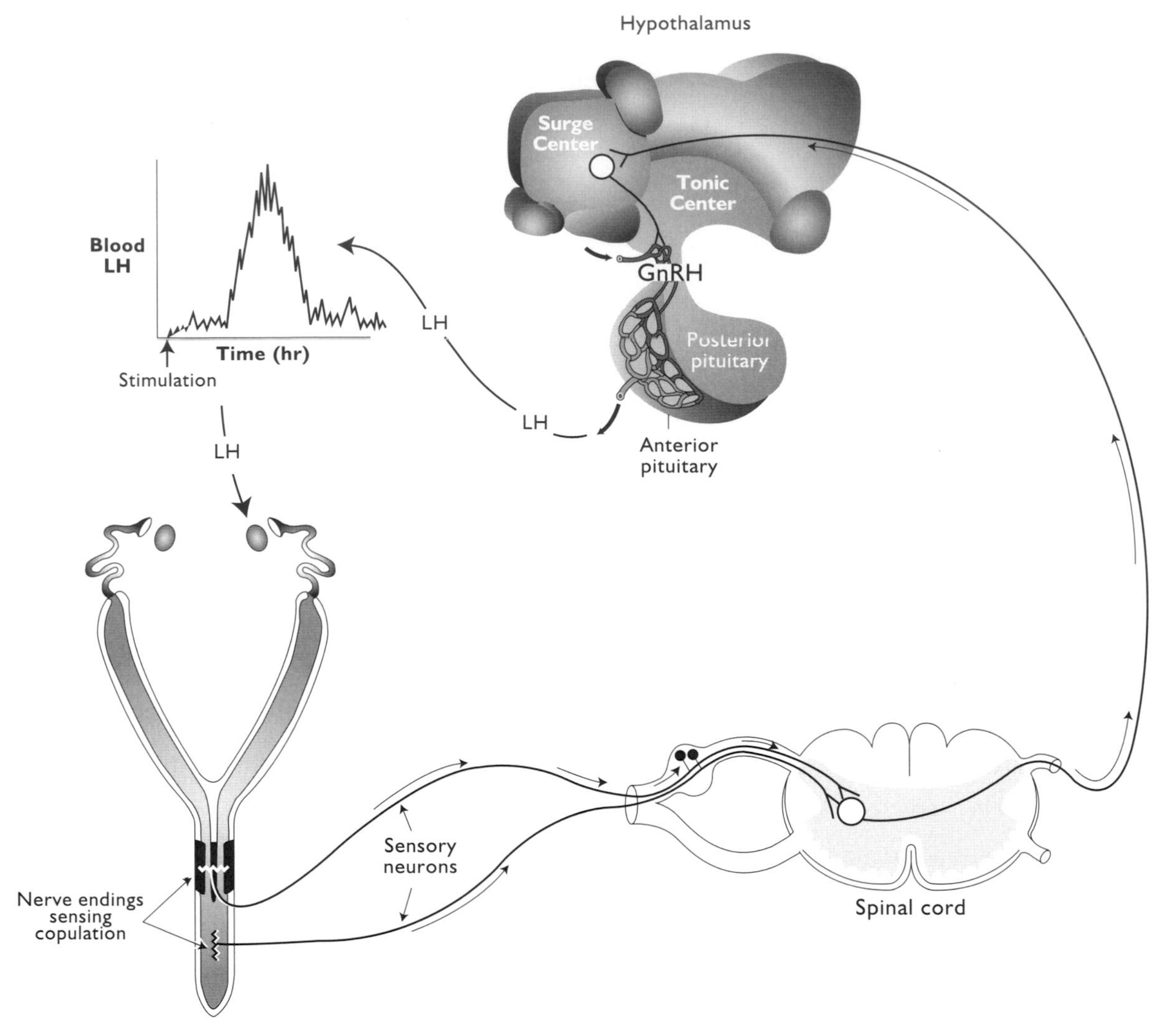

Figure 8-10. Schematic diagram illustrating the pathway for induced ovulation. Tactile stimulation of sensory nerves in the vagina and cervix brought about by copulation is relayed to the spinal cord and eventually to the preovulatory center in the hypothalamus. If the stimulus is of sufficient magnitude, neurons in the preovulatory center fire, causing large quantities of GnRH to be released. (Graphic by Sonja Oei.)

Females that are reflex ovulators can be induced artificially using electrical or mechanical stimulation. The tactile stimulation associated with copulation is converted into action potentials which travel through a pathway from the reproductive organ (the vagina and/or cervix) to the spinal cord. Afferent pathways innervate the hypothalamus. The elevated frequency of action potentials in the sensory nerves in the vagina and cervix causes increased firing of hypothalamic neurons, which then results in a preovulatory surge of GnRH. This release of GnRH in turn causes LH to be released, prompting the cascade of events leading to ovulation. In cats, a single copulation will induce ovulation about 50% of the time. Multiple copulations cause a much higher LH surge amplitude than single copulations. Induced ovulators, particularly the rabbit, make excellent experimental models, since the time of ovulation relative to the onset of reproductive tract stimulation can be controlled. In the rabbit, the timing of ovulation is quite precise relative to stimulation. Thus, if one has the desire to recover embryos or oocytes from the reproductive tract, a higher degree of precision can be achieved in the induced ovulator than with the spontaneous ovulator.

Some spontaneous ovulators (cow) apparently have some residual neural input from the reproductive tract which can alter the timing of the LH surge. For example, research has shown that when heifers (but not cows) are artificially inseminated and the insemination is accompanied by clitoral massage, the LH surge shifts toward the time of stimulation. This manipulation of the LH surge by neural stimulation suggests that the time of ovulation can be altered to some degree in spontaneous ovulators.

Folliculogenesis and Ovulation Can Be Artificially Induced Using Various Hormones

Understanding the basic hormonal requirements for follicular dynamics and ovulation has enabled the manipulation of the timing of ovulation for management and convenience purposes. Two main approaches have been developed. These are hormonally induced ovulation (generally coupled with induced estrus) and **superovulation**. Hormonally induced ovulation requires premature luteolysis or controlled luteolysis. Premature luteolysis can be accomplished using the administration of exogenous prostaglandin $F_{2\alpha}$. Prostaglandin $F_{2\alpha}$ causes luteolysis and therefore causes a decline in blood progesterone. This allows endogenous GnRH to be released, thus stimulating the release of FSH and LH from the anterior pituitary.

Another method to induce ovulation is to treat the animal with progestational (progesterone-like) compounds. Norgestomet is a synthetic progestogen which is used to control ovulation. Females are administered norgestomet in the form of an ear implant (a small capsule injected under the skin of the ear). The norgestomet releasing implant acts as an artificial corpus luteum. Thus, progesterone is high and therefore prevents FSH and LH from being released from the anterior pituitary in sufficient amounts for development and maintenance of the dominant follicle. Norgestomet does not, however, prevent normal luteolysis (Chapter 9). In fact, norgestomet implants are generally administered to cattle along with an injection of both estradiol and norgestomet. Estradiol induces luteolysis in cows, while norgestomet prevents estrus and ovulation. Removal of the norgestomet implant mimics luteolysis and thus follicular growth and ovulation are induced.

Progestational compounds such as 6-chloro-6-dihydro-17-acetoxyprogestrone (CAP), 6-methyl-17-acetoxyprogesterone (MAP) and melengestrol acetate (MGA) have also received intense research with regard to synchronizing estrus and ovulation in cattle. The level of synchrony after animals are treated with these progestational compounds has been quite high. However, fertility has always been suboptimal following use of these compounds.

Superovulation (abnormally high numbers of ovulations) requires the administration of exogenous gonadotropins which cause abnormally high numbers of follicles to be selected. Superovulated females ovulate abnormally high numbers of ova. Methods of superovulation usually include injections of equine chorionic gonadotropin (eCG) or FSH followed by administration of LH, GnRH or human chorionic gonadotropin (hCG) several days later to induce ovulation. The principle of superovulation involves providing the female with higher than normal levels of FSH so that greater numbers of follicles are recruited and selected. Dosages of exogenous gonadotropins required to induce superovulation vary among species.

The four phases of oocyte maturation are:

- ***mitotic division of primordial germ cells (prenatal)***
- ***nuclear arrest (dictyotene)***
- ***cytoplasmic growth***
- ***resumption of meiosis***

Oocyte maturation is not limited to the follicular phase, but occurs throughout the lifetime of the female. Maturation of oocytes occurs in four phases beginning during embryonic development of the female and continuing throughout her reproductive lifetime.

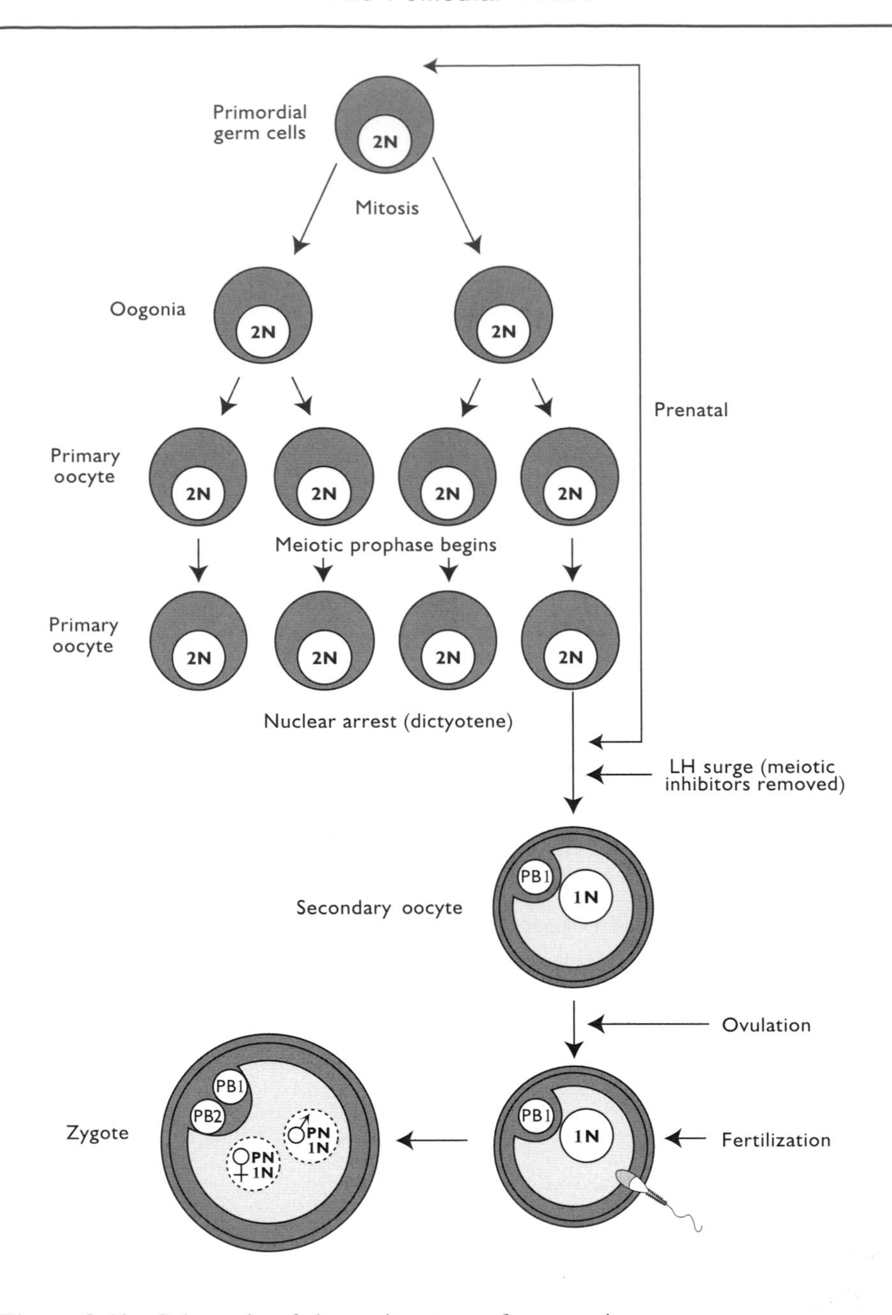

Figure 8-11. Schematic of the major steps of oogenesis.

Mitotic divisions occur prenatally (Chapter 4) and insure that the female is born with a complete supply of germ cells that will provide a future follicular reservoir. Further mitotic activity does not take place postnatally except for a few postnatal days in the rabbit. The last mitotic division from the oogonia to the primary oocyte constitutes an important step because the primary oocyte enters the first meiotic prophase (Figure 8-11). The meiotic prophase is then arrested and the nucleus of the oocyte becomes dormant and will remain so until stimulated by gonadotropins after puberty. This nuclear arrest condition is referred to as the **dictyate (dictyotene) phase** of meiotic prophase. This dictyotene phase is a state of meiosis in which the nucleus of the primary oocyte is arrested. The oocyte remains arrested for a prolonged period of time from late fetal life through birth and puberty. Oocytes remain in this period of dictyotene arrest until ovulation occurs or even later with some species. The purpose of this nuclear arrest is to inactivate the DNA in the female gamete so that it is not vulnerable to possible insult during the lifetime of the female. Insults, or damage to DNA of the female gamete could compromise reproduction because embryo death would likely occur after fertilization.

Oocyte Growth Involves Formation of a Large Cytoplasm and the Zona Pellucida

The neonatal female enters a period of somatic growth and development in which body growth increases but the gonad remains relatively dormant. During this period of growth, however, some of the primary oocytes begin to accumulate larger volumes of cytoplasm and develop a translucent band around this cytoplasm known as the **zona pellucida,** which is formed during the secondary follicle stage. An important development during this stage of maturation is the establishment of **junctional complexes** between neighboring follicular cells and the oocyte, which permit ionic and electronic coupling between different cell types. These cell contacts are important for communication between the oocyte and the adjacent granulosal cells. These junctions are known as **gap junctions** and are illustrated in Figure 8-12. Their presence is especially important after the formation of the zona pellucida which would serve as a barrier limiting diffusion of materials into the oocyte.

Oocyte growth is believed to be mediated primarily by granulosal cells of the follicle. Indeed, *in vitro* experiments have shown that oocytes cannot develop unless follicular cells and the existence of functional gap junctions are present. Gap junctions between granulosal cells and the plasma membrane of the oocyte remain intact until the time of the preovulatory LH surge. During the growth phase, the volume of oocyte cytoplasm increases about 50 times. Presumably, the ability of the oocyte cytoplasm to develop is a direct function of the ability of the cell to maintain functional contact with the granulosal cell.

It was once thought that the zona pellucida was formed exclusively by the follicle cells adjacent to the oocyte. It is now evident that the oocyte itself is primarily responsible for the synthesis of the zona pellucida. The substrates for this **mucopolysaccharide** material are moved from the granulosal cells through their finger-like projections into the oocyte. The components of the final zona pellucida are synthesized by the oocyte

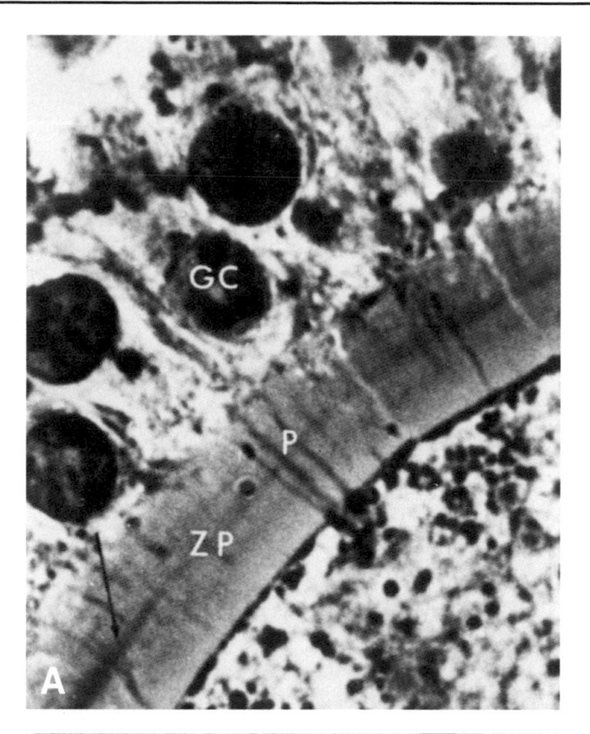

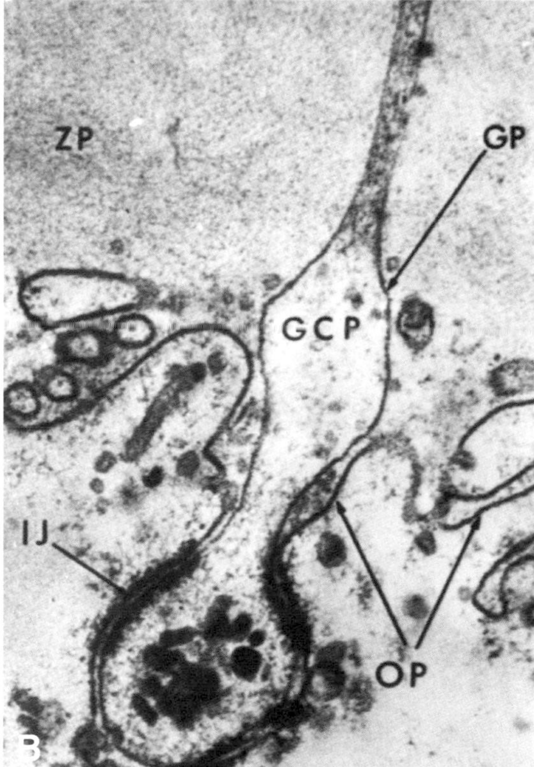

Figure 8-12. Relationship between granulosal cells and the developing bovine oocyte. **A**. Light micrograph showing granulosal cells (GC) with their projections (P) penetrating the zona pellucida (ZP). **B**. Electron micrograph of granulosal cell process (GCP) coursing the zona pellucida (ZP). The plasma membrane of the granulosal cells (GP) is intact and forms junctions (IJ) with the oocyte plasma membrane (OP). These granulosal cells are believed to govern the development of the oocyte. (Micrographs courtesy of R.G. Saacke, Dept. of Dairy Science VPI and SU, Blacksburg, VA.)

itself and then transferred out of the oocyte to form the thick, translucent layer surrounding the cytoplasm (Figure 8-12). At the time of antrum formation in the follicle, the oocyte has attained its full cytoplasmic size and these oocytes presumably have the potential to undergo a nuclear maturation provided that atresia has not been initiated.

Final Maturation and Resumption of Meiosis Occur Near the Time of Ovulation

Once the follicle has entered the dominance phase, the oocyte becomes poised to resume meiosis. It is believed that when the oocyte reaches a critical minimum size, it gains the ability to resume meiosis when the ovulatory LH discharge occurs. Shortly after the LH surge, the gap junctions between the granulosal cells and the oocyte deteriorate. This deterioration precedes meiotic resumption and it is thought that this disruption of communication between the granulosal cells and the oocyte cytoplasm removes the inhibition upon meiosis. The timing of the deterioration of gap junctions varies among species. Therefore, the resumption of meiosis cannot be explained totally by the breakdown of these cellular junctions. For example, in the sheep, pig, mouse and hamster the relationship between the follicle cells and the oocyte is the main factor controlling resumption of meiosis. It is clear that this event takes place in the dominant follicle just prior to ovulation in most mammals. In the dog and the fox, ovulation occurs before meiosis is resumed.

The dictyate stage meiotic block must be interrupted to permit final oocyte maturation. The discharge of gonadotropins is necessary to release the oocyte from inhibitors, presumably provided by the granulosal cells. Cyclic AMP (cAMP) provided by granulosal cells is proposed as the primary inhibitor of meiotic resumption. When granulosal projections dissociate from the cytoplasm of the oocyte, cAMP is no longer available to the oocyte. Another substance called **oocyte meiotic inhibitor** (OMI) has been implicated in controlling the resumption of meiosis. However, this substance has not been purified and its exact role remains uncertain. Once these inhibitors have been removed, the oocyte is free to proceed with the first meiotic division.

The resumption of meiosis is complex and can be described using a number of criteria. In the dominant follicle, the nucleus of the oocyte begins to migrate towards the periphery and flattens against the oocyte plasma membrane. The peripheral migration of the nucleus constitutes an early morphologic sign of the initiation of final oocyte maturation. This migration takes place after the ovulatory surge of LH in rodents and carnivores. In ruminants, the nucleus becomes polymorphic with many folds. This lobulation is then followed by a dissociation of the nuclear membrane. The bivalent chromosomes then line up and the chromatids are then separated by a microtubule system which pulls the chromosome apart, forming the **first polar body**. This meiotic division generally occurs slightly before ovulation. After fertilization, the second meiotic division will occur, producing the **second polar body**. In some cases, the first polar body will divide, producing two additional "daughter" polar bodies. In this case, three polar bodies can be observed.

Further Phenomena for Fertility

Aristotle reported that "Camels copulate with the female in a sitting posture and the male straddles over and covers her...and they pass the whole day long in the operation." The practical significance of this relates to the use of camels as pack animals during military operations. Aristotle reported that camels were spayed (removal of ovaries) to prevent pregnancy. An equally important reason for spaying the female camel was to prevent estrus so that excessive time spent copulating would not interfere with military operations. Tribesmen also discovered that placing stones in the uterus prevented copulation during traveling and wars.

During estrus (2 to 4 days), lions can copulate more than a hundred times, with mating occurring every 15 minutes. It has been estimated that lions copulate 3,000 times for every cub that survives to the yearling stage. One male copulated 157 times in 55 hours with 2 different females. (Lions are induced ovulators.)

In the domestic chicken, ovarian progesterone induces the preovulatory surge of LH, not estradiol.

The elephant shrew and tenrec are natural superovulators. In fact, in the tenrec more than 40 follicles may ovulate, but litters of greater than 10 have not been observed. About 75% of the embryos die and are reabsorbed during gestation.

Female elephants in estrus attract males by releasing a pheromone which is excreted in the urine. This pheromone is potent and can attract bull elephants from miles away.

Female Old World monkeys have a "sex skin" (perianal skin). Under the influence of estrogen the "sex skin" becomes hyperemic and swells. This serves as a visual signal to males, "announcing" the optimum time for copulation.

Additional Reading

Lucy, W. C., J.D. Savio, L. Badinga, R.L. de la Sota and W.W. Thatcher, 1992. Factors that affect ovarian follicular dynamics in cattle. *J. Anim. Sci.* 70:3615.

Thibault, C., M.C. Levasseur, and H.F. Hunter, eds., 1993. *Reproduction in Mammals and Man.* Chapters 15, 16, 17.

9 The Luteal Phase of the Estrous Cycle

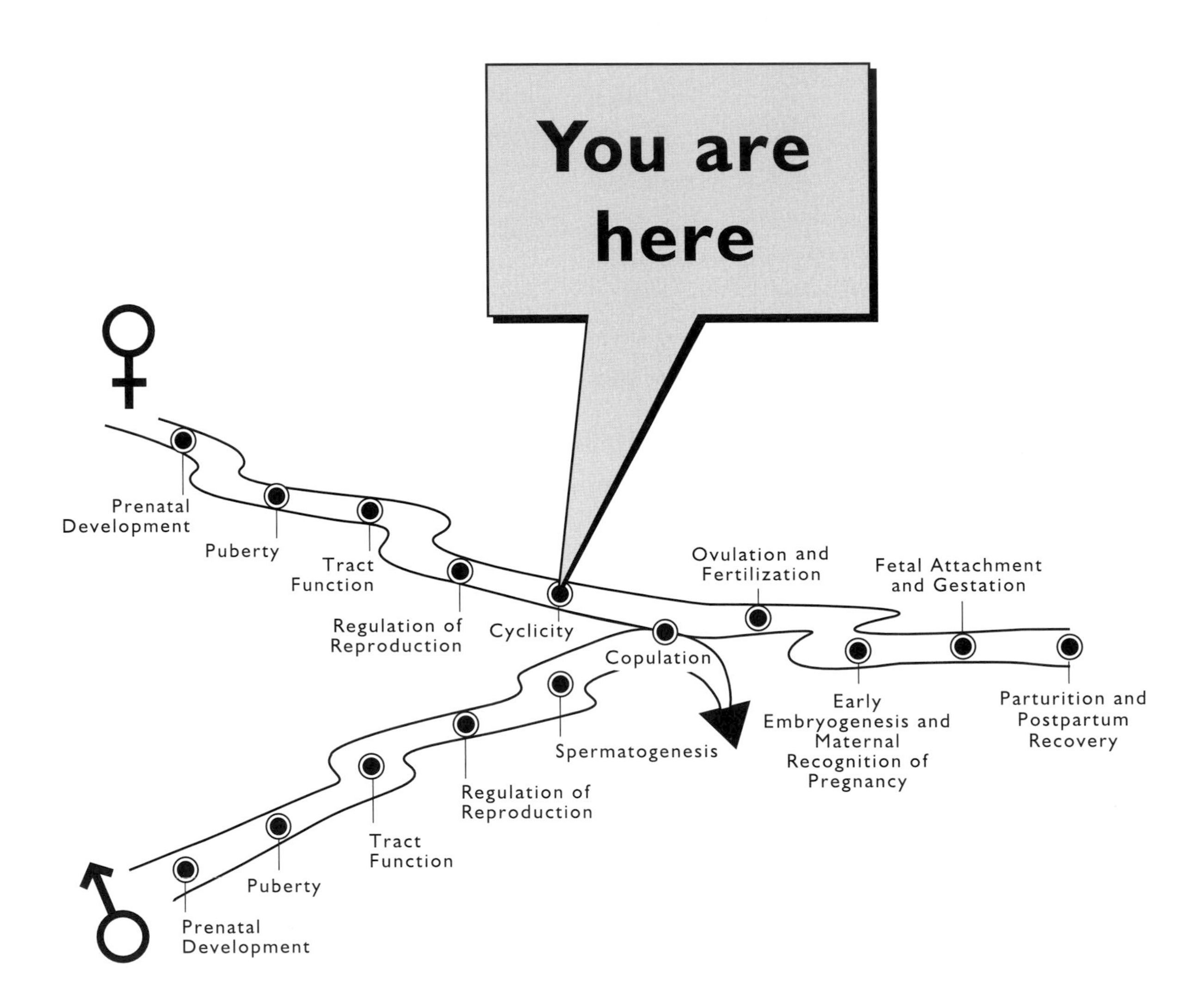

Take-Home Message

During the early luteal phase (metestrus), corpora lutea are formed from follicular cells. In the mid-luteal phase (diestrus), they produce large quantities of progesterone. During the late luteal phase, corpora lutea are destroyed (lysed) by prostaglandin $F_{2\alpha}$ which is produced by the uterine endometrium. Lysis of corpora lutea (luteolysis) is followed by a marked reduction in blood progesterone. The negative feedback exerted by progesterone on the hypothalamus is removed and the female enters a new follicular phase because GnRH increases.

The luteal phase lasts from the time of ovulation until regression (**luteolysis**) of the corpus luteum (CL) near the end of the estrous cycle. It includes **metestrus** and **diestrus** (Figure 9-1). The dominant ovarian hormone during the luteal phase is progesterone.

The luteal phase consists of:
- ***corpora lutea formation***
- ***production of progesterone***
- ***luteolysis***

When the follicle ruptures at ovulation, blood vessels within the follicular wall also rupture. This vascular breakage results in a structure with a "bloody" clot-like appearance. This structure is called the **corpus hemorrhagicum** because of its hemorrhagic (bloody) appearance when viewed from the surface of the ovary. Corpora hemorrhagica can be observed from the time of ovulation until about day 1 to 3 of the estrous cycle (Figures 9-3 through 9-6). Immediately after ovulation, corpora hemorrhagica appear as small, pimple-like structures on the surface of the ovary. At about day 3 to 5, the CL begins to increase in size and lose its hemorrhagic appearance. It increases in mass until the middle of the cycle, when its size is maximal

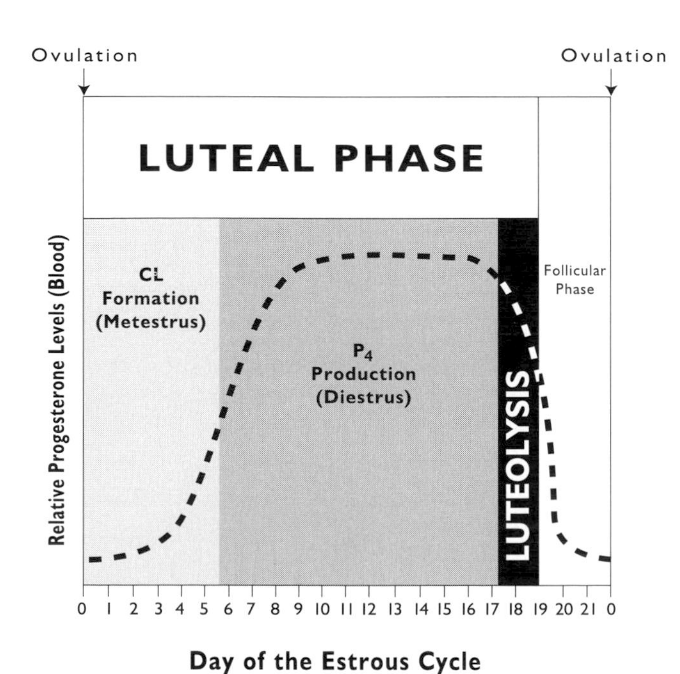

Figure 9-1. The luteal phase begins immediately after ovulation. During the early luteal phase, the corpus luteum (CL) develops (metestrus) and progesterone levels begin to increase. During the mid-luteal phase (diestrus) the corpus luteum is fully functional and progesterone (P_4) plateaus at relatively high levels. During the last 2 to 3 days of the luteal phase, destruction of the corpus luteum occurs (luteolysis) and the luteal phase terminates. Following luteolysis, a new follicular phase is initiated.

and coincides with the maximum production of progesterone during diestrus. Near the end of the luteal phase, luteolysis occurs and the CL loses its functional integrity and decreases in size. Luteolysis causes an irreversible structural degradation of the corpus luteum. A lysed corpus luteum will become a corpus albicans. In general, a corpus albicans can be observed for a substantial period of time (several estrous cycles) after luteolysis. This remnant of the corpus luteum appears as a white scar-like structure because of the connective tissue that remains after the glandular tissue disappears.

The corpus luteum originates from the ovulatory follicle.

After ovulation the **theca interna** and the **granulosal cells** of the follicle undergo a dramatic transformation known as **luteinization**. Luteinization is the process whereby cells of the ovulatory follicle are transformed into luteal tissue. This transformation is governed by LH. Shortly before ovulation the basement membrane of the follicle undergoes partial disintegration and the physical separation of the thecal and granulosal cells becomes incomplete (Figure 9-2). Immediately after ovulation the walls of the follicle collapse (implode) into many folds (Figure 9-2). These folds begin to interdigitate, allowing thecal cells and the granulosal cells to mix, thus forming a gland consisting of connective tissue cells, thecal cells and granulosal cells. In general, the cells of thecal origin and the cells of granulosal origin mix uniformly with one another (Figure 9-2). An exception to this is found in the corpora lutea of the human and other primates, where thecal and granulosal cells are clustered into distinct "islets." It is easy to distinguish microscopically between luteal cells that originate from the granulosal cells and those which originate from the thecal cells. Portions of the basement membrane which separated the thecal cells from the granulosal cells remain and constitute the connective tissue network of the corpus luteum (Figure 9-2).

In general, the corpus luteum increases in size until about midway through the luteal phase (Figures 9-3 through 9-6). In cattle, the corpus luteum can be palpated transrectally. However, the functional status of the corpus luteum is difficult to ascertain by transrectal palpation because the size of the corpus luteum is not always related to its progesterone producing ability. For example, a skilled examiner can almost always determine whether a corpus luteum is present or absent in cows. In mares it is almost impossible to ascertain the functional status of the corpus luteum because it does not protrude from the surface of the ovary.

In the cow, palpation cannot predict with accuracy the degree to which a corpus luteum is functional. In four separate studies cows were transrectally palpated by experienced diagnosticians. Corpora lutea were classified as functional (producing high levels of progesterone) or nonfunctional (regressing or producing low levels of progesterone) by the diagnosticians. Using measurements of blood progesterone as the indicator of corpus luteum function, it was found that 25% to 39% of cows classified as having a functional corpus luteum were not producing high levels of progesterone. Furthermore, 15% to 21% of cows classified as having a nonfunctional corpus luteum had high progesterone levels. Clearly, the use of transrectal palpation to assess the functional status of the corpus luteum has limitations. From a practical reproductive management perspective, this problem limits the effectiveness of treating animals with luteolytic agents to induce estrus and ovulation. In other words, administering luteolytic agents (prostaglandin $F_{2\alpha}$) on the basis of transrectal palpation alone will usually provide suboptimal results.

Recently, the use of real-time ultrasonography has proven effective for the examination of corpora lutea, as well as ovarian follicles. Veterinarians routinely use this technique in cows and mares to determine ovarian status.

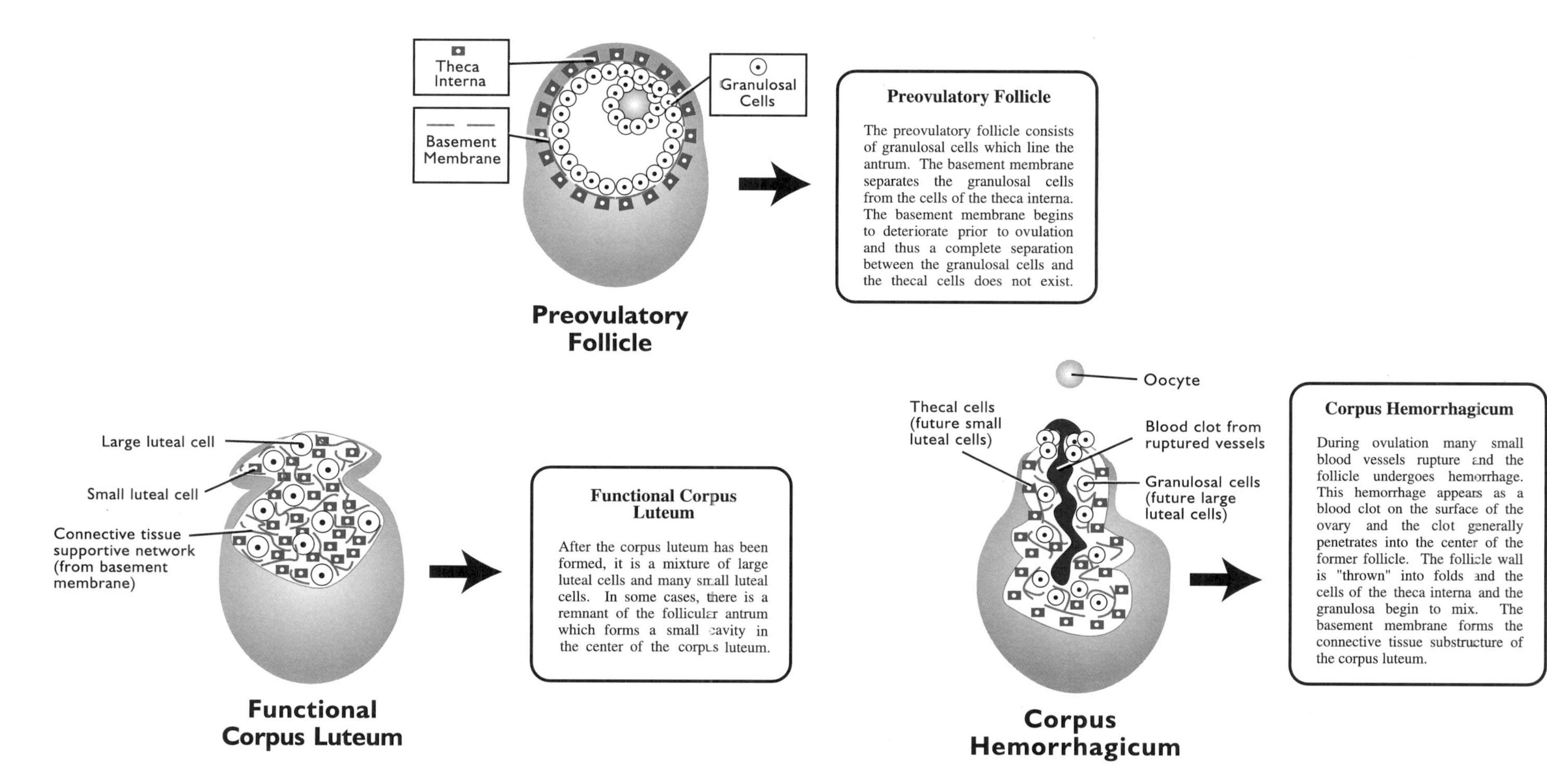

Theca Interna
Basement Membrane
Granulosal Cells
Preovulatory Follicle
Preovulatory Follicle
The preovulatory follicle consists of granulosal cells which line the antrum. The basement membrane separates the granulosal cells from the cells of the theca interna. The basement membrane begins to deteriorate prior to ovulation and thus a complete separation between the granulosal cells and the thecal cells does not exist.
Oocyte
Thecal cells (future small luteal cells)
Blood clot from ruptured vessels
Granulosal cells (future large luteal cells)
Corpus Hemorrhagicum
Corpus Hemorrhagicum
During ovulation many small blood vessels rupture and the follicle undergoes hemorrhage. This hemorrhage appears as a blood clot on the surface of the ovary and the clot generally penetrates into the center of the former follicle. The follicle wall is "thrown" into folds and the cells of the theca interna and the granulosa begin to mix. The basement membrane forms the connective tissue substructure of the corpus luteum.
Large luteal cell
Small luteal cell
Connective tissue supportive network (from basement membrane)
Functional Corpus Luteum
Functional Corpus Luteum
After the corpus luteum has been formed, it is a mixture of large luteal cells and many small luteal cells. In some cases, there is a remnant of the follicular antrum which forms a small cavity in the center of the corpus luteum.

Figure 9-2. Corpus luteum formation. (Graphic by Sonja Oei.)

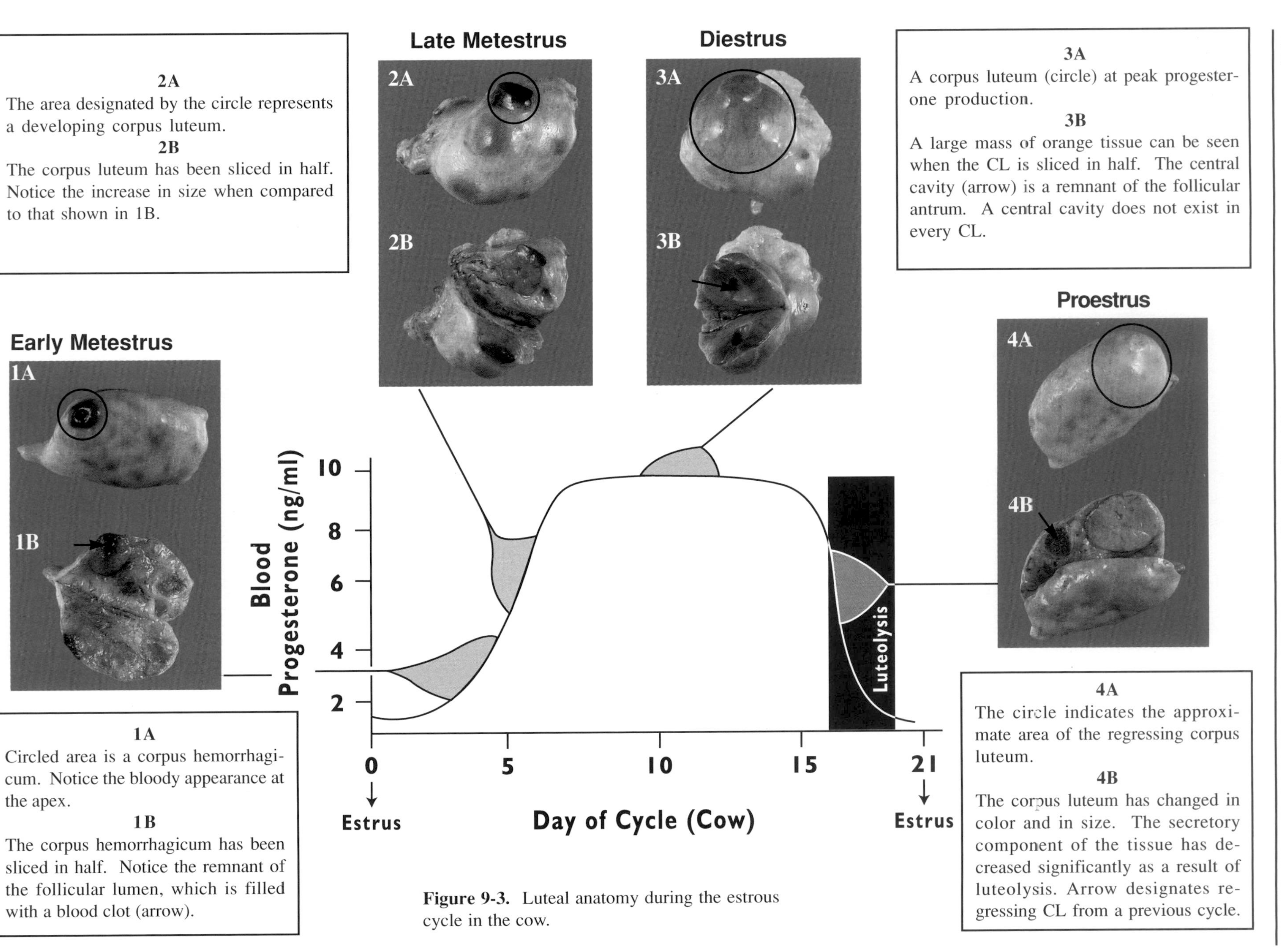

Early Metestrus
1A
1B
Late Metestrus
2A
2B
Diestrus
3A
3B
Proestrus
4A
4B
Blood Progesterone (ng/ml)
10
8
6
4
2
0
5
10
15
21
Estrus
Estrus
Day of Cycle (Cow)
Luteolysis
1A
Circled area is a corpus hemorrhagicum. Notice the bloody appearance at the apex.
1B
The corpus hemorrhagicum has been sliced in half. Notice the remnant of the follicular lumen, which is filled with a blood clot (arrow).
2A
The area designated by the circle represents a developing corpus luteum.
2B
The corpus luteum has been sliced in half. Notice the increase in size when compared to that shown in 1B.
3A
A corpus luteum (circle) at peak progesterone production.
3B
A large mass of orange tissue can be seen when the CL is sliced in half. The central cavity (arrow) is a remnant of the follicular antrum. A central cavity does not exist in every CL.
4A
The circle indicates the approximate area of the regressing corpus luteum.
4B
The corpus luteum has changed in color and in size. The secretory component of the tissue has decreased significantly as a result of luteolysis. Arrow designates regressing CL from a previous cycle.

Figure 9-3. Luteal anatomy during the estrous cycle in the cow.

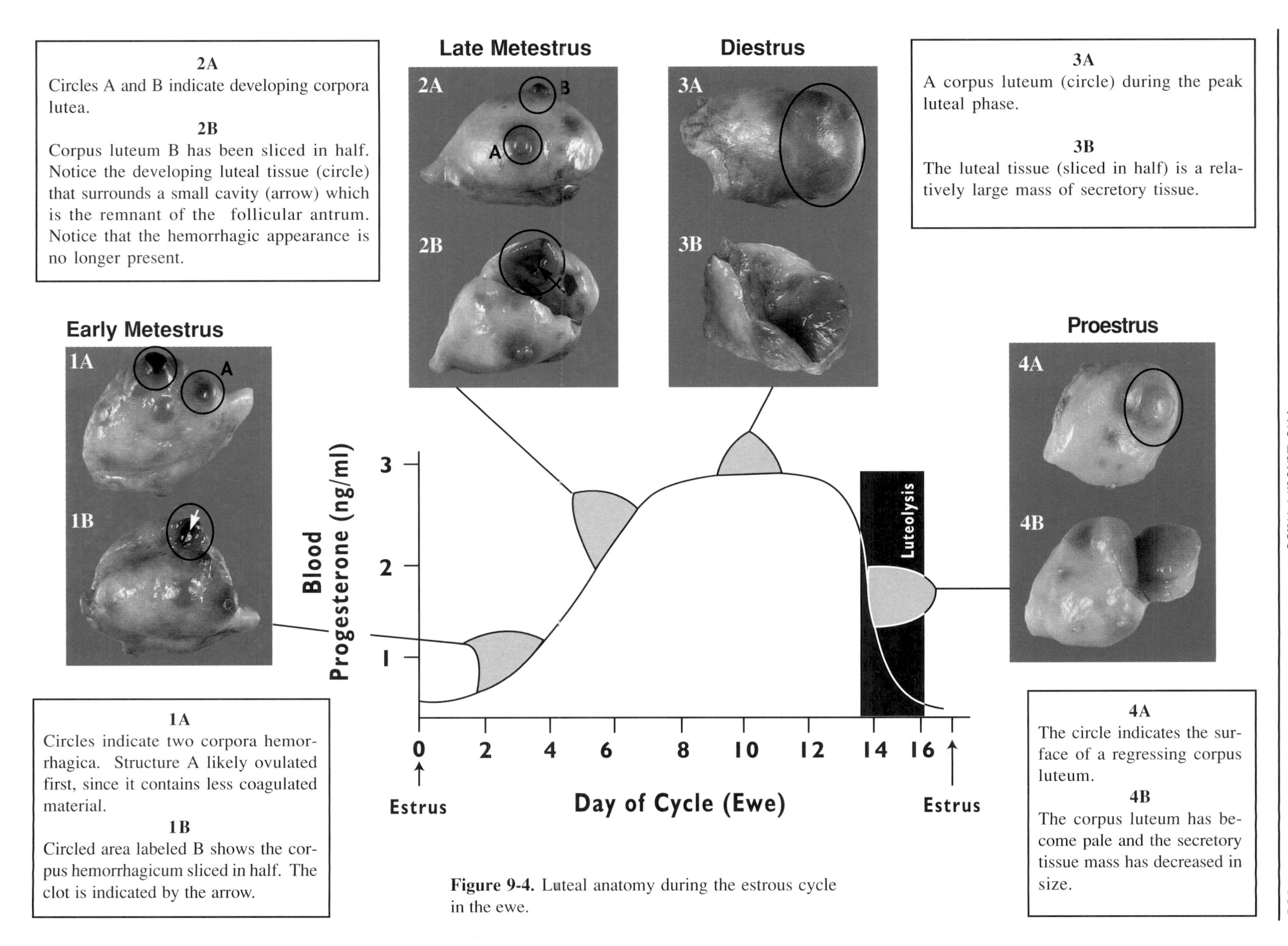

2A
Circles A and B indicate developing corpora lutea.
2B
Corpus luteum B has been sliced in half. Notice the developing luteal tissue (circle) that surrounds a small cavity (arrow) which is the remnant of the follicular antrum. Notice that the hemorrhagic appearance is no longer present.
Late Metestrus
2A
B
A
2B
Diestrus
3A
3B
3A
A corpus luteum (circle) during the peak luteal phase.
3B
The luteal tissue (sliced in half) is a relatively large mass of secretory tissue.
Early Metestrus
1A
A
1B
Proestrus
4A
4B
Blood Progesterone (ng/ml)
3
2
1
Luteolysis
0
2
4
6
8
10
12
14
16
Estrus
Day of Cycle (Ewe)
Estrus
1A
Circles indicate two corpora hemorrhagica. Structure A likely ovulated first, since it contains less coagulated material.
1B
Circled area labeled B shows the corpus hemorrhagicum sliced in half. The clot is indicated by the arrow.
4A
The circle indicates the surface of a regressing corpus luteum.
4B
The corpus luteum has become pale and the secretory tissue mass has decreased in size.

Figure 9-4. Luteal anatomy during the estrous cycle in the ewe.

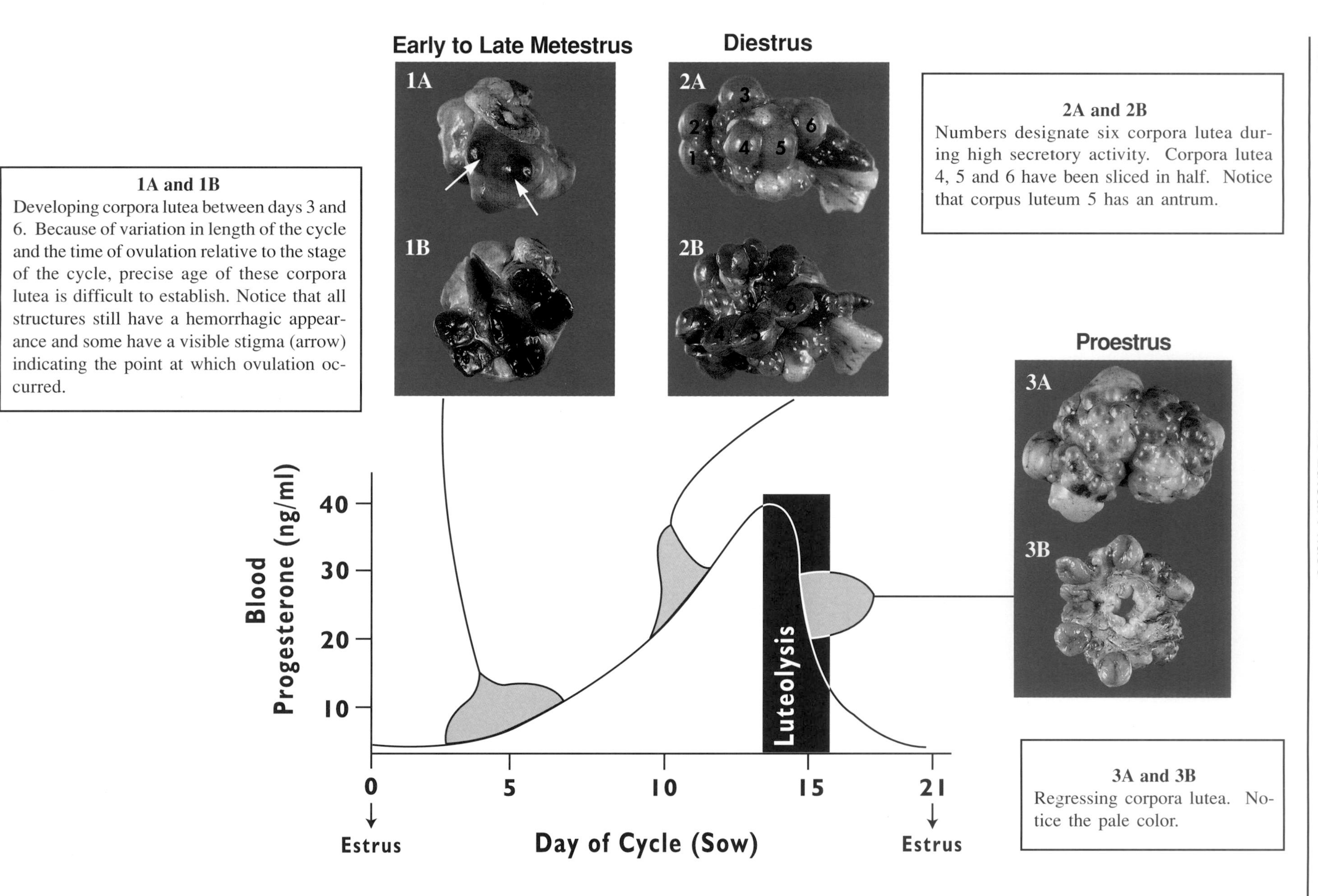

1A and 1B
Developing corpora lutea between days 3 and 6. Because of variation in length of the cycle and the time of ovulation relative to the stage of the cycle, precise age of these corpora lutea is difficult to establish. Notice that all structures still have a hemorrhagic appearance and some have a visible stigma (arrow) indicating the point at which ovulation occurred.
Early to Late Metestrus
1A
1B
Diestrus
2A
2B
1
2
3
4
5
6
2A and 2B
Numbers designate six corpora lutea during high secretory activity. Corpora lutea 4, 5 and 6 have been sliced in half. Notice that corpus luteum 5 has an antrum.
Proestrus
3A
3B
3A and 3B
Regressing corpora lutea. Notice the pale color.
Blood Progesterone (ng/ml)
40
30
20
10
Luteolysis
0
5
10
15
21
Estrus
Day of Cycle (Sow)
Estrus

Figure 9-5. Luteal anatomy during the estrous cycle in the sow.

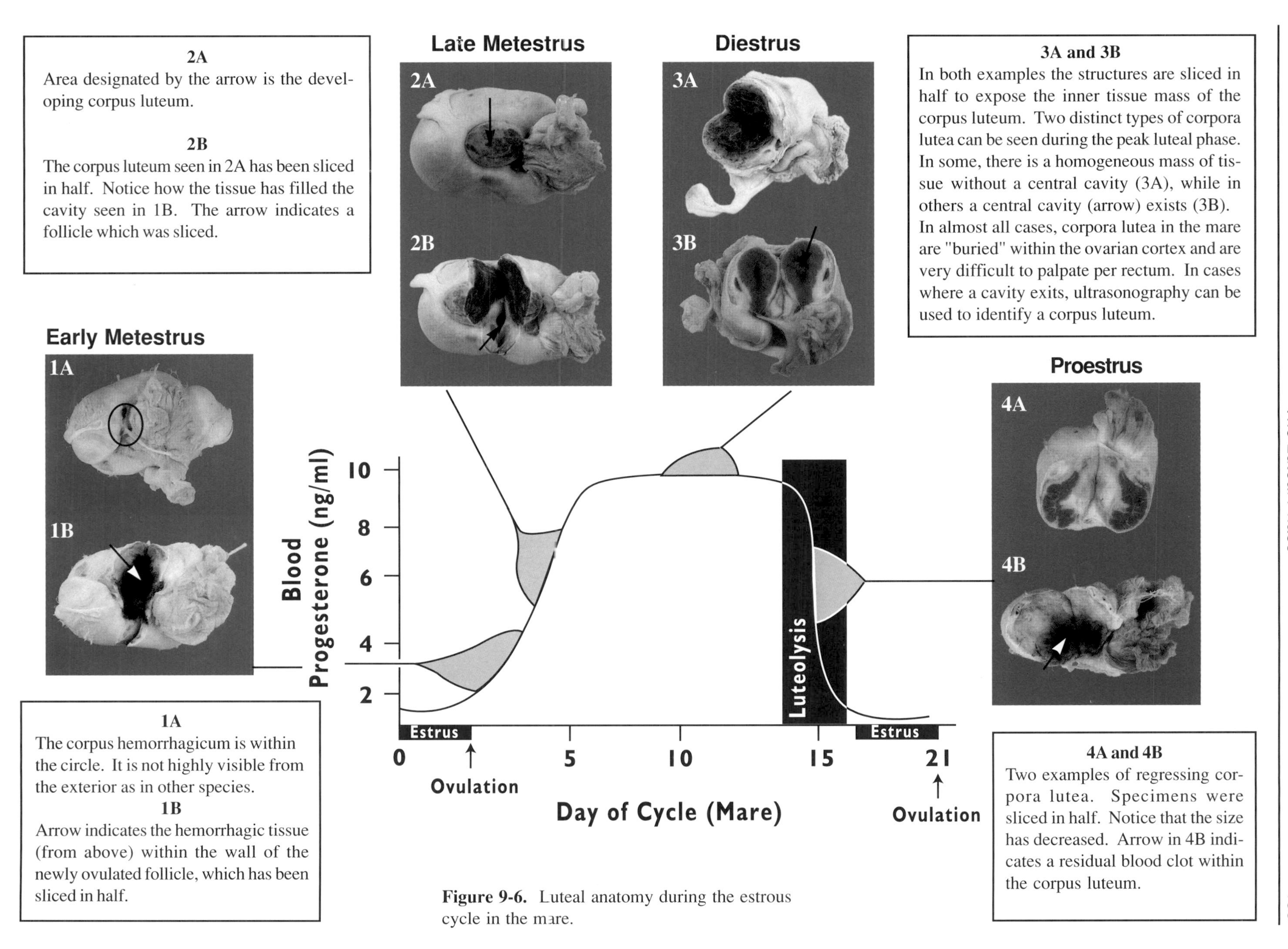

2A
Area designated by the arrow is the developing corpus luteum.
2B
The corpus luteum seen in 2A has been sliced in half. Notice how the tissue has filled the cavity seen in 1B. The arrow indicates a follicle which was sliced.
Late Metestrus
2A
2B
Diestrus
3A
3B
3A and 3B
In both examples the structures are sliced in half to expose the inner tissue mass of the corpus luteum. Two distinct types of corpora lutea can be seen during the peak luteal phase. In some, there is a homogeneous mass of tissue without a central cavity (3A), while in others a central cavity (arrow) exists (3B). In almost all cases, corpora lutea in the mare are "buried" within the ovarian cortex and are very difficult to palpate per rectum. In cases where a cavity exits, ultrasonography can be used to identify a corpus luteum.
Early Metestrus
1A
1B
Proestrus
4A
4B
Blood Progesterone (ng/ml)
10
8
6
4
2
Luteolysis
Estrus
Estrus
0
5
10
15
21
Ovulation
Ovulation
Day of Cycle (Mare)
1A
The corpus hemorrhagicum is within the circle. It is not highly visible from the exterior as in other species.
1B
Arrow indicates the hemorrhagic tissue (from above) within the wall of the newly ovulated follicle, which has been sliced in half.
4A and 4B
Two examples of regressing corpora lutea. Specimens were sliced in half. Notice that the size has decreased. Arrow in 4B indicates a residual blood clot within the corpus luteum.

Figure 9-6. Luteal anatomy during the estrous cycle in the mare.

> ***Luteal tissue consists of large and small luteal cells:***
> - ***large cells originate from the granulosal cells***
> - ***small cells originate from the cells of the theca interna***

Large luteal cells (sometimes called granulosal-lutein cells) vary in diameter from 20-40 micrometers (μm), depending on species. In some species (ruminants), there are a large number of dense secretory granules close to the plasma membrane (Figure 9-7B). These secretory granules contain **oxytocin** in the corpus luteum of the cycle and are believed to contain **relaxin** in the corpus luteum of pregnancy.

Small luteal cells (sometimes called thecal-lutein cells) are less than 20 μm in diameter, have an irregular shape and possess numerous lipid droplets in their cytoplasm (Figure 9-7). They do not contain secretory granules as do the large luteal cells. Both small and large luteal cells are **steroidogenic** (possessing the ability to produce steroids), in this case progesterone.

Large luteal cells rarely multiply after ovulation. Therefore, the total number of granulosal cells "donated" by the follicle determines the number of steroidogenic cells, and thus the steroidogenic potential of the newly formed corpora lutea. In other words, luteal function may be related to the vigor (as judged by the number of granulosal cells) of the follicle prior to ovulation. In the ewe (and presumably other species), an increase in corpus luteum size and weight is due to a threefold increase in volume of large luteal cells coupled with a fivefold increase in the number of small luteal cells. Thus, large luteal cells undergo **hypertrophy** (increase in size), while small luteal cells undergo **hyperplasia** (increase in cell numbers) as they progress toward luteolysis. In addition to changes in steroidogenic cells, non-steroidogenic cells (fibroblasts, capillary cells

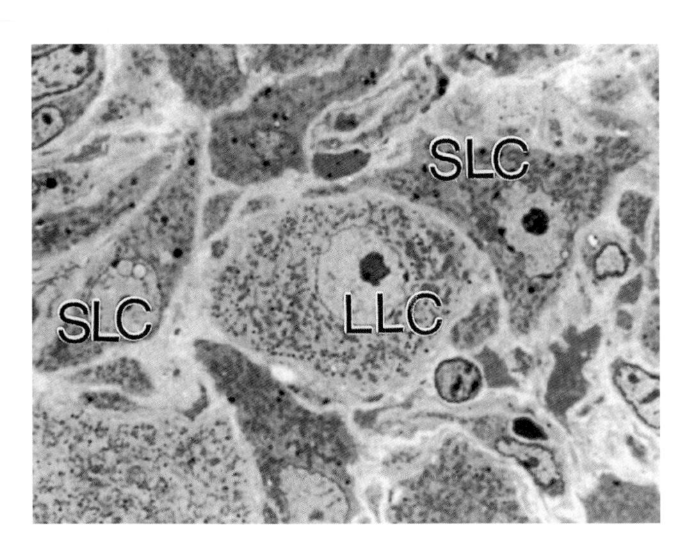

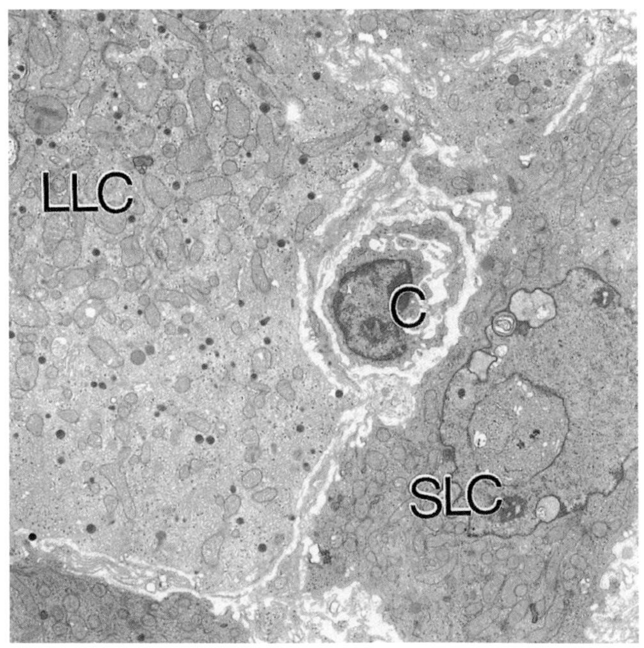

A **B**

Figure 9-7. Light (A) and electron micrograph (B) of ovine luteal cells at day 12 of the estrous cycle. Large luteal cells (LLC) are round, plump cells with a large spherical nucleus. These cells (LLC) are derived from granulosal cells. Small luteal cells (SLC), derived from the cells of the theca interna, are stellate in shape. The cytoplasm of small luteal cells is darker than in the large cells. Note the capillary (C) in B. Progesterone, produced by both cell types has ready access to the blood. (Micrographs courtesy of Dr. Heywood R. Sawyer, Department of Physiology, Colorado State University, Fort Collins.)

and eosinophils) increase in number during the estrous cycle. The net effect of these cellular changes is a marked enlargement of the corpus luteum.

> ***The "vigor" of the corpus luteum probably depends on:***
> - ***the number of luteal cells***
> - ***the degree to which the CL becomes vascularized***

The functional capability (ability to produce progesterone) of the newly developed corpus luteum may also depend on the degree of vascularity in the cellular layers of the follicle. The ability of the corpus luteum to vascularize may relate to its ability to synthesize and deliver hormones. As presented in the previous chapter, follicular fluid is known to contain angiogenic factors. The degree to which these angiogenic factors promote vascularization of the corpus luteum is probably related to the quantity of angiogenic factors present in the follicular tissue.

Insufficient luteal function (poor progesterone synthesis and secretion) is believed to be an important contributor to reproductive failure in food producing animals. A corpus luteum producing suboptimal levels of progesterone probably results in the inability of the dam's uterus to support development of the early embryo.

The primary target organs for progesterone are

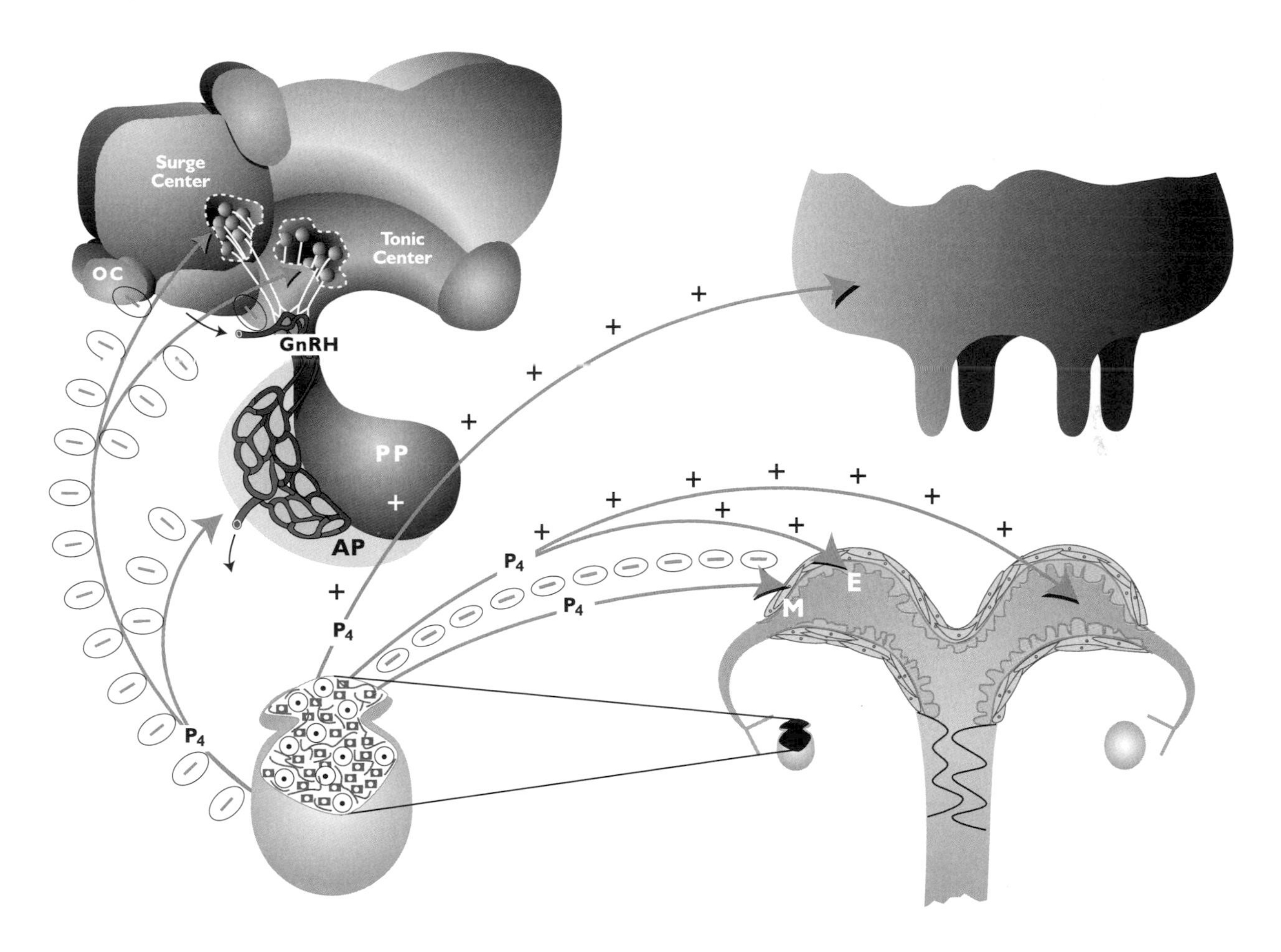

Figure 9-8. Progesterone (P_4) produced by the CL exerts a negative (-) feedback on the GnRH neurons of the hypothalamus. Therefore, GnRH, LH and FSH are suppressed and estrogen cannot be produced. Progesterone is also thought to decrease the number of GnRH receptors in the anterior pituitary. Progesterone exerts a strong positive (+) influence on the endometrium (E) of the uterus. Under the influence of progesterone the uterine glands perform an active secretory function. Progesterone inhibits the myometrium (M) and thus reduces its tone. Progesterone also promotes alveolar development in the mammary gland. (Graphic by Sonja Oei.)

the hypothalamus, the uterus and the mammary gland (Figure 9-8). The uterus has two target components. These two uterine tissues are the glandular endometrium and the muscular myometrium. Progesterone stimulates maximal secretion by the endometrial glands. Secretory products from the endometrial glands contribute to an environment that supports the development of the "free-floating" conceptus after it enters the uterine lumen. An important inhibitory role of progesterone is to reduce the motility (contractions) of the myometrium.

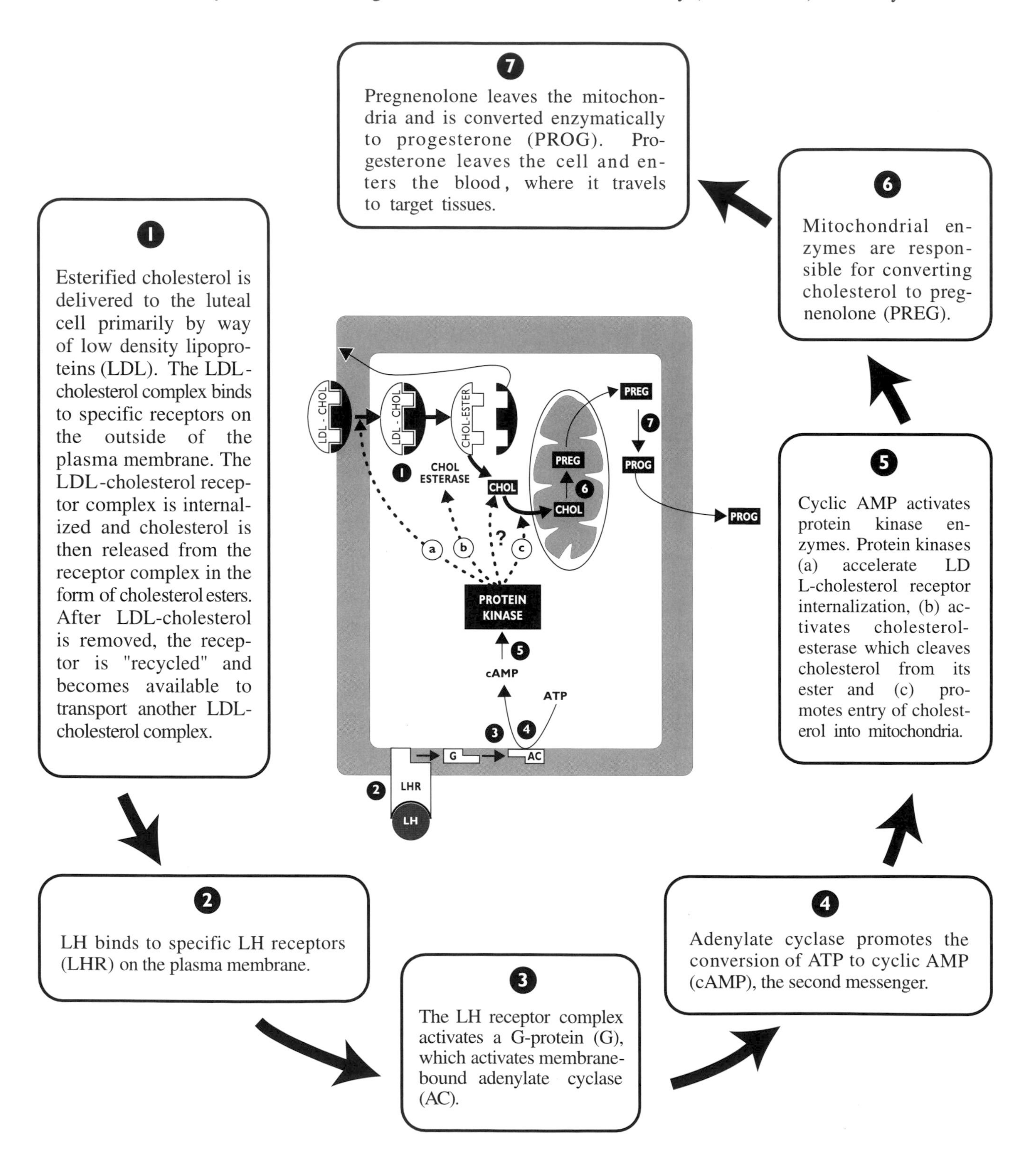

7
Pregnenolone leaves the mitochondria and is converted enzymatically to progesterone (PROG). Progesterone leaves the cell and enters the blood, where it travels to target tissues.
6
Mitochondrial enzymes are responsible for converting cholesterol to pregnenolone (PREG).
1
Esterified cholesterol is delivered to the luteal cell primarily by way of low density lipoproteins (LDL). The LDL-cholesterol complex binds to specific receptors on the outside of the plasma membrane. The LDL-cholesterol receptor complex is internalized and cholesterol is then released from the receptor complex in the form of cholesterol esters. After LDL-cholesterol is removed, the receptor is "recycled" and becomes available to transport another LDL-cholesterol complex.
LDL - CHOL
LDL - CHOL
CHOL-ESTER
CHOL ESTERASE
CHOL
PREG
CHOL
PREG
PROG
PROG
a
b
?
c
PROTEIN KINASE
cAMP
ATP
G
AC
LHR
LH
5
Cyclic AMP activates protein kinase enzymes. Protein kinases (a) accelerate LD L-cholesterol receptor internalization, (b) activates cholesterol-esterase which cleaves cholesterol from its ester and (c) promotes entry of cholesterol into mitochondria.
2
LH binds to specific LH receptors (LHR) on the plasma membrane.
3
The LH receptor complex activates a G-protein (G), which activates membrane-bound adenylate cyclase (AC).
4
Adenylate cyclase promotes the conversion of ATP to cyclic AMP (cAMP), the second messenger.

Figure 9-9. Mechanism of progesterone synthesis by luteal steroidogenic cells.

Such a role causes a "quieting" effect on the myometrium in the cow, pig and ewe, but not in the mare. Myometrial inhibition is believed to be important because it provides a set of "calm" conditions for attachment of the conceptus to the uterine endometrium. In the mare, the conceptus is moved about in the uterine lumen by contractions of the myometrium. This phenomenon will be discussed in more detail in Chapter 13. Progesterone causes final alveolar development of the mammary gland prior to parturition, thereby allowing lactation to be initiated.

Progesterone Synthesis Requires Cholesterol and LH

The presence of basal (tonic) LH and cholesterol is necessary for progesterone to be produced by luteal cells. The mechanism whereby LH causes production of progesterone in luteal cells is illustrated in Figure 9-9.

Progesterone is of major importance in the endocrine control of reproduction because it exerts a strong **negative feedback** on the hypothalamus (Figure 9-8). Elevated progesterone reduces the frequency of the basal episodic secretion of GnRH by the tonic GnRH center. The amplitude of the pulses is relatively high. Such a pattern of LH secretion along with tonic FSH secretion allows follicles to develop during the luteal phase. These follicles do not reach preovulatory status until progesterone decreases and the frequency of LH pulses increases. High progesterone therefore prevents development of preovulatory follicles, production of estrogen, behavioral estrus and the preovulatory surge of GnRH and LH.

Progesterone is an inhibitor because it:
- ***reduces basal GnRH amplitude and frequency***
- ***prevents behavioral estrus***
- ***stops the preovulatory LH surge***
- ***reduces myometrial tone***

Progesterone almost totally inhibits estrual behavior. In general, females under the influence of progesterone do not display estrus and will not accept the male for copulation. However, as pointed out in Chapter 7, progesterone exerts a positive priming effect on the brain to enhance the behavioral effects of estrogen. For example, if cows are **ovariectomized** (removal of ovaries) and treated with estrogen, they will display behavioral characteristics of estrus. These traits will be amplified in both intensity and duration if cows are treated with progesterone for about 5 to 7 days before they receive estrogen.

Lysis of the Corpus Luteum Must Occur Before the Female Can Enter the Follicular Phase

Luteolysis means disintegration or decomposition (lysis) of the corpus luteum. It occurs during a one to three day period at the end of the luteal phase. Luteolysis is a process whereby the corpus luteum undergoes irreversible degeneration characterized by a dramatic drop in blood levels of progesterone (Figures 9-1, 9-3 through 9-6). The two main hormones controlling luteolysis are oxytocin from the corpus luteum and $PGF_{2\alpha}$ produced by the uterine endometrium. Communication between the corpus luteum and the uterine endometrium is necessary in order to bring about successful luteolysis. The uterus, functioning as an endocrine organ, is responsible for producing $PGF_{2\alpha}$, which causes luteolysis. If luteolysis does not occur, the animal will remain in a sustained luteal phase, because progesterone from the corpus luteum inhibits gonadotropin se-

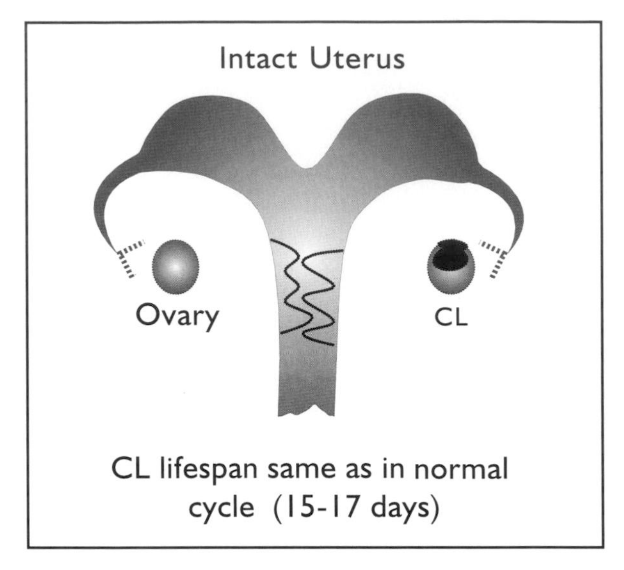

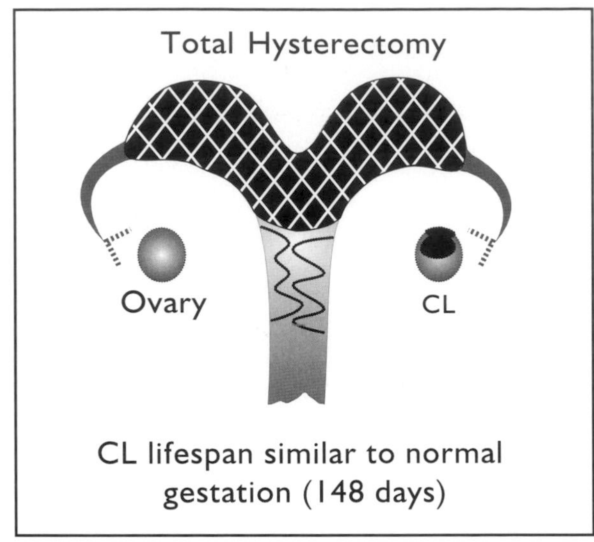

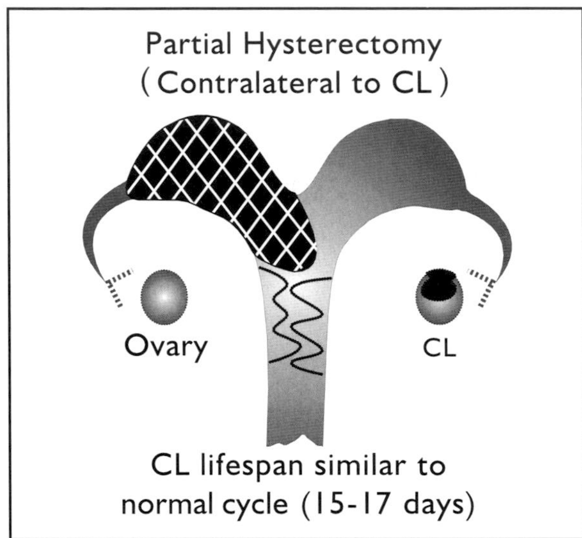

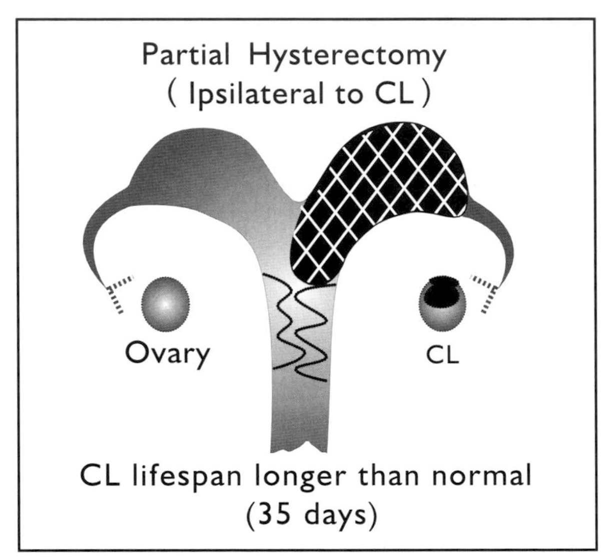

Figure 9-10. Effect of partial and complete hysterectomy upon duration of the estrous cycle in the ewe. Hatched regions represent portions of the uterus that were removed surgically.

cretion (Figure 9-8). The importance of the uterus in controlling the lifespan of the corpus luteum is illustrated in Figure 9-10. In mammals other than primates complete removal of the uterus (**hysterectomy**) after ovulation causes the corpus luteum to be maintained just as if the female were pregnant.

In ewes with an intact uterus the lifespan of the corpus luteum is identical to that seen in the normal cycle (17 days). However, when the entire uterus is removed (total hysterectomy), the lifespan of the corpus luteum is prolonged for months and is similar to a normal gestation period (148 days). Clearly, removal of the entire uterus sustains the lifespan of the corpus luteum dramatically.

The uterus is required for successful luteolysis.

When a partial hysterectomy is performed, a less dramatic effect can be seen. For example, when the uterine horn **ipsilateral** (on the same side) to the corpus luteum is removed, the lifespan of the corpus luteum is almost twice as long (about 35 days) as the normal cycle. In contrast, when the **contralateral** (opposite side) uterine horn is removed, there is little, if any, effect on the lifespan of the corpus luteum. The response to complete and partial hysterectomy is summarized in Figure 9-10. Several important findings have

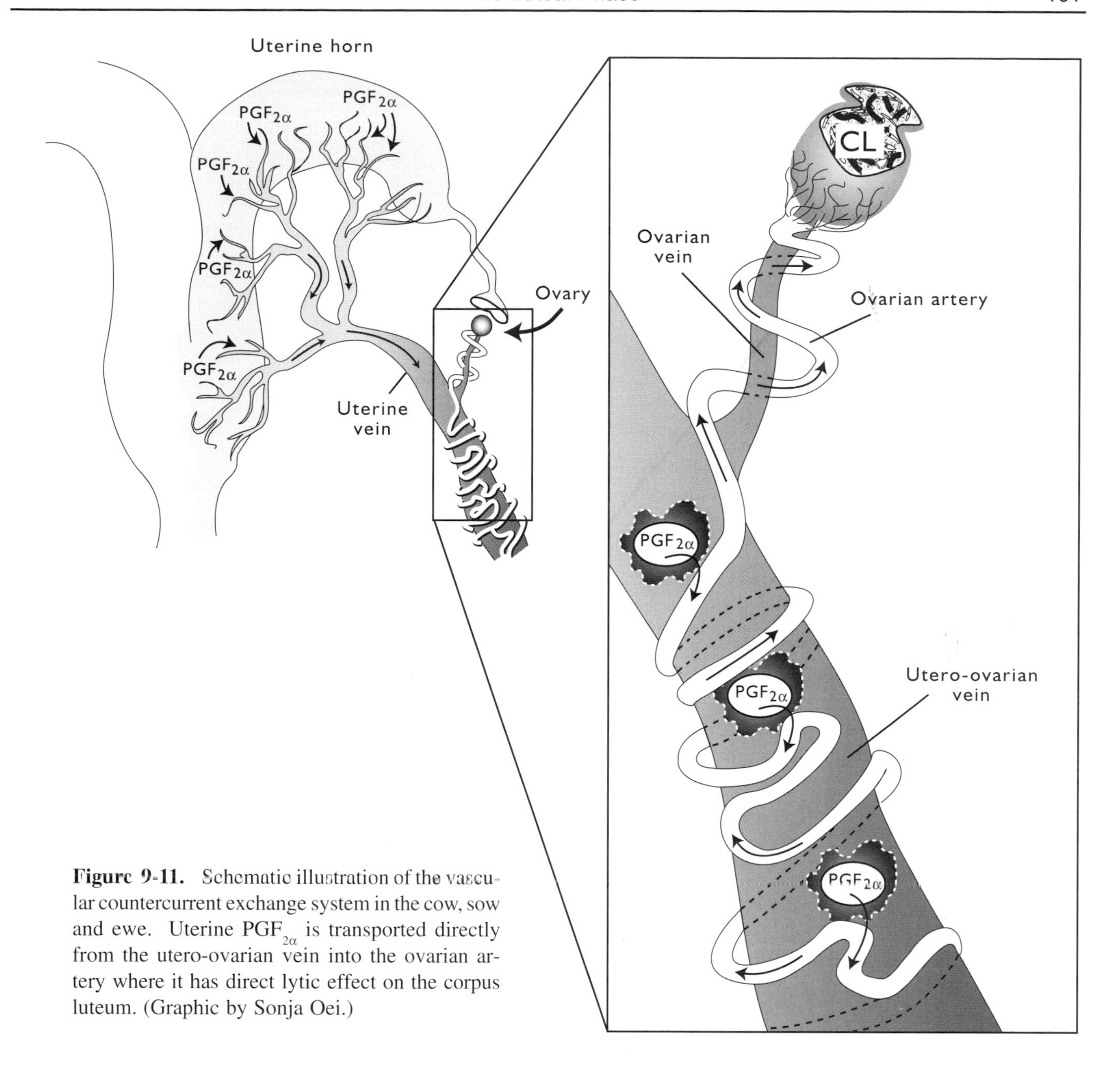

Figure 9-11. Schematic illustration of the vascular countercurrent exchange system in the cow, sow and ewe. Uterine $PGF_{2\alpha}$ is transported directly from the utero-ovarian vein into the ovarian artery where it has direct lytic effect on the corpus luteum. (Graphic by Sonja Oei.)

emerged from the classic experiments illustrated in Figure 9-10. First, the uterus is required for lysis of the corpus luteum. Therefore, the uterus produces a substance(s) that causes luteolysis. Second, removal of the uterus ipsilateral to the corpus luteum increases its lifespan, while removal of the uterine horn contralateral to the corpus luteum does not. A local effect of the uterus directly upon the ipsilateral ovary containing the corpus luteum is obvious. A local effect can be further supported by the fact that when the ovary is transplanted into the neck of the female, but the uterus remains intact, the corpus luteum lifespan is prolonged by many weeks. Collectively, what these experiments have told us is: 1) the uterus is responsible for luteolysis and 2) the uterus must be near the ovary.

You should now understand from the above discussion that the uterus is needed in order to cause luteolysis. Clearly, the uterus must secrete a substance which can cause destruction of the corpus luteum. After years of intensive and heavily focused research, it has been conclusively demonstrated that prostaglandin $F_{2\alpha}$ was the luteolysin in livestock.

> ***A vascular countercurrent exchange system insures that $PGF_{2\alpha}$ will reach the ovary in sufficient quantities to cause luteolysis.***

How does $PGF_{2\alpha}$ get from the uterus to the ovary, where it causes luteolysis? Prostaglandin $F_{2\alpha}$ from the uterus is transported to the ipsilateral ovary through a **vascular countercurrent exchange mechanism.** A countercurrent exchange system involves two closely associated blood vessels in which blood from one vessel flows in the opposite direction to that of the adjacent vessel. Low molecular weight substances in high concentrations in one vessel easily cross over into the adjacent vessel, where they are in low concentration. The $PGF_{2\alpha}$ produced by the endometrium enters the uterine vein, where it is in relatively high concentration. The ovarian artery lies in close association with the utero-ovarian vein. In fact, it is intimately intertwined with the uterine vein. By countercurrent exchange, $PGF_{2\alpha}$ is transferred across the wall of the uterine vein into the blood of the ovarian artery, where it is relatively low in concentration (Figure 9-11). This special anatomical relationship ensures that a high proportion of the $PGF_{2\alpha}$ produced by the uterus will be transported directly to the ovary and the corpus luteum without dilution in the systemic circulation. This mechanism is particularly important since $PGF_{2\alpha}$ is almost completely denatured during one circulatory pass through the pulmonary system in the ewe and the cow (98% to 99%). In the sow, only about 40% of the $PGF_{2\alpha}$ is denatured in the pulmonary circulation. By entering the ovarian artery, $PGF_{2\alpha}$ can exert its lytic effect directly on the corpus luteum before it enters the systemic circulation. The countercurrent exchange system is present in the cow, sow and ewe, but not in the mare. The mare does not metabolize $PGF_{2\alpha}$ as rapidly as other species, so the need for a local transport specialization is not important in the mare. In addition, the mare CL is believed to be more sensitive to $PGF_{2\alpha}$ than the CL of the sow.

Exogenous $PGF_{2\alpha}$ causes luteolysis during about 60% of the cycle in most species. For example, it exerts its most potent effect after day six of the cycle and will almost always cause luteolysis if administered after this time in the cow. In contrast, $PGF_{2\alpha}$ has a negligible effect during the first two to four days after ovulation. In the pig, the corpus luteum does not become responsive to the luteolytic action of a single dose of $PGF_{2\alpha}$ until day 12 to 14 of the cycle. Prostaglandin $F_{2\alpha}$, as well as its analogs, is used widely to cause regression of the corpus luteum and thus synchronize estrus and ovulation, induce abortion and sometimes induce parturition.

> ***Luteal oxytocin stimulates $PGF_{2\alpha}$ synthesis.***

What stimulates the production of $PGF_{2\alpha}$ during the late luteal phase? In addition to progesterone, large luteal cells synthesize and secrete oxytocin. In fact, in the cow and the ewe the corpus luteum contains very large quantities of oxytocin. Luteal oxytocin is stored in secretory granules analogous to those observed in the nerve terminals of the posterior pituitary gland. When oxytocin is injected into ewes near the end of the luteal phase, episodes of $PGF_{2\alpha}$ appear in the circulating blood in response to these injections. The episodes of $PGF_{2\alpha}$ cause luteolysis. In contrast, immunization against oxytocin (developing antibodies that destroy oxytocin) increases the duration of the luteal phase in the ewe. Luteal oxytocin has been shown to be synthesized by the same messenger RNA that is found in the nerves of the posterior pituitary gland. The pattern of luteal oxytocin secretion, along with $PGF_{2\alpha}$ metabolite secretion during the last 6 days of the estrous cycle, is shown in Figure 9-12. It is obvious that luteal oxytocin pulses are nearly coincident with pulses of prostaglan-

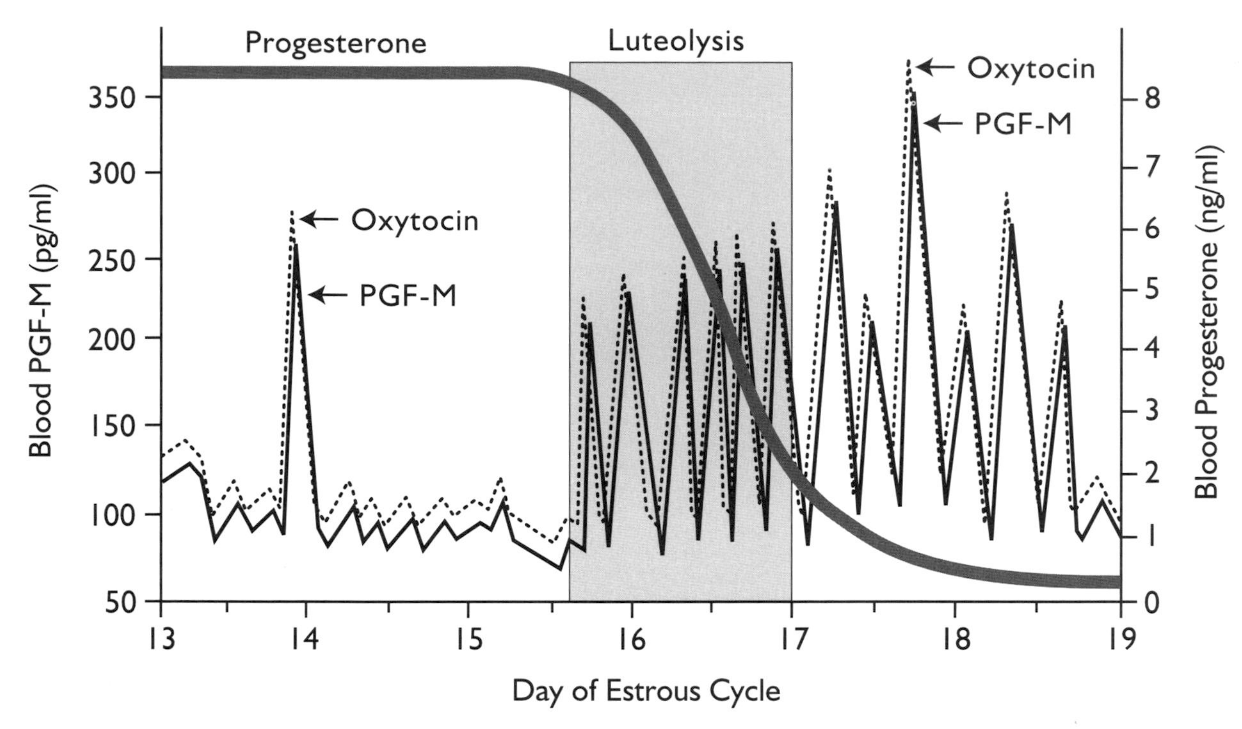

Figure 9-12. Changes in $PGF_{2\alpha}$ secretion during the last 6 days of the estrous cycle as reflected by prostaglandin $F_{2\alpha}$ metabolites (PGF-M). Luteal oxytocin episodes coincide almost perfectly with episodes of PGF-M. When about five pulses of $PGF_{2\alpha}$ occur in a 24-hour period, luteolysis will occur.

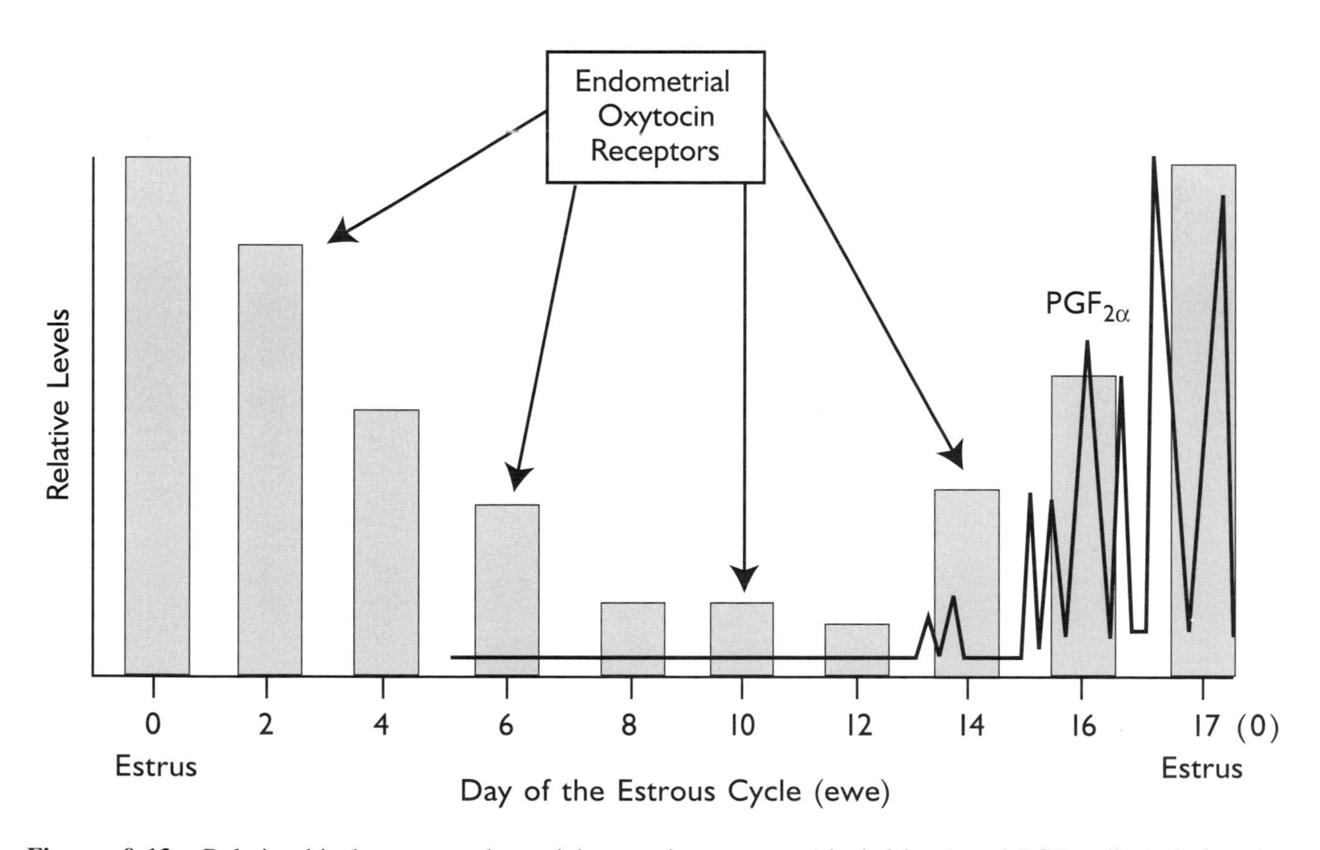

Figure 9-13. Relationship between endometrial oxytocin receptors (shaded bars) and $PGF_{2\alpha}$ (line) during the estrous cycle in the ewe. As the receptors to oxytocin increase, so does the sensitivity to oxytocin. $PGF_{2\alpha}$ is then synthesized in greater and greater quantities during days 13 to 17 of the estrous cycle.

din $F_{2\alpha}$ metabolites. The reason metabolites of $PGF_{2\alpha}$ are measured instead of $PGF_{2\alpha}$ is that the metabolites are longer-lived and are easier to measure. Metabolite levels of $PGF_{2\alpha}$ in the blood are a direct reflection of $PGF_{2\alpha}$ levels.

During the first half of the luteal phase, prostaglandin secretion by the endometrium of the uterus is almost nonexistent. However, during the late luteal phase, secretion of $PGF_{2\alpha}$ begins to occur in pulses (Figures 9-12 and 9-13). The pulses increase in frequency and amplitude as the end of the luteal phase approaches. It has been established that a critical number of $PGF_{2\alpha}$ pulses within a given time span is required to induce complete luteolysis. The exact number of pulses required has not been defined for all species. However, based on data from the ewe, about five pulses in a 24 hour period are required to induce complete luteolysis. Pulsatile release of $PGF_{2\alpha}$ is apparently not required under conditions of exogenous $PGF_{2\alpha}$ administration.

The uterus must be exposed to elevated progesterone for a period of days before it can synthesize and release $PGF_{2\alpha}$ in sufficient quantities to cause luteolysis. During the first half of the estrous cycle progesterone prevents secretion of $PGF_{2\alpha}$ by blocking the formation of oxytocin receptors in the uterus (Figure 9-13). After 10 to 12 days progesterone loses its ability to block formation of oxytocin receptors, although it is not known how this occurs. During the late luteal phase exogenous oxytocin causes the secretion of $PGF_{2\alpha}$ by the uterus. Injections of $PGF_{2\alpha}$ during the late luteal phase lead to a rapid release of ovarian oxytocin. Thus, oxytocin and $PGF_{2\alpha}$ stimulate each other in a positive feedback manner. As you have seen in Figure 9-12, at the end of the luteal phase there are episodes of nearly simultaneous secretion of oxytocin and $PGF_{2\alpha}$ in the circulating blood. In the ewe, oxytocinepisodes precede $PGF_{2\alpha}$ episodes. At this time during the luteal phase uterine responsiveness to oxytocin is increased by the rise in the number of oxytocin receptors in the endometrium (Figure 9-13). The higher the number of endometrial oxytocin receptors, the greater the ability of oxytocin to stimulate the synthesis of $PGF_{2\alpha}$.

Luteolysis results in:

- ***cessation of progesterone production***
- ***structural regression to form a corpus albicans***
- ***follicular development and entrance into a new follicular phase***

The intracellular mechanisms that cause luteolysis have been the subject of intense research during the last 10 years. One of the original theories to explain the demise of the corpus luteum was that $PGF_{2\alpha}$ caused reduction in blood flow to the corpus luteum by causing vasoconstriction (contraction) of arterioles supplying the luteal tissue. While blood flow to the corpus luteum does decrease during luteolysis, the blood flow to the corpus luteum is still 5 to 20 times greater than to the surrounding ovarian tissue. Thus, **ischemia** (reduced blood flow) as a primary mode for luteolysis seems unlikely. It is known that capillaries in the corpus luteum undergo degeneration during luteolysis. It is possible that this capillary degeneration is more responsible for reducing blood flow than vasoconstriction associated with $PGF_{2\alpha}$. Nevertheless, a degree of circulatory disruption is associated with the luteolytic process. However, it is unlikely that this disruption to the luteal vasculature can totally account for luteolysis.

A second line of thinking is the theory that $PGF_{2\alpha}$ binds to specific receptors on large luteal cells and triggers a cascade of events resulting in the death of these cells and, thus, cessation of steroidogenesis. These events are presented in Figure 9-14.

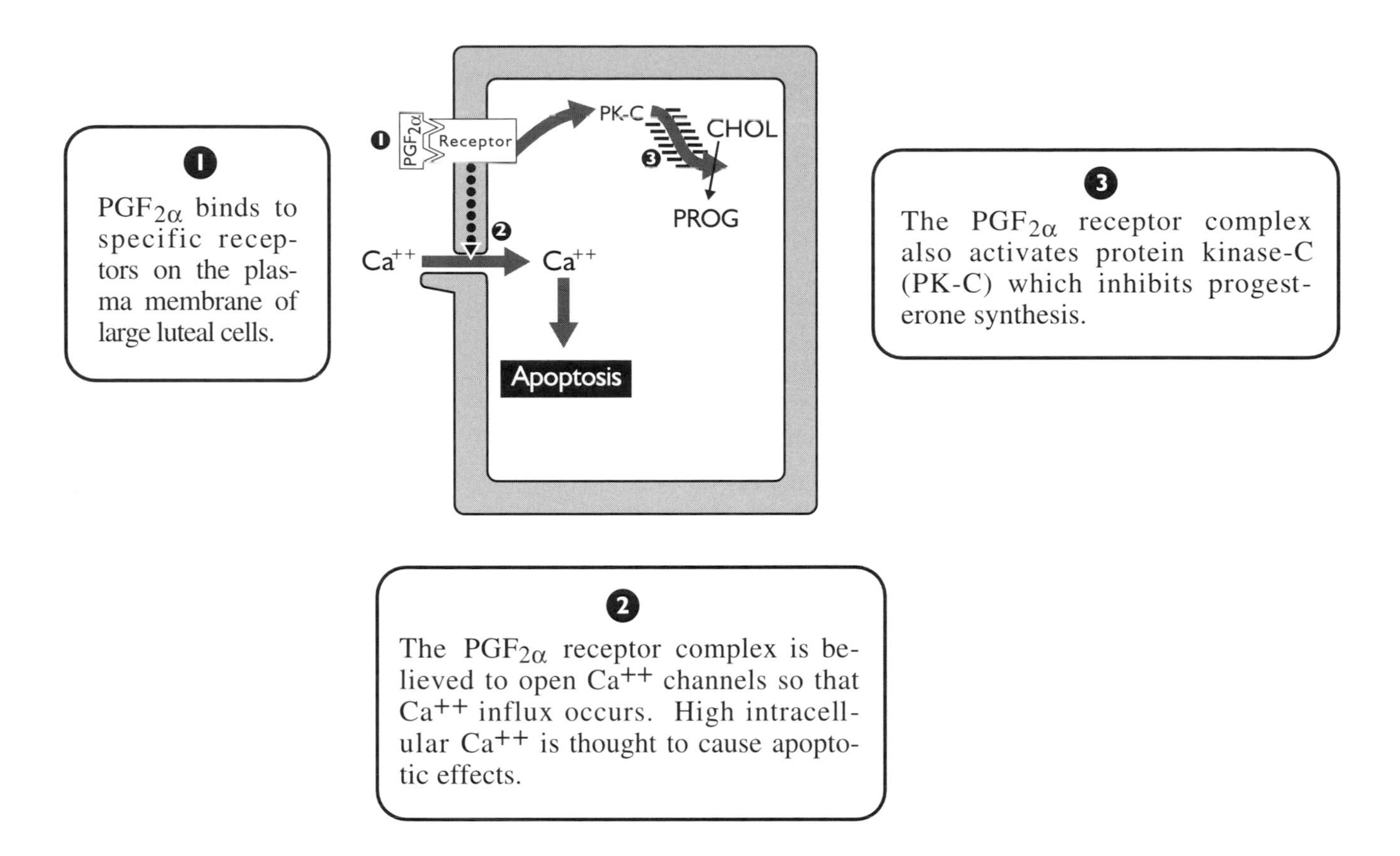

Figure 9-14. Proposed steps resulting in the loss of progesterone production from steroidogenic cells.

The Immune System May Be Responsible for Structural Regression of the Corpus Luteum

It is well known that macrophages and lymphocytes are present in the corpus luteum at the time of luteolysis. These cells are capable of performing phagocytosis of luteal cells. Phagocytic cells increase prior to the onset of luteolysis. The chemotactic stimulus attracting these phagocytic cells to the luteal tissue has not been identified. Macrophages and lymphocytes produce materials known as **cytokines**. Cytokines are non-antibody proteins produced by a variety of immune cells (macrophages, lymphocytes and leukocytes) that act as intercellular mediators of the immune response. Examples of cytokines are interferons, interleukins and tumor necrosis factor. Cytokines have been shown to cause luteal cell death *in vitro*. They also inhibit progesterone synthesis by luteal cells. While the mechanism involving the roles of cytokines in luteolysis is far from clear, it appears that normal morphologic and functional integrity of the corpus luteum can be reduced when these cytokines are present.

In addition to a direct effect on the luteal cell, cytokines may serve as triggering agents for a process called apoptosis. **Apoptosis** (pronounced "a-pa-toe-sis") is a phenomenon which has been described as "programmed cell death." It is quite normal for cells throughout the body to die on a daily basis. Cell death occurs by one of two processes. The first, cell **necrosis,** is brought about by pathologic damage. The second type of cell death, apoptosis, is an ordered biochemical process. This process involves distinct biochemical and morphologic changes in the cell. The process of apoptosis is probably the final step resulting in the death of the luteal cell. Final destruction and "clean-up" of the luteal cells *per se* is probably performed by macrophages which phagocytize damaged luteal cells. Over time the luteal cells disappear completely, leaving only connective tissue behind. Thus, the scar-like **corpus albicans** is formed.

Further Phenomena for Fertility

Female elephants have a uniquely long estrous cycle (16 weeks) and a gestation of 22 months. What does this say about elephant CL?

The regression of the corpus luteum in humans and other primates is not controlled by the uterus. However, $PGF_{2\alpha}$ will induce luteolysis in primates. It is believed that $PGF_{2\alpha}$ of ovarian origin is responsible for causing luteal regression.

The corpus luteum of most rodents (rats, mice, hamsters and gerbils) does not develop unless copulation occurs. Penile stimulation of the cervix causes prolactin release from the female. Prolactin is luteotropic and causes the formation of corpora lutea.

The luteal phase of the estrous cycle of the kangaroo is longer than pregnancy.

Researchers at N.C. State University observed a sow that had 128 corpora lutea on both of her ovaries. This is ten times the normal number of corpora lutea. The cause of such a high number of ovulations is unknown.

Additional Reading

Leymarie, P. and Martal, J. 1993. "The corpus luteum from cycle to gestation" in *Reproduction in Mammals and Man.* 413-433. C. Thibault, M.C. Levasseur and R.H.F. Hunter, eds., Ellipses, Paris.

Niswender, G.D. and T.M. Nett. 1994. "Corpus luteum and its control in infraprimate species." in *The Physiology of Reproduction* 2nd Edition. 781-816. E. Knobil and J.D. Neil, eds., Raven Press, Ltd., New York.

Pate, J.L. and D.H. Townsend. 1994. "Novel local regulators in luteal regression." XXI Biennial Symposium on Animal Reproduction. *J Anim Sci* 72 Suppl. 3:31-42.

10 Endocrinology of the Male and Spermatogenesis

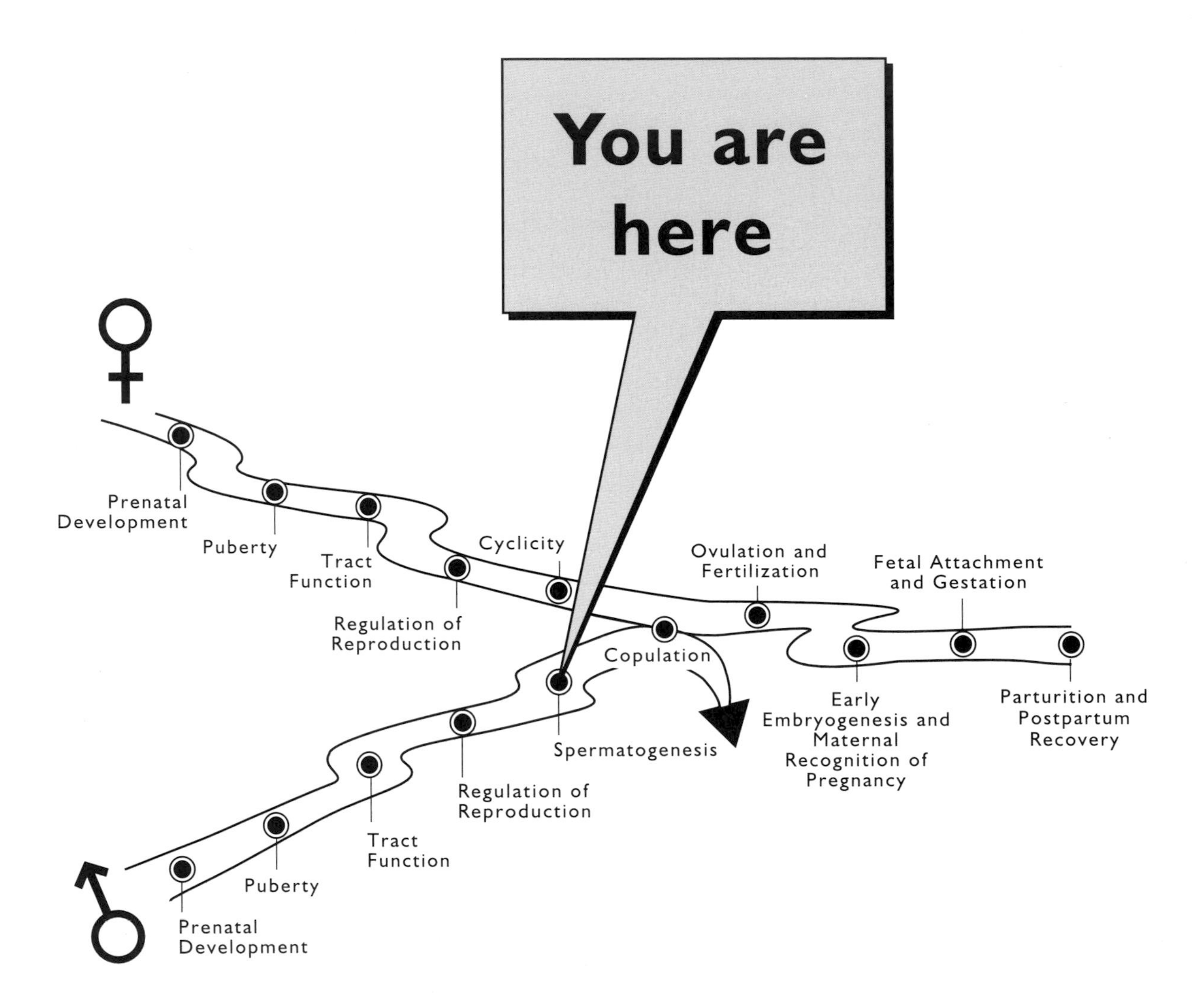

Take Home Message

In the male, GnRH, LH and testosterone are released in pulses that occur every several hours. Follicle stimulating hormone is released in smaller pulses of longer duration. Spermatozoa are produced by the testes by a process called spermatogenesis which requires 5 to 9 weeks, depending on the species. Spermatozoa are released constantly from the testes. Spermatogenesis is the result of all mitotic and meiotic divisions and is concluded by a process called spermiogenesis. Spermiogenesis is the process whereby spherical spermatids are transformed into spermatozoa.

The Endocrine Control/Regulation is Different Than in the Female

Before spermatozoa can be produced, certain endocrine requirements must be met. They are: 1) adequate production of GnRH from the hypothalamus; 2) FSH and LH secretion from the anterior pituitary; and 3) secretion of gonadal steroids, in this case testosterone and some progesterone. Recall from Chapter 6 that the hypothalamus in the male does not develop a surge center. Instead of a period of basal release, followed by a preovulatory surge of GnRH every few weeks, as in the female, the discharge of GnRH from the hypothalamus in the male occurs in frequent, intermittent bursts. These bursts of GnRH last for a few minutes, and cause discharges of LH which follow almost immediately after the GnRH episode. The episodes of LH last from between 10 and 20 minutes and occur between 4 to more than 8 times throughout the day. Concentrations of FSH are lower, but the pulses are of longer duration than LH because of the relatively constant secretion of inhibin by the adult testis (Figure 10-1).

Luteinizing hormone acts on the **Leydig** cells within the testes. These cells, named after the German anatomist Franz von Leydig, are analogous to the cells of the theca interna of the antral follicles in the ovary. They contain membrane-bound receptors for LH. When LH binds to their receptors, Leydig cells produce progesterone, most of which is converted to testosterone. The production of testosterone takes place by the same intracellular mechanism as in the female (Chapters 5 and 8). The Leydig cells synthesize and secrete testosterone less than 30 minutes after the onset of an LH episode. Blood LH is elevated for about 30 to 75 minutes. Response (testosterone secretion) by Leydig cells is short, and secretion is pulsatile and lasts for a period of 20 to 30 minutes (Figure 10-2).

Production of fertile spermatozoa requires:

- ***endocrine regulation of the testis***
- ***mitotic divisions of spermatogonia***
- ***meiotic divisions resulting in haploid spermatids***
- ***morphologic transformation of spermatids into spermatozoa***

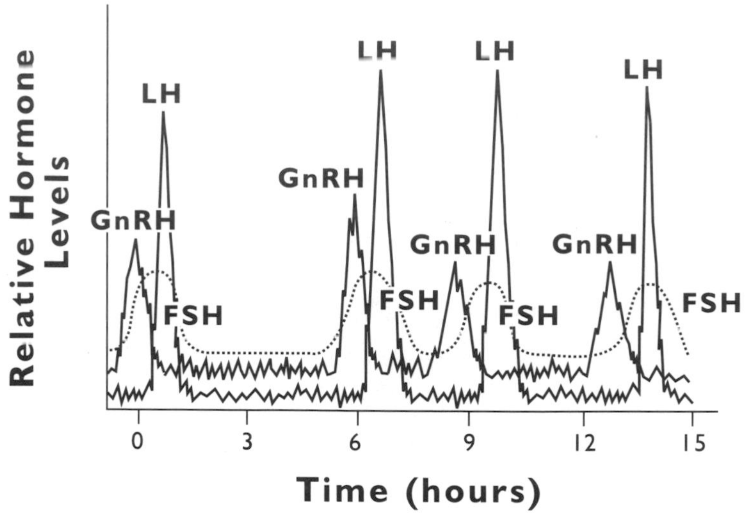

Figure 10-1. Relationship between GnRH, LH and FSH secretion. GnRH causes the release of LH and FSH. Episodes of all three hormones occur between 4 and 8 times in 24 hours. The lower FSH profile when compared to LH is due to inhibin production by Sertoli cells. Also, the greater duration of the FSH episode is probably due to its longer half-life (100 min) when compared to LH (30 min).

> ***Leydig cells are the male equivalent of the follicular theca interna cells.***
>
> ***Sertoli cells are the male equivalent of the follicular granulosal cells.***

It is believed that the pulsatile discharge of LH is important for two reasons. First, high interstitial concentrations of testosterone are essential for spermatogenesis, but high concentrations need not be present continually. Second, Leydig cells become **refractory** to sustained high levels of LH. In fact, continual high concentrations of LH result in reduced secretion of testosterone. From a physiologic perspective the term refractory means unresponsive, or not yielding to treatment. The refractory condition brought about by sustained high concentrations of LH is believed to be caused by a reduction in the number of LH receptors in the Leydig cell. Thus, there is a marked reduction in progesterone

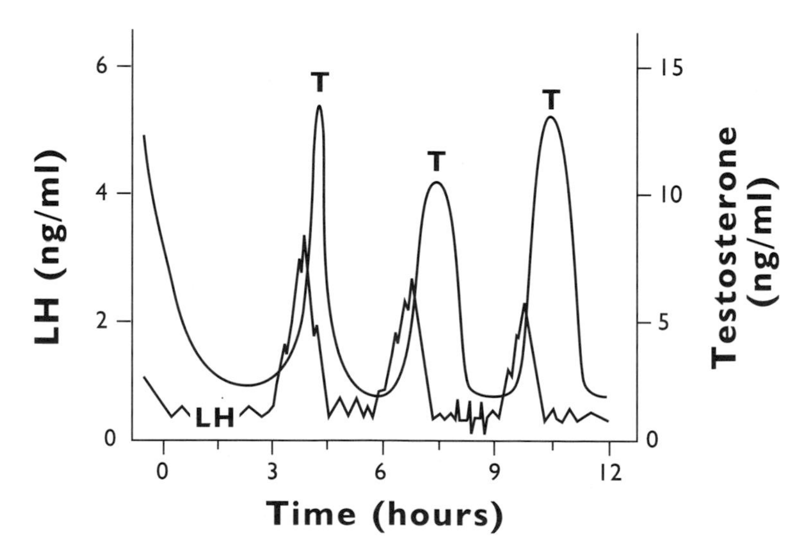

Figure 10-2. Relationship between concentrations of peripheral blood LH and testosterone (T). LH is elevated for .5 to 1.25 hours, while the subsequent testosterone episode lasts for .5 to 1.5 hours.

and testosterone secretion when LH remains high for a sustained period. Intratesticular levels of testosterone must be higher than blood levels of testosterone for successful spermatogenesis. The role of the pulsatile nature of testosterone is not fully understood. It is believed however, that chronically high testosterone concentrations suppress FSH levels. Sertoli cell function is FSH dependent; thus, their function is compromised when FSH is reduced. The periodic reduction in testosterone allows the negative feedback on FSH to be removed (Figure 10-3).

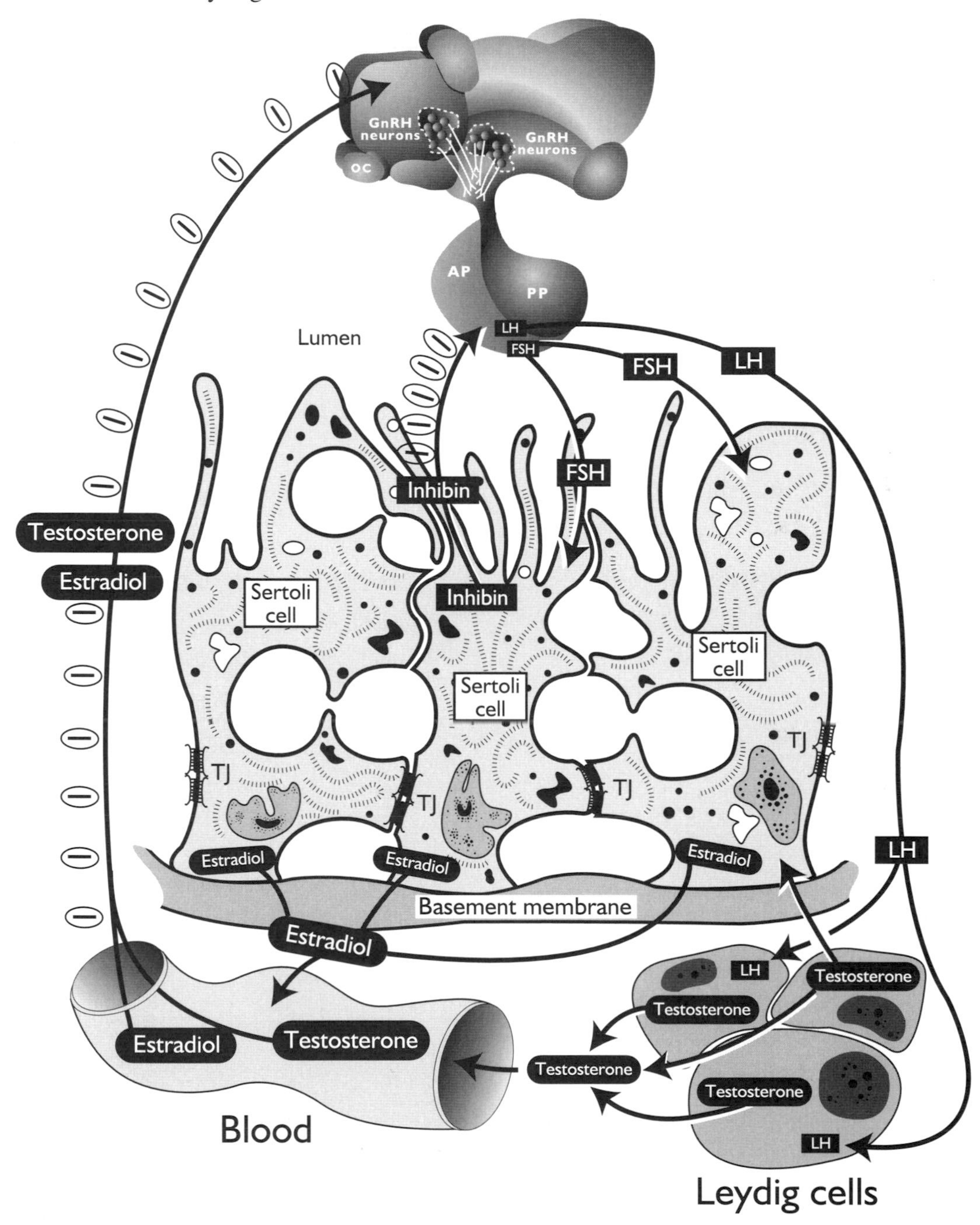

Figure 10-3. Interrelationships among hormone production by Leydig cells, Sertoli cells, the hypothalamus and the anterior pituitary. Luteinizing hormone binds to receptors in the interstitial cells of Leydig and FSH binds to Sertoli cells. Leydig cells produce testosterone which is transported to the adjacent vasculature. Also, testosterone produced by the Leydig cells is transported into the Sertoli cells where it is converted to estradiol. Testosterone and estradiol are transported by the blood, where they exert a negative feedback on the GnRH neurons in the hypothalamus. The Sertoli cells also produce inhibin, which exerts a negative feedback on the anterior pituitary to suppress FSH. Open spaces between adjacent Sertoli cells house developing germ cells. TJ = Tight Junctions. (Graphic by Sonja Oei.)

In addition to production of testosterone by the Leydig cells, the testes also produce estradiol and other estrogens. The stallion and the boar secrete large amounts of estrogens (both free and in conjugated form). In fact, urinary estrogens in the male are significantly higher than urinary estrogens in pregnant mares and sows. These high levels of estrogen seem to be of little consequence, since they are secreted in an inactive conjugated form.

Sertoli cells convert testosterone to estradiol utilizing a mechanism identical to the granulosal cells of the antral follicle in the female. The exact role of estradiol in male reproduction is poorly understood, but there is little doubt that this hormone plays a negative feedback role on the hypothalamus. Testosterone and estradiol in the blood act on the hypothalamus and exert a negative feedback on the production of GnRH and, in turn, LH and FSH are reduced. Therefore, high concentrations of estradiol result in suppression of GnRH and LH discharges (Figure 10-3). In addition to converting testosterone to estradiol, Sertoli cells also produce inhibin which, as in the female, suppresses FSH secretion from the anterior pituitary. The importance of inhibin and suppressed FSH release is not clear.

Spermatogenesis takes place in the seminiferous tubule (Figure 10-4) and consists of the sum of all cellular transformations in developing germ cells that occur in the seminiferous epithelium (Figure 10-5). **Spermatocytogenesis** consists of the mitotic divisions involving proliferation and maintenance of **spermatogonia. Meiosis** insures genetic diversity and involves **primary** and **secondary spermatocytes** which give rise to **spermatids. Spermiogenesis** is the morphologic transformation of **spherical spermatids** into fully differentiated, highly specialized spermatozoa.

The most immature germ cells (spermatogonia) are located at the periphery of the seminiferous tubule

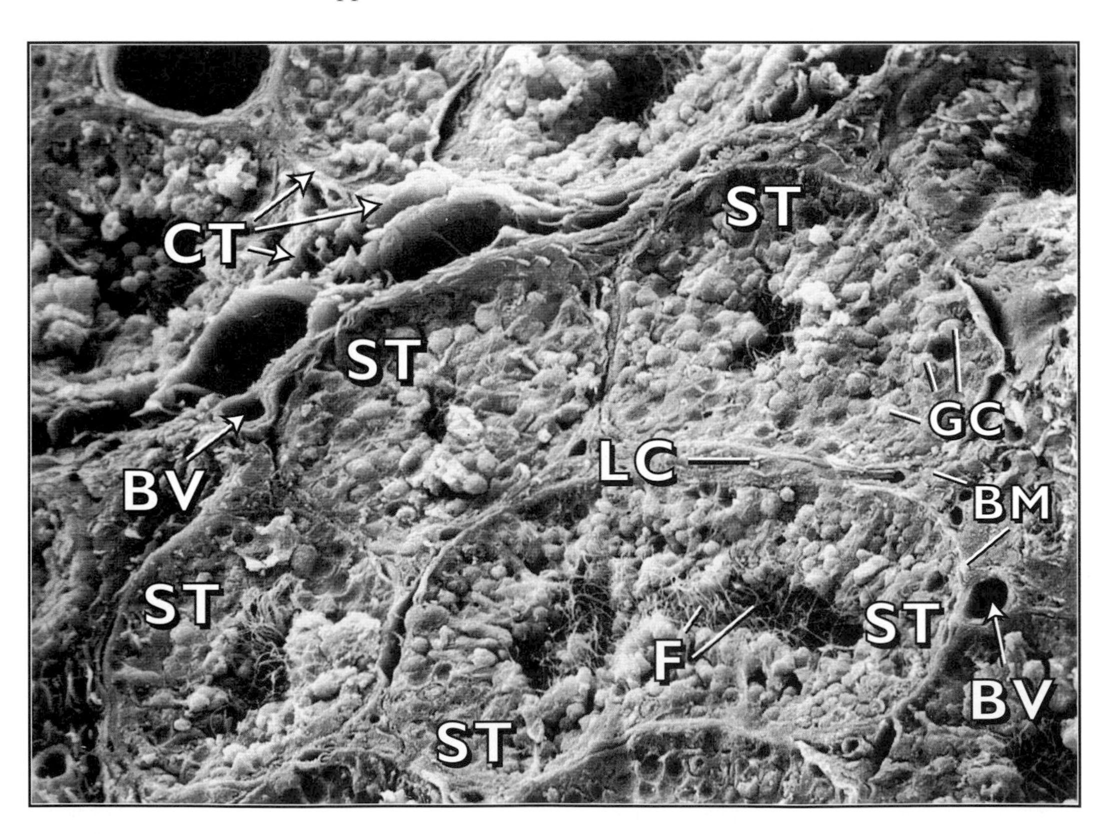

Figure 10-4. Scanning electron micrograph of testicular parenchyma in the stallion. Seminiferous tubules (ST) containing developing germ cells (GC) are surrounded by a basement membrane (BM). Flagella (F) from developing spermatids can be observed protruding into the lumen of some tubules. The interstitial compartment contains Leydig cells (LC), blood vessels (BV) and connective tissue (CT). (Micrograph courtesy of Dr. Larry Johnson, Texas A&M University, with permission from The American Society for Reproductive Medicine - *Fertil. and Steril.*, 1978, 29:208-215.)

Spermatogenesis = spermatocytogenesis + meiosis + spermiogenesis

near the basement membrane. As these germ cells become more mature they are moved toward the lumen. The cell types in the seminiferous epithelium from the basement membrane to the lumen are illustrated in Figure 10-5. Developing germ cells are interconnected by **intercellular bridges** (Figure 10-5). Groups of spermatogonia, spermatocytes and spermatids are connected by bridges, so that the cytoplasm of an entire group or cohort cells is interconnected. The exact number of germ cells that are interconnected is not known, but might approach 100. The significance of these intercellular bridges is not fully understood; however, it is believed that they provide communication between cells that allows for synchronized development among cells of a cohort (groups cells of the same type).

Spermatocytogenesis Generates Spermatogonia That Are Committed to Become More Advanced Cell Types

The most primitive cells encountered in the seminiferous epithelium are the spermatogonia. These specialized diploid (2N chromosomal content) cells are located in the **basal compartment** of the seminiferous epithelium. Spermatogonia undergo several mitotic divisions, with the last division resulting in primary spermatocytes (Figure 10-5). There are three types of spermatogonia: **A-spermatogonia**, **I-spermatogonia** (intermediate) and **B-spermatogonia**. A-spermatogonia undergo several mitotic divisions in which they progress mitotically from A_1 through A_4. A pool of stem cells is maintained so that the process can continue indefinitely.

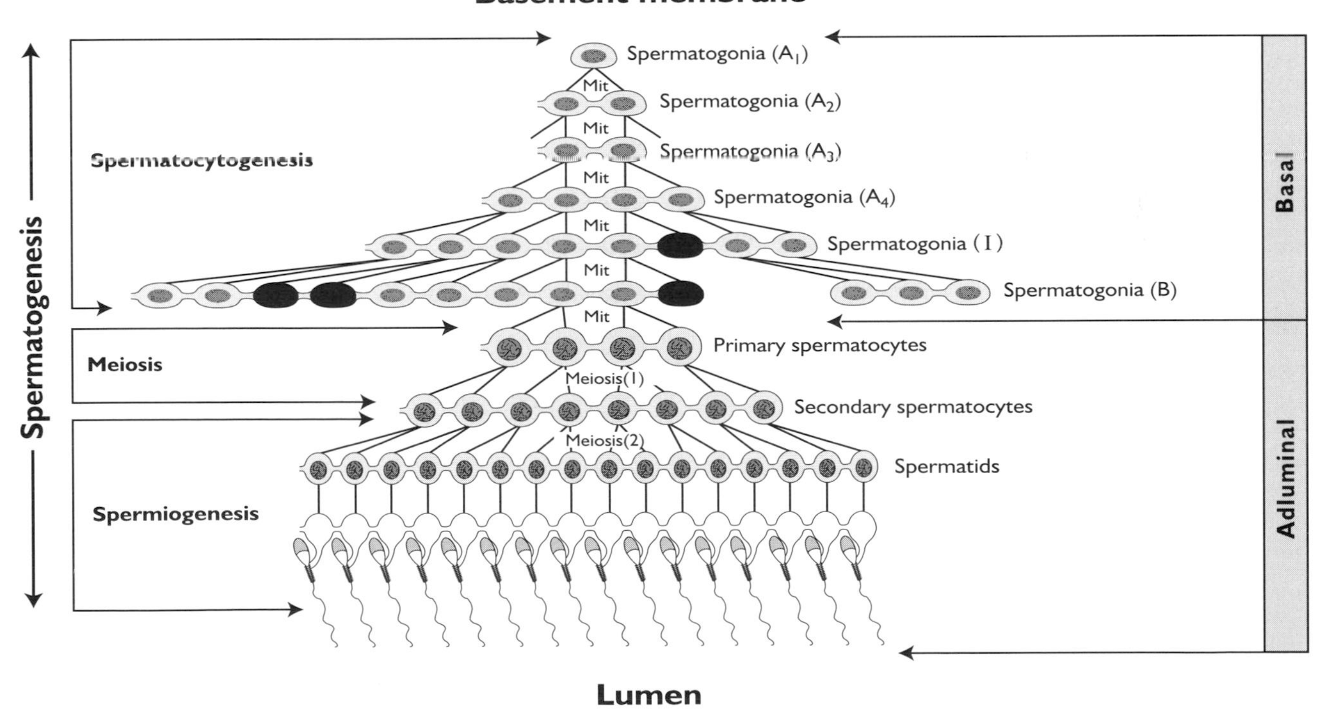

Figure 10-5. Typical cellular sequence of spermatogenesis in mammals. Spermatogonia (A_1 - A_4) undergo a series of mitotic divisions (mit) until B-spermatogonia are formed. The last mitotic division gives rise to primary spermatocytes which enter meiosis. This series of mitotic divisions constitutes spermatocytogenesis and takes place in the basal compartment. After meiosis, haploid spherical spermatids are generated. Spermiogenesis is the morphologic transformation of spherical spermatids into fully differentiated spermatozoa. Meiosis and spermiogenesis take place in the adluminal compartment. Notice that each generation of cells is attached by intercellular bridges. Thus, each generation divides synchronously in cohorts. Black cells designate degeneration.

Stem cells divide mitotically to provide a continual source of A-spermatogonia.

Meiotic Divisions Form Haploid Germ Cells

One of the goals of spermatogenesis is to reduce the number of chromosomes in the gamete to the haploid state. This is accomplished by meiosis. The mitotic divisions of B-spermatogonia result in the formation of primary spermatocytes. These primary spermatocytes immediately enter the first meiotic prophase. As you should recall, meiotic prophase consists of five stages: preleptotene, leptotene, zygotene, pachytene and diplotene. Each of these stages represents a different progression in DNA synthesis and replication. Primary spermatocytes must progress from interphase, immediately after their division, through this series of changes before the first meiotic division can occur. The important event of the preleptotene phase is complete DNA replication forming tetrads without separation. These tetrads then fuse at random points known as chiasmata, and crossing-over of DNA material takes place. The term "crossing-over" refers to segments of one chromosome crossing over to a homologous chromosome when the chromatids separate. Crossing-over results in a random assortment of different segments of each chromosome. Thus, the prophase of the first meiotic division insures that genetic heterogeneity will exist and that each secondary spermatocyte and spermatid will be genetically unique. It should be recognized that the prophase of the first meiotic division is a lengthy process. In fact, the lifespan of the primary spermatocyte is the longest of all germ cell types found in the seminiferous epithelium. For example, in the bull the lifespan of the primary spermatocyte is 18 to 19 days. The total spermatogenic time is 61 days. Thus, the prophase of the first meiotic division (primary spermatocyte) occupies about 30% of the time required for the entire spermatogenic process.

After the first division of meiosis the primary spermatocyte becomes a secondary spermatocyte. The secondary spermatocyte is quite short-lived, existing for only 1.1 to 1.7 days depending on the species. The secondary spermatocyte rapidly undergoes the second meiotic division, resulting in the production of haploid spherical spermatids.

Spermiogenesis Produces a Highly Sophisticated, Self-Propelled Package of Enzymes and DNA

The role of spermatozoa is to deliver the male genetic material to the oocyte during fertilization. To form cells which are capable of fertilization, spherical spermatids must undergo a series of changes in which the nucleus becomes highly condensed, the acrosome is formed and the cell becomes potentially motile. The ability to swim (motility) requires the development of a **flagellum** and a metabolic "powerplant" known as the **mitochondrial helix.**

Spermiogenesis consists of the:

- ***Golgi phase***
- ***cap phase***
- ***acrosomal phase***
- ***maturation phase***

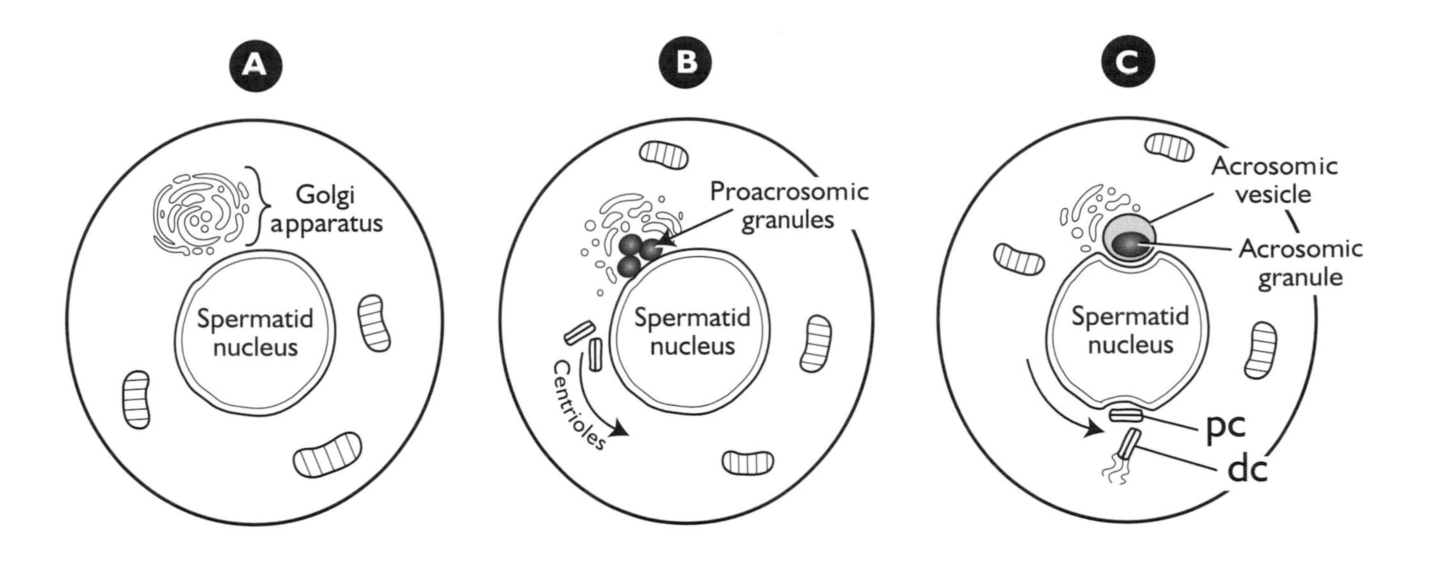

Figure 10-6. The Golgi phase of spermiogenesis. The newly formed spermatid (A) has a well developed Golgi apparatus. Small vesicles of the Golgi fuse, giving rise to larger secretory granules called proacrosomic granules (B). Vesicle fusion continues until a large acrosomic vesicle is formed that contains a dense acrosomic granule (C). During the last half of the Golgi phase the centrioles migrate to a position opposite the acrosomic vesicle. The proximal centriole (PC) will give rise to the attachment point for the tail. The distal centriole (DC) will give rise to the developing axoneme inside the cytoplasm of the spermatid. (Graphic by Sonja Oei.)

The Golgi phase = acrosomic vesicle formation

The **Golgi phase** is characterized by the first steps in the development of the **acrosome**. The newly formed spermatid contains a large, highly-developed Golgi apparatus located above the nucleus which gives rise to many small vesicles (Figure 10-6). The Golgi apparatus is not unique to the spermatid, but is the intracellular "packaging" system for secretory cells in general. In a spermatid, the Golgi will give rise to an important subcellular organelle known as the acrosome. First, proacrosomic vesicles are formed and fuse to generate a large vesicle which resides on one side of the nucleus. This vesicle is called the **acrosomic vesicle** and contains a dense **acrosomic granule** (Figure 10-6). Smaller Golgi vesicles are continually added to the larger vesicle, thus causing an increase in its size.

While the acrosomic vesicle is being formed, the centrioles migrate from the cytoplasm to the base of the nucleus (Figure 10-6). The proximal centriole will give rise to an implantation apparatus that allows the flagellum to be anchored to the nucleus (Figure 10-11). The distal centriole gives rise to the developing **axoneme**. The axoneme is the central portion of a flagellum, in this case the sperm tail.

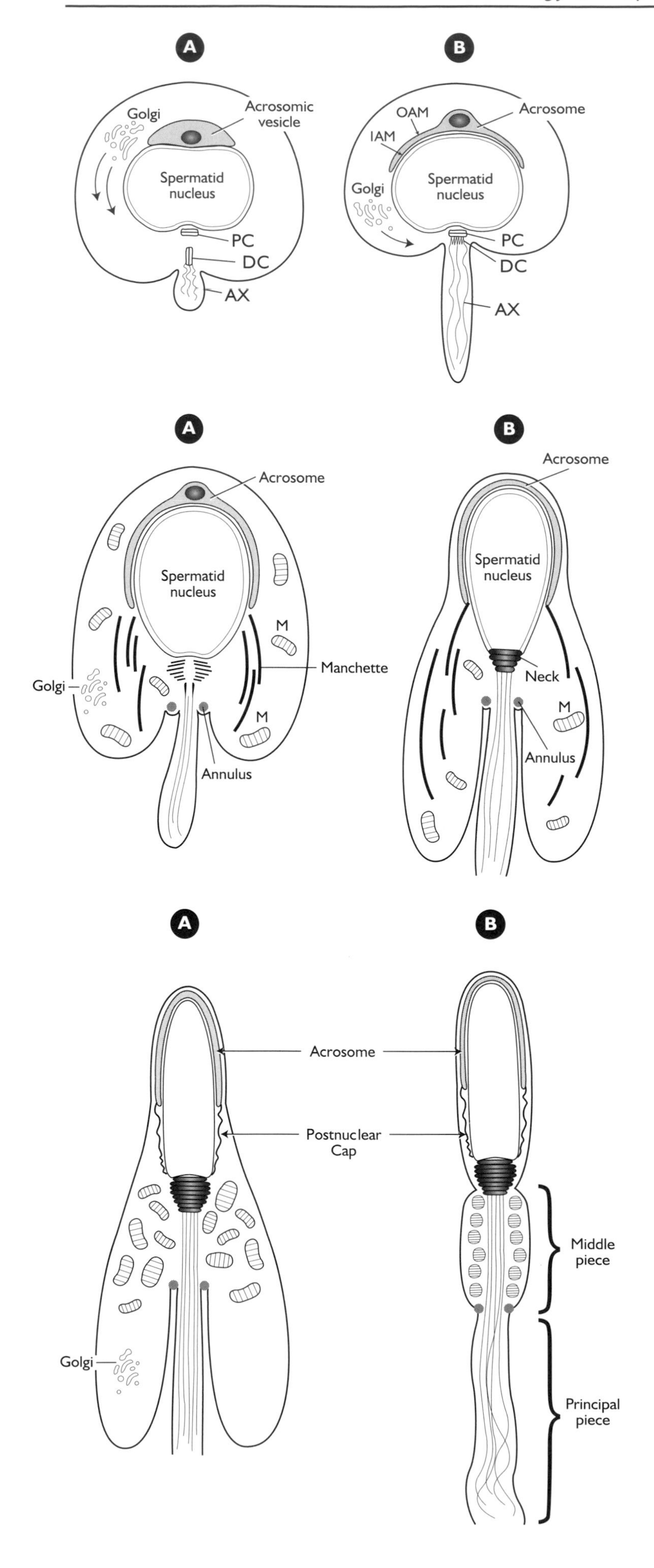

Figure 10-7. The Cap Phase of Spermiogenesis. The acrosomic vesicle flattens and begins to form a distinct cap (B) consisting of an outer acrosomal membrane (OAM) and an inner acrosomal membrane (IAM). The Golgi (A) migrates toward the caudal part of the cell (B) and the distal centriole (DC) forms the axoneme (AX) or flagellum which projects away from the nucleus toward the lumen of the seminiferous tubule. (Graphic by Sonja Oei.)

Figure 10-8. The Acrosomal Phase of Spermiogenesis. The spermatid nucleus begins to elongate (A) and the acrosome eventually covers the majority of the anterior nucleus (B). The manchette forms in the region of the caudal half of the nucleus and extends down toward the developing flagellum. The neck and the annulus are formed, which will become the juncture between the middle piece and the principal piece. Notice that all components of the developing spermatid are completely surrounded by a plasma membrane. M = mitochondria. (Graphic by Sonja Oei.)

Figure 10-9. The Maturation Phase of Spermiogenesis. Mitochondria are assembled around the flagellum to form the middle piece. Dense outer fibers form around the flagellum. The postnuclear cap is formed from the manchette microtubules. The annulus forms the juncture between the middle piece and the principal piece. (Graphic by Sonja Oei.)

The cap phase = acrosomic vesicle spreading over the nucleus

During the **cap phase** the acrosome forms a distinct, easily recognized cap over the anterior portion of the nucleus (Figure 10-7). The Golgi, which now has performed its function by packaging the acrosomal contents and membranes, moves away from the nucleus toward the caudal end of the spermatid. The primitive flagellum (tail), formed from the distal centriole, begins to project from the spermatid toward the lumen (Figure 10-7) of the seminiferous tubule.

The acrosomal phase = nuclear and cytoplasmic elongation

During the **acrosomal phase** the acrosome continues to spread until it covers about 2/3 of the anterior nucleus (Figure 10-8). The nucleus and cytoplasm begins to elongate. A unique system of microtubules known as the **manchette** extends from the area of the posterior nucleus, and portions of the manchette attach to the region of the nucleus just posterior to the acrosome (Figure 10-8). Some of the **microtubules** of the manchette will become the **postnuclear cap** (Figure 10-9). During the acrosomal phase, spermatids become deeply embedded in Sertoli cells with their tails protruding toward the lumen of the seminiferous tubule (Figure 10-4).

The maturation phase = final assembly to form a spermatozoon

During the **maturation phase** portions of the manchette migrate towards the tail and begin to disappear, while portions of it remain to form the final postnuclear cap. Mitochondria migrate toward and cluster around the flagellum in the region posterior to the nucleus. Mitochondria are quickly assembled around the flagellum from the base of the nucleus to approximately the anterior one-third of the tail. They are assembled in a helical fashion (Figure 10-11) and form the middle piece in fully differentiated spermatozoa. Coarse outer fibers of the flagellum and the fibrous sheath are produced and final assembly is complete. It should be emphasized that, as in any cell, the entire spermatozoon is covered with a plasma membrane. Integrity of the plasma membrane is required for the survival and function of spermatozoa.

Finally, release of spermatozoa from the Sertoli cells into the lumen of the seminiferous tubule occurs. This release is referred to as **spermiation** and is analogous to ovulation in the female, except that spermiation occurs continuously throughout the testis.

Spermatozoa = head + tail

Head = nucleus + acrosome + post-nuclear cap

Tail = middle piece + principal piece + terminal piece

The head of a mammalian spermatozoon has a shape characteristic for each species. In food producing mammals the nucleus is oval and flattened and is surrounded by a nuclear membrane. The chromatin is compacted and is almost inert because it is highly **keratinized**. Keratinoid proteins (hair, claws, hoofs and feathers) have a high degree of disulfide cross-linking and are quite insoluble.

The anterior two-thirds of the nucleus is covered by the acrosome. The acrosome is a membrane-bound lysosome that contains hydrolytic enzymes. These enzymes, **acrosin, hyaluronidase, zona lysin, esterases** and **acid hydrolases,** are required for penetration of the cellular investments and the zona pellucida of the ovulated oocyte. During fertilization the

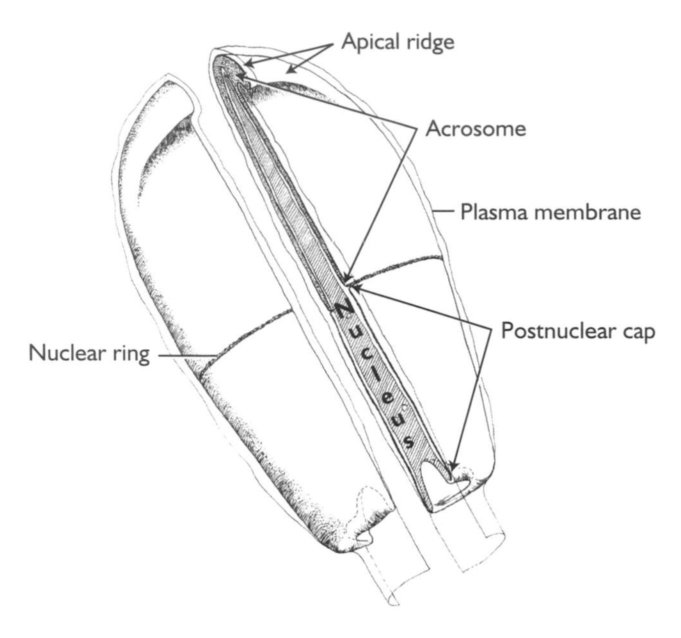

Figure 10-10. The head of a bovine spermatozoon. (Figure courtesy of Dr. R.G. Saacke, Virginia Polytechnic Institute and State University with permission from John Wiley and Sons, Inc. *Am. J. Anat.* 115:143.)

acrosome undergoes an ordered, highly specialized exocytosis, known as the acrosome reaction, which allows release of the enzymes that are packaged in it to digest or penetrate the zona pellucida. These reactions will be described in more detail in Chapter 12. Acrosomal morphology varies among species, but in the boar, ram, bull and stallion the acrosome is similar to that shown in Figure 10-10. The membrane component posterior to the acrosome is the postnuclear cap.

The sperm tail is a self-powered flagellum.

The tail is composed of the **capitulum,** the **middle piece**, the **principal piece** and the **terminal piece**. The capitulum fits into the implantation socket, a depression in the posterior nucleus. The anterior portion of the tail consists of laminated columns that give the neck region flexibility when it becomes motile, so the tail can move laterally from side to side during the flagellar beat. The axonemal component of the tail originates from the distal centriole and is composed of 9 pairs of microtubules that are arranged radially around two central filaments. Surrounding this 9+9+2 arrangement of microtubules are 9 dense fibers that are unique to the flagellum of spermatozoa. This arrangement of tubules in the tail of the spermatozoa is illustrated in Figure 10-11.

The mitochondrial sheath is arranged in a helical pattern (Figure 10-11) around the outer dense fibers of the tail and contributes to the middle piece. The middle piece terminates at the annulus, which demarcates the juncture between it and the principal piece. The principal piece makes up the majority of the tail and continues almost to the end of the flagellum, where it connects to the terminal piece.

Spermatozoa Are Released Continually into the Lumen of the Seminiferous Tubules

One of the major differences between gamete production in the female and the male is that the female produces gametes in a pulsatile manner, occurring every several weeks. In contrast, the male produces gametes continually and uniformly throughout his reproductive lifespan. An exception to this is the seasonal breeder that produces spermatozoa during the breeding season only. Understanding the mechanisms responsible for the continual production of spermatozoa by the seminiferous epithelium represents a major challenge for students of reproductive physiology.

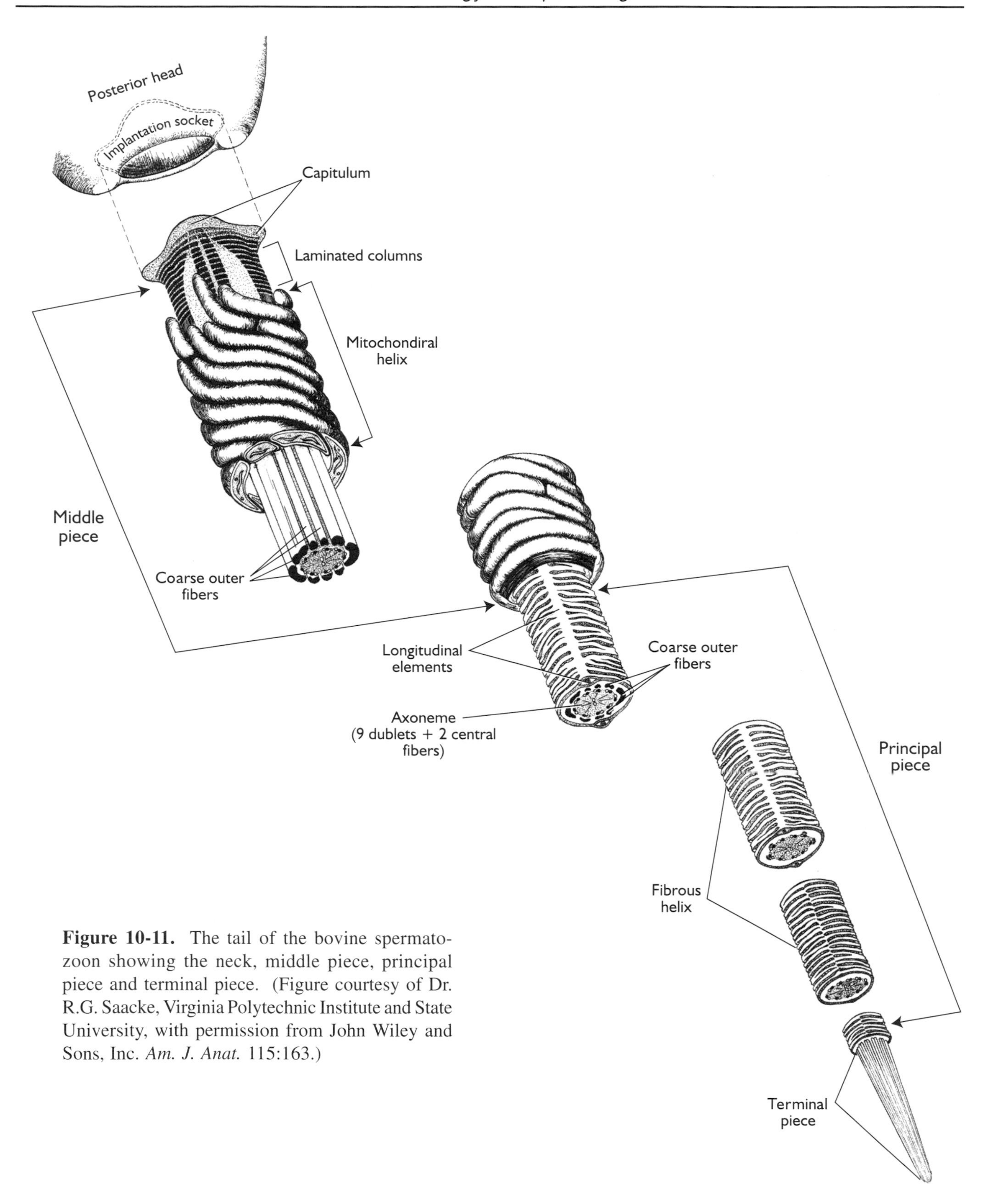

Figure 10-11. The tail of the bovine spermatozoon showing the neck, middle piece, principal piece and terminal piece. (Figure courtesy of Dr. R.G. Saacke, Virginia Polytechnic Institute and State University, with permission from John Wiley and Sons, Inc. *Am. J. Anat.* 115:163.)

In order to comprehend the cycle of the seminiferous epithelium you must first understand:

- ***cellular generations***
- ***stages of the cycle***
- ***duration of each stage***

The **cycle of the seminiferous epithelium** is the progression through a complete series of cellular associations (stages) at one location along the seminiferous tubule. The time required for this progression is the duration of the cycle of the seminiferous epithelium and is unique for each species.

Germ cell generations are cells of the same type located within the seminiferous epithelium.

Within any given cross-section of a seminiferous tubule, one can observe four or five "layers" of germ cells. Cells in each layer comprise a generation. A generation is a cohort of cells that develops as a synchronous group. Each generation of cells (each concentric layer) has a similar appearance and function. Cross-sections along the course of a seminiferous tubule will have a slightly different appearance. For example, while viewing cross section I in Figure 10-12, you will observe four generations of germ cells. Each generation will give rise to a succeeding, more advanced generation. Observe in Figure 10-12 that there is a generation of A-spermatogonia near the basement membrane in the section of the tubule labeled Stage I. Just above the A-spermatogonia is a young generation of primary spermatocytes. Above it lies a third generation consisting of more mature primary spermatocytes. Finally, near the lumen, is a fourth generation of cells. This generation consists of spherical immature spermatids. Remember that the more immature cell types are located near the basement membrane (basal compartment) and the more advanced cell types reside in the adluminal compartment.

In cross-section IV of Figure 10-12, there are five generations of germ cells. You will observe a generation of A-spermatogonia, one generation of intermediate spermatogonia, one generation of primary spermatocytes, one generation of secondary spermatocytes and one generation of spermatids. The spermatids in stage IV are elongated and, thus, are more advanced than the spermatids in stage I.

In cross-section VIII, there are also five generations of germ cells. Observe two generations of spermatogonia (one generation of A and one generation of B-spermatogonia) one generation of primary spermatocytes and two generations of spermatids. One generation of spermatids is quite immature and spherical, while the more advanced generation are mature spermatids ready to be released from Sertoli cells into the lumen of the seminiferous tubule (see Figure 10-4).

To summarize the above example, three cross-sections at different locations along the seminiferous tubule show different generations of cells at different stages of maturity. All sections are actively engaged in spermatogenesis, but only one cross-section (VIII) is ready to release spermatozoa into the lumen. Thus, along the length of any seminiferous tubule there are only certain zones (cross-sections) where spermatozoa are released. All other zones or stages are preparing to release spermatozoa, but the cells in those zones have not reached the appropriate stage of maturity for spermiation to occur.

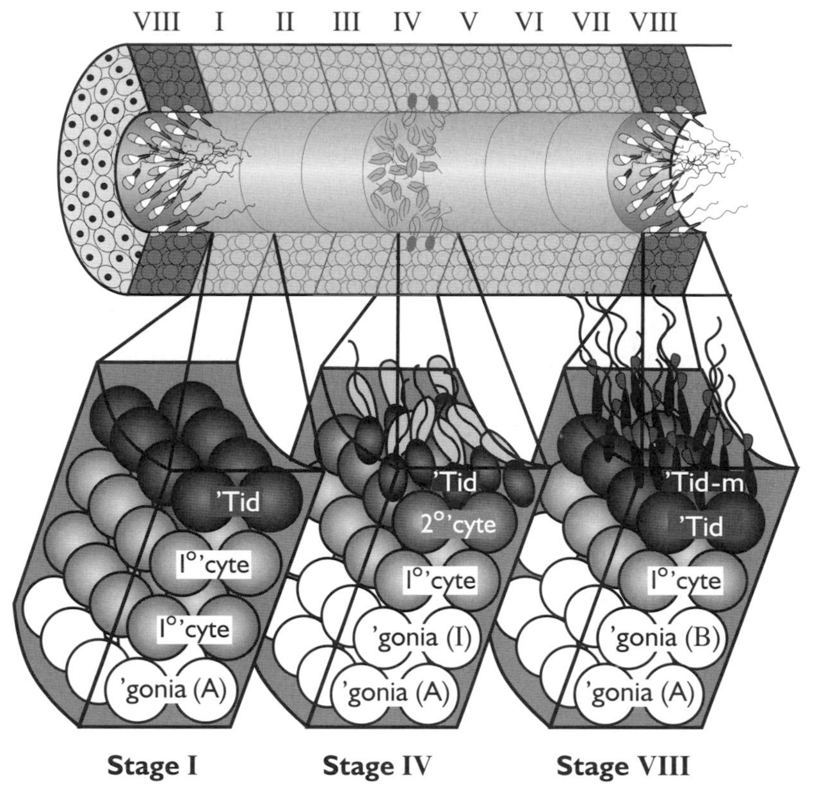

Figure 10-12. At any given location (cross-section) along a seminiferous tubule one can observe different stages (associations of developing germ cells). In this example, we see three sections (Stage I, IV and VIII) with three different cellular associations. 'gonia = spermatogonium, 1°'cyte = primary spermatocytes, 2°'cyte = secondary spermatocytes, Tid = immature spermatid, Tid-m = mature spermatid. (Graphic by Sonja Oei.)

Stages of the cycle are arbitrarily defined cellular associations which disappear and reappear at predictable intervals.

As explained above, sections or zones along a seminiferous tubule contain different cellular associations. These cellular associations, or **stages of the cycle of the seminiferous epithelium,** have been defined arbitrarily by researchers who have made thousands and thousands of observations of the seminiferous epithelium using light microscopy.

If you were to microscopically scan a number of tubules in the testicular parenchyma, you would see tubule cross-sections that contain exactly the same cell types and relationships as other tubules. In fact, with enough observation you would begin to encounter different cross-sections with definable cellular compositions at predictable frequencies. For the purposes of this text, we will describe eight stages in the cycle of the seminiferous epithelium, even though other schemes are available with as many as 14 stages.

Figure 10-13 illustrates the cellular composition of each stage of the seminiferous epithelium. For example, stage I contains one generation of A-spermatogonia, two generations of primary spermatocytes and one generation of spermatids. By scanning from the basement membrane (bottom of diagram) toward the lumen, you can quickly determine which cell types are present at each of the eight stages.

Time requirements of the cycle vary among species.

The entire progression of one cycle of the seminiferous epithelium from stage I through stage VIII

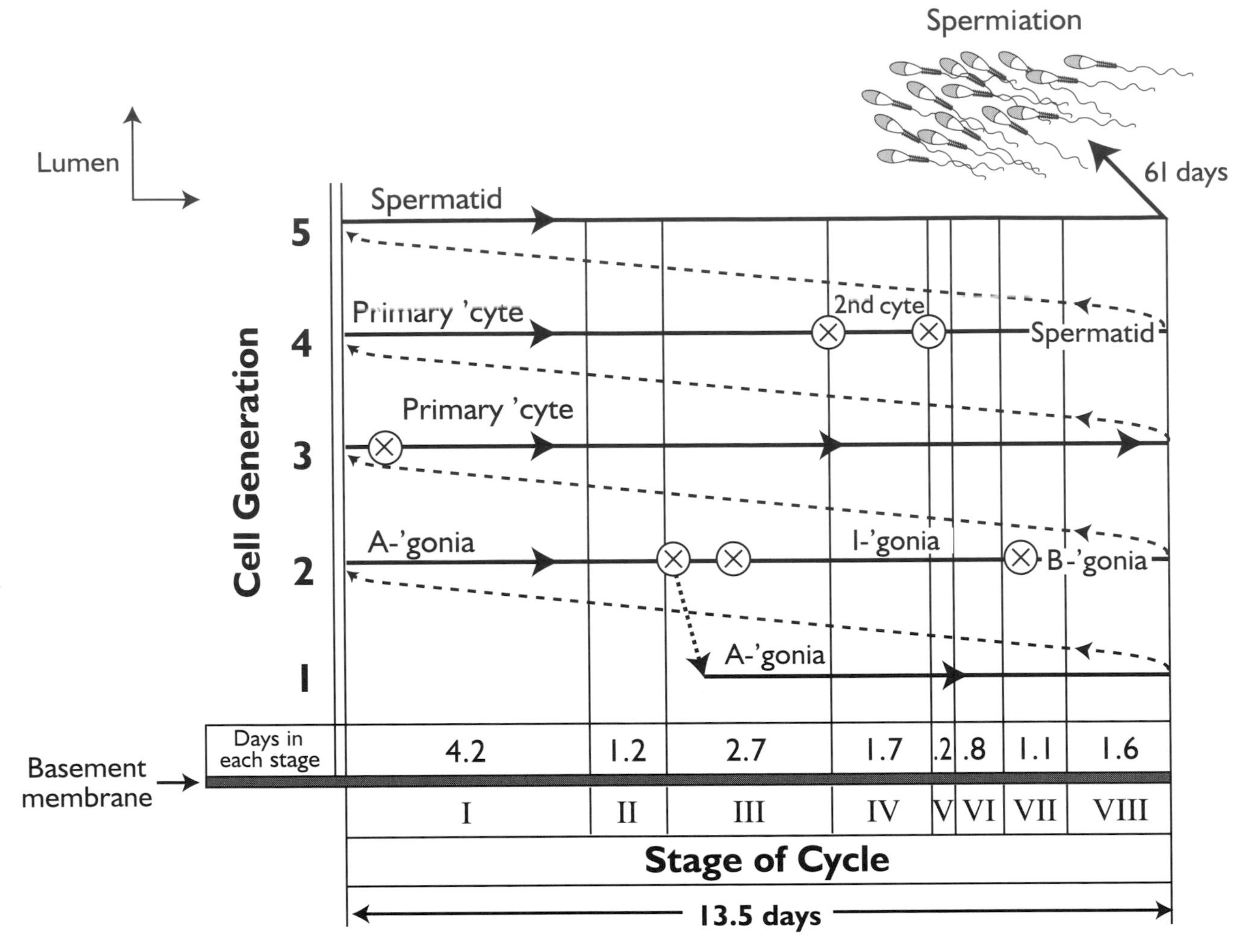

Figure 10-13. The 4.5 cycles of the seminiferous epithelium that make up the spermatogenic cycle in the bull. Along the horizontal axis are the stages (I-VIII) of the cycle. Notice that the width of the column designating each stage varies. This reflects the relative duration of each stage of the cycle. The vertical axis designates each cellular generation. Cell types are designated above the bold line. The X indicates a cell division. (Modified from Amann.)

requires 13.5 days in the bull (for other species see Table 10-1). That is, if you could observe one cross-section of a seminiferous tubule continually, starting at the beginning of stage I, it would require 13.5 days before you would observe spermiation (the end of a stage VIII). After spermiation (end of stage VIII), the cross-section you were observing would again have the same cellular association as it did on the day you started watching (stage I). Thus, one cycle of the seminiferous epithelium would have been completed.

The complete process of spermatogenesis from A-spermatogonia to the formation of fully differentiated spermatozoa takes 60.75 days in the bull. During the 60.75 days, cells at a given area of the seminiferous epithelium proceed through 4.5 cycles of the seminiferous epithelium (13.5 days/cycle X 4.5 cycles = 60.75 days).

This process is analogous to a traditional university timetable. Every year a new class of freshmen enters the university in the fall. These freshmen are analogous to committed A-spermatogonia entering the spermatogenic pathway. The freshmen (A-spermatogonia) undergo noticeable changes during the first year, and after one year they become sophomores. Sophomores are analogous to primary spermatocytes. The sophomores (primary spermatocytes) also undergo maturational changes and become juniors (secondary spermatocytes). Finally, they become seniors (spermatids) and graduate after four years (Figure 10-14).

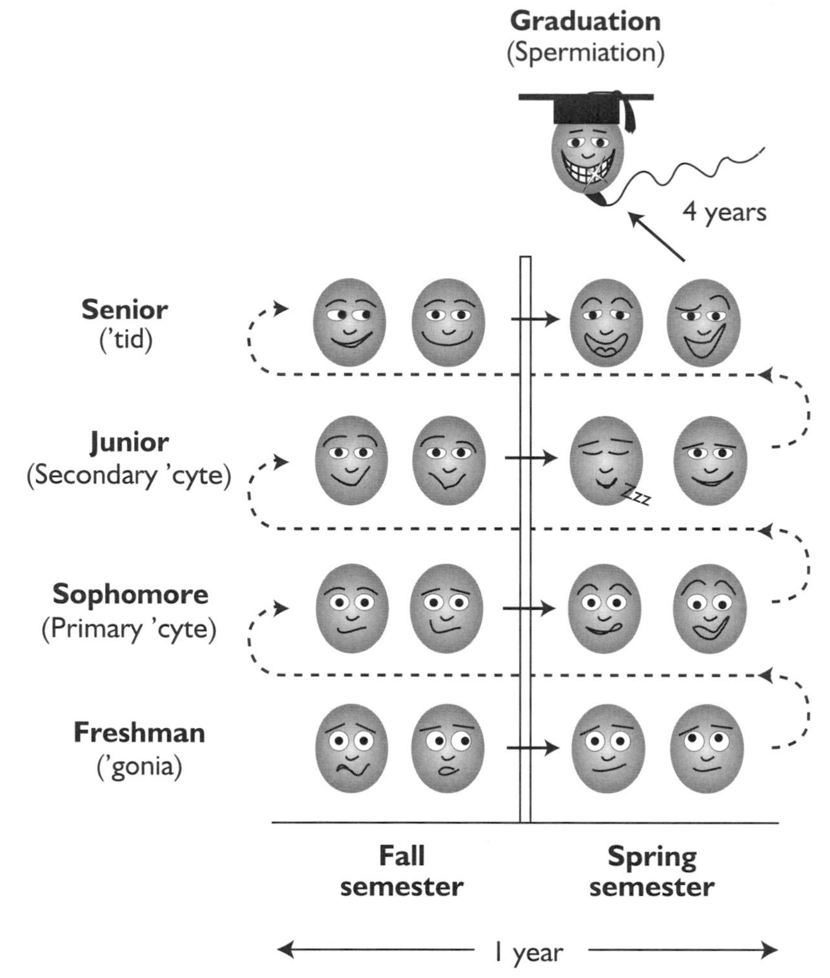

Figure 10-14. The cycle of the seminiferous epithelium is analogous to a university. Every year, freshmen (spermatogonia) enter and seniors (spermatozoa) graduate. However, four years are required for a freshman to progress through the various classes to become a graduating senior. Each class (freshman - senior) is analogous to a generation of germ cells found in the seminiferous epithelium. (Modified from Johnson; see additional reading.) (Graphic by Sonja Oei.)

The cycle of the seminiferous epithelium is almost identical in concept to the university situation, except the school year is only 13.5 days (1 cycle of the seminiferous epithelium). Every 13.5 days a new generation of freshmen (A-spermatogonia) enter and a generation of seniors (spermatids) leave. Graduation by the seniors is analogous to spermiation. Remember, it takes four years to graduate from the university. Similarly, it takes 4.5 cycles for an A-spermatogonium (freshman) to become a fully differentiated spermatozoon (senior). A major difference between the university example and the actual cycle of the seminiferous epithelium is that the germinal elements have different lifespans. For example, a primary spermatocyte exists

Stage ***= specific cellular associations***

Stage duration ***= time required for completion of one stage (cell association)***

Cycle ***= progression through sequence of all stages***

Cycle duration ***= time required to complete one cycle***

Table 10-1. Duration of the Stages of the Cycle of the Seminiferous Epithelium in Various Species.

Stage	Bull	Ram	Boar	Stallion	Rabbit
I	4.2	2.2	1.1	2.0	3.1
II	1.2	1.1	1.4	1.8	1.5
III	2.7	1.9	0.4	0.4	0.8
IV	1.7	1.1	1.2	1.9	1.2
V	0.2	0.4	0.8	0.9	0.5
VI	0.8	1.3	1.6	1.7	1.7
VII	1.1	1.1	1.0	1.6	1.3
VIII	1.7	1.0	0.8	1.9	0.9
TOTAL[A]	13.5	10.4	8.3	12.2	10.7
SPERMATOGENESIS[B]	61	47	39	55	48

[A]Total days required for 1 cycle of the seminiferous epithelium.
[B]Approximate days to complete spermatogenesis (spermatogonia to spermatozoa).

for about 21 days while a secondary spermatocyte exists for only 1.7 days in the bull. In the university, freshman, sophomores, junior and seniors have similar durations.

The duration of each stage of the cycle of the seminiferous epithelium varies with species, as does the length of the cycle of the seminiferous epithelium. Variations in stage, cycle length and total time required for spermatogenesis are presented in Table 10-1.

The spermatogenic wave is the sequential ordering of stages along the length of the seminiferous tubule.

The cycle of the seminiferous epithelium within a given zone of the seminiferous tubule depicts changes over time. The **spermatogenic wave** refers to the distribution of stages along the length of the seminiferous tubule at any given instant in time (i.e. location or site). Imagine that you could walk down the lumen of the seminiferous tubule. As you walk down the tubule, you will encounter zones that are near spermiation (stage VIII). The distance between these spermiation sites is relatively constant. During the wave, each stage of the seminiferous epithelium changes to a successively more advanced stage. For example, a stage I tubule will later become a stage II and stage II will later become a III and so on. Thus, the site of spermiation along the tubule is constantly changing, creating a "wave" of sperm release down the length of the tubule. This "wave" is like the wave conducted by football fans in a stadium. When the fans stand up, they mimic spermiation. They sit back down and don't stand up again until they have had a period of rest. The time spent sitting (stages I - VII) is much longer than the time spent standing. As the wave in the stadium continues, repeated standing and sitting takes place at a relatively constant rate. So does spermiation. The physiologic importance of the spermatogenic wave is to provide a relatively constant supply of spermatozoa to the epididymis, creating a pool for ejaculation.

Sperm production rates by food producing animals are immense.

Man has selected food producing animals with large testes and high sperm producing rates. There is a strong correlation between the size (circumference) of the testicles and their ability to produce spermatozoa. In fact, measurement of scrotal circumference is a common technique used to determine whether or not a bull or ram meets minimum criteria for sperm production when used

Table 10-2. Testicular characteristics and sperm production estimates of selected sexually mature mammals.

Species	Gross weight of paired testes (grams)	Sperm produced per gram of testicular parenchyma	Daily spermatozoal production
Dairy Bull	650	$18x10^6$	$10x10^9$
Beef Bull	500	$18x10^6$	$8x10^9$
Ram	550*	$26x10^6$	$14x10^9$
Boar	750	$30x10^6$	$25x10^9$
Stallion	165	$18x10^6$	$3x10^9$
Rooster	25		
Rabbit	6	$41x10^6$	$.254x10^9$
Man	40	$4.25x10^6$	$45\text{-}207x10^6$

*in breeding season (short day length)

in natural service. Scrotal width is used for the boar and stallion. A measurement of scrotal circumference is simple, non-invasive and a good indicator of sperm producing ability.

Daily sperm production (DSP) is defined as the total number of spermatozoa produced per day by the two testicles. Accurate measurement of DSP requires removal of all or a portion of the testicle and, thus, DSP cannot be measured using non-invasive techniques. However, non-invasive measures such as scrotal circumference or width, or spermatozoa ejaculated into an artificial vagina at high ejaculation frequencies are good estimates of DSP. Interspecies variation in testicular weights, sperm produced per gram of testicular parenchyma and daily sperm production is presented in Table 10-2.

Spermatozoa produced per gram of tissue is sometimes referred to as **spermatogenic efficiency**. The degree to which the testes can produce spermatozoa is dependent, at least in part, on the number of Sertoli cells that populate the testes. For example, the higher the number of Sertoli cells, the higher the spermatozoal production rates. Numbers of Sertoli cells also have been positively correlated with spermatogonial and spermatid numbers. The exact reason that Sertoli cells control spermatozoal production rates is not understood.

Manipulation of Sperm Production

While certain endocrine conditions must be met for spermatogenesis to occur, it is not possible to increase the DSP by administration of exogenous gonadotropins. Thus, until recently there has been no good option for increasing sperm producing ability in mammals. Exciting work being conducted at the University of Illinois has provided the first evidence that sperm production rates can be enhanced in rats by inducing **hypothyroidism** in neonatal rats for a period of about 20 days after birth. If the dams of neonatal rats are fed a **goitrogen** called polypropylthiouracil, it will pass from the maternal blood into the milk, which is consumed by the neonatal rats, that in turn become hypothyroid. When these rats were removed from their dam and allowed to mature, it was discovered that testicular sizes of almost twice their non-treated counterparts occurred. In addition, these animals had significantly higher DSP when compared to controls. Male rats that were hypothyroid for 20 days after birth had higher Sertoli cell numbers than did the controls, and this has been shown to account for the elevated spermatogenic ability. If such an approach proves fruitful in food producing animals, it may be possible to significantly improve spermatogenic potential in animals in which artificial insemination is employed.

Further Phenomena for Fertility

Spermatozoa of the American opossum are ejaculated in doublets. They are formed in the seminiferous epithelium as single cells with an acrosome. During epididymal transit the acrosome of two spermatozoa attach to each other, so that a pair of spermatozoa exists. These doublets apparently have more progressive motility than do single cells. When motility ceases they apparently separate.

Some spiders have no penis. They eject sperm from their abdomen onto their web. The male spider picks up the ejaculate with a special set of antennae and searches for a receptive female who produces a pheromone. The male has to be very careful and deposit the semen by surprise because the female will eat him if she catches him.

In some regions of the world, testes are prized as gourmet treats. In Japan, testicles of dolphins are highly valued hors d'oeuvres. In Spain, bull testicles are served at social events surrounding the occasion of a bull fight. Bull testicles are also consumed by hungry American cowboys at castration time. In all cases, they are cooked.

Additional Reading

Johnson, L. 1991. "Spermatogenesis," in *Reproduction in Domestic Animals* 4th edition, Perry T. Cupps, ed. Academic Press, Inc. San Diego, CA.

Lamming, G.E. ed. 1990. *Marshall's Physiology of Reproduction Vol. 2 - Reproduction in the Male.* Churchill Livingstone, New York.

Russel, L. D. and M. D. Griswold, eds. 1993. *The Sertoli Cell.* Cache River Press, Clearwater, FL.

Dadoune, J.P. and A. Demoulin. 1993. "Structure and functions of the testis" in *Reproduction in Mammals and Man.* C. Thibault, M.C. Levasseur and R. H. F. Hunter, eds. Ellipses, Paris.

11 Reproductive Behavior

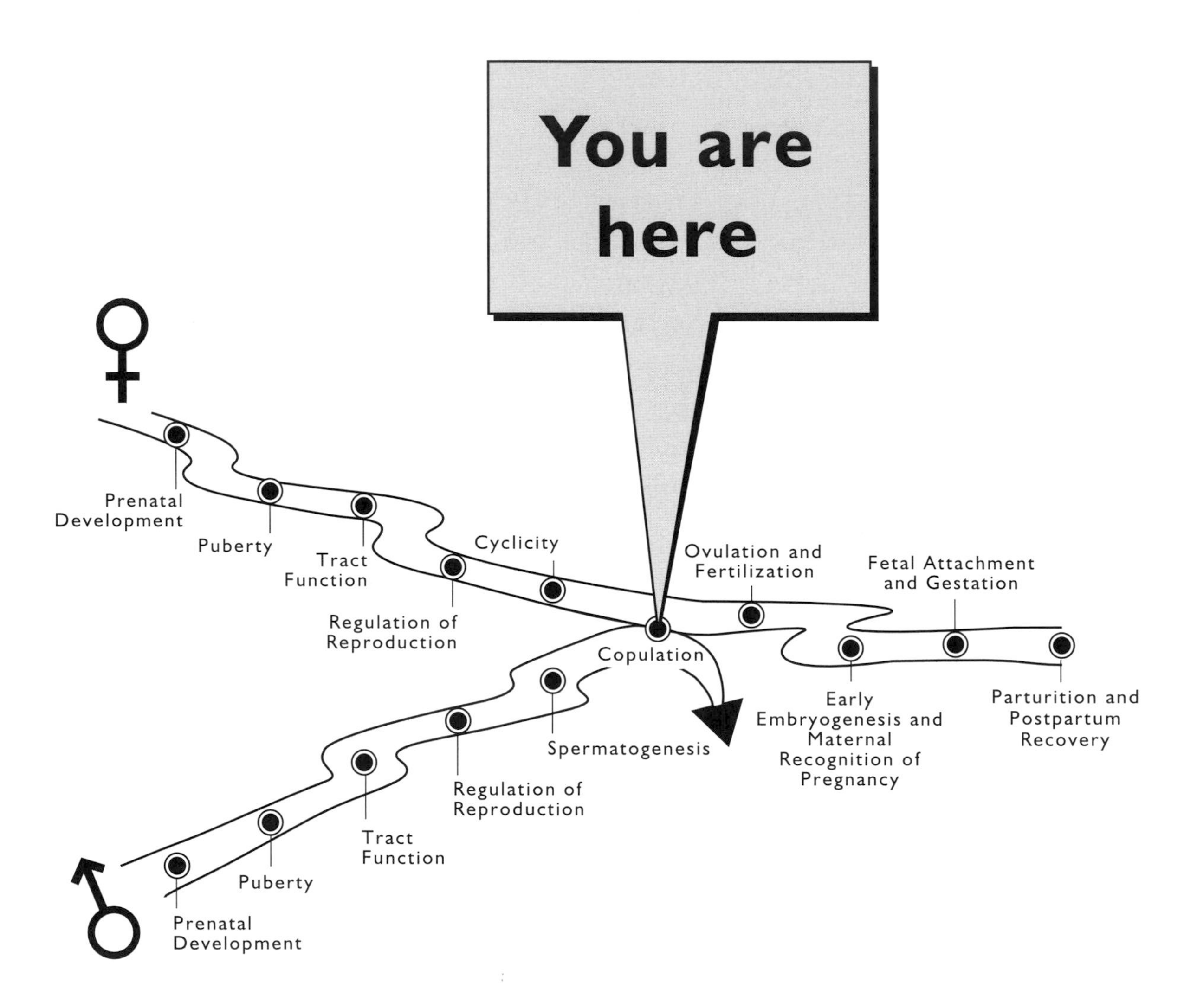

Take Home Message

Reproductive behavior consists of precopulatory, copulatory and postcopulatory stages. In the female sexual receptivity occurs only during estrus and is characterized by distinct behavior and mating posture (lordosis). In the male, reproductive behavior can occur at any time. Sexual arousal in the male involves a cascade of endocrine and neural events that result in erection of the penis, mounting of the sexually receptive female, intromission and ejaculation. Ejaculation is a reflex which is initiated by stimulation of the glans penis and concludes with expulsion of semen.

Reproductive behavior has evolved as one of the strongest drives in the animal kingdom and usually takes precedence over all other forms of activity such as eating, resting and sleeping. The purpose of reproductive behavior is to promote the opportunity for copulation and thus increase the probability that the sperm and the egg will meet. The ultimate goal of reproductive behavior is pregnancy, successful embryogenesis and parturition.

Reproductive behavior consists of three distinct stages:
- ***the precopulatory stage***
- ***the copulatory stage***
- ***the postcopulatory stage***

Reproductive behavior can be divided into three distinct stages. These stages are: the **precopulatory stage**; the **copulatory stage**; and the **postcopulatory stage**. The specific events that occur during each of these stages are presented in Figure 11-1.

Precopulatory behavior is a search for a sexual partner.

As you have already learned, sexual activity of the postpubertal female is confined to estrus (heat). This short period of sexual receptivity limits the time during which precopulatory behavior occurs in the female. In contrast, the male is potentially capable of initiating reproductive behavior at any time after puberty. The initiation of courtship-specific behavior is generally under the influence of the female. She will send subtle, or sometimes overt, signals to the male to initiate courtship behavior. Factors such as sexual signaling pheromones, vocalization, increased physical activity and subtle postural changes are signals provided by the female, which will initiate more aggressive courtship behavior on the part of the male. In addition, it has been hypothesized that female-female interactions such as homosexual mounting activity among cattle may serve as signals to initiate male-female courtship behavior. In general, the male is frequently searching for signals sent by the female to indicate that she is sexually receptive.

Identification of a sexual partner probably requires most of the senses (olfactory, visual, auditory and tactile). The relative importance of these sensory stimuli has not been described critically in most species.

Females of almost all species appear to show marked increase in general physical activity when they come into estrus. Elevated physical activity is generally manifested by increased locomotion. In addition, milling around, exploration, increased phonation and agonistic behavior towards other females can be observed.

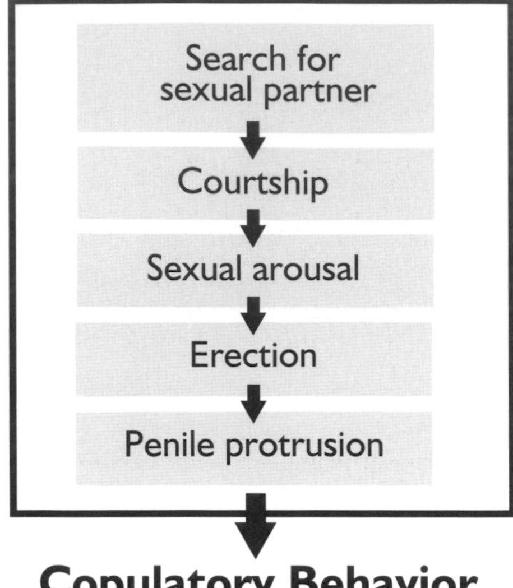

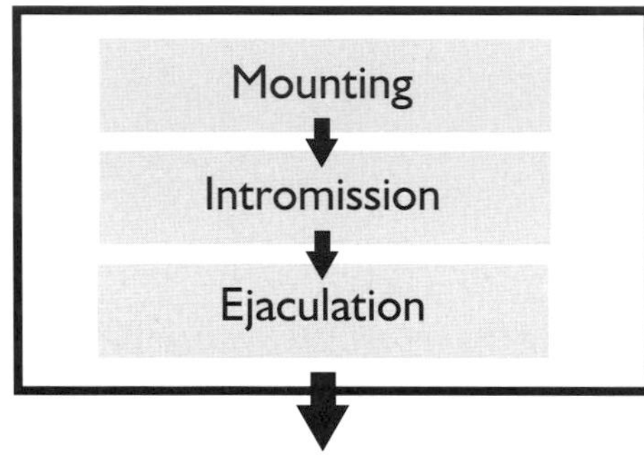

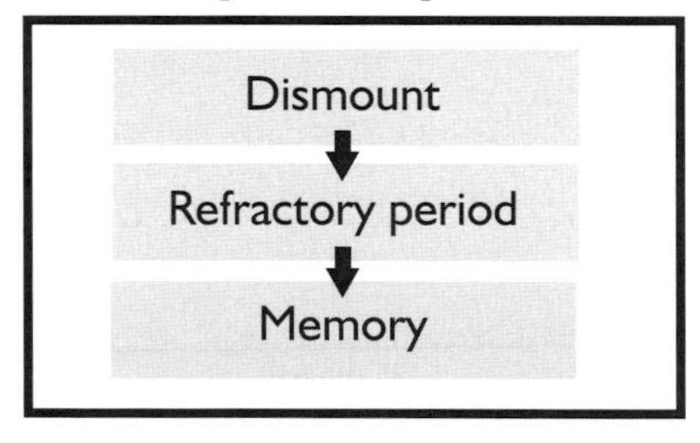

Figure 11-1. The stages of reproductive behavior and the events occurring within each stage.

In almost all species studied, including humans (see ***Further Phenomena for Fertility***) there is a marked increase in physical activity which accompanies the time of ovulation. Presumably, this physical activity is associated with searching for a mate. This increased physical activity can be measured by equipping females with pedometers. Pedometers are devices that monitor and quantitate steps taken by the animal and are currently used in commercial dairy enterprises for detection of estrus.

Courtship-specific behavior is initiated after a sexual partner has been identified.

Once a sexual partner has been identified, a series of highly specific courtship behaviors begin. Courtship-specific behaviors include sniffing of the vulva by the male, urination in the presence of the male by the female, exhibiting **flehmen** behavior (see Figure 11-4), chin resting, circling and increased phonation. In many species the sense of sight appears to be the most important with regard to sexual arousal in the male. This should not be interpreted to mean that other stimuli, such as auditory or olfactory are not important.

Lordosis (mating posture) by the female triggers significant sexual arousal behavior on the part of the male. Once the male has discovered that the female will display lordosis, he will generally become sexually stimulated. It should be emphasized that lordosis is a highly specific female motor response associated with the "willingness" to mate.

Sexual arousal is followed by erection and penile protrusion.

Following exposure to the appropriate arousal stimuli, erection and protrusion of the penis occur. These highly specific motor events are controlled by the central nervous system. The mechanisms of penile protrusion and erection will be presented later. Typical behavior during search, courtship and sexual arousal for the bovine, ovine, porcine and equine is presented in Table 11-1.

Copulatory behavior varies significantly among species with regard to duration.

After significant sexual stimulation has taken place, mounting, intromission and ejaculation follow. In general, mammals can be defined as sustained copulators and short copulators. The bull and the ram are short copulators while the boar is a sustained copulator. The stallion is intermediate with regard to duration of copulation.

Mounting behavior requires immobilization on the part of the female and elevation of the front legs of the male to straddle the posterior region of the female (Figure 11-6). **Intromission** is the entrance of the penis into the vagina. **Ejaculation** is the expulsion of semen from the penis into the female reproductive tract.

FEMALE			
Species	**Search**	**Courtship**	**Arousal**
Cow	Increased locomotion, increased vocalization, twitching & elevation of the tail	Increased grooming, mounting attempts with other females	Homosexual mounting & standing to be mounted
Mare	Increased locomotion, tail erected ("flagging")	Urination stance, urination in presence of stallion	Presents hindquarters to male, clitoral exposure by labial eversion, pulsatile contractions of labia
Ewe	Short period of restlessness	Urination in presence of ram	Immobile stance
Sow	Mild restlessness	Immobile stance	Immobile stance

MALE			
Species	**Search**	**Courtship**	**Arousal**
Bull	Chin resting, testing for lordosis	Flehmen, nuzzling, and licking of perineal region	Penile protrusion with dribbling of seminal fluid with few spermatozoa, erection and attempted mounts
Stallion	Visual search	Flehmen and high degree of excitement	Penile protrusion with no pre-ejaculatory expulsion of seminal fluid
Ram	Neck outstretched and head held horizontally	Flehmen, sniffing and licking of vulva, nudging ewe	Repeated dorsal elevation of scrotum, penile protrusion with no dribbling of seminal fluid
Boar	Moving among females	Nuzzling, grinding of teeth, foams at mouth	Penile protrusion, shallow pelvic thrusts, attempted mounting

Table 11-1. Typical behavior during search, courtship and arousal by female and male food producing mammals.

Copulatory behavior on the part of the male requires a certain degree of learning. Past sexual experiences are important in order for the male to develop appropriate reproductive behavior. For example, negative experiences during the precopulatory and copulatory stages will generally result in less enthusiasm on the part of the male. From a practical standpoint, management of the breeding male should always be directed towards providing the male with a totally positive experience. Utilizing non-estrous females to collect semen from stallions, boars, rams and bulls should be avoided because these females do not willingly stand to be mounted (lordosis). Injury to both the female and the male can occur under these circumstances.

Postcopulatory behavior is a period of refractoriness.

Postcopulatory behavior involves dismounting and a period during which either the male, the female or both will not engage in another period of copulatory behavior. This **refractory period** is a period of time during which a second copulation will not take place. Memory is important in both a positive and negative way. Positive mating experiences promote reproductive behavior and negative experiences do not. When semen is collected for artificial insemination, it is important to reduce the refractory period when multiple ejaculations need to be collected in the shortest possible time. Techniques to reduce the refractory period will be presented later in the chapter. Both males and females often display specific postcopulatory behavior such as vocal emissions, genital grooming, changing postural relationships and various tactile behaviors, such as licking and nuzzling.

Reproductive Behavior Is Programmed During Prenatal Development

During embryogenesis, sexual differentiation occurs, during which the brain is programmed to be either male or female. Recent findings suggest that the very early embryo is neutral with regard to sex (gender). Under the influence of extremely small quantities of estradiol the brain becomes feminized. **Feminization** is the development of female-like behavior. During development, α-fetoprotein is produced which prevents most fetal and maternal estradiol from crossing the blood-brain barrier and entering the brain. When this happens, the embryo becomes "fully feminized," because it has not been exposed to estrogen (see Figure 6-4). Alpha-fetoprotein does not bind to testosterone, which can then enter the brain and be converted to estradiol. In developing males this high concentration of estradiol in the brain causes **masculinization** of the brain. Masculinization results in the ability of the embryo to develop male-like behavior postnatally.

Sex differences in specific brain structures for the control of reproductive behavior have been observed. For example, in the male, the preoptic area of the hypothalamus is larger than in females. In the male, the size of neurons, the neuronal nuclei and the dendritic arborizations are greater. In the female, the ventromedial hypothalamus is more important with regard to reproductive behavior.

Females will display male reproductive behavior following injections of testosterone.

In most mammals, reproductive behaviors are sexually differentiated. For example, mounting, erection and ejaculation are typically male behaviors, while standing to be mounted (lordosis), crouching and elevated locomotion are typically female behaviors. These behaviors are endocrine controlled. For example, sequential treatment with progesterone and estradiol induces sexual receptivity in ovariectomized females and testosterone will restore reproductive behavior in castrated males. In some species, injections of testosterone into castrated females will even induce male-like reproductive behavior. Female fetuses exposed to androgens prenatally will display significantly reduced female behavior and acquire male-like behavior postnatally. In contrast, males exposed to estrogen or progesterone prenatally are unaffected. A classic example illustrating the behavioral manifestations of prenatal exposure to androgens is the freemartin heifer. As previously discussed (Chapter 4), this animal has abnormal development of the reproductive tract because of prenatal exposure to testosterone. In addition, the freemartin displays more male-like behavior than does her normal heifer counterparts. Figure 11-2 summarizes the influence of reproductive steroids on postnatal behavior in the male and the female.

Male reproductive behavior cannot be reversed by estradiol.

The presence of gonadal steroids (estrogen and testosterone) is obligatory for normal reproductive behavior in both the male and the female. For example, ovariectomized females display no estrous behavior (Figure 11-2). Likewise, castrated males have significantly reduced reproductive behavior. But, the abolition of reproductive behavior depends on the duration of time between castration and the opportunity to copulate. For example, males which have reached puberty and established a sustained pattern of reproductive behavior require a longer period of time between abolition of sexual behavior after castration than do males which have not established a sustained pattern of reproductive behavior.

When ovariectomized females receive injections of estradiol, estrous behavior is reestablished, but at a

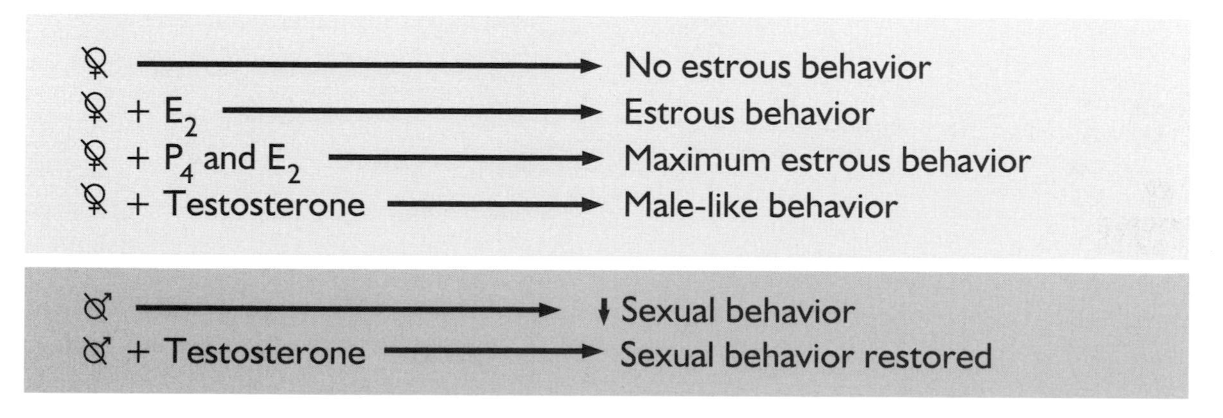

PRENATAL

♀ Fetus + E_2 →	↓ Estrous behavior + male-like behavior
♀ Fetus + Testosterone →	↓ Estrous behavior + male-like behavior
♂ Fetus + E_2 or P_4 →	No effect (normal ♂ behavior)
♂ Fetus + Testosterone →	No effect (normal ♂ behavior)

POSTNATAL

♀\ →	No estrous behavior
♀\ + E_2 →	Estrous behavior
♀\ + P_4 and E_2 →	Maximum estrous behavior
♀\ + Testosterone →	Male-like behavior
♂\ →	↓ Sexual behavior
♂\ + Testosterone →	Sexual behavior restored

Figure 11-2. Influence of various steroid treatments upon reproductive behavior. ("\" = castrated or ovariectomized)

less than maximum level. Among farm animals , ovariectomized females that are treated first with progesterone (to mimic the luteal phase of the cycle) and then treated with estradiol display maximum estrous behavior. In other species estradiol must precede progesterone to produce maximal behavior. It is not clear why progesterone "priming" of the central nervous system for maximal stimulation is necessary. Ovariectomized females that are treated with testosterone develop male-like behavior. They will even develop secondary sex characteristics (reduced pitch of voice, hump on the back of the neck and atrophy of the female reproductive tract).

Reproductive Behavior Is Controlled by the Central Nervous System

The neural pathways and key anatomical components for the control of reproductive behavior are presented in Figure 11-3. Reproductive behavior can take place only if the neurons in the hypothalamus have been sensitized to respond to sensory signals. Testosterone in the male is aromatized to estradiol in the brain and estradiol promotes reproductive behavior. Recall that testosterone is produced in small episodes every 4 to 6 hours. Therefore, there is a relatively constant supply of testosterone, and thus estradiol, to the hypothalamus in the male. This allows the male to initiate reproductive behavior at any time. In contrast, the female experiences high estradiol during the follicular phase only and will display sexual receptivity during estrus only. Under the influence of estrogen, sensory inputs such as olfaction, audition, vision and tactility send neural messages to the hypothalamus. These neurons synapse directly on neurons in the ventromedial hypothalamus as well as the preoptic and anterior hypothalamic regions. These sensory inputs cause neurons in the hypothalamus to release behavior specific peptides which serve as neurotransmitters. These neurotransmitters act on neurons in the midbrain. The neurons in the midbrain serve as receiving zones for the peptides produced by the hypothalamic neurons. The midbrain translates

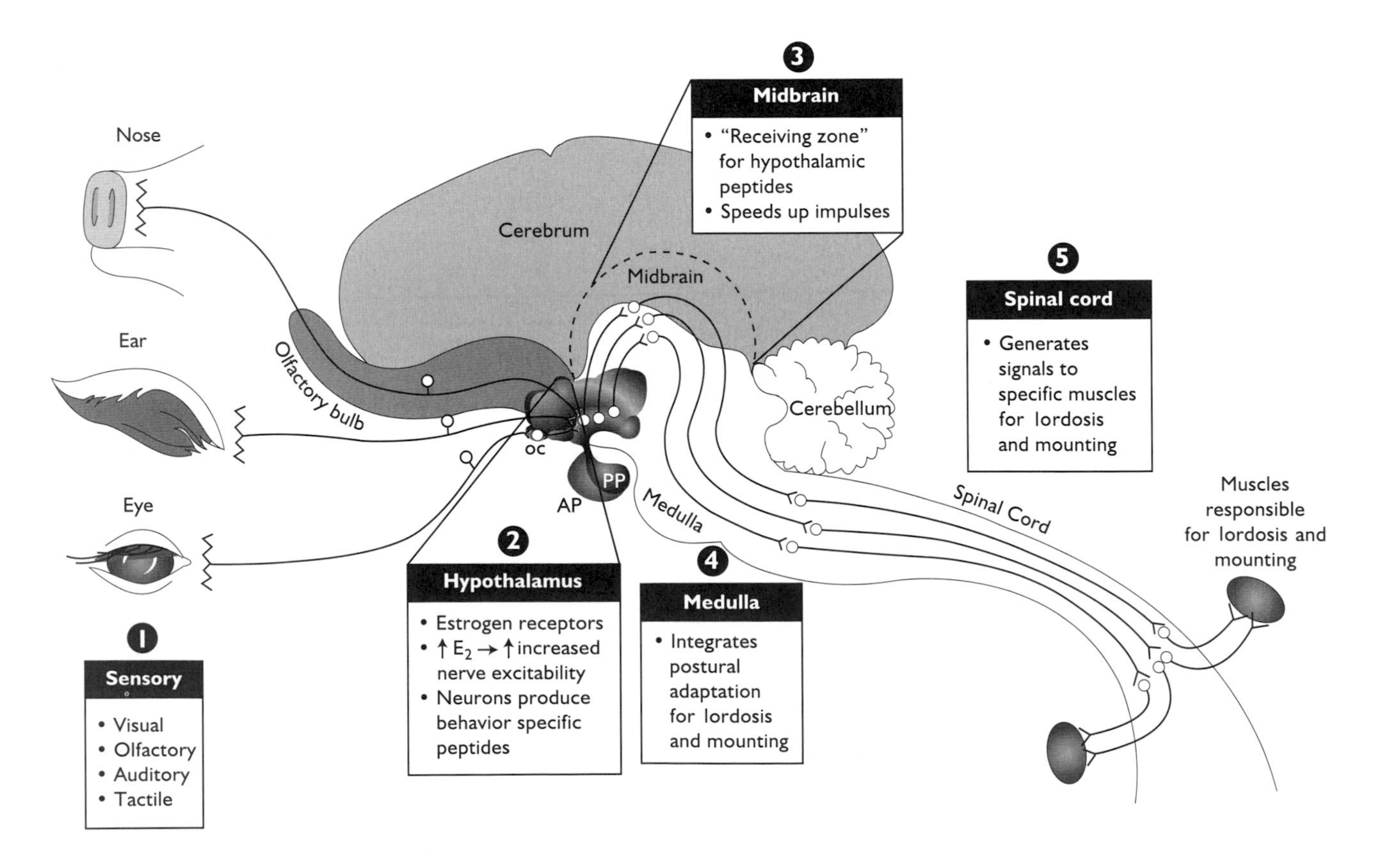

Figure 11-3. Hypothetical nervous pathway eliciting reproductive-specific motor behavior. (Graphic by Sonja Oei.)

signals generated by neuropeptides released by hypothalamic neurons into a fast response. Neurons in the midbrain synapse with neurons in the brain stem (medulla). These nervous signals are integrated in the medulla. From the medulla, nerve tracts extend to the spinal cord where the nerves synapse with motor neurons which innervate muscles that cause lordosis and mounting. It should be emphasized that the model presented in Figure 11-3 does not account for all of the nerve pathways involved in reproductive behavior.

Reproductive behavior is initiated by:
- ***olfaction***
- ***vision***
- ***audition***
- ***tactility***

The primary sensory inputs for reproductive behavior are olfaction, audition, vision and tactility. The degree to which these sensory inputs influence reproductive behavior, particularly precopulatory behavior, varies significantly among species.

The olfactory and the vomeronasal systems respond to pheromones which trigger reproductive behavior.

Secretions from the female reproductive tract serve as sexual attractants that sexually stimulate and attract the male to the female. Vaginal and urinary secretions from females in estrus smell different than secretions from females not in estrus. There is good scientific evidence that females produce pheromonal substances which are identifiable both within species and among species. Recall that a **pheromone** is a volatile substance secreted or released to the outside of the body and perceived by the olfactory system of other individuals of the same species. Pheromones cause specific behavior in the percipient.

Males also produce sex pheromones which attract and stimulate females. Among food producing animals, the best documentation for a male sex pheromone is in swine. Boars produce specific substances which cause sows and gilts to become sexually aroused when they are in estrus. Two sexual attractants are produced by boars. One of these attractants is a secretion of the preputial pouch. The second pheromonal-like substance is present in saliva secreted by the submaxillary salivary glands. During sexual excitement and precopulatory interactions, the boar produces copious quantities of foamy saliva. The active components in saliva are the androgen metabolites 3α-androstenol and 5α-androstenone. Both compounds have a musk-like odor.

It has been demonstrated that dogs have the ability to identify cows in estrus by olfactory discrimination. In addition, rats can be trained to press a lever in response to air bubbled through urine from cows in estrus. Rats did not press the lever when air was bubbled through urine from nonestrous cows. Clearly, urine from cows in estrus contains a material which can be identified by olfaction by other species (dogs and rats).

Some pheromones appear to be less volatile and need to be detected by the **vomeronasal organ** in the bull, ram, stallion and, to some extent, the boar. The male needs to closely approach the source of pheromones, and he will nuzzle the genital region of the female. The vomeronasal organ (Figure 11-4) is an accessory olfactory organ. It is connected to two small openings in the anterior roof of the mouth just behind the upper lip. Fluid-borne, less volatile chemicals can enter the vomeronasal organ through the oral cavity by means of the **nasopalatine** (incisive) **ducts**. Many species, such as bulls, rams and stallions, perform a special investigative maneuver when in close proximity to a female. Vaginal secretions and urine evoke an investigative behavior known as the **flehmen response**. Flehmen behavior allows less volatile materials to be "examined" by sensory neurons in the vomeronasal organ. Flehmen behavior is characterized by head elevation and curling

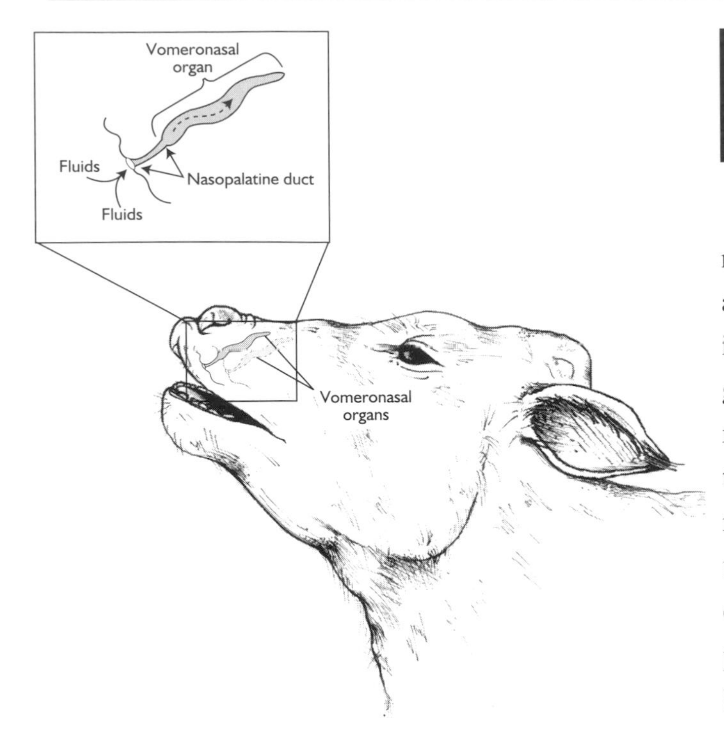

Figure 11-4. Morphology of the vomeronasal organ. Fluids are aspirated into the oral cavity and enter the vomeronasal organ through the nasopalatine duct. The flehmen response is believed to close the nostrils so that a vacuum in the nasopalatine duct sucks fluid into the vomeronasal organ. (Graphic by Sonja Oei.)

of the upper lip (Figure 11-4). Curling of the upper lip closes the nostrils and allows a sucking response to occur in the nasopalatine duct. Thus, less volatile materials can be aspirated through the duct into the vomeronasal organ where they can be evaluated by sensory neurons in the organ. Olfactory bulbectomy in goats inhibits the flehmen response. Flehmen behavior in males is likely to be performed whether the material is from an estrous or nonestrous female. It is believed that the flehmen behavior is used to help a male identify mating opportunities. Flehmen is sometimes performed by females during sexual encounters with males. They occasionally perform the maneuver when sniffing other cows that are in estrus or proestrus. As in the male, females will display flehmen to novel compounds, including fluids associated with the placenta, newborn animals and other volatile materials.

Auditory stimulation can serve as a long-range signal.

In many species, sexual readiness is accompanied by some form of unique vocalization. For example, cows are known to increase their bellowing during the time of estrus. Sows display a characteristic grunting sound associated with estrus. By comparison, mares and ewes are relatively silent. Elevated vocalization serves to alert or send a signal to males that sexual readiness is imminent. The auditory stimulus is more useful in long-range discrimination, rather than close discrimination. The classic example of reproductive driven phonation is the bugling of the bull elk during rut (the breeding season).

Visual signals are valuable for close encounters.

All females display a form of sexual posturing that can be perceived by males. While posturing can be quite subtle, the identification of postures probably takes place easily among members of the same species.

Almost all males experience a degree of sexual stimulation when they observe mating behavior among other animals. It is well documented that in bulls, visual observation of mating behavior enhances sexual stimulation. This observation has led to the common practice of placing bulls used for artificial insemination in "warm-up" stalls. Bulls are brought to the "warm-up" stalls and are allowed to observe the mounting behavior and collection of semen from other bulls prior to entering the collection area themselves. This causes an elevated level of sexual excitement and reduces the time required for final sexual stimulation and collection of semen. This is important because labor requirements for semen collection are significant.

> ***Tactile stimulation is generally the final stimulus before copulation.***

Tactile stimuli from males appears to be important in evoking sexual postures or standing postures by females. For example, biting on the neck and the withers of mares by stallions appears to be important for sexual stimulation. Rubbing of the flanks and genitalia of mares, whether done by the stallion or by a human handler, evokes behavior signals of estrus from the mare that otherwise would not be displayed. Chin resting by a bull on the back of a cow just prior to mounting may have some stimulatory effect on the cow.

> ***Erection of the penis requires:***
> - ***elevated arterial blood inflow***
> - ***restricted venous outflow***
> - ***elevated intrapenile pressure***
> - ***relaxation of the retractor penis muscle***

Erection of the penis is necessary for copulation and deposition of semen in the female reproductive tract. Erection is characterized by a marked increase in the rigidity of the penis. The increased rigidity is the result of a strong increase in arterial inflow of blood when compared to the venous outflow of blood. Erection requires that blood become trapped within the cavernous sinuses of the penis. Increased blood inflow to the penis is brought about by vasodilation of the arteries supplying it. In the bull, ram and boar erection not only involves increased blood flow and a subsequent increase in pressure, but a simultaneous relaxation of the retractor penis muscles. Thus, erection and protrusion also involves straightening of the penis to eliminate the sigmoid flexure. The penis of the bull, boar and ram is fibroelastic in nature and therefore does not increase significantly in diameter during erection and protrusion. In contrast, the penis of the stallion increases significantly in diameter during erection. The stallion has a retractor penis muscle which, as in other species, relaxes during erection. However, the stallion does not have a sigmoid flexure. Engorgement with blood plays a much more significant role in the highly vascular penis of the stallion than in the bull, ram and boar.

Engorgement of the cavernous tissues results from a blockage of venous return from the penis. Contractions of the ischiocavernosus muscles cause compression of the penile veins. As you will recall, the ischiocavernosus muscles surround the two crura. Intermittent contractions of the muscles creates a pump-like action at the base of the penis. These contractions result in a buildup of blood within the corpus cavernosum of the penis and exceptionally high pressures result. For example, during the final stages of erection, the pressures within the cavernous tissue of the goat penis can reach 7,000 mm Hg. When the penis is flaccid, pressures within the corpus cavernosum are only 19 mm Hg. Pressures in the bull penis are around 1700 mm Hg during peak erection and about 30 mm Hg when the cavernous spaces are collapsed. Figure 11-5 summarizes the steps of penile erection and intrapenile pressures as they relate to contraction of the ischiocavernosus and bulbospongiosus muscles.

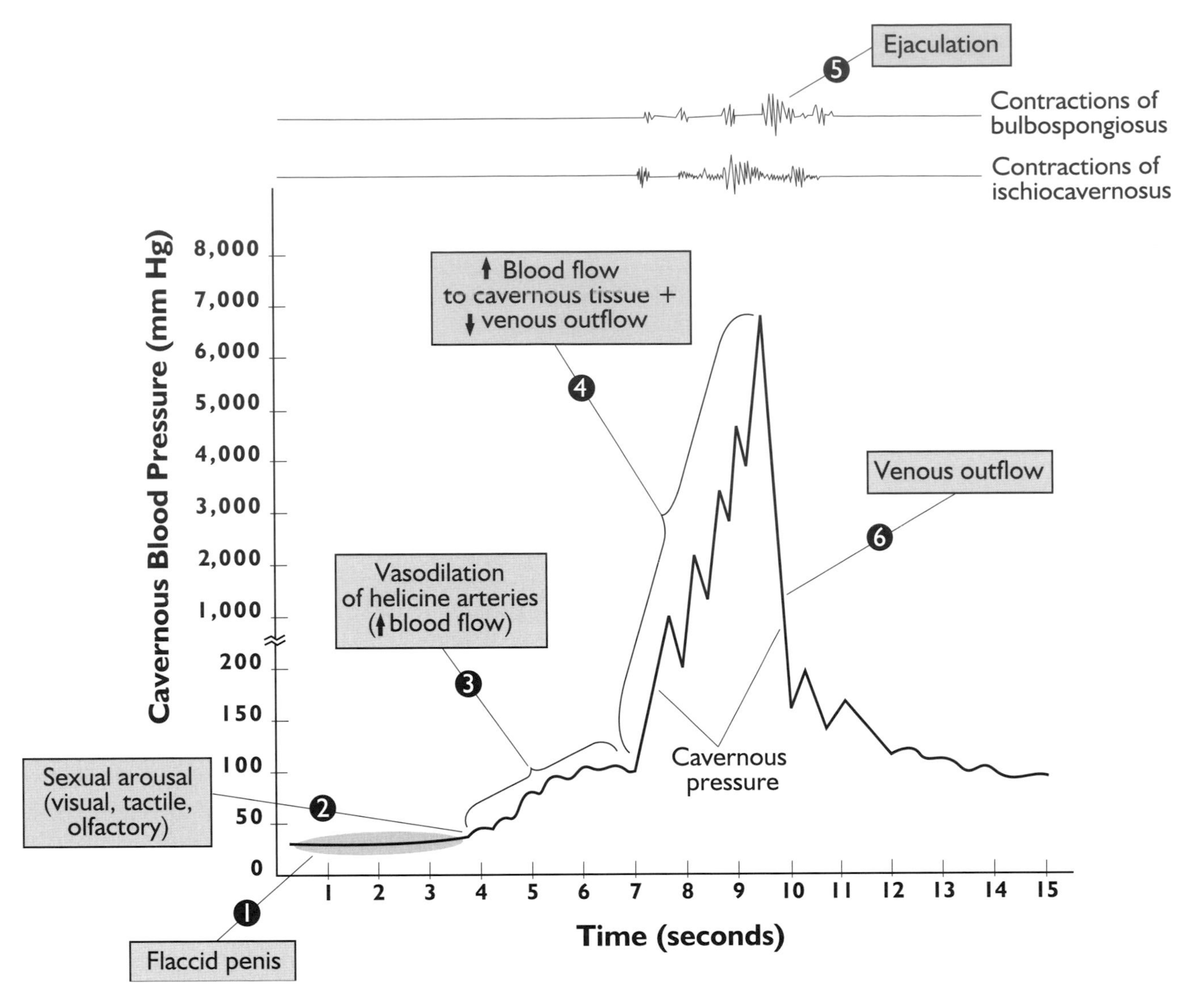

Figure 11-5. Steps in penile erection as they relate to cavernous blood pressure and contraction of the bulbospongiosus and ischiocavernosus muscles. (Modified from Beckett et. al. 1972. *Biol. of Reprod.* 7:359.)

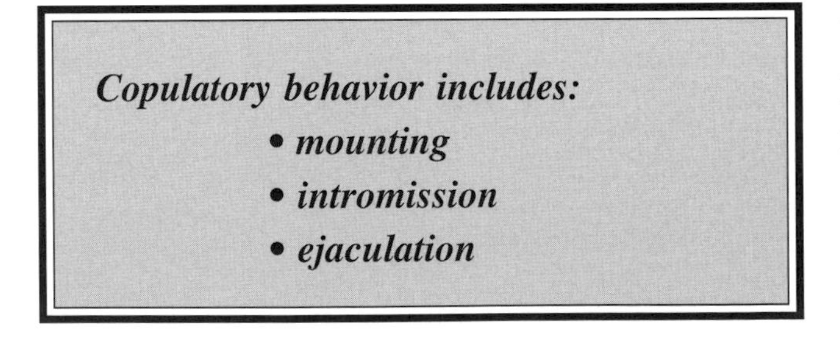

Mounting postures and characteristics of copulatory behavior for various species are presented in Figure 11-6. The purpose of mounting is for the male to position himself so that **intromission** can occur. Intromission is the successful entrance of the penis into the vagina. Following intromission, ejaculation takes place in response to sensory stimulation of the glans penis. The time of ejaculation relative to intromission varies significantly among species (Figure 11-6). For example, in the bull and the ram ejaculation occurs within one or two seconds after intromission. In these species ejaculation is stimulated by the warm temperature of the vagina. Vaginal pressure is relatively unimportant in inducing ejaculation in the ram and bull. In contrast, the boar may have a sustained ejaculation for periods of up to 30 minutes. The stallion has a mating duration of between 30 seconds and one minute.

Mating pair	Duration of copulation	Volume of ejaculate* (range)	Site of semen deposition	Average number of ejaculations to satiation	Maximum number of ejaculations to exhaustion
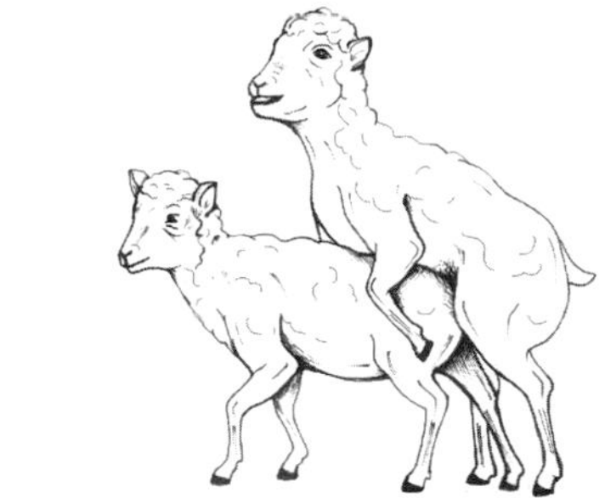	1 to 2 seconds (1 pelvic thrust with foreleg clasping)	.8 to 1 ml (.1 to 2 ml)	External cervical os	10	30 to 40
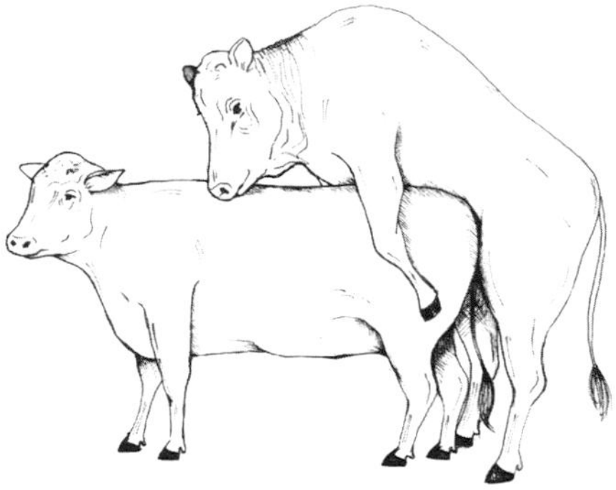	1 to 3 seconds (1 pelvic thrust with foreleg clasp)	3 to 5 ml (.5 to 12 ml)	Fornix vagina	20	60 to 80
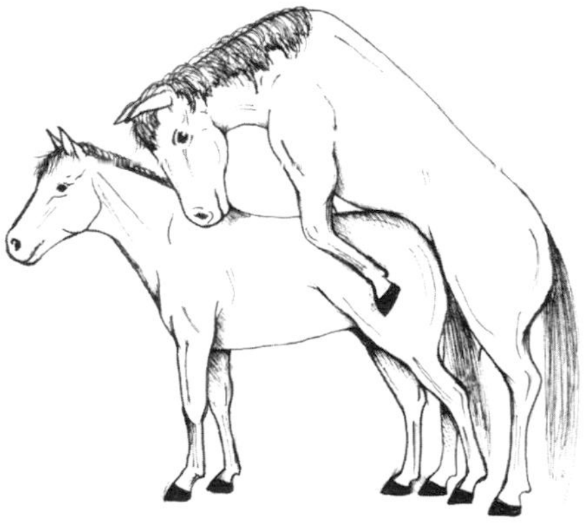	20 to 60 seconds (multiple pelvic thrusting. flagging of tail followed by inactive phase)	75 to 120 ml	External cervical os but semen enters uterus at high pressure	3	20
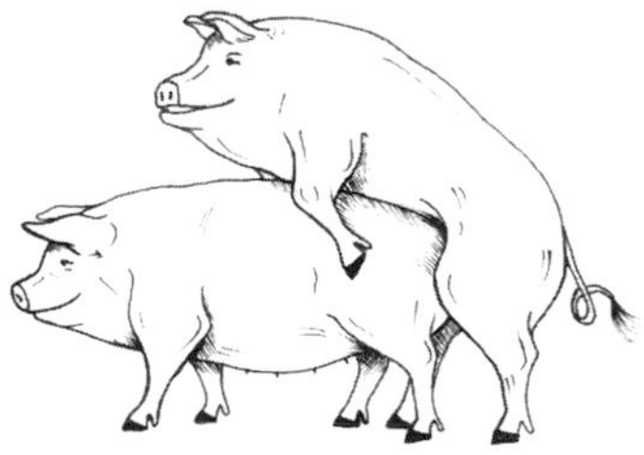	5 to 20 minutes (Rapid pelvic thrusting to engage penis in cervical folds. when penis engaged, thrusting stops and ejaculation commences which is accompanied by somnolence	200 to 250 ml	Cervix and uterus	3	8

* most commonly experienced volumes

Figure 11-6. Characteristics of copulation, site of semen deposition and number of ejaculations to satiation and exhaustion in the ram, bull, stallion and boar. (Graphic by Sonja Oei.)

> ***Ejaculation is a simple neural reflex caused by:***
> - ***intromission***
> - ***stimulation of the glans penis***
> - ***forceful muscle contraction***
> - ***expulsion of semen***

Ejaculation is defined as the reflex expulsion of spermatozoa and seminal plasma from the male reproductive tract. The basic mechanism for ejaculation of semen is quite similar among all mammals. Expulsion of semen is the result of sensory stimulation, primarily to the glans penis which causes a series of coordinated muscular contractions. Once intromission has been achieved, reflex impulses are initiated. These neural impulses are derived mainly from sensory nerves in the glans penis. Upon threshold stimulation, impulses are transmitted from the glans penis by way of the internal pudic nerve to the lumbosacral region of the spinal cord (Figure 11-7). The sensory impulses result in firing of nerves in the spinal cord and the forcing of semen into the urethra is accomplished by nerves in the hypogastric plexus which innervate the target muscles. Of primary importance for ejaculation is the urethralis muscle (which surrounds the pelvic urethra), the ischiocavernosus and the bulbospongiosus muscles.

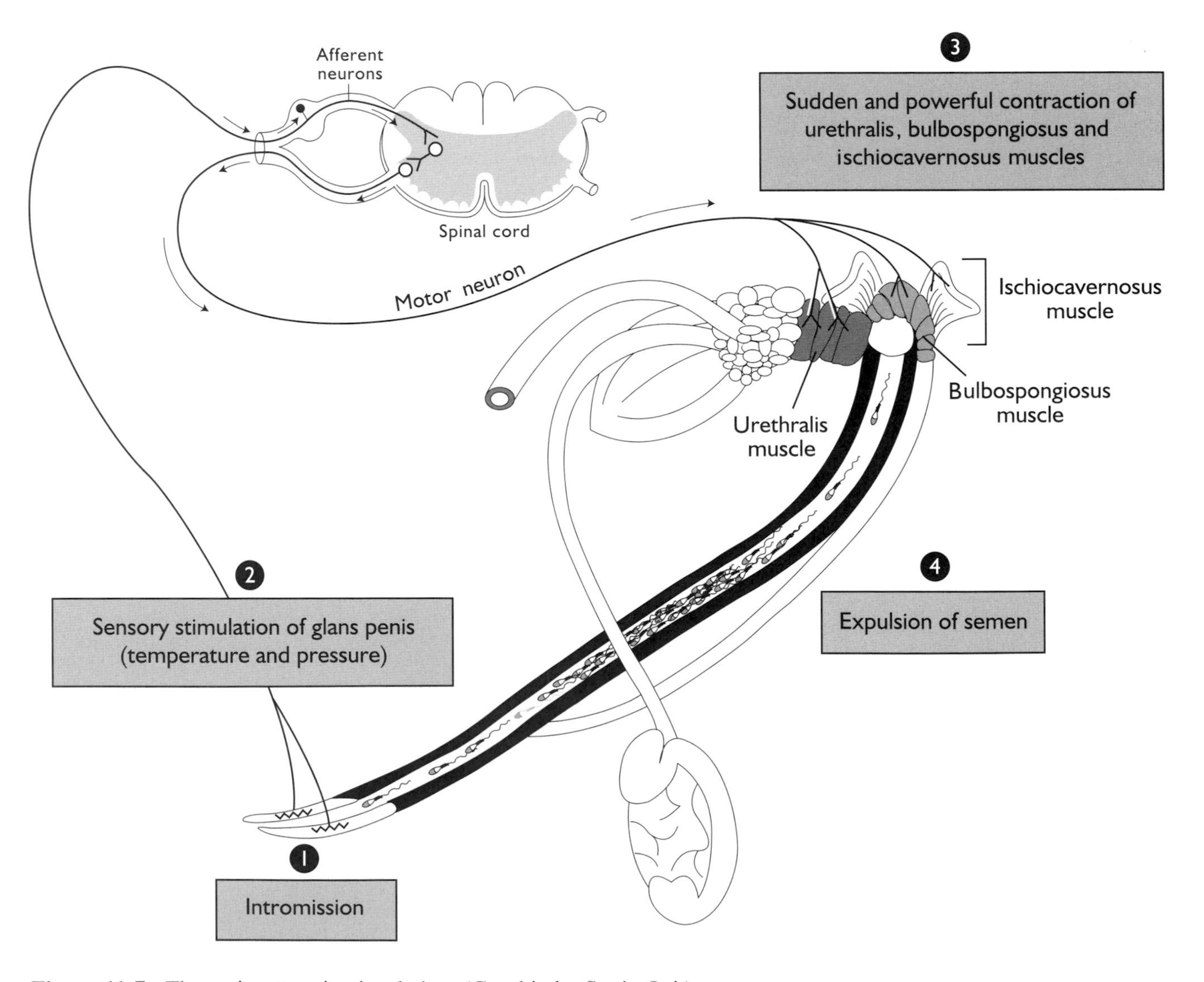

Figure 11-7. The major steps in ejaculation. (Graphic by Sonja Oei.)

Figure 11-7 summarizes the nerve pathways resulting in **emission** and ejaculation. It should be emphasized that emission is defined as the movement of seminal fluids from the accessory sex glands into the pelvic urethra so they can mix with spermatozoa. Emission occurs before and during ejaculation. In some species, such as the boar, emission occurs in a sequence resulting in an ejaculate which consists of various fluid fractions (see Chapter 12).

Postcopulatory behavior involves refractoriness and recovery.

Following ejaculation, all males experience a refractory period before a second ejaculation can occur. The length of time of this refractory period depends on several factors. These factors are: degree of sexual rest prior to copulation, age of the male, species of the male, degree of female novelty and number of previous ejaculations. The postcopulatory refractory period is sometimes erroneously referred to as sexual exhaustion. The refractory period should be considered as part of satiation rather than exhaustion. With natural service, it is quite normal for a male to copulate repeatedly with the same female. For example, a stallion will breed a mare in heat 5 to 10 times during one estrous period. Rams are noted to remate with the same ewe 4 to 5 times. Bulls also remate with estrous cows repeatedly. In fact, it has been noted in most species that if more than one female is in heat at the same time, the male will generally copulate preferentially with one, and sometimes will not copulate with a second female. Boars normally serve sows several times over a period of 1 to 2 days.

Sexual satiation refers to a condition in which further stimuli will not cause immediate responsiveness or motivation under a given set of stimulus conditions. Restimulation may occur after the refractory period. Figure 11-6 compares the normal number of ejaculations to satiety and the number of ejaculations to exhaustion among species. Exhaustion is the condition whereby no further sexual behavior can be induced even if sufficient stimuli are present. As you can see from Figure 11-6, there is a large variation in the behavioral reserves (the behavioral capacity, or **libido**) among farm species. There is also a large variation in libido within species. For example, beef bulls have significantly lower behavioral reserves than dairy bulls. While the factors that control the degree of reproductive behavior among males are poorly understood, they are almost certainly governed by genetic factors.

Reproductive Behavior and Spermatozoal Output Can Be Manipulated

Reproductive behavior can be enhanced by:
- ***introducing novel stimulus animals***
- ***changing stimulus settings***

The degree of novelty of both the copulatory partner and the copulatory environment can be of great importance when managing reproductive behavior in breeding males. Under conditions of artificial insemination, where repeated seminal collection is necessary to maximize the harvest of spermatozoa, an understanding of the influence of novelty and mating situations is important. The **"Coolidge Effect"** can be defined as the restoration of mating behavior in males (that have reached sexual satiation) when the original female is replaced by a novel female. In other words, a sexually satiated male can be restimulated if exposed to a novel female. (For derivation of the term "Coolidge Effect" see ***Further Phenomena for Fertility***.)

In bulls, semen collection can occur as frequently as 4 to 6 ejaculations per week. In order for this collection frequency to be successful, the male must first be sexually stimulated. Sexual stimulation is defined as the

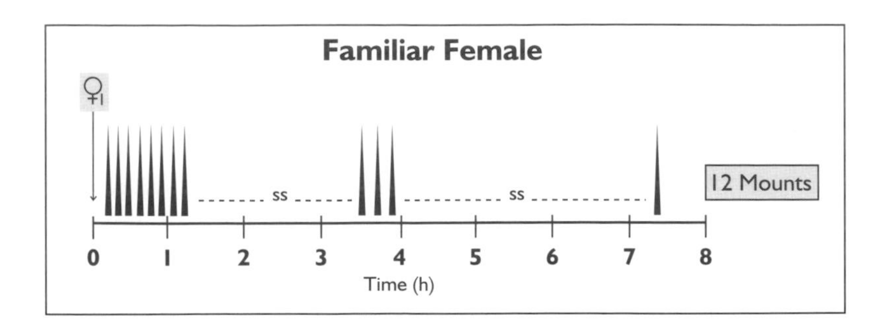

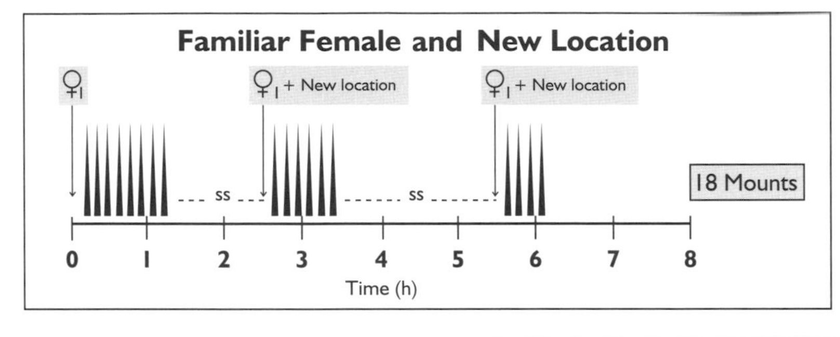

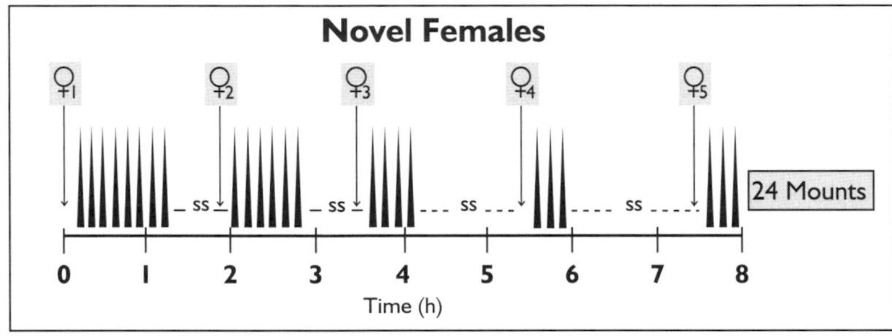

Figure 11-8. The relative influence of introduction of novel females and changing locations upon mounting behavior in bulls. SS = Sexual satiation.

presentation of a stimulus situation which will achieve mounting and ejaculation. The purpose of sexual stimulation is to obtain ejaculation or mating in the shortest time possible so that manpower involved in managing the mating of animals can be minimized. There are three approaches used to induce sexual stimulation in bulls used for artificial insemination. These approaches are: to introduce a novel stimulus animal; to change the stimulus setting; or both. Presentation of novel stimulus animals reinitiates sexual behavior after sexual satiation in bulls (Figure 11-8, "Novel Females") A second approach to achieve sexual stimulation after satiation is to present familiar stimulus animals in new stimulus situations. In other words, changing the location or setting has a stimulatory effect on the satiated male (Figure 11-8 "New Location"). In cases where sexual stimulation is difficult to achieve, presenting a novel stimulus animal, coupled with changing locations, often has positive effects.

There has been little research conducted on the effect of introducing novel animals upon stimulation in the female. However, it has been shown that dairy cows will mount novel cows with a greater frequency than they do familiar cows. As you might expect, the effect of novelty is confounded with the stage of the cycle.

Sexual preparation prolongs sexual stimulation and increases spermatozoa per ejaculation.

In order to maximize the output of spermatozoa per ejaculate, sexual preparation is necessary. **Sexual preparation** is the prolongation of the period of sexual stimulation beyond that needed for mounting and ejaculation. Sexual preparation prolongs the precopulatory stage of reproductive behavior. The purpose of sexual preparation is to collect semen containing the greatest possible number of spermatozoa per ejaculation. Figure 11-9 illustrates the physiologic mechanisms believed to be responsible for enhancing spermatozoal numbers in the ejaculate. Three approaches are used to sexually prepare a male. These are: false-mounting; restraint; and false-mounting plus restraint.

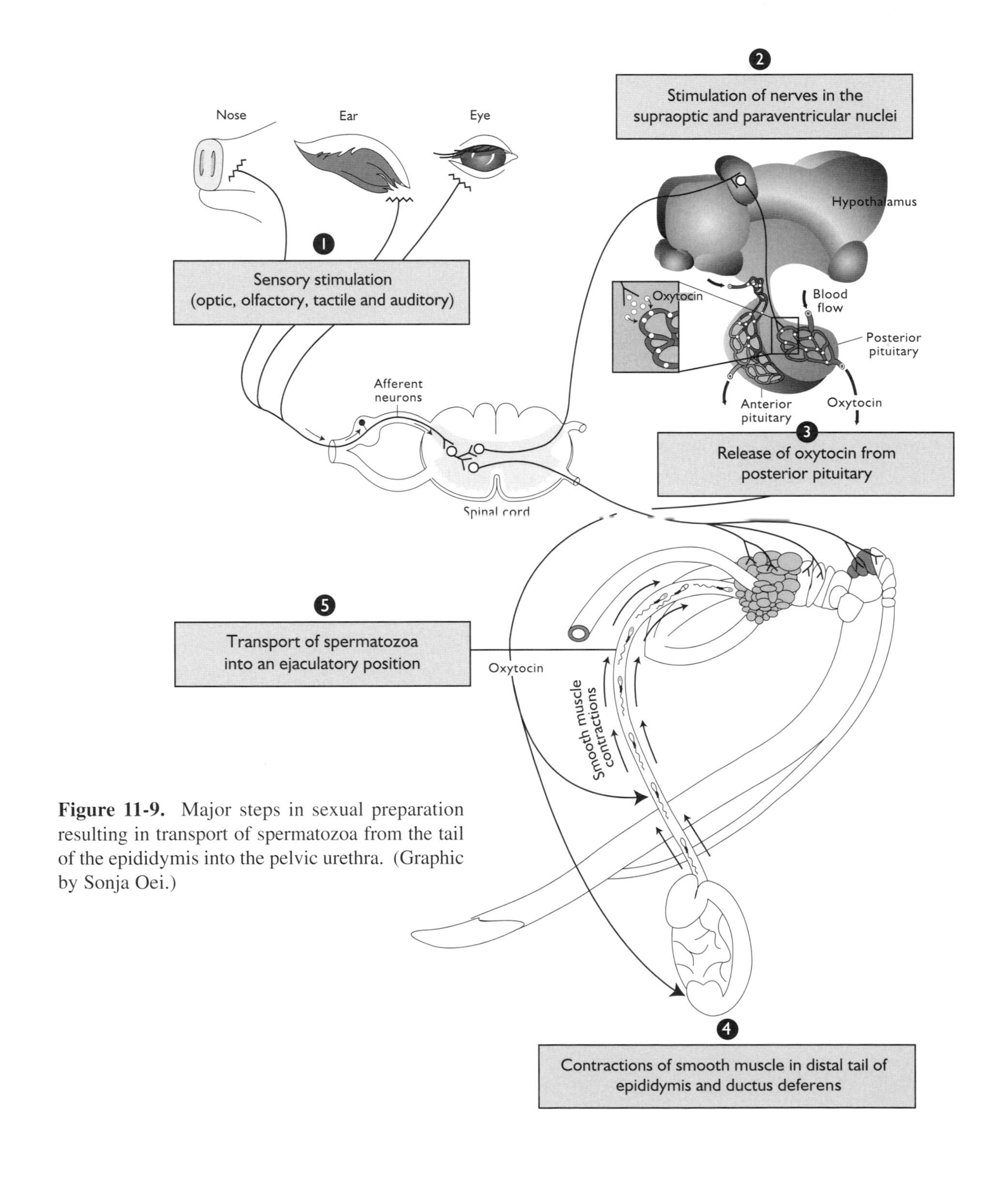

Figure 11-9. Major steps in sexual preparation resulting in transport of spermatozoa from the tail of the epididymis into the pelvic urethra. (Graphic by Sonja Oei.)

> ***Sexual preparation may include:***
> - ***false-mounting***
> - ***restraint***
> - ***false-mounting plus restraint***

False mounting consists of manually deviating the penis during a mount so that intromission cannot occur. If intromission does not occur, ejaculation usually does not occur. **Restraint** prevents the male from mounting even though he wishes to do so. Generally, restraint is for two to three minutes within two or three feet of the stimulus animal. A combination of false mounting and restraint will result in the greatest improvement of spermatozoal output.

In dairy bulls, the recommended procedures for sexual preparation are: one false mount, plus two minutes of restraint, plus two false mounts before each ejaculation. In beef bulls, three false mounts with no restraint is used. In general, beef bulls have lower behavioral reserves (libido) than dairy bulls, and thus have a less rigorous sexual preparation regimen.

While sexual preparation is taking place, release of oxytocin from the posterior pituitary occurs. Oxytocin causes contraction of the smooth musculature surrounding the tail of the epididymis and the ductus deferens. These contractions transport spermatozoa from the tail of the epididymis into the ductus deferens and eventually into the pelvic urethra. Once sperm gain entrance into the pelvic urethra, they begin to mix with secretions from the accessory sex glands.

Homosexual Behavior

Homosexual behavior is common among farm animals and is particularly common in cattle. Similar behavior is seen in sheep and, to a lesser extent, in swine and horses. Such behavior has profound usefulness for detecting cattle in estrus. When a female stands to be mounted by another cow, this alerts the management team that the cow is in estrus, and artificial insemination can be performed. A favorite question of managers and students of reproductive physiology alike is, "What is the evolutionary advantage of animals displaying this kind of behavior?" While a definitive answer is not known, two theories exist to explain female-female mounting behavior in the bovine.

The first explanation theorizes that cows mounting one another provide a visual signal which attracts a bull to the cow in heat. In other words, when a bull sees other cows mounting one another he will further investigate and, if the cow is in standing heat, he will breed her.

The second theory explaining the evolution of homosexual behavior among cows involves inadvertent genetic selection by man for this behavior. It has been proposed that cattle of European descent were selected by humans for their estrous behavior. In Medieval Europe, cattle husbandry practices involved the use of a few cows by each peasant farmer for three purposes: draft, milk and meat. Peasant farmers could not afford to maintain a bull for breeding purposes since the bulls gave no milk, gave birth to no calves and had obnoxious behavior that made them unsuitable for everyday management. In addition, most bulls apparently were owned by wealthy land holders who probably controlled the breeding, as well as the financial aspects of cattle management. Since most cows were kept in groups without intact males, the herdsmen needed some sign to tell him when his cows should be bred. Obviously, the cow that showed the most intense mounting behavior was the one most likely to be observed by the peasant and most likely to be bred by the nobleman's bull. Those that showed little mounting behavior did not become pregnant in a reasonable amount of time. This theory suggests that cows with a high degree of mounting behavior were inadvertently selected because they were noticed by man and offered a greater opportunity to become pregnant. Thus, this behavioral trait was transmitted to their offspring.

Further Phenomena for Fertility

One day President and Mrs. Coolidge were visiting a government farm. Soon after their arrival they were taken off on separate tours. When Mrs. Coolidge passed the chicken pens, she paused to ask the man in charge if the rooster copulated more than once each day. "Dozens of times," was the reply. "Please tell that to the President," Mrs. Coolidge requested. When the President passed the pens and was told about the rooster, he asked, "Same hen every day?" "Oh no, Mr. President, a different one each time." The President nodded slowly and then said, "Please tell that to Mrs. Coolidge."

The praying mantis has unusual reproductive behavior. As soon as the male mounts the female and accomplishes intromission, the female bites his head off. She immediately eats the top half of his body while intromission still exists. The reason for this behavior is because ejaculation is permanently inhibited in the male and can take place only after the head has been removed. It is not known whether the slang phrase "bite-your-head-off" was derived from this behavior.

To mate, the queen bee leaves the hive and performs a mating flight in an area where drones are congregated. The fastest drone is the first to copulate with the queen. Copulation is an in-flight event which lasts from 1 to 3 seconds. When the copulating bees separate, the entire male genitalia is ripped from the male and stays with the queen. The male soon dies and another male will then mate with the queen. Up to 17 matings in one mating flight have been observed.

Some male insects (certain flies and mosquitoes) want to insure that their genetics will be passed on. Males have a sharp, specialized penis which can enter a pupa. The male inseminates the unborn female.

Antelope actually copulate while running. (Some bats copulate in flight.) When the female antelope runs at a steady pace (rather than jumping and darting) it is a signal that she is in estrus. The male runs behind her, mounts, accomplishes intromission and ejaculates while on the run. A steady gait on the part of the female is important!

Females of some species are quite choosy about who gets to fertilize their eggs. In these cases, mate choice is determined by nuptial gifts presented by the male. The female black-tipped hangfly accepts nuptial gifts in the form of food in exchange for copulation. When edible food is presented by the male, the duration of copulation is dependent on the size of the gift. If the gift is small and can be consumed in 5 minutes or less, the female will not allow mating. If the gift is large (cannot be consumed in 20 minutes), the female will allow mating to take place. If the gift provides a meal of only 12 minutes she will leave the gift-giver prematurely and seek another gift-giver as a mate.

Women have periods of elevated physical activity associated with their menstrual cycles. Episodes of increased activity (steps taken during the day) have been observed on day 14 (ovulation), day 5 (menses) and on day 24.

Additional Reading

Albright, J.L., and C.W. Arave. 1997. *The Behaviour of Cattle*. CAB International, Wallingford, UK.

Craig, James V. 1981. *Domestic Animal Behavior: causes and implications for animal care and management.* Prentice-Hall, Inc. New Jersey.

Hart, Benjamin L. 1985. *The Behavior of Domestic Animals*. W.H. Freeman and Co., New York.

Signoret, J.P. and J. Balthazart. 1993 "Sexual Behavior" in *Reproduction in Mammals and Man*. C. Thibault, M.C. Levasseur and R.H.F. Hunder, eds. Ellipses, Paris.

12 Spermatozoa in the Female Tract - Transport, Capacitation and Fertilization

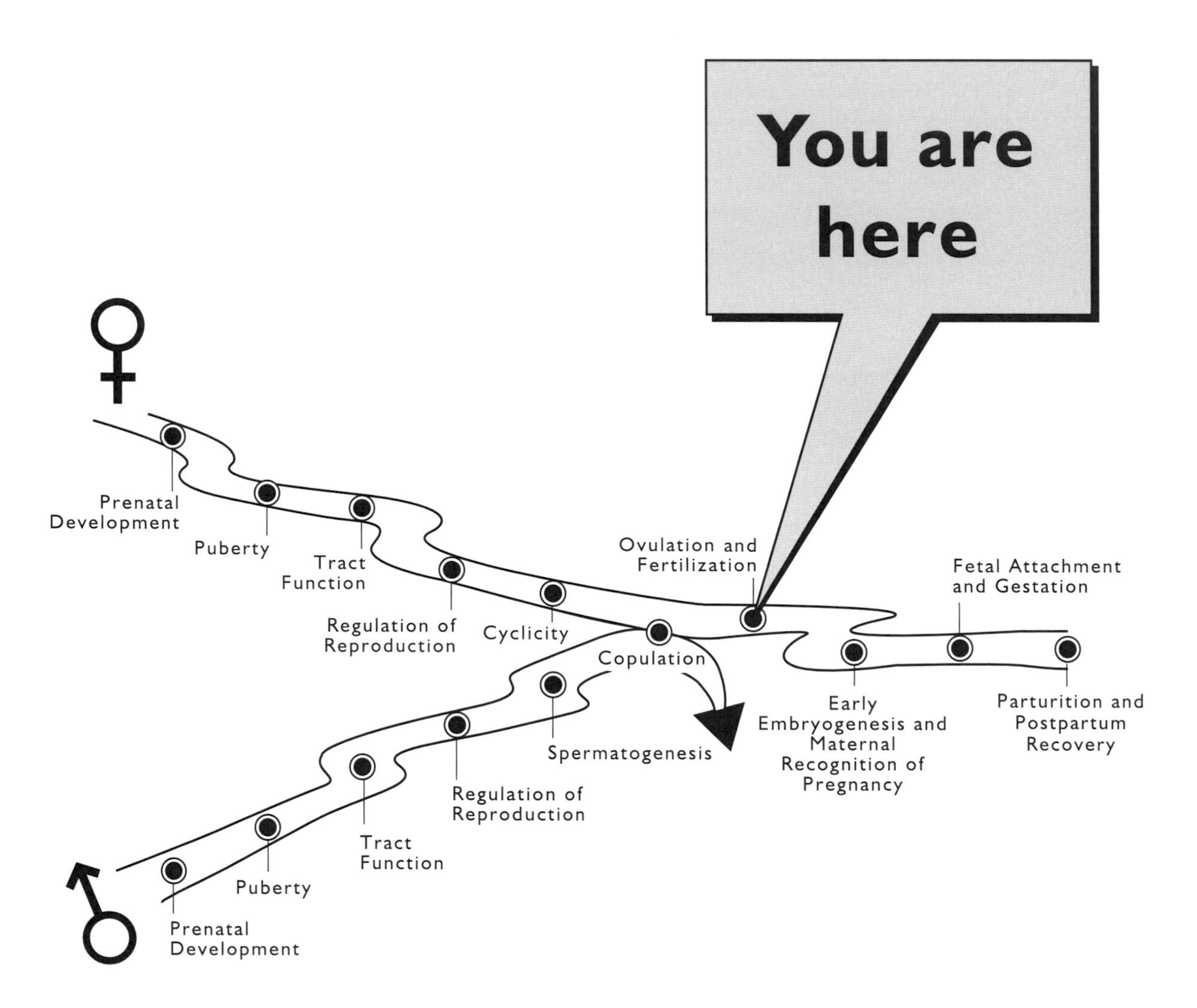

> ### *Take Home Message*
>
> ***Following insemination, viable spermatozoa that are retained in the female reproductive tract must 1) ascend the cervix, 2) be transported to the oviduct, 3) undergo capacitation, 4) bind to the oocyte, 5) undergo the acrosome reaction and 6) penetrate the zona pellucida and fuse with the oocyte plasma membrane. After fusion with the plasma membrane, the fertilizing spermatazoon enters the oocyte cytoplasm and the nucleus decondenses. The male pronucleus is formed, thus signifying successful fertilization.***

Following deposition of semen during copulation, spermatozoa are exposed to a series of different environments which significantly alter their numbers and their function. After insemination, spermatozoa are lost from the female reproductive tract by retrograde transport and many are phagocytized. The remaining spermatozoa must traverse the cervix, enter and traverse the uterus and enter the oviduct. They must undergo capacitation before they can fertilize the oocyte. When sperm encounter the egg they undergo the acrosome reaction and fertilization takes place. This series of events is summarized in Figure 12-1.

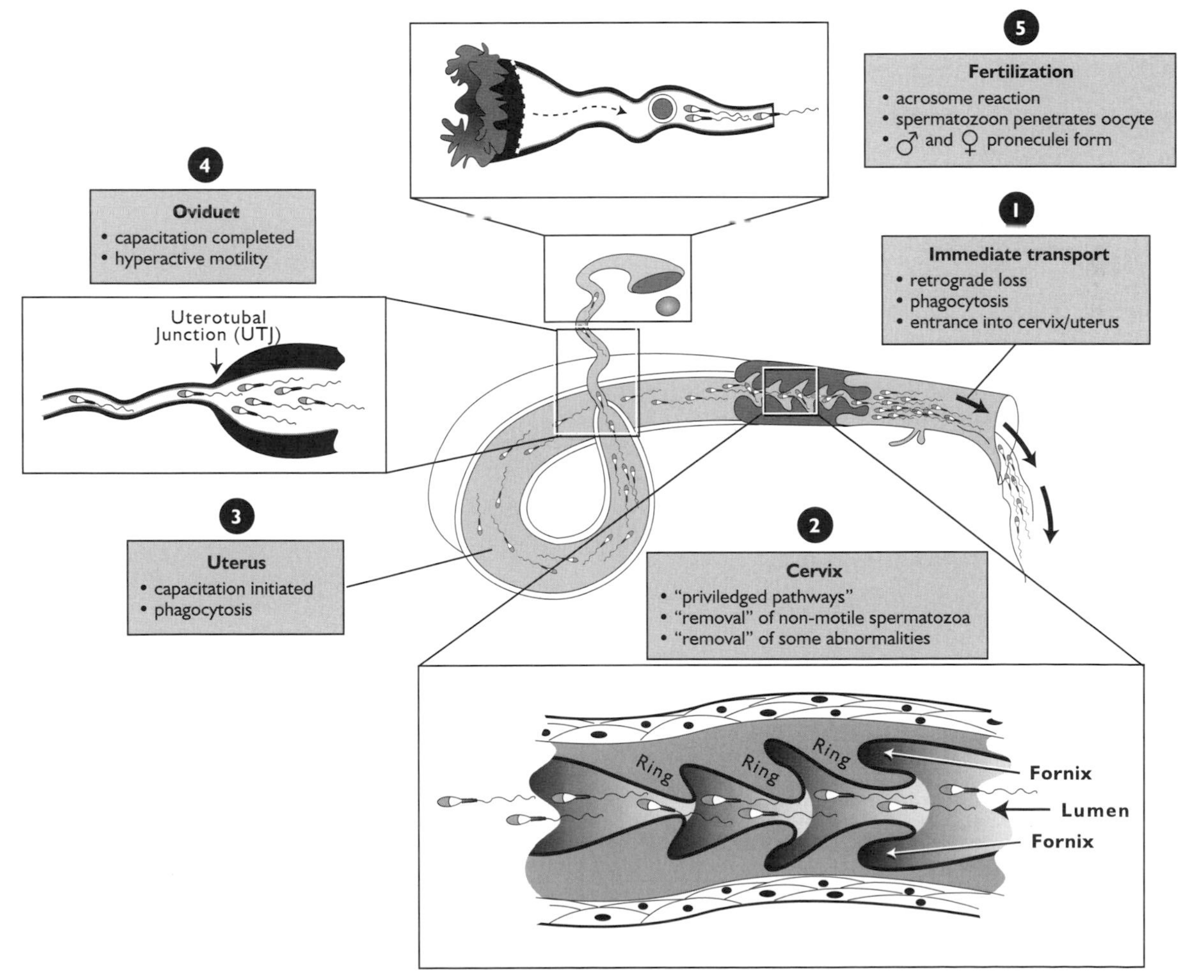

Figure 12-1. Major sequence of events following deposition of spermatozoa in the female reproductive tract. (Graphic by Sonja Oei.)

> ***Spermatozoa are lost from the female tract by:***
> ***• retrograde transport***
> ***• phagocytosis by neutrophils***

In some animals (cow, sheep, rabbit and primates), the male deposits semen in the anterior vagina. In others, (pigs and horses) semen is either deposited directly in the cervix (pig) or is squirted through the cervical lumen during copulation (horse). The stallion ejaculates in a series of "jets" in which a sperm-rich fraction is ejaculated first in a series of 3 to 4 high pressure squirts. This fraction contains about 80% of the spermatozoa. The last 5 to 8 "jets" are of lower pressure and contain fewer sperm. The seminal plasma in the final "jets" is highly viscous and may serve to minimize retrograde sperm loss from the mare's tract. Because of the large volume (200 to 400 ml) of boar ejaculate, most of the semen flows from the cervix into the uterine lumen. As in the stallion, the boar ejaculates a series of seminal fractions with different characteristics as ejaculation progresses. The first fraction consists of accessory fluids and gelatinous pellets. This fraction contains few sperm. The second fraction is rich in spermatozoa and this sperm-rich fraction is followed by a final fraction that forms a coagulum that resembles rice pudding. This coagulum reduces retrograde sperm loss. Immediately after insemination, semen undergoes varying degrees of retrograde transport (from the cervix towards the vulva). The degree to which spermatozoa is lost depends upon the physical nature of the ejaculate and the site of seminal deposition. In some species, the seminal plasma contains a coagulating protein(s) which forms a conspicuous vaginal plug to prevent spermatozoa from undergoing retrograde flow to the exterior. Female rodents (mice and rats) have a relatively solid vaginal plug that is visible following copulation. The presence of the vaginal plug can be used to determine when mating occurred. Food producing animals do not have a conspicuous vaginal plug.

When the female reproductive tract is under the influence of estradiol during estrus, neutrophils (powerful phagocytic white blood cells) sequester in the mucosa of the tract, especially in the vagina and uterus. These neutrophils are poised to attack foreign materials which are introduced into the female reproductive tract at insemination. It should be recognized that, in addition to spermatozoa, microorganisms are introduced into the tract during copulation. Thus, the neutrophil population is important in preventing these microorganisms from colonizing in the female tract. From an immunologic perspective, spermatozoa are foreign to the female. As a result, neutrophils actively phagocytize spermatozoa. They do not discriminate between live and dead spermatozoa. In fact, a single neutrophil is capable of engulfing several spermatozoa even though they are motile. Studies have shown that within 6 to 12 hours after the introduction of spermatozoa into the uterus, there is a large infiltration of neutrophils from the uterine mucosa into the uterine lumen (Figure 12-2). While leukocyte infiltration is an important contributor to post-insemination spermatozoal losses, this infiltration is important for the prevention of reproductive tract infection.

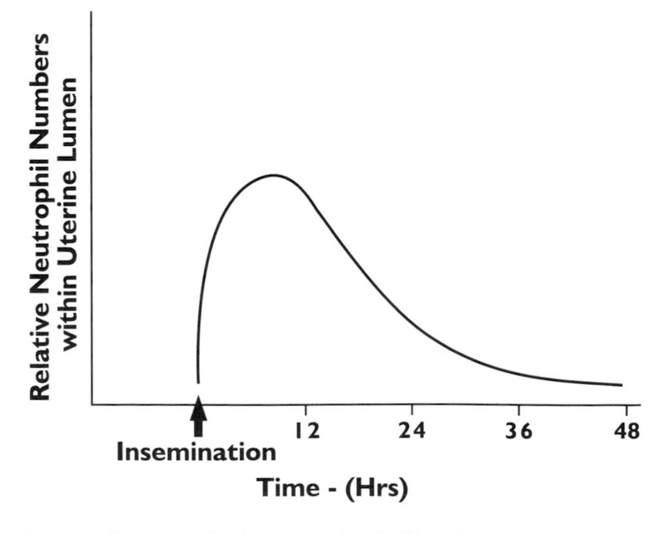

Figure 12-2. Typical neutrophil infiltration pattern into the uterine lumen following insemination in the cow.

Spermatozoal transport consists of a rapid phase and a sustained phase.

Among the least understood phenomena in reproductive physiology are factors that regulate loss and/or retention of spermatozoa from the female tract. The ability of the female to retain viable spermatozoa may influence the fertility of a given mating. Transport of spermatozoa following copulation can be divided into two distinct phases. These are the **rapid transport phase** and the **sustained transport phase**. Within a few minutes after copulation, spermatozoa can be found in the oviducts. Originally, the rapid phase of transport was considered to be important because it delivered spermatozoa to the site of the fertilization very shortly after copulation, where they "postured" themselves for the arrival of oocytes. However, further research showed that spermatozoa arriving in the oviducts within minutes after copulation were non-viable. The functional importance of the rapid phase of sperm transport is not obvious. It may simply represent a short burst of transport activity brought about by contraction of the muscularis of the female tract in conjunction with copulation.

The more important component of transport is the sustained phase in which spermatozoa are transported distally to the oviducts in a trickle-like effect from so-called reservoirs in the cervix and the uterotubal junction. The sustained sperm transport phase delivers spermatozoa to the ampulla of the oviduct in a more uniform manner over a sustained period of time.

It had been erroneously assumed for years that most spermatozoa ascend toward the oviduct soon after they are deposited in the cow uterus by artificial insemination. However, recent studies have shown that a high proportion of spermatozoa deposited in the uterus of the cow or ewe are lost from the tract by retrograde transport. In most cows, over 60% of spermatozoa artificially inseminated into the uterus are lost to the exterior of the tract within 12 hours after deposition. Given these findings, a logical interpretation would be that artificial insemination of spermatozoa deep into the uterus would result in reduced retrograde loss. This assumption is not true because when sperm are deposited deep into both uterine horns (as opposed to the uterine body) the degree of sperm recovered from the vagina (an indication of retrograde loss) is quite similar between the two sites of deposition (Figure 12-3). However, when sperm are deposited in the mid-cervix, a significantly higher degree of retrograde loss of spermatozoa is encountered (Figure 12-4).

Spermatozoa deposited into only one uterine horn of the cow experience intercornual transport. That is, when spermatozoa are deposited into one uterine horn (either right or left), they subsequently are redistributed over time so that both uterine horns eventually contain substantial numbers of spermatozoa. This phenomenon also occurs in swine. In cows, fertility is similar when sperm are deposited within the uterine body or in either of the right or left uterine horn.

The important message from the above discussion is that when artificial insemination is performed in the cow and semen is deposited in the cervix, a greater proportion of spermatozoa are lost to the exterior than when deposition is in the uterus. Thus, when the insemination procedure involves cervical deposition, fertility may be compromised because of greater spermatozoal loss.

Transport of spermatozoa is primarily the result of elevated tone and motility of the muscularis of the female tract.

As you already know, estradiol is high during the follicular phase when insemination occurs. Estradiol stimulates contractions of the muscularis, particularly the myometrium. Also, prostaglandins in semen ($PGF_{2\alpha}$ and PGE_1) cause increased tone and motility of the uterus and/or the oviduct. Intermittent contractions of the muscularis propel spermatozoa in both an anterior and a posterior direction. Fluids secreted into

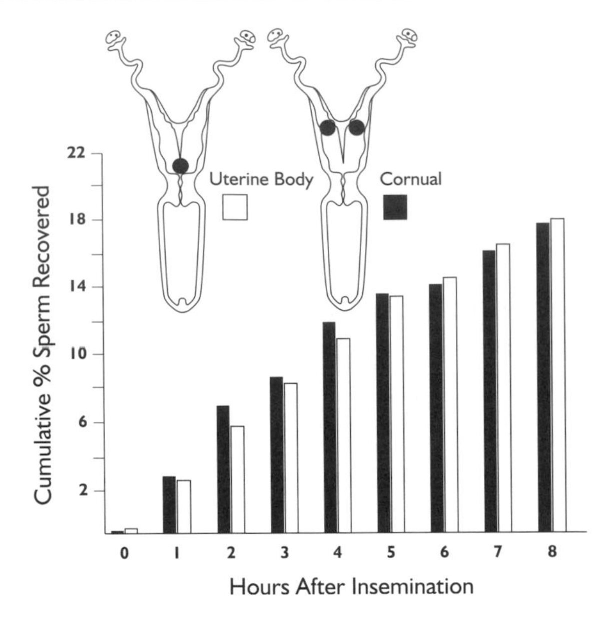

Figure 12-3. Cumulative percent of sperm recovered from the vagina of the cow during an 8 hour period after insemination. In one group of animals, sperm was deposited in the uterine body, while in a second group of animals, sperm was deposited deep in each uterine horn. The cumulative percent of sperm recovered from the vagina did not differ between the two treatment groups (Modified from Gallagher and Senger, 1989, *J. Reprod. Fert. 86:19.*)

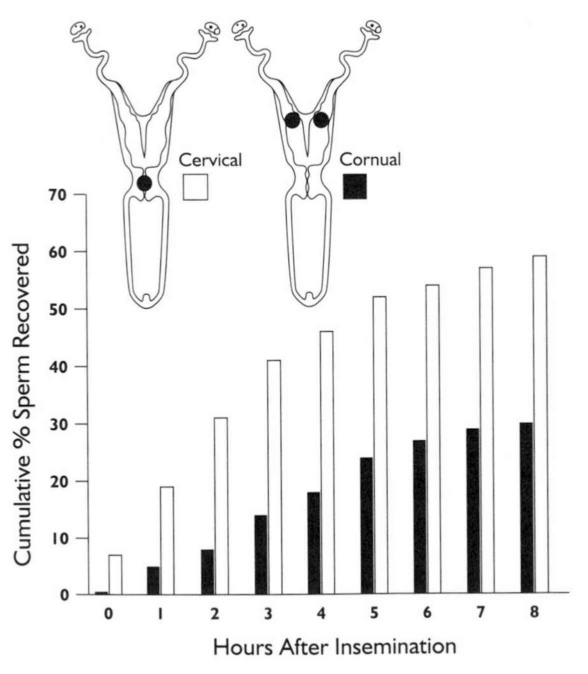

Figure 12-4. Cumulative percent of sperm recovered from the vagina of the cow during an 8 hour recovery period following insemination. Comparisons were made between cervical deposition and cornual deposition. A significantly higher number of sperm were found in the vagina at all hours after insemination when sperm was deposited at mid-cervix when compared to cornual deposition (Modified from Gallagher and Senger, 1989, *J. Reprod. Fert.* 86:19.)

the lumen of the female tract also serve as a vehicle for transport. Control of the directionality, while not understood, is probably under the collective influence of muscular contractions and fluid distribution/characteristics.

In addition to alteration of tract motility, seminal plasma from boars has been shown by German researchers to advance the time of ovulation in gilts. For example, when seminal plasma was infused into the right uterine horn, ovulation occurred about 11 hours earlier in the right ovary than in the left ovary. The left uterine horn did not receive seminal plasma. The specific material in boar seminal plasma provoking early ovulation

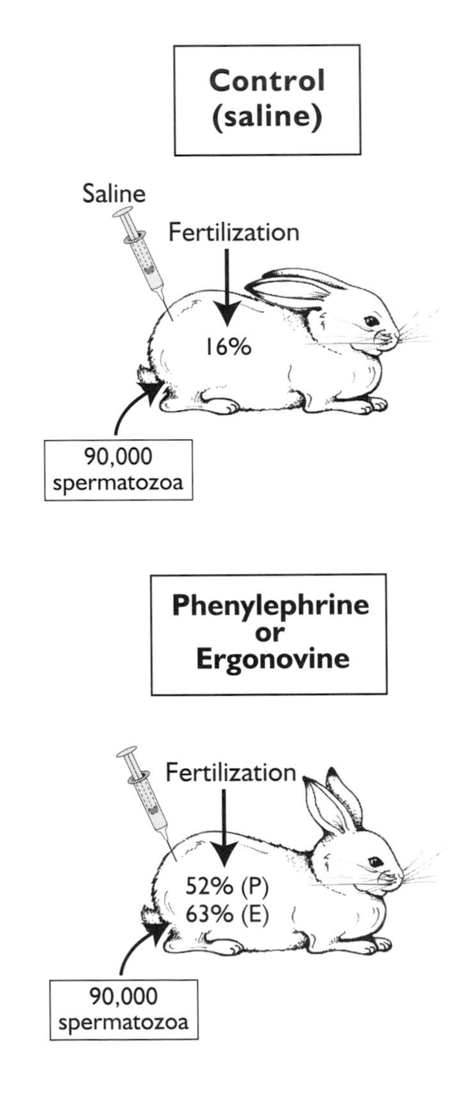

Figure 12-5. Influence of intramuscular phenylephrine (P) and ergonovine (E) on fertilization rate (%) when small numbers of spermatozoa were inseminated. About 200 x 10^6 spermatozoa are deposited by natural service. (Illustration from data of Hawk, et al., 1982 *J. Anim. Sci.* 55:878.) (Graphic by Sonja Oei.)

has not been identified, but it appears to be a protein. Identification of these factors could provide an avenue to control more precisely the time of ovulation in swine.

A logical approach to alter or to minimize the retrograde sperm loss that accompanies natural and artificial insemination would be to treat the female with pharmaceuticals that alter smooth muscle motility in the female tract and thus alter sperm transport. Pharmaceutical manipulation of the uterine myometrium may represent an avenue whereby fewer numbers of spermatozoa can be inseminated with acceptable fertility.

In one test, when rabbits were injected with phenylephrine or ergonovine, two smooth muscle stimulants, the number of sperm reaching the oviducts was significantly elevated. In does inseminated with very low sperm numbers (around 90,000), an intramuscular injection of either phenylephrine or ergonovine resulted in a significantly increased fertilization rate when compared to controls which received neither phenylephrine nor ergonovine (Figure 12-5). This finding suggests that a reduction in numbers of spermatozoa, if accompanied by proper stimulators of smooth muscle motility, can result in acceptable fertilization rates. This would be particulary important if pharmaceuticals could be added to semen used in artificial insemination. If "transport conservation" could be accomplished, fewer sperm could be used in each dose of semen and spermatozoa from genetically superior sires could be distributed on a wider basis.

The cervix is a major barrier to spermatozoal transport. It also serves as a reservoir of spermatozoa.

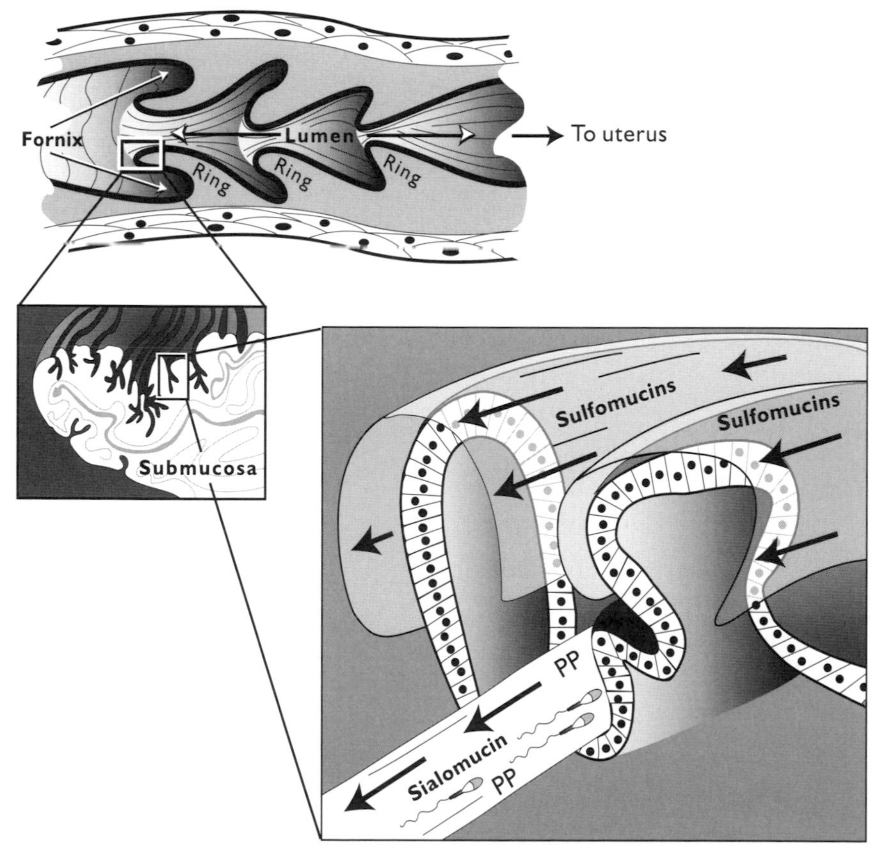

Figure 12-6. Summary of the current concept explaining the mechanism whereby spermatozoa negotiate the cervix in the cow following natural service. Secretion of sulfomucins from the apical portion of the cervical folds produces sheets of viscous mucus which are secreted toward the central lumen and flow in a vaginal direction. Less viscous sialomucins are produced in the basal areas and also flow in a vaginal direction. Spermatozoa found in the basal regions are oriented in a similar direction and traverse the cervix toward the uterus through these "privileged pathways" (PP). (Modified from Mullins and Saacke 1989, *Anat. Rec.* 225:106.) (Graphic by Sonja Oei.)

Following natural service in the cow and ewe and, to some degree, the mare, spermatozoa must negotiate the highly convoluted system of grooves making up the cervix (Figure 12-6). During estrus, the cervix produces mucus. In the cow, cervical mucus consists of two types. One type is a **sialomucin**, which is a mucus of low viscosity. It is produced by cells in the basal areas of the cervical crypts (Figure 12-6). A second type, **sulfomucin** is produced in the apical areas of the cervical epithelium, and this type of mucus is quite viscous. The production of two types of mucus (one of low viscosity and one of high viscosity) creates two distinct environments within the cervix. Spermatozoa encountering the viscous sulfomucin are washed out of the tract. Those that encounter the low viscosity sialomucin in the environment of the crypts of the cervix swim into it. Thus, the low viscosity environment of the deeper cervical crypts creates "priviledged pathways" through which spermatozoa can move.

The ability of spermatozoa to traverse these "privileged pathways" is believed to depend on their ability to swim through the basal channels of the cervix. In this context, the cervix may be a filter which eliminates non-motile spermatozoa. The time required for motile sperm to gain access and traverse these "privileged pathways" probably contributes significantly to the time required for the sustained phase of sperm transport. The specific role of the cervix in spermatozoal transport and/or retention awaits further clarification in the sow and the mare, where a high proportion of spermatozoa are ejaculated into the uterus.

Spermatozoa must reside in the female tract before they acquire maximum fertility.

As you recall from Chapter 3, spermatozoa acquire maturity during epididymal transit. However, the maturational changes that occur in the epidiymis do not render spermatozoa completely fertile. For maximum fertility to be achieved, spermatozoa must reside in the female reproductive tract for a minimum period of time. During the time in the female reproductive tract, some

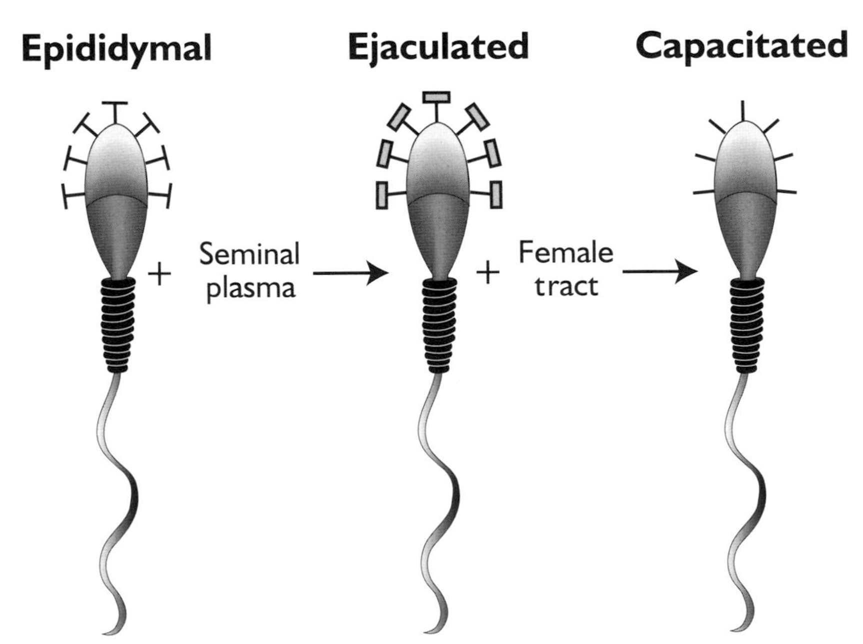

Figure 12-7. A conceptual version of mammalian capacitation. The plasma membrane of epididymal spermatozoa contains a complement of surface molecules (proteins and carbohydrates). These become coated with seminal plasma proteins which mask existing molecules. When sperm become exposed to the female tract environment, these seminal plasma coatings, along with some of the surface molecules, are removed, thus rendering the sperm capable of binding to the oocyte. (Graphic by Sonja Oei.)

spermatozoa will undergo changes that allow them to become fertile. These changes are referred to as spermatozoal **capacitation**. The site for capacitation varies among species. In species where spermatozoa are deposited in the anterior vagina, capacitation may begin as sperm ascend and pass through the cervix. In species where semen is deposited in the uterus, capacitation is probably initiated in the uterus and likely is completed in the isthmus of the oviduct. All spermatozoa are not capacitated at the same rate. Instead, they are capacitated over a relatively long period of time (several hours) and this reflects individual sperm differences as well as location within the tract. Capacitation can occur in fluids other than those found in the luminal compartment of the female reproductive tract. For example, *in vitro* capacitation has been accomplished in a wide variety of species using blood serum, a variety of commercial tissue culture media, Krebs Ringer solutions and Tyrodes solutions. No single *in vitro* environment will support capacitation for all species.

There is little doubt that the plasma membrane of the sperm (particularly the head) undergoes marked biochemical changes during capacitation. One way to envision the process of capacitation is presented in Figure 12-7. The coating of seminal plasma proteins is stripped away by the female tract environment. The exact nature of the stripping process of capacitation is not understood.

An important concept with regard to capacitation is that the process can be reversed by returning capacitated spermatozoa to seminal plasma. For example, when capacitated spermatozoa are removed from the female reproductive tract and returned to seminal plasma, they become **decapacitated** and require additional capacitation time in the female reproductive tract before they can regain their fertility. It appears that the seminal plasma components coat the plasma membrane with surface substances that prevent or inhibit interaction of spermatozoa with the egg.

Fertilization Is a Complex Process and Involves a Cascade of Events

The process of fertilization involves a series of specific interactions between spermatozoa and the oocyte. These are outlined in Figure 12-8.

Acquisition of hyperactive motility occurs in the oviduct.

In the oviduct the motility patterns of spermatozoa become hyperactive. The motility pattern changes from a progressive, linear motility in which they swim in a relatively straight line, into a frenzied, dancing motion that is not linear and is localized in a small area. In general, hyperactive motility occurs in the ampulla of the oviduct and is believed to be brought about by specific molecules produced by the epithelium there. Hyperactive motility is believed to facilitate sperm-oocyte contact.

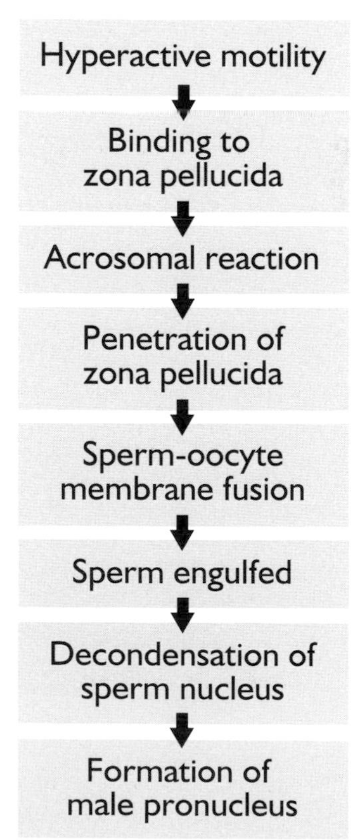

Figure 12-8. Postcapacitation sequence of events leading to fertilization and pronuclei formation.

Binding to the zona pellucida requires specific zona-binding proteins on the spermatozoal membrane.

Spermatozoa are known to contain specific proteins on the membrane surface overlying the acrosome which bind specifically to zona pellucida proteins. These zona binding proteins on the plasma membrane must be exposed during the capacitation process before binding to the zona pellucida can occur. Before zona binding can be understood fully, the molecular makeup of the zona must be described. The zona pellucida of the oocyte consists of three glycoproteins. These glycoproteins have been named **zona protein 1**, **2** and **3** (**ZP1, ZP2** and **ZP3**). Zona proteins 1 and 2 are structural proteins maintaining the structural integrity of the zona. Zona protein 3 is much like a receptor for a hormone. It binds to proteins found on the spermatozoal membrane. Binding of spermatozoa to the zona pellucida is believed to require between 10,000 and 50,000 ZP3 molecules. The current understanding is that the sperm plasma membrane contains two zona binding sites. The first binding site, referred to as the **primary zona binding region** has the responsibility of causing spermatozoa to adhere to the zona pellucida. The second binding site on the spermatozoal plasma membrane is believed to be an **acrosome reaction promoting** ligand. When binding occurs between this region and the ZP3 molecule, a signal transduction occurs. This is much like a typical hormone-receptor binding complex. Binding initiates the acrosome reaction. The relationship between ZP3 and the spermatozoal plasma membrane during binding is illustrated in Figure 12-9.

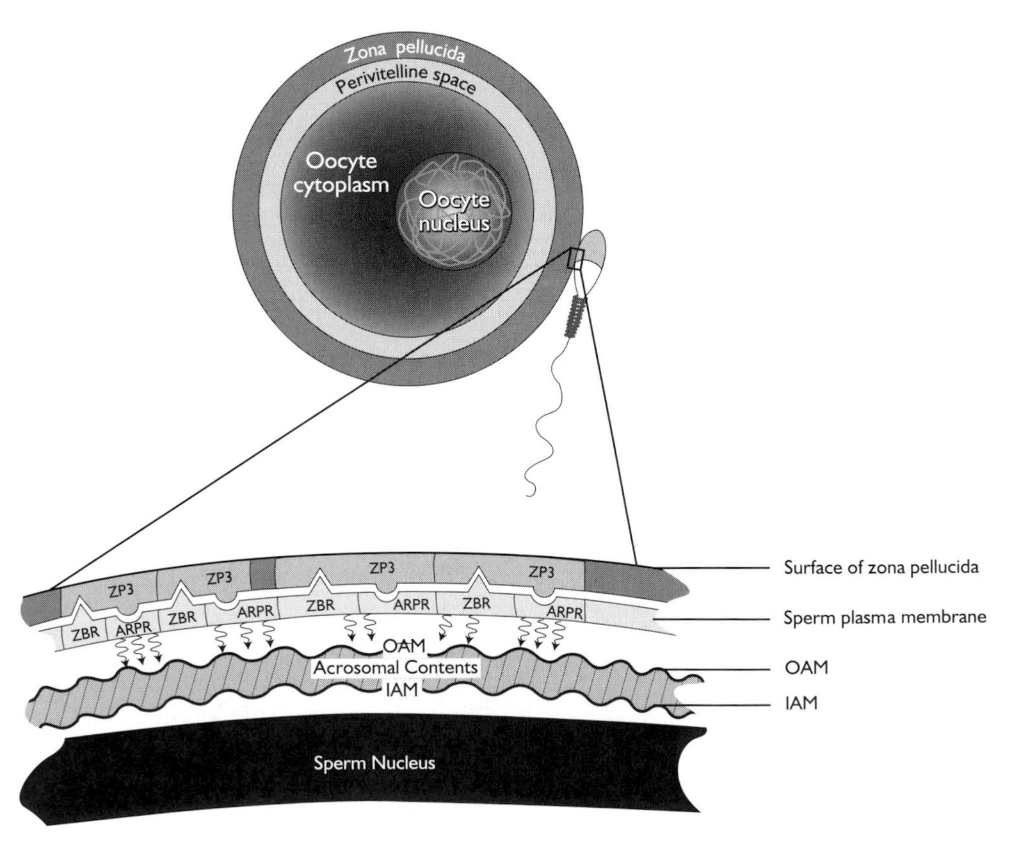

Figure 12-9. Proposed model for zona binding and acrosome reaction initiation in mammalian spermatozoa. The plasma membrane overlying the acrosome contains two receptor-like regions. The first, called the zona binding region (ZBR) reacts with ZP3 to cause physical attachment of the sperm to the zona. A second membrane region, the acrosome reaction promoting region (ARPR) binds to ZP3 and initiates the acrosome reaction by causing the plasma membrane to fuse (arrows) with the outer acrosomal membrane. ARPR= Acrosome Reaction Promoting Region; IAM= Inner Acrosomal Membrane; OAM= Outer Acrosomal Membrane; ZBR= Zona Binding Region. (Graphic by Sonja Oei.)

The acrosomal reaction is an orderly fusion of the spermatozoal plasma membrane and the outer acrosomal membrane.

The purpose of the acrosomal reaction is two-fold. First, the reaction enables spermatozoa to penetrate the zona pellucida. Second, it exposes the equatorial segment so that it can later fuse with the plasma membrane of the oocyte.

The acrosomal reaction begins when the plasma membrane of the spermatozoon forms multiple fusion sites with the outer acrosomal membrane. When the two membranes fuse, many small vesicles are formed (Figure 12-10) and this process is called **vesiculation.** After vesiculation has occurred, the acrosomal contents are dispersed and the sperm nucleus is left with the inner acrosomal membrane surrounding it. Vesiculation characterizes the acrosome reaction and morphologically distinguishes it from a damaged acrosome. Damage to the acrosome brought about by changes in osmotic pressure, cooling or heating is irreversible, and renders spermatozoa incapable of fertilization. Damaged acrosomes do not vesiculate in an orderly fashion, but rupture all at once.

Release of acrosomal enzymes allows the spermatozoon to digest its way through the zona pellucida.

The penetration of the zona pellucida by a spermatozoon is believed to be a rapid process and probably takes no more than a few minutes. Following attachment, the acrosome reaction allows the release of a variety of enzymes. **Acrosin** is one enzyme that is released from spermatozoa during the acrosomal reaction. It hydrolyzes zona proteins as well as enhances the sperm's ability to bind to the zona. In the inactive form, acrosin is known as **proacrosin,** which has a strong affinity for the zona. Thus, proacrosin aids in binding the spermatozoon to the zona as the acrosomal reaction proceeds. As proacrosin is converted to acrosin, the sperm begins to penetrate and make its way through the zona pellucida. The mechanical force generated by the flagellar action of the tail may be sufficient to push the sperm through the zona. It is important to note that the

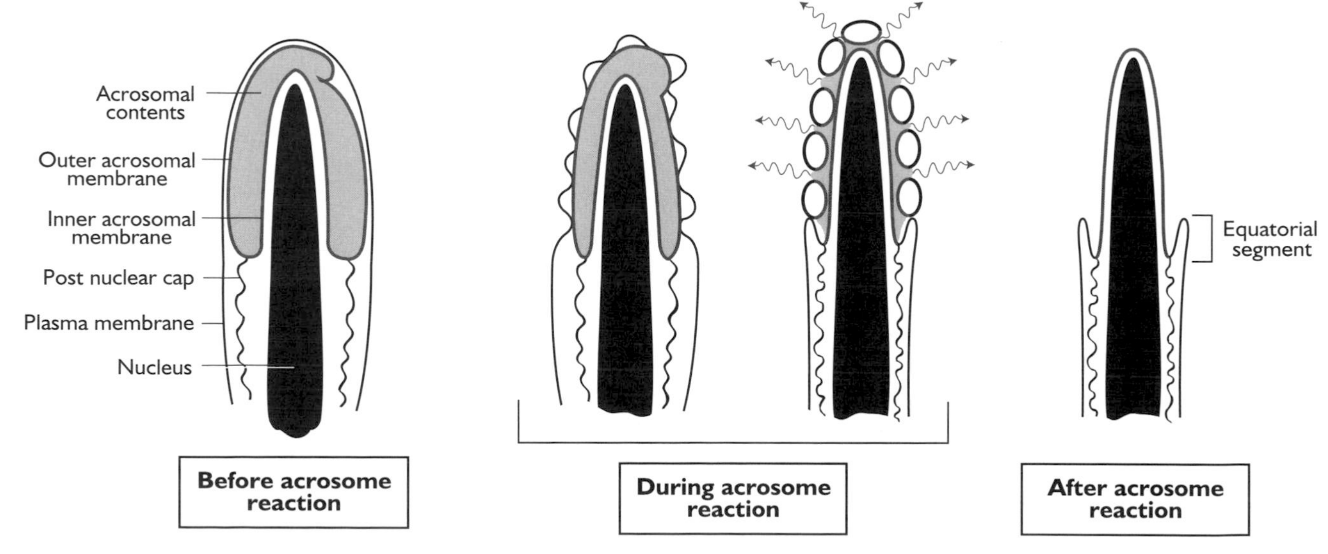

Figure 12-10. Schematic illustration of the acrosomal reaction. Before the reaction begins, all membranes of the head are intact. During the reaction, the plasma membrane overlying the acrosome begins to fuse with the outer acrosomal membrane. The fusion of the two membranes leads to vesiculation which creates tiny pores through which the acrosomal enzymes escape. Release of acrosomal enzymes allows penetration through the zona pellucida. After the reaction, the vesicles are sloughed, leaving the inner acrosomal membrane and the equatorial segment intact. (Graphic by Sonja Oei.)

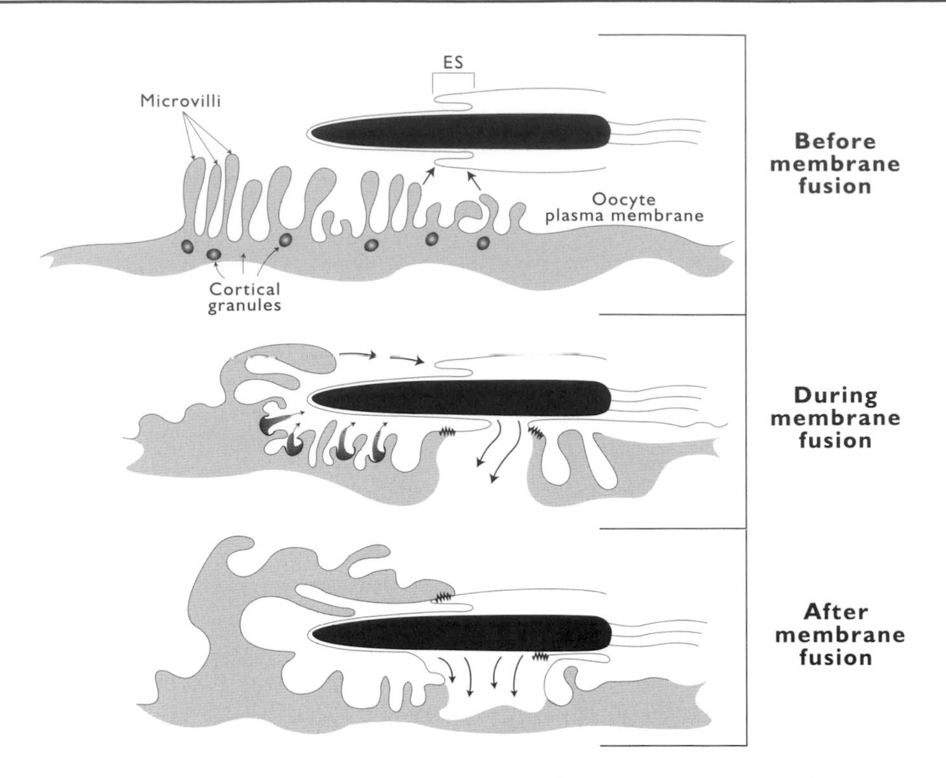

Figure 12-11. Diagram illustrating the sperm-oocyte membrane fusion. The oocyte membrane fuses in the equatorial segment (ES). Once fusion has taken place, the nucleus of the sperm is inside the cytoplasm of the oocyte. (Modified from Yanagimachi, *Physiology of Reproduction*; Knobil and Neill, eds., Vol. 1, pg. 246.) (Graphic by Sonja Oei.)

acrosomal reaction allows the spermatozoon to digest a small hole through the zona through which it can pass. Placing a hot marble on the surface of a block of chilled butter would be an appropriate analogy. The hot marble would move through the butter in a small regional hole, but the butter in most of the block would be unchanged. This small regional dissolution leaves the zona predominately intact. Maintenance of an intact zona pellucida is believed to be important because it prevents blastomeres in the early embryo from separating during embryogenesis.

Fertilization requires fusion of the equatorial segment and the oocyte plasma membrane.

When the spermatozoon completely penetrates the zona and reaches the perivitelline space (the space between the zona and the oocyte plasma membrane), it settles into a bed of microvilli formed from the oocyte plasma membrane. The plasma membrane of the oocyte fuses with the membrane of the equatorial segment and the fertilizing spermatozoon is engulfed. The actual fusion of the oocyte plasma membrane with the equatorial segment is believed to be brought about by a so-called **fusion protein** located on this portion of the membrane. Prior to the acrosome reaction, this fusion protein is in an inactive state. After vesiculation and release of the acrosomal contents, the fusion protein is activated, thus enabling the sperm membrane to fuse or bind with the oocyte membrane. This process is illustrated in Figure 12-11.

The cortical reaction prevents penetration by additional spermatozoa.

After membrane fusion, the oocyte undergoes a series of changes which prepare it for early embryogenesis. The most easily recognizable is the **cortical reaction.** During the first and second meiotic divisions of oogenesis, small, dense granules called cortical granules move to the periphery of the oocyte cytoplasm. The contents of the cortical granules consist of mucopolysacharides, proteases, plasminogen activator, acid phosphatase and peroxidase. After membrane fusion between the oocyte and spermatozoon, the cortical granules undergo **exocytosis** and their contents are released into the perivitelline space (Figure 12-11). Exocytosis of the cortical granules results in the **zona block,** a process whereby the zona pellucida changes biochemically so that further sperm cannot penetrate it. As a result of the zona block, **polyspermy** cannot take place.

Polyspermy is the fertilization of an oocyte by more than one spermatozoon which results in embryo death. In addition to alteration of the zona pellucida, the cortical reaction is believed to reduce the ability of the oocyte plasma membrane to fuse with additional spermatozoa, thus causing the **vitelline block**, another mechanism to prevent polspermy. Some species have both a zona block to polyspermy as well as a vitelline block, while others have either a zona or a vitelline block.

Pronuclei formation allows the male and female DNA to form a single nucleus.

After the sperm nucleus has entered the cytoplasm of the egg, it becomes the male pronucleus. Before the pronucleus can be formed, however, the nucleus of the sperm must undergo marked changes within the oocyte cytoplasm. As you will recall, one of the maturational changes that occurs in the epididymis is the acquisition of large numbers of disulfide crosslinks in the sperm nucleus. Thus, the nucleus of the mammalian sperm is almost inert. The keratinoid-like quality of insolubility is considered to be important during exposure to the female tract environment, during sperm transport and during the penetration through the zona pellucida. After the fertilizing spermatozoon enters the oocyte cytoplasm the nucleus must "decondense" so that the chromosomes may pair up with the chromosomes of the female pronucleus. The decondensation of the sperm nucleus requires that the disulfide crosslinks (which are abundant) be reduced. In the cytoplasm of the oocyte, disulfide crosslinks in the sperm nucleus are reduced quickly. The primary reducing agent is glutathione. When disulfide bond reduction occurs, the sperm nucleus decondenses and the nuclear material is available for interaction with the female nuclear material. The final step of fertilization is the fusion of the male and female pronuclei. This fusion is referred to as **syngamy**. Following syngamy, the zygote enters the first stages of embryogenesis.

Further Phenomena for Fertility

Some species have delayed fertilization. This is a process whereby the male inseminates the female and spermatozoa remain viable in the female tract for a sustained period of time. When a rooster inseminates a hen she can lay fertile eggs for over 20 days. Sperm are stored in special utero-vaginal glands. Some bats mate in the autumn before hibernation. The female does not ovulate until spring. Sperm are stored in her tract during the winter. Fertilizing life of bat sperm has been reported to range from 68 to 198 days depending on the species of bat. Snakes have been reported to store sperm that are fertile for up to 6 years.

The bifurcation of the glans penis of the opossum led to the widespread Appalacian folk belief that opossums mated through the nose, with one fork of the glans penis penetrating each nostril. Little scientific consideration was given to the issues of sperm transport.

Prostitutes encounter spermatozoa on a frequent basis. It is known that prostitutes have blood titers of antisperm antibodies. Some prostitutes even have severe allergic reactions.

Mammals deliver sperm to the female in seminal plasma. However, many lower forms of animals make use of special packages for delivering spermatozoa to the female reproductive tract. These packages are called spermatophores. These spermatophores are produced within the male reproductive tract and are stored there until copulation. In some cephalopods (octopus and squid) the male deposits the spermatophore in the female tract or into the buccal cavity (cheek pouch), from which it can be conviently transferred to the female tract. In some annelids, spermatophores are "injected" subcutaneously, after which the spermatozoa spread throughout the female's body before contacting eggs.

Motility of trout spermatozoa is induced by the fresh water into which it is ejaculated. Motility lasts for only about 30 seconds. During this time the sperm must locate a single tiny hole in the egg (called a micropyle) through which it enters before fertilization can occur. All this happens while being swept about by moving water.

Additional Reading

Yanagimachi, R. 1996. "Mammalian Fertilization." In *Physiology of Reproduction, 2nd Ed.* E. Knobil and J.D. Neil, eds. Raven Press, Ltd., New York.

Anderson, G.B., 1991. "Fertilization, Early Development and Embryo Transfer." In *Reproduction in Domestic Animals,4th ed.* P.T. Cupps, ed. Academic Press, Inc., New York.

Crozet, N. 1993. "Fertilization *in-vivo* and *in-vitro."* In *Reproduction in Mammals and Man.* C. Thibault, M.C. Levasseur and R.H.F. Hunter, eds. Ellipses, Paris.

Mullins, K.J. and R.G. Saacke. 1989. Study of the functional anatomy of bovine cervical mucosa with special reference to mucus secretion and sperm transport. *Anat. Rec.* 255:106.

13 Early Embryogenesis and Maternal Recognition of Pregnancy

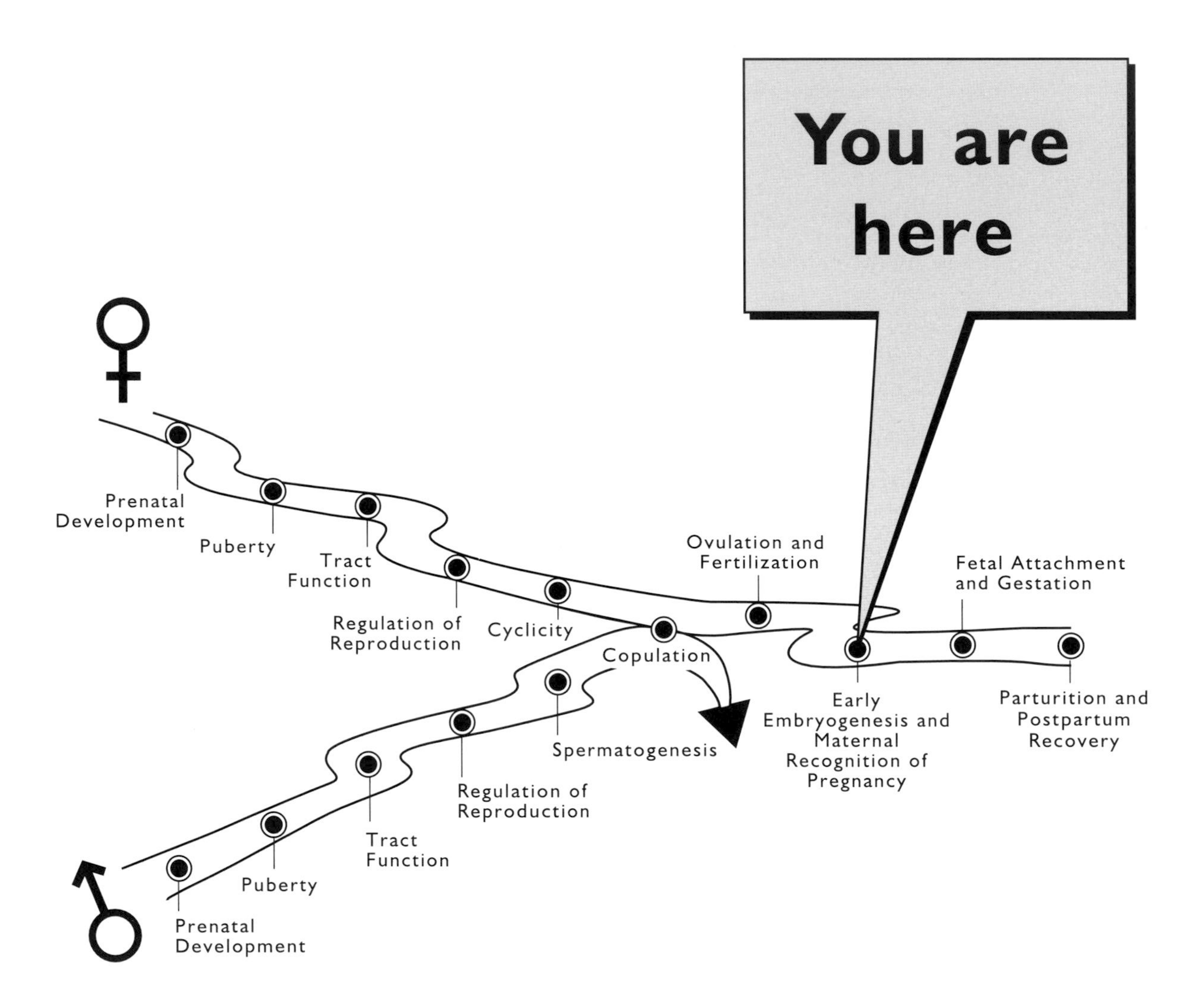

Take Home Message

A successful preattachment pregnancy requires that the embryo develop into a blastocyst, hatch from the zona pellucida, develop a functional trophoblast and produce materials that prevent luteolysis or that enhance luteal function.

Before describing the important events of early embryogenesis, several potentially confusing terms with overlapping meanings need to be defined. It should be emphasized that these terms have subtly different uses depending on the species and the context in which they are used. After **syngamy** (fusion of the male and female pronuclei), the zygote becomes an **embryo.** An embryo is defined as an organism in the early stages of development. In general, an embryo has not acquired an anatomical form which is readily recognizable in appearance as a member of the specific species. For example, at early stages of development, the pig embryo cannot be distinguished from the cow embryo except by skilled embryologists. As a matter of fact, at certain stages, the human embryo cannot be distinguished from the embryos of lower species.

A **fetus** is defined as a potential offspring that is still within the uterus, but is generally recognizable as a member of a given species. Most physiologists think of a fetus as the more advanced form of an embryo. The terms embryo, conceptus and fetus are often used interchangeably to describe the developing organism.

A **conceptus** is defined as the product of conception. It includes 1) the embryo during the early embryonic stage, 2) the embryo and extraembryonic membranes during the preimplantation stage and 3) the fetus and placenta during the post-attachment phase.

After fertilization, four important developmental events must occur before the embryo attaches to the uterus. Only after these milestones have been achieved will the embryo be eligible to develop a more intimate semipermanent relationship with the uterus.

Four steps must be achieved before the embryo can attach to the uterus. They are:

- ***development within the confines of the zona pellucida***
- ***hatching of the blastocyst from the zona***
- ***formation of the extraembryonic membranes***
- ***maternal recognition of pregnancy***

The presence of male and female pronuclei within the cytoplasm of the oocyte characterizes a developmental stage of the newly fertilized oocyte (Figure 13-1). When male and female pronuclei can be observed, the cell is called an **ootid.** The ootid is one of the largest single cells in the body and is characterized by having an enormous cytoplasmic volume relative to nuclear volume. This characteristic is important, since subsequent cell divisions within the confines of the zona pellucida will involve partitioning of the cytoplasm into smaller and smaller cellular units (Figure 13-1).

Following fusion of the male and female pronuclei, the single-celled embryo, now called a **zygote,** undergoes a series of mitotic divisions called **cleavage divisions.** The first cleavage division generates a two-celled embryo, the cells of which are called **blastomeres**. Each blastomere in the two-celled embryo is about the same size and represents almost exactly one-half of the single-celled zygote. Each blastomere undergoes subsequent divisions, yielding 4, 8 and then 16 daughter cells.

In the early stages of embryogenesis, each blastomere has the potential to develop into separate healthy offspring. Identical twins are derived from blastomeres of a two-celled embryo which divide independently to form two separate embryos. Blastomeres from the 2-, 4- and 8- celled embryos are **totipotent.** Totipotency is a term used to describe when a single cell (blastomere) gives rise to a complete, fully formed individual. Identical twins can be artificially produced in the laboratory by separating individual blastomeres, placing each blastomere inside a surrogate zona pellucida and allowing it to develop within the uterus of a host female. The individual blastomeres isolated from 4- and 8- celled stages can develop into normal embryos in the rabbit, horse, cow and sheep. Totipotency has not been demonstrated when whole blastomeres beyond the 16-cell stage are used. Recently, nuclei from somatic cells from the adult sheep have been transplanted into enucleated oocytes. These oocytes have developed into normal lambs. Therefore, it appears that all cells may have the potential for totipotency if exposed to the appropriate environmental conditions.

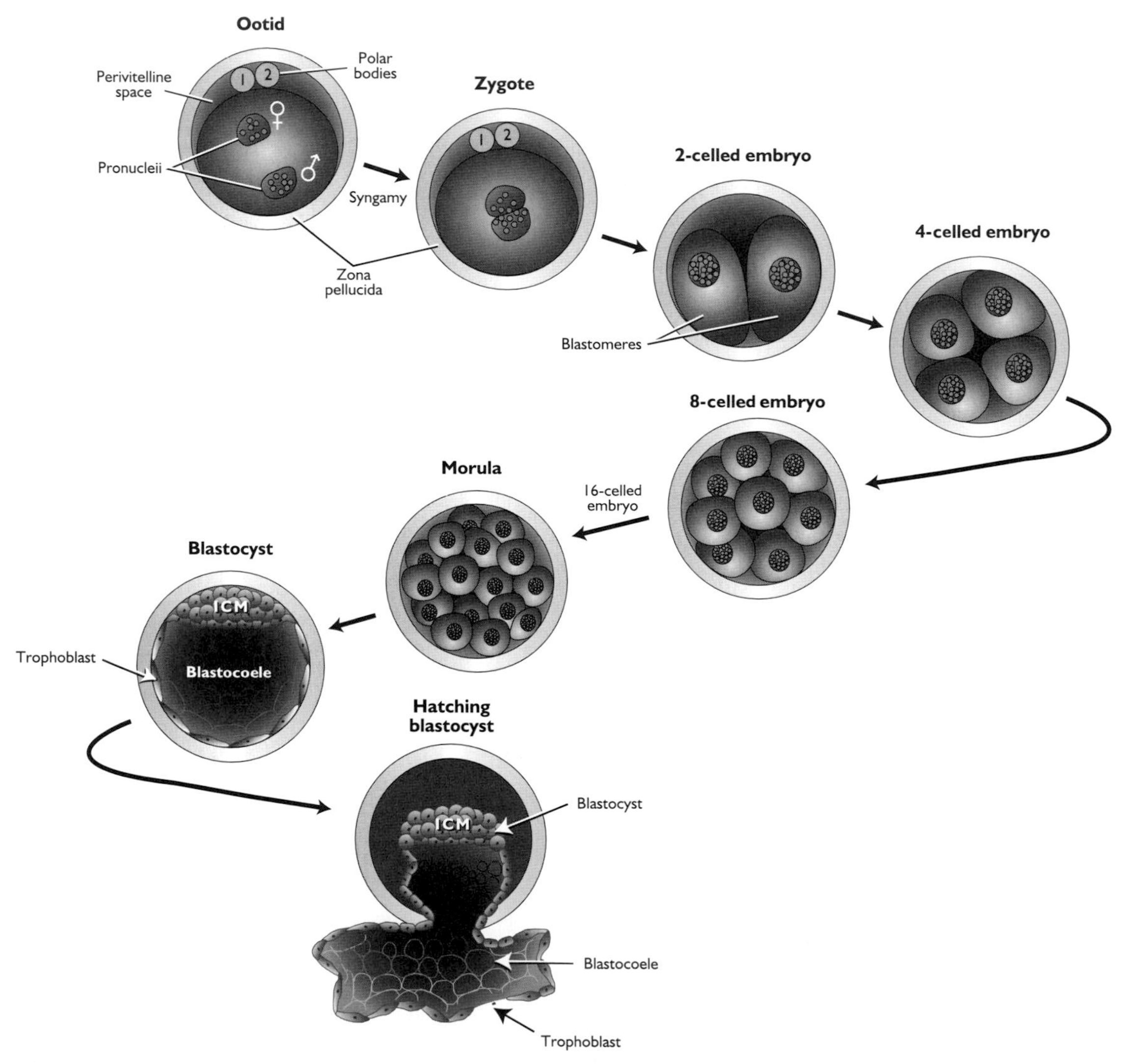

Figure 13-1. Development of a preimplantation embryo within the confines of the zona pellucida. In the ootid, male and female pronuclei, along with the first and second polar bodies are present. The fusion of the male and female pronuclei into a single diploid nucleus constitutes syngamy. The single-celled embryo (zygote) undergoes cleavage (mitotic division) to give rise to 2 daughter cells called blastomeres . Mitotic divisions continue until a ball of cells (morula) is formed. From the morula a blastocyst develops which consists of an inner cell mass (ICM), a cavity called a blastocoele and a trophoblast. Finally, the rapidly growing blastocyst "hatches" from the zona pellucida. (Graphic by Sonja Oei.)

The mitotic divisions of each blastomere generally occur simultaneously. Throughout this successive mitotic activity, the cells become progressively smaller and smaller with no net increase in size of the embryo, because the divisions take place inside the zona pellucida, which has a fixed volume.

When a solid ball of cells is formed and individual blastomeres can no longer be counted accurately, the early embryo is called a **morula** (Figure 13-1). When the morula is formed, the cells in the center begin to be compacted more than the cells in the outer region. Thus, during the morula stage, cells begin to separate into two distinct populations, the inner and outer cells. Cells in the inner portion of the morula develop **gap junctions** (Figure 13-2) which allow for intercellular communication and may enable the inner cells to remain in a defined cluster. The outer cells of the morula develop cell-to-cell adhesions known as **tight junctions** (Figure 13-2). These tight junctions are believed to alter the permeability characteristics of the outer cells. After the tight junctions are formed, fluid begins to accumulate inside the embryo. This fluid accumulation is believed to be brought about by an active sodium pump in the outer cells of the morula which pump ions into the center portion of the morula. This buildup of ions causes the ionic concentration of the fluid surrounding the cells of the morula to increase. As the ionic strength inside the morula increases, water diffuses into the embryo and begins to form a fluid filled cavity (Figure 13-2).

Hatching of the blastocyst is governed by three forces. They are:

- ***growth and fluid accumulation within the blastocyst***
- ***production of enzymes by the trophoblastic cells***
- ***contraction of the blastocyst***

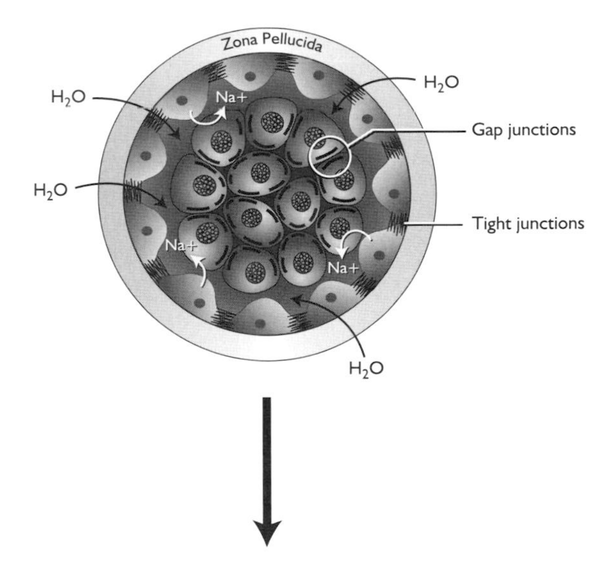

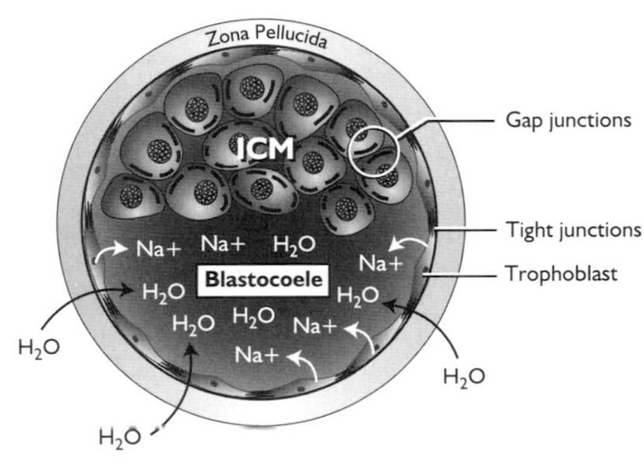

Figure 13-2. Proposed mechanism of blastocoele formation and cell regionalization in the transition from a morula to a blastocyst. Sodium is pumped into the intercellular spaces by the outer cells of the morula and water follows osmotically. Thus, fluid accumulates and a cavity known as the blastocoele is formed. As a result of the two types of intercellular connections (gap junctions and tight junctions), cells of the morula polarize to form two distinct tissues, the trophoblast and the inner cell mass (ICM). (Graphic by Sonja Oei.)

When a distinct cavity is recognizable, the embryo is called a **blastocyst**. Because of the nature of the tight junctions (found in the outer cells) and the gap junctions (found among the inner cells), the embryo is partitioned into two distinct cellular populations. These are known as the **inner cell mass** and the **trophoblast.** The inner cell mass will develop into the embryo proper and the trophoblastic cells will eventually give rise to the **chorion**. The chorion will become the fetal component of the placenta, which will be described later.

Table 13-1. Timing of preattachment embryogenesis relative to ovulation in various species.

Species	2-cell	4-cell	8-cell	Morula	Blastocyst	Hatching
cow	24h	1.5d	3d	**4-7d**	**7-12d**	**9-11d**
horse	24h	1.5d	**3d**	**4-5d**	**6-8d**	**7-8d**
sheep	24h	1.3d	2.5d	**3-4d**	**4-10d**	**7-8d**
pig	14-16h	1.0d	**2d**	**3.5d**	**4-5d**	**6d**

Values in non-shaded portion = development in the oviduct
Values in shaded portion = development in the uterus

As the blastocyst continues to undergo mitosis, fluid continues to fill the blastocoele, and the pressure within the embryo begins to increase. Concurrent with growth and fluid accumulation is the production of proteolytic enzymes by the trophoblastic cells. These enzymes weaken the zona pellucida so that it ruptures easily as growth of the blastocyst continues. Finally, the blastocyst itself begins to contract and relax. Such behavior causes intermittent pressure pulses. These pressure pulses coupled with continued growth and enzymatic degradation cause the zona pellucida to rupture.

When a small crack or fissure in the zona pellucida develops, the cells of the blastocyst squeeze out of the opening escaping, from its confines (Figure 13-1). The blastocyst now becomes a free-floating embryo within the lumen of the uterus.

Development of the Extraembryonic Membranes Represents an Explosion of Embryonic Tissue Growth Prior to Attachment

After hatching, the conceptus undergoes massive growth. For example, in the cow at day 13 the blastocyst is about 3 mm in diameter. In the next four days (day 17), the cow blastocyst will become 250 mm in length (about the length of the printed portion of this page) and will appear as a filamentous thread. By day 18 of gestation, the blastocyst occupies space in both uterine horns. While the blastocyst of the cow (and the ewe) grows quite rapidly during this early preattachment stage, the development of the pig blastocyst is even more dramatic. On day 10 of pregnancy, pig blastocysts are 2 mm spheres. During the next 24 to 48 hours, these 2 mm blastocysts will grow to about 200 mm in length (about the width of this page). This means that the blastocyst is growing at a rate of 4 to 8 mm per hour. By day 16, the pig blastocyst reaches lengths of 800 to 1000 mm. The dramatic growth of the conceptus is due largely to the development of a set of membranes called the **extraembryonic membranes**. The pig, sheep and cow are characterized as having filamentous or threadlike blastocysts prior to attachment. In the mare, however, blastocysts do not change into a threadlike structure but remain spherical.

The extraembryonic membranes of the preattachment embryo consist of the:

- ***yolk sac***
- ***chorion***
- ***amnion***
- ***allantois***

Formation of the extraembryonic membranes is an obligatory step in the acquisition of the embryo's ability to attach to the uterus of the dam. The extraembryonic membranes are a set of four anatomically distinct membranes which originate from the trophoblast, the primitive endoderm and the embryo.

The trophoblast, along with the **primitive endoderm,** gives rise to the **chorion** and the **amnion** (Figure 13-3). The yolk sac develops from the primitive endoderm. The chorion will eventually attach to the uterus, while the amnion will provide a fluid filled protective sac for the developing fetus.

As the hatched blastocyst begins to grow, it develops an additional layer just beneath, but in contact with, the inner cell mass. This layer of cells is called the primitive endoderm (Figure 13-3) and will continue to grow in a downward direction, eventually lining the trophoblast. At the same time the primitive endoderm is growing to become the inside lining of the trophoblast, it also forms an evagination at the ventral portion of the inner cell mass. This evagination forms the yolk sac (Figure 13-3). The yolk sac in domestic animal embryos is a transient extraembryonic membrane which regresses in size as the conceptus develops. In spite of its regression, you will recall (Chapter 4) that the yolk sac contributes the primitive germ cells which migrate to the genital ridge.

As the blastocyst continues to expand, the newly formed double membrane (the trophoblast and primitive endoderm) is called the **chorion.** As it develops, the chorion pushes upward in the dorsolateral region of the conceptus and begins to surround it. As the chorion begins to send wing-like projections above the embryo, the amnion begins to form (Figure 13-3). When the chorion fuses over the dorsal portion of the embryo, it then forms a complete sac around the embryo which constitutes the amnion. The amnion is filled with fluid and serves to protect the embryo from mechanical perturbations and serves as an anti-adhesion material to prevent tissues in the rapidly developing embryo from adhering to each other. The amnionic vesicle can be palpated in the cow between days 30 and 45 and feels like a small, turgid balloon inside the uterus. The embryo, however, is quite fragile during this early period and amnionic vesicle palpation should be conducted with caution.

During the same time that the amnion is developing, a small evagination from the posterior region of the primitive gut begins to form (Figure 13-3). This sac-like evagination is referred to as the **allantois.** The allantois is a fluid filled sac that collects liquid waste from the embryo. As the embryo grows, the allantois continues to expand and eventually will make contact with the chorion (Figure 13-3). When the allantois reaches a certain volume, it presses against the chorion and eventually fuses with it. When fusion takes place the two membranes are called the **chorioallantoic membrane** (Figure 13-3). The chorioallantoic membrane is the fetal contribution to the **placenta** and will provide the surface for attachments to the endometrium.

Table 13-2. Pregnancy recognition factor, critical days of pregnancy recognition and time of conceptus attachment in food producing mammals.

Species	Pregnancy Recognition Factors	Critical Period for Recognition (days after ovulation)	Time of Attachment (days after ovulation)
Cow	bIFN-τ (bTP-1)	15-18	18-22
Ewe	oIFN-τ (oTP-1)	12-14	15-18
Sow	Estradiol (E_2)	11-12	14-18
Mare	3 Proteins/Estrogens?	12-14	36-38

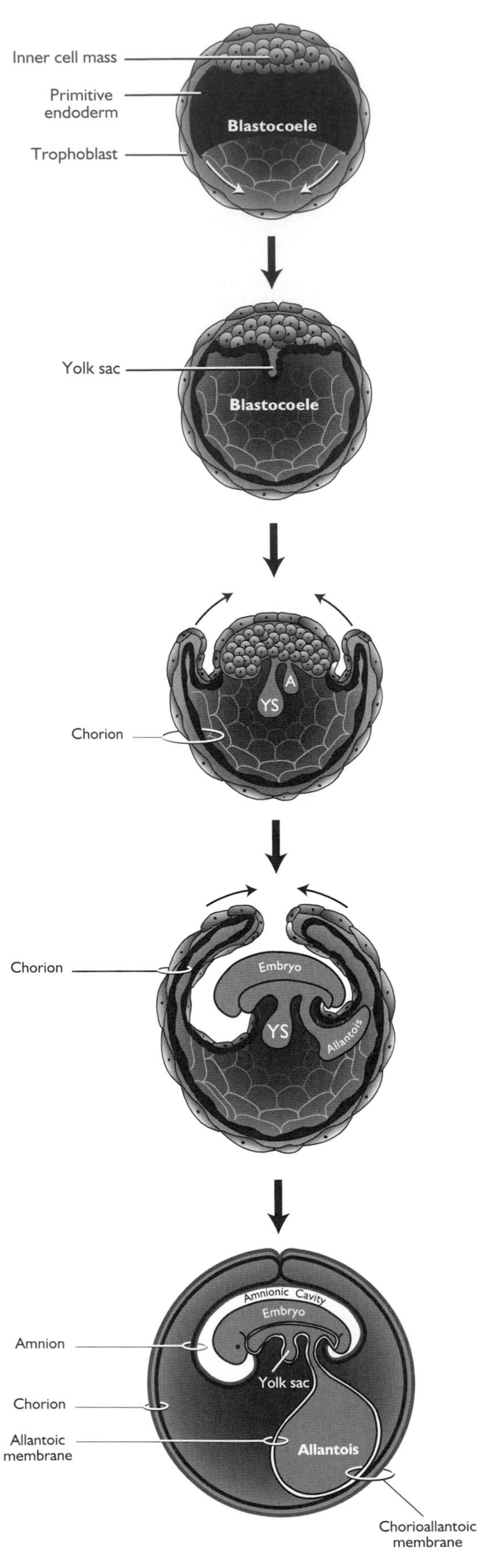

The primitive endoderm forms beneath the inner cell mass and begins to grow downward (arrows).

As the primitive endoderm grows, an evagination in the ventral inner cell mass forms the yolk sac.

The newly formed primitive endoderm fuses with the trophoblast to form a double membrane called the chorion. The chorion pushes upward and begins to surround the embryo. At the same time a new sac, called the allantois (A), begins to form from the primitive gut.

The yolk sac (YS) regresses and the allantois expands. The chorion nearly surrounds the embryo.

When the leading edges of the chorion fuse, a complete sac, called the amnion, surrounds the embryo and forms the amnionic cavity. The yolk sac continues to regress while the allantois expands, making contact with the chorion. The allantois and the chorion eventually fuse, forming the chorioallantoic membrane.

Figure 13-3. Schematic illustration of the general developmental course of the extraembryonic membranes in domestic animals. The sequence shown occurs between about day 10 and day 20 after ovulation. (Graphic by Sonja Oei.)

The conceptus must provide a timely biochemical signal or a pregnancy will terminate.

In order for the events of early embryogenesis to continue into an established pregnancy, luteolysis must be prevented. Progesterone must be maintained at sufficiently high levels so that embryogenesis and attachment of the developing conceptus to the endometrium can take place. The embryo enters the uterus between days 2 and 5 after ovulation, depending on the species (Table 13-1). The critical series of events by which the conceptus initially signals its presence to the dam and enables pregnancy to continue is referred to as **maternal recognition of pregnancy**. If an adequate signal is not delivered in a timely manner, the dam will experience luteolysis, progesterone concentrations will decline and pregnancy will be terminated (Figure 13-4). Signals are provided by the conceptus and recognition factors as they relate to the critical recognition period are presented in Table 13-2.

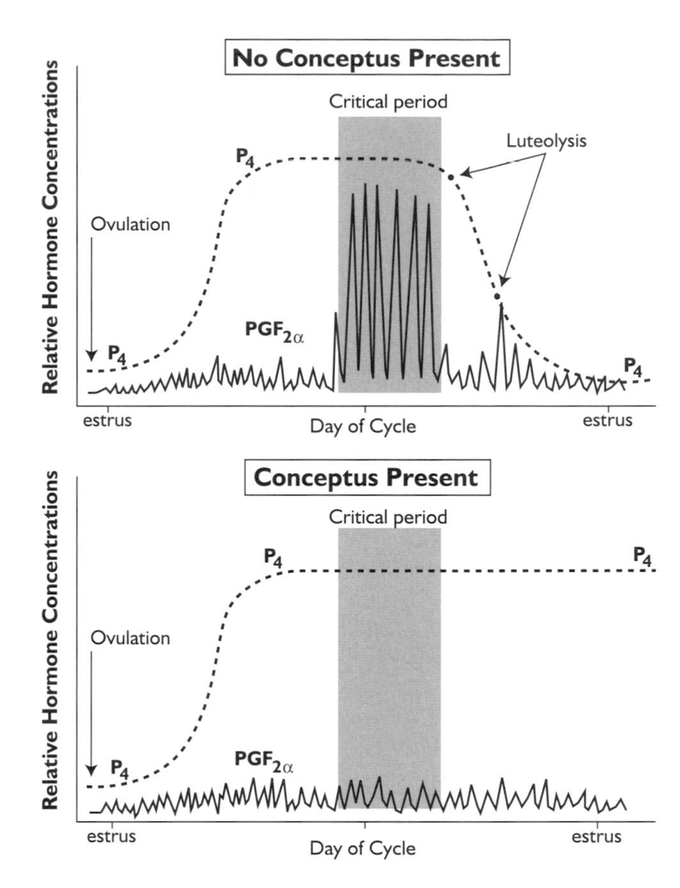

Figure 13-4. Comparison between the endocrine condition of a female with conceptus present and a female with no conceptus. Maternal recognition of pregnancy must occur prior to luteolysis if the pregnancy is to be maintained.

Maternal recognition of pregnancy must occur prior to luteolysis.

Recall from Chapter 9, that the corpus luteum of ruminants produces oxytocin which stimulates endometrial cells to synthesize $PGF_{2\alpha}$. The production of $PGF_{2\alpha}$ is dependent upon a threshold number of oxytocin receptors that are synthesized by endometrial cells at a critical time during the estrous cycle. When these receptors are available in sufficient numbers, pulsatile secretion of $PGF_{2\alpha}$ occurs in response to luteal oxytocin secretion and luteolysis follows (Figure 13-4). Clearly, this mechanism must be prevented if a successful pregnancy is to proceed.

In the ewe and cow, the blastocyst blocks the synthesis of endometrial oxytocin receptors.

In the ewe and the cow, the free-floating blastocyst produces specific proteins that provide the signal for prevention of luteolysis. The specific proteins were once called **ovine trophoblastic protein 1** (oTP-1) and **bovine trophoblastic protein 1** (bTP-1). Both of these proteins belong to a class of materials known as **interferons.** Most interferons are nonspecific glycoproteins produced by leukocytes, fibroblasts, lymphocytes and trophoblastic cells. Interferons have antiviral action and alter the function of target cells. Because trophoblastic proteins (oTP-1 and bTP-1) constitute a separate class of interferons, they are now

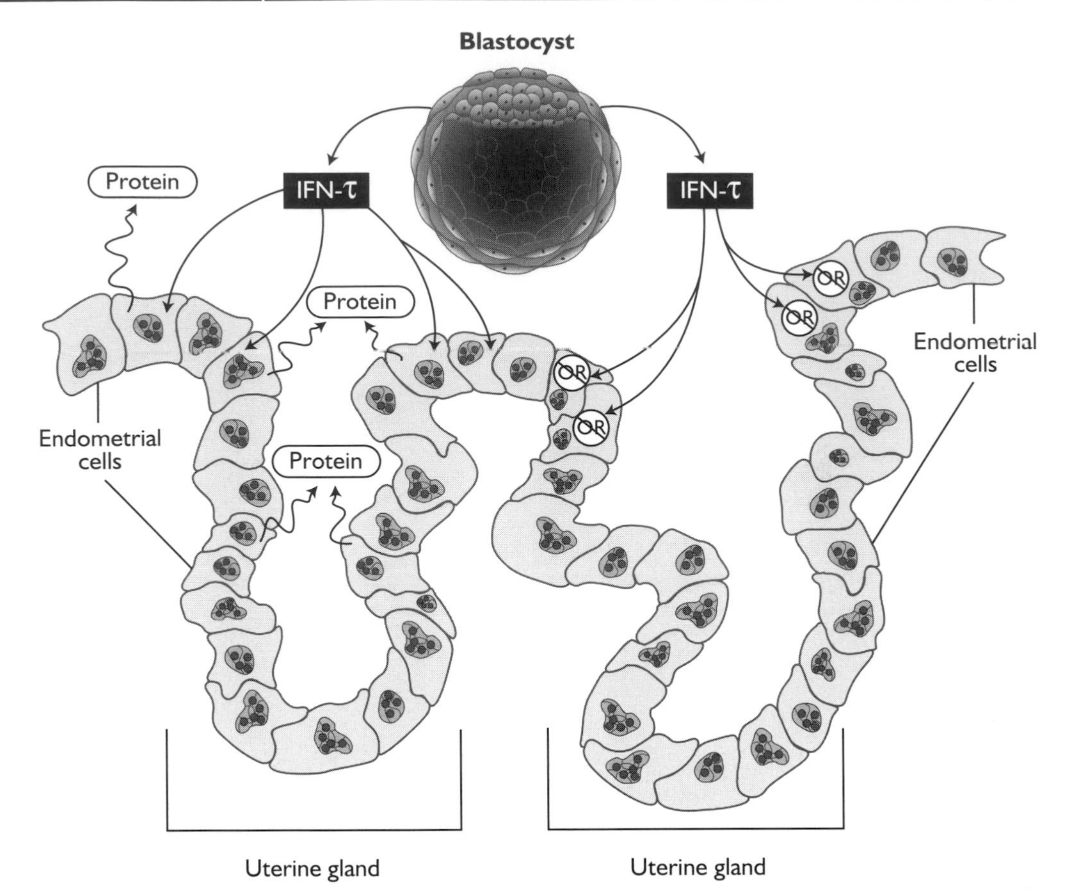

Figure 13-5. IFN-τ is produced by the trophoblastic cells of the blastocyst (cow and ewe). IFN-τ acts on the endometrial cells of the uterus to inhibit the production of oxytocin receptors (OR) so that oxytocin cannot stimulate $PGF_{2\alpha}$ synthesis. In addition, IFN-τ causes production of proteins from the uterine glands. (Graphic by Sonja Oei.)

referred to as **ovine Interferon τ (oIFN-τ)** and **bovine Interferon τ (bIFN-τ)**. The use of the Greek letter τ designates the trophoblastic origin of these proteins.

A relatively small protein (18,000 to 20,000 daltons), oIFN-τ is produced by the trophoblastic cells of the blastocyst and is present in the uterus from about day 13 to 21 after ovulation. Production of progesterone by the corpus luteum cannot be enhanced by oIFN-τ and therefore it is not luteotropic. Instead, oIFN-τ binds to the endometrium and inhibits oxytocin receptor synthesis by endometrial cells. Figure 13-5 summarizes the proposed effect of oIFN-τ and bIFN-τ on endometrial production of oxytocin receptors. In addition to blocking oxytocin receptor synthesis, IFN-τ also binds to the apical portion (Figure 13-5) of the uterine glands and promotes protein synthesis believed to be critical to preimplantation embryonic survival.

In the sow, estradiol reroutes $PGF_{2\alpha}$ secretion by the endometrium.

In the sow, two major differences exist in maternal recognition of pregnancy, compared to the ewe and cow. First, the conceptus of the pig produces estradiol which serves as the signal for maternal recognition of pregnancy. Second, $PGF_{2\alpha}$ is produced in significant quantities, but is rerouted into the uterine lumen. The conceptus begins to produce estradiol between days 11 and 12 after ovulation. The production of estrogen does not inhibit the production of $PGF_{2\alpha}$, but causes the $PGF_{2\alpha}$ to be secreted in a different direction than in the cycling sow. The direction of secretion is away from the submucosal capillaries and toward the uterine lumen. Luminal $PGF_{2\alpha}$ has little access to the circulation and thus cannot cause luteolysis. The precise mechanism of rerouting of $PGF_{2\alpha}$ is not completely understood.

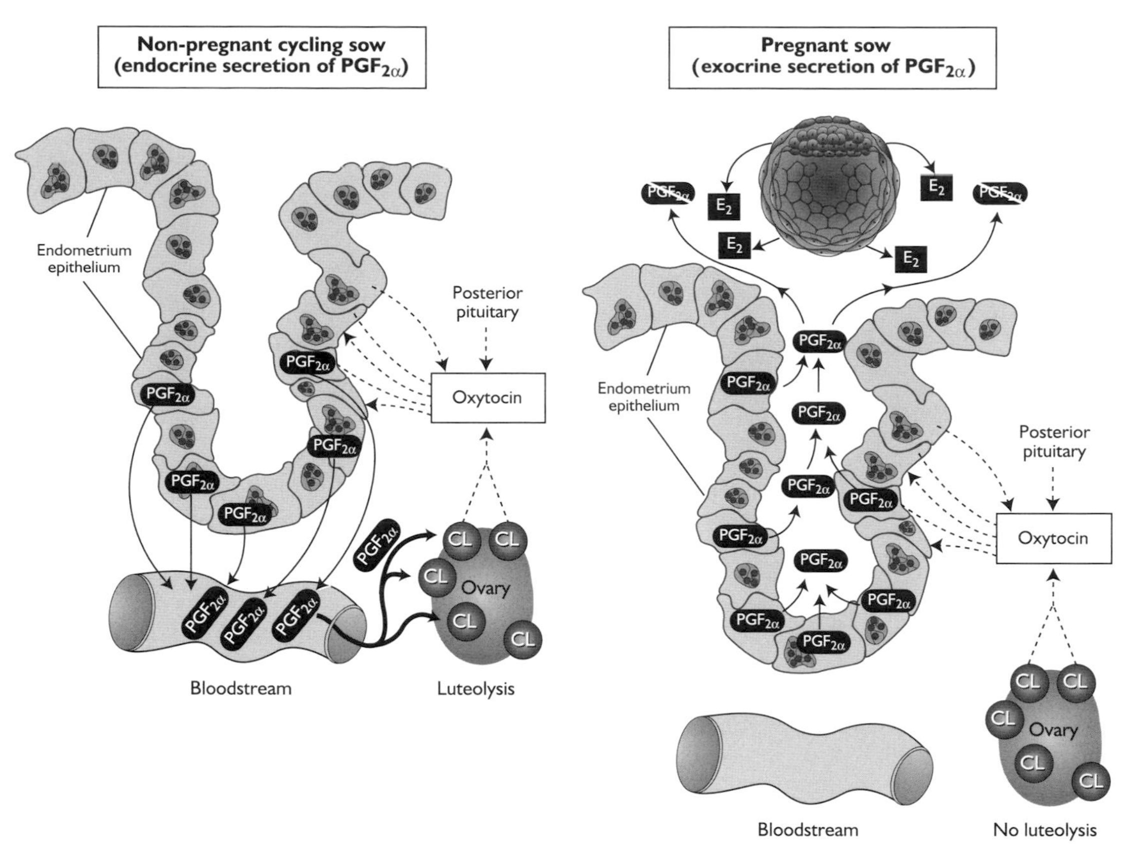

Figure 13-6. In the non-pregnant sow, oxytocin from the endometrium, posterior pituitary and CL promotes $PGF_{2\alpha}$ synthesis by the uterine endometrium. $PGF_{2\alpha}$ diffuses by concentration gradient towards the endometrial capillaries, where it drains into the uterine vein and is transported to the ovary and causes luteolysis. In the pregnant sow, the blastocyst produces estradiol which causes the $PGF_{2\alpha}$ to be rerouted into the uterine lumen, where it is destroyed, thus preventing luteolysis. In the pregnant sow, oxytocin is also produced by the CL and posterior pituitary like in the cycling sow. (Graphic by Sonja Oei.)

However, it is believed that estrogen causes increased receptor production for prolactin in the endometrium. Prolactin changes the ionic flux for calcium. This is thought to promote the **exocrine** secretion of $PGF_{2\alpha}$ (into the uterine lumen) rather than an **endocrine** secretion (into the uterine vasculature). Porcine conceptuses produce interferons, but these materials do not affect corpora lutea longevity or function.

Another important feature of maternal recognition of pregnancy in the sow is that there must be at least two conceptuses present in each uterine horn for pregnancy to be maintained. If conceptuses are not present in one uterine horn, $PGF_{2\alpha}$ will be secreted in an endocrine fashion, luteolysis will occur and the pregnancy will be terminated. Figure 13-6 summarizes the proposed mechanism for maternal recognition of pregnancy in the sow.

The equine conceptus must migrate over the endometrial surface to establish maternal recognition of pregnancy.

In the mare, the presence of the conceptus causes prevention of luteolysis. Also, in the presence of the conceptus, the endometrial production of $PGF_{2\alpha}$ is significantly reduced. A unique feature of maternal recognition of pregnancy in the mare is that the conceptus must migrate within the uterus from one uterine horn to the other. This migration must occur between 12 and 14 times per day during days 12, 13 and 14 of pregnancy in order to inhibit $PGF_{2\alpha}$ (Figure 13-7). The intrauterine migration of the equine conceptus appears necessary because the conceptus does not elongate as in other species. Therefore, there is less contact between the

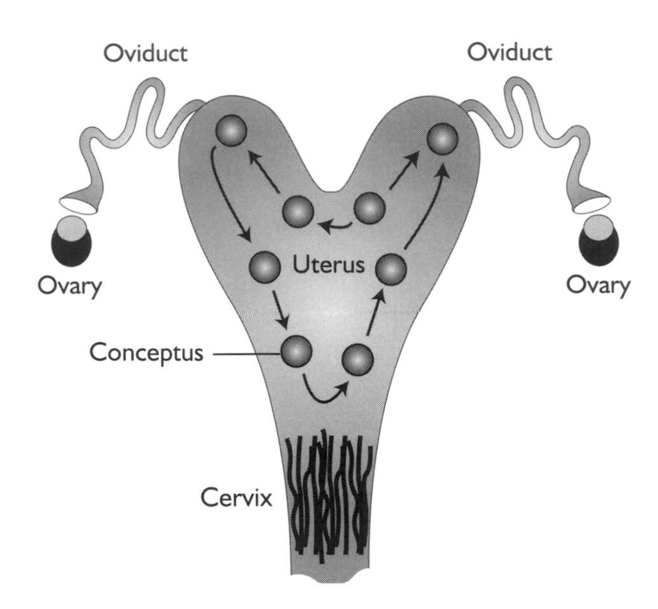

Figure 13-7. Illustration showing the pathway of transuterine migration of the horse conceptus. Each bold dot represents a "stopping spot" in which the embryo will spend between 5 and 20 minutes within a given uterine zone. (Graphic by Sonja Oei.)

conceptus and the endometrial surface. In other words, the migration of the conceptus is probably necessary to distribute pregnancy recognition factors to the endometrial cells.

Like the other species, the conceptus of the horse produces proteins which apparently have some effect on the recognition of pregnancy (Table 13-2); however, the specific roles are yet unknown.

> ***The net effect of successful pregnancy recognition is maintenance of high blood progesterone concentrations.***

If pregnancy recognition signals are provided, progesterone will be maintained at sufficiently high concentrations and the conceptus will continue to grow and develop. The extraembryonic membranes will form an attachment with the endometrium to provide a semipermanent link between the dam and the fetus. This semipermanent link is known as the **placenta** and will be discussed in the next chapter.

Further Phenomena for Fertility

Some species have delayed implantation (attachment to the uterus) in which a viable embryo floats within the uterus for a sustained period of time. Martins (a mink-like animal) copulate in July or August and the embryo develops to the blastocyst stage, but attachment does not occur until January. The young are born about 50 days after attachment.

The presence of the marsupial embryo within the uterus does not interrupt the estrous cycle. Therefore, pregnancy recognition in this species is apparently not caused by a substance(s) produced by the embryo. Instead, the semipermanent attachment of the prematurely born fetus to the teat provides a pregnancy recognition mechanism, because it arrests cyclicity.

The female nine-banded armadillo has several unique features. First, the female has a simplex uterus (like primates), in spite of being a primitive life form. She has no vagina, but retains a urogenital sinus. She spontaneously ovulates a single oocyte in the summer which enters embryonic diapause (delayed attachment) for about 3 to 4 months. Soon after implantation, cells of the inner cell mass give rise to four separate identical embryos. Thus, the female armadillo gives birth to identical quadruplets. In spite of what the news media tells us, cloning is not new and is not an unnatural process. The genetic implications of identical offspring in this species are not known.

The human blastocyst (along with guinea pigs, hedgehogs and chimpanzees) first attaches to the endometrium, passes through the endometrial epithelium and becomes completely imbedded in the endometrium. Thus, the embryo is isolated from the uterine lumen. Knowledge of this phenomenon led to the term "implantation." True implantation does not occur in domestic animals.

In rodents, a successful pregnancy can be terminated if an alien male (one that did not cause the pregnancy) shows up and hangs out with the pregnant female. This is known as the "Bruce Effect."

Additional Reading

Bazer, F.W., T.L. Ott and T.E. Spencer. 1994. Pregnancy recognition in ruminants, pigs and horses: Signals from the trophoblast. *Theriogenology*. 41:79.

Ginther, O.J. 1992. *Reproductive Biology of the Mare*. 2nd ed. Equiservices, Cross Plains, WI.

Flint, A.P.F. 1995. Interferon, the oxytocin receptor and the maternal recognition of pregnancy in ruminants and non-ruminants: A comparative approach. *Reprod. Fertil. Dev.* 7:313.

Mirando, M.A., M.U. Zumcu, K.G. Carnahan and T.E. Ludwig. 1996. A role for oxytocin during luteolysis and early pregnancy in swine. *Reprod. Dom. Anim.* 31:455.

Roberts, R.M., D.W. Leaman and J.C. Cross. 1992. Role of interferons in maternal recognition of pregnancy in ruminants. *P.S.E.B.M.* 200:7.

Thatcher, W.W., C.R. Staples, G. Danet-Desnoyers, B. Oldick and E.P. Schmitt. 1994. Embryo health and mortality in sheep and cattle. *J. Anim. Sci.* 72(suppl. 3):16.

14 Placentation, the Endocrinology of Gestation and Parturition

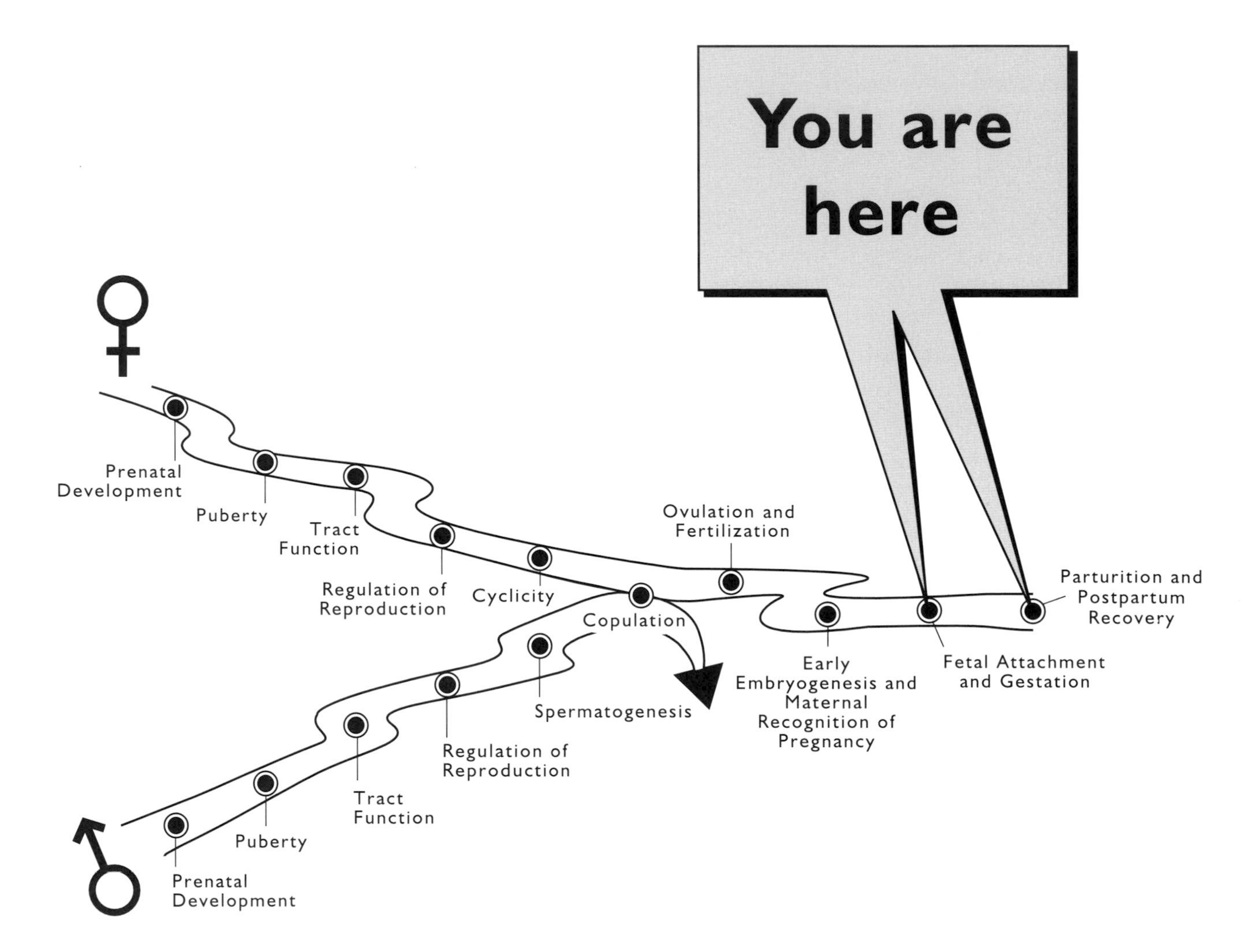

Take Home Message

The placenta is an organ which provides an interface for metabolic exchange between the dam and the fetus. Placentas are described morphologically according to the distribution of chorionic villi on their surface as well as the degree of intimacy between the maternal and the fetal interface. The placenta is a transitional endocrine organ which produces hormones that are responsible for: 1) maintenance of pregnancy; 2) stimulation of the maternal mammary gland; and 3) promotion of fetal growth. Parturition is brought about by a production of fetal corticoids and requires removal of the progesterone block. Parturition consists of three stages. They are: 1) initiation of myometrial contractions; 2) expulsion of the fetus; and 3) expulsion of the fetal membranes.

Attachment of the conceptus to form an intimate, but temporary, relationship with the uterus is an evolutionary step which provides significant advantage to the conceptus. The phenomenon of intrauterine development ensures that the developing conceptus will be provided with adequate nutrition and protection during its development. In contrast, lower forms of animals lay eggs (**oviparous**). The safety of potential offspring of oviparous animals is jeopardized because the female cannot completely protect the eggs from environmental and predatory danger. Thus, **eutherian mammals** (mammals with a placenta), have a strong reproductive advantage over oviparous animals.

The final steps of reproduction are:
- ***formation of a placenta***
- ***acquisition of endocrine function of the placenta***
- ***parturition***

The placenta is a transient organ of metabolic interchange between the conceptus and the dam. It is also a transient endocrine organ. The placenta is composed of a fetal component derived from the chorion and a maternal component derived from modifications of the uterine endometrium. The discrete regions of contact between the chorion and the endometrium form specific zones of metabolic exchange. The placenta also produces a variety of hormones. This transient endocrine function is important for the maintenance of a successful pregnancy.

Parturition (giving birth to the young) is the final step in the reproductive process. It is initiated by the fetus and involves a complex cascade of endocrine events that promote myometrial contractions, dilation of the cervix, expulsion of the fetus and expulsion of the extraembryonic membranes.

Placentas Have Different Distributions of Chorionic Villi and Varying Degrees of Intimacy

As you have learned in the previous chapter, the conceptus consists of the embryo and the extraembryonic membranes (amnion, allantois and chorion). The chorion is the fetal contribution to the placenta. The functional unit of the fetal placenta is the **chorionic villus**. Chorionic villi are small, finger-like projections that appear on the surface of the chorion. These tiny villi protrude away from the chorion toward the uterine endometrium. Placentas are classified according to the distribution of chorionic villi on their surfaces, giving each type a distinct anatomical appearance. Placentas may also be classified by the intimacy of the tissues at the maternal-fetal interface. In other words, placentas are classified based on the degree of separation of the fetal and maternal blood supplies.

Chorionic villi distribution is classified as:
- ***diffuse***
- ***cotyledonary***
- ***zonary***
- ***discoid***

The diffuse placenta of the pig has a velvet-like surface with many closely spaced chorionic villi that are distributed over the entire surface of the chorion (Figure 14-1). Initial attachment occurs around day 12 and is well established by day 18 to 20 after ovulation (Table 13-2).

Diffuse placentas have uniform distribution of chorionic villi which cover the surface of the chorion.

The mare placenta is also classified as diffuse, but it is characterized as having many specialized "microzones" of chorionic villi known as **microcotyledons** (Figure 14-1). These microcotyledons are microscopically discrete regions at the fetal-maternal interface. As in the pig, they are also distributed over the entire chorionic surface.

The mare placenta also contains unique transitory structures known as **endometrial cups.** These are discrete areas ranging from a few millimeters to several centimeters in diameter. The endometrial cups are of both trophoblastic and endometrial origin. There are 5 to 10 endometrial cups distributed over the surface of the placenta. Endometrial cups produce **equine chorionic gonadotropin (eCG)** and develop between day 35 and 60 of pregnancy. Following day 60, the endometrial cups are sloughed into the uterine lumen and are no longer functional. Attachment of the conceptus to the endometrium is initiated at about day 24 and becomes well established by 36 to 38 days (Table 13-2).

Cotyledonary placentas have a large number of discrete button-like structures called cotyledons.

Ruminants have a **cotyledonary** placenta (Figure 14-1). A cotyledon is defined as a unit of the placenta of trophoblastic origin consisting of abundant blood vessels and connective tissue. In sheep, there are between 90 and 100 cotyledons distributed across the surface of the chorion and, in cattle, 70 to 120 cotyledons have been observed. The **placentome** (point of interface) in the cotyledonary placenta consists of a **fetal cotyledon** contributed by the fetus and a **maternal caruncle** originating from the **caruncular regions** of the uterus. At about day 16 in sheep and day 25 in cattle, the chorion initiates attachment to the caruncles of the uterus. Prior to this time the placenta is essentially diffuse. During the formation of the placentomes, chorionic villi protrude into crypts in the caruncular tissue. Attachment is well established by day 30 in ewes and day 40 in cows (Table 13-2).

In the cow, the placentomes form a convex structure, while in the ewe they are concave (Figure 14-1). During gestation, the cotyledons will increase many-fold in diameter. In fact, cotyledons in the cow near the end of gestation may measure 5 to 6 centimeters in diameter. Such growth provides enormous surface area to support placental transfer of nutrients from the dam and metabolic wastes from the fetus.

Zonary placentas have a band-like zone of chorionic villi.

The **zonary placenta** (found in dogs and cats) includes a prominent region of exchange that forms a broad zone around the chorion near the middle of the conceptus (Figure 14-1). A second region consists of a highly pigmented ring at either end of the central zone. This pigmented zone consists of small hematomas (blood clots). The function of this zone is not understood. A third

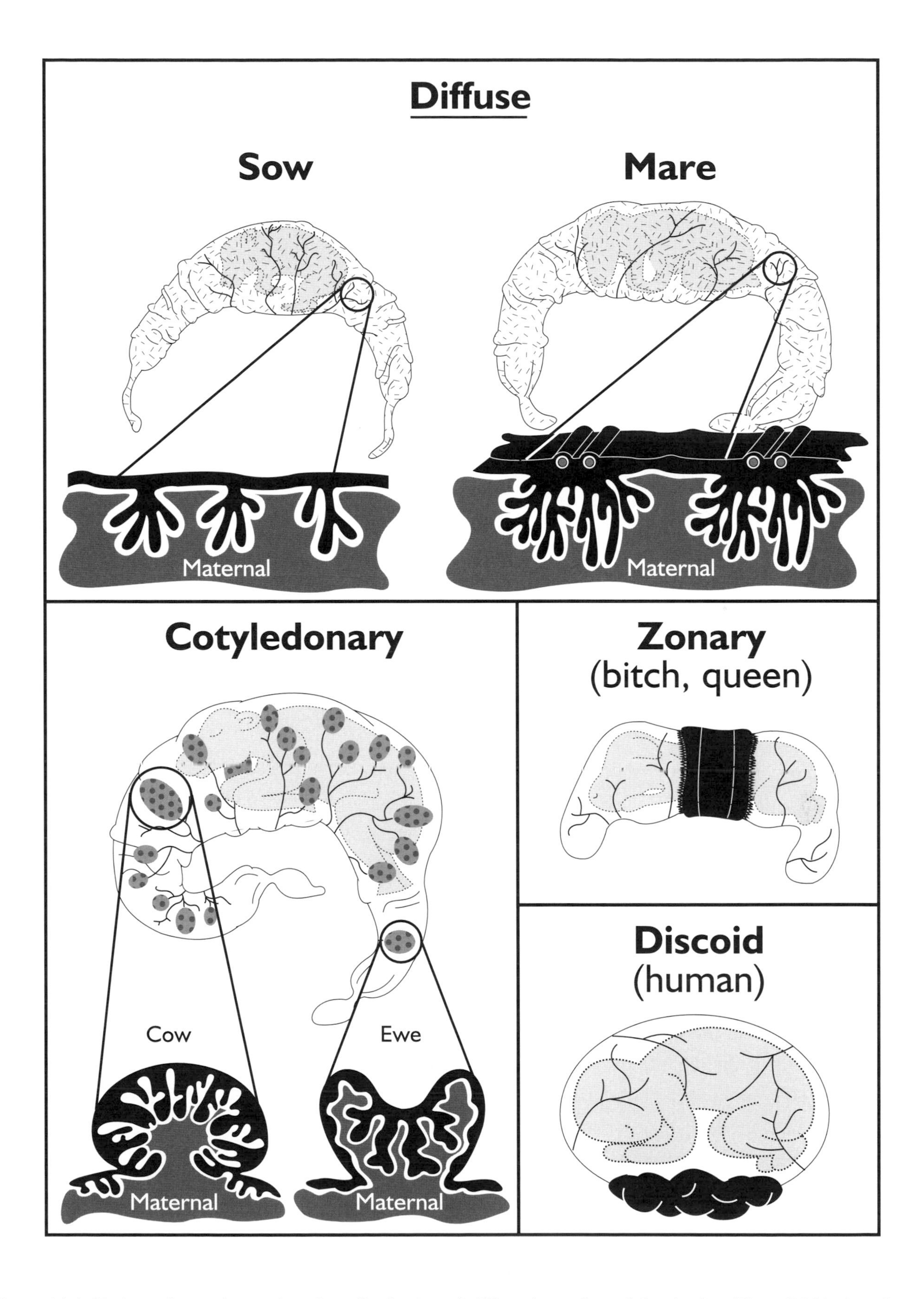

Figure 14-1. Various placental types based on distribution of villi on the surface of the chorion. The solid black regions are the chorion. (Graphic by Sonja Oei.)

region is a transparent zone on the distal ends of the chorion which has poor vascularity. This zone may be involved in absorption of materials directly from the uterine lumen.

> ***Discoid placentas form a regionalized disc.***

The **discoid** placenta (Figure 14-1) is found in rodents and primates. It is characterized as having one or two distinct disks on one region of the chorion. These discs contain chorionic villi which interface with the endometrium and provide the region for nutrient and metabolic waste exchange.

Placental Classification by Microscopic Appearance Is Based on the Number of Placental Layers That Separate the Fetal Blood from the Maternal Blood

The nomenclature for describing placental intimacy is derived by first describing the tissues of the maternal placenta in the prefix of the word. The tissues of the fetal placenta constitute the suffix. Exchange can occur through as many as seven tissue layers and as few as one. The name of the prefix and suffix of each type of placenta changes depending on the number of tissue layers that exist.

> ***Prefix =maternal side Suffix =fetal side***
> ***"epithelio" "chorial"***
> ***epitheliochorial***

The **epitheliochorial** placenta (Figure 14-3) is the least intimate among the placental types. In the epitheliochorial placenta, both the endometrial epithelium (maternal side) and epithelium of the chorionic villi are intact. The epitheliochorial placenta is found in the sow and the mare. Recall that the placentas of the sow and the mare are diffuse and occupy a large proportion of the surface area of the chorion. Thus, the need for a highly intimate relationship is offset by the large total surface area of the diffuse placenta.

Ruminants also have an epitheliochorial placenta. However, the endometrial epithelium sometimes erodes, causing intermittent exposure of the maternal capillaries to the chorionic epithelium. This type of placenta has been termed the **syndesmochorial** placenta.

In addition to the feature of partial erosion of the endometrial epithelium, a unique cell type is found in the ruminant placenta. These cells are called **binucleate giant cells.** As their name implies, they are characterized as being quite large and have two nuclei. Binucleate giant cells appear at about day 14 in the sheep and between days 18 and 20 in the cow. These cells originate from trophoblastic cells and are believed to be formed continuously throughout gestation. Binucleate giant cells constitute around 20% of the fetal placenta. During development, the binucleate giant cells migrate from the chorionic epithelium and invade the endometrial epithelium (Figure 14-2). The binucleate giant cells are believed to transfer complex molecules from the fetal to the maternal placenta. There is evidence that they secrete **placental lactogen**. Also, these cells secrete **pregnancy specific protein B (PSPB)**, a protein unique to pregnancy in ruminants. The binucleate giant cells are also important sights of steroidogenesis, producing progesterone and estrogen. These cells will no doubt emerge as increasingly important players in the function of the ruminant placenta as further research is completed.

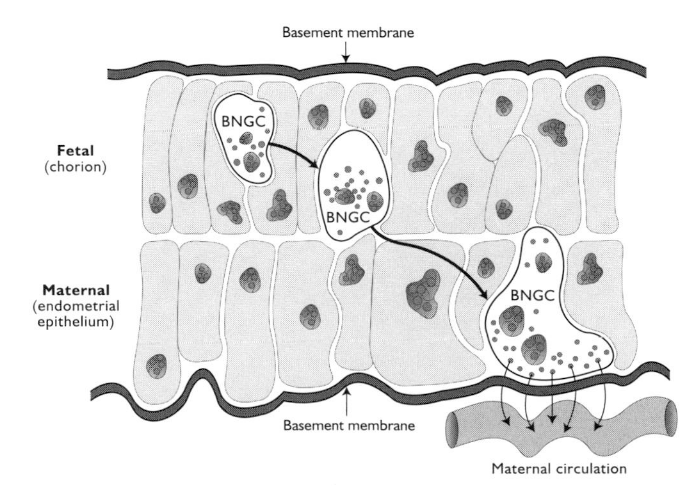

Figure 14-2. The migration of binucleate giant cells (BNGC) from the chorion to the endometrial epithelium. (Graphic by Sonja Oei.)

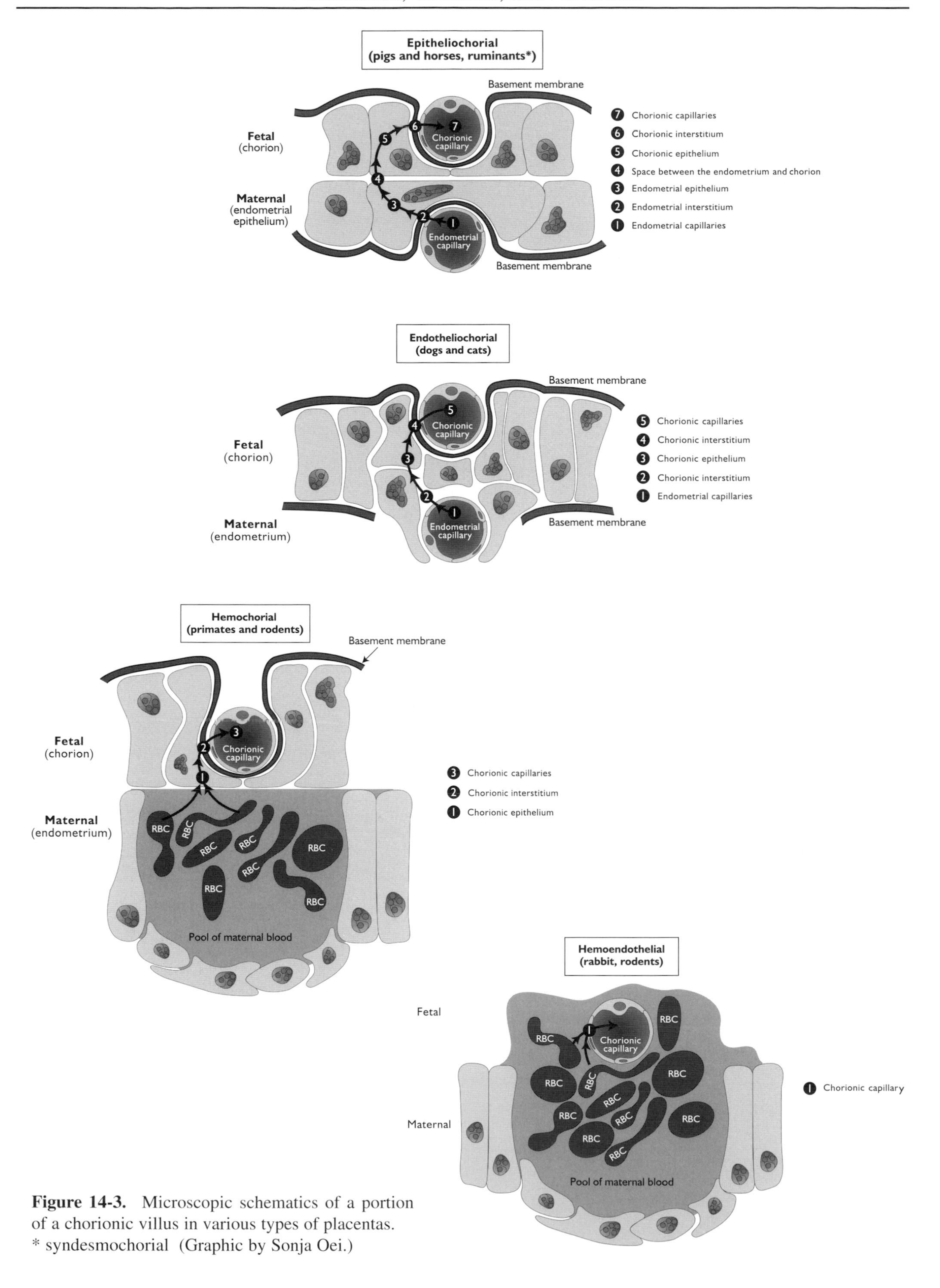

Figure 14-3. Microscopic schematics of a portion of a chorionic villus in various types of placentas. * syndesmochorial (Graphic by Sonja Oei.)

The **endotheliochorial placenta** is characterized as having complete erosion of the endometrial epithelium and underlying interstitium. Thus, maternal capillaries are directly exposed to epithelial cells of the chorion (Figure 14-3). The chorionic epithelium packs around the vessels on the maternal side. Note in Figure 14-3 that this type of placenta is more intimate than the epitheliochorial placenta because the endometrial epithelium no longer exists. Dogs and cats possess the endotheliochorial placenta.

The **hemochorial placenta** (Figure 14-3) is characterized as having the chorionic epithelium in direct apposition to maternal pools of blood. Thus, nutrients and gases are exchanged directly from maternal blood and must move through only three tissue layers. This highly intimate relationship is found in primates (Figure 14-3).

The most intimate placenta is the **hemoendothelial** type (Figure 14-3). The barriers to waste, nutrient and gaseous transfer are almost nonexistent. This type of placenta is found in the rabbit, rat and guinea pig. The chorionic capillaries are immersed directly in pools of blood and materials are transferred directly from maternal blood pools through a single layer of chorionic capillary endothelium. Even though the hemoendothelial placenta is quite intimate, there is no direct exchange of the blood components (cells, proteins) between the maternal and fetal sides.

The Placenta Regulates the Exchange Between the Fetus and Dam

Placental exchange involves a number of mechanisms found in other tissues. These are **simple diffusion**, **facilitated diffusion** and **active transport**. Gases and water pass from high to low concentrations by simple diffusion. The placenta contains active transport pumps for sodium and potassium, as well as calcium. Glucose and other metabolically important materials such as amino acids are transported by facilitated diffusion utilizing specific carrier molecules.

Glucose is the major source of energy for the fetus. The majority of glucose is derived from the maternal circulation. Near the end of gestation, glucose consumption by the fetus is exceptionally high and can lead to a metabolic drain of glucose away from the dam. Such a glucose drain favors the development of ketosis in the dam. Ketosis results from the metabolism of body fat, which generate ketones for energy when glucose is limited. Periparturient ketosis is common in dairy cows where postpartum metabolic demands are exceptionally high because of high milk production.

Some materials cannot be transported across the placenta. With the exception of some immunoglobulins, maternal proteins do not cross the placental barrier. Immunoglobulins can be transported from the maternal to the fetal side in a hemochorial or an endotheliochorial placenta. However, the fetus synthesizes the majority of its own proteins from amino acids contributed by the dam. Lipids do not cross the placenta. Instead, the placenta hydrolyzes triglycerides and maternal phospholipids and synthesizes new lipid materials to be used by the fetus. Large peptide hormones such as thyroid stimulating hormone, adrenal cortical stimulating hormone, growth hormone, insulin and glucagon do not cross the placenta. Smaller molecular weight hormones such as steroids, thyroid hormone and the catecholamines (epinephrine and norepinephrine) cross the placenta with relative ease. Vitamins and minerals are transferred to the fetus at variable rates. Fat soluble vitamins do not cross the placenta with ease, while water soluble vitamins pass across the placenta with relative ease.

Of significant importance is the ability of the placenta to transfer toxic and potentially pathogenic materials. Many toxic substances easily cross the placental barrier. These include ethyl alcohol, lead, phosphorus and mercury. Also, opiate drugs and numerous common pharmaceuticals such as barbiturates and antibiotics can cross the placental barrier. Some substances may be highly **teratogenic.** Teratogenic means inducing abnormal development (birth defects). These substances include LSD, amphetamines, lithium, diethylstilbestrol and thalidomide. It is well documented that these materials induce abnormal fetal development and cause serious birth defects.

It is known that a wide range of microorganisms can contaminate the fetus. Viruses can cross the placental barrier with ease and thus many viral diseases can be transmitted from the dam to the fetus. Such human diseases as German measles, Herpesvirus and HIV can be transmitted from the pregnant mother to the fetus. Bacteria such as syphilis can also be transmitted to the fetus.

The Placenta Is a Major Endocrine Organ During Pregnancy

In addition to serving as a metabolic exchange organ, the placenta serves as a transitory endocrine organ. Hormones from the placenta gain access to both the fetal and the maternal circulation.

> ***The placenta produces hormones that can:***
> - ***stimulate ovarian function***
> - ***maintain pregnancy***
> - ***influence fetal growth***
> - ***stimulate mammary function***
> - ***assist in parturition***

The placenta of the mare produces a gonadotropin called **equine chorionic gonadotropin (eCG)**. Equine chorionic gonadotropin is also called **pregnant mare serum gonadotropin (PMSG).** Equine chorionic gonadotropin is produced by the endometrial cups of the placenta. Endometrial cups are a transient placental endocrine gland. They begin producing eCG at the time of attachment of the conceptus to the endometrium. The relationship between the formation of the endometrial cups in the mare and the synthesis of eCG is presented in Figure 14-4. As you can see, the production of eCG is closely related to the weight of the endometrial cups.

Equine chorionic gonadotropin acts as a luteotropin and provides a stimulus for maintenance of the **primary corpus luteum**. The primary corpus luteum in the mare is defined as the corpus luteum formed from the ovulated follicle. In addition, eCG is responsible for controlling the formation and maintenance of **supplementary (accessory) corpora lutea**. As eCG increases, the pregnant mare will often ovulate, thus generating accessory corpora lutea. The eCG-induced ovulations occur between days 40 and 70 of pregnancy. Luteinization (promoted by eCG) also occurs in antral follicles which do not ovulate. Thus, eCG has a significant positive impact on the ability of the ovary to

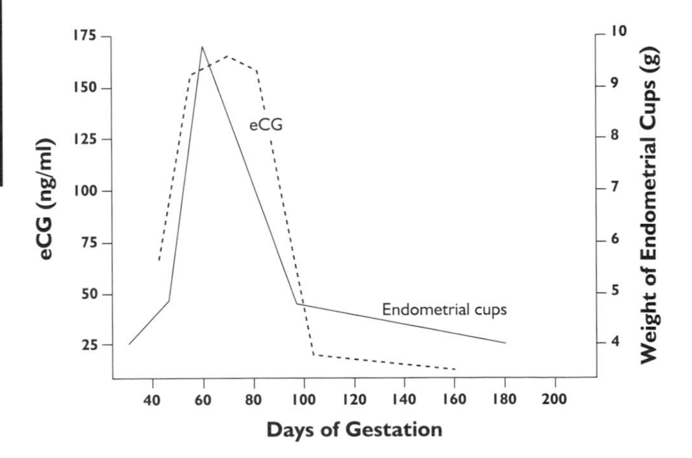

Figure 14-4. Relationship between growth of the endometrial cups and concentration of eCG in blood of the dam as a function of stage of gestation. (From Ginther *Reproductive Biology of the Mare.)*

produce progesterone. Indeed, if one examines the progesterone profile, it can be seen that there is a close relationship between the progesterone and the production of accessory corpora lutea (Figure 14-5).

In addition to its luteotropic action, eCG has powerful FSH-like actions when administered to females of other species. In fact, eCG will cause marked follicular development in most species. It is used commonly to induce superovulation where embryo transfer is performed (cow, sheep, rabbit). In mares, however, eCG does not exert significant FSH-like action.

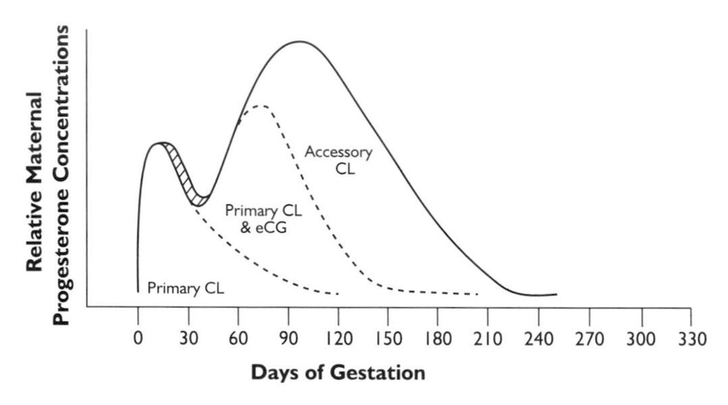

Figure 14-5. Luteal progesterone output during the first half of gestation in the mare. Progesterone from the primary corpus luteum (CL) increases rapidly after ovulation and then fades (hatched region of the curve). Upon stimulation by eCG the primary CL is stimulated and progesterone concentration in the maternal blood again increases (middle curve). As eCG continues to increase accessory CL develop and progesterone increases until about day 100. After about day 100 the placenta assumes a progesterone producing role. See Figure 14-6. (Modified from Ginther *Reproductive Biology of the Mare*.)

The second major gonadotropin of placental origin is **human chorionic gonadotropin (hCG)**. This hormone is not only found in the human but in many other primates. Often hCG (and eCG) may simply be referred to as a "CG." It originates from the trophoblastic cells of the chorion and is secreted as soon as the blastocyst hatches from the zona pellucida. Human chorionic gonadotropin can be detected in the blood and urine of the pregnant woman as early as days 8 to 10 of gestation. It increases rapidly in the urine of the pregnant woman, reaching a maximum value at about 2.5 months. Its presence in the urine constitutes the basis for over-the-counter pregnancy diagnosis kits.

The primary role of hCG during early pregnancy is to provide a luteotropic stimulus for the transition of the ovulatory corpus luteum to the CL of pregnancy. Luteal LH receptors also bind hCG, resulting in sustained progesterone production. The administration of hCG into non-primate females can cause ovulation. In fact, hCG is used commonly to induce ovulation.

The Placenta Secretes Progesterone and Estrogen

Progesterone is obligatory for early embryonic development by providing the stimulus for elevated secretion by the endometrial glands. High progesterone is also responsible for the so-called "**progesterone block**" that inhibits myometrial contractions. Progesterone increases in the blood of the pregnant female and peaks at different stages of gestation for different species. The absolute levels of progesterone also vary significantly among species (Figure 14-6). While progesterone is always produced by the corpus luteum in early pregnancy, the role of the corpus luteum in maintenance of pregnancy varies among species. In some species (ewe, mare and woman), the corpus luteum is not needed for the entire gestational period because the placenta takes over production of progesterone. For example, in the ewe the corpus luteum is responsible for initial production of progesterone, but the placenta assumes responsibility for its production after only 50 days of gestation (Table 14-1). In other species, lutectomy (surgical removal of corpora lutea) will terminate pregnancy regardless of when this occurs during gestation (sow or rabbit). Lutectomy in the cow up to 8 months of gestation will result in abortion. It should be pointed out that even though the placenta takes over for the corpus luteum of pregnancy, the corpus luteum produces progesterone throughout gestation.

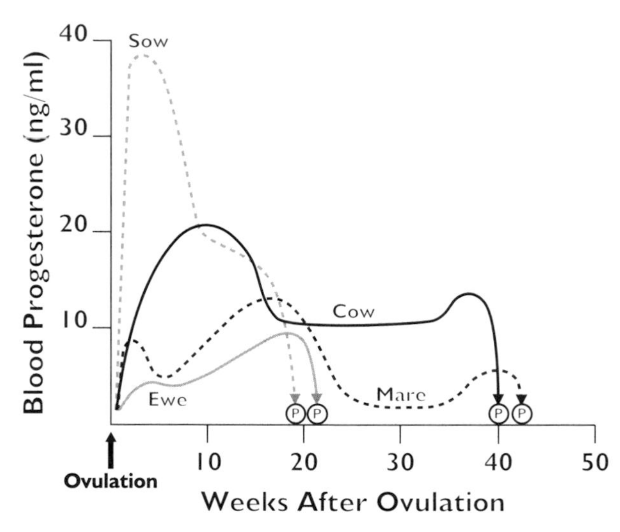

Figure 14-6. Progesterone profiles in females of various species. P= Parturition.

They are believed to be similar to growth hormone, thus promoting the growth of the fetus. Placental lactogen also stimulates the mammary gland (lactogenic) of the dam. The degree to which fetal somatotropic (growth) versus lactogenic effects occur depends on the species (Figure 14-7). For example, in the ewe **ovine placental lactogen (oPL)** has a more potent lactogenic activity than somatotropic activity. A similar condition exists in humans, but not in the cow. Placental lactogens have been studied most intensely in the ewe. They are produced and secreted by the binucleate giant cells of the placenta. The secretory products of the binucleate cells are transferred into the maternal circulation.

In addition to progesterone, estrogens are also an important product of the placenta, particularly during the last part of gestation. In fact, the peak of estrogen in most species signals the early preparturient period. The profiles of estrogen during the gestation period will be presented in the subsequent section on parturition.

Certain Placental Hormones Stimulate Mammary Function of the Dam and Fetal Growth

The placenta is known to produce a polypeptide hormone known as **placental lactogen** that is also called **somatomammotropin**. Placental lactogens have been found in rats, mice, sheep, cows and humans.

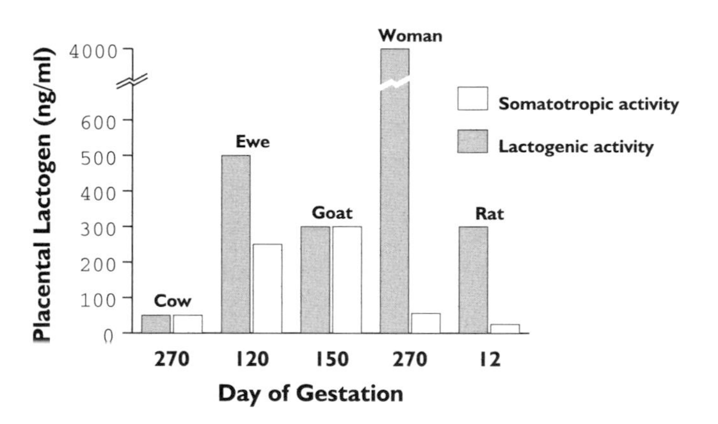

Figure 14-7. Placental lactogen in blood of pregnant females near termination of gestation. Lactogenic activity of placental lactogen promotes mammary function in the dam. Somatotropic activity promotes fetal growth. (Modified from Martal in *Reproduction in Man and Mammals.*)

Table 14-1. Gestational length and time of placental takeover for progesterone production in various species.

SPECIES	GESTATION LENGTH	TIME OF PLACENTAL TAKEOVER
Cow	9 mo	6-8 mo
Ewe	5 mo	50 d
Goat	5 mo	5 mo
Mare	11 mo	70 d
Rabbit	1 mo	1 mo
Sow	3.8 mo	3.8 mo
Woman	9 mo	50 d

It has been hypothesized that the sire may have an effect on the degree to which the fetus can produce placental lactogen. Such an effect could cause elevated concentrations of placental lactogen by the fetus. Increased placental lactogen secretion would cause enhanced stimulation of the maternal mammary gland and thus promote elevated milk production. This theory suggests that it might be possible for the sire to influence fetal placental lactogen and enhance milk production in the dam. This **sire-on-fetus-hypothesis** has not been tested critically, but could hold promise for enhancing genetic improvement in dairy and beef cattle.

Relaxin Is Also a Product of the Placenta

Relaxin of placental origin has been shown to exist in humans, mares, cats, pigs, rabbits and monkeys. In the rabbit, relaxin may be produced entirely by the placenta and not at all by the ovary. Relaxin is not present in the bovine placenta during any stage of gestation. It is likely (with the exception of the rabbit) that relaxin, during the time of parturition, originates from both the ovary and the placenta. A possible exception to this may be the cow, because ovariectomy does not result in calving difficulties. The role of relaxin is therefore questionable in the cow.

Parturition Is a Complex Cascade of Physiologic Events

The three stages of parturition are:
- ***initiation of myometrial contractions (removal of progesterone block)***
- ***expulsion of the fetus***
- ***expulsion of the fetal membranes***

The fetus initiates stage I of parturition.

The fetus triggers the onset of parturition by initiating a cascade of complex endocrine/biochemical events. The fetal pituitary-adrenal axis is obligatory for the initiation of parturition. During the conclusion of gestation, the fetal mass approaches the inherent space limitations of the uterus. As a result, it is believed that the fetus becomes stressed. Such stress causes the fetal anterior pituitary to release **adrenocorticotropic hormone (ACTH)**. ACTH is a peptide hormone which is produced in response to various forms of stress. It stimu-

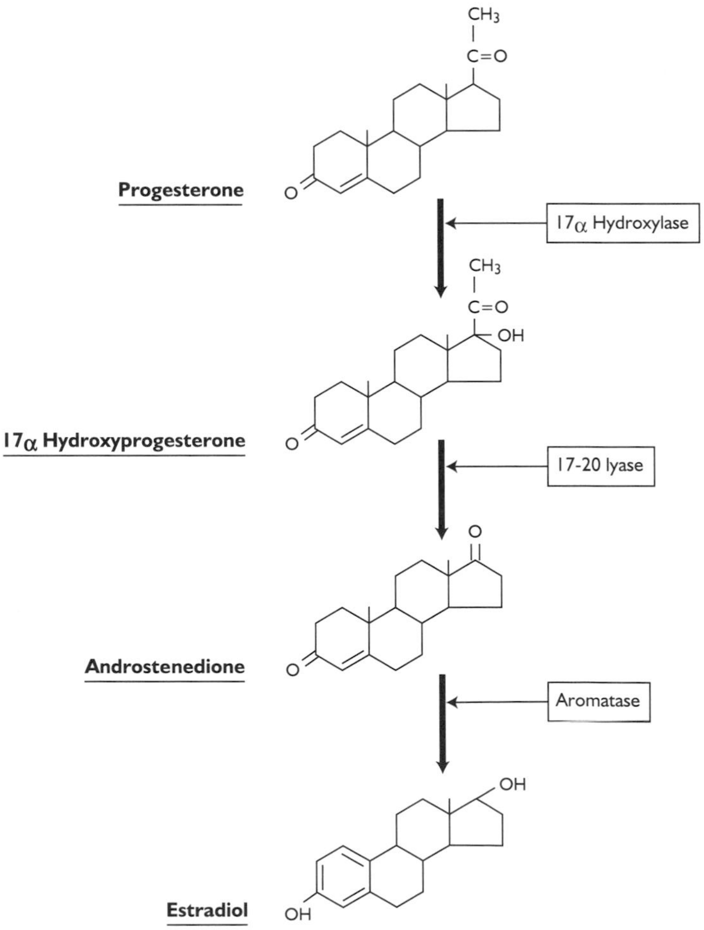

Progesterone → (17α Hydroxylase) → 17α Hydroxyprogesterone → (17-20 lyase) → Androstenedione → (Aromatase) → Estradiol

Figure 14-8. Conversion of progesterone to estradiol by fetal corticoid activation of 17α-hydroxylase, 17-20 lyase and aromatase. This conversion removes the "progesterone block" to myometrial activity.

lates the fetal adrenal cortex to produce corticoids. The elevation of fetal corticoids initiates a cascade of events which cause dramatic changes in the endocrine condition of the dam. These endocrine changes cause two major events to occur: 1) removal of the myometrial "progesterone block," enabling myometrial contractions to begin; and 2) elevation of reproductive tract secretions, particularly by the cervix.

Removal of the "progesterone block" occurs because fetal cortisol promotes the synthesis of three enzymes that convert progesterone to estradiol. The conversion pathway is illustrated in Figure 14-8. Progesterone, which is high at the placental interface, is converted to 17α-hydroxyprogesterone by the enzyme 17α-hydroxylase. Fetal cortisol also triggers the enzyme 17 to 20 lyase to convert 17α-hydroxyprogesterone to androstenedione. Androstenedione is converted to estrogen by activation of an aromatase enzyme. This involves aromatization of the A ring of the steroid and removal of the 19 carbon. The conversion of progesterone to estradiol accounts, at least in part, for the dramatic drop in progesterone and dramatic elevation of estradiol. The relationship between progesterone and estradiol during gestation is presented in Figure 14-9.

In addition to converting progesterone to estradiol, fetal corticoids also cause the placenta to synthesize $PGF_{2\alpha}$. The synthesis of $PGF_{2\alpha}$ helps abolish the "progesterone block." As both estradiol and prostaglandin become elevated, the myometrium becomes increasingly more motile and begins to display noticeable contractions. Also, $PGF_{2\alpha}$ causes the CL of pregnancy to regress, facilitating the decline in progesterone. The drop in progesterone in some species is brought about both by the conversion of progesterone into estradiol and by the luteolytic process brought about by PGF_{2a}. Endocrine events associated with parturition are summarized in Figures 14-10 and 14-11.

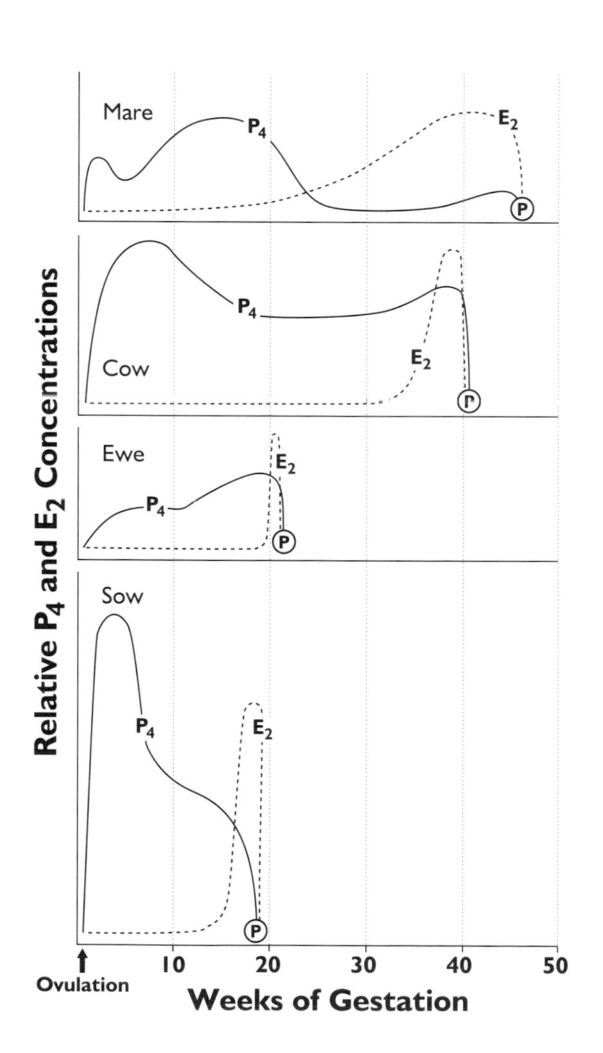

Figure 14-9. Estrogen (E_2) and progesterone (P_4) profiles during gestation in the cow, sow, mare and ewe. P = Parturition.

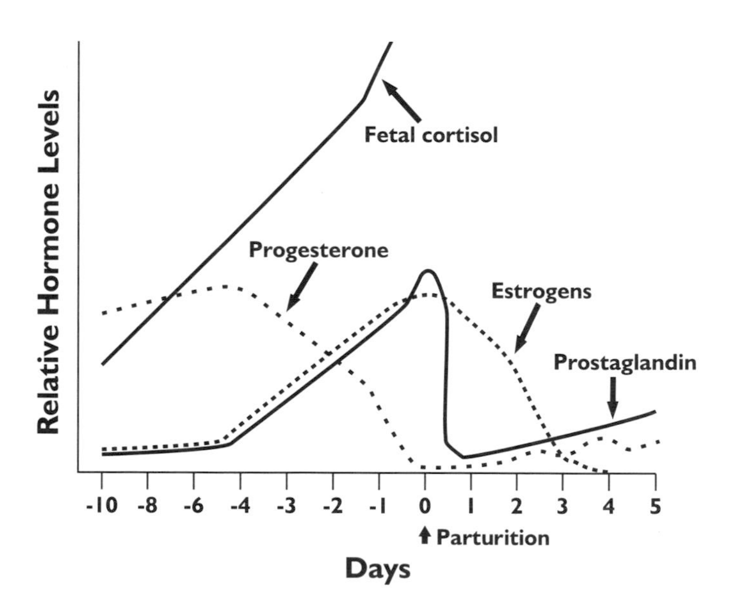

Figure 14-10. Relative hormone profiles in the cow during the periparturient period.

As the pressure inside the uterus continues to increase, the fetus in the cow, mare and ewe rotates so that the front feet and head are positioned to the posterior of the dam. Such a rotation is important to insure a proper delivery (Figure 14-12). If the fetus fails to position itself correctly, **dystocia** (difficult birth) will occur.

As the levels of estradiol increase, coupled with the elevation in levels of $PGF_{2\alpha}$, the contracting uterus begins to push the fetus toward the cervix, applying pressure to the cervix. The endocrine events that promote the first stage of parturition (dilation of the cervix and entry of the fetus into the cervical canal) are summarized in Figure 14-11.

Pressure on the cervix brought about by increased myometrial contractions activates pressure-sensitive neurons located in the cervix, that synapse in the spinal cord and eventually synapse with oxytocin producing neurons in the hypothalamus (Figure 14-12). Oxytocin released into the systemic circulation acts to facilitate the myometrial contractility initiated by estradiol and by $PGF_{2\alpha}$. As the pressure against the cervix continues to increase, so does the oxytocin secretion, and thus the force of contraction of the myometrial smooth muscle begins to peak. When this occurs, the fetus enters the cervical canal and the first stage of parturition is complete.

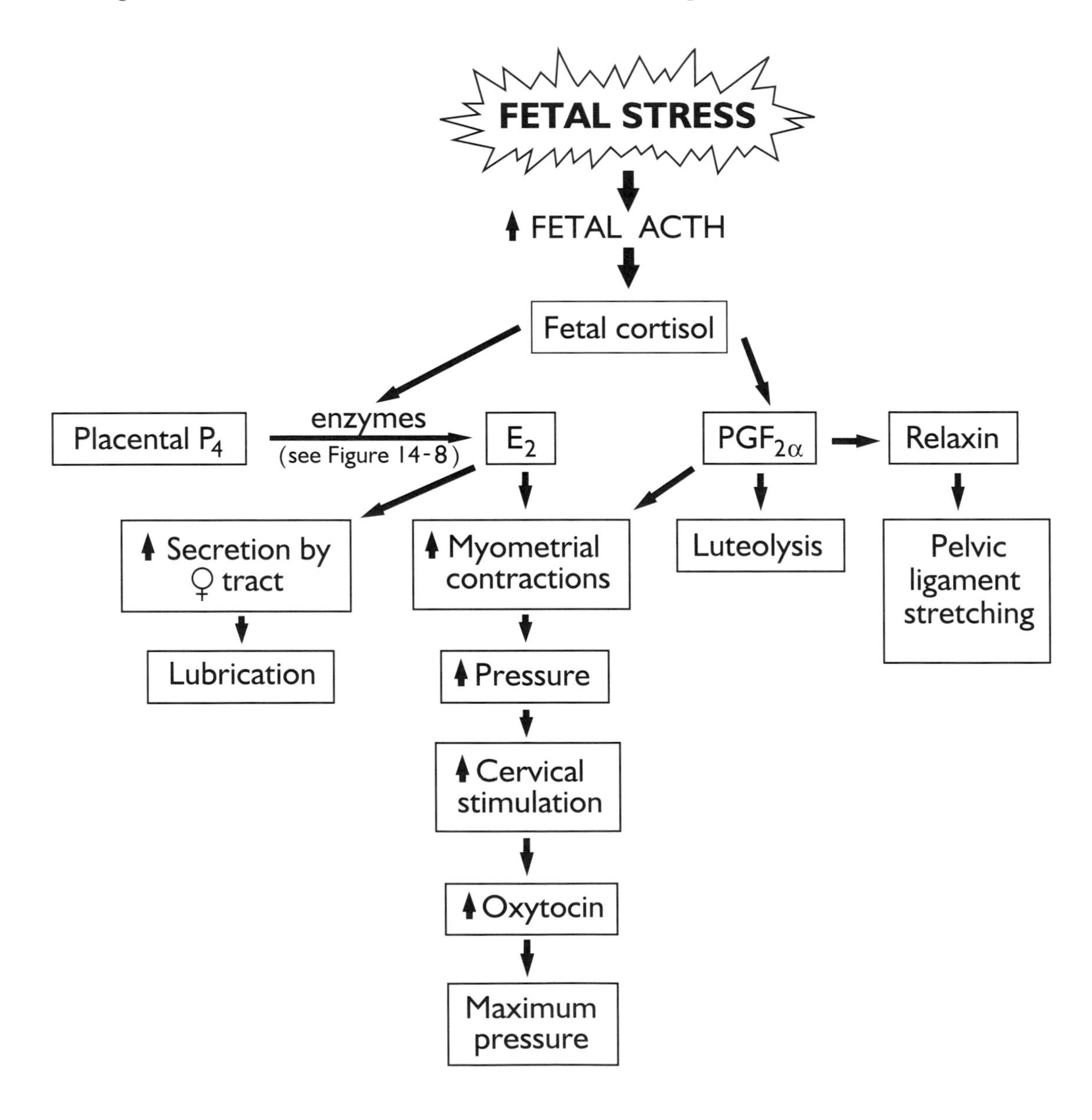

Figure 14-11. Pathway of events prompted by fetal cortisol.

Expulsion of fetus (Stage II) requires strong myometrial and abdominal muscle contractions.

Another important hormone involved in successful parturition is **relaxin.** Relaxin is a glycoprotein that is produced by either the corpus luteum or the placenta, depending upon the species. The synthesis of relaxin is stimulated by $PGF_{2\alpha}$. It causes a softening of the connective tissue in the cervix and promotes elasticity of the pelvic ligaments. Thus, this hormone prepares the birth canal by loosening the supportive tissues so that passage of the fetus can occur with relative ease.

One of the dramatic effects of estradiol elevation prior to parturition is that it initiates secretory activity of the reproductive tract in general, and particularly the cervix. As estradiol increases, the cervix and vagina begin to produce mucus. This mucus washes out the cervical seal of pregnancy and thoroughly lubricates the cervical canal and the vagina. Mucus reduces friction and enables the fetus to exit the reproductive tract with relative ease. As myometrial contractions continue to increase, the animal's feet and head begin to put pressure on the fetal membranes. When the pressure reaches a certain level, the membranes rupture, with subsequent loss of amniotic and allantoic fluid. This fluid also serves to lubricate the birth canal. As the fetus enters the birth canal, it becomes hypoxic (deprived of adequate levels

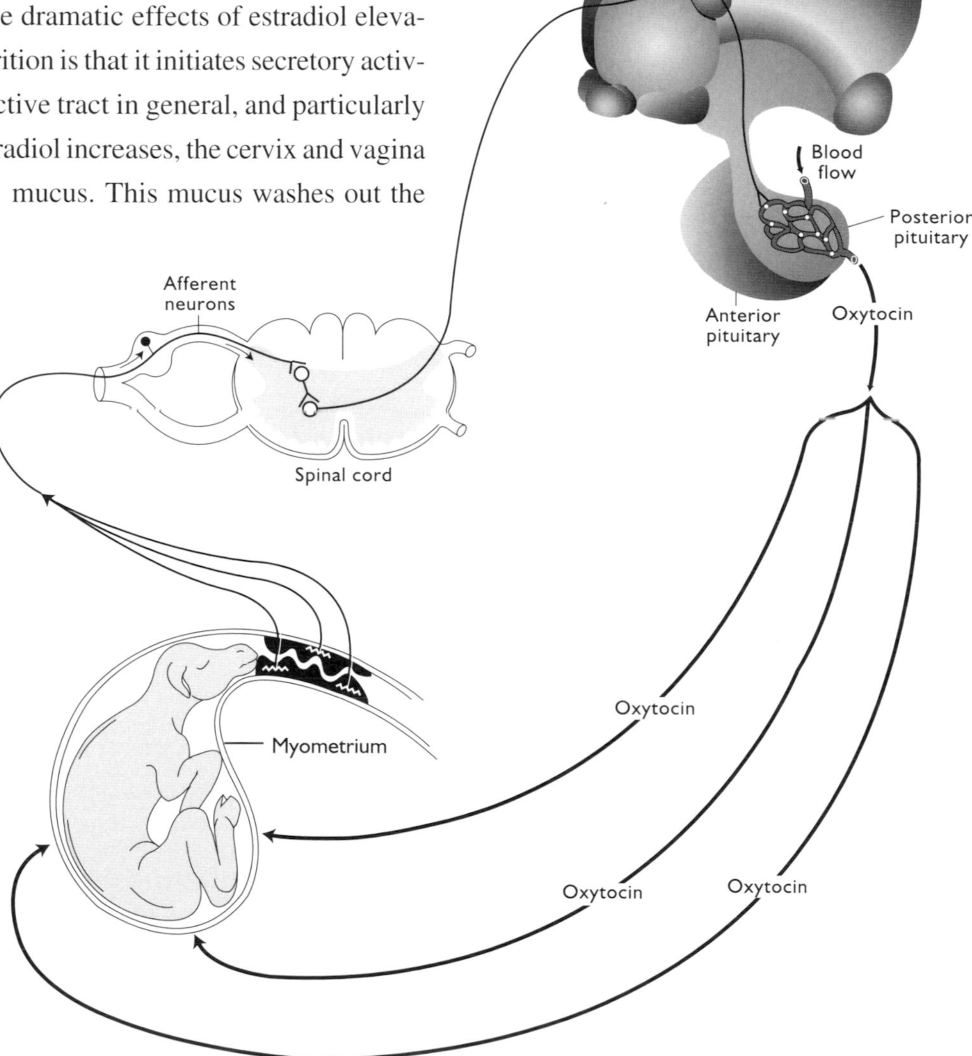

Figure 14-12. Pathway of sensory activation of oxytocin secretion by the posterior pituitary. As the fetus moves into the birth canal, elevated pressure on the cervix stimulates sensory neurons. A neural pathway terminates in the paraventricular nucleus (PVN) and causes oxytocin to be secreted from the posterior pituitary. Oxytocin causes contraction of the myometrium. (Graphic by Sonja Oei.)

Table 14-2. Duration of stages of parturition among various species.

Species	Stage I (Myometrial Contractions/ Cervical Dilation)	Stage II (Fetal Expulsion)	Stage III (Fetal Membrane Expulsion)
Cow	2 to 6h	30 to 60 min	6 to 12h
Ewe	2 to 6h	30 to 120 min	5 to 8h
Mare	1 to 4h	12 to 30 min	1h
Sow	2 to 12h	150 to 180 min	1 to 4h

of oxygen). This hypoxia promotes fetal movement which, in turn, promotes further myometrial contraction. This positive feedback system creates a set of conditions where the time of parturition is reduced, since an increased strength of contraction follows fetal movement. In a sense, the fetus is controlling its exit from the uterus. The uterine contractions are accompanied by abdominal muscle contractions of the dam, which further aid in expulsion of the fetus.

Expulsion of fetal membranes (Stage III) is important for successful parturition.

In most species, expulsion of the fetal membranes quickly follows expulsion of the fetus. Expulsion of the fetal membranes requires that the chorionic villi become dislodged from the crypts of the maternal side of the placenta. This release of the chorionic villi is believed to be brought about by powerful vasoconstriction of arteries in the villi. Vasoconstriction reduces the pressure and thus allows the villi to be released from the crypt. Obviously in some forms of placentation, there must be some maternal vasoconstriction. For example, in animals which have hemochorial and hemoendothelial placentation, the blood on the maternal side is adjacent to the fetal placenta. Thus, if vasoconstriction does not occur at the maternal level, hemorrhage is likely.

The duration of parturition is variable among species and this variation is summarized in Table 14-2. Extension beyond what is considered to be the normal upper-end duration of parturition constitutes a difficult birth (**dystocia**). Such prolonged parturition can result in serious complications to both the fetus and the dam. Difficulties in parturition usually occur in the second stage (expulsion of the fetus). One cause of dystocia is excessive size of the fetus. Fetal size is controlled by both the dam and the sire. In primiparous dams, it is always advisable to breed females to a male of small body size so that fetal size does not exceed the ability of the female to give birth successfully.

A second cause of dystocia is failure of proper fetal rotation. About 5% of all births in cattle are characterized by abnormal positioning of the fetus during parturition. Such abnormal positioning results in difficult and sometimes impossible births and requires Caesarean section.

A third cause of dystocia is multiple births in monotocous species. Twins generally cause dystocia. This is because 1) both twins may be presented simultaneously, 2) the first fetus is positioned abnormally and therefore blocks the second and 3) the uterus becomes fatigued by difficult and sustained contractions.

A discussion of obstetrical procedures used to correct these problems is beyond the scope of this book, but can be researched by consulting references at the conclusion of this chapter.

Further Phenomena for Fertility

The term "Caesarean" was derived from the false notion that Julius Caesar himself was born by removing him from his mother through an incision in the abdominal and uterine wall. His family name, Caesar was derived from the belief that Julius' ancestors (centuries before him) were born in such a way. The name Caesar is derived from the Latin word "caesus" which means "to cut." The name also fits the way Julius died.

In a number of teleost fishes (fishes with a more or less ossified skeleton) the female incubates the eggs in her mouth, and in some species the male does the same. The term "keep your mouth shut" has a special meaning in this species.

In pipe fishes and seahorses the female lays her eggs in a brood pouch of the male and he is responsible for gestation. In fact, several females may lay eggs in one male's brood pouch. The brood pouch offers a special environment for developing offspring and is under the control of prolactin.

Lampreys (a predatory eel) build nests over sandy bottomed streams. They assemble rock walls to slow the water running over the nest. At spawning, they stir up the sand which sticks to the eggs. The sand weights the eggs and prevents them from floating downstream. It also reduces predation. This is another form of attachment that enables successful embryogenesis.

The female African elephant has a gestation period of 1.8 years. The calf weighs about 300 pounds at birth and nurses for about three years.

Additional Reading

Arther, G.H., D.E. Noakes, H. Pearson and T.J. Perkinson. 1996. *Veterinary Reproduction and Obstetrics.* 7th ed. W.B. Saunders Co. Philadelphia.

Catchpole, H.R. 1991. "Hormonal Mechanisms in Pregnancy and Parturition." In *Reproduction in Domestic Animals.* 4th ed., P.T. Cupps, ed., Academic Press, San Diego.

Flood, P.F. 1991. "The Development of the Conceptus and its Relationship to the Uterus." In *Reproduction in Domestic Animals.* 4th ed., P.T. Cupps, ed., Academic Press, San Diego.

Ginther, O.J. 1992. *Reproductive Biology of the Mare.* 2nd ed. Equiservices, Cross Plains, WI.

Morrow, D.A. 1986. *Current Therapy in Theriogenology- Diagnosis, Treatment and Prevention of Reproductive Diseases in Small and Large Animals.* 2nd ed. W.B. Saunders Co. Philadelphia.

Thibault, C., M.C. Levasseur and R.H.F. Hunter. 1993. *Reproduction in Man and Mammals.* Ellipses, Paris.

Glossary

A

accessory sex glands. Glands of the male reproductive system surrounding the pelvic urethra that produce seminal plasma. The accessory sex glands are the vesicular glands (seminal vesicles), prostate, bulbourethral glands (Cowper's Glands) and the ampullae.

acrosin. A proteolytic enzyme specific to the acrosome of spermatozoa. Acrosin causes zona pellucida dissociation during sperm penetration.

acrosomal granule. An intracellular granule within the young spermatid resulting from the condensation of Golgi products within the confines of the acrosomal membrane that will give rise to the acrosomal contents.

acrosomal phase. A specific developmental phase of spermiogenesis in which the acrosome extends toward the posterior of the nucleus.

acrosomal reaction. An orderly fusion of the spermatozoal plasma membrane and the outer acrosomal membrane that enables the release of acrosomal enzymes so that spermatozoa can penetrate the zona pellucida. The acrosomal reaction exposes the equatorial segment so that it can later fuse with the plasma membrane of the oocyte.

acrosomal vesicle. A vesicle within the young spermatid resulting from fusion of smaller vesicles; the precursor to the acrosome.

acrosome. A membrane-bound organelle of the spermatozoon that covers the anterior one-third to one-half of the nucleus. It contains proteolytic enzymes required for penetration of the zona pellucida.

action potential. The rapid, all-or-none depolarization of a nerve cell membrane that is propagated from a nerve cell body to the axon and to another nerve or to an effector organ.

active transport. Transport of materials across a cell membrane against a concentration gradient (from low concentration to high). Energy in the form of ATP is required to "pump" materials into or out of the cell.

activin. A nonsteroidal regulator synthesized in the pituitary gland and gonads, which stimulates the secretion of follicle stimulating hormone.

adeno-. A prefix designating a glandular organ or tissue. For example, the adenohypophysis is the glandular portion of the hypophysis.

adenohypophysis. The anterior pituitary gland.

adenosine triphosphate (ATP). The energy source of the cell. It is synthesized from adenosine diphosphate (ADP).

adenylate cyclase. A membrane-bound enzyme activated by a hormone-receptor complex, the activation of which is mediated by G-protein. Adenylate cyclase promotes conversion of ATP to cyclic AMP.

adluminal compartment. The compartment or zone of a seminiferous tubule defined at its lower boundary by the tight junctions of Sertoli cells and at its upper boundary by the lumen of the seminiferous tubule.

adrenal corticoids. A class of steroid hormones produced by the adrenal cortex, they govern mineral metabolism, induce parturition and mediate response to stress.

adrenal corticotropin (ACTH). A glycoprotein hormone produced by the anterior pituitary that controls the release of adrenal corticoids.

agonist. Any substance capable of binding to receptors for the native substance that causes action identical to the native substance. Degree of response varies depending on the agonist.

allantois. One of the extraembryonic membranes formed from the embryonic ectoderm that serves as a liquid waste storage reservoir for the developing fetus.

alpha fetoprotein (AFP). A fetal protein that binds estradiol and prevents it from crossing the blood-brain barrier.

alpha subunit. The protein component of a glycoprotein hormone common to all gonadotropins.

amnion. One of the extraembryonic membranes formed from the chorion and surrounding and enclosing the fetus. It is filled with fluid and serves to protect the embryo against mechanical damage and to prevent tissue adhesions during embryonic development.

Glossary

ampulla (plural: ampullae). In the female, the ovarian one-third of the oviduct characterized by a large diameter and many mucosal folds. In the male, enlargements in the ductus deferens that open directly into the pelvic urethra.

ampullary-isthmic junction. The region of the oviduct where the isthmus makes an anatomical transition into the ampulla.

analog. A substance having a similar structure to a native hormone, and which causes similar or opposite physiologic response.

androgen binding protein (ABP). A protein secreted by the Sertoli cells. It binds testosterone in the seminiferous tubules and delivers testosterone to the epididymis.

androgens. A class of substances (usually steroids) that promote development of male secondary sex characteristics and function of the male reproductive tract.

anestrus. When a female does not experience estrous cycles.

angiogenic factors. Substances that promote angiogenesis (the growth of blood vessels).

annulus. A ring-like structure at the posterior end of the middle piece of a spermatozoon.

anosmic. Without the sense of smell.

antagonist. A material that blocks or inhibits the action of a hormone.

anterior pituitary (adenohypophysis). The glandular portion of the pituitary that is derived from the stomodeal ectoderm of the embryo. The anterior pituitary produces gonadotropins (FSH and LH), adrenocorticotropin (ACTH), thyroid stimulating hormone (TSH), growth hormone (GH) and prolactin.

antidiuretic hormone (ADH). A hormone synthesized within the cell bodies of neurons of the hypothalamus and released from the posterior pituitary. ADH promotes the reabsorption of water in the distal tubule and collecting duct of the kidney.

anti-müllarian hormone (AMH). A hormone produced by embryonic Sertoli cells in the male. It causes degeneration of the paramesonephric ducts (Müllerian ducts) and probably causes the differentiation of Leydig cells within the fetal testis.

antral follicle (tertiary follicle). An ovarian follicle that contains an antrum (cavity). Antral follicles consist of an oocyte, follicular fluid, granulosal cells, the theca interna and the theca externa.

antrum. A cavity or chamber.

apical ridge. A ridge created by the folding of the anterior acrosome.

apoptosis. A process of organized cell death distinguishable from necrosis because it involves the nuclear control of cell degeneration.

artificial insemination. Mechanical placement of semen containing viable spermatozoa into the female reproductive tract. In most species, seminal deposition is made into the uterus.

atresia. Degeneration and resorption of ovarian follicles before ovulation.

atretogenic. Promoting or causing the process of atresia.

axoneme. The core of the spermatozoal flagellum consisting of a complex of hollow fibrils arranged in a 9+9+2 architecture typical of all flagella. Two single fibrils are centrally positioned and are surrounded by 9 pairs of fibrils.

B

basal compartment. The compartment of the seminiferous tubule containing spermatogonia between the basement membrane and the tight junctions of adjacent Sertoli cells.

basal secretion. Base line secretion of hormones or other substances.

beta subunit. The component of a glycoprotein hormone which gives the hormone its specificity or uniqueness.

bicornuate uterus. A uterus consisting of distinct uterine horns (cornua).

binucleate giant cells. Cells originating in the chorion of the ruminant placenta that migrate toward the endometrial epithelium and produce pregnancy-specific substances.

blastocoele. The cavity in the central portion of the blastocyst.

blastocyst. An early embryo consisting of an inner cell mass, a blastocoele and a trophoblast.

blastomere. A cell produced by the cleavage divisions of the early embryo.

blood-testis barrier. The specialized permeability barrier consisting primarily of multiple junctional complexes (tight junctions) between Sertoli cells that divides the seminiferous epithelium into the basal compartment and the adluminal compartment. Two separate environments exist between these two compartments.

bovine interferon tau (bIFN-τ). A glycoprotein (formerly called bovine trophoblastic protein 1) produced by the preimplantation bovine conceptus that allows maternal recognition of pregnancy by inhibiting oxytocin receptor synthesis by the endometrial cells.

broad ligament. The ligament (continuous with the peritoneum) which supports the female reproductive tract consisting of the mesometrium, the mesosalpinx and the mesovarium.

bulbospongiosus muscle. A thick, circular, striated muscle that is continuous with the urethralis muscle at the position of the bulbourethral glands. It covers the bulb of the penis and attaches to the proximal shaft of the penis. In the stallion, it extends on the ventrolateral surfaces of the penis to the glans penis.

bulbourethral glands (Cowper's glands). Paired glands that lie on the dorsal surface of the caudal end of the pelvic urethra. These glands are so named because they are associated with the bulb of the penis and the pelvic urethra.

C

canalization. Formation of canals of tube-like structures within a tissue.

cap phase. The phase of spermiogenesis in which the acrosomic vesicle begins to spread over the anterior portion of the spermatid nucleus.

capacitation. The process whereby spermatozoa acquire fertility in the female reproductive tract.

capitulum. The bulbous protuberance at the anterior portion of the flagellum of the spermatozoon, which fits into the implantation socket (a depression in the posterior nucleus).

caput epididymis. The head of the epididymis.

caruncular regions. Highly vascular and non-glandular regions of the ruminant uterus which protrude from the endometrial surface. They will form the maternal cotyledon.

cauda epididymis. The tail of the epididymis; the primary sperm storage reservoir of the extragonadal duct system.

centrioles. Cylindrical organelles located in the centrosome and containing 9 triplets of microtubules arranged around the edges. The centrioles migrate to a position opposite the acrosomic vesicle and give rise to the capitulum and axoneme of the spermatid.

cervical (annular) rings. Circular, ring-shaped protrusions present in the cervix of the cow and ewe.

cervical seal of pregnancy. A highly viscous plug that cements the folds of the cervix together during pregnancy, thus isolating the developing fetus from the exterior environment.

cervix. A structure consisting of dense connective tissue with varying degrees of foldings and protrusions covering the mucosal epithelium. The cervix connects the uterus to the vagina.

chorioallantois. The extraembryonic membrane resulting from the fusion of the chorion and the allantois.

chorion. The outermost extraembryonic membrane, derived from the trophoblastic ectoderm. It will develop villi which will form the fetal sites of placental attachment.

chorionic girdle. A specialized region of the chorion in the equine fetus that forms the initial attachment to the endometrium.

chorionic villi. Small fingerlike projections that appear on the surface of the chorion protruding toward the uterine endometrium and which compose the functional unit of the fetal placenta.

cleavage divisions. The series of mitotic divisions of the early embryo within the confines of the zona pellucida giving rise to equally sized daughter cells, called blastomeres.

clitoris. A small body of highly innervated erectile tissue located in the posterior extremity of the ventral vaginal floor. It is the homologue of the penis.

collagenase. An enzyme that hydrolyzes collagen, a component of connective tissue.

columnar epithelium. An epithelial type consisting of cells which are taller than they are wide, thus resembling columns.

commissure. A seam or a line resulting from the site of union of two components of an organ system.

conception. The union of an oocyte with a spermatozoon; fertilization; to become pregnant.

conceptus. The products of conception, including the embryo, the extraembryonic membranes and the placenta.

constrictor vulvae. The bundles of skeletal muscle embedded in the labia that maintain closure of the labial commissure.

Coolidge Effect. Renewal of sexual stimulation in the sexually satiated male by the introduction of a novel female into the stimulus setting.

conception. The union of an oocyte with a spermatozoon; fertilization; to become pregnant.

copulation. Sexual intercourse; union of the male and female by means of their genitalia.

copulatory stage. The second stage of reproductive behavior consisting of mounting, intromission and ejaculation.

cornua. A structure resembling a horn.

corpus albicans (plural: corpora albicantia). A white scar-like fibrous ovarian structure that replaces the regressing corpus luteum.

corpus cavernosum. The cavernous erectile tissue in the central portion of the penis that allows for influx of blood during erection of the penis.

corpus epididymis. The body of the epididymis.

corpus hemorrhagicum. A small, bloody clot-like structure that results from rupture of blood vessels during ovulation.

corpus luteum (CL) (plural: corpora lutea). An orange to yellow colored transient endocrine structure formed after ovulation from granulosal and thecal cells of the ovarian follicle. The corpus luteum is responsible for producing progesterone and oxytocin.

corpus prostate. The body of the prostate, located dorsal to the anterior pelvic urethra.

corpus spongiosum. The portion of erectile tissue in the penis that surrounds the penile urethra.

cortex. The outer portion of an organ in contrast to the inner portion or medulla.

cortical reaction. A reaction following spermatozoal penetration of the oocyte in which the membrane surrounding the cortical granule in the oocyte cytoplasm fuses with the oocyte plasma membrane. Their contents are expelled into the perivitelline space. The cortical reaction is believed to prevent polyspermy.

corticoids. A class of steroid hormones secreted by the adrenal cortex.

cortisol (hydrocortisone). An anti-inflammatory steroid secreted by the adrenal cortex.

cotyledonary. A term referring to the presence of cotyledons (found in ruminants) as the functional unit of the placenta.

cotyledons. The points of attachment between the fetal and maternal placenta, consisting of a maternal cotyledon contributed by the caruncular areas of the uterus and the fetal cotyledon contributed by the chorion of the conceptus.

cremaster muscle. A striated muscle continuous with the internal oblique muscle that partially surrounds the spermatic cord and attaches to the dorsal pole of the testis.

crus penis (pl. crura). One of two lateral spongy areas surrounded by the ischiocavernosus muscle, through which blood passes as it enters the penis. The crura fuse distally to form the corpus cavernoseum penis.

cryptorchid. An individual in which one or both of the testes have failed to descend into the scrotum.

cycle of seminiferous epithelium. The progression through a complete series of cellular associations at one location along a seminiferous tubule.

cyclic AMP. Cyclic adenosine monophosphate; a cyclic nucleotide that serves as a "second messenger" for protein hormone action.

cyclicity. The condition in which a female displays estrus (or menstrual) cycles with a predictable duration.

cyclopentanoperhydrophenanthrene. The common nucleus of steroid hormones consisting of three 6-membered rings (A, B and C), and one 5-membered ring (D).

cytokines. Materials released by immune cells which act as intercellular mediators of the immune response.

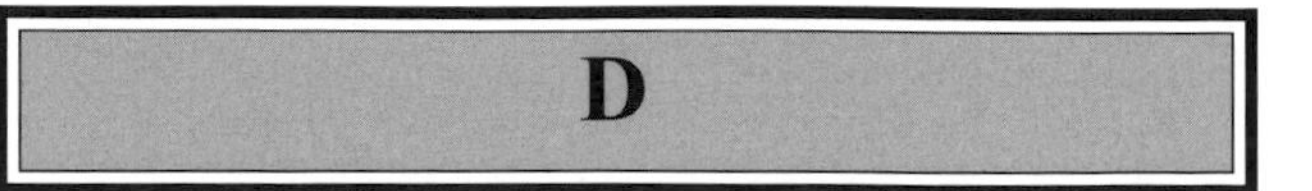

daily sperm production (DSP). The quantity of spermatozoa produced by both testicles in one day.

dartos muscle. See tunica dartos.

decapacitation. The exposure of spermatozoa to seminal plasma after capacitation has occurred, thus requiring additional capacitation time before fertility can be acquired.

depolarization. A change in nerve cell electrical potential caused by sodium influx.

descendin. A material believed to be produced by the fetal testis that promotes rapid growth of the gubernaculum, thus promoting descent of the testis into the scrotum.

diastolic pressure. The minimum arterial blood pressure associated with diastole (relaxation) of the heart.

dictyotene phase. A phase of meiosis unique to the primary oocyte in which the nuclear material is arrested or rendered inactive until final stages of oogenesis. Oocytes remain in the dictyotene phase in the fetal ovary until final folliculogenesis.

diestrus. The stage of the estrous cycle characterized by a dominance of progesterone from the corpora lutea and periods of relative quiescence of reproductive behavior.

differentiation. The development of structure and function that is more specialized than the original cells or tissue.

diffuse placenta. A placenta characterized by uniform distribution of chorionic villi across the surface of the chorion (e.g. pig, mare).

diplotene. The stage of the first meiotic prophase in which two chromosomes in each bivalent begin to repel one another and move apart.

discoid. Placenta characterized by a regional disk that attaches to the endometrium. Primates have a discoid placenta.

disseminate prostate. Prostatic tissue diffusely distributed within the walls of the pelvic urethra.

distal cytoplasmic droplet. A remnant cytoplasm located just posterior to the middle piece of the spermatozoon.

diverticulum (plural: diverticula). A blind tube, or outpocketing, that diverts from a main tubular organ or cavity.

dominant follicle. The final maturational stage of folliculogenesis resulting in the production of relatively high concentrations of estradiol and inhibin.

down-regulation. Reduced receptor density.

ductus deferens. The duct derived from the mesonephric duct that connects the tail of the epididymis to the ampulla and transports sperm into the pelvic urethra.

duplex uterus. A uterus containing two cervices.

dystocia. Abnormal or difficult parturition.

E

ectoderm. The outer layer of cells in the embryo.

efferent ducts. Ducts that are embryologically derived from the mesonephric tubules connecting the rete testis to the head of the epididymis.

efferent neurons. Neurons originating in the central nervous system and travelling to effector organs.

ejaculation. The expulsion of semen from the pelvic and penile urethra.

elongated blastocyst. A blastocyst that has undergone rapid growth after hatching from the zona pellucida, but before attachment to the uterus to form a long, filamentous structure.

embryo. An animal in the early stages of development which has not taken an anatomical form that is recognizable as a member of a species.

emission. The discharge of accessory sex gland secretions into the pelvic urethra.

endocrine. Pertaining to the secretion by an internal gland, the products of which are most commonly secreted into the blood.

endoderm. The innermost layer of cells in the embryo.

endometrial cups. Discrete raised areas (ranging from a few millimeters to a few centimeters) found in the gravid uterine horn of the mare that produce equine chorionic gonadotropin (eCG). These structures slough from the endometrial surface at about day 100 of gestation.

endometrium. The mucosal lining of the uterus

endotheliochorial placenta. A form of placenta found in dogs and cats in which the endometrial epithelium has completely eroded and the maternal capillaries are almost directly exposed to the chorionic epithelium.

epididymal transit. The transport of spermatozoa from the proximal head of the epididymis to the distal tail.

Glossary

epididymal transit time. The time required for spermatozoa to move from the proximal head of the epididymis to the distal tail.

epididymis (ductus epididymis). A duct derived embryologically from the mesonephric duct, which connects the efferent ducts to the vas deferens. It serves as a transport, storage and maturation site for spermatozoa.

episodic. A pattern of secretion in which a hormone is released in bursts of varying duration and quantity.

epitheliochorial placenta. A form of placenta found in the sow and mare in which the endometrial epithelium is directly apposed to the epithelium of the chorion.

epithelium. The layer of cells resting on a basement membrane that form the epidermis of the skin and the surface layer of mucous and serous membranes. The epithelium may be simple, consisting of a single layer, or stratified, consisting of several layers. Cells making up the epithelium may be flat (squamous), cube-shaped (cuboidal), or cylindrical (columnar), with modifications including ciliated, pseudostratified, glandular and neuroepithelium.

epoöphoron. Rudimentary tubules located in the mesosalpinx region that are remnants of the mesonephric duct.

equatorial segment. The segment of the acrosome which remains after the acrosomal reaction. The equatorial segment fuses with the oocyte membrane during fertilization.

equine chorionic gonadotropin (eCG). A luteotropic hormone produced by the endometrial cups of the mare. It also has powerful FSH-like actions when administered to females of other species.

erection. The rigid state of the penis caused when blood enters the cavernous tissue of the penis. Relaxation of the retractor penis muscles allows complete erection.

esterases. A generic classification of enzymes that catalyze the hydrolases of esters.

estradiol. The predominant estrogen produced by the dominant follicles during the follicular phase of the estrus cycle.

estrogen. A generic term used to describe a substance (natural or synthetic) that exerts biologic effects characteristic of estrogenic hormones.

estrous. Adjective used to describe phenomena associated with the estrous cycle.

estrous cycle. The reproductive cycle of the female, generally defined as the period from one estrus (heat) to the next. Ovulation can also signify the beginning and end of the estrous cycle. The estrous cycle consists of two phases, the follicular phase and the luteal phase.

estrous synchronization. The use of exogenous hormones to cause more than one femGlossary252Glossaryale to display estrus and ovulate during a similar time.

estrual. An adjective used to describe phenomena associated with estrus (heat).

estrus. The period of sexual receptivity in the female.

eutherian mammal. Mammals that develop a placenta.

excitatory neurotransmitter. A neurotransmitter that causes increases in sodium permeability in the postsynaptic neuron.

excurrent duct system. The efferent ducts, epididymis and vas deferens.

exocrine. A glandular secretion that is delivered to a surface, into a lumen or through a duct.

exocytosis. Process whereby secretory materials too large to diffuse through the cell membrane are released from the cell. During exocytosis the membrane surrounding the secretory product fuses with the plasma membrane of the cell and releases the contents to the exterior.

exogenous. Originating or produced outside the body.

external cremaster muscle. A striated muscle originating from the internal abdominal oblique muscle, traveling down the spermatic chord and attaching to the dorsal tunica vaginalis.

external genitalia. Portion of the male or female reproductive tract that can be viewed externally.

external uterine bifurcation. The external point of separation (forking) of the two uterine horns.

extracellular domain. The portion of a hormone receptor that protrudes from the surface of the plasma membrane and binds the hormone.

extraembryonic membranes. Membranes formed by the embryo, and which are peripheral to it. The three extraembryonic membranes are the amnion, the chorion and the allantois.

extragonadal spermatozoal reserves (EGR). The spermatozoa stored within the extragonadal duct system.

F

facilitated diffusion. A type of diffusion requiring a carrier molecule that moves materials from a region of high concentration to a region of low concentration.

fallopian tube. The oviduct.

false mount. A mount in which intromission is prevented.

feminization. A condition promoting the development of female appearance and behavior.

fetal cotyledon. The fetal contribution to the cotyledonary placenta derived from the chorion.

fetus. The unborn young of a eutherian mammal that is considered to have identifiable features of a given species.

fimbria (plural: fimbriae). A fringe-like structure at the distal end of the infundibulum of the oviduct.

flagellum (plural: flagella). A long, whip-like appendage of the spermatozoa responsible for propelling it.

flehmen. A response commonly made by male cattle, sheep, goats and horses to urine and secretions of the female tract, characterized by elevation of the head, closing of the nostrils and curling of the upper lip. This response is sometimes displayed by females.

follicle. The egg and its encasing cells at any stage of its development.

follicle stimulating hormone (FSH). A glycoprotein hormone secreted by the anterior pituitary in response to GnRH. FSH promotes follicular development in the female and Sertoli cell function in the male.

follicular dynamics. The sum of the intraovarian processes involved in follicular development and degeneration.

follicular fluid. A fluid produced by the granulosal cells that fills the antrum of the follicle.

follicular phase. The phase of the estrous cycle characterized by the presence of a dominant follicle that produces estradiol. Females display behavioral estrus and ovulate during the follicular phase.

follicular selection. The emergence of ovulatory follicles from a cohort of previously recruited antral follicles.

folliculogenesis. The process whereby ovarian follicles develop from primary into secondary and eventually into antral follicles, which become eligible for ovulation.

fornix vagina. The anterior portion of the vagina that forms a crypt that extends anterior to the cervix.

freemartin. The sterile heifer twin to a bull. It has incomplete development of the reproductive tract and male-like behavior.

fusion protein. A protein believed to be located on the equatorial segment of a spermatozoon that allows the plasma membrane of the oocyte to fuse with the equatorial segment.

G

G-protein. A membrane-bound protein that responds to a hormone-receptor complex by activating membrane-bound adenylate cyclase.

gamete. A mature oocyte or spermatozoon.

gap junctions. The membrane specializations that provide continuity between two adjacent cells, allowing passage of small molecular weight materials from one cell to another.

Gartner's cysts (ducts). The remnants of the mesonephric ducts that can be found in the vagina as blind cysts or ducts.

genital ridge. The swellings in the dorsal body wall of the developing embryo into which primordial germ cells migrate. These form the gonad.

germ cells. Spermatozoa or oocytes.

germ layers. The ectoderm, mesoderm and endoderm. These are the earliest recognizable forms of tissue structure of the early embryo.

germinal epithelium. The epithelium of the seminiferous tubule that produces spermatozoa.

gestation. The length of time between conception and birth of the offspring.

glans penis. The anatomically specialized, highly sensitive distal end of the penis.

glycoprotein. A type of protein characterized as having carbohydrate molecules attached to the main protein chain.

goitrogen. A substance that inhibits thyroid function.

Glossary

golgi apparatus. A membranous structure located near the nucleus of almost all cells, consisting of a parallel stack of flattened sacs whose function is to concentrate and package intracellular products.

Golgi phase. The phase of spermiogenesis in which the Golgi vesicles fuse to form larger vesicles which reside on one side of the nucleus.

gonad. The organ that produces gametes; the testis in the male and the ovary in the female.

gonadal hormones. Any hormone produced by the male or female gonad.

gonadotroph. A cell type in the anterior pituitary that produces gonadotropins.

gonadotropin. The hormones (FSH and LH) of anterior pituitary origin that stimulate gonadal function.

gonadotropin releasing hormone (GnRH). A decapeptide released from terminals of neurons in the surge and tonic LH centers of the hypothalamus which causes the release of gonadotropins from the anterior pituitary.

Graafian follicle. A large, dominant preovulatory follicle.

granulosal cells (membrana granulosa). The cellular layer lining the antrum of an antral follicle.

growth hormone (somatotropin). A hormone produced by the anterior pituitary. It promotes growth and lactogenesis.

gubernaculum. A connective tissue cord attaching the testes to the base of the scrotum. It governs testicular descent.

H

half-life (T1/2). The period of time required for one-half of a substance to be destroyed or removed from the body.

heat. See estrus.

hemochorial placenta. A placenta characterized as having the chorionic epithelium in direct apposition to pools of maternal blood.

hemoendothelial placenta. A placenta characterized as having chorionic capillaries immersed directly in pools of maternal blood.

hilus. A region housing blood and lymphatic vessels and nerves which enter and leave an organ.

hormone. A substance produced by one or more glands that is transported by the blood to exert a specific effect upon another organ.

hormone receptor. A molecule located in the cells of the target tissues that have a specific affinity or attraction for a specific hormone, causing the cell to perform a new function.

human chorionic gonadotropin (hCG). A hormone produced by the human placenta that has strong luteotropic activity.

hyaluronidase. A group of enzymes that hydrolyze hyaluronic acid. One or more of these enzymes is present in the acrosome of the spermatozoa.

hyperemia. Excessive blood flow to an organ or region of the body.

hyperplasia. An increase in the number of cells in a tissue or organ.

hypertrophy. An increase in organ or gland size not related to elevated cell numbers.

hypothalamic hormones. Hormones produced by neurons located in the hypothalamus.

hypothalamic nuclei. Anatomically specific groupings or clusters of nerve cell bodies in the hypothalamus.

hypothalamo-hypophyseal portal system. A unique circulatory network that delivers minute quantities of releasing hormones from the pituitary stalk directly to the anterior pituitary without dilution by the systemic circulation.

hypothalamus. The specialized ventral portion of the brain surrounding the third ventricle consisting of distinct clusters of cell bodies called hypothalamic nuclei which are responsible for synthesis of releasing hormones oxytocin and antiduretic hormone.

hypothyroidism. A deficiency of thyroid activity characterized by decreased metabolic rate, fatigue and lethargy.

hysterectomy. Surgical removal of the uterus.

I

implantation. Attachment of the embryo to the uterus.

incisive duct. The duct that connects the oral cavity to the nasal cavity and receives the ducts of the vomeronasal organ.

infrared thermography. A technique that enables the surface temperature of a physical body to be determined.

infundibulum. A hollow funnel-shaped structure or passage.

inguinal canal. A narrow, elongated opening in the lower lateral portion of the abdominal cavity through which the spermatic cord passes.

inguinal hernia. A condition whereby portions of the gut enter the inguinal canal and even the scrotum.

inhibin. A glycoprotein hormone produced by Sertoli cells in the male and granulosal cells in the female that specifically inhibits the release of FSH from the anterior pituitary.

inhibitory neuron. A neuron that produces a neurotransmitter which causes hyperpolarization of a postsynaptic neuron.

inhibitory neurotransmitter. A specific chemical released by an inhibitory neuron causing the post synaptic membrane to become more permeable to potassium, thus lowering the resting membrane potential.

inner cell mass. A cluster of cells located at one pole of the blastocyst from which the embryo will develop.

intercellular bridges. The connections between adjacent developing male germ cells that form a cohort of cells of similar developmental type.

intercornual spermatozoal transport. A phenomenon where the spermatozoa that are deposited into only one uterine horn through artificial insemination are subsequently redistributed over time so that both horns eventually contain substantial numbers of spermatozoa.

interdigitating prominences. Interlocking finger-like processes found in the cervix of the sow, analogous to the rings of the bovine or ovine cervix.

interferons (IFN). Glycoproteins produced by a variety of cells that exert antiviral, antiproliferative and immunosuppressant effects. They are classified as α (from leukocytes), β (from fibroblasts), γ and Ω (from lymphocytes), and τ. IFN-τ is produced by the trophoblast in the ruminant embryo. It is antiluteolytic in addition to possessing the characteristics of the other classifications of IFNs.

internal uterine bifurcation. The internal point of separation (forking) of the two uterine horns.

interneuron. Any neuron in a chain of neurons that is situated between a sensory neuron and the efferent neuron.

interstitial cells of Leydig. Cells found in the interstitial compartment of the testes that produce testosterone.

interstitial compartment. The compartment of the testicular parenchyma which surrounds the seminiferous tubules.

intracellular domain. The component of a hormone receptor located inside the cell that is attached to the transmembrane domain of the receptor.

intromission. The insertion of one part into another. The insertion of the penis into the vagina.

in-utero. Within the uterus.

in-vitro. Within glass, as in a test tube.

in-vivo. Within the living body or organism.

ipsilateral. On the same side.

ischemia. A local reduction in blood flow resulting in accumulation of metabolites.

ischiocavernosus muscle. A paired, powerful, striated muscle originating on the medial surface of the ischium, covering the crura of the penis and inserting on the proximal shaft of the penis.

isthmus. A narrow passage connecting two larger cavities. The isthmus of the oviduct is of small diameter and connects the large diameter ampulla of the oviduct to the uterus.

J

junctional complex. The specialized region of cell to cell attachment consisting of tight junctions, intermediate junctions and desmosomes.

K

keratinization. The development of an insoluble protein containing a high degree of disulfide cross-linking (hair, feathers, nails, sperm heads).

keratinoid protein. Any of a family of proteins characterized as having a high degree of dissulfide crosslinking that form the primary constituents of epidermis, hair, nails and horny tissues.

L

labia. The lip-shaped structures forming the lateral boundaries of the female external genitalia.

labial commissure. The point of junction between the two labia of the female external genitalia.

lactational anestrus. A lack of cyclicity brought about by nursing and presence of the young.

lactogenic. A condition in which lactation is promoted.

lateral ventricle. A cavity within the brain through which cerebrospinal fluid moves. Lateral ventricles are attached to the third ventricle.

Leydig cells. Cells found in the interstitial compartment of the testis that produce testosterone.

libido. The behavioral drive associated with the desire to copulate.

long-day breeder. A seasonal breeder in which reproductive activity and cyclicity peaks during long photoperiods (spring and summer).

longitudinal cervical folds. Longitudinal creases that protrude into the lumen of the cervix of the mare and are continuous with the endometrial folds of the uterus.

lordosis. A condition in which the lumbar position of the spine is unusually curved, forming a convex or hollowed-out appearance. The lumbar curvature is characteristic as a mating posture of females in estrus.

luteal phase. The phase of the estrous cycle characterized by progesterone dominance and the presence of a functional corpus luteum. The luteal phase begins immediately after ovulation and ends after lysis of the corpus luteum.

luteinization. The process whereby granulosal and thecal cells are transformed into luteal cells. Luteinization is brought about by the hormone LH.

luteinizing hormone (LH). A glycoprotein hormone secreted by the anterior pituitary which causes ovulation and subsequent development and maintenance of the corpus luteum. In the male, it causes Leydig cells to produce testosterone.

luteolysis. The process whereby luteal tissue is rendered nonfunctional.

luteolytic. A material that promotes luteolysis.

luteotropic. Having an affinity for or stimulating the corpus luteum.

M

mammary glands. Glands of the female capable of secreting milk during lactation.

manchette. The specialized microtubules which appear in the cytoplasm of developing spermatids around the posterior portion of the nucleus. They become closely apposed to the nuclear membranes and contribute to the postnuclear cap region.

masculinization. A condition promoting the development of male appearance and behavior.

maternal cotyledon. The maternal contribution to a cotyledonary placenta derived from the uterine caruncles.

maternal recognition of pregnancy. The process whereby the female physiologically recognizes the presence of a conceptus, and therefore luteolysis does not occur.

maturation phase. The final phase of spermiogenesis in which the developing spermatid resembles a spermatozoon. During this phase the flagellum is completely formed and the mitochondria cluster around the flagellum to form a complete middle piece.

median eminence. The most ventral part of the hypothalamus which forms a stalk connecting the hypothalamus to the pituitary. Nerve terminals from neurons originating in various hypothalamic nuclei populate this region and secrete releasing hormone into the primary capillary of the hypothalamo-hypophyseal portal system which is located in the median eminence.

mediastinum. The connective tissue core of the testes which houses the rete tubules.

medulla. The inner or central portion of an organ in contrast to the outer portion or cortex.

meiosis. The cell divisions occurring in developing germ cells in which the daughter cell nucleus receives half the number of chromosomes (haploid) found in somatic cells.

meiotic prophase. The first stage of meiosis in which the nuclear or chromosomal material duplicates. Meiotic prophase occurs in primary spermatocytes.

melatonin. A hormone secreted by the pineal gland predominantly during darkness that alters GnRH and gonadotropin secretion.

membrane granulosa. See granulosal cells.

mesoderm. The middle germ layer of the embryo.

mesometrium. The portion of the broad ligament that supports the uterus

mesonephric ducts (Wolffian ducts). The ducts which provide an outlet for the fluid produced by the mesonephros in the developing embryo. They will be retained and form the epididymis and the ductus deferens in the male and will become vestigial in the female.

mesonephric kidney (mesonephros). One of three renal systems appearing in the mammalian embryo. The mesonephros undergoes regression and does not serve an excretory function in the postnatal animal.

mesonephric tubules. The tubules of the mesonephric kidney that connect the capillary tufts of the mesonephros to the mesonephric duct. These tubules will be retained as the efferent ducts in the male.

mesosalpinx. A portion of the broad ligament which surrounds and supports the oviduct.

mesovarium. A portion of the broad ligament which attaches the ovary to the mesometrium.

metanephros kidney. The most advanced form of the three renal types found in the developing mammalian embryo that is retained and becomes the permanent and functional kidney.

metestrus. A stage of the estrous cycle between ovulation and formation of a functional corpus luteum.

microcotyledons. Unique forms of chorionic villi which characterize the mare placenta.

microtubules. Cylindrical cytoplasmic elements associated with mitosis and meiosis and related to the movement of chromosomes on the nuclear spindle during cell division.

middle piece (midpiece). A portion of the sperm flagellum around which the mitochondrial helix is entwined.

mitochondrial helix. The helical arrangement of mitochondria around the flagellum of mammalian sperm.

moiety. A component or part of a molecule.

monoestrus. Animals which display only one period of sexual receptivity (estrus) during a year.

monotocous. Mammals which typically give birth to a single offspring.

morula. A stage of early embryonic development within the confines of the zona pellucida characterized by a round mass of blastomeres resulting from cleavage divisions of the zygote.

motility. The ability to move or contract. (Sperm motility, swimming; uterine motility, contracting).

motor neuron. Myelinated neuron conveying action potentials from the spinal cord to skeletal muscles.

mucopolysaccharide. A complex protein-polysaccharide complex that functions as protective coating.

mucosa. An epithelial lining or coating of a structure.

Müllerian ducts. See paramesonephric ducts.

muscularis. The smooth muscular layer covering a tubular or hollow organ.

myoid layer. A smooth muscle layer (e.g. surrounding the seminiferous tubule, epididymis or oviduct).

myometrium. The smooth muscle layer of the uterus consisting of an inner circular layer and an outer longitudinal layer.

N

nasopalatine ducts. A pair of ducts opening into the oral cavity and continuous with the ducts of the vomeronasal organ. Fluid-born, less volatile chemicals can enter the vomeronasal organ by means of these ducts during the Flehmen response.

necrosis. The death of cells, tissues or organs, usually resulting from damage to the tissue or lack of circulation.

negative feedback. The set of conditions whereby a hormone exerts an inhibitory effect on another gland or organ suppressing the level of hormone secretion. For example, progesterone exerts a negative feedback on the hypothalamus and thus limits the release of GnRH.

neuroendocrine reflex. A reflex initiated by stimulation of sensory neurons that causes the release of a neurohormone from neurosecretory cells.

neurohormone. A material released from a neuron directly into the blood that causes a response on a remote tissue.

neurohypophysis. The posterior pituitary gland.

neuropeptides. A variety of materials produced by neurons which exert specific effects on other neurons or tissues.

neurosecretory cell. A neuron that secretes a substance into the blood.

neurotransmitter. A specific chemical released from the terminal boutons of neurons which causes either excitation or inhibition of postsynaptic neurons.

nuclear receptors. The specialized molecules within the nucleus of the cell that combine with a drug, steroid, hormone or chemical mediator to alter the function of the cell.

oestrous. British spelling of estrous.

oestrus. British spelling of estrus (heat).

oocyte. A developing egg cell in one of two stages. The primary oocyte is derived from an oogonium by differentiation near the time of birth and has begun, but not completed, the first maturation division. The secondary oocyte is derived from a primary oocyte shortly before ovulation by a division that produces the first polar body.

oocyte meiotic inhibitor. A substance implicated in controlling the resumption of meiosis in the oocyte. Once it has been removed, the oocyte can proceed with the first meiotic division.

ootid. The oocyte after the first meiotic division in which the first polar body is present.

optic chiasm. An x-shaped crossing of the optic nerve fibers in the floor of the brain.

ostium. A small opening in a tubular organ.

ovarian cortex. The outer portion of the ovary which contains developing and atretic follicles as well as functional and regressing corpora lutea.

ovarian follicles. Spherical structures which contain the oocyte classified as primary, secondary or antral, depending on the number and type of cellular layers present.

ovarian medulla. The inner portion of the ovary that houses blood vessels, lymphatics and nerves.

ovariectomy. Surgical removal of one or both ovaries.

ovary. The female gonad.

oviducts. The small, usually convoluted ducts (Fallopian tubes or uterine tubes) originating embryologically from the paramesonephric ducts that transport ova and sperm. The oviduct consists of the ampullary and posterior isthmic regions.

ovine interferon T (oIFN-T). A specific protein produced by the ovine trophoblast that is antiluteolytic. It contributes to maternal recognition of pregnancy in the ewe. The original name for this material was ovine trophoblastic protein 1.

ovine placental lactogen (oPL). A polypeptide hormone produced by the ovine placenta with both lactogenic and somatotropic effects.

oviparous. Animals that produce eggs which are hatched outside the body of the ovulatory animal, as in birds.

ovulation. The periodic rupture of mature ovarian follicles resulting in the discharge of an oocyte.

ovulation fossa. A conspicuous depression in the ovarian surface that is the site of each ovulation in the mare.

oxytocin. A nonapeptide synthesized by neurons in the hypothalamus and released by nerve terminals in the posterior pituitary. It is also produced by the corpus luteum. It causes contractions in smooth muscle in the male and female reproductive tract and regulates luteolysis.

P

pachytene. The stage of meiotic prophase following zygotene in which the paired homologous chromosome threads shorten, thicken and twist about each other. Longitudinal cleavage occurs to form two sister chromatids. Each homologous chromosome pair becomes a set of four chromatids. Crossing-over occurs during this phase.

pampiniform plexus. A specialized vascular plexus beginning in the spermatic cord and terminating on the dorsal pole of the testis. It consists of the testicular artery and vein, which are elaborately intertwined. The pampiniform plexus provides a countercurrent heat exchange mechanism for the testes.

paramesonephric ducts (Müllerian ducts). The ducts that originate lateral to the mesonephric ducts in the female embryo. They develop into the oviducts, uterus, cervix and sometimes portions of the vagina.

paraventricular nucleus (PVN). A hypothalamic nuclus that synthesizes oxytocin.

parenchyma. The cells of a gland or organ supported by a connective tissue framework.

parturition. To give birth.

pelvic urethra. The region of the urethra extending from the point of entry of the urethra into a single canal which extends to the base of the penis. Surrounding the pelvic urethra is a specialized muscle known as the urethralis muscle and the accessory sex glands which secrete their products via ducts directly into the canal.

penile shaft. The principle cylindrical portion of the penis.

penile urethra. The portion of the urethra inside the penis.

penis. The male organ of copulation consisting of a shaft and the glans penis.

perimetrium. The serous outer covering of the uterus that is continuous with the peritoneum.

perineum. The external surface surrounding the vulva and the anus in the female and between the scrotum and the anus in the male.

peritoneum. The serous membrane reflected over the viscera and lining the abdominal cavity.

perivitelline space. The space separating the oocyte plasma membrane from the zona pellucida.

phagocytic cells. Cells that perform endocytosis of particulate material, wherein the engulfed material is killed and digested. Example; neutrophils and macrophages.

pheromone. A volatile material secreted externally that is recognized by the olfactory system. Pheromones stimulate or inhibit reproduction.

photoperiod. The period of time during the day when there is daylight.

pineal gland. A pigmented outgrowth of the dorsal brain that secretes melatonin and is thought to act in controlling biological systems, including seasonal reproduction.

pinealocyte. The cell of the pineal gland that secretes melatonin.

pituitary hormones. Hormones that are released into the blood from the anterior and posterior pituitary. The primary reproductive hormones from the anterior pituitary are follicle stimulating hormone (FSH), luteinizing hormone (LH) and prolactin. Oxytocin is the primary reproductive hormone released from the posterior pituitary.

placenta. The organ of metabolic exchange between the fetus and the dam consisting of a portion of embryonic origin (chorion) and a portion of maternal origin (endometrium). The placenta is also a temporary endocrine organ.

placental lactogen (somatomammotropin). A hormone produced by the placenta which stimulates lactogenesis in the dam and fetal growth.

placentome. The specific anatomical region of attachment between the fetal and maternal placenta.

plasmin. An enzyme that dissolves blood clots by converting fibrin into soluble products.

plasminogen. An inactive form of plasmin found in blood plasma.

polar body. A small portion of oocyte cytoplasm containing one-half of the female genetic material that is removed by exocytosis into the perivitelline space during the first and second meiotic divisions.

polyestrus. Females experience multiple estrous cycles that are uniformly distributed throughout the year.

polypnea. Very rapid respiratory frequency; panting.

polyspermy. A condition in which more than one spermatozoon fertilizes the oocyte.

polytocous. Mammals which give birth to multiple offspring (litter-bearers).

positive feedback. A condition whereby a hormone exerts a stimulatory effect on another gland or tissue.

postcopulatory stage. The third (last) stage of reproductive behavior consisting of a dismount, a refractory period and memory.

posterior pituitary (neurohypophysis). The portion of the pituitary gland that originates from the infundibulum of the brain during embryogenesis. The posterior pituitary is neural tissue that houses terminals from neurons located in specific hypothalamic nuclei.

postnuclear cap. The membranous portion surrounding the posterior one-half to one-third of the sperm cell. The postnuclear cap originates from the manchette during spermiogenesis.

postsynaptic neuron. A neuron onto which the terminals of presynaptic neurons synapse.

precopulatory stage. The first stage of reproductive behavior consisting of search, courtship, sexual arousal, erection and penile protrusion.

pregnancy specific protein B. A protein unique to pregnancy in ruminants that is produced by binucleate giant cells in the chorion.

pregnant mare serum gonadotropin (PSMG). See equine chorionic gonadotropin.

preovulatory follicle. The egg (oocyte) and its encasing cells through all stages of development within the ovary prior to ovulation.

preovulatory GnRH center (surge center). A group of specific hypothalamic nuclei in the female that respond to high levels of estradiol by secreting high concentrations of GnRH during a relatively short period of time.

presynaptic neuron. A neuron which secretes neurotransmitters that cause excitation or inhibition in the postsynaptic neuron.

primary corpus luteum. The corpus luteum formed from the ovulatory follicle in the mare.

primary follicle. An ovarian follicle characterized as having a single layer of spindle shaped cells surrounding the oocyte. The nucleus of oocytes contained within the primary follicles is arrested in the dictyate stage (dictyotene).

primary portal plexus. The arterial capillary plexus of the hypothalamo-hypophyseal portal system into which releasing hormones are secreted.

primary spermatocyte. The daughter cells of spermatogonia that enter the first meiotic prophase and will give rise to a secondary spermatocytes.

Primary zona binding region. A specific site on the sperm plasma membrane that allows spermatozoa to adhere to the zona pellucida.

primiparous. Referring to the first parity or pregnancy of a female.

primitive endoderm. The innermost cellular layer of the embryo in the first stages of embryogenesis which gives rise to the yolk sac and, along with the trophoblast, give rise to the chorion and amnion.

primitive sex cords. Cords of cells that penetrate to the interior of the embryonic gonad that incorporate primordial germ cells. These cords will give rise to the seminiferous tubules.

primordial follicles. The most primitive stage of the ovarian follicle.

principal piece. The portion of the sperm tail that extends from the middle piece to the terminal piece.

privileged pathways. The deeper crypts of the cervix that are filled with low viscosity sialomucin through which the spermatozoa can move toward the uterus.

proacrosomal granule. Any of the small dense bodies found inside one of the vacuoles of the golgi body. These granules fuse to form the acrosomic granule.

proacrosin. An inactive form of acrosin found in the acrosome of mammalian spermatozoa.

proestrus. The stage of the estrous cycle between luteolysis and the onset of estrus.

progesterone. A steroid hormone produced by corpora lutea and the placenta that is required for the maintenance of pregnancy.

progesterone block. The inhibition of myometrial contractions during gestation due to high progesterone levels.

progestin. Any substance that produces an effect similar to progesterone.

prolactin. A hormone secreted by the anterior pituitary which stimulates lactogenesis and initiates maternal behavior.

pronephros. The most primitive form of kidney found in developing mammalian embryos that degenerates and gives way to the function of the mesonephros.

pronucleus. The nuclear material derived from the oocyte (female pronucleus) and the fertilizing spermatozoon (male pronucleus). Each pronucleus contains a haploid number of chromosomes.

proper ligament of the ovary. See utero-ovarian ligament.

prostaglandin $F_{2\alpha}$. A prostaglandin produced by the uterine endometrium that stimulates the contraction of the uterine myometrium, causes vasoconstriction in some vessels and causes luteolysis.

prostaglandin (PG). A class of physiologically active substances (designated as PGE, PGF, PGA and PGB) that are present in most tissues of the body. Prostaglandins are derived from arachidonic acid and have a wide variety of functions.

prostate gland. One of the accessory sex glands of the male consisting of a body (sometimes paired) which is outside of the pelvic urethra and/or a disseminate portion which forms a glandular layer in the wall of the pelvic urethra.

protein kinases. A class of control enzymes which phosphorylate proteins.

proteolytic enzymes. Enzymes which catalyze the splitting of proteins by hydrolysis of the peptide bonds with the formation of smaller peptides.

proximal cytoplasmic droplet. A cytoplasmic remnant in the neck region of a newly formed spermatozoon.

puberty. A developmental process in which endocrine and morphologic changes transform the animal into an individual capable of reproducing. Puberty involves the acquisition of gonadotropin secretion, gametogenesis, gonadal steroid secretion, development of secondary sex characteristics and reproductive behavior.

R

Rathke's pocket (pouch). An invagination of the stomodeal ectoderm in the developing embryo that gives rise to the anterior pituitary.

receptor. See hormone receptor.

recruitment. A stage of antral follicle development in which small antral follicles begin to develop into larger follicles.

rectogenital pouch. The pouch (space) between the rectum and the reproductive organs.

reflex ovulation (induced). A condition whereby the female must experience cervical and/or vaginal stimulation (usually in the form of mating) before ovulation can occur.

refractory. Temporarily unresponsive to nervous or sexual stimuli.

relaxin. A polypeptide hormone secreted by the placenta and/or the corpus luteum of pregnancy that causes the cervix to dilate and softens the ligaments in the pelvic region, thus tending to widen the birth canal during parturition.

releasing hormones. Small peptides produced by neurons in hypothalamic nuclei that cause the release of anterior pituitary hormones.

renewable stem cells. Cells in the seminiferous epithelium which provide a continual supply of stem cells so that spermatogenesis can continue indefinitely.

rete testis. A network of tubules housed within the mediastinum that are connected to the straight portions (tubuli recti) of the seminiferous tubules and merging into the efferent ducts.

rete tubules. A series of tubules in the mediastinum which serve to transport spermatozoa from the seminiferous tubules to the efferent ducts.

retractor penis muscles. A pair of smooth muscles originating on the ventral surface of the first few caudal vertebrae. The muscles circumvent the rectum and continue to their attachment on the lateral and urethral surfaces of the penis. Relaxation of this muscle is required for full penile protrusion and erection.

retroperitoneal. Located behind or outside of the peritoneum. The reproductive tracts of both the male and the female are retroperitoneal.

S

salpinx. Oviduct.

scrotum. A sac consisting of skin, sweat glands, a layer of smooth muscle (tunica dartos) and connective tissue that houses the testes.

season. A term used in reference to the breeding season in females.

seasonal anestrus. A period of anestrus induced by either long (ewe) or short (mare) photoperiods.

seasonal polyestrus. A condition in which females exhibit multiple estrous cycles during a specific season of the year.

second messenger. An intracellular material which responds to a hormone-receptor complex and initiates a specific set of intracellular reactions.

secondary follicle. An ovarian follicle characterized by having two or more layers of cells surrounding the oocyte, but without an antrum.

secondary spermatocyte. The daughter cells of primary spermatocytes that will complete the second meiotic division and give rise to spermatids.

sella turcica. A vault-like depression in the sphenoid bone that houses the anterior and posterior pituitary. The sella turcica is so named because it resembles, in side view, a Turkish saddle.

seminal plasma. The noncellular liquid portion of semen produced by the accessory sex glands.

seminiferous epithelium. The epithelium between the basement membrane and the lumen of the seminiferous tubules consisting of developing germ cells and Sertoli cells.

seminiferous tubules. The highly tortuous tubules within the testes that produce spermatozoa.

serosa. A serous membrane making up the outermost covering of an organ or serving as a lining of a cavity.

Sertoli cells. Somatic cells in the seminiferous epithelium that are believed to govern spermatogenesis. Sertoli cells contain FSH receptors and produce a wide variety of materials and hormones. They are named after the famous Italian scientist Enrico Sertoli.

sexual preparation. The prolongation of the period of sexual stimulation beyond that needed for mounting and ejaculation. Sexual preparation serves to maximize the number of spermatozoa per ejaculate by stimulating the release of oxytocin, causing contraction of the smooth muscle in the distal tail of the epididymis and ductus deferens, thus moving spermatozoa into an ejaculatory position.

sexual satiation. A condition in which further stimuli will not cause immediate sexual responsiveness or motivation.

sexually indifferent stage. The stage of embryogenesis when the sex of the embryo cannot be determined based on morphologic features.

short-day breeders. Females which begin to exhibit estrous cycles during times of short photoperiods (short days).

sialomucin. A mucus of low viscosity produced by the mucosa of the basal cervical crypts.

sigmoid flexure. The s-shaped curvature of the penis in the boar, ram and bull when it is not erect and is retracted into the body. During sexual excitation and erection, the sigmoid flexure disappears when the penis straightens.

silent ovulation. A condition whereby ovulation occurs without behavioral estrus. Silent ovulation frequently occurs in the first postpartum estrous cycle of dairy cows and the first estrous cycle after seasonal anestrus in ewes.

simple diffusion. The movement of water and other materials across a membrane along a concentration gradient.

simple neural reflex. A reflex which employs a series of nerves to translate a stimulus into a physical response through direct innervation of the target tissue (effector organ).

simplex uterus. A uterus found in primates, consisting of a large uterine body without uterine horns.

smooth muscle. A type of muscle without striations which surrounds most organs of the reproductive tract; often referred to as the muscularis.

somatic cells. Any of the body cells other than germ cells.

somatomammotropin. See placental lactogen.

somatotropic. Having an affinity for or stimulating the body or body cells. Having a stimulating effect on body nutrition and growth.

spay. The removal of the ovaries (ovariectomy).

spermatic artery. The artery supplying blood to the testes that originates from the aorta and travels into the spermatic cord.

spermatic cord. A collection of tissues that suspends the testis in a pendular fashion. The spermatic cord contains the testicular artery and vein, lymphatics, the pampiniform plexus, nerves, the cremaster muscle and the ductus deferens.

spermatids. Haploid male germ cells derived from secondary spermatocytes that undergo a transformation from a spherical cell to a fully specialized and differentiated spermatozoon with a head and a tail.

spermatocytes. The male germ cells derived from the final mitotic division of spermatogonia (primary spermatocyte) and giving rise to a haploid spermatid (secondary spermatocyte).

spermatocytogenesis. A series of mitotic divisions of the spermatogonia that produce primary spermatocytes.

spermatogenesis. The process whereby spermatozoa are formed. It consists of spermatocytogenesis (mitosis), meiosis and spermiogenesis.

spermatogenic efficiency. The number of spermatozoa produced per gram of testicular parenchyma.

spermatogenic wave. A sequential ordering of stages of the cycle of the seminiferous epithelium along the length of the seminiferous tubule.

spermatogonia. The most primitive of the male germ cell types located in the broad compartment of the seminiferous tubule that give rise to primary spermatocytes after a series of mitotic divisions.

spermatozoa. The male gamete consisting of a head (nucleus) and a tail (flagellum) which exhibits motility when exposed to the appropriate physiologic environment.

spermiation. The release of mature spermatozoa from Sertoli cells into the lumen of the seminiferous tubule.

spermiogenesis. A subcategory of spermatogenesis during which spermatids undergo morphologic transformation into highly specialized spermatozoa. Spermiogenesis consists of the Golgi phase, the cap phase, the acrosomal phase and the maturation phase.

sphenoid bone. A bone forming the floor of the cranial cavity that houses the sella turcica into which the hypophysis fits.

spontaneous ovulation. A condition whereby ovulation is brought about by changing endocrine conditions without the need for cervical or vaginal stimulation.

steroid. A generic term referring to closely related compounds that contain a common ring structure.

steroidogenic. Producing or synthesizing steroid hormones.

stigma. The small protrusion at the apex of a follicle which represents a site of deterioration of the follicular wall prior to ovulation.

stomodeal ectoderm. A layer lining the stomodeum or embryonic mouth (oral cavity).

stomodeum. A depression in the oral region of the embryo which will form the mouth and become continuous with the gut.

stratified squamous epithelium. A type of epithelium characterized by flattened cells in multiple layers lining portions of the vagina.

submucosa. A region of tissue lying just beneath the mucosal layer housing the vasculature, nerve supply and lymphatics.

suburethral diverticulum. An outpocketing of tissue located just beneath the urethra which forms a blind pouch that probably has no significance.

sulfated glycoproteins 1 and 2. The products of Sertoli cells believed to be related to fertility acquisition (SGP-1) and to provide a detergent effect which allows spermatozoa and fluids to move through the tubular network of the testis with ease (SPG-2).

sulfomucin. A type of mucus characterized as being highly viscous produced by cells that line the lumen in the bovine cervix.

superior cervical ganglion. A group of nerve cell bodies that serve as a relay point for the neural impulses involved in seasonal cyclicity.

superior hypophyseal artery. The primary artery supplying the hypothalamo-hypophyseal portal system.

superovulation. Ovulation of abnormally high numbers of ova.

supplementary corpora lutea. The corpora lutea produced by the pregnant mare as a result of ovulation and/or luteinization induced by equine chorionic gonadotropin.

suprachiasmatic nucleus. A hypothalamic nucleus located just above the optic chiasm which is believed to be part of the GnRH surge center.

surge center. See preovulatory center.

synapse. The functional junction between two nerve cells characterized by close apposition of the membrane of the presynaptic terminal (teledendrite) with the postsynaptic membrane (dendrite). Nerve terminals can also synapse with blood vessels, in the case of the hypothalamic portal system, or in the case of oxytocin producing neurons in the posterior pituitary.

syncytiotrophoblast. Cells comprising the outer layer of the trophoblast which make contact with the endometrium of the uterus to form attachment with the endometrium.

syndesmochorial placenta. A type of epitheliochorial placenta in which the endometrial epithelium locally erodes, causing intermittent exposure of the maternal capillaries to the chorionic epithelium.

syngamy. The fusion of the male and female pronuclei within the cytoplasm of the newly fertilized oocyte, giving rise to the zygote.

systolic pressure. Blood pressure occurring during ventricular systole (contraction). Systolic pressure is the highest pressure during the cardiac cycle.

T

target tissue. A tissue containing receptors to a specific hormone or neurotransmitter that elicits a response to the hormone or neurotransmitter.

teratogenic. Causing abnormal development.

tertiary follicle. See antral follicle.

testicular capsule. The tunica albuginea.

testis (plural: testes). One of the two male gonads .

testis determining factor (TDF). A substance synthesized by the primitive sex cords that causes the development of the male gonad and the male reproductive tract. The absence of TDF results in the development of the female reproductive tract.

testosterone. The male sex hormone and the most potent naturally occurring androgen produced by the interstitial cells of Leydig.

theca externa. The outermost layer of an antral follicle that provides structural integrity and support for the follicle.

theca interna. The layer of flattened spindle-shaped cells just outside the basement membrane of an antral follicle with receptors to LH.

third ventricle. One of the ventricles of the brain that is attached to the right and left lateral ventricles and to the cerebral aqueduct. It is surrounded by the hypothalamus.

thyroxin. Hormone produced by the thyroid gland that governs metabolic rate.

tight junction. See junctional complex.

tonic GnRH center. A term used to describe the hypothalamic nuclei which control the tonic release of GnRH. The tonic center collectively consists of the ventromedial nucleus, the arcuate nucleus and the median eminence.

totipotency. The ability of a single cell to differentiate and develop into a complete organism.

transferrin. A plasma globulin responsible for transporting iron. Some transferrin is produced by Sertoli cells. Relatively high concentrations are found in fluid of the seminiferous tubules and the rete tubules.

translocating cytoplasmic droplet. The residual cytoplasm from spermiogenesis that is relocating from the neck to the distal middle piece of the spermatozoa. Sperm containing translocating droplets are characterized as having the flagellum bent back toward the head of the sperm forming a crook containing the droplet.

transmembrane domain. The portion of a hormone receptor within the plasma membrane that connects the extracellular and intracellular domains.

transrectal palpation. Manual palpation of the reproductive tract via the rectum. This technique is used to artificially inseminate the cow and mare. It is also used to ascertain pregnancy, ovarian status and uterine/ cervical conditions in these species.

trophoblast. The cell layer covering the blastocyst which will form the chorion.

-tropin. A suffix referring to nourishment or having an affinity for.

tubular compartment. The compartment of the testicular parenchyma consisting of the seminiferous tubules.

tubulus contortus. The highly convoluted tortuous component of a seminiferous tubule contributing to the majority of its length. It is attached to a straight portion (tubulus rectus) that connects to the rete tubule. The tubulus contortus is the primary site of spermatogenesis.

tubulus rectus. The straight portion of the seminiferous tubule through which mature spermatids pass before entering the rete tubules.

tunica albuginea. A dense, whitish connective tissue covering an organ (testis, ovary, penis).

tunica dartos. The layer of smooth muscle which is a component of the scrotum that controls contraction and relaxation of the scrotum.

tunica vaginalis. An extension of the peritoneum which surrounds the spermatic cord and the testes. It consists of an outer parietal layer and an inner visceral layer.

tunica vasculosa. A layer well supplied with blood vessels. The vascular lining of the connective tissue septa within the testis.

up-regulate. A condition whereby receptor density is elevated.

urethra. The canal for the discharge of urine from the bladder to the exterior of the animal. In the female, it exits in the floor of the posterior vagina. In the male, it conveys urine from the bladder into the pelvic urethra and then into the penile urethra. The pelvic and penile urethra transports semen as well as urine.

urethralis muscle. The striated, circular muscle surrounding the pelvic urethra, the contractions of which cause semen to move into the penile urethra.

urogenital sinus. An embryonic cavity in the posterior of the animal that will give rise to the bladder, the pelvic urethra (male), the vagina (female) and the external genitalia of both the male and female.

uterine body. The anatomical region of the uterus anterior to the cervix and posterior to the internal uterine bifurcation.

uterine glands. The tubular glands in the endometrium of the uterus that secrete materials that are believed to be important to the survival and function of the pre-implantation embryo.

uterine horns (cornua). The portions of the uterus that are the result of the incomplete fusion of paramesonephric ducts.

utero-ovarian ligament. A portion of the broad ligament which attaches the ovary to the uterus.

uterotubal junction. The site where the oviduct joins the uterus.

uterus. A hollow, tubular organ surrounded by smooth muscle and lined with epithelium that connects the cervix to the oviducts. It is responsible for sperm transport, early embryonic development, formation of maternal placenta and parturition. The uterus produces prostaglandin $F_{2\alpha}$.

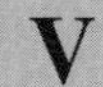

vagina. The female copulatory organ that connects the external genitalia to the cervix.

vaginal process. The space (cavity) formed between the visceral and parietal tunica vaginalis during descent of the testes.

vas deferens (ductus deferens). A small, muscular tube that connects the distal tail of the epididymis to the ampulla.

vascular countercurrent exchange. A process whereby exchange of substances and/or heat occurs in an artery and a vein that are intimately associated.

vesicular glands. The seminal vesicles.

vesiculation. A process whereby membrane vesicles are formed. Vesiculation occurs during the acrosome reaction when the plasma membrane of the sperm fuses with the outer acrosomal membrane, forming many small vesicles.

vestibular glands. Glands located in the posterior portion of the vestibule, which actively secrete a mucus-like material during estrus.

vestibule. The portion of the vagina anterior to the clitoris extending to and including the urethral opening. It is common to both the urinary and reproductive systems.

visceral tunica vaginalis. See tunica vaginalis.

vitelline block. A phenomenon which prevents polyspermy by rendering the plasma membrane of the oocyte incapable of further binding with the sperm membrane.

vomeronasal organ. An accessory olfactory organ consisting of a pair of blind ducts located in the floor of the nasal cavity. The ducts open into the oral cavity through the incisive duct. They are believed to be associated with identification of nonvolatile pheromones.

vulva. The external genitalia of the female.

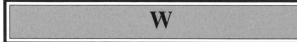

W

Wolffian duct. See mesonephric duct.

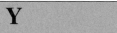

Y

yolk sac. A transient extraembryonic membrane derived from the primitive endoderm that regresses in size as the conceptus develops. The yolk sac contributes red blood cells, primitive germ cells and some nutrients to the fetus.

Z

zona block. A mechanism to prevent polyspermy which renders the zona pellucida incapable of binding additional spermatozoa.

zona lysin. An enzyme in the acrosome which aids in penetration of the zona pellucida.

zona pellucida. A thick, translucent mucoprotein surrounding the oocyte and early embryo.

zona proteins (ZP). Specific proteins of the zona pellucida which provide structure (ZP1 and ZP2) and bind spermatozoa (ZP3).

zonary placenta. A placenta of dogs and cats in which chorionic villi attach to the uterus in a well defined zone or band.

zygote. The diploid cell resulting from the fusion of the male and female pronuclei.

Index

B

C

Index

F

FB = Fact Box

G

FB = Fact Box

J

K

L

M

FB = Fact Box

R

S

T

FB = Fact Box

Collision Repair FUNDAMENTALS

Collision Repair FUNDAMENTALS

James E. Duffy

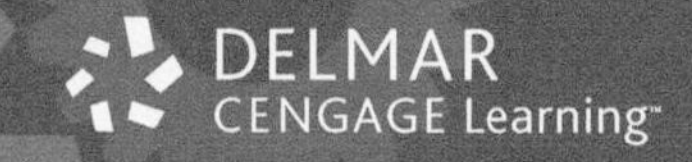

Australia • Brazil • Japan • Korea • Mexico • Singapore • Spain • United Kingdom • United States

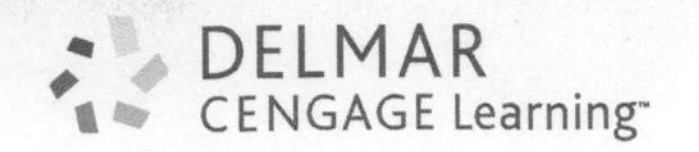

Collision Repair Fundamentals
James E. Duffy

Vice President, Technology and Trades ABU: David Garza

Director of Learning Solutions: Sandy Clark

Managing Editor: Larry Main

Senior Acquisitions Editor: David Boelio

Product Manager: Matthew Thouin

Marketing Director: Deborah S. Yarnell

Marketing Manager: Erin coffin

Marketing Coordinator: Patti Garrison

Director of Production: Patty Stephan

Content Project Manager: Barbara L. Diaz

Content Project Manager: Cheri Plasse

Editorial Assistant: Lauren Stone

Library of Congress Control Number: 2007001719

ISBN-13: 978-1-4180-1336-3

ISBN-10: 1-4180-1336-6

Delmar
Executive Woods
5 Maxwell Drive
Clifton Park, NY 12065
USA

Cengage Learning is a leading provider of customized learning solutions with office locations around the globe, including Singapore, the United Kingdom, Australia, Mexico, Brazil, and Japan. Locate your local office at **www.cengage.com/global**

Cengage Learning products are represented in Canada by Nelson Education, Ltd.

To learn more about Delmar, visit **www.cengage.com/delmar**

Purchase any of our products at your local bookstore or at our preferred online store **www.cengagebrain.com**

Printed in the United States of America
4 5 6 7 22 21 20 19 18

CONTENTS

SECTION 7 Estimating and Entrepreneurship 471

CHAPTER 28 Estimating Repair Costs 471

CHAPTER 29 Entrepreneurship and Job Success 487

PREFACE

ABOUT THE BOOK

Delmar Cengage Learning is pleased to present *Collision Repair Fundamentals*. The primary goal of this book is to address the wide range of skills that students must master to become successful automotive collision repair technicians. Designed for a student's first exposure to collision repair, this text presents complex topics in an easy-to-understand format. The writing level, page layout, use of color, and large number of illustrations help engage students who are visual learners. The text provides explanations of the theories behind a successful repair and information on the latest collision repair tools, equipment, and techniques. Safety is emphasized throughout the book, and tips and strategies are highlighted for students to use in protecting themselves and the environment. *Collision Repair Fundamentals* offers insight into what it takes to become a successful, well-rounded collision repair technician. We hope that this text becomes an important tool in your classroom. Good luck!

FEATURES OF THE TEXT

Learning how to repair collision damage on today's vehicles can be a challenge. To guide readers through this complex material, we have included a series of features that will ease the teaching and learning processes.

OBJECTIVES

Each chapter begins with a list of objectives. The objectives state the expected outcome that will result from completing a thorough study of the contents of the chapter.

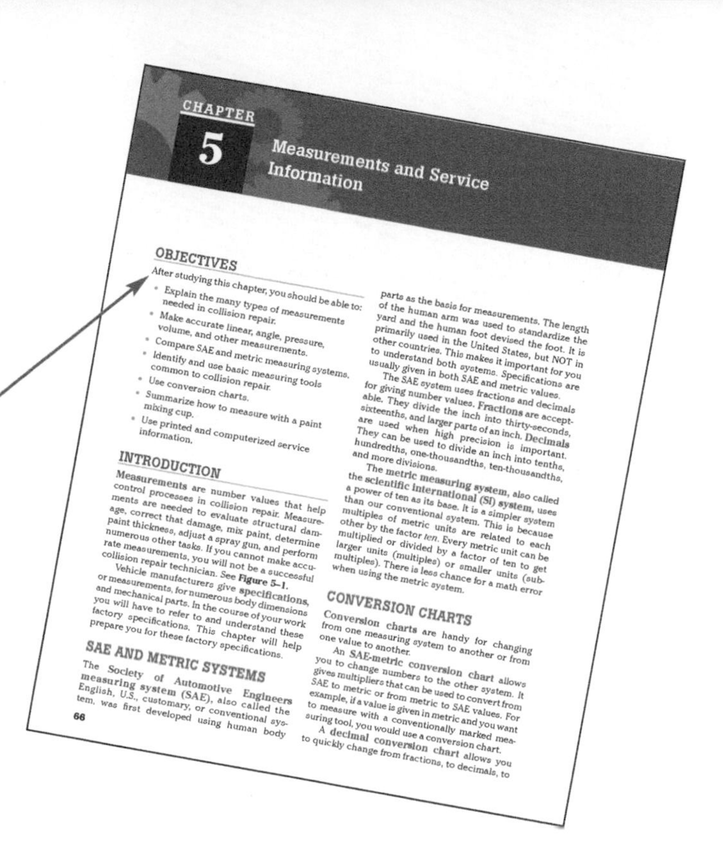

CHAPTER 5

Measurements and Service Information

OBJECTIVES

After studying this chapter, you should be able to:

- Explain the many types of measurements needed in collision repair.
- Make accurate linear, angle, pressure, volume, and other measurements.
- Compare SAE and metric measuring systems.
- Identify and use basic measuring tools common to collision repair.
- Use conversion charts.
- Summarize how to measure with a paint mixing cup.
- Use printed and computerized service information.

INTRODUCTION

Measurements are number values that help control processes in collision repair. Measurements are needed to evaluate structural damage, correct that damage, mix paint, determine paint thickness, adjust a spray gun, and perform numerous other tasks. If you cannot make accurate measurements, you will not be a successful collision repair technician. See **Figure 5–1.**

Vehicle manufacturers give **specifications,** or measurements, for numerous body dimensions and mechanical parts. In the course of your work you will have to refer to and understand these factory specifications. This chapter will help prepare you for these factory specifications.

SAE AND METRIC SYSTEMS

The **Society of Automotive Engineers measuring system (SAE),** also called the English, U.S., customary, or conventional system, was first developed using human body parts as the basis for measurements. The length of the human arm was used to standardize the yard and the human foot devised the foot. It is primarily used in the United States, but NOT in other countries. This makes it important for you to understand both systems. Specifications are usually given in both SAE and metric values.

The SAE system uses fractions and decimals for giving number values. **Fractions** are acceptable. They divide the inch into thirty-seconds, sixteenths, and larger parts of an inch. **Decimals** are used when high precision is important. They can be used to divide an inch into tenths, hundredths, one-thousandths, ten-thousandths, and more divisions.

The **metric measuring system,** also called the **scientific international (SI) system,** uses a power of ten as its base. It is a simpler system than our conventional system. This is because multiples of metric units are related to each other by the factor *ten*. Every metric unit can be multiplied or divided by a factor of ten to get larger units (multiples) or smaller units (sub-multiples). There is less chance for a math error when using the metric system.

CONVERSION CHARTS

Conversion charts are handy for changing from one measuring system to another or from one value to another.

An **SAE-metric conversion chart** allows you to change numbers to the other system. It gives multipliers that can be used to convert from SAE to metric or from metric to SAE values. For example, if a value is given in metric and you want to measure with a conventionally marked measuring tool, you would use a conversion chart.

A **decimal conversion chart** allows you to quickly change from fractions, to decimals, to

66

232 SECTION 3 Prepainting Preparation

when these chemicals are absorbed by rain water and form acids. When it rains or snows, these acids settle on the paint surface. They can become stronger as the water evaporates.

Acid rain damage may cause craters to be etched into the paint film, changes in pigment colors, and fading or dulling.

Acid rain damage can be identified with a magnifying glass while feeling the surface for depressions.

Industrial fallout is when metallic particles are released into the atmosphere from steel mills, foundries, and railroad operations. This is another source of paint damage. The metallic particles fall onto the vehicle's surface. They then corrode when exposed to moisture. The resulting damage will appear as black or brown spots or rust-colored rings on the paint surface. The particles can etch into the surface, causing a coarse or sandy surface.

Industrial fallout damage can be identified by feel or wiping a terry cloth towel over the surface. The metallic particles will catch on the cloth and can be easily seen.

Hard water spotting damage forms when rain or tap water dries on the paint surface. The water evaporates, leaving hard minerals on the paint surface. Hard water spotting leaves a round white ring on the paint surface. It is often repairable because the mineral deposits are on top of the paint film.

UV radiation damage results from excessive exposure of the paint film to the sun's radiation. Exposure to UV radiation can cause discoloration, cracking, checking, dulling, or yellowing.

When paint is badly aged or damaged, the finish should be completely removed. There are three common ways of stripping paint from metal surfaces: chemical stripping, abrasive blasting, and sanding or grinding.

CHEMICAL STRIPPING

Chemical stripping uses a chemical action to dissolve and remove paint down to bare metal. A chemical paint remover is often used for stripping large areas of paint. Chemical stripping is effective in those places where a power sander cannot reach.

Before applying paint remover, mask off the area to ensure that the remover does NOT dissolve any paint NOT meant to be stripped. Use two or three thicknesses of masking paper to give adequate protection. Cover any crevices to prevent the paint remover from seeping to the bottom of a panel.

DANGER

Paint remover (stripper) should be applied following the manufacturer's instructions. Pay attention to warnings regarding ventilation and smoking. Also wear protective clothing such as rubber gloves, long sleeve shirts, and goggles. If paint remover comes in contact with your skin or eyes, it can cause serious chemical burns.

WARNING

Some paint removers can harm body filler beneath the paint. The chemical residue can be difficult to remove completely. If the chemical residue is NOT cleaned properly, it can cause paint adhesion problems.

Before applying the paint remover, slightly sand the surface of the paint to be stripped. This will help the chemical stripper penetrate and dissolve the paint more quickly.

To apply paint remover, brush on a heavy coat in one direction only, to the entire area being treated. Use a soft bristle brush. Do NOT brush the material out. Allow the paint remover to stand and soak until the finish is softened.

Although paint remover is quickly effective on most paints, some surfaces can prove stubborn. More than one application of remover may be needed.

Caution should be taken when removing the loosened paint coatings. Some paint removers are designed to be neutralized by water. Others are more easily removed with a squeegee or scraper. See **Figure 14–3.**

Be sure to rinse off any residue that remains by using a cleaning solvent and abrasive pad. Follow immediately by wiping with a clean rag. This rinsing operation is essential. Many paint removers contain wax. If left on the surface, the residue will prevent the paint from adhering, drying, and hardening properly.

After chemical stripping, you will sometimes have to remove small patches of remaining

DANGER

Instructors often tell us that safety is their most important concern. Danger notes appear throughout the text to alert students to important personal safety information.

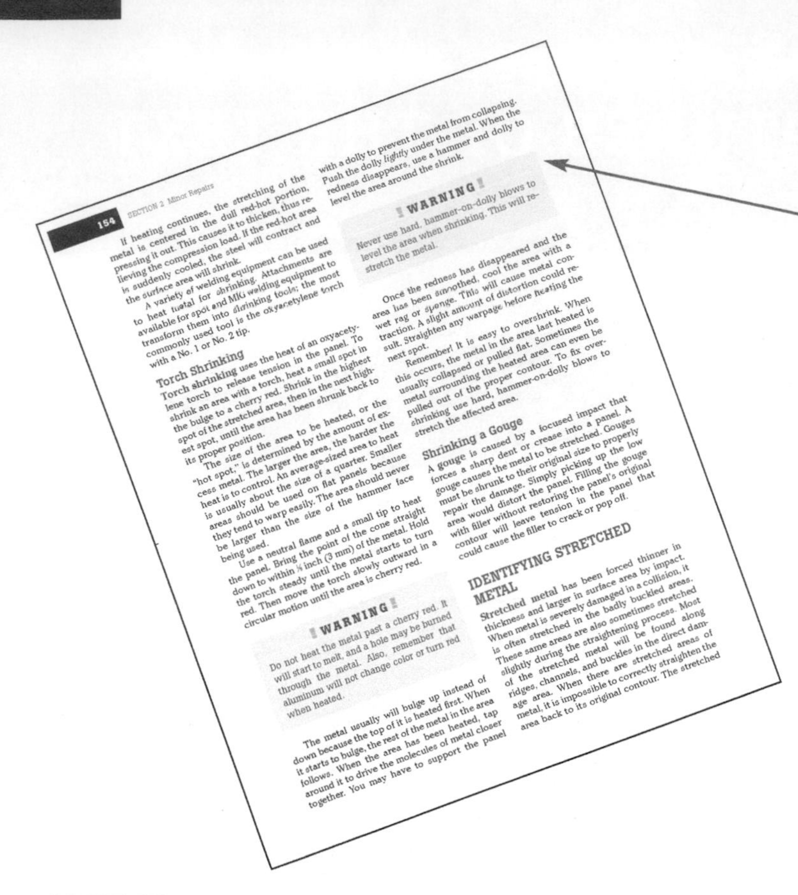

154 SECTION 2 Minor Repairs

If heating continues, the stretching of the metal is centered in the dull red-hot portion, pressing it out. This causes it to thicken, thus relieving the compression load. If the red-hot area is suddenly cooled, the steel will contract and the surface area will shrink.

A variety of welding equipment can be used to heat metal for shrinking. Attachments are available for spot and MIG welding equipment to transform them into shrinking tools; the most commonly used tool is the oxyacetylene torch with a No. 1 or No. 2 tip.

Torch Shrinking

Torch shrinking uses the heat of an oxyacetylene torch to release tension in the panel. To shrink an area with a torch, heat a small spot in the bulge to a cherry red. Shrink in the highest spot of the stretched area, then in the next highest spot, until the area has been shrunk back to its proper position.

The size of the area to be heated, or the "hot spot," is determined by the amount of excess metal. The larger the area, the harder the heat is to control. An average-sized area to heat is usually about the size of a quarter. Smaller areas should be used on flat panels because they tend to warp easily. The area should never be larger than the size of the hammer face being used.

Use a neutral flame and a small tip to heat the panel. Bring the point of the cone straight down to within ⅛ inch (3 mm) of the metal. Hold the torch steady until the metal starts to turn red. Then move the torch slowly outward in a circular motion until the area is cherry red.

WARNING

Do not heat the metal past a cherry red. It will start to melt, and a hole may be burned through the metal. Also, remember that aluminum will not change color or turn red when heated.

The metal usually will bulge up instead of down because the top of it is heated first. When it starts to bulge, the rest of the metal in the area follows. When the area has been heated, tap around it to drive the molecules of metal closer together. You may have to support the panel with a dolly to prevent the metal from collapsing. Push the dolly *lightly* under the metal. When the redness disappears, use a hammer and dolly to level the area around the shrink.

WARNING

Never use hard, hammer-on-dolly blows to level the area when shrinking. This will restretch the metal.

Once the redness has disappeared and the area has been smoothed, cool the area with a wet rag or sponge. This will cause metal contraction. A slight amount of distortion could result. Straighten any warpage before heating the next spot.

Remember! It is easy to overshrink. When this occurs, the metal in the area last heated is usually collapsed or pulled flat. Sometimes the metal surrounding the heated area can even be pulled out of the proper contour. To fix overshrinking use hard, hammer-on-dolly blows to stretch the affected area.

Shrinking a Gouge

A **gouge** is caused by a focused impact that forces a sharp dent or crease into a panel. A gouge causes the metal to be stretched. Gouges must be shrunk to their original size to properly repair the damage. Simply picking up the low area would distort the panel. Filling the gouge with filler without restoring the panel's original contour will leave tension in the panel that could cause the filler to crack or pop off.

IDENTIFYING STRETCHED METAL

Stretched metal has been forced thinner in thickness and larger in surface area by impact. When metal is severely damaged in a collision, it is often stretched in the badly buckled areas. These same areas are also sometimes stretched slightly during the straightening process. Most of the stretched metal will be found along ridges, channels, and buckles in the direct damage area. When there are stretched areas of metal, it is impossible to correctly straighten the area back to its original contour. The stretched

WARNINGS

Warnings provide students with important guidelines to follow to prevent damage to tools, equipment, the vehicle, or the repair.

NOTES

The notes sprinkled throughout the text emphasize key points or refer students to related information in other chapters.

CHAPTER 14 Vehicle Surface Preparation 237

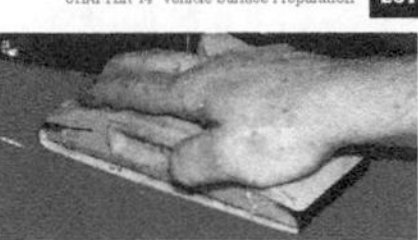

Figure 14–9. When wet sanding, water is applied to the body surface to carry away particles and to avoid clogging of finer paper grits. Again, use a sanding block to support the sandpaper on larger flat or slightly curved surfaces.

Figure 14–8. A soft, flexible block or sanding sponge should be used on very curved surfaces. The soft block will flex to match the surface profile. Here the technician is sponge sanding the louvers in a custom fiberglass hood.

4. To sand convex or concave panels, use a flexible backing pad. See **Figure 14–8.** You can also use the side of your hand to hand sand concave (curved inward) surfaces. You can use the palm of your hand to hand sand convex (curved outward) surfaces. You must hold your hand to match the shape of the surface.

WARNING

Never try to sand a flat surface while holding the sandpaper in your hand. An irregular surface will result.

5. Carefully find and sand scratches using a finer grit paper.
6. When block sanding primer or filler, make certain to sand the area until it feels smooth and level. Rub your hand or a clean cloth over the surface to check for rough spots.

Remember! If you can feel the slightest bump or dip in the surface, it will show up after painting. A surface will look smooth when sanded dull or when in primer. However, a shiny, reflective paint will exaggerate or magnify any surface roughness.

Block sanding can be done wet or dry. **Dry sanding** is often done with coarser nonwaterproof sandpaper, without using water. It is commonly done to remove material quickly. The majority of two-component primer-surfacers can be sanded dry.

Wet sanding is done with finer waterproof sandpaper, using water to flush away sanded particles. Some primers are wet sanded. Clearcoats are sanded with sandpaper as fine as No. 2,000 grit. Wet sanding reduces the problem of paper clogging.

Wax and silicone can penetrate beneath the surface. Because this contamination is NOT easily detected, you might want to add wax and grease remover or soap to the water when wet sanding. Look at **Figure 14–9.**

Scuff Pads

Scuff padding is done with a nylon pad on hard-to-reach areas to clean and scuff the surface. Scuff padding is often done inside door jambs, around hood and trunk openings, and other restricted areas. Since the scuff pad is flexible, it will scuff irregular surfaces easily.

Paint scuffing is needed to make sure the new paint bonds properly. If you paint over a smooth, hard surface, the new paint will not have anything to bond to and it will peel off. Paint scuffing can be done with fine sandpaper or a scuff pad, wet or dry.

When scuff pad sanding, you can place the pad over a sanding block on flat surfaces. You can also use your hand to hold and shape the pad on curved or restricted areas. See **Figure 14–10.**

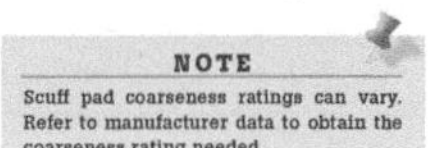

NOTE

Scuff pad coarseness ratings can vary. Refer to manufacturer data to obtain the coarseness rating needed.

Abrasive grinding discs are used for jobs such as grinding off rust and removing paint. They are available in many grit sizes and in diameters of 3 to 9 inches (76 to 229 mm). The

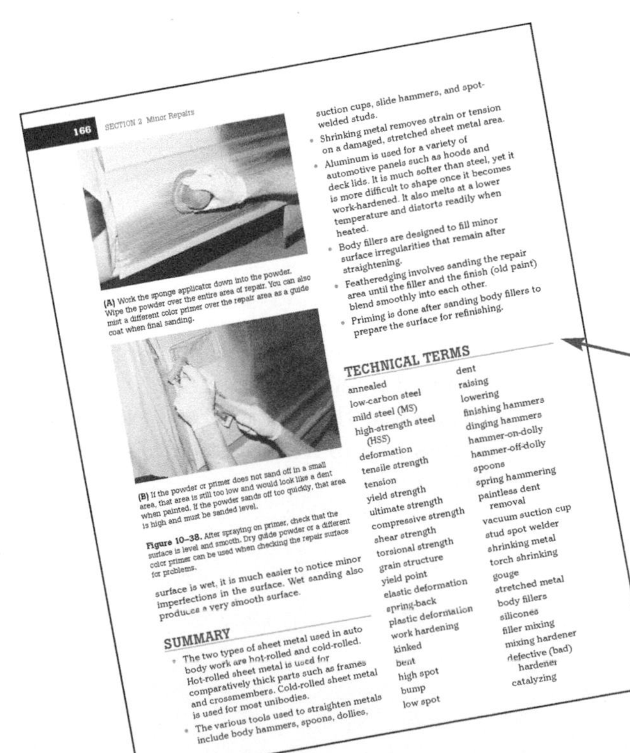

166 SECTION 2 Minor Repairs

(A) Work the sponge applicator down into the powder. Wipe the powder over the entire area of repair. You can also mist a different color primer over the repair area as a guide coat when final sanding.

(B) If the powder or primer does not sand off in a small area, that area is still too low and would look like a dent when painted. If the powder sands off too quickly, that area is high and must be sanded level.

Figure 10–38. After spraying on primer, check that the surface is level and smooth. Dry guide powder or a different color primer can be used when checking the repair surface for problems.

surface is wet, it is much easier to notice minor imperfections in the surface. Wet sanding also produces a very smooth surface.

SUMMARY

- The two types of sheet metal used in auto body work are hot-rolled and cold-rolled. Hot-rolled sheet metal is used for comparatively thick parts such as frames and crossmembers. Cold-rolled sheet metal is used for most unibodies.
- The various tools used to straighten metals include body hammers, spoons, dollies, suction cups, slide hammers, and spot-welded studs.
- Shrinking metal removes strain or tension on a damaged, stretched sheet metal area.
- Aluminum is used for a variety of automotive panels such as hoods and deck lids. It is much softer than steel, yet it is more difficult to shape once it becomes work-hardened. It also melts at a lower temperature and distorts readily when heated.
- Body fillers are designed to fill minor surface irregularities that remain after straightening.
- Featheredging involves sanding the repair area until the filler and the finish (old paint) blend smoothly into each other.
- Priming is done after sanding body fillers to prepare the surface for refinishing.

TECHNICAL TERMS

annealed
low-carbon steel
mild steel (MS)
high-strength steel (HSS)
deformation
tensile strength
tension
yield strength
ultimate strength
compressive strength
shear strength
torsional strength
grain structure
yield point
elastic deformation
spring-back
plastic deformation
work hardening
kinked
bent
high spot
bump
low spot
dent
raising
lowering
finishing hammers
dinging hammers
hammer-on-dolly
hammer-off-dolly
spoons
spring hammering
paintless dent removal
vacuum suction cup
stud spot welder
shrinking metal
torch shrinking
gouge
stretched metal
body fillers
silicones
filler mixing
mixing hardener
defective (bad) hardener
catalyzing

TECHNICAL TERMS

Each chapter ends with a list of the terms that were introduced in the chapter. These terms are defined in the glossary and are highlighted in the text upon first use. Students can be assigned to write definitions of these terms.

SUMMARY

Highlights and key bits of information are listed at the end of each chapter. This list can be used as a refresher and as a study tool.

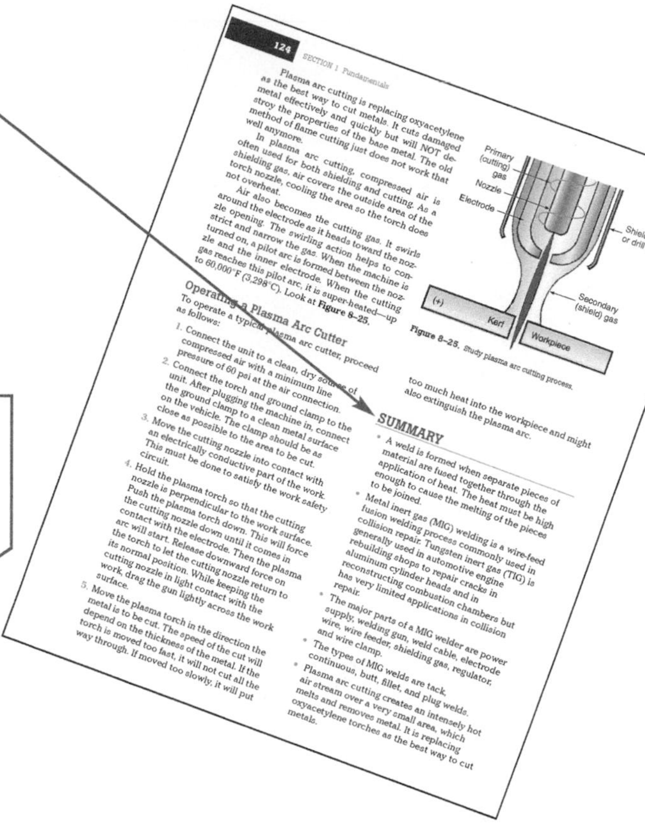

REVIEW QUESTIONS

A combination of true/false, short-answer, fill-in-the-blank, multiple-choice, and ASE-style questions make up the end-of-chapter review questions. Different question types are used to challenge the reader's understanding of the chapter content.

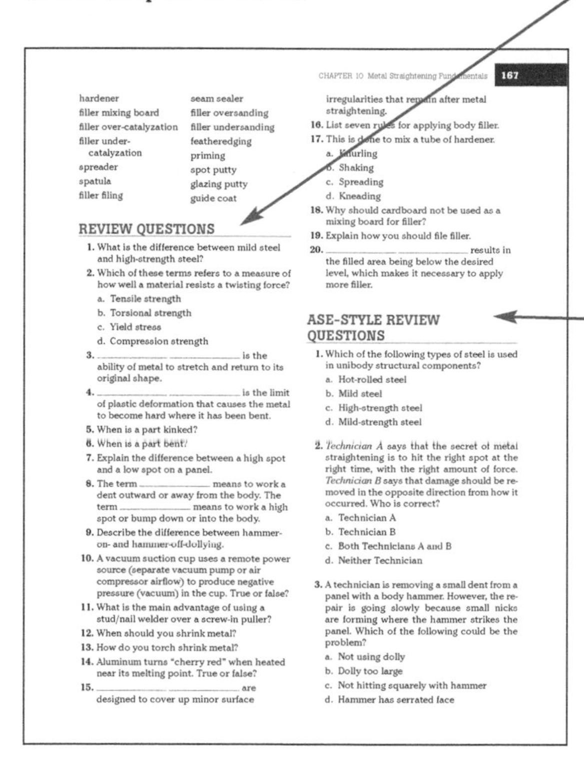

CHAPTER 10 Metal Straightening Fundamentals 167

hardener
filler mixing board
filler over-catalyzation
filler under-catalyzation
spreader
spatula
filler filing
seam sealer
filler oversanding
filler undersanding
featheredging
priming
spot putty
glazing putty
guide coat

REVIEW QUESTIONS

1. What is the difference between mild steel and high-strength steel?
2. Which of these terms refers to a measure of how well a material resists a twisting force?
   a. Tensile strength
   b. Torsional strength
   c. Yield stress
   d. Compression strength
3. ______ is the ability of metal to stretch and return to its original shape.
4. ______ is the limit of plastic deformation that causes the metal to become hard where it has been bent.
5. When is a part kinked?
6. When is a part bent?
7. Explain the difference between a high spot and a low spot on a panel.
8. The term ______ means to work a dent outward or away from the body. The term ______ means to work a high spot or bump down or into the body.
9. Describe the difference between hammer-on- and hammer-off-dollying.
10. A vacuum suction cup uses a remote power source (separate vacuum pump or air compressor airflow) to produce negative pressure (vacuum) in the cup. True or false?
11. What is the main advantage of using a stud/nail welder over a screw-in puller?
12. When should you shrink metal?
13. How do you torch shrink metal?
14. Aluminum turns "cherry red" when heated near its melting point. True or false?
15. ______ are designed to cover up minor surface irregularities that remain after metal straightening.
16. List seven rules for applying body filler.
17. This is done to mix a tube of hardener.
   a. Knurling
   b. Shaking
   c. Spreading
   d. Kneading
18. Why should cardboard not be used as a mixing board for filler?
19. Explain how you should file filler.
20. ______ results in the filled area being below the desired level, which makes it necessary to apply more filler.

ASE-STYLE REVIEW QUESTIONS

1. Which of the following types of steel is used in unibody structural components?
   a. Hot-rolled steel
   b. Mild steel
   c. High-strength steel
   d. Mild-strength steel
2. *Technician A* says that the secret of metal straightening is to hit the right spot at the right time, with the right amount of force. *Technician B* says that damage should be removed in the opposite direction from how it occurred. Who is correct?
   a. Technician A
   b. Technician B
   c. Both Technicians A and B
   d. Neither Technician
3. A technician is removing a small dent from a panel with a body hammer. However, the repair is going slowly because small nicks are forming where the hammer strikes the panel. Which of the following could be the problem?
   a. Not using dolly
   b. Dolly too large
   c. Not hitting squarely with hammer
   d. Hammer has serrated face

ASE-STYLE REVIEW QUESTIONS

Each chapter ends with a series of ASE-style questions that will expose students to the types of questions that are found on the ASE Certification Exams.

ACTIVITIES

Activities are included at the end of each chapter. These activities offer the readers the opportunity to apply what they have learned.

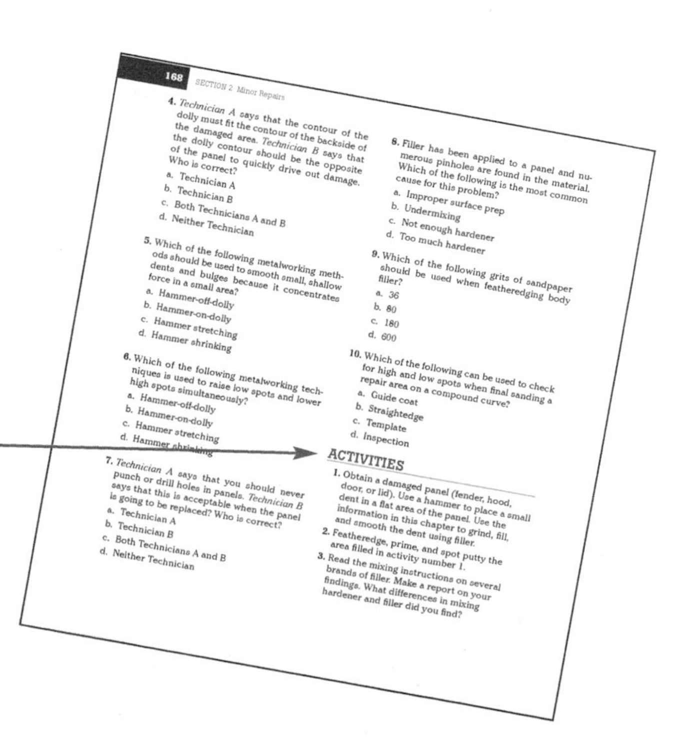

168 SECTION 2 Minor Repairs

4. *Technician A* says that the contour of the dolly must fit the contour of the backside of the damaged area. *Technician B* says that the dolly contour should be the opposite of the panel to quickly drive out damage. Who is correct?
   a. Technician A
   b. Technician B
   c. Both Technicians A and B
   d. Neither Technician
5. Which of the following metalworking methods should be used to smooth small, shallow dents and bulges because it concentrates force in a small area?
   a. Hammer-off-dolly
   b. Hammer-on-dolly
   c. Hammer stretching
   d. Hammer shrinking
6. Which of the following metalworking techniques is used to raise low spots and lower high spots simultaneously?
   a. Hammer-off-dolly
   b. Hammer-on-dolly
   c. Hammer stretching
   d. Hammer shrinking
7. *Technician A* says that you should never punch or drill holes in panels. *Technician B* says that this is acceptable when the panel is going to be replaced? Who is correct?
   a. Technician A
   b. Technician B
   c. Both Technicians A and B
   d. Neither Technician
8. Filler has been applied to a panel and numerous pinholes are found in the material. Which of the following is the most common cause for this problem?
   a. Improper surface prep
   b. Undermixing
   c. Not enough hardener
   d. Too much hardener
9. Which of the following grits of sandpaper should be used when featheredging body filler?
   a. 36
   b. 80
   c. 180
   d. 600
10. Which of the following can be used to check for high and low spots when final sanding a repair area on a compound curve?
   a. Guide coat
   b. Straightedge
   c. Template
   d. Inspection

ACTIVITIES

1. Obtain a damaged panel (fender, hood, door, or lid). Use a hammer to place a small dent in a flat area of the panel. Use the information in this chapter to grind, fill, and smooth the dent using filler.
2. Featheredge, prime, and spot putty the area filled in activity number 1.
3. Read the mixing instructions on several brands of filler. Make a report on your findings. What differences in mixing hardener and filler did you find?

SUPPLEMENTS

INSTRUCTOR'S CD

A supplementary disc is available to instructors who want to make classroom lectures as efficient and engaging as possible. This CD-ROM includes PowerPoint™ presentations with images, an Image Library, and a Computerized Test Bank with hundreds of modifiable questions and answers.

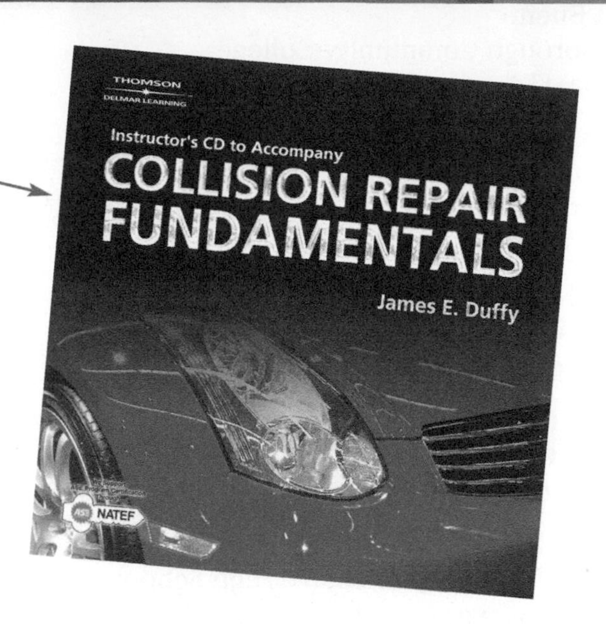

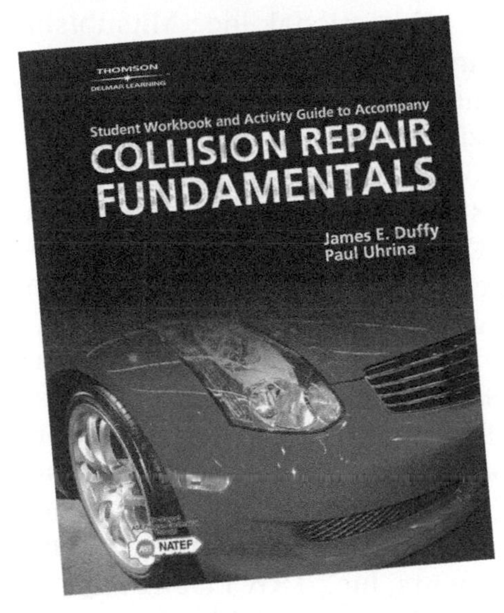

STUDENT WORKBOOK AND ACTIVITY GUIDE

The accompanying Student Workbook provides chapter-by-chapter shop activities and job sheets to reinforce the chapter content and have students put the information to work. Chapter review activities are also included to reinforce key chapter concepts and offer ideal homework or classroom work for students.

INSTRUCTOR'S GUIDE

An Instructor's Guide provides chapter outlines to support classroom lectures, and answers to the end-of-chapter questions found in the core text.

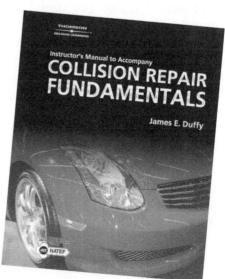

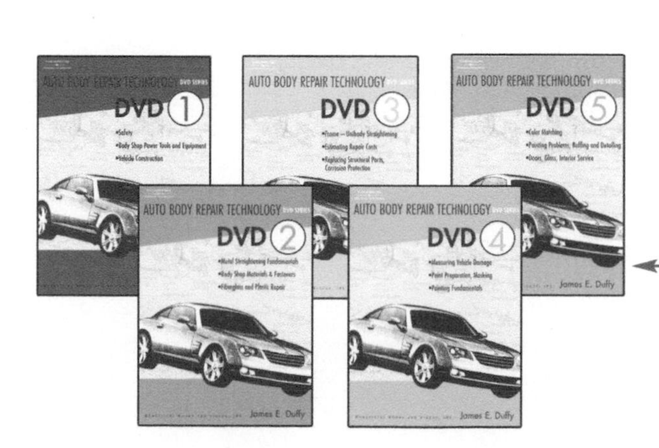

DVD SERIES

Interactive DVDs bring text alive with digital video footage on all major repair areas. The DVDs include buttons for viewing specific subjects, closed captioning for the hearing impaired, and on-screen test questions for self-evaluation.

ACKNOWLEDGMENTS

We would like to acknowledge and thank the following dedicated and knowledgeable educators for their comments, cricitisms, and suggestions during the review process:

John Bueno
Hillsborough Community College
Tampa, FL

Frank L. Damazo
Frederick County Public Schools
Career and Technology Center
Frederick, MD

Kevin Kubat
James Valley Career and Technical Center
Jamestown, ND

Robert Magee
Bergen County Technical High School
Teterboro, NJ

Frederick T. Steeves
Oxford Hills Comprehensive High School
South Paris, MN

CONTRIBUTING COMPANIES

We would like to thank the following companies who provided technical information and art for this edition:

3M Automotive Trades Division; American Honda Motor Co., Inc.; American Isuzu Motors Inc.; American Suzuki; NIASE; Audi of America; Babcox Publications; Badger Air Brush Co.; BASF; Bee Line Co.; BlackHawk Collision Repair, Inc.; BMW of North America; Carborundum Abrasives North America; Car-O-Liner; Chief Automotive Systems; Cooper Tools; DaimlerChrysler Corporation; Danaher Tool Group; Dataliner AB; DeVilbiss Automotive Refinishing Products; Dorman Products; Dynabrade, Inc.; Edelmann; Equalizer Industries; Evercoat Fibreglass Co., Inc.; FMC Automotive Equipment Division; Ford Motor Company; Fred V. Vowler Co., Inc.; Service Operations; Hein-Werner; Helicoil, Fastening Systems Division; Hopkins Manufacturing Corporation; HTP America, Inc.; Hunter Engineering Company; I-CAR; ITW Automotive Refinishing; Kansas Jack; Klein Tools, Inc.; L.S. Starrett Company; Lab Safety Supply Inc., Janseville, WI; Lincoln Electric Co.; MAACO Enterprises, Inc.; Marson Corp.; Mazda Motor of America, Inc.; McQuay-Norris; Mercedes-Benz of North America, Inc.; Mitchell International, Inc.; Mitsubishi Motor Sales of America, Inc.; Morgan Manufacturing Inc.; Munsell Color Group; Mustang Monthly Magazine; NATEF; NCG Company/Spotle Distributor; Nissan North America, Inc.; Norco Industries, Inc.; Oatey Bond Tite; OTC, a Division of SPX Corporation; Palnut Co.; PBR Industries; Perfect Circle/Dana Corp.; Porsche Cars North America, Inc.; PPG Industries, Inc.; Riverdale Body Shop; Rotary Lift/A Dover Industries Co.; Saab Cars USA, Inc.; Sartorius; Seelye, Inc.; Sellstrom Mfg.; Snap-on Tools Corporation; Stanley Tools; Subaru of America and Fuji Industries, Ltd.; Talsol Corporation; Team Blowtherm; Tech-Cor, Inc.; The Eastwood Company; TIF Instruments, Inc.; TRW Plastic Fasteners and Retainers Division; U.S. Chemicals and Plastics, Inc.; Volkswagen of America; Wedge Clamp International, Inc.

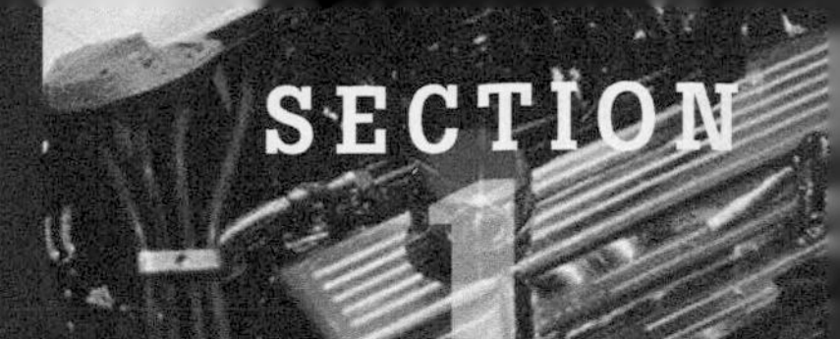

Fundamentals

CHAPTER 1

Careers in Collision Repair

OBJECTIVES

After studying this chapter, you should be able to:

- Summarize the collision repair industry.
- List the related skills needed to become a good collision repair technician.
- Explain the typical movement of a vehicle through a collision repair facility.
- Summarize the major areas of repair in a body shop.
- Describe basic procedures for repairing a collision damaged vehicle.

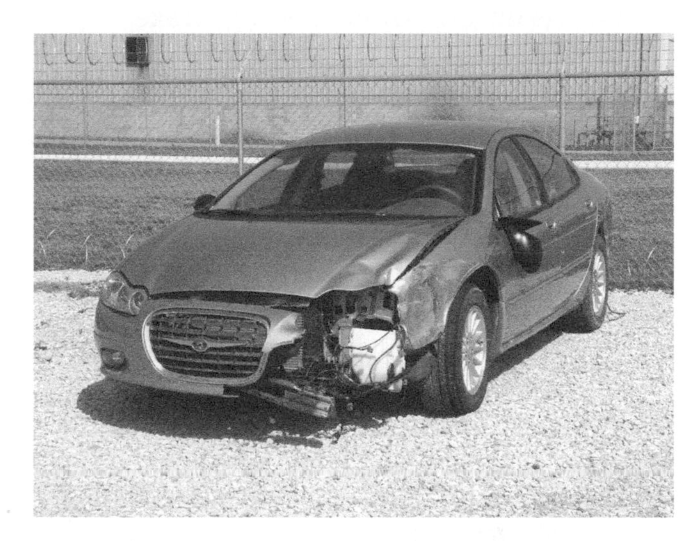

Figure 1–1. When a car is damaged in a collision, great skill and knowledge are needed to fix it properly.

INTRODUCTION

Considering that we are a "nation on wheels," you have selected an excellent area of employment to study. The skills you learn will be in high demand as long as there are people driving cars and trucks.

If you are just beginning your study of collision repair, you have much to learn. Only highly skilled, knowledgeable professionals can properly repair collision damaged vehicles. Study the material in this textbook carefully and you will be on your way to a successful career in collision repair. See **Figure 1–1.**

HISTORY NOTE

Did you know that the first self-propelled vehicle was in a collision the very first time it was driven? The huge steam engine–powered vehicle, trying to avoid a horse-drawn carriage, crashed into a brick wall. The vehicle, the brick wall, and the driver were all "hurt." As this first crash of the first motor vehicle on its first drive points out, there will always be collisions and a need for well-trained collision repair technicians.

COLLISION REPAIR TECHNICIAN

Collision repair technicians are skilled, knowledgeable people who know how to use specialized equipment and highly technical methods to restore collision damaged vehicles.

They must possess the basic skills in the following areas:

1. *Metalworker*—A collision repair technician must be able to do all types of metalworking to properly form and shape sheet metal car bodies after a collision.
2. *Welder*—A collision repair technician must weld and cut steel, aluminum, composites, and plastics efficiently during body repairs.
3. *Auto repair technician*—A collision repair technician must remove and install mechanical systems, requiring some skill in automotive repair technology.
4. *Plumber*—A collision repair technician must work with numerous lines, hoses, and fittings during power steering, brake system, and fuel system service.
5. *Electrician*—A collision repair technician must be good at testing and repairing wiring and electrical components after damage. Finding shorts, opens, and other wiring problems is essential to today's computer-controlled vehicles.
6. *Air-conditioning technician*—A collision repair technician may be required to work on air-conditioning systems.
7. *Computer technician*—A collision repair technician should be able to scan and repair computer problems stemming from collision damage.
8. *Painter/refinishing technician*—A collision repair technician should know how to restore vehicle finishes to their original condition after collision repairs are made.

As this points out, today's collision repair technician must be a highly skilled professional. (Refer to **Figure 1–2.**) Low-skilled technicians can no longer survive and earn a living with modern, complex automotive technology.

OTHER PERSONNEL

The collision repair and paint technicians are the principals in any collision repair business. However, there are other jobs that must be done as well. The following describes other personnel who work in and with the collision repair shop.

The **shop owner** must be concerned with all phases of work performed. In smaller shops, the owner and shop manager are usually the same person. In large operations or dealerships, the owner might hire a shop manager. In all cases, the person in charge should understand all of the work done in the shop as well as its business operations.

The **shop supervisor** is in charge of the everyday operation of the shop. This job involves communication with all personnel who contribute to the facility's success.

The **parts manager** is in charge of ordering all parts (both new and salvaged), receiving all parts, and seeing that they are delivered to the ordering technician. Since not every collision repair shop has an actual parts manager, the task of ordering parts can fall on each employee at one time or another.

The **bookkeeper** keeps the shop's books, prepares invoices, writes checks, pays bills, makes bank deposits, checks bank statements, and takes care of tax payments. Many shops hire an outside accountant to perform these tasks.

The **office manager's** duties include various aspects of the business such as handling letters, estimates, and receipts. In many small shops, the office manager also acts as the parts manager and bookkeeper.

A *receptionist* is sometimes employed to greet customers, answer the phone, route messages, and do other tasks.

A **helper** or **apprentice** learns new jobs while assisting experienced personnel. He or she might help a technician mask a car before painting, install parts, or help clean up the work area at the end of the day.

THE PROFESSIONAL

The term "professional" refers to the attitude, work quality, and image that a business and its workers project to customers. It is interesting to note that in Europe a shop cannot open without the presence of a "Meister" or "master" craftsperson. A **professional:**

1. is customer oriented.
2. is up to date on vehicle developments.
3. keeps up with advancements in the repair industry.
4. pays attention to detail.
5. ensures that his or her work is up to specifications.
6. participates in trade associations.

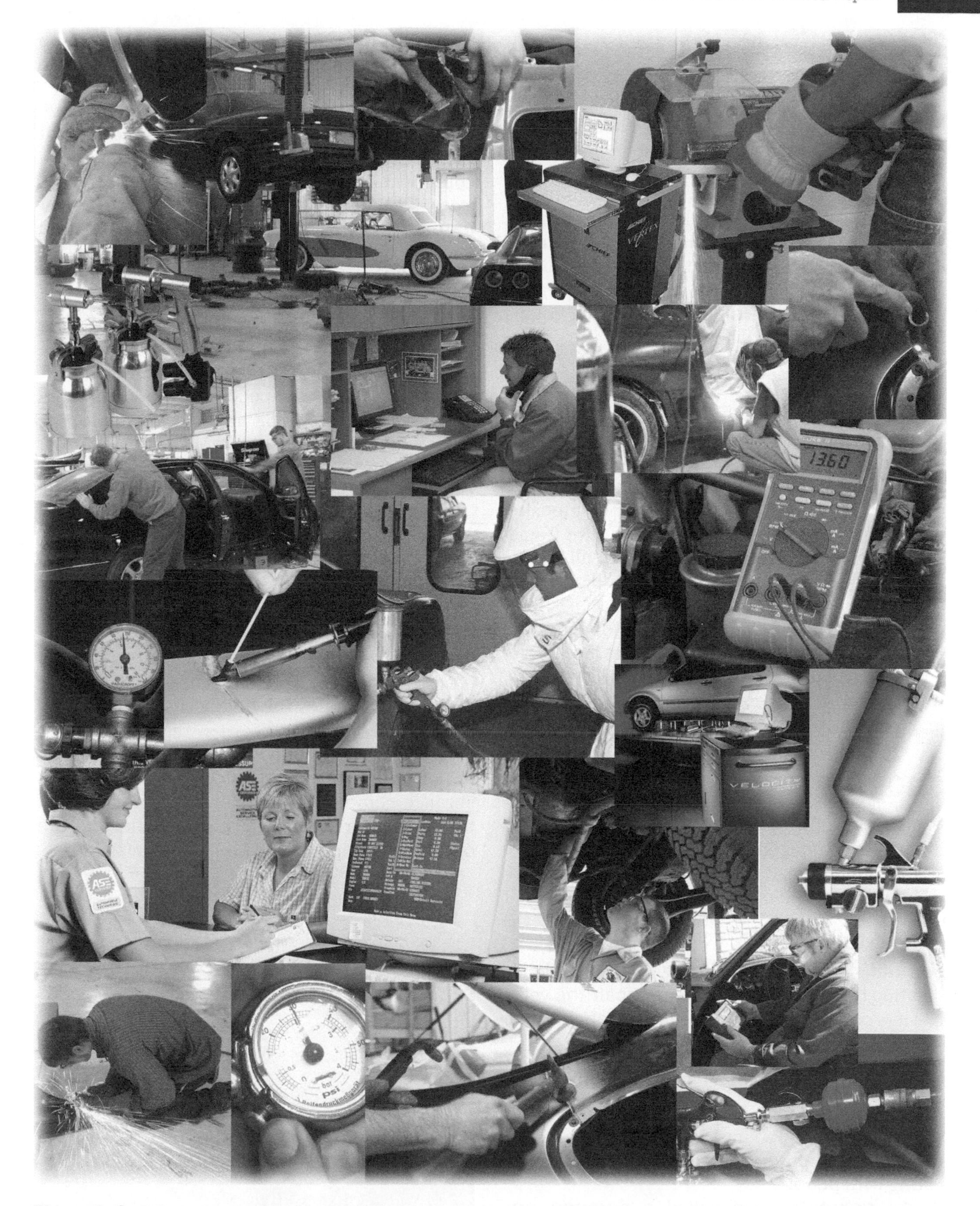

Figure 1–2. To be a good auto body technician, you must have some of the skills of a welder, sculptor, metalworker, auto mechanic, electrician, painter, and other tradespeople.

WHAT IS COLLISION REPAIR?

Collision repair is the process of restoring a damaged vehicle back to a "like new" condition by repairing both structural and cosmetic damage. Another term for collision repair is "auto body repair."

With minor damage, this can be as simple as replacing a bumper or a grille, or fixing a small dent. With major damage, this can be a complicated process, requiring that you partially disassemble the vehicle and use frame straightening equipment, welding equipment, spraying equipment, and other specialized tools.

WHAT IS A COLLISION?

A **collision** is an impact that causes damage to the vehicle body and chassis. Since vehicles can weigh more than a ton, metal parts can be crushed, bent, and torn. Plastic or composite parts can be broken and deformed. The frame might even be forced out of alignment, all resulting from the tremendous force of a collision.

A collision might be as minor as a "door ding" where someone accidentally opened the door and hit another car. Or, it might be severe enough to cause a **total loss,** where repairs would be more expensive than the cost of buying another vehicle.

SHOP OPERATIONS

Many types of workers are involved in repairing a collision damaged vehicle. It is important to have a general idea of the duties of everyone in a shop to succeed on the job.

Estimating

Estimating involves analyzing damage and calculating how much it will cost to repair the vehicle. It is critical that the quote on the repair is not too high nor too low.

In most shops, a trained **estimator** makes an appraisal of vehicle damage and determines the parts, materials, and labor needed to repair the vehicle. Estimators must be good with repair methods, computers, numbers, and communicating with people.

An **estimate,** also called a **damage appraisal or physical damage report,** is a written or printed form that explains what must be done to repair the vehicle. The estimate must explain which parts can be repaired and which will require replacement, summarizing all aspects of the repair and costs.

Manual estimating involves using an estimating sheet for writing out information about the vehicle, using crash estimating guides, and collision damage manuals to make the repair estimate. **Crash estimating books** and **collision damage manuals** contain vehicle identification information, the price of new parts, time needed to install the parts, refinishing or painting data, and other information.

Computer estimating involves using electronic **hardware** (computer, printers, hard drives, CD-ROM drives) and **software** (computer programs, CDs) to speed up the estimating process. The estimator might use a laptop to input which parts must be replaced or repaired. See **Figure 1–3.** This saves time over writing the estimate out longhand. When this information is entered, the computer can streamline the estimating processes by automating many steps of writing the estimate.

When making an estimate, the estimator must make sure no damage is overlooked. For example, with a major impact, he or she must check for damage to the suspension, engine, electrical system, and interior of the vehicle. Many parts besides the body can be affected by a collision.

The estimate is usually given to the customer, who gives the repair estimate to the insurance company. The insurance company will then select a repair shop or give a check to the owner for completing the repair.

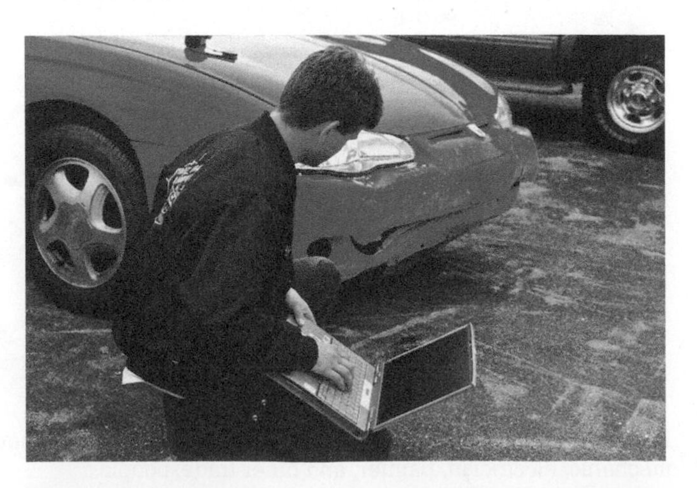

Figure 1–3. Here an estimator is using a laptop computer and estimating software to calculate costs of damage repair.

The **insurance adjuster/appraiser** reviews the estimates and determines which one best reflects how the vehicle should be repaired. He or she may inspect the collision damaged vehicle to make sure the repairs will be done cost effectively.

Once the owner and/or the insurance company approves the repairs, the vehicle is turned over to the shop supervisor. The supervisor and sometimes a technician will then review the estimate to determine how to proceed with the repair.

Washup

Washup involves a thorough cleaning of the automobile before beginning work. Mud, dirt, wax, and other contaminants must be cleaned off before starting body work. They could contaminate the work area and the new paint. The vehicle must be completely dry before being moved to the metalworking area.

Bodywork

The *bodywork area* is where the car is repaired in the shop. The damage can be the result of either a collision or deterioration. The repair tasks in this area of the facility are performed by collision repair technicians and their helpers. See **Figure 1–4.**

Depending upon the severity of the damage, the technician may have to remove and replace parts or simply use hand tools to work out small sheet metal dents.

Minor Repairs

Minor repairs are those that require minimum time and effort. Small dents, paint scratches, and damaged trim are typical examples. They require moderate skill and the use of hand tools, power tools, and collision repair tools. Refer to **Figure 1–5.**

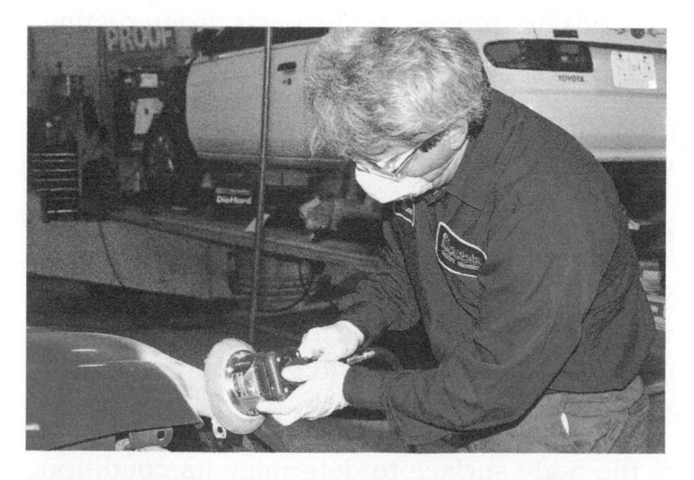

Figure 1–4. Here the auto body technician is using an air sander to level body filler on the dented body part.

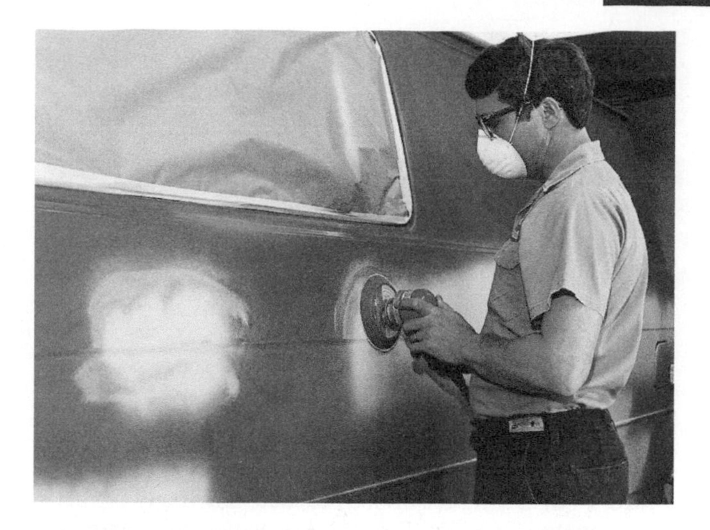

(A) Many kinds of sanders are used in collision repair. (Courtesy of PPG Industries, Inc.)

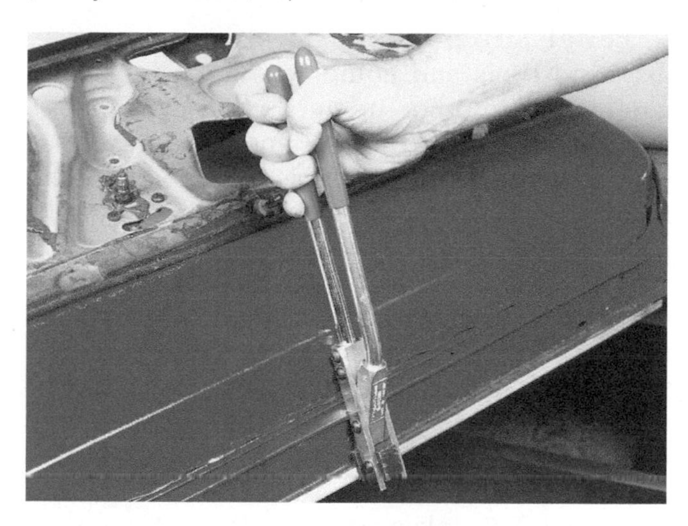

(B) Special pliers are designed to fold metal over a door frame during door skin replacement.

Figure 1–5. Many kinds of tools and equipment must be mastered by a collision repair technician.

Hand tools generally include tools used by both auto mechanics and collision repair technicians, such as wrenches, screwdrivers, and pliers. They are commonly used to remove parts, fenders, doors, and similar assemblies.

Power tools use air pressure or electrical energy to aid repairs. This classification includes air wrenches, air and electric drills, sanders, and similar tools.

Body shop tools are the most specialized tools designed for working with body parts. They can be used to cut metal, straighten small dents, and do similar tasks.

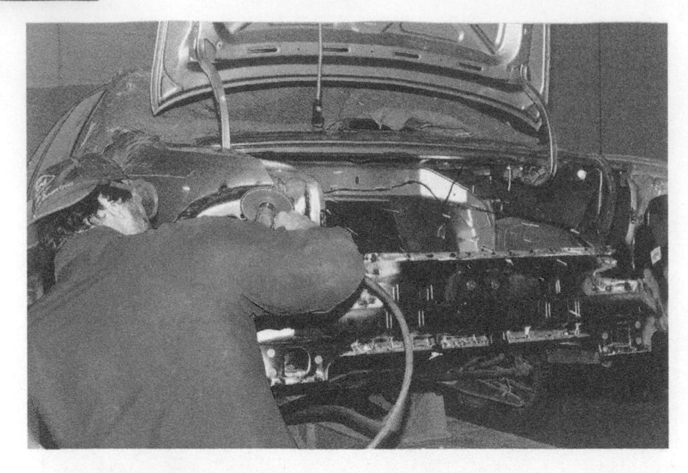

Figure 1–6. During major body repairs, new body panels must be welded in place. Note the rear panels that were replaced on this car.

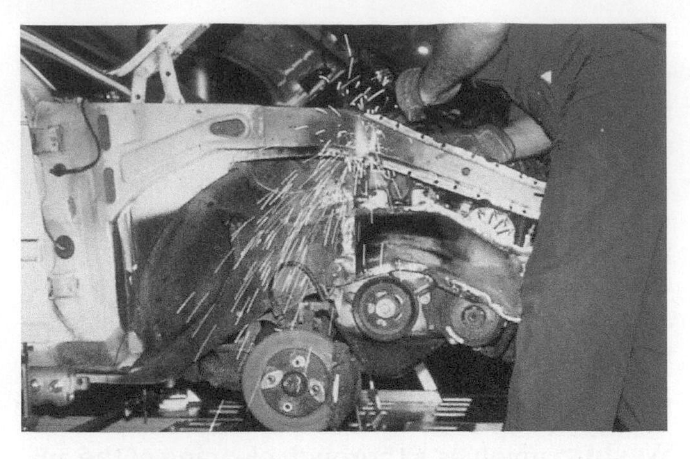

Figure 1–7. When straightening with a rack, you may have to use heat to aid component straightening. If a unibody structural component cannot be straightened, it must be cut off and a new piece must be welded into place. (Courtesy of Chief Automotive Systems, Inc.)

Panel straightening involves using various hand tools and equipment to reshape the panel back into its original contour. Dollies, body hammers, body filler, and sanders are a few of the tools and materials used to fix metal panel damage. Similar tools are needed with plastic or composite panels.

Panel replacement involves removing and installing a new panel or body part. It may be necessary to unbolt and replace a fender, door, or spoiler, for example, **Figure 1–6.** With quarter panels and other welded body sections, the technician has to cut off the damaged panel with power tools and then use a welder to install the new panel. This takes considerable skill.

Major Repairs

Major repairs is a general category that typically involves replacement of large body sections and frame or unibody straightening. To begin a major repair, the technician must normally remove severely damaged body parts, like fenders, bumpers, etc. Then measurements are taken at specific body points to analyze the damage. See **Figure 1–7.**

Measuring Systems allow you to check for frame or unibody misalignment resulting from a collision. Various types of gauges and measuring devices can be used to compare known good body specifications with the actual measurements. The measurements will help determine what must be done to straighten any frame or unibody misalignment. See **Figure 1–8.**

Once you have measured to determine the extent and direction of frame or unibody misalignment, you can use straightening equipment to straighten the frame back into alignment.

Frame straightening equipment, also called a **frame rack,** uses a large steel framework, pulling chains, and hydraulic power to pull or push the frame back into its original position. The vehicle frame or unibody is clamped down onto the frame-straightening equipment so it cannot move. Pulling chains are fastened to the damaged portion of the vehicle. Then tremendous hydraulic force is applied to the chains to pull the frame or body in the direction opposite the deformation.

After straightening, more measurements are taken to determine if everything is returned to specifications. If not, frame rails and other unibody sections may have to be replaced.

CORROSION PROTECTION

Corrosion protection involves using various methods to protect body parts from rusting. When doing repairs, you must always use recommended methods of protecting repair areas from rust. Discussed later in this book, there are various methods of corrosion protection.

SURFACE PREPARATION

Surface preparation, or "surface prep," involves getting the surface ready for painting. It is needed to make sure the repairs and new paint will hold up over time.

Begin with **surface inspection;** look closely at the body surface to determine its condition. This will let you decide what must be done to the surface to prepare it for new paint.

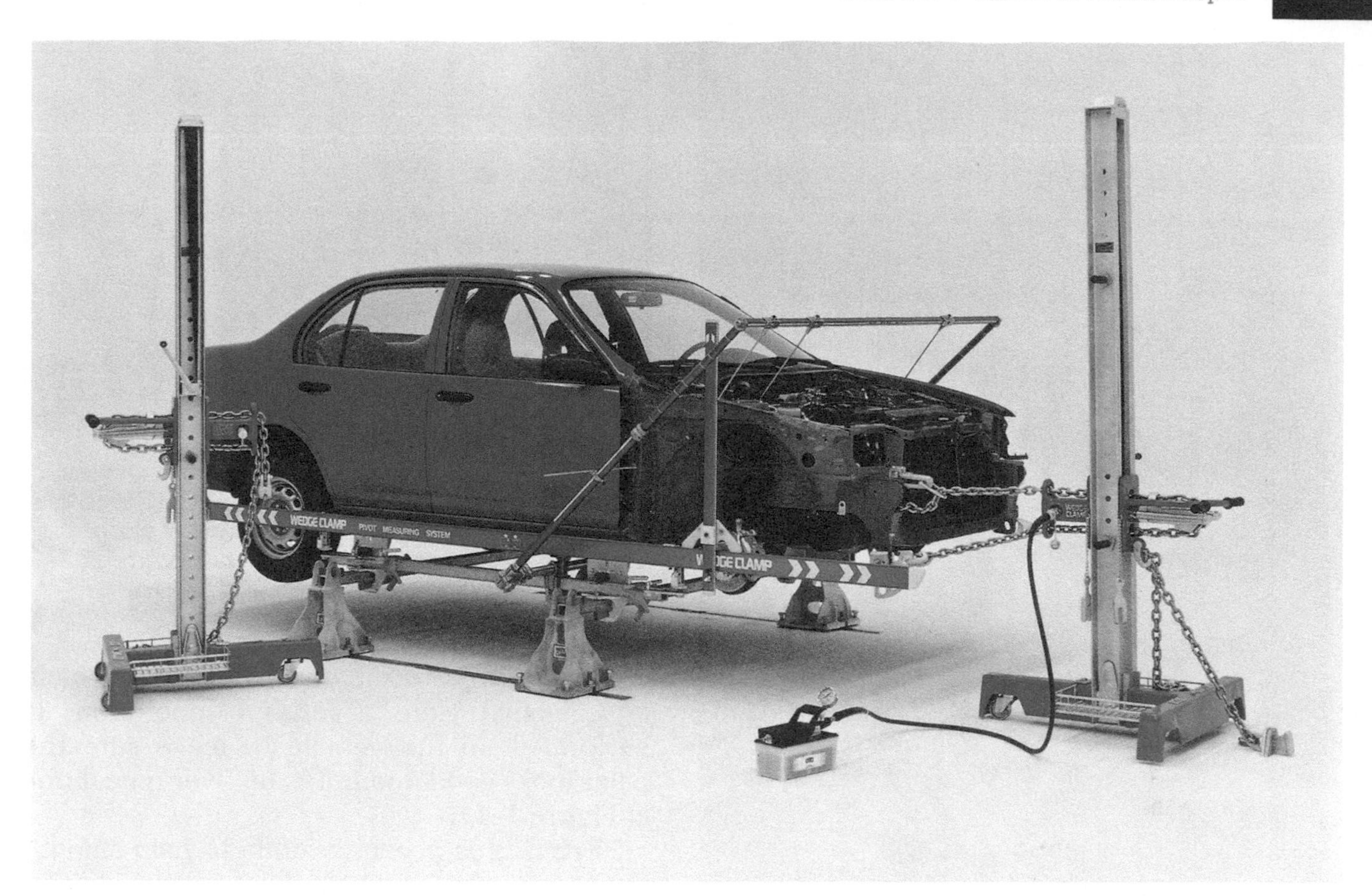

Figure 1–8. If the frame or unibody of the car has been damaged, a frame rack is often needed to pull out the structural damage. The frame or unibody is clamped down and large hydraulic tower chains are used to pull the vehicle back into its original shape. (Courtesy of Wedge Clamp)

You might only have to lightly scuff sand the surface to ready it for painting. If the paint is cracked and peeling, you may need to remove the paint. **Stripping** can be done by applying a chemical remover to soften and lift off the paint. Stripping can also be done using air-powered blasting equipment.

Sanding uses an abrasive coated paper or plastic backing to level and smooth a body surface being repaired. Sanding with coarse, rough paper may be done to level body filler. Sanding with fine, smooth paper may also be done to lightly scuff the surface so the new paint will stick.

Masking

Masking protects surfaces and parts from paint overspray. Masking protects the parts of the vehicle such as windows, trim, and lights. Masking is done by placing special tape, paper, or plastic over areas NOT to be painted.

Masking can also be done by spraying a special water-soluble material over surfaces not to be painted. The masking material can then be washed off with soap and water after painting. See **Figure 1–9.**

The **masking area** in the shop is usually equipped with masking paper and tape dispensers, tire covers, and other needed materials.

Paint overspray is an unwanted paint mist that spreads away from the surface being painted. It can stick to any uncovered or unmasked surface. Considerable time can then be wasted trying to clean off surfaces coated with a paint overspray. Masking is an important step before priming and painting.

REFINISHING (PAINTING)

Refinishing or **painting** basically involves applying primer and paint over the properly prepared vehicle body. It is the most visible aspect of collision repair. Although it does not affect vehicle safety, it does affect the customer's evaluation of the repair because it is easy to see paint defects. See **Figure 1–10.**

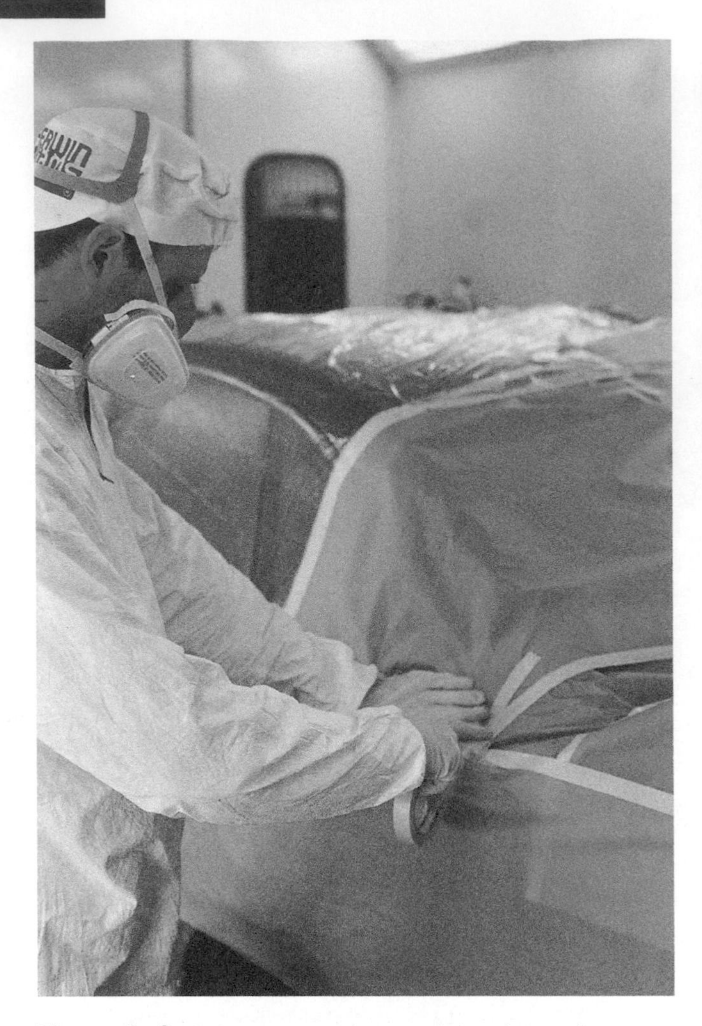

Figure 1–9. Paint prep involves readying the car for spraying by final sanding and masking to cover the parts not to be painted.

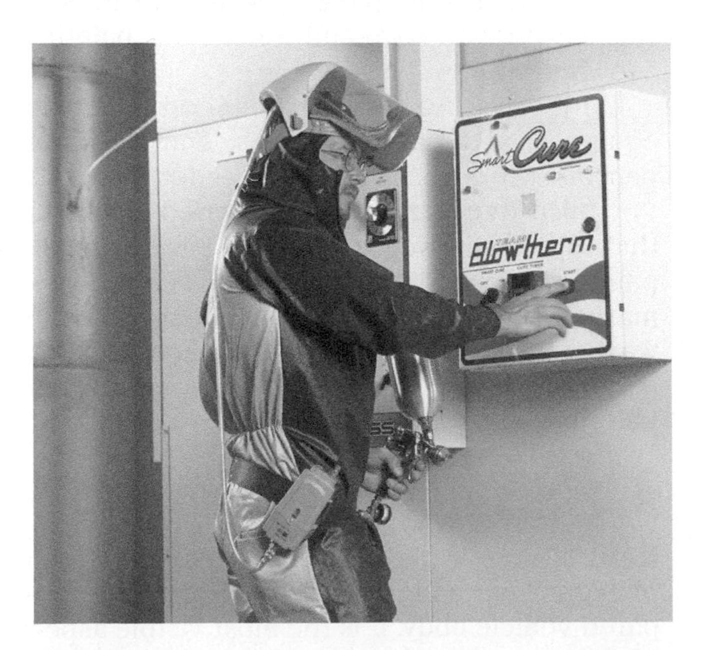

Figure 1–10. Collision repair facility personnel, if properly trained, can earn a good living. If you study and learn the contents of this book, you are on your way to a solid career in collision repair. (Courtesy of Team Blowtherm)

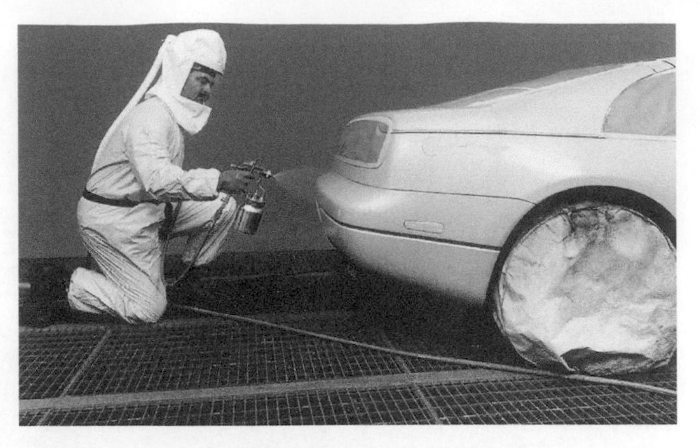

Figure 1–11. When painting, the technician must wear safety gear to protect the skin and the lungs from chemicals. A spray gun is used to apply thin, even coats of primer first and then color. Note how the lights and tire have been masked to prevent overspray. (Courtesy of PPG Industries, Inc.)

The **paint shop area** is where the vehicle is refinished. Here, a series of operations is performed on the vehicle to make sure the paint looks good and holds up over time. Look at **Figure 1–11.**

Priming is primarily done to help smooth the body surface and help the top coats of paint adhere or stick to the body. It is done before painting. Discussed in later chapters, various types of primer and other prepainting steps may be required.

Paint selection involves finding out what type of paint materials must be used on the specific vehicle. It must be done properly to make sure the paint matches the rest of the vehicle and to ensure long paint life. The technician must determine what kind of paint is on the car and then select the right paint for the job.

Paint mixing usually involves adding solvents to give the paint the right "thickness" or viscosity for spraying. It also may involve mixing in a recommended amount of catalyst (hardener) to make the paint cure. Instructions on the container will give information about the type of materials and ratio of paint-to-solvent or thinner required. Proper paint mixing is critical to how the paint flows out of the spray gun and onto the vehicle body. Incorrect mixing makes it impossible to do a good paint job.

Spraying is the physical application of color or primer using a paint spray gun. The technician methodically moves the spray gun next to the vehicle body while spraying accurate layers of paint onto it. This requires a high degree of skill to prevent **paint runs** (excess paint thickness that flows down or "runs") and other painting problems.

When the vehicle moves into the spray booth, the painting technician takes over. Final cleaning is done at this point. Masking is removed after the paint has completely dried.

Custom painting involves forming various designs in the paint. Precut mask designs, airbrush work, pinstriping, and other techniques can be used with custom painting.

Drying

Drying involves using different methods to cure the fresh paint. If only partially dry when returned to the customer, the new paint can be easily damaged.

Air drying is done by simply letting the paint dry in the atmosphere.

Forced drying uses special heat lamps or other equipment to speed the paint curing process. Most shops use drying equipment to speed up drying. This is especially useful in drying today's paints. Drying equipment designs vary.

Postpainting Operations

Postpainting operations include the tasks that must be done before returning the vehicle to the customer. This would include removal of masking tape, reinstalling parts, and cleaning. Any paint flaws or problems must also be repaired.

Wet sanding involves using a water-resistant, ultrafine sandpaper and water to level the paint. It can sometimes be done to fix small imperfections (orange peel, runs, etc.) in the paint. Wet sanding and buffing can also be done to a good paint job to make it even better looking.

Compounding or *buffing* is done to smooth newly painted surfaces, after wet sanding, for example, or to remove a thin layer of old, dull paint. See **Figure 1–12.** It will make the paint smooth and shiny. An air or electric buffing machine equipped with a pad is used to apply buffing compound to the finish. The abrasive action cuts off a thin layer of topcoat to brighten the color and shine the paint.

Detailing is a final cleanup and touch-up on the vehicle. It involves washing body sections, cleaning and vacuuming the interior, touching up any chips in sections not painted, and other tasks to improve vehicle cosmetics. Detailing can also involve other tasks such as polishing trim, cleaning glass, installing trim, and cleaning the tires. This will ready the vehicle for return to the customer.

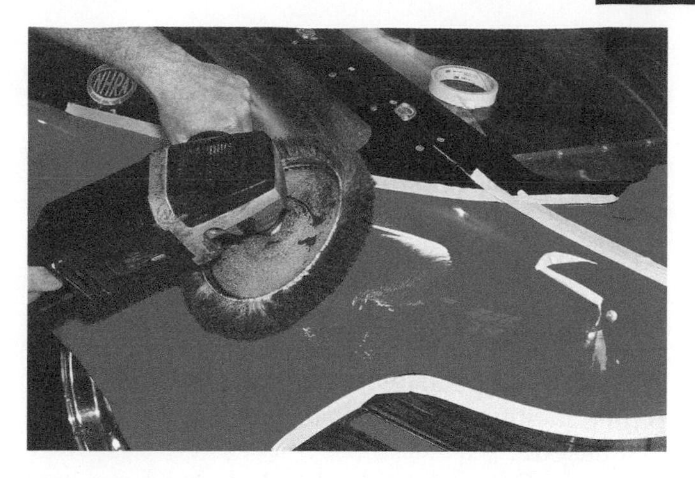

Figure 1–12. Buffing is done to restore gloss or shine to paint. If the paint is old, it can be buffed with a compound and buffing machine to restore shine. If new paint has minor problems, it can be wet sanded and buffed to remove minor flaws.

Mechanical-Electrical Repairs

Mechanical repairs include tasks like replacing a damaged water pump, radiator, or engine bracket, for example. Mechanical components like these are often damaged in a collision. Many mechanical parts are easy to replace and can be done by the collision repair technician. However, other mechanical repairs may require special skills and tools. In this case, the vehicle would be sent to a professional mechanic. See **Figure 1–13.**

Electrical repairs include tasks like repairing severed wiring, replacing engine sensors,

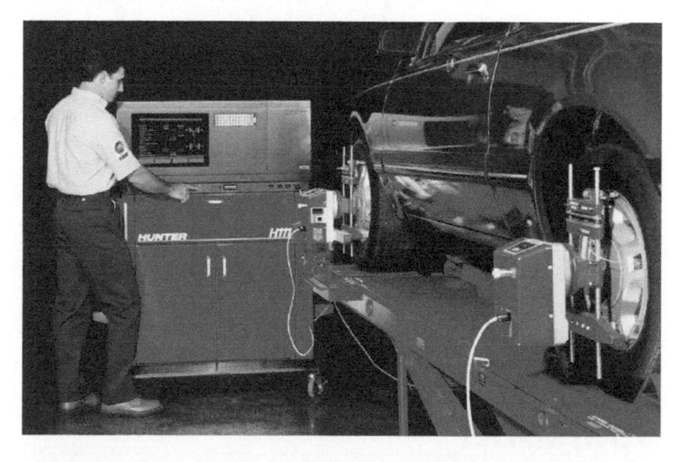

Figure 1–13. Mechanical repairs are sometimes done in larger collision repair shops. An alignment rack has all of the equipment needed to check and correct alignment of wheels. This is often needed after collision repairs. (Courtesy Hunter Engineering Company)

and scanning for computer or wiring problems. During a collision, the impact on the vehicle and the resulting metal deformation can easily crush wires and electrical components. For this reason, today's collision repair technician must have the basic skills needed to work with and repair electrical/electronic components.

COLLISION REPAIR FACILITIES

There are several ways to classify a collision repair facility. A few of the most common are discussed.

An **independent body shop** is one owned and operated by a private individual. The shop is NOT associated with other shops or companies.

A **franchise facility** is tied to a main headquarters that regulates and aids the operation of the business. The shop logo, materials used, pricing, and the like are all set by the headquarters, and the franchise must follow these guidelines.

A **dealership body shop** is owned and managed under the guidance of a new car dealership—Ford, GM, Chrysler, Toyota, etc. This type of shop often concentrates on repairs of the specific make of vehicles sold by the dealership.

A **progression shop** is often organized like an assembly line with specialists in each area of repair. One person might do nothing but "frame" work. Another technician might be good at "building the body" or installing parts and panels. The shop might have a wheel alignment technician, prep people, painter, and cleanup specialists. The vehicle will move from one area and specialist to the next until fully repaired.

A **specialty shop** concentrates on and only does specific types of repairs. For example, a collision repair facility might send a radiator with a small hole in it to a specialty radiator shop for repair with their specialized equipment.

Complete collision services means the facility might do wheel alignments, cooling system repairs, electrical system diagnosis and repair, suspension system work, and other repairs. Today, more and more collision repair shops are offering complete collision services.

SUMMARY

- Collision repair involves repairing damage after a vehicle has been in an accident. Another term for "collision repair" is *auto body repair.*
- A collision is an impact that causes damage to the vehicle body and chassis.
- There are several ways to classify a collision repair facility. A few of the most common are: independent, franchise, dealership, progression, specialty, and complete collision services.

TECHNICAL TERMS

collision repair technicians
shop owner
shop supervisor
parts manager
bookkeeper
office manager
helper
apprentice
professional
collision repair
collision
total loss
estimating
estimator
estimate
damage appraisal
physical damage report
manual estimating
crash estimating books
collision damage manuals
computer estimating
hardware
software
insurance adjuster/appraiser
washup
minor repairs
hand tools
power tools
body shop tools
panel straightening
panel replacement
major repairs
frame straightening equipment
frame rack
corrosion protection
surface preparation
surface inspection
stripping
sanding
masking
masking area
paint overspray
refinishing
painting
paint shop area
priming
paint selection
paint mixing
spraying
paint runs
custom painting
drying
air drying
forced drying
postpainting operations
wet sanding
compounding
detailing
mechanical repairs
electrical repairs
independent body shop

franchise facility
dealership body shop
progression shop
specialty shop
complete collision services

REVIEW QUESTIONS

1. What happened to the first self-propelled vehicle?
2. ________ ________ ________ are skilled, knowledgeable people who know how to use specialized equipment and highly technical methods to restore collision damaged vehicles.
3. List and explain the basic skills often required of a repair technician.
4. The term "professional" refers to the ________, ________, and ________ that a business and its workers project to customers.
5. List six traits of a professional technician.
6. Define the term "collision repair."
7. What is a "total loss?"
8. ________ involves analyzing damage and calculating how much it will cost to repair the vehicle.
9. What is the job of an insurance adjuster/ appraiser?
10. ________ ________ involves using various hand tools and equipment to bend or shape the panel back into its original contour.
11. Why would you use a measurement system?
12. ________ ________ ________, also called a ________ ________, uses a large steel framework, pulling chains, and hydraulic power to pull or push the frame back into its original position.
13. Explain two ways to strip off deteriorated paint quickly.
14. Give two reasons for sanding a body surface.
15. Basically, how and why do you mask a car?
16. ________ ________ ________ means the facility might do wheel alignments, cooling system repairs, electrical system repairs, suspension system work, and other repairs.

ASE-STYLE REVIEW QUESTIONS

1. Which of the following jobs is NOT part of the collision repair industry?
   a. Metalwork
   b. Auto repair technician
   c. Finance agent
   d. Welder

2. *Technician A* says that collision damage is caused by an impact on the vehicle body and/or chassis. *Technician B* says that opening a car door and accidentally hitting another vehicle is a collision. Who is correct?
   a. Technician A
   b. Technician B
   c. Both Technicians A and B
   d. Neither Technician

3. *Technician A* says that an estimate is the analyzing of damage and a calculation of the repair cost. *Technician B* says that the estimate is a guide for the repair of the vehicle. Who is correct?
   a. Technician A
   b. Technician B
   c. Both Technicians A and B
   d. Neither Technician

4. *Technician A* says that the first step in collision repair is disassembly of the vehicle. *Technician B* says that the first step is washing the vehicle. Who is correct?
   a. Technician A
   b. Technician B
   c. Both Technicians A and B
   d. Neither Technician

5. *Technician A* says that major repair is a general term that refers to repairs that involve replacement of large body parts. *Technician B* says that corrosion protection involves using various methods to protect body parts from rusting. Who is correct?
   a. Technician A
   b. Technician B
   c. Both Technicians A and B
   d. Neither Technician

6. *Technician A* says that masking is a job done by the frame repair technician. *Technician B* says that masking is a job done in the paint department. Who is correct?
   a. Technician A
   b. Technician B
   c. Both Technicians A and B
   d. Neither Technician

7. *Technician A* says that detailing is a job done by the office manager. *Technician B* says that detailing is the final cleanup and touch-up to the vehicle. Who is correct?
   a. Technician A
   b. Technician B
   c. Both Technicians A and B
   d. Neither Technician

ACTIVITIES

1. Ask a technician or shop owner to visit your classroom. Ask him or her to describe the duties of his or her position.
2. Make a field trip to a collision repair facility. Have the shop owner or supervisor give you a guided tour of the shop. Discuss the field trip in class the next day.

CHAPTER

2 Safety, ASE Certification

OBJECTIVES

After studying this chapter, you should be able to:

- List the types of dangers and accidents common to a collision repair facility.
- Explain how to avoid shop accidents.
- Outline the control measures needed when working with hazardous substances.
- Summarize hand and power tool safety.
- Describe safety practices designed to avoid fire and explosions.
- Explain the benefits of ASE certification.
- Summarize the purpose of I-CAR.
- Know the sources of professional training and certification available to collision repair facility personnel.

INTRODUCTION

Safety involves working intelligently to prevent personal injury and property damage. A collision repair facility can be a very dangerous place to work if safety rules are not followed. Carelessness and safety mistakes can be deadly.

It is up to you to learn and follow accepted safety rules. Remember that you must still read all tool, equipment, and material instructions because they will give more specific details than this chapter.

Most injuries are caused by ignoring accepted safety rules. Smart technicians never gamble with their well-being by ignoring safety practices. See **Figure 2–1.** They know that shop safety does not waste time. It protects the most important investment—your health.

Some injuries happen instantly, while others result from prolonged exposure over time. For example, if you fail to wear leather gloves when welding, you can be burned in a split second. If you fail to wear a dust mask or respirator when sanding filler, you may not have symptoms of injury until years later when you are diagnosed with lung cancer.

WHAT CAUSES ACCIDENTS?

Accidents are unplanned events that hurt people, break tools, damage vehicles, or have other adverse effects on the business and its employees. Since a collision repair facility has so many potential sources of danger, safety must be your number one concern.

Remember! Accidents do not just happen; people cause accidents!

TYPES OF ACCIDENTS

Care must be taken to prevent several kinds of accidents, including asphyxiation, chemical burns, electrocution, fires, and explosions.

Asphyxiation refers to anything that prevents normal breathing. There are many mists, gases, and fumes in a collision repair facility that can damage your lungs and affect your ability to breathe.

Chemical burns result when a corrosive chemical such as paint remover injures your skin or eyes.

Electrocution results when electricity passes through your body. Severe injury or death can result.

A **fire** is rapid oxidation of a flammable material, producing high temperatures. A burn from a fire can cause painful injuries and permanent scar tissue. There are numerous **combustibles** (paints, solvents, reducers, gasoline, dirty rags)

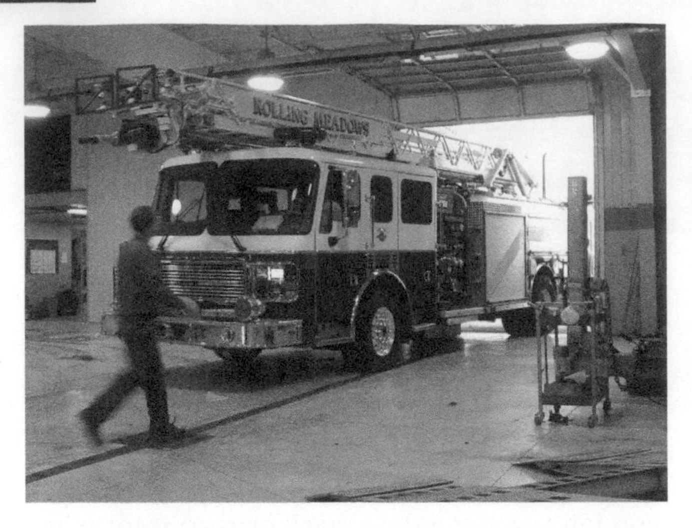

(A) The technician is slowly and safely pulling a huge fire truck into the body shop for minor paint work.

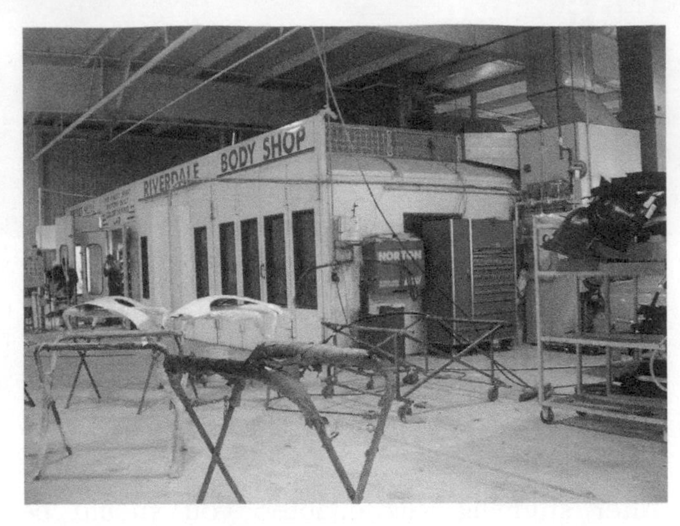

(C) The prep area outside the paint booth is used for final sanding and masking work prior to painting.

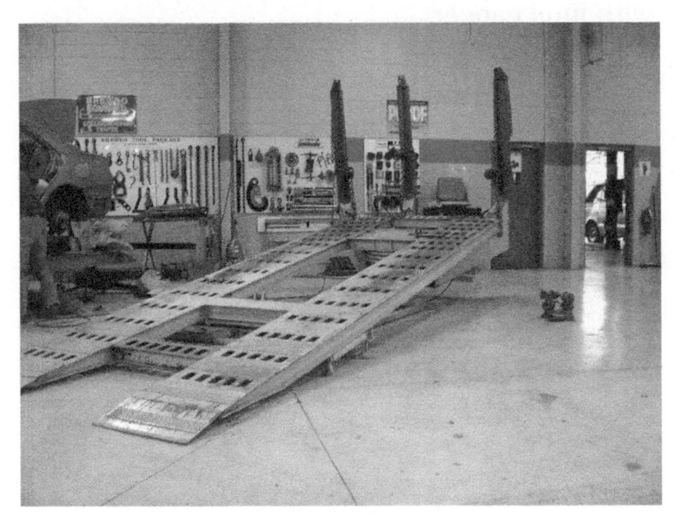

(B) The metal working area has tools and equipment for repairing the body-frame structure of a vehicle. The frame rack can exert tons of pulling traction and can be very dangerous if misused.

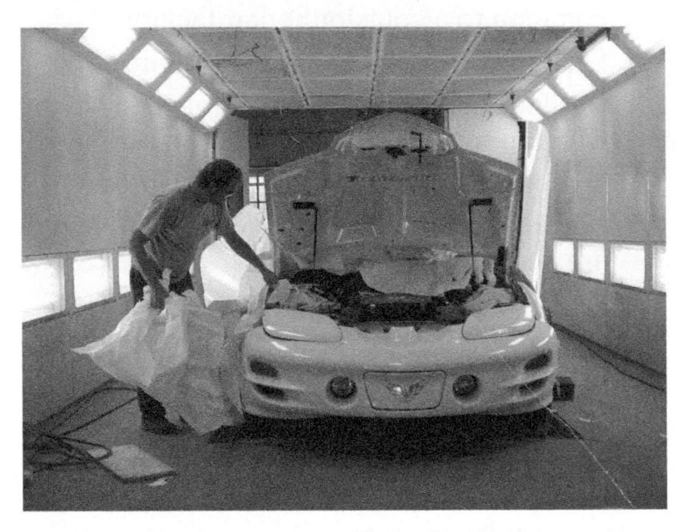

(D) The technician has just finished baking the paint job in the drying room of the paint booth.

Figure 2–1. A body shop or collision repair facility can be a safe and rewarding place to work if everyone follows established safety rules. If anyone fails to follow these rules, it can be a dangerous place of employment.

in a collision repair facility. Any one of these can quickly cause a fire.

Explosions are air pressure waves that result from extremely rapid burning. For example, if you were to weld near a gas tank, it could explode. The fumes in the tank could ignite and the tank could blow open.

Physical injury is a general category that includes cuts, broken bones, strained backs, and similar injuries. To prevent these painful injuries, constantly think and evaluate each step. Always think about what you are doing and try to do it safely.

TEXTBOOK SAFETY

Thousands of collision repair technicians are injured or killed every year. Broken safety rules cause most of these accidents.

Do not learn to respect safety rules the difficult way—by experiencing a painful injury. Learn to respect safety the easy way—by studying this book and following known safety practices.

Manufacturer's instructions are very detailed procedures for a specific product. They are written to guide you in the use of the exact item, whether it be a piece of equipment or a certain type of paint.

Always refer to manufacturer's instructions. They may be in the owner's instruction manual for tools and equipment. With paint and chemicals, they are normally printed on the container's label, product information sheet, or material safety data sheet (MSDS).

OVERALL SHOP SAFETY

True professionalism and shop safety begins with how a technician performs given work tasks. A professional understands the ever-present dangers in a collision repair facility and strives to avoid making dangerous mistakes.

You will be using air and electric tools, welders, cutting equipment, hydraulic frame straightening equipment, and hazardous materials. If you do not know or do not follow correct methods, you or someone else may be seriously injured. See **Figure 2–2.**

Accidents have a far-reaching effect, not only on the victim, but also on the victim's family and friends. Therefore, it is the obligation of all employees and the employer to develop a safety program. A **safety program** is a written shop policy designed to protect the health and welfare of personnel and customers. It includes rules on everything from equipment use to disposal of hazardous chemicals.

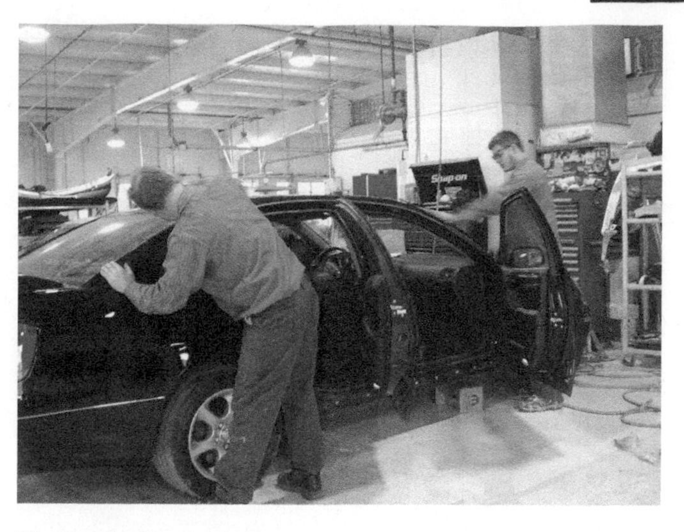

Figure 2–2. Here technicians are helping each other install a long piece of trim. Cooperation among employees is good for everyone in the facility. It increases production, profits, income, and safety.

SHOP LAYOUT AND SAFETY

The **shop layout** is the general organization or arrangement of work areas. For various safety reasons, you should fully understand the layout of your shop. This will help you learn fire exit routes, fire extinguisher locations, storage areas, and other information to make you a better worker. Study the typical collision repair facility layout in **Figure 2–3.**

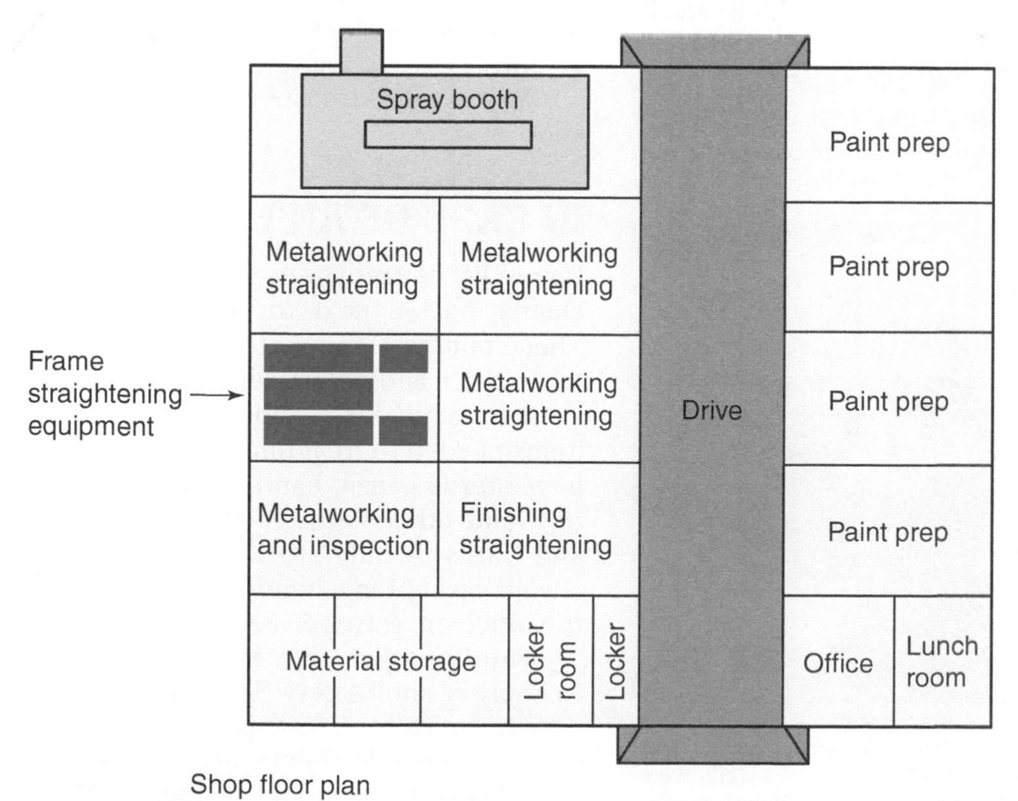

Figure 2–3. Collision repair shop layouts vary. Learn the layout of your shop. Memorize fire extinguisher locations and fire exit routes.

A collision repair facility is typically divided into these work areas:

1. Metalworking area
2. Repair stall
3. Frame straightening equipment
4. Front end rack (alignment rack)
5. Tool and equipment storage room
6. Classroom area
7. Paint preparation area
8. Finishing or spray area
9. Office
10. Locker room

The **metalworking area** is where parts are removed, repaired, and installed. This is the largest area in the shop where many tasks are performed. Dangers in this area are many and varied—cutting metal, welding, grinding, etc. See **Figure 2–4.**

A **repair stall** is a work area for one vehicle. Also termed a **bay,** it is usually marked off with painted lines on the floor. The stall has room in the front, rear, and sides for working on the vehicle. Stalls are often marked off in metalworking and prep areas.

The frame rack is a large piece of equipment designed to straighten damaged vehicle structures. It has powerful hydraulic rams and arms that require skill, training, and safety for use. It can exert tons of pulling force that can injure. If a frame rack chain were to come loose or break, it could fly with a tremendously destructive force. See Figure 2–4.

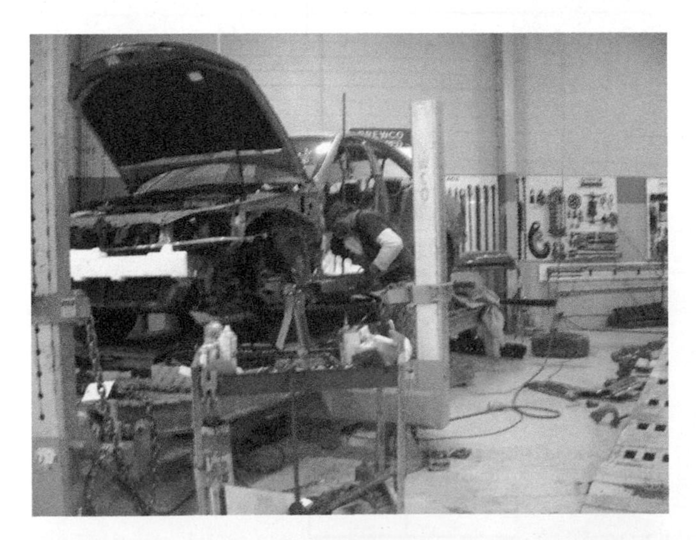

Figure 2–4. The frame rack has potential to cause serious injury. Pulling chains can exert tons of force. If a chain were to break or slip off the vehicle, it could fly back with deadly force.

A **front end rack** or **alignment rack** is used to measure and adjust the steering and suspension of a vehicle before and after repairs. It is needed to make sure the wheels are aligned to factory specifications. Dangers result from driving vehicles up and onto the rack and from using the small **pneumatic** (air) or **hydraulic** (oil-filled) equipment.

The **tool and equipment storage room** is an area for safely keeping specialized tools and equipment. It may have a pegboard wall or shelves for keeping tools that are not in use. Dangers result only if tools are not stored and maintained properly.

A **classroom** may be provided for lectures, demonstrations, and meetings of shop personnel.

The **paint prep area** is where the vehicle is readied for painting or refinishing. The vehicle is cleaned and masked in this area.

The **finishing area** or **spray booth** is where the body is painted. It normally has a large metal enclosure to keep out dirt and circulate clean, fresh air.

The **shop office** contains business equipment. This area keeps the shop financially sound. Office workers keep track of paperwork, making sure estimates are accurate, bills are paid, parts are ordered, and that payroll checks go out.

As you will learn, specific rules apply to each shop area.

IN CASE OF AN EMERGENCY

Have a list of **emergency telephone numbers** clearly posted next to the shop's telephone. These numbers should include a doctor, hospital, and fire and police departments.

A **first aid kit** includes many of the medical items needed to treat minor shop injuries. It will have sterile gauze, bandages, scissors, antiseptics, and other items to help treat minor cuts and burns. A fully stocked first aid kit should always be kept in a handy location, usually near the office or restroom. See **Figure 2–5.**

Safety signs give information that helps to improve shop safety. Signs are often posted to denote fire exits, extinguisher locations, dangerous or flammable chemicals, and other information. Safety signs should be located throughout the shop.

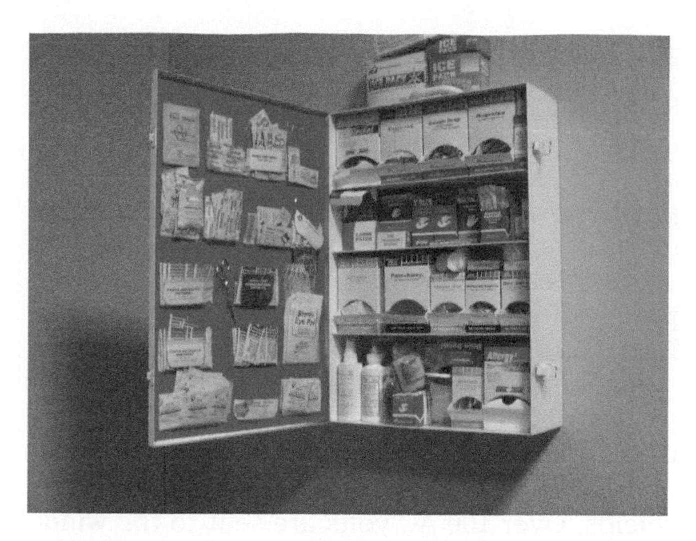

Figure 2–5. Know the location of the shop's first aid kit. The kit should be kept fully stocked with supplies to treat minor injuries.

WORK AREA SAFETY

It is very important that the work area be kept safe. This must be a "team effort" involving everyone working in the shop.

Keep all surfaces clean, dry, and orderly. Wipe up any oil, coolant, or grease on the floor. If someone were to slip and fall, it could result in serious injuries.

Hang tools up or put them away when they are not in use. Roll up idle hoses and air lines so they do not create traffic hazards.

Floor jacks, bumper jacks, jack stands, and creepers should be kept in their designated area, out of aisles and walkways.

FIRE SAFETY

Gasoline is a highly flammable petroleum or crude oil-based liquid that vaporizes and burns rapidly. Always keep gasoline and diesel fuel in approved safety cans. Never use them to wash your hands or tools.

Oily, greasy, or paint-soaked rags should be stored in an approved metal container with a lid. When soiled rags are left lying about improperly, they are prime candidates for **spontaneous combustion** (fire that starts by itself).

Use only approved explosion-proof equipment in hazardous locations. An **Underwriters Laboratories (UL)**–approved drum transfer pump along with a drum vent should be used when working with drums to transfer chemicals.

Keep all solvent containers closed when not in use. Handle all solvents and other liquids with care to avoid spillage.

Store paints, solvents, pressurized containers, and other combustible materials in approved and designated storage cabinets or rooms. Storage rooms should have adequate ventilation.

Never light matches or smoke in the spraying area! The paint mist and fumes are extremely explosive.

Vehicle batteries often explode! Hydrogen gas in the air near vehicle batteries can cause the battery to go off like a small bomb. Flying chunks of plastic and sulfuric acid can cause serious injury. Charge batteries only in a well-ventilated area.

Do not use torches or welding equipment at the mixing bench or in the paint area.

Never use automotive-type paints on household items such as toys or furniture. This could pose a dangerous health hazard to anyone who might ingest the paint.

Trash and rubbish should be removed from the shop area regularly. If it is not, serious fire and work area dangers can result.

Hold a rag around a fuel line fitting when disconnecting it.

You must release fuel pressure on many fuel injected vehicles before working on them because they can retain fuel pressure. Disconnect the battery before working on a fuel system.

Keep gas cylinders away from sources of heat like a furnace or room heater.

Never drop a gas cylinder. The head could break off and cause serious injury. Shut off the main gas valve on top of the tank after use—if a hose leak develops, this can prevent an explosion.

Electrical Fires

Electrical fires result when excess current causes wiring to overheat, melt, and burn. This often results when a wire or wires are short to ground while doing electrical work or after the collision cuts through wire insulation. To prevent electrical fires, always disconnect the battery when doing electrical work or when damage may have cut through wires.

Fire Extinguishers

A **fire extinguisher** is designed to quickly smother a fire. There are several types available for putting out different kinds of fires. See **Figure 2–6.**

Know where the fire extinguishers are located in your shop. During a fire, a few seconds can be a "lifetime" for someone.

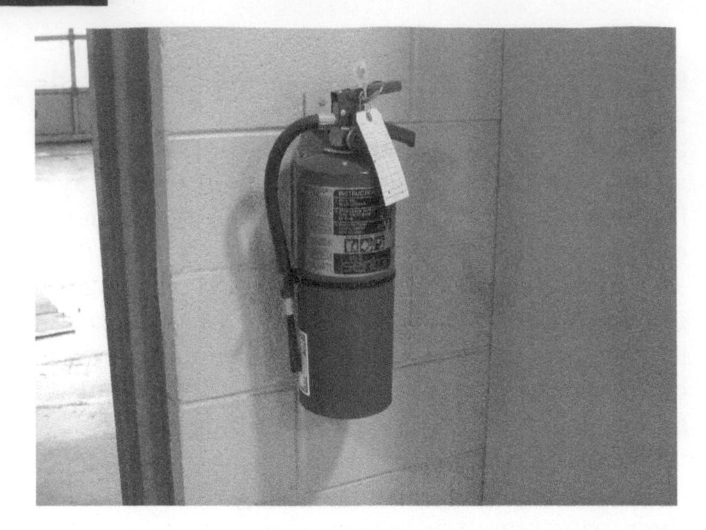

Figure 2–6. Memorize the location of all fire extinguishers in your shop. A few seconds during a fire can be a lifetime.

Never smoke while working on any vehicle or machine in the shop. There are too many flammables that could start a fire.

In case of a gasoline fire, do not use water. Water will spread the fire. Use a fire extinguisher to smother the flames. Never open doors or windows unless it is absolutely necessary. The draft will only make the fire worse.

A good rule is to call the fire department first and then attempt to extinguish the fire. Standing 6 to 10 feet (2 to 3 meters) from the fire, hold the extinguisher firmly in the recommended position. Aim the nozzle at the base of the fire and use a side-to-side motion, sweeping the entire width of the fire.

Stay low to avoid inhaling the smoke. If it gets too hot or too smoky, get out. Remember, never go back into a burning building.

AVOIDING FALLS

Keep all shop floor drain covers snugly in place. Open drains have caused many toe, ankle, and leg injuries.

To clean up oil, use a commercial oil absorbent. Spread the absorbent on the spill. Rub it with your broom in a circular motion. Then use a dust pan and broom to pick up the absorbent.

Make sure that aisles and walkways are kept clean and wide enough for safe movement. Provide for adequate work space around all machines. Cluttered walking areas contain items waiting to cause injury. Never leave tools or a creeper lying on the floor.

AVOIDING ELECTROCUTION

Keep all water off the floor. Remember that water is a conductor of electricity. A serious shock hazard will result if a live wire happens to fall into a puddle in which a person is standing. The floor must be dry when using electric power tools.

Electrocution results when electric current passes through the human body. This can affect heart and brain functions, possibly causing serious injury or death.

Disconnect electrical power before performing any service on a machine or tool.

Some late model vehicles have heated windshields. Over 100 AC volts are sent to the windshield to quickly warm the glass for melting ice and snow. This can be enough voltage and current to cause serious injury. Hybrid vehicles can also have high voltage/current devices that can cause electrical shock.

AVOIDING ASPHYXIATION

Make certain the work area is well lit and **ventilated** (that it has good supply of fresh air flowing through it).

Vehicle engine exhaust produces deadly **carbon monoxide (CO)** gas, which is odorless and invisible. Connect a shop vent hose to the tailpipe of any vehicle being operated in the shop.

Check and service furnaces and water heaters in the shop at least once every 6 months.

Asbestos dust used in the manufacture of older brake and clutch assemblies is a cancer-causing agent. Never blow this dust into the shop. Use a vacuum system while wearing a filter mask to clean off asbestos dust safely.

Proper ventilation is also important in areas where caustics, degreasers, undercoats, and finishes are used. Ventilation can be by means of an air-changing system, extraction floors, or a central dust extraction system.

Set the parking brake when working on a vehicle with the engine running. If the vehicle has an **automatic transmission** (shifts through gears automatically using hydraulic system), place it in park.

With a **manual transmission** (must be hand shifted through each forward gear), the vehicle should be in reverse (engine off) or neutral (engine on) unless instructed otherwise for a specific service operation.

AVOIDING EYE INJURIES

Remember that your eyes are irreplaceable. They are very delicate and can be permanently damaged in a split second. Human eyes are sensitive to dust, flying particles from grinding, and mists or vapors from spraying. Such exposure could cause severe eye injury and possibly the loss of sight.

When risks to your eyes exist, wear appropriate eye or face protection. See **Figure 2–7.**

A good pair of **safety glasses** is suitable with only minor danger, as when blowing off dust or sanding with an air sander.

Wear a **full-face shield** when there is more danger from flying particles, as when grinding.

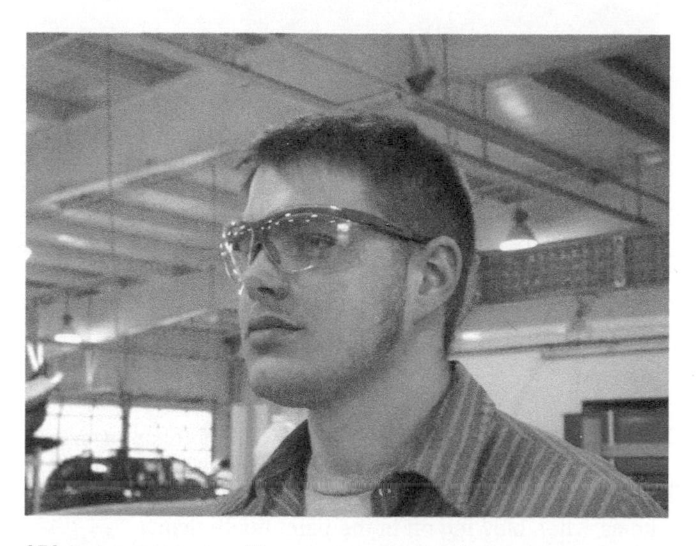

(A) Safety glasses will protect your eyes but not your face.

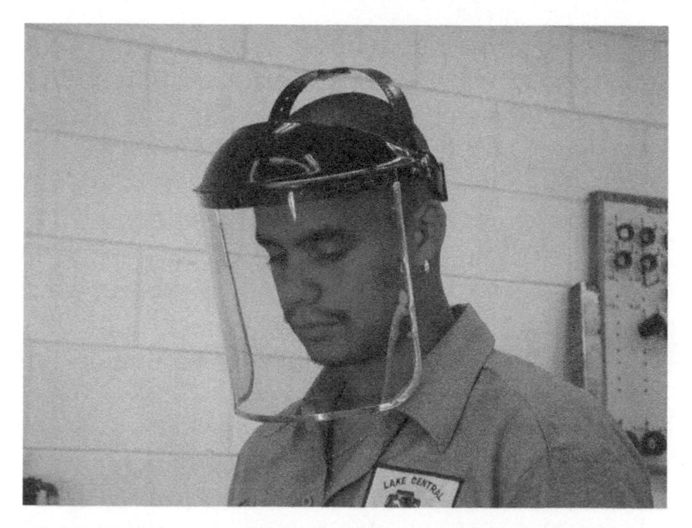

(B) A full-face shield is better when grinding or doing repair operations that can throw material out violently.

Figure 2–7. Your eyes cannot be replaced. Always wear appropriate eye protection for the job you are working on.

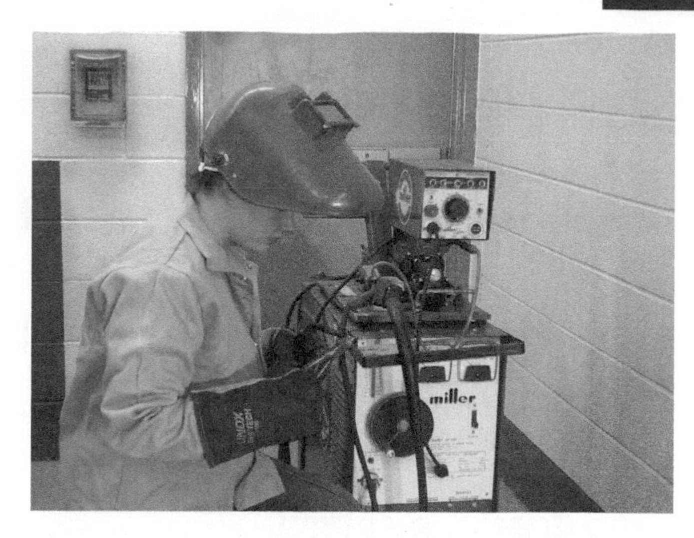

Figure 2–8. When electric welding, the arc is bright enough to burn your eyes and cause permanent damage. Wear a welding helmet, leather gloves, and nonflammable clothing.

Wear chemical splash **goggles** when handling solvents, thinners, reducers, and other similar liquids. Because the eyes are very susceptible to irritation, approved safety goggles should also be worn when paint mists are present.

A welding helmet or welding goggles with the proper shade lens must be worn when welding. These will protect your eyes and face from flying molten metal and harmful light rays. See **Figure 2–8.**

AVOIDING CHEMICAL BURNS

There are many sources of chemical burns in a collision repair facility. Cleaners, some paints, refrigerants, and solvents can cause skin and eye burns. A few rules to follow to prevent chemical burns include:

- Remove solvent-soaked clothing. The cloth will hold these chemicals against the skin, causing skin irritation or a chemical burn. Wear long sleeves for added protection.
- Wear **rubber** or **plastic gloves** to protect yourself from the harmful effects of corrosive liquids, undercoats, and finishes. Use impervious gloves when working with solvents or two-component primers and topcoats. These gloves offer special protection from the chemicals found in two-component systems.

DANGER

Chemical paint remover is very powerful. When using it, use extreme caution and protective gear.

When washing hands, use a proper **hand cleaner.** Never use thinner as a hand cleaner. Many chemicals can be absorbed into the skin, eventually causing long-term illnesses.

PERSONAL SAFETY

Personal appearance and conduct can help prevent accidents. Follow these general guidelines for personal safety.

Loose clothing, unbuttoned shirt sleeves, dangling ties, loose jewelry, and shirts hanging out are very dangerous. Instead, wear approved shop coveralls or jumpsuits. Pants should be long enough to cover the top of the shoes.

A clean **jumpsuit** or **lint-free coveralls** should be worn when in the spraying area. Dirty clothing can transfer dirt to freshly painted surfaces. See **Figure 2–9.**

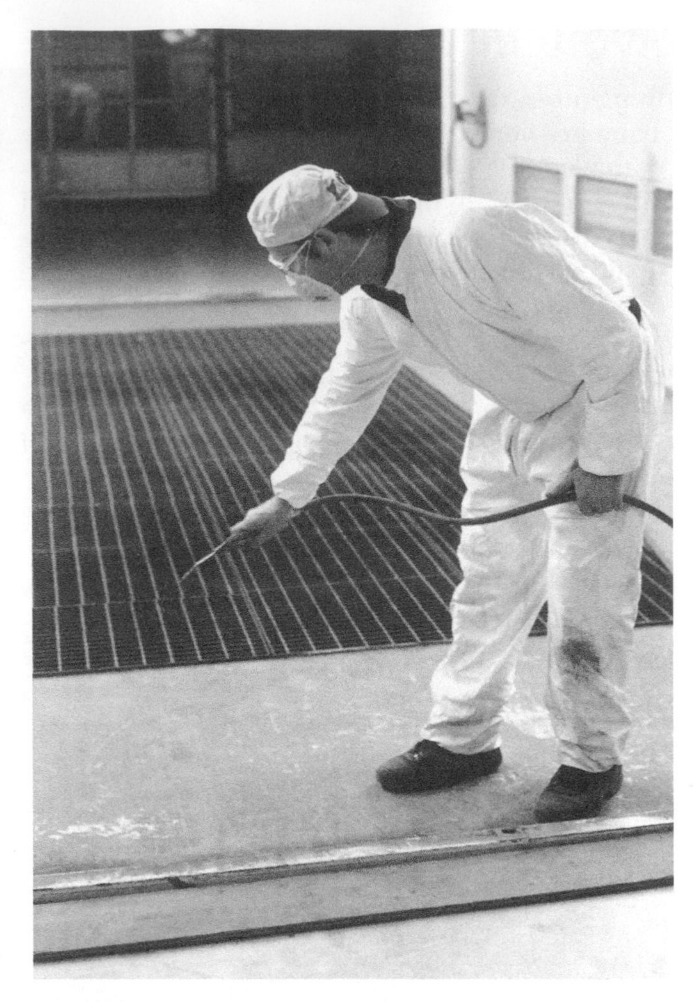

Figure 2–9. Note the safety gear worn by this professional painting technician. Clean coveralls, a painter's cap, safety glasses, and a dust respirator are "common sense" safety items when blowing off in the paint booth floor.

Wear thick **leather shoes** that have nonslip soles to prevent falls and foot injuries. Good work shoes provide support and comfort for someone who is standing for a long time. Never wear athletic shoes or sandals in the shop. Toes can be broken or severed if a heavy object falls on them.

To keep hair safe and clean, wear a **cap** or hat when sanding, grinding, and doing similar jobs. Wear a protective **painter's stretch hood** in the spray booth; this is a cloth head covering with a see-through lens for protection from overspray or airborne materials. When working beneath the hood or under the vehicle, wear a head covering known as a **bump cap;** this is a thick cloth hat without a bill that protects your head from minor injuries while working. Keep clothing away from moving parts when an engine or a machine is running.

Tie long hair securely behind your head before beginning to work. If hair becomes tangled in moving parts or air tools, it can cause serious injury.

Any loose or hanging clothing, such as shirttails, ties, cuffs, or scarves, creates a risk of getting wrapped up in moving parts of the vehicle or machinery, causing serious bodily injury. Remove all jewelry before working.

Use a portable shop light when working in dark areas, such as under a vehicle. This will increase work speed, quality, and safety.

When lifting and carrying objects, bend at your knees, not your back. Do not bend your waist when lifting. Remember, heavy objects should be lifted and moved with the proper equipment for the job. Get someone to help you.

Never overreach! Maintain a balanced stance to avoid slipping and falling while working.

Proper conduct can also help prevent accidents. Horseplay is dangerous and very unprofessional.

Do not risk injury through the lack of knowledge. Use shop equipment or machinery only after receiving proper instruction.

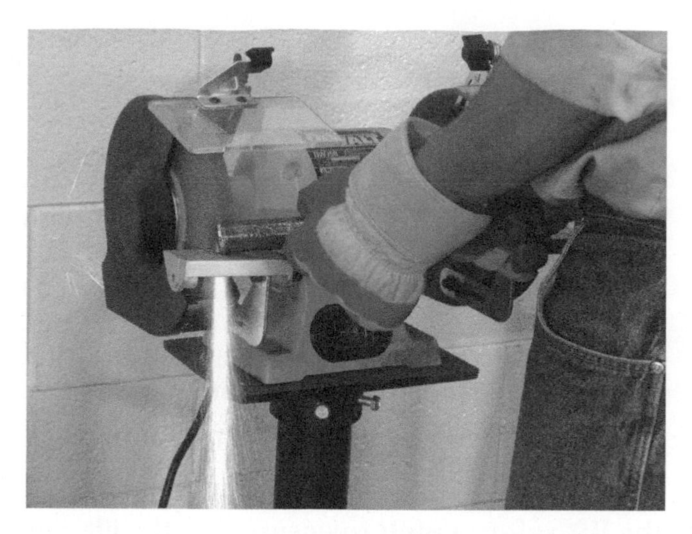

Figure 2–10. Leather gloves will protect your hands from painful cuts and gouges when working around bench and air grinders. A spinning abrasive wheel will cut into skin and bones like a "hot knife through butter."

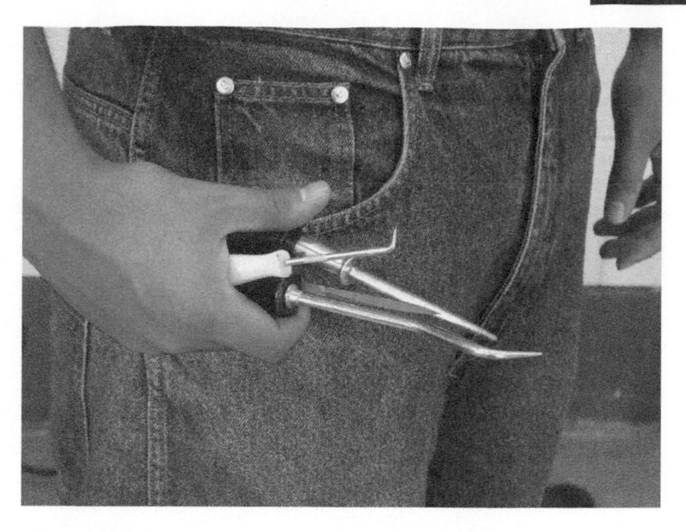

Figure 2–11. Never accidentally place sharp tools into your pockets. The first time you bend over, the sharp tools can jab deeply into your flesh.

Metalworking air hammers, the piercing noise of grinding, and the radio blaring full blast can all make it difficult to hear anything else. Some shop noise is enough to cause permanent hearing loss.

When in metalworking areas, wear **earplugs** or **earmuffs** to protect your eardrums from damaging noise levels.

To prevent serious burns, avoid contact with hot metal parts such as the radiator, exhaust manifold, tailpipe, catalytic converter, and muffler.

During metalworking, it is very easy to be cut by sharp, jagged metal on a spinning grinding wheels. Use caution. See **Figure 2–10.**

When driving a vehicle into a shop, watch out for other vehicles and people. It is best to have someone act as a guide. Leave the window open and the radio off, so that the helper's directions can be heard.

TOOL AND MACHINE SAFETY

Collision repair tools and equipment can cause serious injuries if basic safety rules are NOT observed. Some general tool rules include the following:

Keep tools clean and in working condition. Greasy or oily tools can easily slip out of your grasp, possibly causing injury.

Be careful when using sharp or pointed tools that can cause injury. If a tool should be sharp, keep it sharp.

Do not use any hand tools for any job other than that for which they were specifically designed.

Never carry screwdrivers, punches, or other sharp items in your pockets. You could be injured or damage the vehicle. See **Figure 2–11.**

When using an electric power tool, make sure that it is properly grounded. The third round ground prong sends electricity flow to the ground if the tool shorts out, not through your body.

Check the wiring insulation for cracks and bare wires. To avoid serious injury when using electric tools, never stand on a wet or damp floor.

Do not operate a power tool or machine without its safety guard(s) in place.

When power grinding, cutting, or sanding, or doing similar operations, always wear safety glasses.

When using power equipment on small parts, never hold the part in your hand. It could slip and you could injure your hand. Use a bench vise instead.

Before plugging in any electric tool, make sure the switch is OFF to prevent serious injury. When you are through, turn the tool off to ready it for the next person.

Use **jack stands** or **safety stands** to support a vehicle whenever you must work underneath it. Jack stands are strong steel pieces of equipment designed to support a vehicle; they have four legs to hold them steady and an

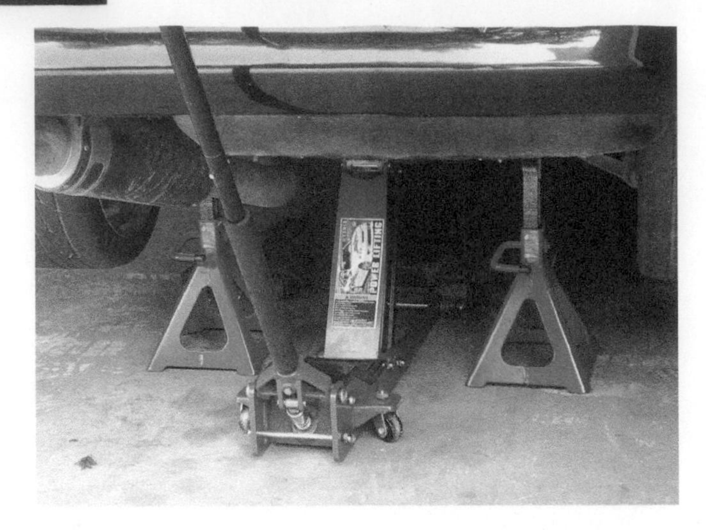

Figure 2–12. Thousands of workers have been seriously injured or killed when a car fell on them. After raising a car with a floor jack, install jack stands before working under the vehicle. Make sure the jack and stands are placed under recommended lift points to avoid damaging the thin sheetmetal floor pan.

extendible shoe on which the vehicle rests. **Hydraulic jacks** are used to raise a vehicle before placing jack stands and to lower it after working. Never trust hydraulic jacks alone; they are for raising the vehicle, not holding it. Many people have been seriously injured when a vehicle fell on them. See **Figure 2–12.**

Use a tool or machine only for its designed task. Never misuse or modify equipment.

Keep hands away from moving parts when the machine or tool is under power. Running vehicle engines often cause injuries. Never clear debris from a machine when it is under power, and never use your hands.

Use caution with compressed air. Pneumatic tools must be operated at the pressure recommended by their manufacturer. The downstream pressure of compressed air used for cleaning purposes must remain at a pressure level below 30 psi (2.1 kg/cm^2).

Do not use compressed air to clean clothes. Even at low pressure, compressed air can cause dirt particles to become embedded in your skin, which can result in infection. Air entering an artery could cause death.

Store all parts and tools properly by putting them away neatly. This practice not only cuts down on injuries, it also reduces time wasted looking for a misplaced part or tool.

When working with a hydraulic press or power unit, apply hydraulic pressure in a safe manner. It is generally wise to stand to the side when operating hydraulic tools. Always wear safety glasses.

If the shop has a hydraulic lift, be sure to read the instruction manual. Check the pads to see that they are making proper contact with the frame. Then raise the vehicle about 6 inches (15 centimeters) and check to make sure it is well balanced on the lift.

Any rattling or scraping sounds mean that the vehicle is not positioned properly. If this happens, lower the lift and realign the pads. Test it again. See **Figure 2–13.**

After lifting the vehicle to full height, engage the **lift safety catch** to ensure that the lift cannot lower while you are working underneath the vehicle.

Never permit anyone—technician or customer—to remain in the vehicle while it is being lifted.

When welding or cutting near vehicle interiors, remove the seats and carpets to prevent a fire. Always have water and a fire extinguisher nearby.

PAINT SHOP SAFETY

Many paints and paint-related products present serious health hazards unless proper precautions are taken. More vehicles are now being refinished with urethane enamels, which contain harmful chemicals. These chemicals can cause nose, throat, and lung irritation. They can also cause serious respiratory problems. Symptoms can include shortness of breath, tightness in the chest, dizziness, nausea, abdominal pain, and vomiting.

RESPIRATORS

Respirators are needed in the paint shop to keep airborne materials from being inhaled. They must be used even when adequate ventilation is provided. See **Figure 2–14.**

Respirator Types

A **dust or particle respirator** is a filter that fits over your nose and mouth to block small airborne particles. It is not designed to stop paint mist and fumes. A dust respirator is used when sanding or grinding to keep the dangerous materials out of your lungs.

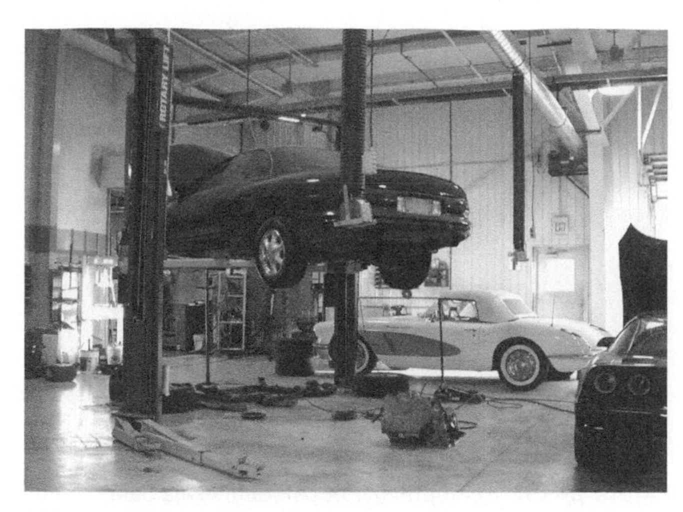

(A) Always make sure that the center of gravity of the vehicle is centered on the lift. For example, a front engine vehicle has the center of gravity slightly forward of the center. A rear engine vehicle has the center of gravity slightly behind the center.

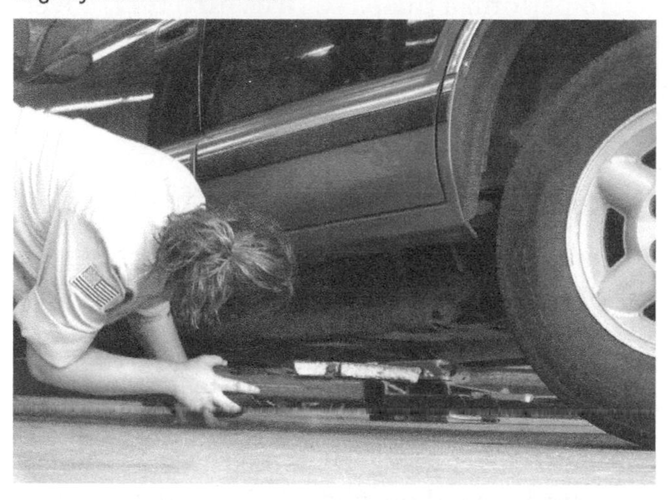

(B) Position the arms on a lift at factory recommended lift points. Double-check their locations before raising the car in the air.

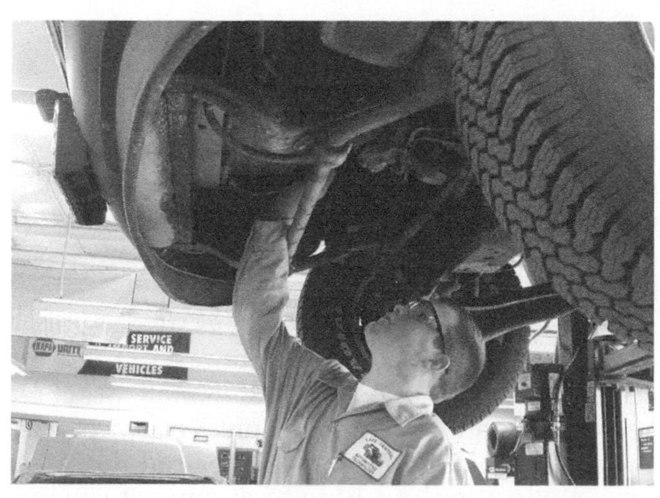

(C) Make sure the mechanical safety catch is engaged on the lift before working under the vehicle.

Figure 2–13. Thousands of cars and trucks have fallen off lifts, with deadly results.

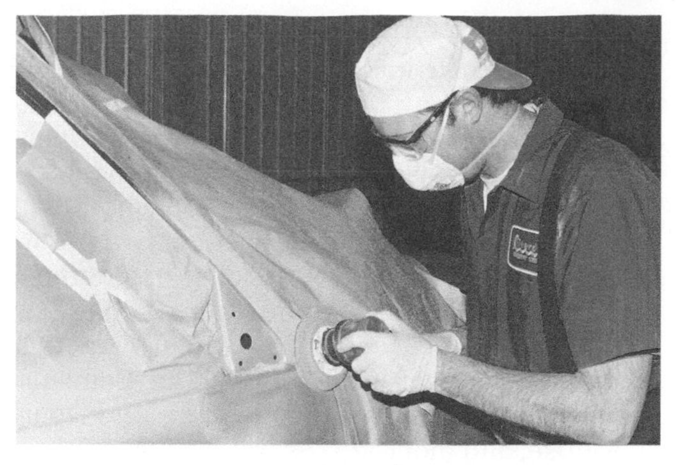

(A) A dust respirator will help keep airborne particles from entering your lungs when sanding, grinding, or blowing off paint and primer. Without a respirator, your nose, throat, and lungs will collect paint and primer.

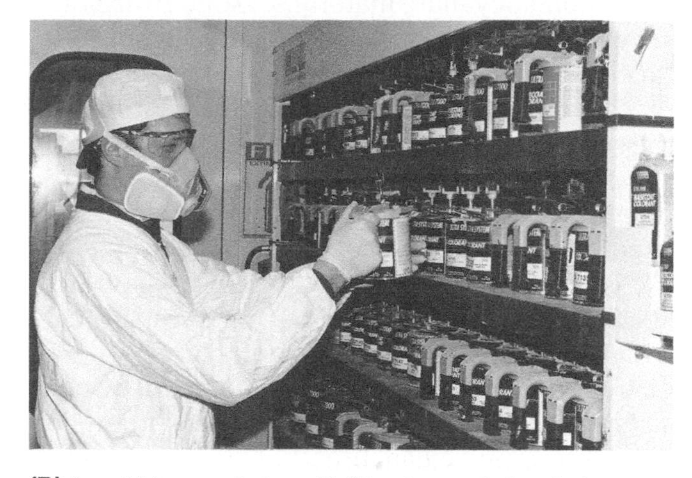

(B) A cartridge respirator will filter dust and chemical vapors. It provides a better level of protection when working with painting chemicals.

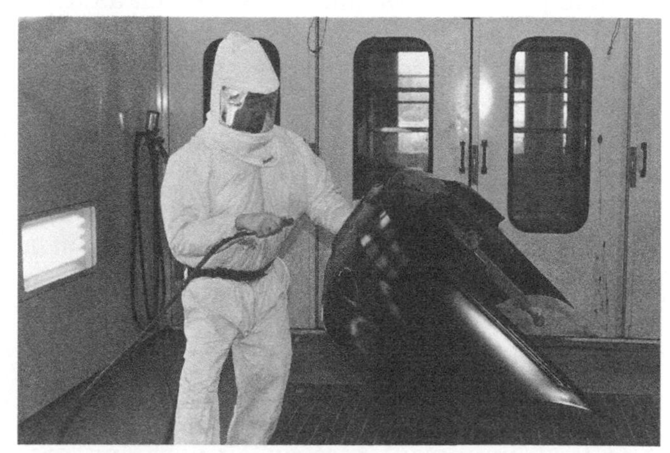

(C) An air-supplied respirator is essential when painting vehicles. Air is pumped from outside the shop and into the painter's helmet. Cool, clean air is circulated inside the painter's helmet to provide maximum protection from toxic paint materials.

Figure 2–14. Study and use the three types of respirators to protect your respiratory system (mouth, throat, and lungs).

Sanding operations create dust that can cause bronchial irritation and possible long-term lung damage. Protection from this health hazard is often overlooked. Just because the sanding dust does not cause immediate symptoms does not mean that it will not cause problems when you get older. An approved dust respirator should be worn whenever sanding or grinding operations are performed. See Figure 2–14A.

Follow the instructions provided with the dust respirator to ensure proper fit. Bend or shape it so that air cannot leak around your face, nose, and mouth.

Cartridge filter respirators protect against vapors and spray mists of nonactivated enamels (no hardener added), lacquers, and other nonisocyanate materials. **Isocyanates** are very hazardous materials that are often used to "accelerate" (speed-up/shorten) drying times, or to "activate/harden" refinishing material. If the refinishing materials contain no isocyanates, an air-purifying cartridge filter respirator with organic vapor cartridges and prefilters can be used (see Figure 2–14B).

To maintain the cartridge filter respirator, keep it clean and change the prefilters and cartridges as directed by the manufacturer.

An approved **air-supplied respirator** consists of a half-mask, full-face piece, hood, or helmet to which clean, breathable air is supplied through a hose from a separate air source. It provides protection from the dangers of inhaling isocyanate paint vapors and mists, as well as from hazardous solvent vapors. See Figure 2–14C.

The fresh-air-supply respirator is cool to wear and does not require fit testing. The fresh-air-supply respirator may include a self-contained oilless pump to supply air to either one hood or two half-mask respirators. Refer to **Figure 2–15.**

The pump's air inlet must be located in a clean air area. Some shops mount the pumps on an outside wall, away from the dust and dirt generated by shop operations.

Respirator Testing and Maintenance

It is very important that an air-purifying cartridge filter respirator fits securely around your face. This will prevent contaminated air from entering your lungs. To check for respirator air leaks, a **fit test** should be performed prior to using the respirator, making both negative and positive pressure checks.

To make a **negative pressure test,** place the palms of your hands over the cartridges and inhale. A good fit will be evident if the face piece collapses onto your face.

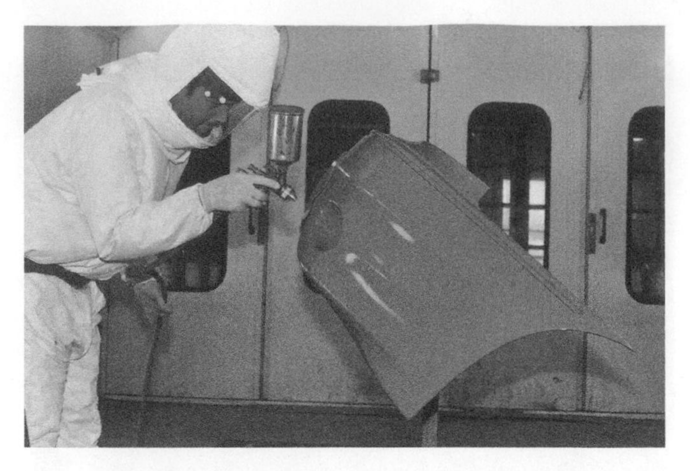

Figure 2–15. When priming or painting, use a paint booth and air-supplied respirator for your long-term health.

To perform a **positive pressure test,** cover up the exhalation valve and exhale. A proper fit is evident if the face piece billows out without air escaping from the mask.

DUSTLESS SANDING SYSTEMS

A **dustless sanding system** uses a blower or air pump to draw airborne dust into a storage container, much like a vacuum cleaner. Depending on the system, vacuum pumps, vacuum pullers, brush motors, or turbine motors can be used to provide sufficient air volume. This action pulls airborne sanding dust through holes in a special sanding pad or through a shroud that surrounds the sanding pad.

AIR BAG SAFETY

Air bags can be very dangerous because they deploy with tremendous force. Air bags can reach speeds of over 100 miles per hour during deployment. They can break arms, hands, fingers, or cause even more serious injury if you are near the bag during accidental deployment.

When working around air bags, use caution and follow service manual directions to prevent accidental deployment. Never install or connect a new air bag module until all wiring is checked with a scan tool and repaired if necessary. A short in the wiring to an impact sensor or to the air bag module could make the new air bag deploy as soon as it is connected to its control circuit.

Refer to the vehicle's service manual to learn the precautions that must be followed when servicing an air bag. It will give the details needed to work safely. For details on air bag service, refer to Chapter 27.

MANUFACTURER'S WARNINGS

Manufacturer's warnings give important procedures for the safe use of products. Study and follow instructions and warnings given by product and equipment manufacturers. Follow them to the letter.

Most of the products used in a collision repair shop carry warning and caution information that must be read and understood by users. Likewise, all federal (including Occupational Safety and Health Administration [OSHA], Mine Safety and Health Administration [MSHA], and National Institute for Occupational Safety and Health [NIOSH]), state, and local safety regulations should not only be fully understood, but also strictly observed.

Material safety data sheets (MSDS), available from all product manufacturers, detail chemical composition and precautionary information for all products that can present a health or safety hazard.

Employers must know the general uses, protective equipment, accident or spill procedures, and other information for safe handling of hazardous material. They must provide training to employees as part of their job orientation.

The best way to protect yourself when using paint and body products is to be familiar with the correct application procedures. Follow all safety and health precautions found on MSDS and on product labels.

RIGHT-TO-KNOW LAWS

In collision repair and refinishing shops, hazardous wastes are generated. As a result, every employee is protected by right-to-know laws.

Right-to-know laws give essential information and stipulations for safely working with hazardous materials. They began with OSHA's Hazard Communication Standard. This document was originally intended for chemical companies and manufacturers that require employees to handle potentially hazardous materials in the workshop. Since then, the majority of states have enacted their own right-to-know laws. The federal courts have decided that these regulations should apply to all companies, including the auto collision repair and refinishing professions.

WASTE DISPOSAL

Many shops use "full-service" haulers to test and remove hazardous waste from the property. Besides hauling the hazardous waste away, the hauler will also take care of all the paperwork, deal with the various government agencies, even advise the shop on how to recover disposal costs.

The collision repair shop is ultimately responsible for the safe disposal of hazardous wastes, even after they leave the shop. Be sure that any hauling contract is in writing.

In the event of an emergency hazardous waste spill, you or the shop owner must contact the National Response Center (1-800-424-8802) immediately. Failure to do so can result in a $10,000 fine or a year in jail, or both.

ASE CERTIFICATION

Just as doctors, accountants, electricians, and other professionals are licensed or certified to practice their professions, collision repair and refinishing technicians can also be certified. The National Institute for Automotive Service Excellence (ASE) offers a certificate program. **ASE certification** is a testing program to help prove that you are a knowledgeable collision repair or refinishing technician. See **Figure 2–16.**

Certification protects the general public and the professional. It assures the general public and the prospective employer that certain minimum standards of performance have been met.

ASE tests include multiple-choice questions pertaining to the service and repair of a vehicle. They do not include theoretical questions. To prepare for ASE collision repair or refinishing tests, study the material in this book carefully.

To help you prepare for the Collision Repair and/or Painting and Refinishing tests, some test questions at the end of service chapters in this text are similar to those used by ASE.

Collision repair and refinishing technicians can get certified in one or more technical areas by taking and passing written certification tests. The **National Institute for Automotive Service Excellence (ASE)** offers a voluntary certification program that is recommended by the major vehicle manufacturers in the United States. The Collision Repair and Painting and Refinishing tests contain 40 questions in various areas.

Technicians who pass the written tests are awarded a certificate and a shoulder emblem for their work clothes. See **Figure 2–17.**

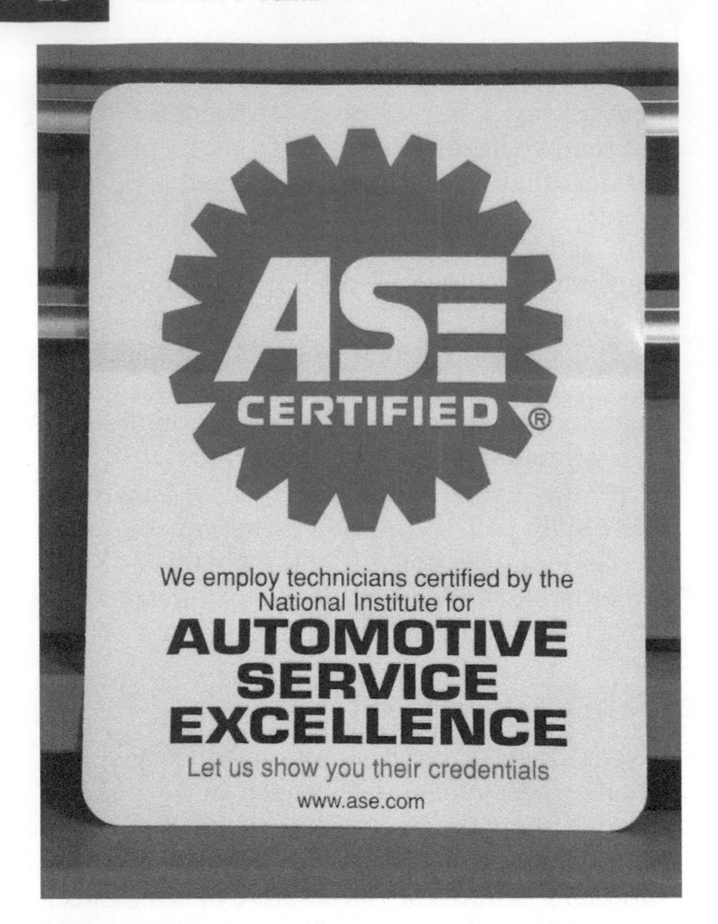
ASE
CERTIFIED
We employ technicians certified by the National Institute for
AUTOMOTIVE SERVICE EXCELLENCE
Let us show you their credentials
www.ase.com

Figure 2–16. ASE certification is the standard for collision repair. Most modern shops require their body and paint technicians to pass ASE certification tests. This shows potential customers that the shop takes pride in having qualified technicians repair their cars.

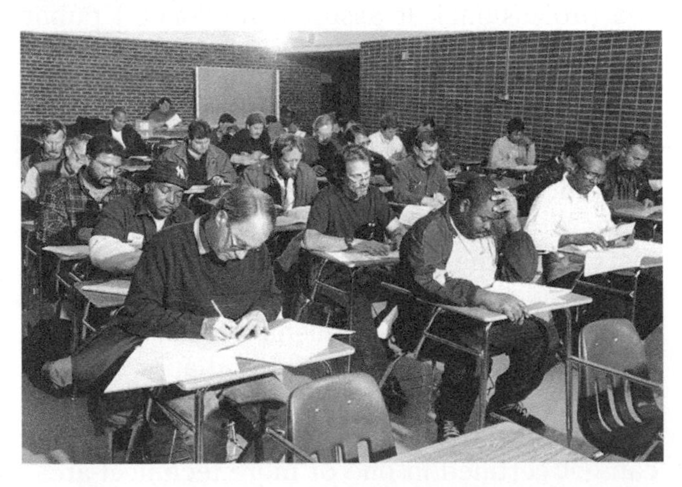

Figure 2–17. These technicians are taking the ASE exams to become certified technicians in their respective fields of expertise.

Many employers now expect their collision repair and refinishing technicians to be certified. The certified technician is recognized as a professional by the public, employers, and peers. For this reason, the certified technician usually receives higher pay than one who is not certified. Look at **Figure 2–18.**

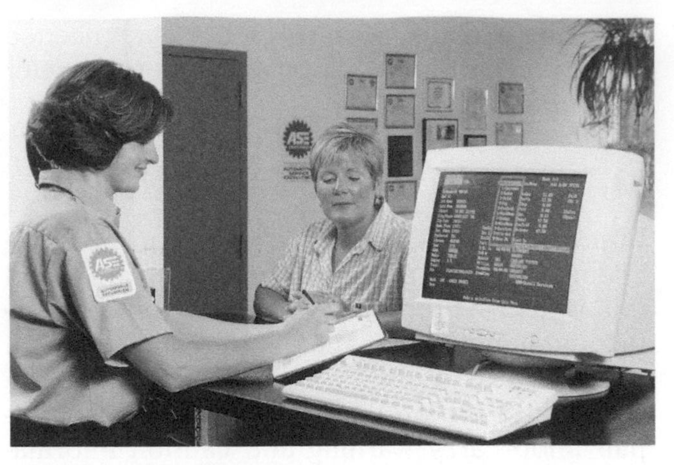

Figure 2–18. ASE certification shows customers and your employer that you have passed standardized tests and know how to do your work properly. (http://www.ase.com)

For further information on the ASE certification program, write:

ASE
13505 Dulles Technology Drive
Herndon, VA 22071-3145
703-713-3800

Or contact ASE on the World Wide Web at http://www.asecert.org

SUMMARY

- Care must be taken to prevent several types of accidents, including asphyxiation, chemical burns, electrocution, fires, and explosions.
- A safety program is a written shop policy designed to protect the health and welfare of personnel and customers. It includes rules on everything from equipment use to disposal of hazardous chemicals.
- In case of an emergency, be sure the following are available and easily seen: emergency telephone numbers, a first aid kit, and safety signs denoting fire exits, fire extinguishers, and dangerous chemical information.
- Certification protects the general public and the technician. ASE certification assures the general public and the prospective employer that certain minimum standards of performance have been met.

TECHNICAL TERMS

safety
accidents
asphyxiation
chemical burns
electrocution
fire
combustibles
explosions
physical injury
manufacturer's instructions
safety program
shop layout
metalworking area
repair stall
bay
front end rack
alignment rack
pneumatic
hydraulic
tool and equipment storage room
classroom
paint prep area
finishing area
spray booth
shop office
emergency telephone numbers
first aid kit
safety signs
gasoline
spontaneous combustion
Underwriters Laboratories (UL)
electrical fires
fire extinguisher
electrocution
ventilated
carbon monoxide (CO)
asbestos dust
automatic transmission
manual transmission
safety glasses
full-face shield
goggles
rubber gloves
plastic gloves
hand cleaner
jumpsuit
lint-free coveralls
leather shoes
cap
painter's stretch hood
bump cap
earplugs
earmuffs
jack stands
safety stands
hydraulic jacks
lift safety catch
respirators
dust respirator
particle respirator
cartridge filter respirator
isocyanates
air-supplied respirator
fit test
negative pressure test
positive pressure test
dustless sanding system
manufacturer's warnings
material safety data sheets (MSDS)
right-to-know laws
ASE certification
ASE tests
National Institute for Automotive Service Excellence (ASE)

REVIEW QUESTIONS

1. Safety involves using proper work habits to prevent ______________ and ______________.

2. List six kinds of accidents that are common in a collision repair facility.

3. What are some combustible materials found in a collision repair facility?

4. Name ten collision repair facility work areas.

5. How is frame straightening equipment dangerous?

6. When soiled rags are left lying about improperly, they can cause:

a. Spontaneous combustion
b. Chemical burns
c. Explosion
d. None of the above

7. Asbestos dust is inert and does not pose a health problem. True or False?

8. Wear ______________ or ______________ to protect yourself from the harmful effects of corrosive liquids, undercoats, and finishes.

9. What can happen if you wear athletic shoes and drop a heavy part on your foot?

10. When using an electric power tool, make sure that it is properly ______________. The ______________ ground ______________ sends electricity flow to the ground, not through your body if the tool shorts out.

11. Numerous people have been seriously injured when a vehicle fell on them. How could this have happened?

12. Which of these are needed in the paint shop to keep paint mists and fumes from being inhaled?

a. Face shield
b. Mouth piece
c. Respirator
d. Shop rag

13. *Technician A* leaves his shirt sleeves unbuttoned in the shop. *Technician B* wears loose clothing instead of coveralls. Who is correct?

a. Technician A
b. Technician B
c. Both Technicians A and B
d. Neither Technician

14. Which of the following is important to shop safety?
    a. Jack stands
    b. Attitude
    c. Approved metal containers
    d. All of the above
15. When running an engine in a vehicle with an automatic transmission, place it in ______________.
    a. Neutral
    b. Reverse
    c. Park
    d. Drive
16. Which of the following statements is correct?
    a. Gasoline is an ideal cleaning solvent.
    b. Never keep more than 10 days' worth of paint outside of approved storage areas.
    c. Oily rags should be stored in approved metal containers.
    d. All of the above.
17. With which type of respirator can facial hair prevent an airtight seal?
    a. Cartridge filter type
    b. Air-supplied type
    c. Full-face type
    d. Hood type
18. Why should you become ASE certified?

ASE-STYLE REVIEW QUESTIONS

1. A technician is going to prime a repaired panel. A catalyzed primer is going to be used. Which of the following should the technician do?
    a. Read the owner's manual for the spray gun.
    b. Read the label on the can of primer.
    c. Wear a dust respirator.
    d. Work in a well-ventilated area.

2. Which one of the following details the chemical composition and precautionary information for products that can present a health or safety hazard and is available from all product manufacturers?
    a. MSDS
    b. DSMS
    c. Instructions
    d. Warnings

3. A technician is transferring flammable materials from bulk storage. Which of the following should be done to prevent an explosion?
    a. Keep the drum(s) grounded.
    b. Pour the material slowly.
    c. Pour the material quickly.
    d. Ground his body.

4. Which of the following should be done before removing fuel lines on a fuel injection system?
    a. Relieve fuel pressure.
    b. Disconnect battery ground.
    c. All of the above.
    d. None of the above.

5. When a battery charger is connected to a vehicle, wires start to smoke and a fuse blows. Which of the following is the most common cause?
    a. Charger set too high
    b. Shorted wires from collision
    c. Open wires from collision
    d. Charger connected backwards

6. A fire has broken out under a vehicle in the shop. *Technician A* says to open all shop doors and windows to let out the smoke. *Technician B* says to keep them closed. Who is correct?
    a. Technician A
    b. Technician B
    c. Both Technicians A and B
    d. Neither Technician

7. A technician is using electrically powered equipment. Which of the following can cause serious injury?
    a. Water on floor
    b. No ground prong
    c. Bad wire insulation
    d. All of the above

8. A technician is refinishing a vehicle with catalyzed paint. What type of respirator should be worn?

a. Dust respirator
b. Cartridge respirator
c. Disposable respirator
d. Air-supplied respirator

9. A vehicle is being raised in the air for working on the underbody. *Technician A* says to mount the vehicle on safety stands. *Technician B* says to leave the vehicle supported by the hydraulic floor jack. Who is correct?

a. Technician A
b. Technician B
c. Both Technicians A and B
d. Neither Technician

ACTIVITIES

1. Ask a parent, relative, or friend who has been in a collision to describe what happened during and after the collision when trying to get the vehicle repaired.

2. Go to the library and look up information on different types of insurance—full coverage, liability, no-fault. Prepare a report on this subject.

CHAPTER

3 Hand Tools

OBJECTIVES

After studying this chapter, you should be able to:

- Identify and explain general purpose hand tools.
- Identify and explain the use for the most important collision repair hand tools.
- Compare the advantages and disadvantages of different tools.
- Properly select the right tool for the job.
- Maintain and store tools properly.

INTRODUCTION

Professional collision repair technicians invest thousands of dollars in their tools. A good set of tools will speed repairs and improve work quality. The importance of having the right tools for the job cannot be overstated.

Remember! Tools serve to increase the abilities of your hands, arms, legs, back, eyes, and ears. They allow you to do things that would be impossible otherwise. Neither you, nor the very best technician, can do quality work using inferior tools. See **Figure 3–1.**

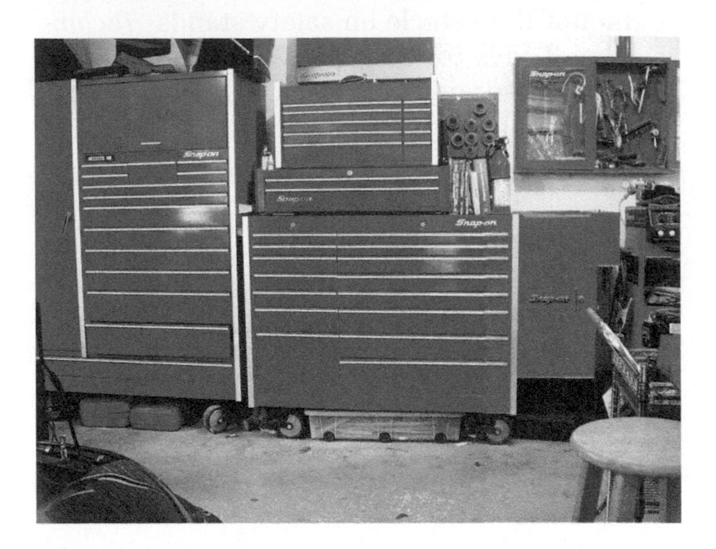

Figure 3–1. A professional set of hand tools is a big investment. Always purchase quality tools with a lifetime guarantee against failure. High-quality tools will save you time, effort, and help you get more work done for more profit. (Courtesy of Snap-on Tools Corp.)

PURCHASE QUALITY TOOLS

Never buy cheap, low-grade tools. Cheap tools slow down your work rate and efficiency because they are heavier, more clumsy, and break more easily. You usually get what you pay for. Good tools will pay for themselves in a short period of time.

A **lifetime tool guarantee** means the tool will be replaced or repaired if it ever fails or breaks. Some guarantees are for the life of the tool; some are NOT. Even though guaranteed tools are more expensive, they will save money in the long run.

TOOL STORAGE

Always store tools properly when they are not in use. This will protect them from damage or loss. It will also speed your work because you will be able to find tools more quickly. Keep related tools together in one drawer. Keep heavy tools in one drawer and small or delicate tools in another. This will keep the delicate tools from being damaged.

After use, wipe oil and grease off tools. A greasy, oily tool can easily slip from a technician's hand and cause injury. Keeping tools clean makes them safer and prolongs their life and usefulness.

Tool holders are clip racks, pouches, or trays that help you organize small tools. Tool holders allow you to carry the tool set to the job easily. This saves you from having to walk back and forth to and from your tool box.

A **tool box** stores and protects your tools. Most tool boxes are made up of a large, bottom roll-around cabinet and an upper tool chest. The **upper chest** often holds commonly used tools at eye level. The **lower cabinet** often stores heavier tools. See Figure 3–1.

DANGER

NEVER open more than one tool box drawer at the same time because the box can flip over. Serious injury could result! Close each drawer before opening the next one.

GENERAL DUTY HAMMERS

Hammers are used for striking and exerting an impact on a part. Always use the right hammer for the task and use it properly. See **Figure 3–2.**

A **ball peen hammer** has a flat face for general striking and a round peen end for shaping sheet metal, rivet heads, or other objects.

The **brass** or **lead hammer** will make heavy blows without marring the metal surface. The soft metal head will dent and protect the part.

A **plastic hammer** is for making light blows where parts can be easily damaged. It is used on delicate parts.

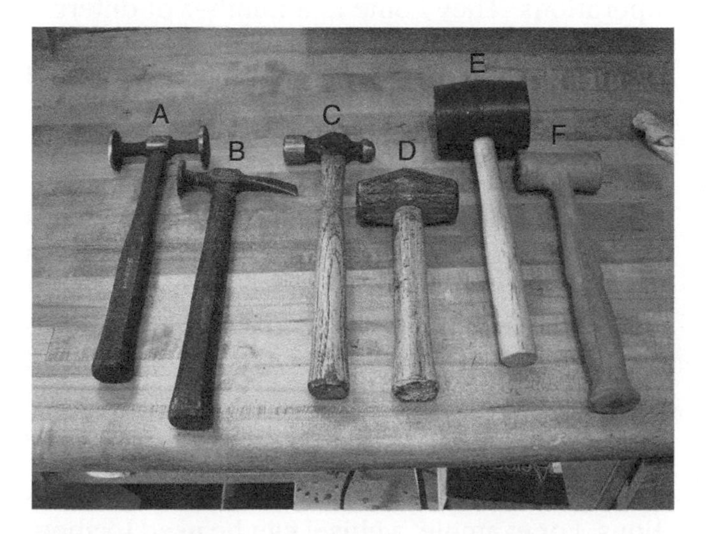

Figure 3–2. Here is an assortment of hammers used in a body shop. Study them! **(A)** Bumping hammer. **(B)** Picking-bumping hammer. **(C)** Ball peen hammer. **(D)** Sledge hammer. **(E)** Rubber mallet. **(F)** Dead blow hammer. (Courtesy of Snap-on Tools Corp.)

A **dead blow hammer** has a metal face filled with lead shot (balls) to prevent rebounding. It will not bounce back up after striking. It is good for driving operations where part damage must be avoided.

A **rubber mallet** has a solid rubber head that is fairly heavy. It is often used to gently bump sheet metal without damaging the painted finish. It is also used to install wheel covers. Rubber mallets can be used in conjunction with a suction cup on soft "cave-in" type dents. While pulling on the cup, the technician uses the mallet to tap lightly all around the surrounding high spots. A "popping sound" occurs as the high spots drop and the low spot springs back to its original contour.

BODY HAMMERS

Body hammers are designed to work with sheet metal. They often have a point on one end and a flat head or a head of an odd shape on the other. They come in many different designs. Each style is designed for a special use. See Figure 3–2.

Picking hammers have a sharply pointed head and will remove many small dents. The pointed end is used to raise small dents from the inside. The flat end is for hammer-and-dolly work to remove high spots and ripples. Picking hammers come in a variety of shapes and sizes. Some have long picks for reaching behind body panels. Some have sharp points; others are blunted.

Bumping hammers are used to bump out large dents. They may have a round or square face. The surfaces of the faces are nearly flat and large enough that the force of the blows are spread over a large area. These hammers are used for initial straightening on damaged panels. They are also used for working inner panels and reinforced sections that require more force but not a finished appearance.

Finishing hammers are used to achieve the final sheet metal contour. The face on a finishing hammer is smaller than that of the heavier bumping hammer. The surface of the face is crowned to concentrate the force on top of the ridge or high spot.

Shrinking hammers are finishing hammers with a serrated or cross-grooved face. They are used to shrink spots that have been stretched by excessive hammering.

DANGER

When using hammers, make sure the head is tight on its handle. Injury could result if the head were to fly off. Try to hit the object squarely and hold the handle securely.

DOLLIES AND SPOONS

A **dolly** or **dolly block** is used like a small, portable anvil. It is generally held on the back side of a panel being struck with a hammer. Together the hammer and dolly straighten high spots down and low spots up to reshape the damaged body panel. See **Figure 3–3.**

Body spoons are used sometimes like a hammer and at other times like a dolly. They are available in a variety of shapes and sizes to match various panel shapes. The flat surfaces of a spoon distribute the striking force over a wide area to prevent hammer dents. They are particularly useful on creases and ridges.

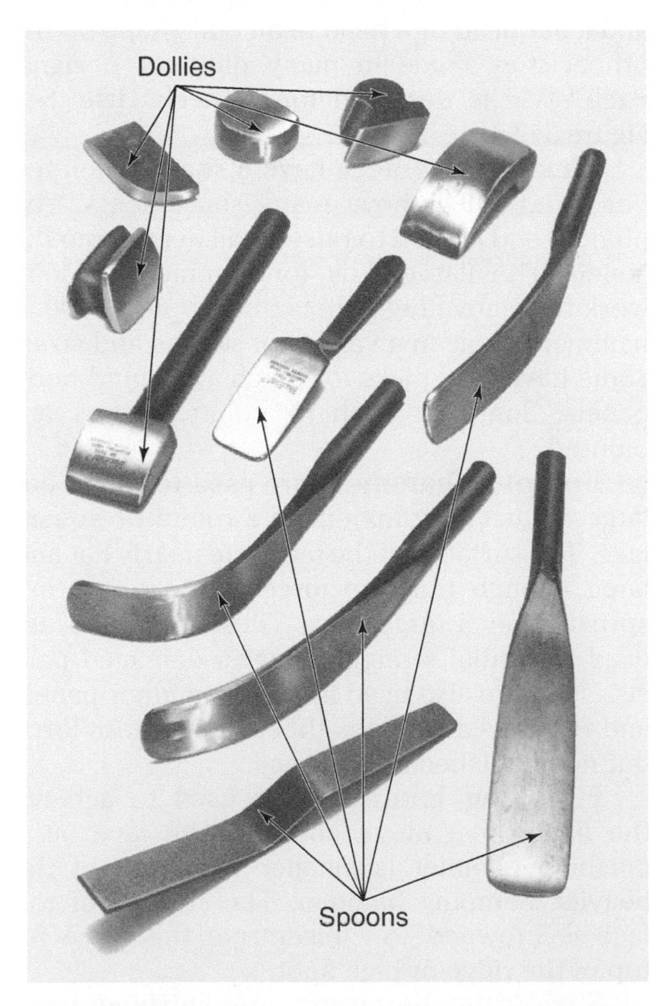

Figure 3–3. Dollies and spoons will help you straighten and repair damaged sheet metal. They are often placed on the back of damaged panels so hammer blows reshape the metal properly. (Courtesy of Snap-on Tools Corp.)

HOLDING TOOLS

A **vise** will secure or hold parts during hammering, cutting, drilling, and pressing operations. It normally bolts onto a workbench.

Vise caps are soft lead, wood, or plastic jaw covers that will protect a part from marring. Vise jaws are often knurled, and the small teeth will damage parts if they are not covered.

WARNING

Never hammer on a vise handle when tightening it. Use only your hands to tighten a vise handle.

A **C-clamp** is a screw attached to a curved frame. It will hold objects on a work surface or drill press while you are working on them.

PUNCHES AND CHISELS

Punches and chisels are necessary in every body repair tool chest. There are several types.

Punches are used for driving and aligning operations. They come in a number of different shapes for different tasks.

A **center punch** is pointed to start a drilled hole or to mark parts. The indentation will keep a drill bit from wandering out of place.

A **drift** or **starting punch** has a fully-tapered shank. It will drive pins, shafts, and rods partially out of holes. A **pin punch** has a straight shank for use after a starting punch. It will push a shaft completely out of a hole.

An **aligning punch** is long and tapered and used to align body panels and other parts. It can be used to line up fender bolt holes and bumpers, for example.

Chisels are handy for some cutting operations. For example, a chisel can be used to shear off rivet heads or separate sheet metal parts. See **Figure 3–4.**

Keep the ends of chisels and punches ground and shaped correctly. If the end becomes

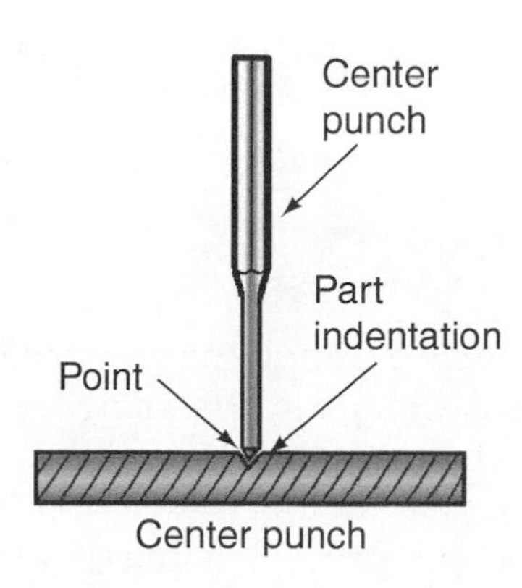

(A) The center punch will make a small dent for drilling a hole in a part.

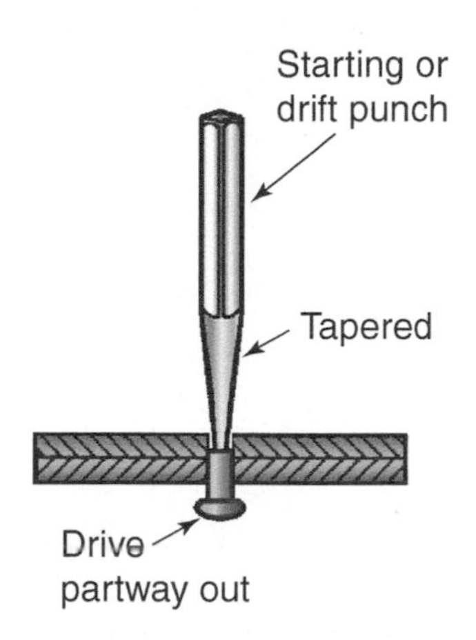

(B) The starting or drift punch is tapered but has a flat tip for driving out bolts or rivets.

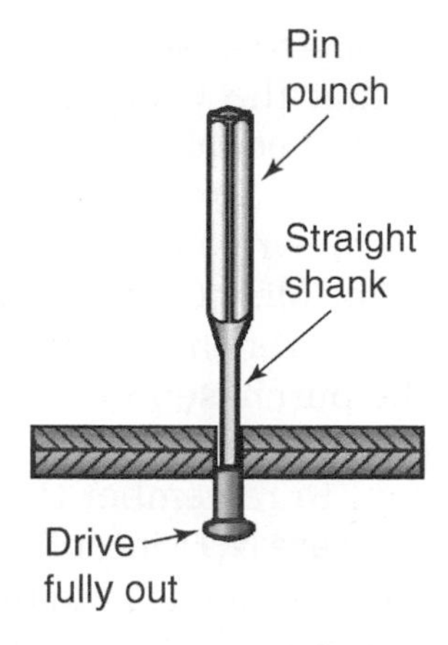

(C) The pin punch has a straight side and will drive the fastener completely out of the hole.

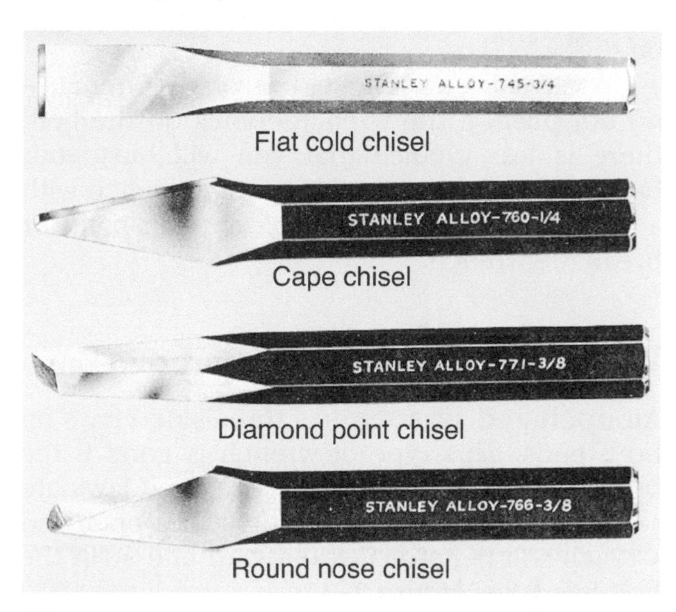

(D) Note the chisel names. They are used for cutting operations.

Figure 3–4. Study the use of punches and chisels. (Courtesy of Stanley Tools)

mushroomed or enlarged, grind it down. The sharp deformed end could cause hand injuries.

WRENCHES

Wrenches are used to loosen or tighten nuts and bolts. Various types of hand wrenches are shown in **Figure 3–5.**

Wrench size is the distance across the wrench jaws. Wrenches come in both standard (inch) and metric (millimeter) sizes. The size is stamped on the side of the wrench. The width of the jaw opening determines the size of a wrench.

For example, a ½-inch wrench has a jaw opening from face to face of approximately

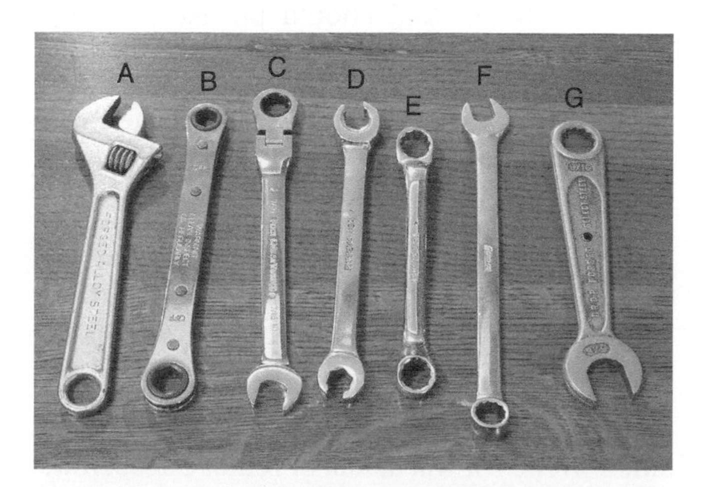

Figure 3–5. Study basic hand wrench types. **(A)** Adjustable or crescent wrench. **(B)** Ratchet wrench. **(C)** Ratchet open-end wrench. **(D)** Tubing or flare nut wrench. **(E)** Offset box wrench. **(F)** Box-end wrench. **(G)** Open-end wrench.

½ inch. The actual size is slightly larger than its normal size so that the wrench can fit around a nut or bolt head of equal size.

Most standard or **Society of Automotive Engineers (SAE)** wrench sets include sizes from 3/16 to 1 inch. Metric sets usually include 6- to 19-millimeter wrenches. Smaller and larger wrenches can be purchased but are rarely used in collision repair.

It is important to remember that metric and SAE size wrenches are NOT interchangeable. For example, a 9/16-inch wrench is 3/10 millimeter larger than a 14-millimeter nut. If the 9/16-inch wrench is used to turn or hold the 14-millimeter nut, the wrench will probably slip, rounding the points on the nut.

When using a wrench, PULL on the wrench—do not push. If the wrench comes off the bolt, there is less chance that you will hurt your hand. Never extend the length of a wrench with a pipe for leverage. Excess force can bend or break the wrench.

WRENCH TYPES

An **open-end wrench** has three-sided jaws on both ends. This type of wrench is good if the bolt or nut is not very tight. The open jaws are weak. If a bolt is extremely tight, the open-end wrench will bend or flex outward and strip the bolt head. See **Figure 3–6.**

A **box-end wrench** has closed ends that surround the bolt or nut head. It is a stronger design than an open-end wrench. It is available in 12-point and 6-point types. A 6-point will grip the head better and should be used on very tight, corroded, or partially stripped fastener heads.

A **combination wrench,** as implied, has both types of ends—box end and open end. It provides the features of two wrench types.

A **tubing, flare nut,** or **line wrench** has a small split in its jaw to fit over lines and tubing. It can be slipped over fuel, brake, and power steering lines. Avoid using an open-end wrench on tubing nuts because they will round off and strip easily. Tubing nuts are very soft.

An **Allen wrench** is a hex, hexagon, or six-sided wrench. It will install or remove set screws. Set screws are often used on pulleys, gears, and knobs.

A **crescent** or **adjustable wrench** has movable jaws to fit different head sizes. It can be

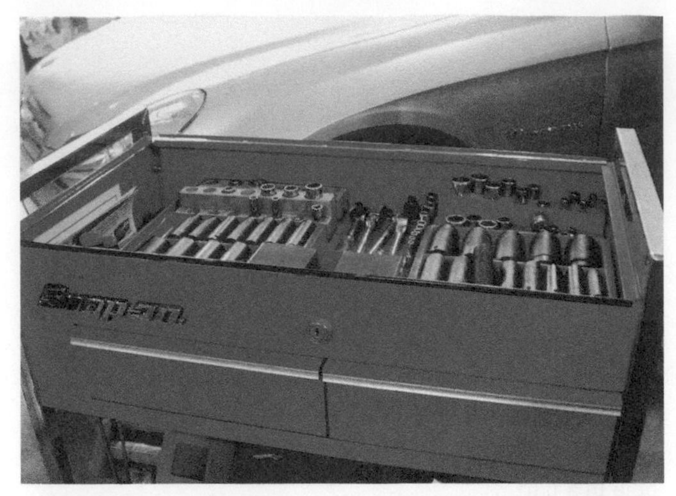

(A) Keeping your socket set in a roll-around cart is handy and will speed your work.

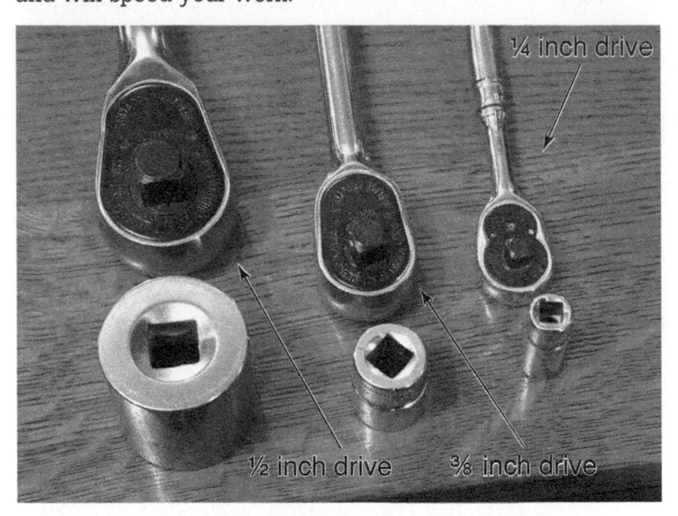

(B) Compare socket drive sizes. On the left is a large ½-inch drive ratchet and socket for use on large fasteners. In the middle is a 3/8-inch drive for medium-size bolts and nuts. On the right is a small ¼-inch drive for removing and installing smaller fasteners.

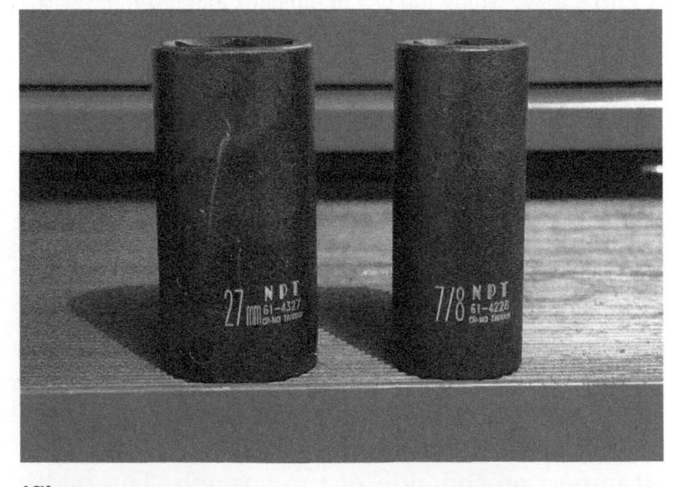

(C) You cannot interchange metric and conventional wrench or socket sizes. Make sure the wrench fits the bolt or nut head properly.

Figure 3–6. A set of socket wrenches and ratchets are essential to a body technician.

used when a correct size wrench is not available. For example, if a bolt is badly corroded, an adjustable wrench may be set to fit the odd head dimension.

A **pipe wrench** is another type of adjustable wrench for holding and turning round objects. Its sharp jaw teeth dig into and grasp the part. A pipe wrench will mar and damage part surfaces and should be used only when necessary.

A **chain wrench** is also used to grasp and turn round objects. It is used to remove stuck or damaged engine oil filters or to adjust exhaust systems.

Specialized body wrenches come in a variety of designs to meet specific demands. For example, the frame wrench is designed to bend the lip of heavy gauge frame rail.

Sockets

Sockets are cylinder-shaped, box-end wrenches for rapid turning of bolts and nuts. They come in a variety of designs—deep sockets, swivel sockets, impact sockets, etc. Refer to Figure 3–6.

Deep sockets are longer for reaching over stud bolts. **Swivel sockets** have a universal joint between the drive end and socket body. **Impact sockets** are thicker and case hardened for use with an air-powered impact wrench. Impact sockets are often black in color. *Conventional sockets,* or nonimpact sockets, are usually chrome plated.

Socket drive size is the size of the square opening for the drive handle. Common drive sizes are ¼, ⅜, ½, and ¾ inch. Small ¼-inch drive sockets are often used when working on an instrument panel with its many small screws. Large ½-inch drive sockets would be needed on larger suspension system parts.

Sockets are also made in 4-point, 6-point, 8-point, and 12-point configurations. Again, a 6-point is the strongest and will not strip the bolt or nut head easily.

A **ratchet** has a small lever that can be moved for either loosening or tightening bolts and nuts. It is a common type of socket drive handle.

A **breaker bar** provides the most powerful way of turning bolts and nuts. Also called a **flex handle,** it will break loose large or extremely tight fasteners.

A **speed handle** can be rotated to quickly remove or install loose bolts and nuts.

Extensions fit between the socket and its drive handle. They allow you to reach in and install the socket when surrounded by obstructions.

A **universal joint** allows you to reach around objects with a socket wrench and extension. It will flex, allowing you to rotate the socket from an angle. Separate universal joints and swivel sockets are available.

A **torque wrench** is used to measure tightening force. **Torque** is a measurement of twisting force. It is given in both inch-pounds and foot-pounds, as well as in metric measurements of Newton-meters. See **Figure 3–7.**

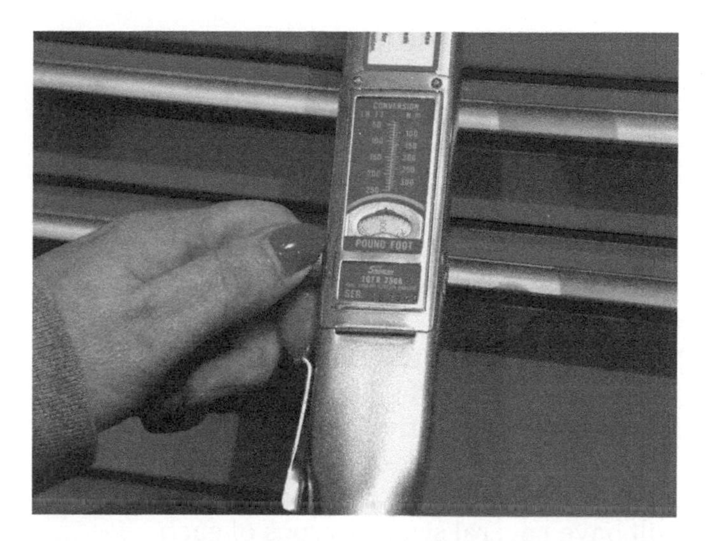

(A) Set the torque wrench for the bolt or nut to be tightened.

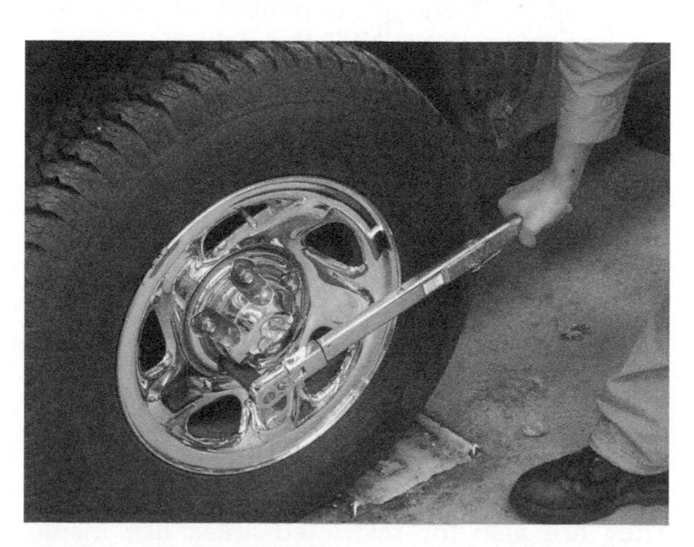

(B) Slowly pull on the wrench until it clicks, which indicates you have reached torque setting.

Figure 3–7. A torque wrench should be used on wheel lug nuts and steering/suspension parts because they are critical to vehicle safety.

If the fastener is tightened to a value less than its specification, the fastener can vibrate loose. If tightened too much, the threads can strip or the fastener can break. In either case, damage to other automobile parts can result. This can also endanger the driver and passengers of the vehicle.

Always torque all bolts and nuts to the **manufacturer's specifications** (factory values given in the service manual). If there are no specifications listed, use the general torque specifications chart. One is given in the back of this book.

PRYBARS

Prybars are used to gain leverage for shifting heavy parts. They are hardened steel bars with various end shapes. Prybars are often used to adjust engine belt tension. They will also shift parts to align holes. This will aid in hand starting bolt threads.

SCREWDRIVERS

Screwdrivers allow you to rotate screws for installation or removal. Many threaded fasteners used in the automotive industry are driven by a screwdriver. Each fastener requires a specific kind of screwdriver. A well-equipped technician will have several sizes or types of each.

When selecting a screwdriver, select a tip wide and thick enough to almost fill the screw head opening. If it is NOT the right size, screwdriver and screw damage will result. See **Figure 3–8.**

A **standard screwdriver** has a tip with a single flat blade for fitting into the slot in the screw. A **Phillips screwdriver** has two crossing blades for a star-shaped screw head. **Torx®** and *square head screwdrivers* have specially shaped tips.

Stubby screwdrivers have a very short shank. They can fit into tight or restricted areas. For example, you might use them to install trim around a wheel opening. **Offset screwdrivers** have the shank at a 90-degree angle to the tip. They are also for restricted areas like inside glove boxes.

An **impact driver** is hit with a hammer to rotate tight or stuck screws. The body of the driver can be rotated to change directions for installing or removing screws.

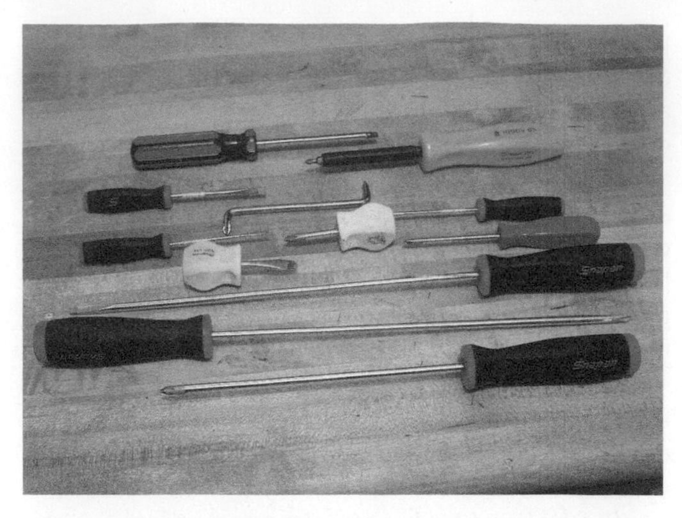

(A) Study screwdriver types.

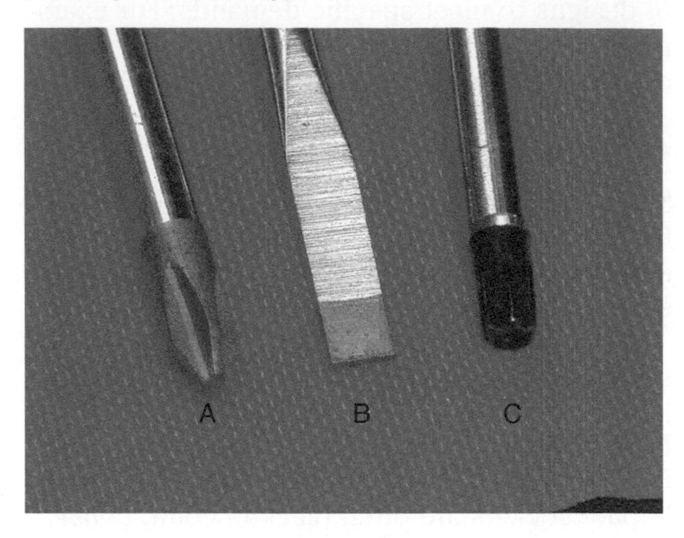

(B) From left to right: **[A]** Phillips; **[B]** Standard; **[C]** Torx.

Figure 3–8. Screwdrivers are used to remove a variety of screws when doing body work.

PLIERS

Pliers are used for working with wires, clips, and pins. They will grasp and hold parts like fingers. The collision repair technician must own several types. See **Figure 3–9.**

! WARNING !

Do NOT use pliers in place of a wrench. They will scar and damage parts like nuts and bolts.

Slip-joint, or **combination, pliers** will adjust for two sizes. They are the most common design used by the collision repair technician.

Rib joint or **Channellock® pliers** have several jaw settings for grasping different size

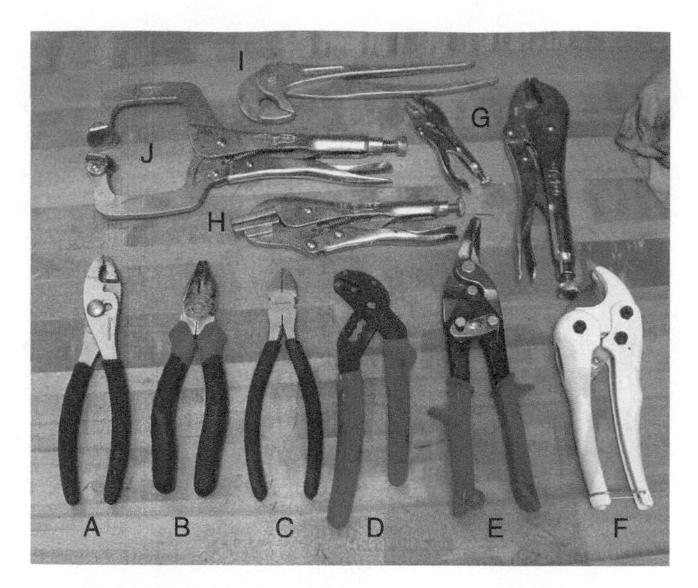

Figure 3–9. Study plier types. **(A)** Slip-joint pliers. **(B)** Electrical pliers. **(C)** Side cut pliers. **(D)** Channellock pliers. **(E)** Tin snips. **(F)** Hose cutting pliers. **(G)** Vise-Grip pliers. **(H)** Metal working flat jaw Vise-Grip pliers. **(I)** Wheel lip pliers. **(J)** Welding Vise-Grip pliers.

objects. They will open wider than combination pliers.

Needlenose pliers have long, thin jaws for reaching in and grasping small parts. Never twist needlenose pliers or you will spring the jaws out of alignment. **Snap ring pliers** have tiny tips for fitting into circlips or snap rings. Both external and internal types are available.

Vise-Grip® or **locking pliers** have jaws that lock into position on parts. The jaws can be adjusted to different widths. Then, when clamped down, they will hold the part and free your hand to do another task. Special locking pliers with extended jaws are available for welding or working with sheet metal.

Diagonal cutting pliers have cutting jaws that will clip off wires flush with a surface. Another name for these is **side cut pliers.**

SHEET METAL TOOLS

Various tools are used by the technician to work body sheet metal. The following are some examples.

A **sheet metal gauge** is used to measure body or repair panel thickness or gauge size. It has small openings with the gauge size stamped next to it. Gauge size is a number system that denotes the thickness of sheet metal.

To use a thickness gauge, find the opening that fits the sheet metal. The number equals sheet metal thickness. Generally, a larger gauge number means thinner sheet metal. Ten gauge sheet metal would be thicker than 20 gauge.

Tin snips are the most common metal cutting tool. They can be used to cut straight or curved shapes in sheet metal. They are also used to trim panels to size.

Panel cutters will precisely cut sheet metal, leaving a clean, straight edge that can be easily welded. They are used to make straight or curved cutoffs in panels, often to repair corrosion.

FILES

Files are used to remove burrs and sharp edges and to do other smoothing tasks. Various shapes and coarsenesses of teeth are available. See **Figure 3–10.**

In general, a **coarse file** works well on soft materials, such as brass, aluminum, and plastics. A **fine file** will give a smoother surface on harder materials. A fine file is normally used to smooth steel.

When using a file, always have a handle securely in place. The sharp tang, if NOT covered, can easily puncture your hand or wrist. Apply filing pressure only on the forward stroke. Lift the file on the backstroke.

Never press too hard or file too rapidly. This will quickly dull the file. Do NOT hammer on a file. Never pry with a file. It is very brittle and can shatter. Clean the file with a stiff wire brush or card brush when it is clogged.

Body files have very large, open teeth for cutting plastic body filler. They often have a

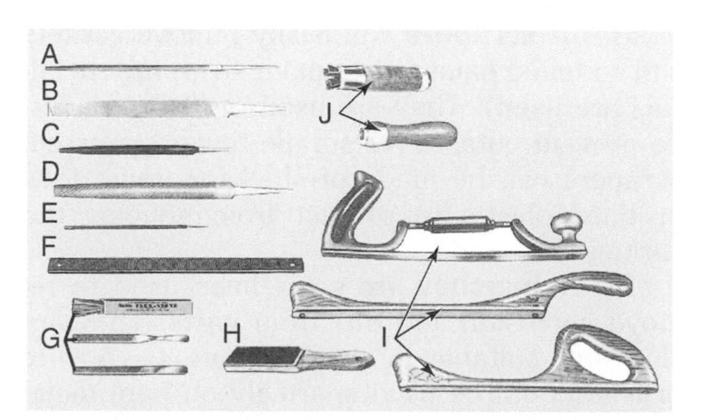

Figure 3–10. Note the names of files and file accessories. **(A)** Round file. **(B)** Flat file. **(C)** Diamond file. **(D)** Half round file. **(E)** Rat tail file. **(F)** Body file. **(G)** Small files. **(H)** File cleaning card. **(I)** Body file handles. **(J)** File handles. (Courtesy of Snap-on Tools Corp.)

separate blade that fits into a handle. They are commonly used when metal finishing damaged areas. See **Figure 3–10.**

SAWS

A **hacksaw** is sometimes needed to cut metal parts in collision repair. Most hacksaws have an adjustable frame that accepts different blade lengths. When installing a hacksaw blade, the blade teeth should point AWAY from the handle.

A reciprocating saw has a handle with the blade extending out one end. No frame is used. After making a starting hole, a jab saw can be used to cut into a blind panel that is not accessible from the back.

Hacksaw blade coarseness is rated in teeth per inch or millimeter. Blades also come in different tooth configurations. Select the correct blade for the material to be cut.

When using a hacksaw, place one hand on the handle and the other on the frame. Push down lightly on the forward stroke and release downward pressure on the backstroke.

As a general rule, count "one thousand one, one thousand two," and so on to time each stroke. If cuts are made too fast, the blade will quickly overheat and become dull. This method of timing stroke speed works for saws and files.

CLEANING TOOLS

Collision repair technicians sometimes have to clean vehicle parts when working. For example, they may need to replace mechanical parts (suspension or steering system parts, for example) that are covered with oil or grease.

Hand scrapers will easily remove gaskets and softened paint (when paint stripping chemicals are used). They are used on flat surfaces. To prevent cuts, never scrape toward yourself. Scrapers can be made of steel for tough jobs or hard plastic to protect from gouging the surface.

Steel brushes are sometimes used to remove corrosion and dirt from parts. They are slow but suitable in some situations. A wire brush should be used sparingly on bare metal because it can leave scratches. Wire brushes are ideal for cleaning weld joints.

Softer bristle brushes are often used with cleaning solvent to remove oil and grease from parts.

CREEPERS, COVERS

A **creeper** allows you to lie and move around on the shop floor while working. It also allows you to slide around and under a vehicle without getting dirty. A **stool creeper** is a small seat with caster wheels. You can lay your tools on the creeper to keep them handy.

Covers protect the vehicle from damage. A **fender cover** is often placed over the body to protect the paint from chips and scratches while you are working.

Seat covers protect the vehicle seats from being stained. Always use covers when needed. One stained seat or paint scratch will teach you the need for protecting the vehicle.

HYDROMETERS

Hydrometers are used to measure the **specific gravity** or density of a liquid. They are used to check antifreeze, battery acid, and other liquids.

An **antifreeze tester** is a hydrometer for testing the strength of the cooling system solution. It detects the water-to-antifreeze concentration. An indicating arrow or the number of floating balls indicates the freeze-up protection of the antifreeze. If the cooling system does not have enough antifreeze, major engine and radiator damage can result during cold weather.

FLUID HANDLING TOOLS

Funnels are needed to pour fluids into small openings. They may be needed when adding oil to an engine or brake fluid to a master cylinder.

Spouts are designed to install into a can for handy pouring. They too are often used when adding oil.

A **grease gun** is used to lubricate high friction points on a vehicle's steering and suspension systems. Some collision repair equipment also requires lubrication.

The grease gun tip is installed over grease fittings so that heavy grease can be injected into the part or fitting. Replaceable *grease cartridges* are often used with a grease gun.

An **oil can** is often used to lubricate parts and air tools. It has a long spout for applying oil to hard-to-reach areas. A **suction gun** can be used to remove or extract liquid. By pulling on the handle, a fluid can be pulled up into the gun.

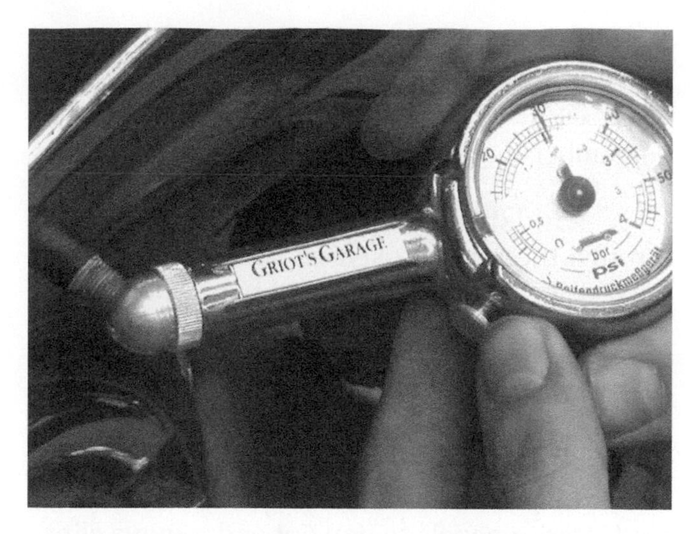

Figure 3–11. Proper tire inflation is important to vehicle safety. To check tire pressure, push the tire gauge over the valve stem tip. Read the gauge and compare it to the maximum pressure rating on the tire sidewall.

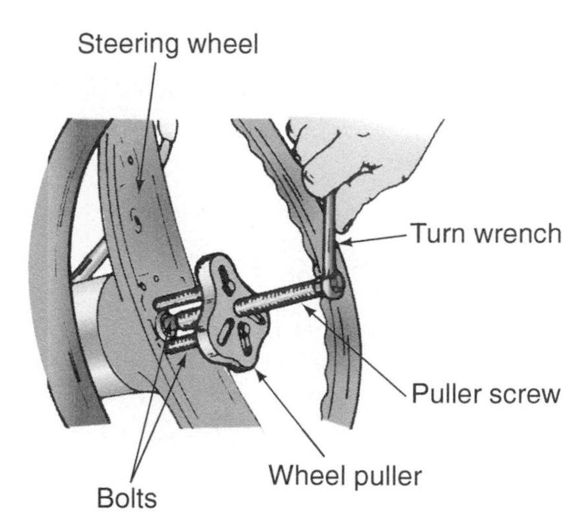

Figure 3–12. Wheel pullers will remove pressed-on parts, like a steering wheel. Wear eye protection! (OTC, a division of SPX Corp.)

TIRE TOOLS

A **tire pressure gauge** will accurately measure tire air pressure when pressed over the tire valve stem. Various designs are available. The gauge will read pressure in pounds per square inch (psi) or kilopascals. You should always check tire air pressures before releasing a vehicle to the customer. Low air pressure is common and can be dangerous. Recommended tire pressure is printed on the sidewall of the tire. Refer to **Figure 3–11.**

A **tread depth gauge** will quickly measure tire wear. The gauge is placed over the most worn area of the tire tread. A small pin on the gauge is pushed down into the tread. The gauge reading equals tire tread depth. The tire should be replaced or recommended for replacement if the tread is worn thinner than about ⅛ of an inch (3 mm).

PULLERS, PICKS

Wheel pullers are used to remove steering wheels, engine pulleys, and similar pressed-on parts. They are often bolted or mounted on the part, then a large screw is tightened to force the part off. See **Figure 3–12.**

A **slide hammer** is another type of puller that uses a hammering action to remove parts. Various ends can be installed on a slide hammer, as shown in **Figure 3–13.**

A **dent puller** is a slide hammer that will accept various pulling tips: a threaded tip, a hook tip, a cutting tip, or a suction cup. With the appropriate tip installed into the damaged panel, the slide hammer is briskly slid along the steel shaft and struck against its handle. This produces a powerful pulling force to help remove dents in sheet metal panels.

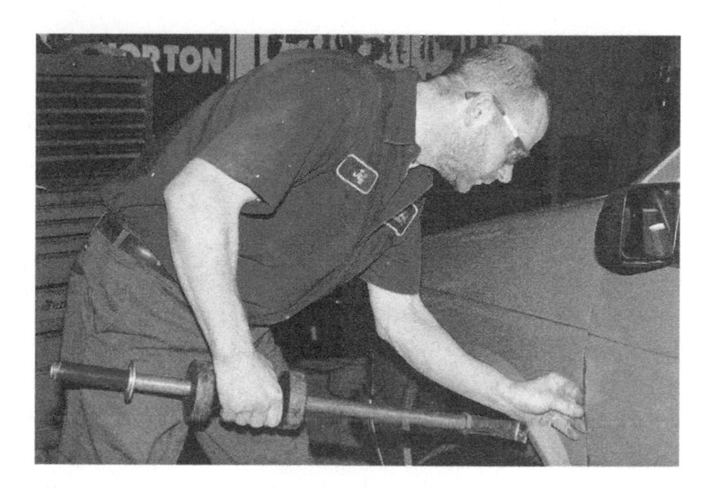

Figure 3–13. A slide hammer will produce power pulling blows to pull dents out of panels.

Pull rods have a handle and curved end for light pulling of dents. A small dent or crease can be pulled up with a single pull rod, but three or four may be used simultaneously to pull up larger dents. A body hammer can also be used with a pull rod. The high crown of a dent can be bumped down, while the low spot is pulled up. Simultaneous bumping and pulling returns the panel to its original shape with less danger of stretching the metal.

Picks are used to reach into confined spaces for removing tiny dents or dings. They are made

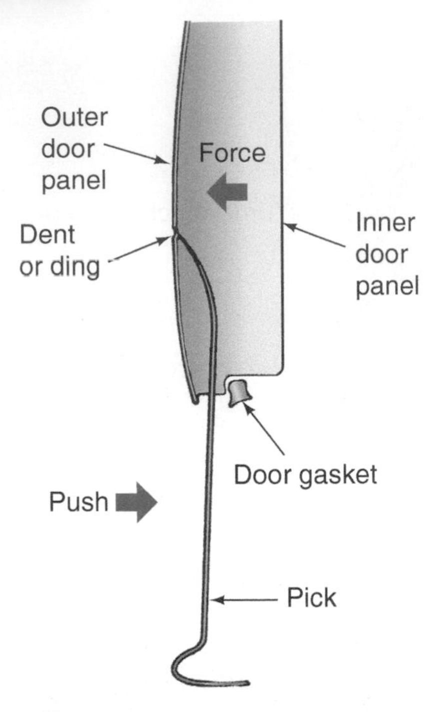

Figure 3–14. A pick tool is often used during dent removal. The pick will reach behind a hidden or blind panel to carefully push out small dents and door dings.

of strong case-hardened, spring steel. The pick is used to push up low spots. Picks vary in length and shape; most have a U-shaped handle. See **Figure 3–14.**

Picks are commonly used to straighten small dents in doors, quarter panels, and other sealed body sections. Picks are often preferred to slide hammers and pull rods because they do not require drilling holes in the sheet metal. They are used during **paintless dent removal** (straightening small body dings or dents without painting the panel).

NOTE

Straightening tools and techniques are discussed more in other text chapters. Refer to the index for additional information.

MISCELLANEOUS COLLISION REPAIR TOOLS

A variety of other miscellaneous hand tools will be useful from time to time. Many are inexpensive and have several uses. A few are very expensive but may be provided by the shop.

A common **utility knife** with a retractable blade is handy for cutting or trimming. Most come with extra blades stored in the handle. Remember that they will cause deep skin lacerations (cuts).

A **windshield knife** is designed to cut through the sealant used on some windshields. It has a sharp cutter blade and two handles. You hold one handle to guide the cutter and pull on the other handle to force the knife through the sealant. An electric heated windshield knife can be used to cut the adhesive. Air or pneumatic windshield cutters are also available.

Trim pad tools are designed to reach behind interior panels to pop out and remove clips. They often have a flat fork end that will surround the clip and push on the trim panel to prevent damage. They are often needed to remove inner door trim panels. See **Figure 3–15.**

A **door hinge spring compressor** is used to remove and install the small spring used on some door hinges. To use this tool, the screw is tightened to compress the spring. The spring is then shortened so that it can be installed or removed.

A **door striker wrench** is a special socket designed to fit over or inside door striker posts. It will allow you to turn and loosen the post for adjustment or replacement.

A **door alignment tool** can be used to slightly bend and adjust sprung doors and hatches. It has steel knurled blocks that fit next to the door hinge. Depending upon the placement of

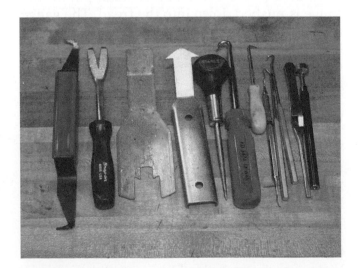

Figure 3–15. An assortment of trim tools is needed with today's cars. They will help you remove and install small plastic or metal clips that secure body molding and trim pieces to the vehicle.

the tool, when the door is partially closed you can quickly realign a door.

A **locksmith tool,** also termed a "slim jim," is used to open locked doors on vehicles. If you do not have a key or the keys are locked in the vehicle, this type of tool will often trip and unlock the door for entry into the passenger compartment. Although designs vary, one type simply slips down between the door glass and door frame to move the lock mechanism.

Suction cup tools have a large synthetic rubber cup for sticking onto parts. They are often used to hold window glass when holding or moving the glass. They can also be used to straighten large surface area dents in panels.

Dispensers or **cartridge guns** are used to apply adhesive or sealer to body panels. They are often spring loaded. When you press the trigger, spring tension acts on the cartridge to force the material out of its tip.

A **smoke gun** can be used to find air leaks around doors and windows. With the vehicle's blower on, one technician blows smoke around all potential leakage points. Another technician stands outside to find smoke coming out of the passenger compartment, locating the leak.

A *body filler dispenser* is used to squeeze the desired amount of body filler and hardener onto the mixing board. The material is forced out of the machine by the turn of a handle. This helps keep debris out of the filler.

Spreaders or **spatulas** are used to apply filler to low spots in body panels. They are usually made of plastic or sometimes of rubber. They come in various widths for different size dents or low spots.

A **masking machine** is designed to feed out masking paper while applying masking tape to one edge of the paper. It speeds the work because the tape is already attached to the paper. You can quickly apply the masking paper to the body with a masking machine. See **Figure 3–16.**

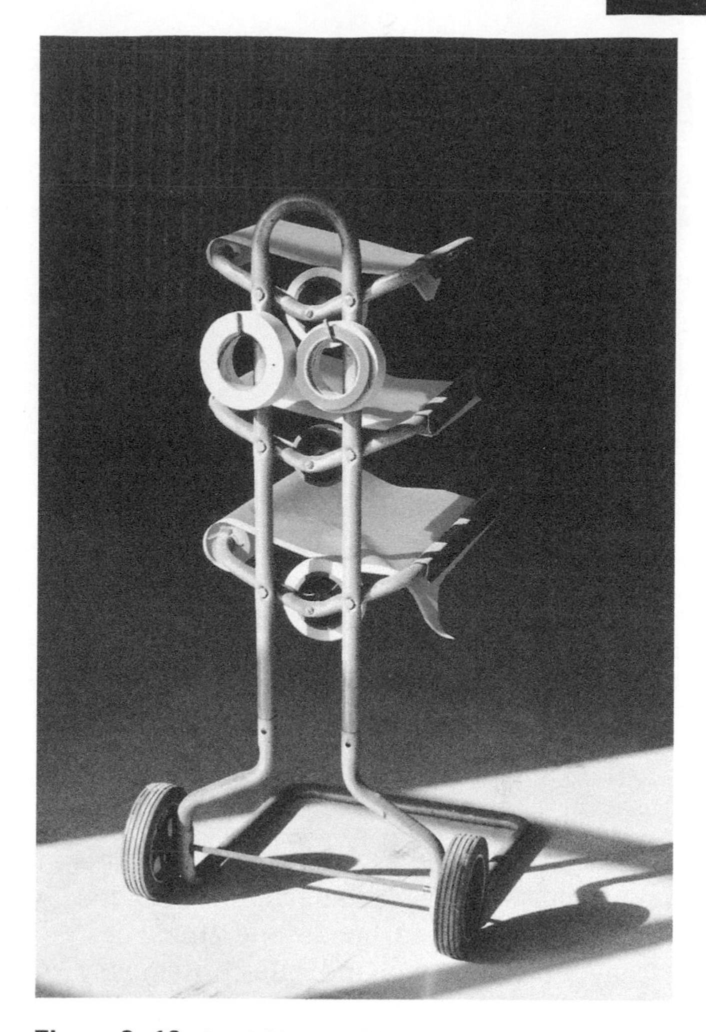

Figure 3–16. A masking machine will apply masking tape to the edges of masking paper so you can cover and protect areas of the car that are not to be painted.

Pinstripe brushes are used to apply paint in small, controlled areas. Small paint brushes can also be used to touch up chips along the lower body panel that were not painted. Pinstripe brushes come in different widths and lengths.

A **hood/trunk tool** is a telescoping rod that can be used to prop open the hood or trunk lid. It has rubber tips that contact the vehicle and panel. The tool will extend out and lock at varying lengths to help hold these panels in place while you are removing or installing fasteners. See **Figure 3–17.**

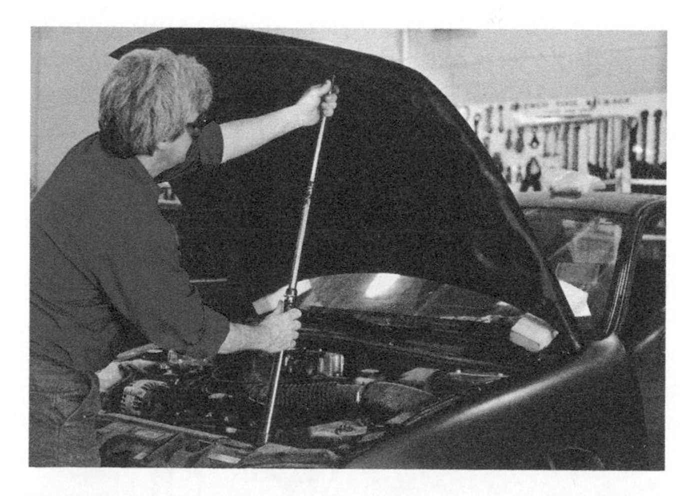

Figure 3–17. A telescoping hood tool is handy when doing major repairs to the front of a vehicle.

Sanding blocks support sand paper when working with body filler. See **Figure 3–18.**

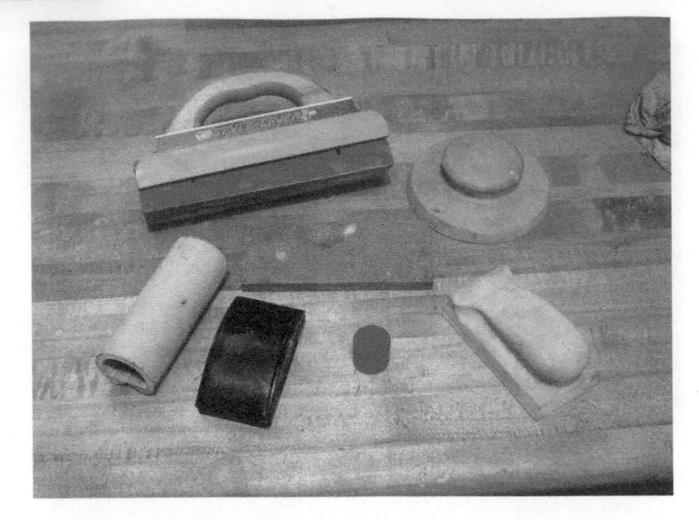

Figure 3–18. Sanding blocks are used when hand sanding body filler. They come in various shapes and sizes. The contour of the sanding block must match the shape of the body part being repaired. Use a flat sanding block on a flat body panel and a round sanding block if the area of the repair is round.

WARNING

Always ask another technician to help you remove and install hoods and trunk lids. They are very heavy and clumsy. Help may be needed to prevent damage to vehicle parts during installation and removal.

Note that many other more specialized hand tools are explained in this textbook. See **Figure 3–19** and refer to the index or specific chapters to gain more information on these specialized hand tools.

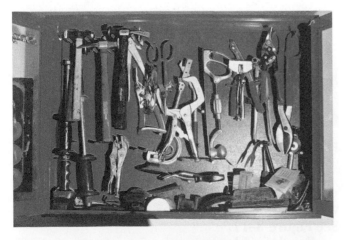

Figure 3–19. There are several other body shop hand tools. They are explained in later chapters. (http://.www.snap-on.com)

SUMMARY

- Purchase quality tools with lifetime guarantees. Quality tools will pay for themselves in a short period of time.
- Proper storage will protect tools and speed your work when they are easy to locate.
- Some of the more widely used tools in collision repair work include general duty hammers, body hammers, dollies and spoons, holding tools, punches and chisels, wrenches, prybars, pliers, sheet metal tools, files, saws, cleaning tools, creepers, covers, hydrometers, fluid handling tools, tire tools, pullers, picks, and knives.

TECHNICAL TERMS

lifetime tool guarantee
tool holders
tool box
upper chest
lower cabinet
hammers
ball peen hammer
brass hammer
lead hammer
plastic hammer
dead blow hammer
rubber mallet
body hammers
picking hammers
bumping hammers
finishing hammers
shrinking hammers
dolly
dolly block
body spoons
vise
vise caps
C-clamp
punches
center punch
drift punch
starting punch
pin punch
aligning punch
chisels
wrenches
wrench size
Society of Automotive Engineers (SAE)
open-end wrench
box-end wrench
combination wrench
tubing wrench
flare nut wrench
line wrench
Allen wrench
crescent wrench
adjustable wrench
pipe wrench
chain wrench
sockets
deep sockets
swivel sockets
impact sockets
socket drive size
ratchet
breaker bar
flex handle
speed handle
extensions
universal joint
torque wrench
torque

manufacturer's specifications
screwdrivers
standard screwdriver
Phillips screwdriver
Torx® screwdriver
stubby screwdriver
offset screwdrivers
impact driver
pliers
slip-joint pliers
combination pliers
rib joint pliers
Channellock® pliers
needlenose pliers
snap ring pliers
Vise-Grip® pliers
locking pliers
diagonal cutting pliers
side cut pliers
sheet metal gauge
tin snips
panel cutters
files
coarse file
fine file
body files
hacksaw
hand scrapers
steel brushes
softer bristle brushes
creeper
stool creeper
covers
fender cover
seat covers
hydrometers
specific gravity
antifreeze tester
funnels
spouts
grease gun
oil can
suction gun
tire pressure gauge
tread depth gauge
wheel pullers
slide hammer
dent puller
pull rods
picks
paintless dent removal
utility knife
windshield knife
trim pad tools
door hinge spring compressor
door striker wrench
door alignment tool
locksmith tool
suction cup tools
cartridge guns
smoke gun
spreaders
spatulas
masking machine
pinstripe brushes
hood/trunk tool
sanding blocks

REVIEW QUESTIONS

1. A good set of tools will speed ____________, and improve ____________.
2. What is a tool guarantee? Why would you want one?
3. Which tools would you put in the top chest of a tool box and which in the lower roll-around cabinet?
4. This type of hammer is often used to install wheel covers.
   a. Lead hammer
   b. Plastic hammer
   c. Dead blow hammer
   d. Rubber mallet
5. ____________ are used to achieve the final contour. The face on a ____________ is smaller than that of the heavier bumping hammer.
6. How are dollies or dolly blocks used?
7. ____________ are used sometimes like a hammer and sometimes like a dolly.
8. Never hammer on a vise handle when tightening it. True or false?
9. This type of punch is pointed to start a drilled hole or mark parts.
   a. Drift punch
   b. Starting punch
   c. Center punch
   d. Aligning punch
10. What is wrench size?
11. A car has damage to the front suspension and a brake line has to be removed. *Technician A* says to use Vise-Grip pliers first to make sure the fitting comes loose. *Technician B* says to use a combination wrench to protect the fitting nut from damage. Who is correct?
    a. Technician A
    b. Technician B
    c. Neither Technician
    d. Both Technicians A and B
12. List the most common socket drive sizes.
13. This tool provides the most powerful way of turning bolts and nuts.
    a. Ratchet
    b. Flex handle
    c. Speed handle
    d. Impact driver
14. Never twist on ____________ pliers or you will spring the jaws out of alignment.
15. Generally, a larger gauge number means a thinner sheet metal. Ten gauge sheet metal would be thicker than 20 gauge. True or false?

16. Explain when you would use a coarse file instead of a fine file.
17. What are body files?
18. A ______________ is a small seat with caster wheels.
19. Explain the use of a slide hammer dent puller.
20. ______________ have a handle and curved end for light pulling of dents.

ASE-STYLE REVIEW QUESTIONS

1. A technician is doing metal work on a panel. There are some ⅛-inch diameter high spots remaining. Which hammer should be used to straighten these small raised areas?
   a. Brass hammer
   b. Bumping hammer
   c. Shrinking hammer
   d. Picking hammer

2. *Technician A* is using a dolly to back up metal straightening with a finishing hammer. *Technician B* is using a dolly as a hammer to raise a low spot from behind. Who is correct?
   a. Technician A
   b. Technician B
   c. Both Technicians A and B
   d. Neither Technician

3. Which of the following is sometimes used as a dolly and sometimes as a hammer?
   a. Sanding block
   b. Pick
   c. Spoon
   d. Slide hammer

4. *Technician A* says to use soft vise caps when clamping a vehicle's control arm in a vise. *Technician B* says that you need the vise jaws to cut into the part for secure clamping. Who is correct?
   a. Technician A
   b. Technician B
   c. Both Technicians A and B
   d. Neither Technician

5. A bolt head is rusted and must be removed. *Technician A* is going to use locking pliers to try to remove the bolt. *Technician B* says to use a six-point wrench first. Who is correct?
   a. Technician A
   b. Technician B
   c. Both Technicians A and B
   d. Neither Technician

6. Which of the following is the best tool to use on a brake line fitting?
   a. Adjustable wrench
   b. Open-end wrench
   c. Closed-end wrench
   d. Tubing wrench

7. A vehicle's lug nuts have been overtightened. Which of the following tools should be used to loosen the lug nuts?
   a. Torque wrench
   b. Ratchet
   c. Locking pliers
   d. Breaker bar

8. A rusted bolt head has rounded off while being loosened. Which of the following tools should be used to remove it?
   a. Locking pliers
   b. Slip-joint pliers
   c. Breaker bar
   d. Speed handle

9. *Technician A* is using a hydrometer to measure the specific gravity of a vehicle's antifreeze solution. *Technician B* is using a hydrometer to check the viscosity of motor oil. Who is correct?
   a. Technician A
   b. Technician B
   c. Both Technicians A and B
   d. Neither Technician

10. A slide hammer is being used to straighten a dent. *Technician A* says that a hooked attachment will grip and pull exposed surfaces. *Technician B* says to weld rods or pins onto the panel for tool attachment. Who is correct?

a. Technician A

b. Technician B

c. Both Technicians A and B

d. Neither Technician

ACTIVITIES

1. Tour your shop. Note the location of all hand tools. Prepare a report on your findings.

2. Visit an outside collision repair shop. Talk with other technicians about the tools they use. Discuss with the class anything you learned about new tools or techniques.

3. Order catalogs from tool manufacturers. Compare the quality, price, and warranty of tools offered by each manufacturer.

CHAPTER

4 Power Tools and Equipment

OBJECTIVES

After studying this chapter, you should be able to:

- Identify power tools found in a collision repair facility.
- Explain the purpose of each type of power tool.
- Summarize how to safely use tools.
- Identify the typical types of equipment used in collision repair.
- Describe how to use collision repair equipment.
- Select the right power tool or piece of equipment for the job.
- Explain low emissions spray equipment and regulations.
- Explain the operation of spray booths and drying rooms.
- Identify the various types of spray guns and explain how each type operates.

INTRODUCTION

From the time of the blacksmith to today's technician, tools have served to increase the abilities of human hands, arms, legs, backs, eyes, and ears. They allow us to do things that would be impossible otherwise.

Power tools and equipment use electrical energy, compressed air, or hydraulic power. Drills, sanders, cut-off tools, scanners, air compressors, spray guns, frame straightening equipment, alignment racks, and some measurement systems all use some form of power to do their work. For you to work efficiently, a sound grasp of the technology and use of power tools and equipment is essential.

DANGER

Power tools and equipment can be very dangerous if NOT used correctly. Always follow the instructions given in the owner's manual for the specific tool or piece of equipment. The information in this chapter is general and cannot cover all tool variations. If in doubt about any tool or piece of equipment, ask your instructor or shop supervisor for a demonstration.

DANGER

The use of air-driven or electric power tools requires safety glasses, goggles, or a face shield. Also, never wear loose clothing that could get caught in a tool. Wear leather gloves when grinding, welding, or doing other tasks that could injure your hands.

AIR SUPPLY SYSTEM

The shop's **air supply system** provides clean, dry air pressure for numerous tools and equipment. It has an air compressor, metal lines, rubber hoses, quick disconnect fittings, a pressure regulator, filters, and other parts.

AIR COMPRESSOR

An **air compressor** is made up of an electric motor, an air pump, and a large air storage tank. The motor spins the air pump, which works like a small, reciprocating piston engine. Piston

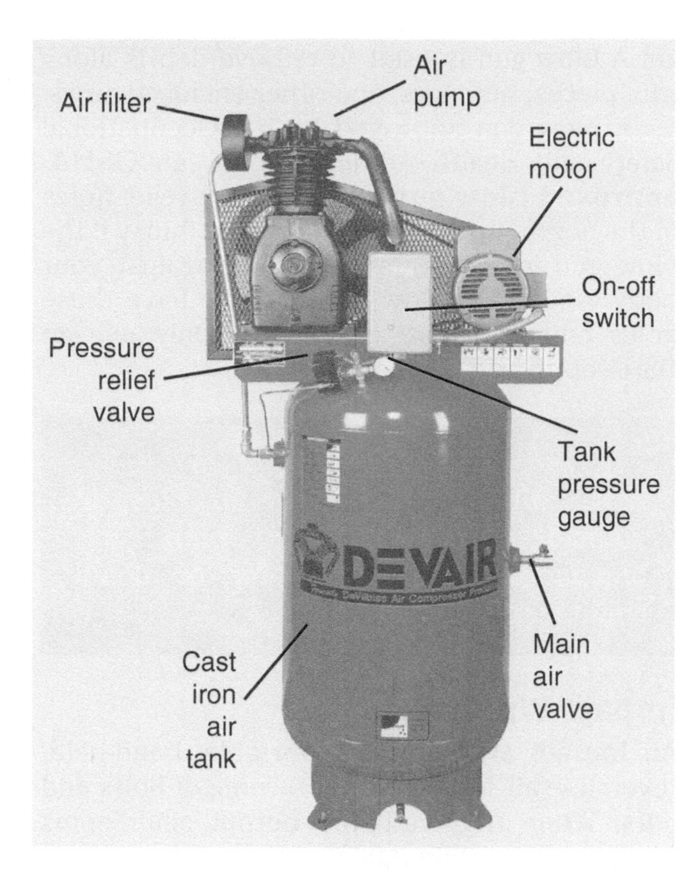

Figure 4–1. Note the major parts of an air compressor. It serves as the air pump or "heart" for the air supply to your air tools. (Courtesy of Team Blowtherm)

action in the air pump pushes the air into a large, thick steel storage tank. The "heart" of any paint shop is its air compressor. See **Figure 4–1.**

A **compressor drain valve** on the bottom of the tank allows you to drain out water. The compression of the air tends to make moisture condense out of the air. This moisture must be drained out periodically to prevent it from entering the air lines.

An **automatic drain valve** periodically opens a solenoid-operated valve on the bottom of the air compressor to remove moisture from the storage tank. This saves you from having to manually open the drain valve every day. The system is commonly found on large industrial air compressors.

A **compressor pressure relief valve** prevents too much pressure from entering the tank. It is a spring-loaded valve that opens at a predetermined pressure, usually around 90 to 120 psi (63 to 84 kg/cm^2).

An **air tank shut-off valve** is a hand valve that isolates the tank pressure from shop line pressure. It should be closed at night or when the compressor is not going to be used. If it is NOT closed, the compressor would run all night if a hose leaked or ruptured.

Compressor oil plugs are provided for filling and changing air pump oil. The oil level in the compressor should be checked regularly and the oil changed periodically. Normally use single weight, nondetergent oil or the oil recommended by the manufacturer.

AIR LINES

Shop air lines are thick steel pipes that feed out from the compressor tank to several locations in the collision repair shop. Flexible synthetic rubber **air hoses** connect the metal pipes to the air tools and equipment.

Air hose sizes are ¼ inch (6 mm), 5⁄16 inch (8 mm) and ⅜ inch (10 mm) inside diameters (ID). There is less restriction using larger hoses. The preferred diameter is 5⁄16 inch (8 mm), and it is used in many shops.

Air couplings allow you to quickly install and remove air hoses and air tools. Couplings should also have a large enough inside diameter to prevent airflow restrictions.

By sliding the outer fitting sleeve back and pushing, you can connect or disconnect a tool and a hose.

AIR PRESSURE REGULATOR AND FILTER

An **air pressure regulator** is used to precisely control the amount of pressure fed to air tools and equipment. A regulator is commonly used to reduce air pressure sent to paint spray guns. However, pressure regulators may NOT be used between the compressor and many air tools, like impact guns. Those tools require the power of full line pressure. See **Figure 4–2.**

The air pressure regulator has a thumb screw, spring-loaded valve, and pressure gauge. By turning the thumb screw while watching the gauge, you can set pressure to the desired level. The regulator pressure gauge often reads in both pounds per square inch (psi) and metric values (kPa, bar, etc.).

An **air line filter-drier** is used in the air line to remove moisture and debris from the air flowing through the air lines. It is designed to trap and hold water and oil that passes out of the compressor air pump. If any of these materials were to enter your paint spray gun, they would ruin the paint job.

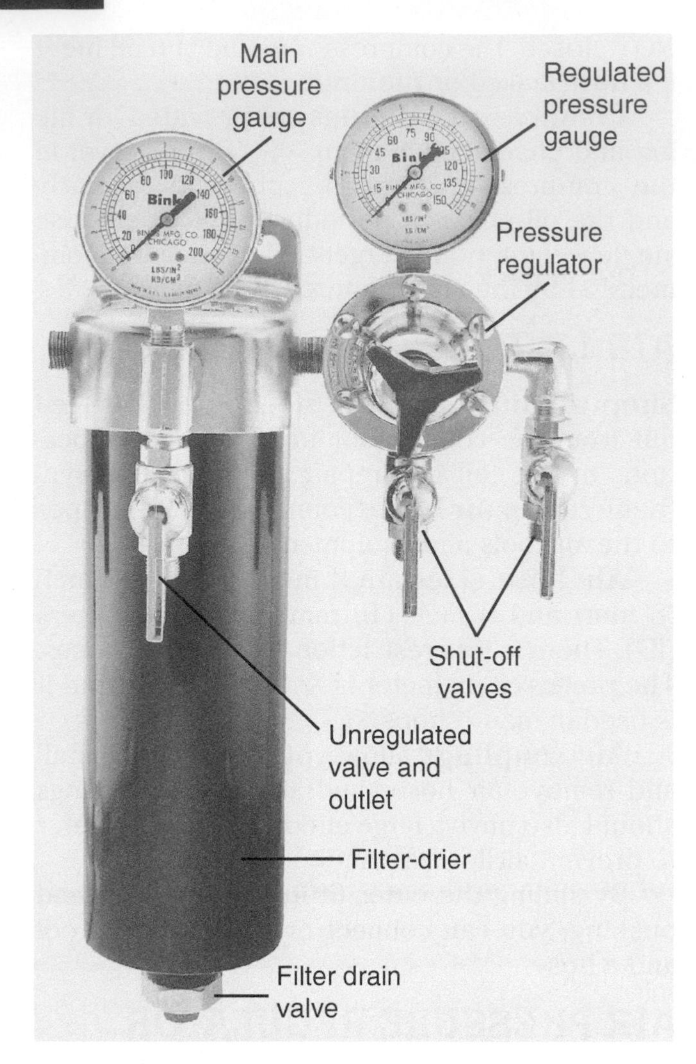

Figure 4–2. A pressure regulator allows you to adjust air line pressure to match the specs for the air tool, such as a spray gun that operates on a lower pressure than most other air tools. (Courtesy of ITW Automotive Refinishing)

An **air filter drain valve** allows you to remove trapped water and oil from the filter. It should be opened every evening to purge this unwanted material.

AIR TOOLS

Air tools include hand-held spray guns, impact guns, and other tools used in the collision repair shop. It is critical that you know how to identify and use them safely. There are various types of air tools. They run cool and are very dependable.

Air Blow Gun

An **air blow gun** is used to blow dust and dirt off the vehicle and its parts. It has a trigger that can be pressed to release a strong stream, or blast, of air. A blow gun is used to remove debris along trim pieces, bumpers, and other enclosed areas.

A blow gun approved by the Occupational Safety and Health Administration (an **OSHA-approved blow gun**) has pressure-relief holes in the nozzle tip. This helps prevent injury if the blow gun is accidentally pressed against your body. Non-OSHA blow guns do not have these holes and are more dangerous. Only use an OSHA-approved blow gun!

DANGER

Never direct a blow gun air blast at yourself or others. If air enters your bloodstream, serious injury or death could result.

Impact Wrenches

An **impact wrench** is a portable, hand-held, reversible air tool for rapid turning of bolts and nuts. When triggered, the output shaft spins freely at more than 2,000 rpm (revolutions per minute). The socket snaps over the square drive head and shaft. See **Figure 4–3.**

When using an air impact wrench, it is important that only *impact sockets* and **impact adapters** (usually black) are used. Other types of sockets and adapters (chrome plated) might shatter and fly off, endangering everyone in the immediate area.

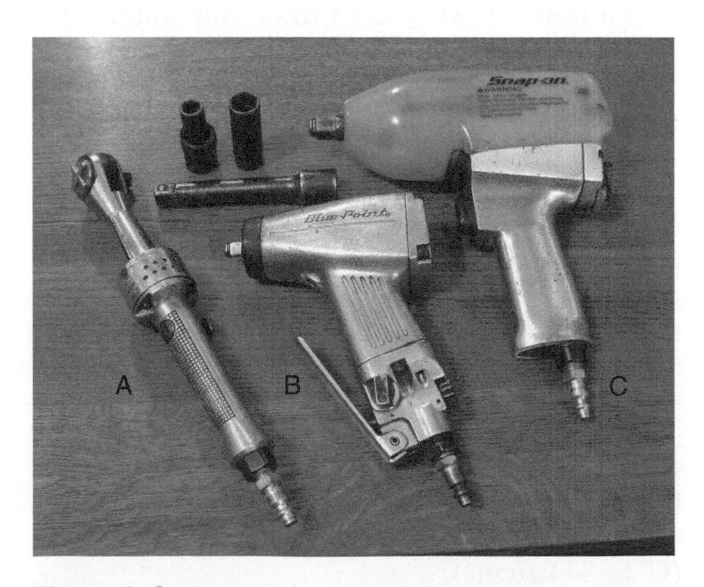

Figure 4–3. Air impact wrenches and ratchets greatly speed your work. **(A)** A ½-inch impact is good for large fasteners. **(B)** ⅜-inch drive impact is for smaller bolts and nuts. **(C)** An air ratchet is handy for turning smaller fasteners in tight quarters.

DANGER

Never use a conventional universal joint on an impact gun. The spinning joint can fly apart and explode. Use only special impact-type swivel joints with an impact wrench.

A ½-*inch impact wrench* has a ½-inch drive head and is shaped like a pistol with a hand grip hanging down. It can tighten fasteners to over 100 foot-pounds of torque. Remember that this is enough to snap off or stretch most bolts. It is commonly used on bolt and nut head sizes over about 9⁄16 inch (14 mm). A ½-inch impact wrench is frequently used to service wheel lug nuts.

A ⅜-*inch impact wrench* has a drive head of a smaller size for working with fastener heads under 9⁄16 inch (14 mm). It is lighter and more handy for working with small bolts and nuts on body panels.

The **air ratchet** wrench, like the hand ratchet, has a special ability to work in hard-to-reach places. Its ⅜-inch angle drive reaches in and loosens or tightens where other hand or power wrenches cannot fit. An air ratchet is handy for working behind panels, in tight quarters. The air ratchet wrench looks like an ordinary ratchet. It has a larger hand grip that contains the air vane motor and drive mechanism.

WARNING

Remember that there is no reliable adjustment with an air ratchet or impact wrench. Where accurate torque is required, use a torque wrench! The air regulator on air-powered wrenches can be employed to adjust torque only to an approximate tightness. Adjust the impact to ensure you do NOT overtighten. Then use the hand torque wrench to tighten the bolt or nut to specs.

Air Hammer

An **air hammer** uses back-and-forth hammer blows to drive a cutter or driver into the work piece. It works like a conventional hammer and chisel or punch but much quicker. Different shaped tools can be installed in the air hammer. For cutting, flat, forked, and curved cutters are useful.

An **air chisel** is similar, but it is smaller and is often equipped with a cold chisel type of cutter.

DANGER

When using an air hammer or chisel, make sure the tool is held against the work before pulling the trigger. This will prevent the cutter from possibly flying out of the tool. Avoid running into hidden hardware, frame rails, and wiring with cutting tools.

Drills

Drills are used to make accurately sized holes in metal and plastic parts. Both air and electric drills are available.

Air drills use shop air pressure to spin a drill bit. They can be adjusted to any speed and are more commonly used than electric drills. Air drills are smaller and lighter than electric drills. This compactness makes them a great deal easier to use for most tasks.

Drill bits of different sizes fit into the chuck on drills for making holes in parts. The size is usually stamped on the upper part of each bit.

A **key** is used to tighten the chuck. The **chuck** has movable jaws that close down and hold the bit. The key has a small gear that turns a gear on the chuck.

Never leave a key in a drill when not tightening. Also, unhook the air hose when installing a bit. Otherwise, injury could result. This also applies to a large drill press.

Hole saws are special cutters for making large holes in body panels. They fit into a drill like a drill bit.

A **spot weld drill** is specially designed for removing spot welded body panels, **Figure 4–4.** It has a clamp-type head and lever arm for accurately drilling through spot welds. The cutter will not deviate from the weld center during cutting.

Air Cutters

An **air nibbler** is used like tin snips to cut sheet metal. It has an air-powered snipping blade that moves up and down to cut straight or curved shapes in sheet metal panels.

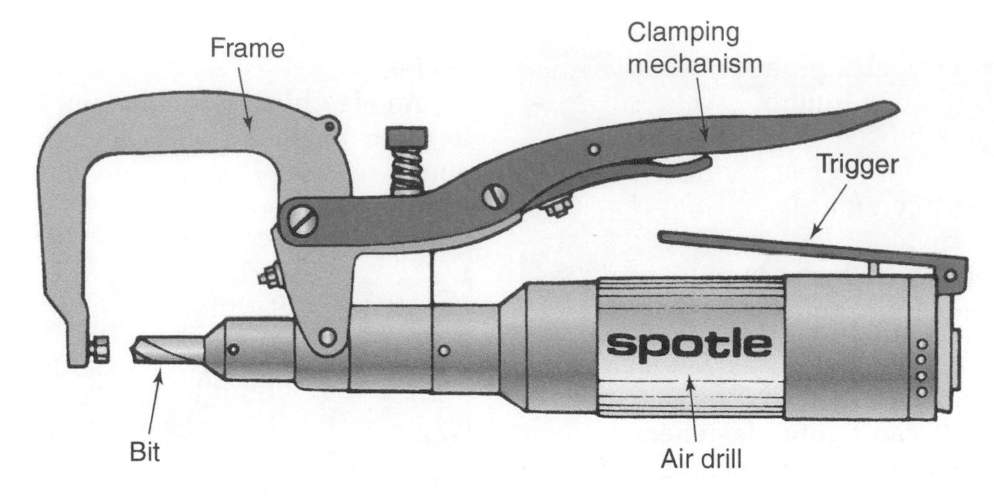

Figure 4–4. A spot weld drill has a special frame mounted over the drill bit so that you can adjust the depth of the drilled hole for removing welded-on body panels. (Courtesy of NCG Company/Spotle Distributor)

An **air cutoff tool** uses a small abrasive wheel to rapidly cut or grind metal. It is handy for cutting when a confinement prevents the use of a nibbler.

An **air saw** uses a reciprocating (back-and-forth) action to move a hacksaw-type blade for cutting parts. It works just like a hacksaw but will cut much more quickly. Look at **Figure 4–5.**

Air Sanders

An **air sander** uses an abrasive action to smooth and shape body surfaces. Different coarseness sandpapers can be attached to the pad on the sander. *Coarser sandpaper* removes material more quickly. *Fine sandpaper* produces a smoother surface finish. Air sanders are one of the most commonly used air tools in collision repair.

A **circular sander** simply spins its pad and paper around and around in a circular motion. This type of sander is seldom used in collision repair. See **Figure 4–6.**

A **safety trigger** is designed to help prevent you from turning the power tool on by accident. The on-off trigger has a spring-loaded arm that locks the trigger off and keeps it from being pushed down. You must pull back on the safety

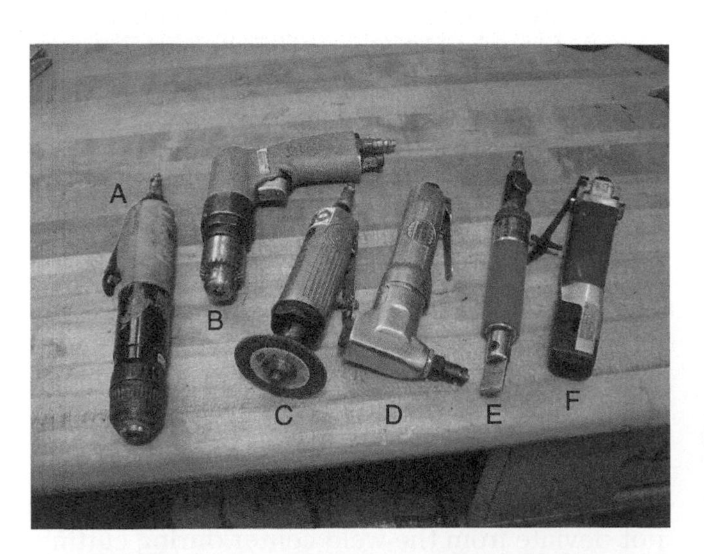

Figure 4–5. These air tools are for drilling, grinding, and cutting operations. **(A)** Air drill/grinder with quick disconnect chuck. **(B)** Air drill with conventional chuck. **(C)** A cutoff wheel is often used to cut and grind metal. **(D)** An air nibbler will quickly cut sheet metal. **(E)** Air chisel with cut and separate spot welds in sheet metal. **(F)** An air saw uses reciprocating action to cut metal.

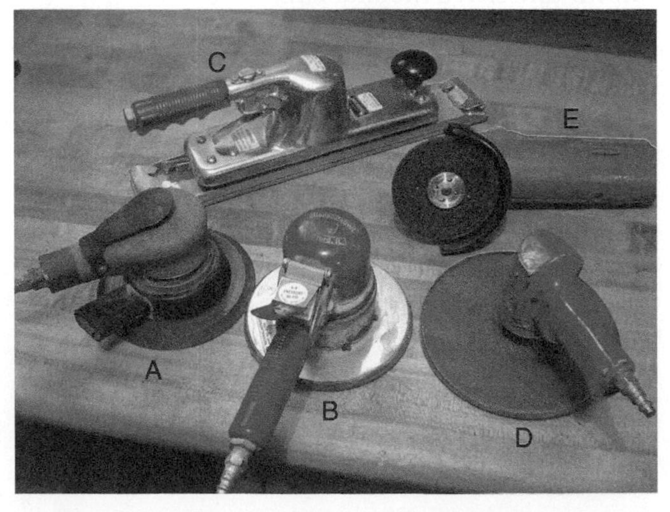

Figure 4–6. Sanders and grinders are very important tools of a body technician. They must be selected and used properly for quality body work. **(A)** A dual-action sander will feather or final sand a repair area. **(B)** A single-action sander will plane down a flat surface efficiently. **(C)** An air file will level down a large flat surface efficiently. **(D)** A small grinder with a flexible abrasive disc rapidly removes material. **(E)** A grinder with thicker disc is often used to grind down spot welds.

lever and then push down on the trigger to energize the tool. Many potentially dangerous power tools are now equipped with a safety trigger.

An **oscillating sander** spins a sanding pad that is mounted to a concentric shaft that also has a counterweight on it. These sanders are used because they sand very smoothly and sand faster than some other sanders.

An **orbital** or **dual-action sander** moves in two directions at the same time. This produces a much smoother surface finish. A dual-action, or DA, sander is used to featheredge a repair area. It is the workhorse of body technicians.

The **sander pad** is a soft synthetic rubber mounting surface for the sandpaper. It normally screws into the sander head.

Sander pads can be designed to use adhesive, self-stick sandpaper, or a Velcro system. The Velcro system is gaining popularity because the sandpaper runs cooler, fine grits do not clog as easily, you can change sandpaper more quickly, and you can reuse the sandpaper if desired. Refer to **Figure 4–7.**

DANGER

Never allow an air sander to freewheel, or spin, without the sandpaper being in contact with the work surface! Due to the high rotation speeds that would result, the sandpaper could fly off the pad and cause serious injury.

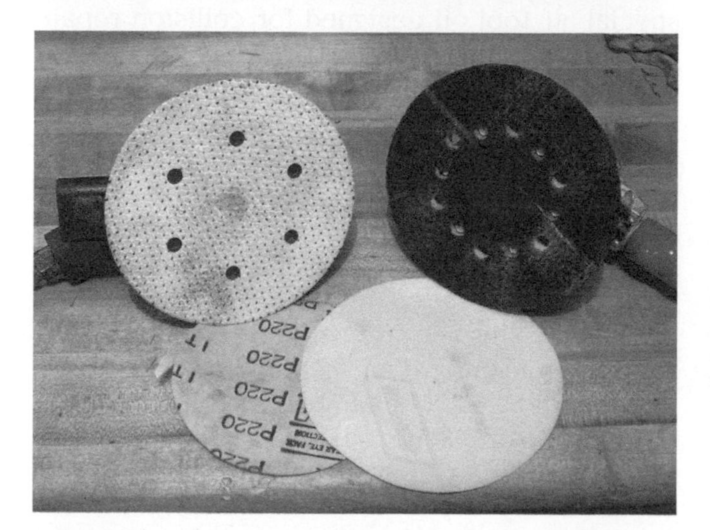

Figure 4–7. Here are the two most common types of air sander pads. (Left) A smooth sander pad requires self-stick sandpaper discs. (Right) A Velcro pad has small fiber hooks that engage small fiber loops on the surface of the sandpaper.

An **air file** is a long, thin air sander for working large surfaces on panels. It is handy when you must true or sand a large repair area. It will plane down filler so that a large area is level or flat. An air file is often used for rough shaping operations on body filler.

GRINDERS

Grinders are used for fast removal of material. They are often used to smooth metal joints after welding and to remove paint and primer. They come in various sizes and shapes. See **Figure 4–8.**

The most commonly used portable air grinder in collision repair and refinishing shops is the **disc-type grinder.** It is operated like the single-action disc sander. An air grinder should be used carefully. It can quickly thin down and cut through body panels, causing major problems.

DANGER

If an air grinder will cut metal, it can certainly cut a technician. Wear leather gloves and a full-face shield when grinding.

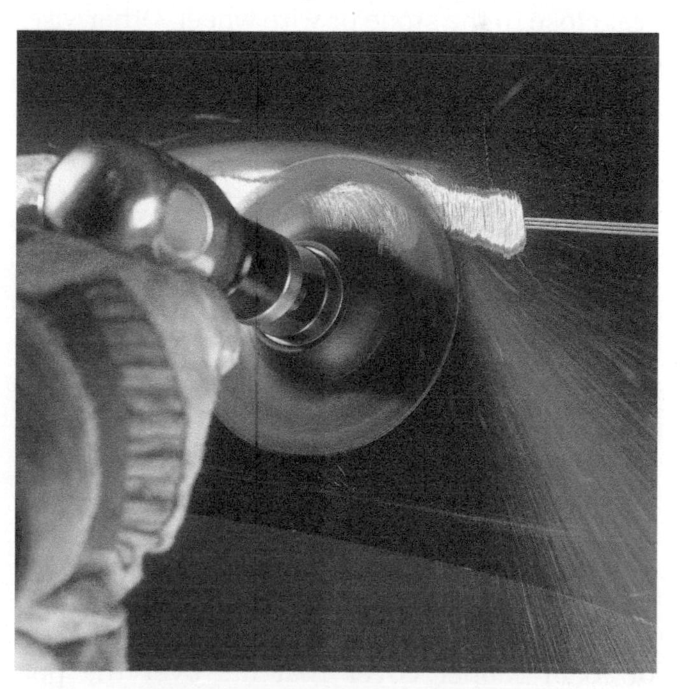

Figure 4–8. A grinder is commonly used to quickly remove old paint or rust from body panels. (Courtesy of Norton)

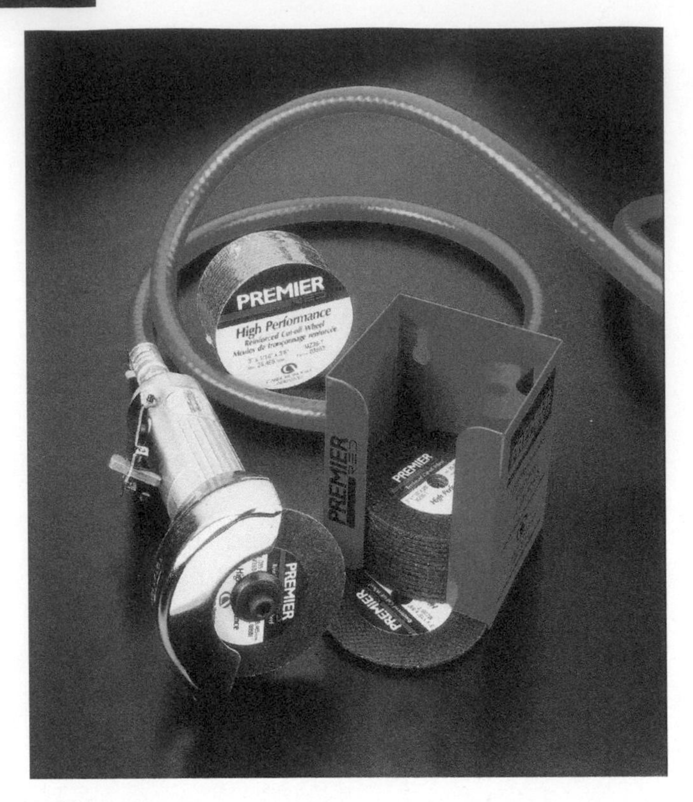

Figure 4–9. A cutoff tool is commonly used to cut sheet metal and grind down spot welds. It will grind quickly and accurately. (Courtesy of Norton)

A **bench grinder** is a stationary, electric grinder mounted on a workbench or pedestal stand. It is used to sharpen chisels and punches and to shape other tool tips.

When using a bench grinder, keep the tool rest close to the stone or wire wheel. Otherwise, the tool or part can be pulled into the grinder. This can force your hand into the wheel or brush, causing a painful injury. Also, keep the shield in place over the top of the stone or brush and wear eye protection.

A cutoff wheel is a small grinder with a very narrow abrasive wheel for cutting metal quickly. See **Figure 4–9.**

POLISHERS

An **air polisher** is used to smooth and shine painted surfaces by spinning a soft buffing pad. Polishing or buffing compound is applied to the paint with the polisher pad. This removes minor imperfections to increase **paint gloss** or shine.

A polishing pad is a cotton, synthetic cloth, or foam rubber cover that fits over the polisher's backing plate or arbor. Sometimes the pad and backing plate are *integral,* or *one piece.*

A **cloth or cotton polishing pad** is often used when heavy polishing is needed. The pad is very tough and will cut paint smoothly and quickly.

A **foam rubber polishing pad** is commonly used for final polishing to remove swirl marks. It is very soft and will produce a higher luster than a cloth pad.

Swirl marks are tiny, unwanted circular marks that can be seen after buffing. They are often caused by using a course polishing compound or a pad that is too hard or dirty. When polishing, swirl marks should be kept to a minimum. Use a foam pad for final polishing.

A **pad cleaning tool** is a metal star wheel and handle that will clear dried polishing compound out of the cloth or cotton pad. The wheel is held onto the spinning pad to clean out and soften the pad material. It will help prevent swirl marks in the paint.

PNEUMATIC TOOL MAINTENANCE

Air tools need little upkeep. However, you will have problems if basic maintenance is not performed. For instance, moisture gathers in the air lines and is blown into tools during use. If a tool is stored with water in it, rust will form and the tool will wear out quickly.

Air tool lubrication involves injecting a few drops of oil into the air inlet of all air tools to prevent corrosion and friction damage. To avoid contamination of vehicle's surfaces, use only special air tool oil designed for collision repair air tools. It is formulated to prevent surface contamination that can result from oil spraying from the air outlet on the tool. Motor oil and transmission fluid should NOT be used to lubricate air tools, because they will contaminate the repair surface and your paint. Refer to **Figure 4–10.**

Put a small amount of oil into the air inlet or into special oil holes on the tool BEFORE AND AFTER use. This will prevent rapid wear and rusting of the vane motor and other parts of the tool. Run the tool after adding the oil. Wipe off excess oil on the tool to keep it off body parts.

An **in-line oiler** is an attachment that will automatically meter oil into air lines for air tools. It can be used on lines used for air tools but NOT for spray guns.

Never forget! Your tools and equipment cannot function correctly without good care. To do

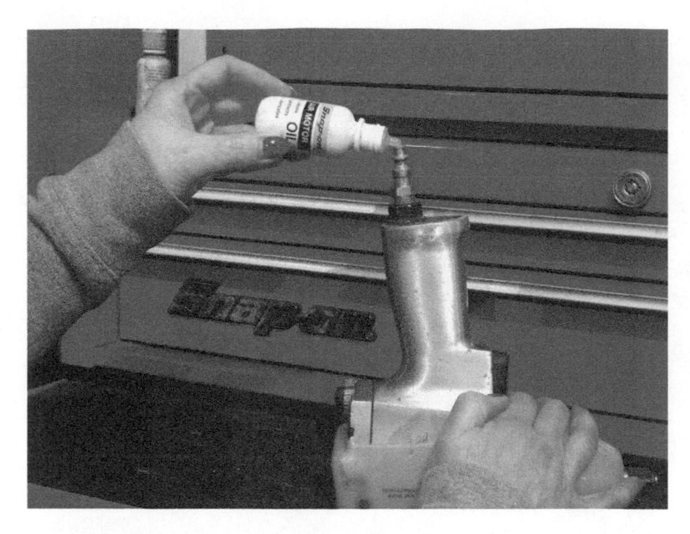

Figure 4–10. Always lubricate your air tools every evening before putting them away. This will keep any moisture from rusting and ruining your air tools. It is best to use non-paint-contaminating spray gun oil in all of your air tools.

high-quality collision repair and refinishing/painting work, maintain your tools and equipment.

BLASTERS

Blasters are air-powered tools for forcing sand, plastic beads, or another material onto surfaces for paint removal. For example, they are handy when trying to remove surface rust or cracking, deteriorating paint from body panels.

With today's thin-gauge, high-strength steel, plastic media blasting is often recommended over grinding. Grinding thins the metal and makes it weaker.

A **hand blaster** is a small, portable tool for blasting parts and panels on the vehicle. Abrasive is installed in the blaster cup or container. Airflow through the tool pulls a metered amount of abrasive out of the tool and forces it against the work piece. This will quickly remove paint, primer, rust, and scale to take the surface down to bare metal.

A **cabinet blaster** is a stationary enclosure equipped with a sand or bead blast tool. A window and rubber gloves in the cabinet allow you to blast parts without being exposed to the abrasive dust. It is often used on small parts removed from a car.

SPRAY GUNS

Spray guns are used to apply sealer, primer, paint, and other materials to the car. Spray guns must atomize the liquid so that it flows onto the vehicle surface smoothly and evenly. The term **atomize** means to break the liquid into very tiny droplets or a fine mist. This will help the material go down smoothly. This requires sufficient air pressure and volume at the spray gun. See **Figure 4–11.**

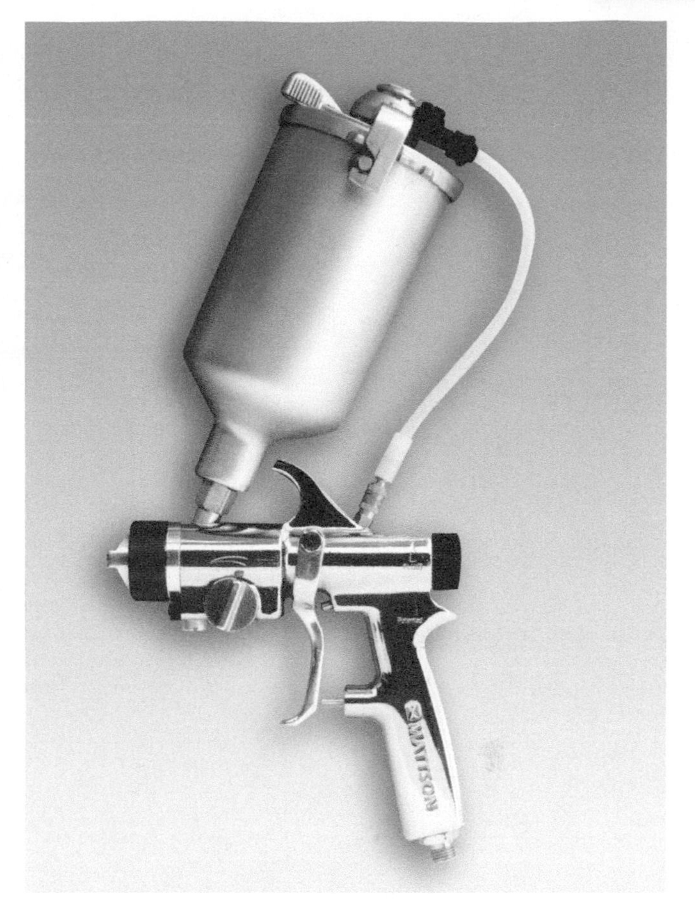

Figure 4–11. Spray guns are used to apply a paper-thin film of primer and paint to the vehicle body. They are precision tools that must be handled and cared for properly. This is a modern, high-efficiency gravity-feed spray gun. (Courtesy of Mattson)

If you plan on being a good painter, you must know your painting equipment inside and out.

Spray Gun Parts

To use, service, and troubleshoot a spray gun properly, you must understand the operation of its major parts. See **Figure 4–12** as each spray gun part is discussed.

The **gun body** holds the parts that meter air and liquid. The body holds the spray pattern adjustment valve, fluid control valve, air cap, fluid tip, trigger, and related parts.

The **spray gun cup** often fits onto the bottom or on top of the body to hold the material to be sprayed. The cup fits against a rubber

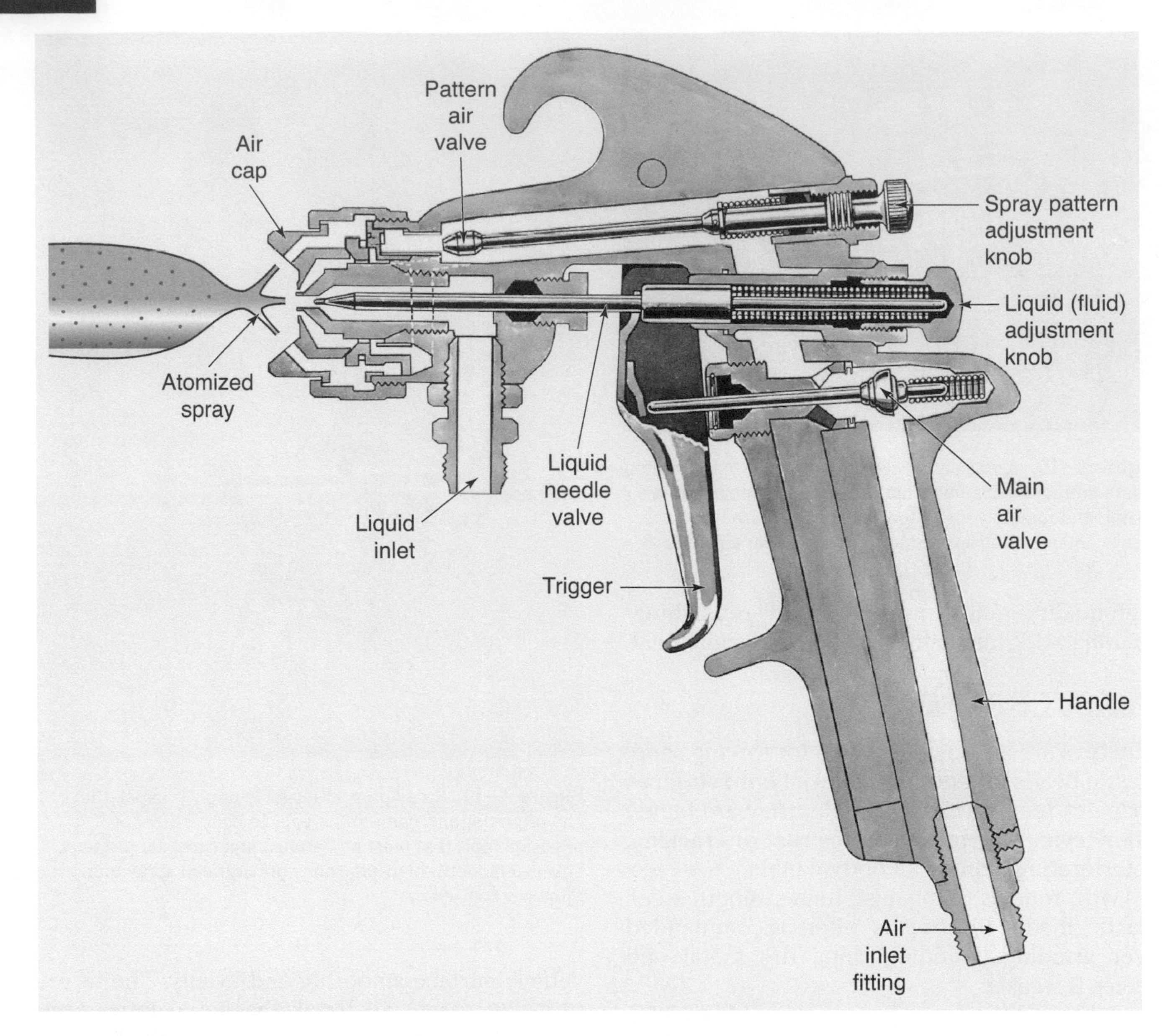

Figure 4–12. Study the cutaway view of this spray gun and learn the part names. (Courtesy of ITW Automotive Refurbishing)

seal to prevent leakage. The seal is mounted in a lid on the gun body.

The spray gun's **fluid control valve** can be turned to adjust the amount of paint or other material emitted. It consists of a thumb screw or knob, needle valve, and spring. Turning the knob affects how far the trigger pulls the needle valve open. The **fluid needle valve** seats in the fluid tip to prevent flow or can be pulled back to allow flow.

The spray gun's **air control valve** controls how much air flows out of the air cap side jets. It has an *air needle* that can be slid back and forth to open or close the air valve.

The *spray gun trigger* can be pulled to open both the fluid and air valves. It uses lever action to pull back on the needle valves.

The **spray gun air cap** works with the air valve to control the spray pattern of the paint. It screws over the front of the gun head.

The **spray pattern** is the shape of the atomized spray when it hits the body. With little airflow out of the side jets on the cap, you would have a very round, concentrated spray pattern. As you adjust airflow up, the cap jets narrow and better atomize the fluid flowing out of the gun.

For more information on this and other related subjects, refer to the text index.

Gravity-Feed Spray Guns

A **gravity-feed spray gun** mounts the cup on top of the spray gun head so that the pull of gravity helps the material flow out of the cup.

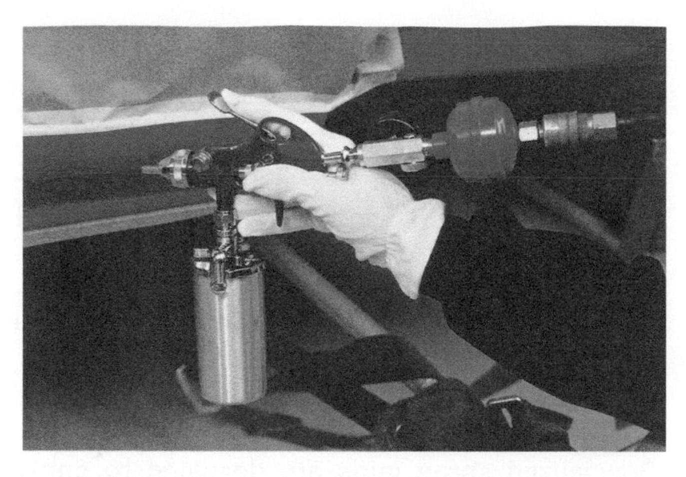

Figure 4–13. This small touch-up spray gun is good for painting small areas or for doing custom paint work.

A gravity-feed design helps eliminate the problem of spitting. All of the liquid will flow down into the pickup hole formed in the bottom of the cup (see **Figure 4–13**). No pickup tube is needed. The gravity-feed spray gun is a very common design with today's high spray efficiency requirements.

Siphon Spray Guns

Siphon spray guns use airflow through the gun head to form a suction or vacuum that pulls paint into the airstream. One is shown in **Figure 4–14.**

An **air vent hole** and hose on the siphon spray gun allow atmospheric pressure to enter the vacuum cup. This vent often becomes clogged with curing or drying primer or paint. If the vent is plugged, paint will not spray out of the gun.

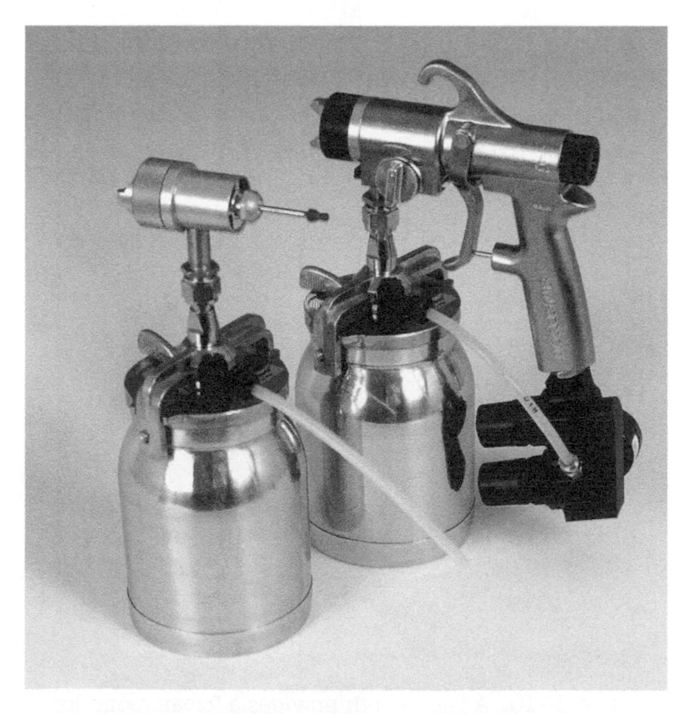

Figure 4–14. Although new suction-feed spray guns are high-efficiency designs, they are being replaced by gravity feed for improved dependability. (Courtesy of Matteson)

Pressure-Feed Spray Guns

Pressure-feed spray guns use shop air pressure inside the paint cup or tank to force the material out of the gun.

Having a remote cup or tank makes the pressure-feed spray gun lighter and easier to handle. It also permits spraying with the gun aiming straight for painting under flared parts without danger of "spitting." Also, with the cup or tank away from the vehicle, the problem of paint dripping from the cup is eliminated.

! WARNING !

Always adjust line pressure to specifications to prevent damage or rupture of the cup or tank. The specifications will be given by the manufacturer.

Pressure guns also hold pressure AFTER being disconnected from the air source. This can be dangerous and messy if you accidentally open the lid and paint shoots all over the shop. Make sure you release cup or tank pressure before opening the lid.

Touch-Up Spray Guns

Touch-up spray guns are very small and are ideal for painting small repair areas. Often called a "door jamb gun," they have a tiny cup for holding a small amount of material. They operate like a conventional spray gun. See Figure 4–13.

VOC Emissions

Volatile organic compounds (VOCs) are harmful substances produced by many painting materials. Some geographic regions require the use of high transfer efficiency spray equipment to cut VOC emissions. These laws are designed to reduce the amount of air pollutants entering the earth's atmosphere.

High-Efficiency Spray Guns

High-efficiency spray guns are designed to reduce VOC emissions by applying more of the material to the vehicle and allowing less into the air. Check local ordinances to find out if you must use these types of guns.

High-efficiency spray guns are called **HVLP** for high volume, low pressure, or **LVLP** for low volume, low pressure. They use 10 psi (68.95 kPa) or less for reducing overspray and emissions.

Transfer efficiency describes the percentage of spray material a spray gun is capable of depositing on the surface. Transfer efficiency for spray guns must be at least 65 percent to meet regulations in some geographic locations. This means that at least 65 percent of the material sprayed must remain on the vehicle.

High transfer efficiency means more paint applied will remain on the surface. There is less spray material wasted as overspray. High transfer efficiency cuts VOC emissions and protects our atmosphere.

Transfer efficiency ratings are affected by the type of gun, gun adjustment, air pressure, spray pattern, and reduction of spray material. See **Figure 4–15.**

Electrostatic spray guns electrically charge the paint particles at the gun to attract them to the vehicle body. They operate on the theory that opposites attract. The charged paint particles are attracted to the grounded metal body of the vehicle. VOC regulations also list electrostatic spray equipment as complying to the minimum 65 percent transfer efficiency requirement.

Electrostatic spray guns are used for spraying finishes in automotive assembly plants and fleet use. They have higher transfer efficiency than other types of spray equipment when spraying complex shaped parts.

Electrostatic spray guns do NOT help attract the paint to nonmetal plastic parts. To spray plastics, an electrically conductive **primer** must be applied. This primer cannot be applied using electrostatic spray equipment. Maintenance and repairs are somewhat expensive. Also, the orientation of metallic flakes may be difficult to manage.

Specialized Spray Guns

Specialized spray guns are designed to apply various materials. They can be used to spray rubberized chip-resistant materials, anticorrosion materials, and other substances.

SPRAY BOOTHS

A spray booth is designed to provide a clean, safe, well-lit enclosure for painting and refinishing. It isolates the painting operation from dirt and dust to keep this debris out of the paint. It also confines the volatile fumes created by spraying and removes them from the shop area. See **Figure 4–16.**

In some areas, automatically operated fire extinguishers are required because of the highly explosive nature of refinishing materials.

The **downdraft spray booth** forces air from the ceiling down through exhaust vents in the floor. The downward flow of air from the ceiling to the floor pit creates an envelope of air passing by the surface of the vehicle.

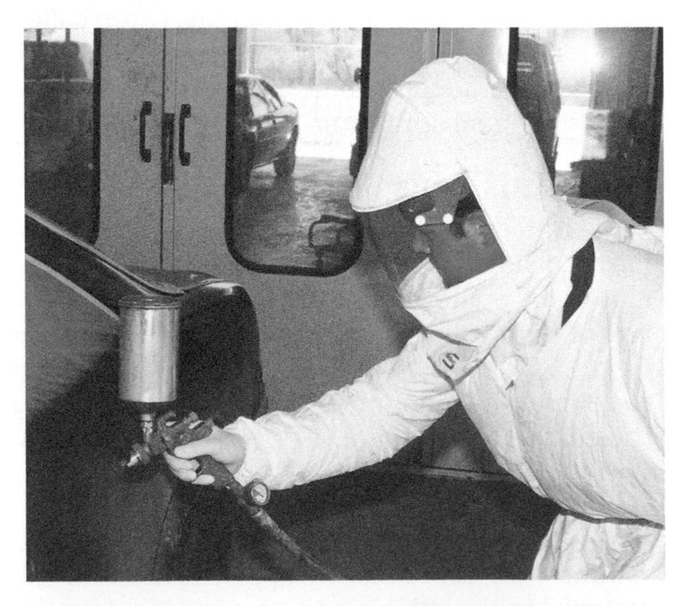

Figure 4–15. Here a paint technician is using a gravity-feed spray gun in the paint booth to refinish this damaged vehicle.

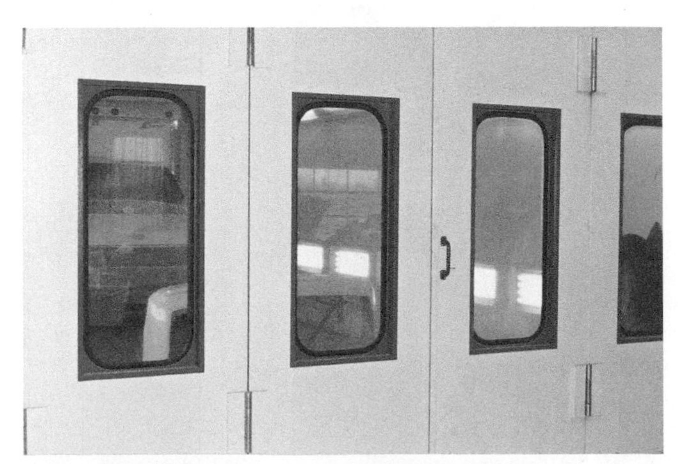

Figure 4–16. A paint booth provides a "clean room" for painting vehicles. Filtered airflow inside the booth pulls any dust or particles out and away from wet paint being applied to the vehicle's body.

By taking clean, heated air and directing it downward, the downdraft prevents contamination and overspray from settling on the freshly painted surface of the vehicle. This air movement also helps to remove toxic vapors from the breathing zone of the painter, providing a safer working environment.

A **side draft** or **crossflow spray booth** moves air sideways over the vehicle. An air inlet in one wall pushes fresh air into the booth. A vent on the opposite wall removes the booth air.

PAINT DRYING EQUIPMENT

A dust-free **paint drying room** will speed up drying/curing, produce cleaner work, and increase the volume of refinishing work. Some drying rooms have forced air or permanent infrared units for the rapid drying of paint and primers. These ovenlike units can speed up the drying time by as much as 75 percent.

Infrared drying equipment uses special bulbs to generate infrared light for fast drying of materials. They can be designed into booth systems. They range from portable panels for partial or sectional drying to large heating units capable of moving automatically along a track next to the vehicle for overall drying. Look at **Figure 4–17.**

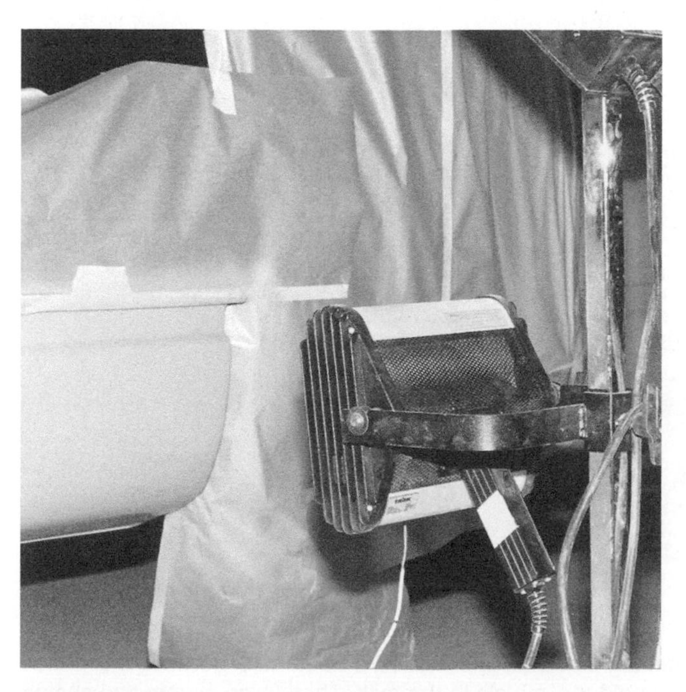

Figure 4–17. Portable or booth-mounted infrared lights will help cure modern paints more quickly.

! WARNING !

When using a drying room, caution must be taken NOT to overheat and destroy the finish. A surface thermometer measures panel temperatures to prevent overheating damage. It also lets you know when the surface is hot enough for complete drying.

MEASURING SYSTEMS

A **measuring system** is used to gauge and check the amount of frame and body damage on the vehicle. It is a special machine for comparing known good measurements with those on the vehicle being repaired. Refer to **Figure 4–18.**

In some designs, the measuring system mounts over the vehicle. Brackets and rods are positioned so that pointers aim at specific reference points on the body. Other systems use laser light to denote properly located reference points. If any reference point does NOT line up with a measuring system, the frame or unibody must be straightened or parts must be replaced.

STRAIGHTENING SYSTEMS

Hydraulic equipment uses a confined fluid or oil to develop the pressure necessary for operation. The pressure is achieved manually (pumping on a handle or lever) or by a small motor (either air or electrically driven) that drives a pump.

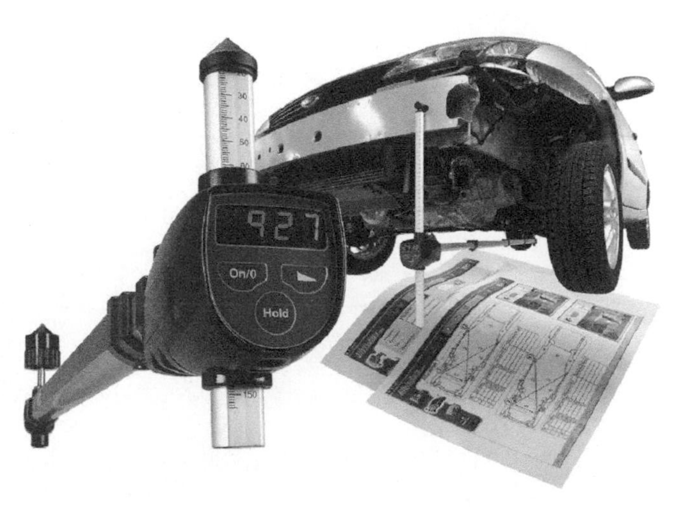

Figure 4–18. A measure system is needed to repair major vehicle damage. It will measure specific points on the vehicle to determine the direction and extent of collision damage to the frame or unibody structure. (Courtesy of Lasermate)

A **straightening system,** sometimes called a **frame rack,** is a hydraulic machine for straightening a damaged frame or unibody structure back into proper alignment. See **Figure 4–19.** The vehicle can be anchored to the shop floor or rack using clamps and chains. Then pulling chains are attached to the bent or damaged areas of the vehicle. One type of frame straightening equipment is shown in **Figure 4–20.**

Pulling posts are vertical uprights on the frame machine that allow the chains to pull in the needed directions to straighten the damage.

There are two basic types of frame/panel straighteners on the market: portable and stationary.

Frame straightening accessories are the many chains, special tools, and other parts needed. They will vary with the equipment

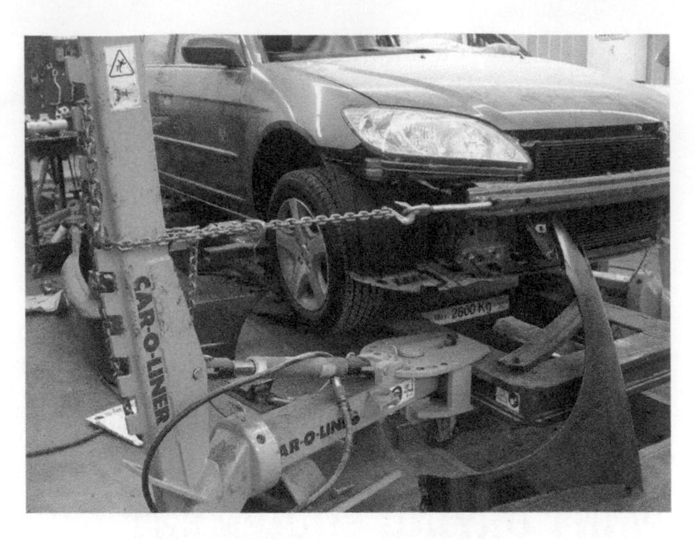

Figure 4–19. A frame rack or pulling equipment uses hydraulic power to force major damage back out of the frame or unibody structure of the vehicle.

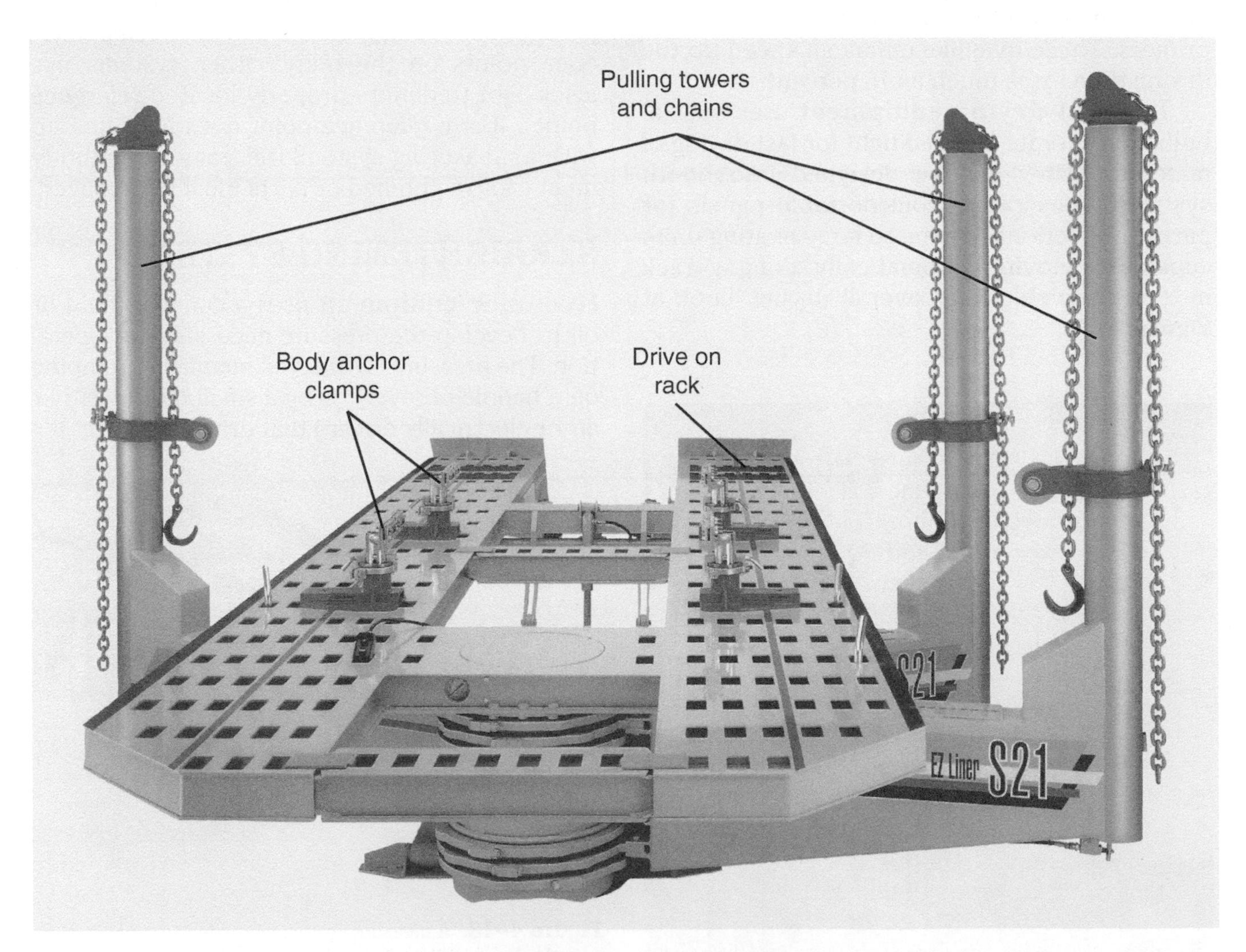

Figure 4–20. Note the major parts of a frame/unibody straightening machine, often called a frame rack because it is a rack that can pull damage out of a frame or unibody structure. Anchors hold the vehicle to the rack. Then large towers and chains can be used to pull the bent or collapsed areas out of the vehicle. (Courtesy of Chief Automotive Systems, Inc.)

manufacturer. To perform the many different straightening operations involving pushing, pulling, or holding a vehicle, a large assortment of adapters is included in a typical kit.

Body jacks, also known as porta-powers, can be used with frame/panel straighteners or by themselves. A body jack has a small hand-operated pump that operates a hydraulic cylinder. Pumping the handle extends the cylinder ram to produce a powerful pushing action.

A **body dolly** is a set of caster wheels that is clamped to the vehicle. It allows you to move the vehicle around the shop during repairs.

LIFTS

The traditional stationary in-ground lift was usually found only in service stations, muffler shops, transmissions shops, and tire dealers. Today, collision repair shops use lifts because it is easier to evaluate underbody damage and make repairs.

Raising a vehicle on a lift or a hoist requires special care. Adapters and hoist plates must be positioned correctly on lifts to prevent damage to the underbody of the vehicle. The exhaust system, tie-rods, and shock absorbers could be damaged if the adapters and hoist plates are incorrectly placed.

For more information on lifts, refer to the text index.

ELECTRIC TOOLS

Electric power tools plug into shop wall alternating current (AC) outlets. Drill presses, heat guns, welders, and vacuum cleaners are all vital electric-only tools. In addition, electric tools such as drills, polishers, and sanders perform the same tasks as their pneumatic counterparts.

Most electric power tools are built with an external grounding system for safety. A wire runs from the motor housing, through the power cord, to the third prong on the power plug. When connected to a grounded, three-hole electrical outlet, the grounding wire will carry any current that leaks past the electrical insulation of the tool. It will carry this current away from you and into the ground of the shop's wiring. See **Figure 4–21.**

Never use an adapter plug that eliminates and disconnects the third ground prong or you could be electrocuted.

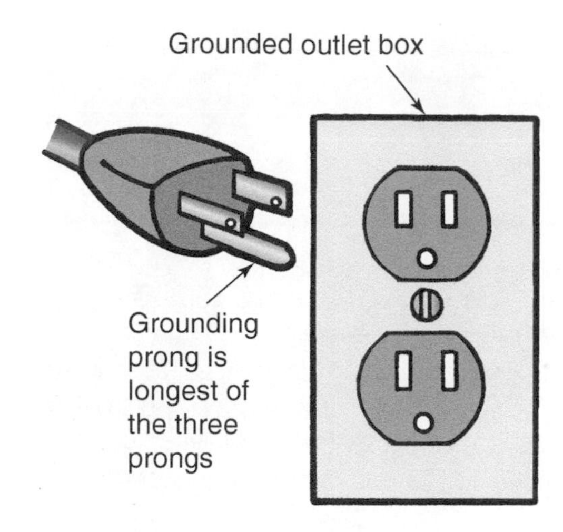

Figure 4–21. Never cut off the third, round ground prong on electrical equipment. It prevents any short in a power tool from causing electrocution.

BATTERY CHARGER

A **battery charger** converts 120 volts AC into 13 to 15 volts direct current (DC) for recharging drained batteries.

To use a battery charger, connect red to positive and black to negative. The red lead on the charger goes to the positive terminal of the battery. The black lead goes to ground or the negative battery terminal.

After connecting the charger, adjust its settings as needed (12-volt battery, fast or slow charge, etc.).

DANGER

A battery explosion could result if charger instructions are not followed. If you connect a charger to a battery while the charger is running, any small spark could ignite explosive gases that are around the battery.

MULTIMETER

A **multimeter** is a voltmeter, ammeter, and ohmmeter combined into one electrical tester. Also called a volt-ohm-milliammeter (VOM), a multimeter is often used for many types of electrical tests. See **Figure 4–22.**

An **analog meter** uses a needle that swings right and left for making measurements. This is

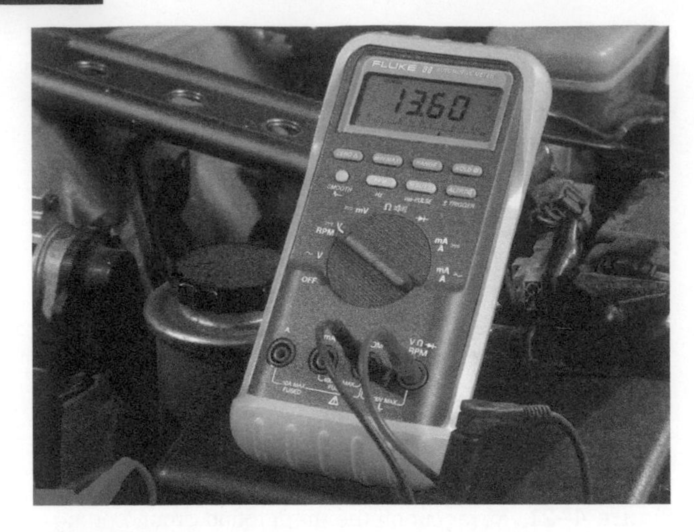

Figure 4–22. A digital multimeter will measure voltage, current, and electrical resistance when doing repairs to damaged wiring. (Courtesy of Fluke)

an older design that is being replaced by digital meters. A **digital meter** uses a number display to show readings.

WARNING

Never use a *low impedance* (low resistance) meter to test modern electronic circuits. The low resistance and high current through the meter can damage and ruin delicate computer and electronic circuits. Use only *high impedance* (high internal resistance) meters.

An **inductive meter** clips around the outside insulation of wiring to take electrical readings. It is time saving when making current (amp) measurements.

SCAN TOOLS

Scanners or **scan tools** are used to diagnose or troubleshoot vehicle computer system and wiring problems. A scanner connects to the vehicle's diagnostic connector or **assembly line diagnostic link (ALDL).** The scanner's electronic circuits can then communicate with the vehicle's on-board computer to help find problems.

A **scanner cartridge** is installed into the scanner for the specific make and model of vehicle being tested. The cartridge holds the information needed for that vehicle.

When there is a circuit problem, the vehicle's computer will illuminate a **malfunction indicator light** in the dash and store a trouble code number in its memory. The **trouble code number** denotes the specific problem circuit with the abnormal electrical operating value.

Modern scan tools will convert this trouble code number into a short word description of the potential problem. Most will also guide the technician through a short list of instructions for troubleshooting the specific problem. The scan tool might say that a circuit has high resistance and you should do ohmmeter tests to check for open wiring. Collision damage often severs wiring and produces trouble codes. See **Figure 4–23.**

Many late model vehicles have standardized **on-board diagnostics II (OBD II)** that monitors the operation of hundreds of circuits and components. The location of the OBD II diagnostic connector should be visible from under the left center of the dash.

Early diagnostic connectors came in various configurations. An adapter was often needed to make the scanner cable fit the vehicle's connector. Adapters are labeled for easy location for each make of vehicle. With OBD II, the standardized connector is a 16-pin connector. For more detailed information on scan tool use, refer to Chapter 26.

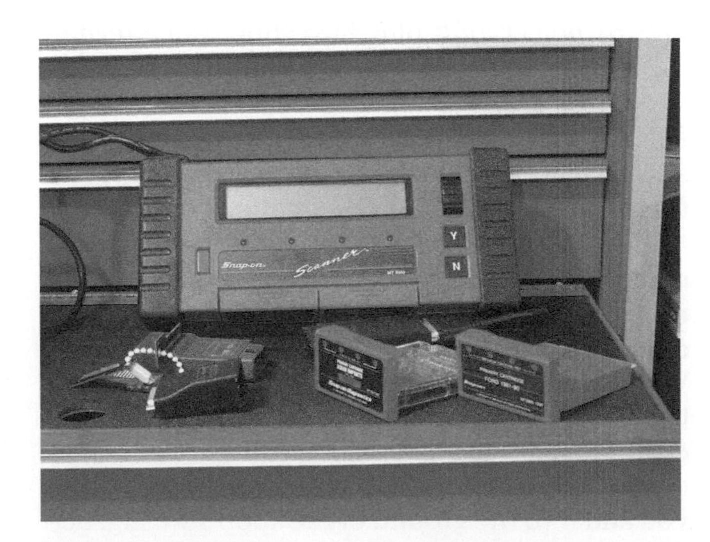

Figure 4–23. A scan tool can be plugged into the vehicle's diagnostic connector to quickly find vehicle problems, to clear trouble codes, and to do other electrical tests. (Courtesy of Snap-on Tool Corp.)

ENGINE ANALYZER

An **engine analyzer** is a large group of test instruments mounted in a roll-around cabinet. It can be used to find various kinds of trouble in the ignition, fuel injection, charging, and other electrical systems.

PERSONAL COMPUTER

The **personal computer,** or **PC,** is now an important tool for doing various collision repair shop tasks. It is used to keep track of business transactions, complete damage reports, and even perform electrical tests on vehicles. See **Figure 4–24.** A computer can find and manipulate huge amounts of data about all aspects of the shop operation. It is finding wider, more varied uses.

Portable or *laptop computers* are small handheld units often used during estimating. They have small keyboards for inputting data.

SOLDERING GUN

A **soldering gun** is used to heat and melt solder for making electrical repairs. It has a transformer that converts AC into DC. DC is sent through the gun tip, heating the tip enough to melt solder.

Solder is a mix of lead and tin for joining electrical wires and components. **Rosin core solder** is designed for doing electrical repairs. The **rosin** serves as a flux to make the melted solder adhere to the parts being joined.

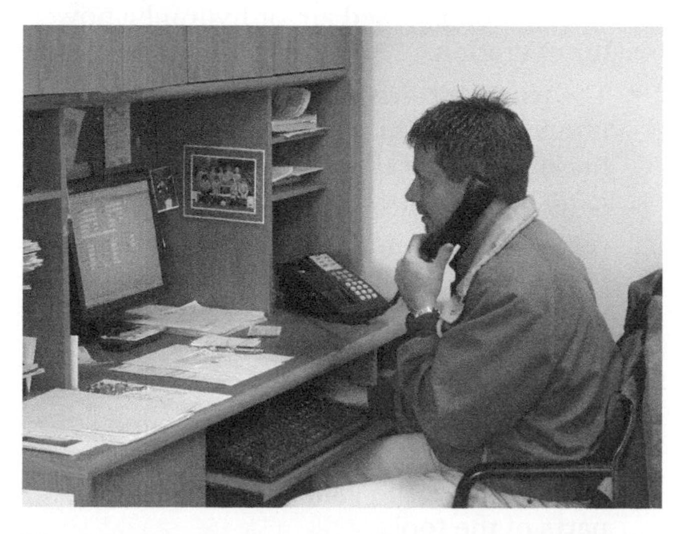

Figure 4–24. Personal computers can be found in several places in a modern auto body repair facility. PCs are used for bookkeeping, estimating damage, as a source of repair information, and when mixing paint.

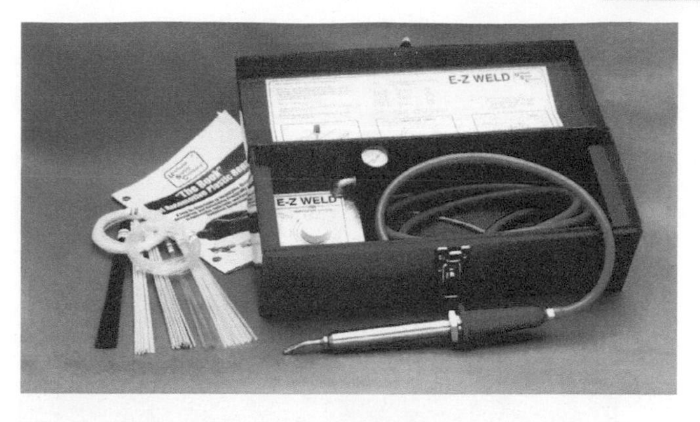

Figure 4–25. A plastic welder will heat plastic welding rods to repair minor damage to plastic panels, like expensive bumper covers. (Courtesy of Urethane Supply Co.)

Acid core solder is used for doing nonelectrical repairs, as on radiators. It should NOT be used for electrical repairs, because the acid can corrode connections and affect their electrical resistance.

PLASTIC WELDER

A **plastic welder** is used to heat and melt plastic and composites for repairing or joining parts made of these materials. It works like a soldering gun but operates at a lower temperature. One is shown in **Figure 4–25.**

AIR-CONDITIONING TOOLS

Because air-conditioning parts are often damaged in frontal collisions, you should understand the use of basic air-conditioning tools and equipment.

Air-conditioning (A/C) gauges are used to measure operating pressures in a vehicle's air conditioning system.

The A/C gauges are connected to **service ports** (small test fittings) in the system. The engine is then started and the A/C is set to maximum cooling. Gauge pressures are compared to known good readings. If pressures are too high or low, refer to troubleshooting charts to help find the problem.

A **leak detector** is a tool for finding refrigerant leaks in lines, hoses, and other parts of an air-conditioning system. The tester is turned on and moved around possible leakage points. Since air-conditioning refrigerant is heavier than air, the probe should be moved below possible leakage points. The tester will emit an

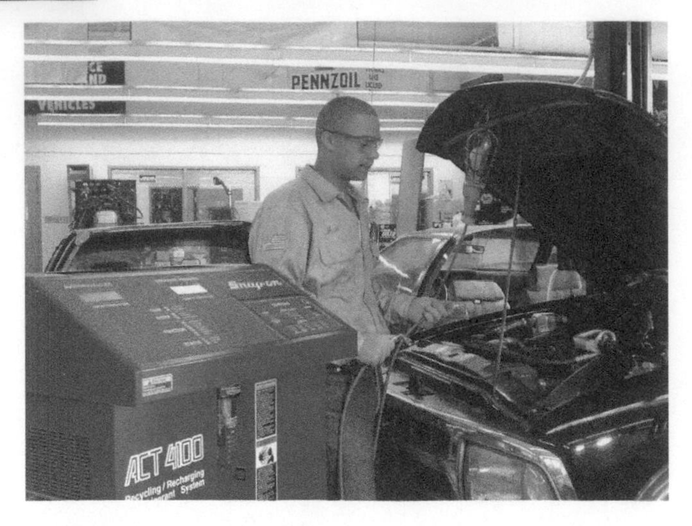

Figure 4–26. An air-conditioning charging station will recover used refrigerant and keep it from leaking into the atmosphere. It will then filter the refrigerant for reuse in the vehicle. Special training is needed to service A/C systems.

audible tone or noise if a leak is present. This helps you find and fix refrigerant leaks more quickly.

A **charging station** is a machine for automatically recharging an air-conditioning system with refrigerant. It has pressure gauges, a tank of refrigerant, and electronic controls for metering the right amount of refrigerant into the system. See **Figure 4–26.**

A **recovery station** is used to capture the old, used refrigerant so that it does not enter and pollute the atmosphere. It consists of a large metal tank and vacuum pump. The recovery station pulls the refrigerant out of the vehicle and forces it into the storage tank. The station will then filter, clean, and dry the used refrigerant so that it can be recycled.

A **recovery-charging station** can recover, evacuate, recycle, and charge a vehicle's air-conditioning system. It combines the features of a recovery station and a charging station in one roll-around cabinet.

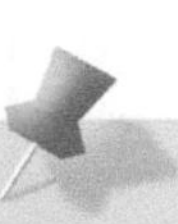

NOTE

For more information on power tools and equipment, refer to the textbook index. This will let you find additional information.

OTHER EQUIPMENT

Many other types of equipment are used in collision repair shops. You should have a basic understanding of their purpose.

A **tire changer** is a machine for quickly dismounting and mounting tires on and off wheels. It uses **pneumatic** (air) pressure to easily force the tire bead off or onto the wheel rim.

A **wheel balancer** is used to locate heavy areas on a wheel and tire assembly. It spins the wheel and tire and measures vibration. It will denote where **wheel weights** should be positioned on the wheel to equalize the weight and prevent vibration.

A **wheel alignment machine** is used to measure wheel alignment angles so they can be adjusted. After collision repairs, the wheels of the vehicle often need realignment. The wheel alignment machine will show actual wheel angles so that they can be adjusted back to specifications.

Headlight aimers are used to adjust the direction of the vehicle headlights. They normally mount over the headlights. Leveling bulbs in the aimers will let you know if each bulb is aiming too high, too low, or correctly. By turning headlight aiming screws on the headlights, you can readjust the beams to aim correctly in front of the vehicle.

SUMMARY

- Power tools and equipment use electrical energy, compressed air, or hydraulic power for operation.
- The use of air-driven or electric power tools requires safety glasses or a face shield. For hazardous operations, wear both.
- Some of the power tools used in collision repair are air compressors, air pressure regulators and filters, air blow guns, impact wrenches, air hammers, drills, air cutters, air sanders, grinders, polishers, blasters, and spray guns.
- Pneumatic tools should be lubricated BEFORE AND AFTER use to prevent wear and rusting of the vane motor and other parts of the tools.
- Volatile organic compounds (VOCs) are harmful substances produced by many painting and refinishing materials. Some geographic regions require the use of high

transfer efficiency spray equipment to cut VOC emissions.

- The personal computer (PC) has become an important tool for accomplishing various collision repair tasks. It is used to keep track of business transactions, complete damage reports, and even perform electrical tests on vehicles.

TECHNICAL TERMS

air supply system
air compressor
compressor drain valve
automatic drain valve
compressor pressure relief valve
air tank shut-off valve
compressor oil plugs
shop air lines
air hoses
air hose sizes
air couplings
air pressure regulator
air line filter-drier
air filter drain valve
air tools
air blow gun
OSHA-approved blow gun
impact wrench
impact adapters
air ratchet
air hammer
air chisel
drills
air drills
drill bits
key
chuck
hole saws
spot weld drill
air nibbler
air cutoff tool
air saw
air sander
circular sander
safety trigger
oscillating sander
orbital sander
dual-action sander
sander pad
air file
grinders
disc-type grinder
bench grinder
air polisher
paint gloss
cloth or cotton polishing pad
foam rubber polishing pad
swirl marks
pad cleaning tool
air tool lubrication
in-line oiler
blasters
hand blaster
cabinet blaster
spray guns
atomize
gun body
spray gun cup
fluid control valve
fluid needle valve
air control valve
spray gun air cap
spray pattern
gravity-feed spray gun
siphon spray gun
air vent hole
pressure-feed spray guns
touch-up spray guns
volatile organic compounds (VOCs)
high-efficiency spray guns
HVLP
LVLP
transfer efficiency
high transfer efficiency
electrostatic spray guns
primer
downdraft spray booth
side draft spray booth
crossflow spray booth
paint drying room
infrared drying equipment
surface thermometer
measuring system
hydraulic equipment
straightening system
frame rack
pulling posts
frame straightening accessories
body jacks
body dolly
AC
battery charger
DC
multimeter
analog meter
digital meter
low impedance
high impedance
inductive meter
scanners
scan tools
assembly line diagnostic link (ALDL)
scanner cartridge
malfunction indicator light
trouble code number
on-board diagnostics II (OBD II)
engine analyzer
personal computer
PC
soldering gun
solder
rosin core solder
rosin
acid core solder
plastic welder
air-conditioning (A/C) gauges
service ports
leak detector
charging station
recovery station
recovery-charging station
tire changer
pneumatic
wheel balancer
wheel weights
wheel alignment machine
headlight aimers

REVIEW QUESTIONS

1. List the major parts in a shop's air supply system.
2. What is a shop air compressor?

3. This valve must be opened every night to remove moisture from the compressor's storage tank.
   a. Pressure relief valve
   b. Drain valve
   c. Bypass valve
   d. Oil valve
4. How do you use air hose couplings?
5. What is the purpose of an air pressure regulator?
6. Why is air tool lubrication important and how do you do it?
7. An ______________ is a portable, hand-held, reversible air-powered wrench for rapid turning of bolts and nuts.
8. It is OK to use conventional, chrome-plated sockets on impact wrenches. True or False, and why?
9. Describe some common uses for a ½-inch impact wrench.
10. A key is used to tighten the ______________. The ______________ has movable jaws that close down and hold the drill bit.
11. This type of sander moves in two directions as it moves, producing a much smoother surface finish.
    a. Circular
    b. Reciprocating
    c. File
    d. Orbital
12. A spray gun must ______________ the liquid, that is, break the liquid into fine mist of droplets.
13. List and describe the major parts of a typical paint spray gun.

ASE-STYLE REVIEW QUESTIONS

1. Which of the following is the most common maintenance task on an air compressor?
   a. Change oil
   b. Change filters
   c. Open tank drain
   d. Adjust belt
2. For safety, normal shop air pressure should not exceed:
   a. 50 psi
   b. 120 psi
   c. 150 psi
   d. 175 psi
3. *Technician A* says you have to unscrew quick disconnect fittings. *Technician B* says to pull back on the fitting sleeve. Who is correct?
   a. Technician A
   b. Technician B
   c. Both Technicians A and B
   d. Neither Technician
4. Small amounts of water come out of the spray gun during refinishing. Which of the following could be the source of the problem?
   a. High humidity
   b. Too much air pressure
   c. Contaminated filter-drier
   d. Contaminated respirator air supply
5. *Technician A* says it is not safe to blow yourself off with an air nozzle. *Technician B* says that serious injury can result if air enters your bloodstream. Who is correct?
   a. Technician A
   b. Technician B
   c. Both Technicians A and B
   d. Neither Technician
6. Large bolts must be tightened to secure a truck bed to the frame. Which drive size should be used?
   a. ⅛ inch
   b. ¼ inch
   c. ⅜ inch
   d. ½ inch
7. *Technician A* says that a foam pad will produce fewer swirl marks than a cotton pad. *Technician B* says that a finer compound will also reduce swirl marks. Who is correct?
   a. Technician A
   b. Technician B

c. Both Technicians A and B
d. Neither Technician

8. *Technician A* says to always store the key in the drill press chuck. *Technician B* says that this practice is dangerous. Who is correct?
a. Technician A
b. Technician B
c. Both Technicians A and B
d. Neither Technician

9. Which type of air sander should be used for initial removal of plastic filler to help quickly level the surface?
a. Orbital sander
b. Circular sander
c. Belt sander
d. Oscillating sander

10. Which sandpaper system allows you to change sandpaper more quickly and also allows you to reuse sandpaper?
a. Velcro system
b. Adhesive system
c. Self-stick system
d. Epoxy system

ACTIVITIES

1. Tour your shop and note the location of all power tools and equipment. Discuss with the class any questions you might have on power tool or equipment use.
2. Visit an outside shop. Watch technicians as they use power tools and equipment. Have a class discussion about how technicians used the tools.
3. Disassemble and reassemble a shop spray gun. Note the condition of all parts. Report on the condition of the gun.
4. Inspect your shop air compressor. Find the tank drain valve, shut-off valve, and other parts.

CHAPTER

5 Measurements and Service Information

OBJECTIVES

After studying this chapter, you should be able to:

- Explain the many types of measurements needed in collision repair.
- Make accurate linear, angle, pressure, volume, and other measurements.
- Compare SAE and metric measuring systems.
- Identify and use basic measuring tools common to collision repair.
- Use conversion charts.
- Summarize how to measure with a paint mixing cup.
- Use printed and computerized service information.

INTRODUCTION

Measurements are number values that help control processes in collision repair. Measurements are needed to evaluate structural damage, correct that damage, mix paint, determine paint thickness, adjust a spray gun, and perform numerous other tasks. If you cannot make accurate measurements, you will not be a successful collision repair technician. See **Figure 5–1.**

Vehicle manufacturers give **specifications,** or measurements, for numerous body dimensions and mechanical parts. In the course of your work you will have to refer to and understand these factory specifications. This chapter will help prepare you for these factory specifications.

SAE AND METRIC SYSTEMS

The **Society of Automotive Engineers (SAE) measuring system,** also called the English, U.S., customary, or conventional system, was first developed using human body parts as the basis for measurements. The length of the human arm was used to standardize the yard and the human foot devised the foot. It is primarily used in the United States, but NOT in other countries. This makes it important for you to understand both systems. Specifications are usually given in both SAE and metric values.

The SAE system uses fractions and decimals for giving number values. **Fractions** are acceptable. They divide the inch into thirty-seconds, sixteenths, and larger parts of an inch. **Decimals** are used when high precision is important. They can be used to divide an inch into tenths, hundredths, one-thousandths, ten-thousandths, and more divisions.

The **metric measuring system,** also called the **scientific international (SI) system,** uses a power of ten as its base. It is a simpler system than our conventional system. This is because multiples of metric units are related to each other by the factor *ten*. Every metric unit can be multiplied or divided by a factor of ten to get larger units (multiples) or smaller units (submultiples). There is less chance for a math error when using the metric system.

CONVERSION CHARTS

Conversion charts are handy for changing from one measuring system to another or from one value to another.

An **SAE-metric conversion chart** allows you to change numbers to the other system. It gives multipliers that can be used to convert from SAE to metric or from metric to SAE values. For example, if a value is given in metric and you want to measure with a conventionally marked measuring tool, you would use a conversion chart.

A **decimal conversion chart** allows you to quickly change from fractions, to decimals, to

Customary	Conversion	Metric
Multiply	by	to get equivalent number of:
	Length	
Inch	25.4	Millimeters (mm)
Foot	0.3048	Meters (m)
Yard	0.9144	Meters
Mile	1.609	Kilometers (km)
	Area	
Inch ^{2}	645.2	Millimeters^2 (mm^2)
Foot ^{2}	6.45	Centimeters^2 (cm^2)
Yard ^{2}	0.0929	Meters^2 (m^2)
	0.8361	Meters^2 (m^2)
	Volume	
Inch ^{3}	16,387.	mm^3
	16.387	cm^3
	0.0164	Liters (l)
Quart	0.9464	Liters
Gallon	3.7854	Liters
Yard ^{3}	0.7646	Meters^3 (m^3)
	Mass	
Pound	0.4536	Kilograms (kg)
Ton	907.18	Kilograms (kg)
Ton	0.907	Tonne (t)
	Temperature	
Fahrenheit	(+F°- 32)÷1.8	Celsius

F° -40 0 32 40 80 98.6 120 160 200 212

C° -40 -20 0 20 37 40 60 80 100

Customary	Conversion	Metric
Multiply	by	to get equivalent number of:
	Acceleration	
Foot/sec ^{2}	0.3048	Meter/sec^2 (m/s^2)
Inch/sec ^{2}	0.0254	Meter/sec^2
	Torque	
Pound-inch	0.11298	Newton/meters (Nm)
Pound-foot	1.3558	Newton/meters
	Power	
Horsepower	0.746	Kilowatts (kw)
	Pressure or stress	
Inches of water	0.2491	Kilopascals (kPa)
Pounds/sq. in.	6.895	Kilopascals
	Energy or work	
BTU	1055.	Joules (j)
Foot-pound	1.3558	Joules
Kilowatt-hour	3,600,000. or 3.6 x 10 ^{6}	Joules (j =1 Ws)
	Light	
Foot candle	1.0764	Lumens/meter^2 (lm/m^2)
	Fuel performance	
Miles/gal	0.4251	Kilometers/liter (km/l)
Gal/mile	2.3527	Liter/kilometer (l/km)
	Velocity	
Miles/hour	1.6093	Kilometers/hr. (km/h)
	Force	
Kilogram	9.807	Newtons (N)
Once	0.2780	Newtons
Pound	4,448	Newtons

Figure 5–1. This chart gives factors for converting from English to metric. Read through and compare values in each system of measurement. (Courtesy of General Motors Corp., Service Operations)

millimeters. This is often used for various tasks, such as selecting drill bits. One is shown in **Figure 5–2.**

LINEAR MEASUREMENTS

Linear measurements are straight line measurements of distance. They are commonly used when evaluating major structural damage after a collision. There are many types of tools used for linear measurements.

SCALES

A **scale** or **ruler** is the most basic tool for linear measurement. It has an accuracy of approximately 1⁄64 in. or 0.5 mm. See **Figure 5–3.**

An **SAE rule** often has markings in fractions of an inch (½, ¼, ⅛, 1⁄16) or in decimal parts of an inch (0.10, 0.20, 0.30, 0.40). Refer to **Figure 5–4.**

A **metric rule** or **meter stick** is marked in millimeters and centimeters. The numbered lines usually equal 10 millimeters (1 centimeter).

Fraction	Decimal	Millimeters
1/64	.01563	.3969
1/32	.03125	.7938
	.03937	1.0000
3/64	.04688	1.1906
1/16	.06250	1.5875
5/64	.07813	1.9844
	.07874	2.0000
3/32	.09375	2.3813
7/64	.10938	2.7781
	.11811	3.0000
1/8	.12500	3.1750
9/64	.14063	3.5719
5/32	.15625	3.9688
	.15748	4.0000
11/64	.17188	4.3656
3/16	.18750	4.7625
	.19685	5.0000
13/64	.20313	5.1594
7/32	.21875	5.5563
15/64	.23438	5.9531
	.23622	6.0000
1/4	.25000	6.3500
17/64	.26563	6.7469
	.27559	7.0000
9/32	.28125	7.1438
19/64	.29688	7.5406
5/16	.31250	7.9375
	.31496	8.0000
21/64	.32813	8.3344
11/32	.34375	8.7313
	.35433	9.0000
23/64	.35938	9.1281
3/8	.37500	9.5250
25/64	.39063	9.9219
	.39370	10.0000
13/32	.40625	10.3188
27/64	.42188	10.7156
	.43307	11.0000
7/16	.43750	11.1125
29/64	.45313	11.5094
15/32	.46875	11.9063
	.47244	12.0000
31/64	.48438	12.3031
1/2	.50000	12.7000

Fraction	Decimal	Millimeters
	.51181	13.0000
33/64	.51563	13.0969
17/32	.53125	13.4938
35/64	.54688	13.8906
	.55118	14.0000
9/16	.56250	14.2875
37/64	.57813	14.6844
	.59055	15.0000
19/32	.59375	15.0813
39/64	.60938	15.4781
5/8	.62500	15.8750
	.62992	16.0000
41/64	.64063	16.2719
21/32	.65625	16.6688
	.66929	17.0000
43/64	.67188	17.0656
11/16	.68750	17.4625
45/64	.70313	17.8594
	.70866	18.0000
23/32	.71875	18.2563
47/64	.73438	18.6531
	.74803	19.0000
3/4	.75000	19.0500
49/64	.76563	19.4469
25/32	.78125	19.8438
	.78740	20.0000
51/64	.79688	20.2406
13/16	.81250	20.6375
	.82677	21.0000
53/64	.82813	21.0344
27/32	.84375	21.4313
55/64	.85938	21.8281
	.86614	22.0000
7/8	.87500	22.2250
57/64	.89063	22.6219
	.90551	23.0000
29/32	.90625	23.0188
59/64	.92188	23.4156
15/16	.93750	23.8125
	.94488	24.0000
61/64	.95313	24.2094
31/32	.96875	24.6063
	.98425	25.0000
63/64	.98438	25.0031
1	1.00000	25.4000

Figure 5–2. A decimal conversion chart will let you quickly change fractions, decimals, and metric equivalents. (Courtesy of Perfect Circle/Dana Corp)

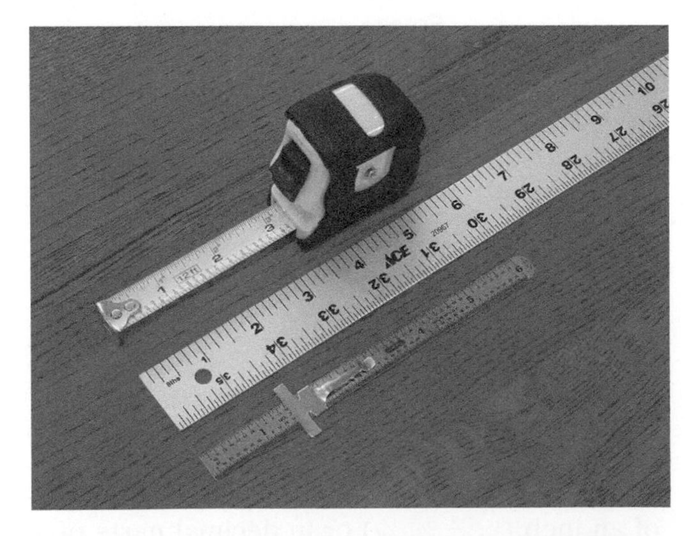

Figure 5–3. A pocket scale, yardstick or meter stick, and a tape measure are commonly used to make linear or straight line measurements in collision repair.

Figure 5–5 compares fractional and metric scales.

Parallax error results when you read a rule or scale from an angle, instead of looking straight down. Viewing at an angle causes you to read the wrong line on the scale. Always look straight down when reading a rule.

A **pocket scale** or rule is very small (typically 6 in. or 152 mm long). It will clip into your shirt pocket and can be handy for numerous small measurements. A **yardstick** or *meter stick* may also be used for some larger linear measurements.

A **tape rule** or **tape measure** will extend out for making very long measurements. A tape measure is commonly used to make large distance measurements during body damage evaluation.

A **tram gauge** is a special body dimension measuring tool (see **Figure 5–6**). It is usually a lightweight frame with pointers. The pointers

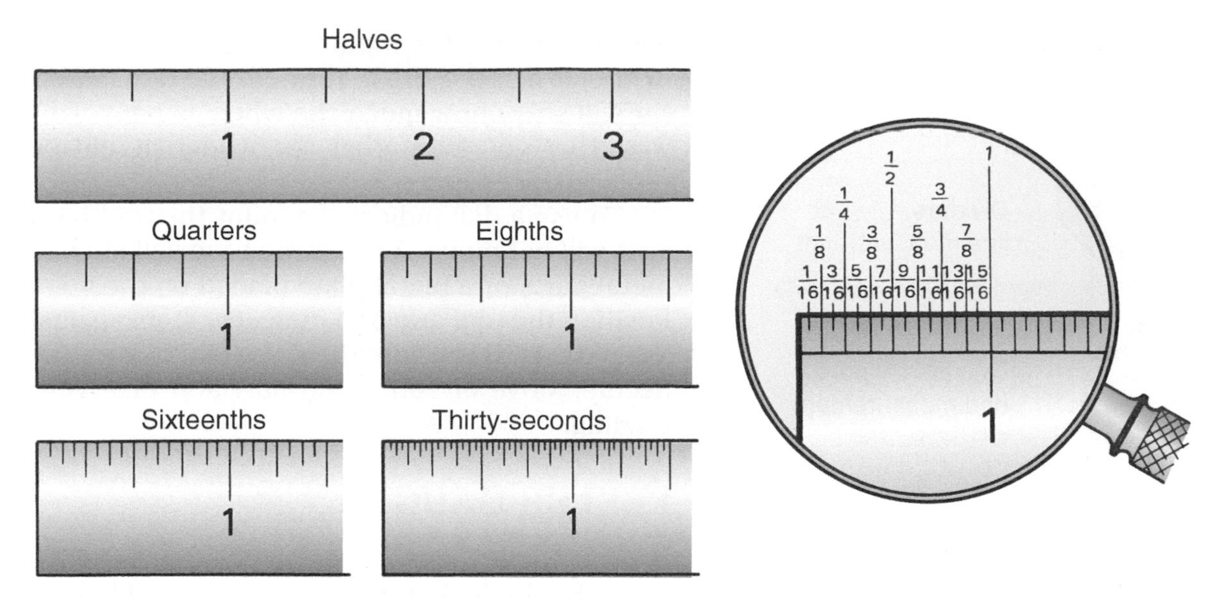

Figure 5–4. Review divisions of a ruler. Memorize each part of an inch, as shown on the left, under a magnifying glass.

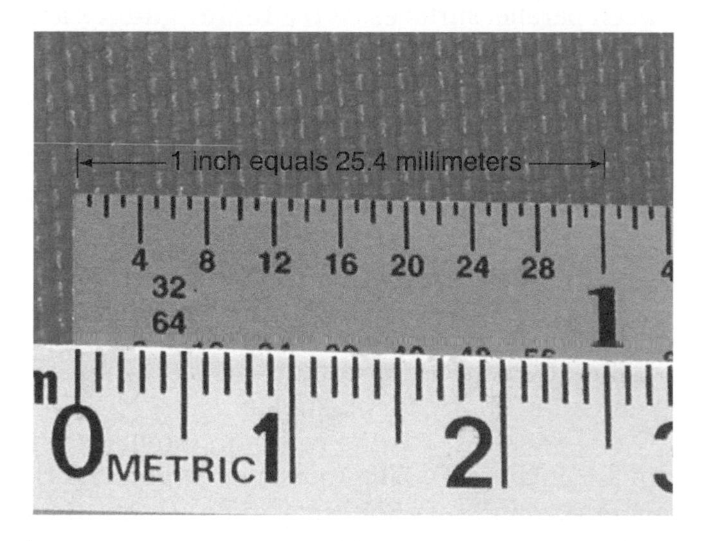

Figure 5–5. Note how 1 inch equals 25.4 millimeters. The metric ruler has been placed over the inch ruler.

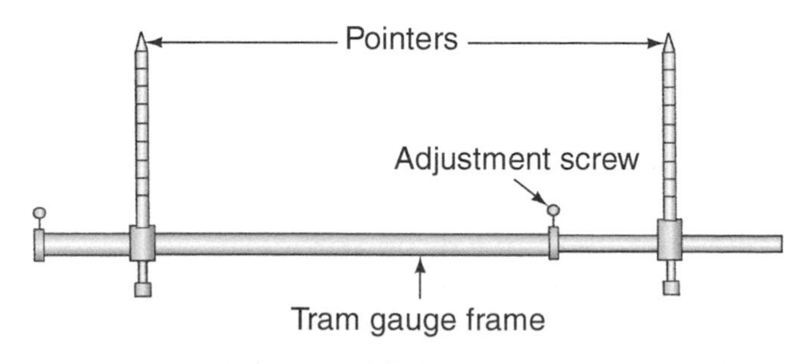

Figure 5–6. A tram gauge is used to measure across points on a damaged vehicle. If point measures are too close or too far apart, the vehicle must be put on a frame rack to pull out the unibody or frame damage.

can be aligned with body dimension reference points to determine the direction and amount of body misalignment damage.

DIVIDERS AND CALIPERS

Dividers have straight, sharp tips for taking measurements or marking parts for cutting. In collision repair work, dividers are sometimes used for layout or marking cut lines. They will scribe circles and lines on sheet metal and plastic. They will also transfer and make surface measurements. Dividers are sometimes used when fabricating repair pieces for corrosion repair. See **Figure 5–7.**

MICROMETERS

Micrometers are sometimes used for measuring mechanical parts when great precision is important. Often called a "mike," it can easily measure one-thousandths of an inch (0.001 in.) or one-hundredths of a millimeter (0.01 mm).

You might use one to measure the thickness of a brake system rotor. If worn too thin, this would tell you to replace the rotor. See **Figure 5–8.**

DIAL INDICATORS

A **dial indicator** is often used to measure part movement and out-of-round in thousandths of an inch (hundredths of a millimeter). For example, the indicator might be used to check for

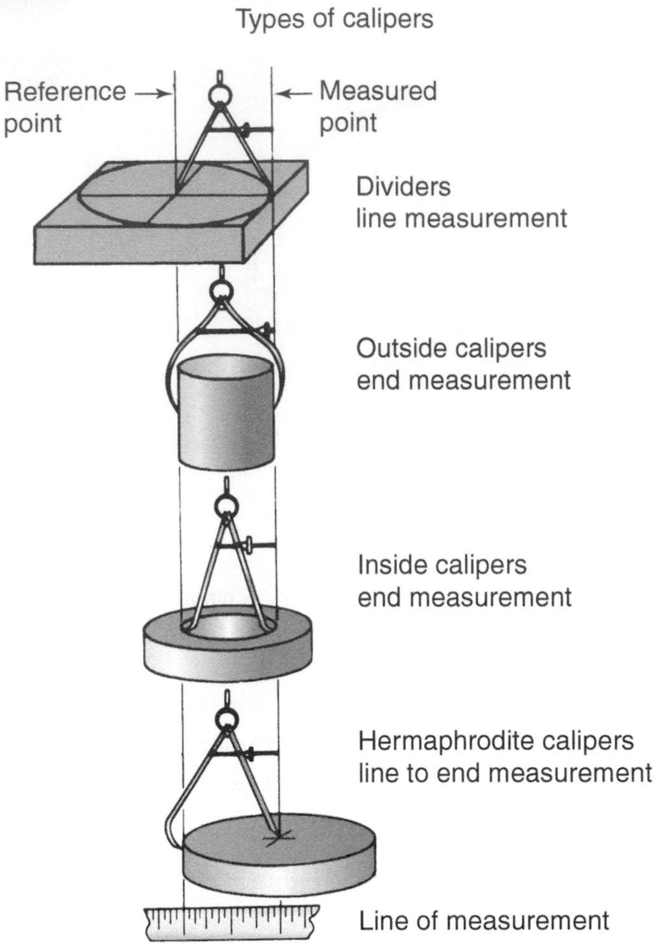

Types of calipers

Reference point

Measured point

Dividers line measurement

Outside calipers end measurement

Inside calipers end measurement

Hermaphrodite calipers line to end measurement

Line of measurement

Figure 5–7. Calipers are used when fabricating sheet metal for custom repairs. Study their use.

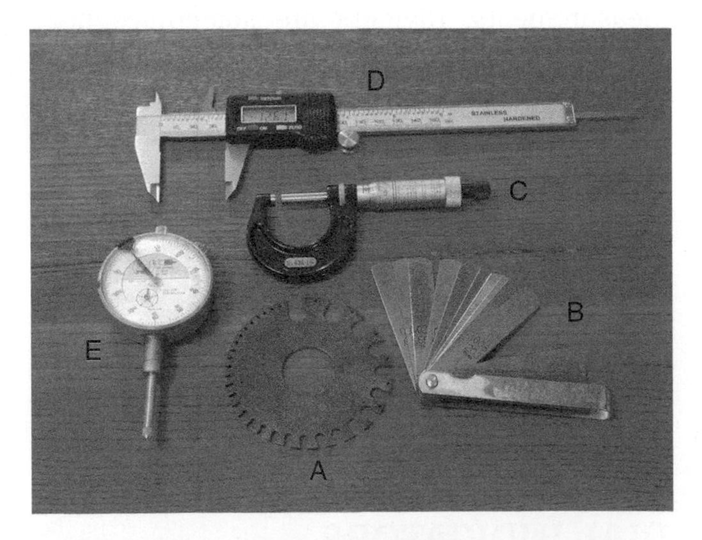

Figure 5–8. Learn the names of these measuring tools. **(A)** Sheet metal thickness gauge. **(B)** Feeler gauge. **(C)** A micrometer will measure to ten-thousandths of an inch. **(D)** A sliding caliper will measure to one thousandths of an inch. **(E)** A dial indicator will measure runout in thousandths of an inch.

wheel damage. It is mounted against the wheel or tire. When the tire is rotated, the dial indicator will show how much the wheel is bent. This would let you know that the wheel should be replaced. See **Figure 5–9.**

To use a dial indicator, mount the tool base so it will not move. A magnetic base will stick to metal parts or a metal plate placed on the floor. Position the tool arm and indicator stem against the part. Turn the outside of the dial to zero the needle. Move or rotate the part and take your reading.

FEELER GAUGES

Feeler gauges measure small clearances inside parts. Blade thickness is given on each blade in thousandths of an inch (0.001, 0.010, 0.020) or in hundredths of a millimeter (0.01, 0.07, 0.10).

Flat feeler gauges are for measuring between parallel surfaces. **Wire feeler gauges** are round and are for measuring slightly larger distances between nonparallel or curved surfaces.

PRESSURE AND FLOW MEASUREMENTS

You will have to make pressure and flow measurements when working. Pressures are important for air tools, spray guns, and other equipment. Adequate airflow is important when working in a paint spray booth, for example.

A **pressure gauge** reads in pounds per square inch (psi), kilograms per square centimeter (kg/cm^2), or kilopascals (kPa). A few pressure gauges also show or measure vacuum. Note the two scales given on the pressure gauge in **Figure 5–10.**

Air pressure gauges are used on the shop's air compressor, on pressure regulators, or at the spray gun. Tire pressure gauges are also needed to check for proper tire inflation. Hydraulic pressure gauges can be found on hydraulic presses and other similar equipment.

Remember! Excessive pressure can be dangerous or damage parts. Low air pressure may keep the tool from working properly.

A **vacuum gauge** reads vacuum, negative pressure, or "suction." It reads in inches of mercury (in. Hg) or kilograms per square centimeter (kg/cm^2).

A **flow meter** measures the movement of air, gas, or liquid past a given point. A **manometer,** or

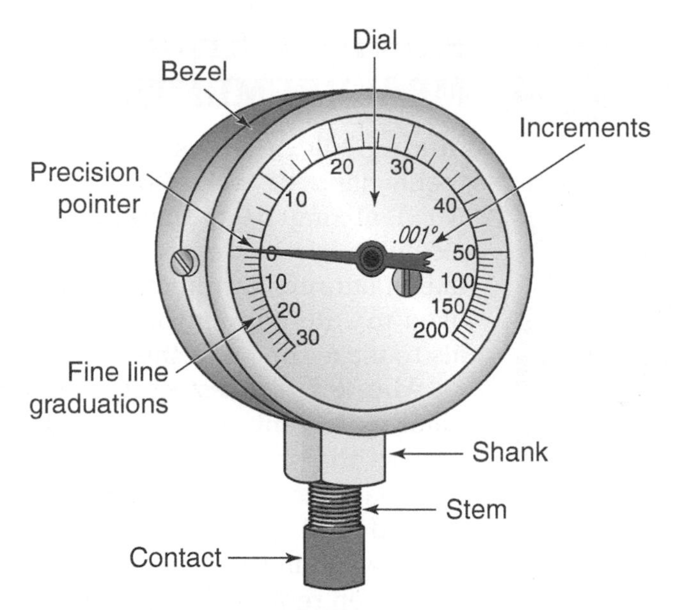

(A) Study parts of a dial indicator. (Courtesy of Danaher Tool Group)

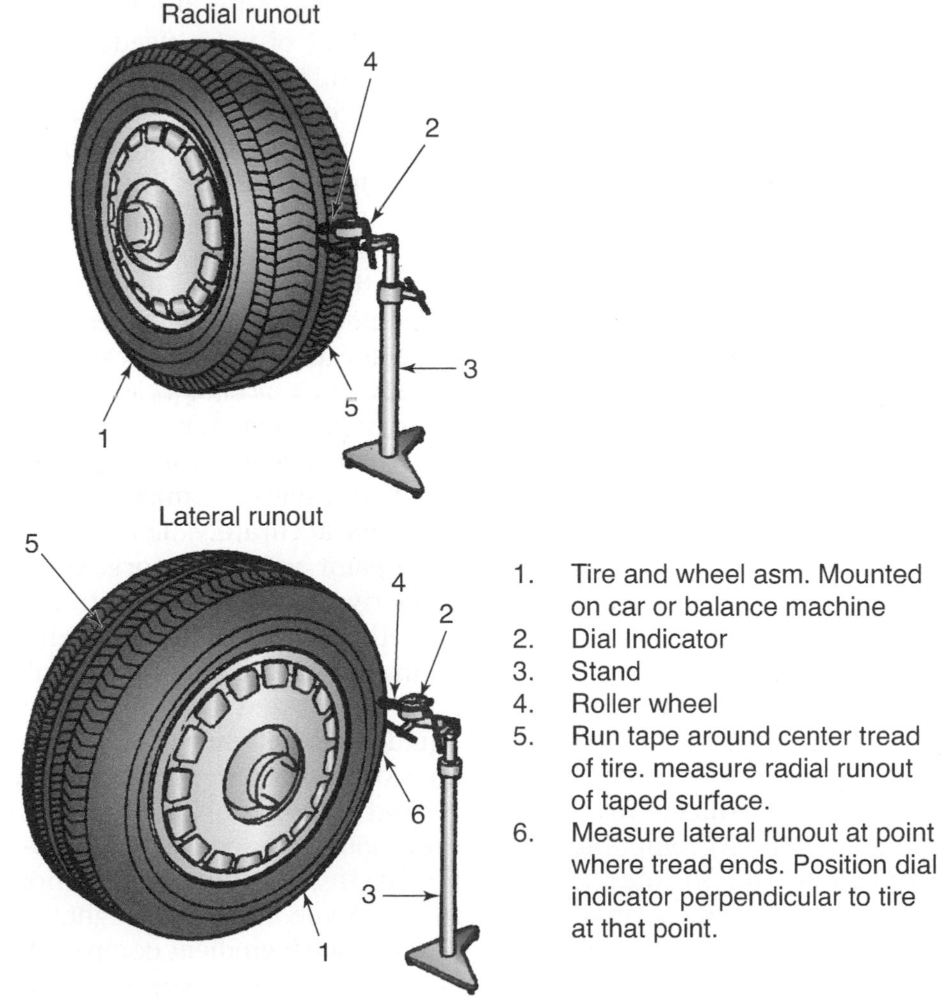

(B) Mount the indicator on a heavy base and adjust its point up against the wheel. Rotate the wheel slowly while reading the dial. If the runout is beyond specs (about 0.020 inch), the wheel must be replaced or straightened.

Figure 5–9. A dial indicator is commonly used for measuring part movement. They are often used to check for bent wheels that were damaged in collision.

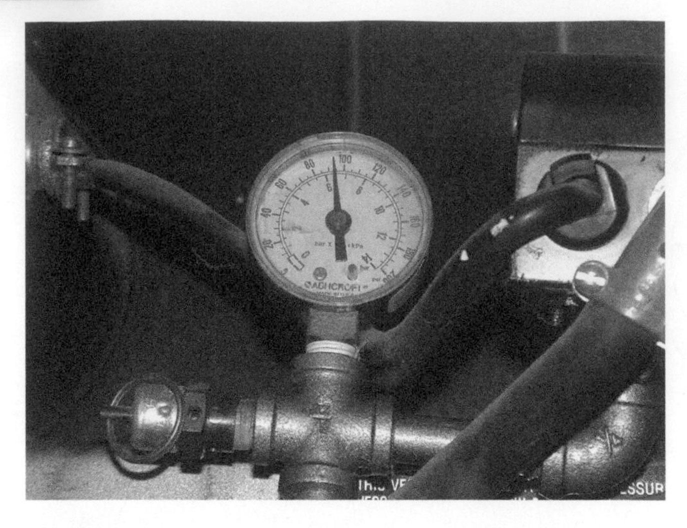

Figure 5–10. Pressure gauges are used to monitor pressure in air or hydraulic systems. They often read in both English and metric. This gauge is on an air compressor tank.

airflow meter, is designed for use in a paint booth. Airflow meters can register in feet per minute or meters per minute. Liquid flow meters often register in gallons per hour or liters per hour.

ANGLE MEASUREMENTS

Angle measurements divides a circle into 360 parts, called *degrees*. You will learn to read angles in degrees when doing wheel alignment, for example. This is explained in later chapters.

TEMPERATURE MEASUREMENTS

Temperature is usually measured in degrees Fahrenheit (F) or Celsius (C). In the collision repair shop, temperatures are important in the drying of various materials such as primers, paints, and adhesives.

Thermometers are used to measure temperature. For example, paint manufacturers often give different mixing values and recommend different thinners and reducers for different **ambient** (outside or room) temperatures.

Surface temperature thermometers are available in several different designs—magnetic thermometers, paper thermometers, digital thermometers.

Before applying any type of material during collision repairs, the vehicle and the material to be used must be at room temperature. A vehicle's surface temperature must be brought to room temperature prior to applying fillers and paint materials. Failure to do so may result in formation of condensation on the surface.

PAINT-RELATED MEASUREMENTS

Mixing scales are used by paint suppliers and technicians to weigh the various ingredients when mixing paint materials. Scales will precisely weigh out each ingredient. Using paint manufacturers formulations, mixing scales are used to add different pigments or other materials to make the paint the desired color.

Manual mixing scales simply weigh each paint ingredient as it is poured into the mixing cup on the scale. You must look up the paint formula to see how much of each material is needed and carefully pour out that amount while watching the scale. Most manual scales have been replaced by computerized scales.

Electronic mixing scales help automate paint mixing. After the technician programs in the amount of paint needed for the area to be refinished, a computerized scale will state how much of each material to pour into the mixing cup. It will state how much pigment, tint, flake, and binder to use by weight. As you pour each ingredient into the cup sitting on the scale, the scale will go to zero. Once zeroed, you have added the correct amount of that ingredient. The computerized scale will then prompt you to add a specific amount of the next ingredient. This will allow you to more quickly produce the correct mix of ingredients for the specific color paint.

When mixing and using paint and solvents or other additives, you must measure and mix their contents accurately. This is essential to doing good paint and body work. You must be able to properly mix reducers or thinners, hardeners, and other additives into the paint. If you do NOT, serious paint problems will result.

A **graduated pail** is often used to measure liquid materials when mixing. It has measurement lines on it like a kitchen measuring cup. Liquid is poured into the pail until it is next to the scale for the amount needed. See **Figure 5–11.**

Mixing instructions are normally given on the material's label. This might be a percentage or parts of one ingredient compared to the other(s).

A **percentage reduction** means that each material must be added in certain proportions or parts. For instance, if a color requires 50 percent reduction, this means that 1 part reducer (solvent) must be mixed with 2 parts of color.

Mixing by parts means that for a specific volume of paint or other material, a specific amount of another material must be added. If

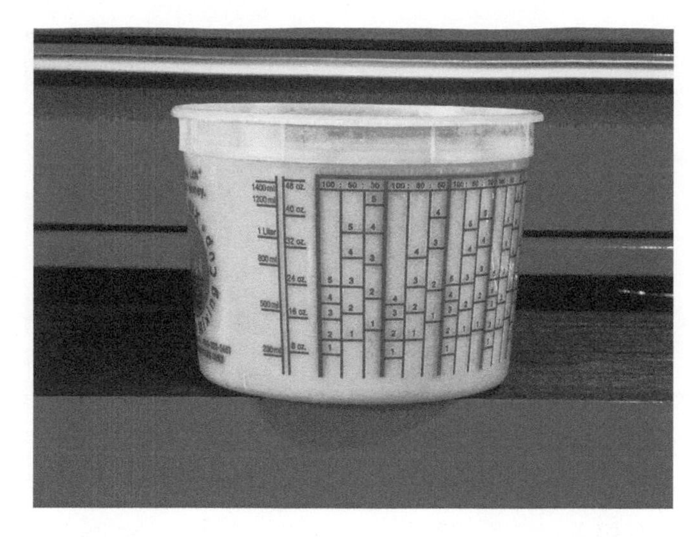

Figure 5–11. This mixing cup has scales on it. You can fill the cup until the paint or other material is even with the correct graduation to quickly mix materials in correct proportions.

you are mixing a gallon of color in a spray gun pressure tank, for example, and directions call for 25 percent reduction, you would add 1 quart of reducer. There are 4 quarts in a gallon and you want 1 part or 25 percent reducer for each 4 parts of color.

Proportional numbers denote the amount of each material needed. The first number is usually the parts of paint needed. The second number is usually the solvent (or reducer). A third number might be used to denote the amount of hardener or other additives required.

For example, the number 2:1:1 might mean add 1 part solvent and 1 part hardener to 2 parts of color. For a half gallon of color, you would add a quart of solvent and a quart of catalyst. This can vary, so always refer to the exact directions on the materials.

A **mixing chart** converts a percentage into how many parts of each material must be mixed. One is given in **Figure 5–12.** Study the percentages and parts of each material that must be mixed.

PAINT MIXING STICKS

Graduated **paint mixing sticks** have conversion scales that allow you to easily convert ingredient percentages into part proportions. They are used by painters to help mix colors, solvents, catalysts, and other additives right before spraying. See **Figure 5–13.**

Paint mixing sticks should NOT be confused with **paint stirring sticks** (wooden sticks) for mixing the contents after they are poured into the spray gun cup or a container.

VISCOSITY CUP MEASUREMENT

A **viscosity cup** is used to measure the thickness or fluidity of the mixed refinishing materials; paints (color), primers, sealers, or even clears. It is a small cup attached to a handle.

Reduction percentage		Reduction proportions	Paint (color)		Solvent
20%	=	5 parts paint / 1 part solvent		20%	
25%	=	4 parts paint / 1 part solvent		25%	
33%	=	3 parts paint / 1 part solvent		33%	
50%	=	2 parts paint / 1 part solvent		50%	
75%	=	4 parts paint / 3 parts solvent		75%	
100%	=	1 part paint / 1 part solvent		100%	
125%	=	4 parts paint / 5 parts solvent		125%	
150%	=	2 parts paint / 3 parts solvent		150%	
200%	=	1 part paint / 2 parts solvent		200%	
250%	=	2 parts paint / 5 parts solvent		250%	

Figure 5–12. This chart shows a range of possible mixing percentages and converts them into parts. Fifty percent would equal 1 part paint to 1 part solvent, for example.

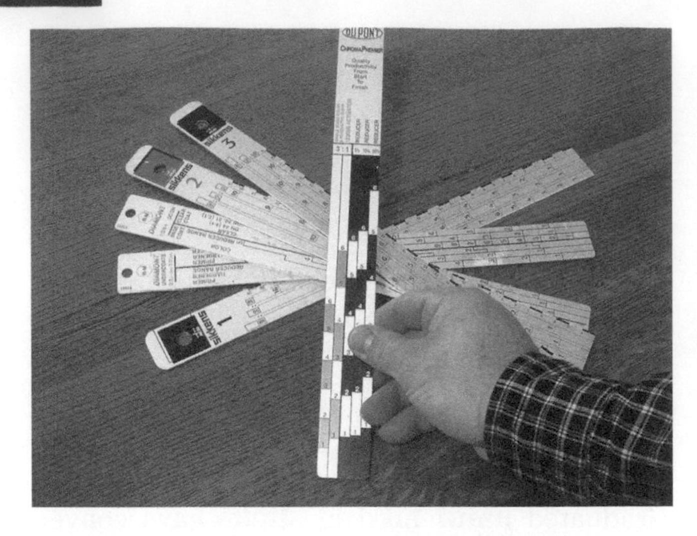

Figure 5–13. Mixing sticks, discussed in detail later, also have graduations so you can mix the ingredients in paint correctly.

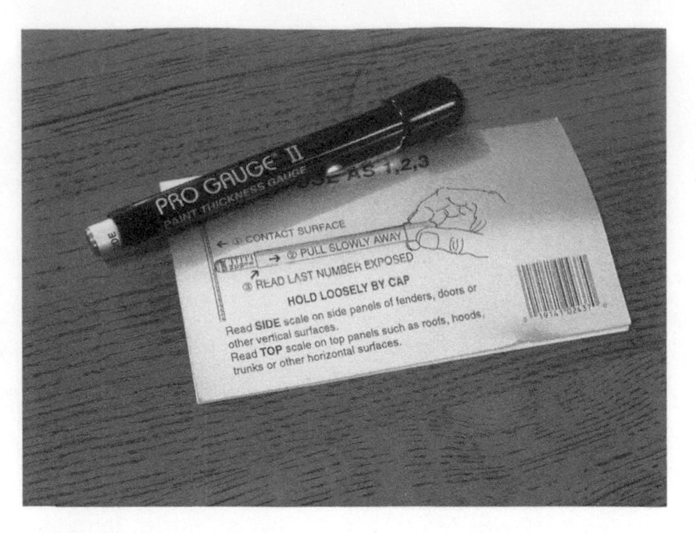

Figure 5–14. A paint thickness or mil gauge will measure the thickness of paint. If a car has been painted several times, paint film thickness will be excessive and the paint must be stripped off before repainting. Its use is explained later.

To use a viscosity cup, dip it into the mixed paint until submerged. Lift the cup out and hold it over the paint container. As soon as the cup is lifted out, start timing how long it takes for the cup to empty. The paint will leak out of a small specific size **orifice** (hole) in the bottom of the cup.

PAINT MATERIAL THICKNESS MEASUREMENT

Paint thickness is measured in **mils** or thousandths of an inch (hundredths of a millimeter). Original equipment manufacture (OEM) finishes are typically about 2 to 6 mils thick. With basecoat/clearcoats, the basecoat is approximately 1 to 2 mils thick. The clearcoat is about 2 to 4 mils thick. This is approximately the thickness of a piece of typing paper.

If a panel has been repainted, paint thickness will increase. If too much paint is already on the vehicle, it may have to be removed prior to painting. Paint/material buildup should be limited to no more than 12 mils. The OEM finish and one refinish usually equal just under 12 mils. Exceeding this thickness could cause cracking in the new finish. Chemical stripping or blasting would be needed to remove the old paint buildup.

A **mil gauge** can be used to measure the thickness of the paint on the vehicle. This can be done before refinishing, after refinishing, and during other finishing operations. See **Figure 5–14.**

There are three types of mil thickness gauges. One type, known as a **pencil mil gauge,** measures paint/refinishing materials with a calibrated magnet and spring setup. The magnet is placed against painted steel components and then slowly pulled away. The tool contains a graduated scale that is exposed as the magnet sticks to the panel. The last number exposed on the scale before the magnet detaches from the panel is the paint film/material thickness in mils.

The **electronic mil gauge** shows mil thickness with a digital readout. Some electronic mil gauges can also measure mil thickness on nonmagnetic materials such as aluminum and composites.

VEHICLE IDENTIFICATION NUMBER (VIN) NUMBERS

A good technician must have a complete understanding of commonly used terms that identify parts and assemblies of a vehicle. If the technician is NOT familiar with this language, it is difficult to order parts and read a repair order.

The **Vehicle Identification Number (VIN) plate** is used to accurately identify the body style, model year, engine, and other data about the vehicle. For years, the VIN plate has been riveted to the upper left corner of the instrument panel, visible through the windshield. See **Figure 5–15.**

Prior to 1981 and on foreign vehicles, check the service manual for the location of the VIN, vehicle certification label, or body plate. Service manuals and collision estimating guides also

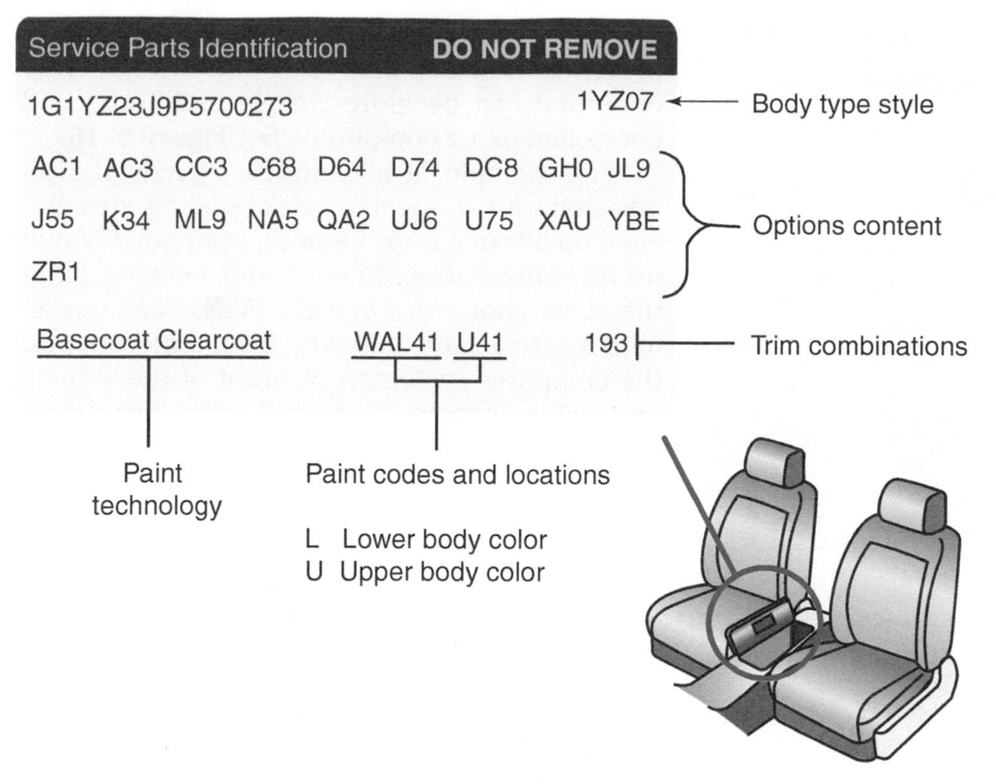

Figure 5–15. Automobile manufacturers place labels on their vehicles with important information on them. The service literature gives label locations and codes for understanding them. (Courtesy of General Motors Corp., Service Operations)

contain all of the necessary VIN number decoding information.

The **body ID number**, or **service part number**, gives information about how the vehicle is equipped. It will give paint codes or numbers for ordering the right type and color paint; lower and upper body colors if the vehicle has two-tone paint. The body ID number also gives trim information. This number will be on the body ID plate on the door, console lid, or elsewhere on the body.

COLLISION REPAIR PUBLICATIONS

Various manuals or publications are used by a collision repair shop. It is important that you understand the purpose and use of each.

All automobile manufacturers publish yearly **service manuals** that describe the construction and repair of their vehicle makes and models. These manuals give important details on repair procedures and parts. Also called shop or repair manuals, they give instructions, specifications, and illustrations for their specific cars and trucks. Service manuals have information on mechanical as well as body repair.

The *contents page* of a service manual lists the broad categories in the manual and gives their page numbers. Each *service manual section* then concentrates on describing that area of repair.

Service manual abbreviations represent technical terms or words and save space. Each manufacturer uses slightly different abbreviations.

Aftermarket repair manuals are published by publishing companies (Mitchell Manuals, Motor Manuals, Chilton Manuals) rather than the manufacturer. They can give enough of the information needed for most repairs.

Repair charts give diagrams that guide you through logical steps for making repairs. They can vary in content and design. Most use arrows and icons (graphic symbols) that represent repair steps.

Diagnosis charts or **troubleshooting charts** give logical steps for finding the source of problems. Mechanical, body, electrical, and other types of troubleshooting charts are provided in service manuals. They give the most common sources of problems for the symptoms being experienced.

Paint reference charts in service manuals give comparable paints manufactured by different

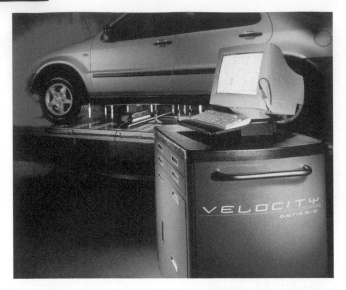

Figure 5–16. Computers are now found throughout a modern body shop: in the office for bookkeeping, estimating, to retrieve service information, on the frame rack, measuring system, and in the paint mixing room. This computer is used for measuring vehicle damage. (Courtesy of Chief Automotive Systems)

companies. This will help you match the color of the new paint with the paint already on the vehicle.

Collision estimating manuals or guides give information for calculating the cost of repairs. They have part numbers, prices, section illustrations, and other data to help the estimator. Discussed in later chapters, electronic or computer-based estimating guides are also available.

A **vehicle dimension manual** gives unibody and frame measurements of undamaged vehicles. Dimensions are given for every make and model car and truck. These known good dimensions can be compared to actual measurements taken off of a damaged vehicle. This will let you know how badly the vehicle is damaged and what must be done to repair it.

COMPUTERIZED SERVICE INFORMATION

Computerized service information places service manuals, dimension manuals, estimating manuals, and other data on compact discs. This allows a personal computer to be used to more quickly look up and print the desired information.

Most shops now have their service information on computer. This allows more efficient handling of shop operations. Estimating, parts ordering, bookkeeping, and the whole shop operation can be more closely monitored and controlled using computers. See **Figure 5–16.**

For example, if a technician needs the dimensions for a specific vehicle being straightened on a frame rack, he or she can quickly pull up this information on computer because all of the data about the vehicle (VIN, year, make, model, etc.) have already been entered into the computer system. A printout of the vehicle dimensions can be made and taken out to the repair area.

COLOR MATCHING MANUALS

Color matching manuals contain information to help you make the old and new paint color look the same or match when painting panels. They have paint code information, color chips, blending and tinting data, tinting procedures, and other information.

SUMMARY

- Vehicle manufacturers give specifications, or measurements, for numerous body dimensions and mechanical parts. In the course of your work you will have to refer to and understand these factory specifications.
- The SAE measuring system is used primarily in the United States, while the metric system, also called the scientific international (SI) system, is used worldwide.
- Pressure measurements are measured in pounds per square inch (psi), kilograms per square centimeter (kg/cm^2), or kilopascals (kPa).
- Temperature is usually measured in degrees Fahrenheit (°F) or Celsius (°C). In the collision repair shop, temperatures are important in the drying of various materials such as primers, paints, and adhesives.
- The Vehicle Identification Number (VIN) is used to accurately identify the body style, model year, engine, and other data pertaining to the vehicle.

TECHNICAL TERMS

measurements
specifications
Society of Automotive Engineers (SAE) measuring system
fractions
decimals
metric measuring system
scientific international (SI) system
conversion charts
SAE-metric conversion chart
decimal conversion chart
linear measurements
scale
ruler
SAE rule
metric rule
meter stick
parallax error
pocket scale
yardstick
tape rule
tape measure
tram gauge
dividers
micrometers
dial indicator
feeler gauges
flat feeler gauges
wire feeler gauges
pressure gauge
vacuum gauge
flow meter
manometer
angle measurements
thermometers
ambient
surface temperature thermometers
mixing scales
manual mixing scales
electronic mixing scales
graduated pail
mixing instructions
percentage reduction
mixing by parts
proportional numbers
mixing chart
paint mixing sticks
paint stirring sticks
viscosity cup
orifice
paint thickness
mils
mil gauge
pencil mil gauge
electronic mil gauge
Vehicle Identification Number (VIN) plate
body ID number
service part number
service manuals
service manual abbreviations
aftermarket repair manuals
repair charts
diagnosis charts
troubleshooting charts
paint reference charts
collision estimating manuals
vehicle dimension manual
computerized service information
color matching manuals

REVIEW QUESTIONS

1. ______________ are number values that help control processes in collision repair.
2. Explain how you might use conversion charts.
3. How do you avoid parallax error when reading a scale?
4. Describe the three types of tips available for digital thermometers.
5. If a paint requires 50 percent reduction, how would you mix the paint and its solvent?
6. When mixing refinishing materials, what might the numbers 2:1:1 mean?
7. A ______________ is used to measure the actual consistency or fluidity of the mixed materials, usually paint.
8. Paint/material buildup should be limited to no more than this amount.
   a. 12 mils
   b. 2 mils
   c. 50 mils
   d. 100 mils
9. What can happen if the paint on the vehicle is too thick?
10. The ______________ is used to accurately identify the body style, model year, engine, and other data about the vehicle.
11. This type of manual gives information for calculating the cost of collision repairs.
    a. Service manual
    b. Dimensions manual
    c. Estimating manual
    d. Paint code manual

ASE-STYLE REVIEW QUESTIONS

1. Which of the following types of error results when you read a rule or scale from an angle?
   a. Compound
   b. Parallax
   c. Conversion
   d. Specification

2. Paint reduction calls for using 1 quart of reducer for each gallon of color. What reduction would this be?

a. 125 percent
b. 75 percent
c. 25 percent
d. 5 percent

3. Paint mixing instructions give the number 2:1:1. What does this mean?

a. 2 parts color, 1 part reducer, 1 part hardener
b. 2 parts hardener, 1 part color, 1 part reducer
c. 2 parts reducer, 1 part color, 1 part hardener
d. 2 hours, 1 minute, 1 second curing time

4. *Technician A* is using a mixing stick to measure out color, reducer, and hardener. *Technician B* is using electronic or computerized scales. Who is correct?

a. Technician A
b. Technician B
c. Both Technicians A and B
d. Neither Technician

5. *Technician A* says that original OEM paints are typically about 6 to 20 mils thick. *Technician B* says that the basecoat is approximately 10 to 12 mils thick. Who is correct?

a. Technician A
b. Technician B
c. Both Technicians A and B
d. Neither Technician

6. Which of the following would be used to verify the actual amount of frame or unibody damage on a vehicle?

a. Dimensions manual
b. Estimating manual
c. Service manual
d. Owner's manual

7. Paint drains too quickly out of a viscosity cup. This means you have added too much:

a. Color
b. Catalyst
c. Reducer
d. Toner

ACTIVITIES

1. Find the VIN on several vehicles. Write down the location of the VIN for several cars. Look up the VIN data in a service manual.

2. Use a paint thickness gauge to check for excess paint layers on several vehicles. Did different panels have more paint than others? How many vehicles had paint thicker than normal? Could you see any paint cracking or other surface problems when the paint was too thick?

CHAPTER

6 Fasteners

OBJECTIVES

After studying this chapter, you should be able to:

- Identify the various fasteners used in vehicle construction.
- Remove and install bolts and nuts properly.
- Explain when specific fasteners are used in vehicle construction.
- Explain bolt and nut torque values.
- Summarize the use of chemical fasteners.
- Identify hose clamps.

INTRODUCTION

Fasteners are the thousands of bolts, nuts, screws, clips, and adhesives that hold a vehicle together.

As a collision repair technician, you will constantly use fasteners when removing and installing body parts. This makes it important for you to be able to identify and use fasteners properly.

Remember that each fastener is engineered for a specific application. Always replace fasteners with exactly the same type that was removed from the *original equipment manufacture (OEM)* assembly.

BOLTS

A **bolt** is a shaft with a head on one end and threads on the other. A **cap screw** is a term that describes a high-strength bolt. Bolts and cap screws are usually named after the body part they hold: fender bolt, hood hinge bolt, etc. Their shape and head drive configuration also helps name them.

Bolt Terminology

To work with bolts properly, you must understand basic bolt terminology. See **Figure 6–1.**

The **bolt head** is used to tighten, or torque, the bolt. A socket or wrench fits over the head,

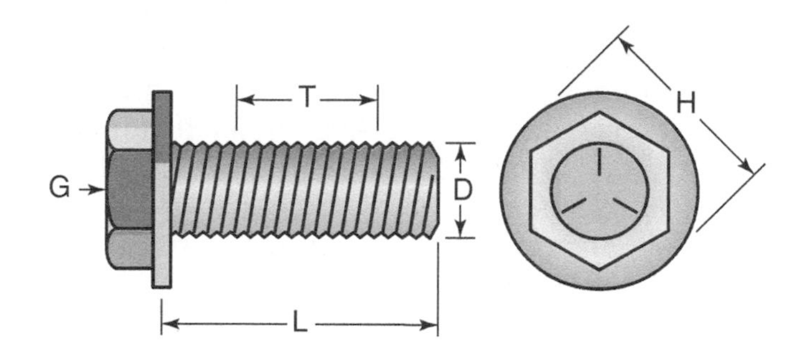

H - Head
G - Grade marking (bolt strength)
L - Length (inches)
T - Thread pitch (thread/inch)
D - Nominal diameter (inches)

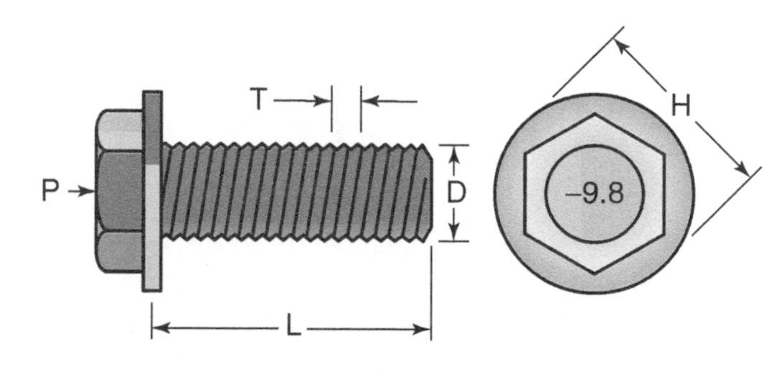

H - Head
P - Property class (bolt strength)
L - Length (millimeters)
T - Thread pitch (millimeters)
D - Nominal diameter (millimeters)

Figure 6–1. Bolt measurements are needed when working. Study each dimension of both USC and metric bolts.

which enables the bolt to be tightened or loosened. Some metric and USC/SAE sockets are very close in size. It is very important to use the correct wrench or socket when tightening or loosening nuts and bolts. The improper wrench or socket could strip or round off the nut or bolt you are working on. This could damage your tools, or even cause you an injury if the tool slips off.

Bolt length is measured from the end of the threads to the bottom of the bolt head. It is NOT the total length including the bolt head.

Bolt diameter, sometimes termed **bolt size,** is measured around the outside of the threads. For example, a ½-inch bolt has a thread diameter of ½ inch, while its head or wrench size would be ¾ inch.

Bolt head size is the distance measured across the flats of the bolt head. In USC, head size is given in fractions, just like wrench size. A few common sizes are 7⁄16, ½, and 9⁄16 inch. In the metric system, 8-, 10-, 13-millimeter head sizes are typical. Common USC and metric bolt head sizes are given in **Figure 6–2.**

Bolt **thread pitch** is a measurement of thread coarseness. Bolts and nuts can have coarse, fine, and metric threads. Bolt threads can be measured with a **thread pitch gauge.** One is shown in **Figure 6–3.**

The two common metric threads are coarse and fine and can be identified by the letters SI (System International or International System of Units) and ISO (International Standards Organization).

Common english USC/SAE head sizes	Common metric head sizes
Wrench size (inches)*	Wrench size (millimeters)*
3/8	9
7/16	10
1/2	11
9/16	12
5/8	13
11/16	14
3/4	15
13/16	16
7/8	17
15/16	18
1	19
1-1/16	20
1-1/8	21
1-3/16	22
1-1/4	23
1-5/16	24
1-3/8	26
7/16	27
1-1/2	29
	30
	32

*The wrench sizes given in this chart are not equivalents, but are standard head sizes found in both inches and millimeters.

Figure 6–2. These are common bolt head and wrench sizes. Never use a USC wrench on metric bolts or vice versa. This will damage the bolt head.

WARNING

Do NOT accidentally interchange thread types or damage will result. It is easy to mistake metric threads for USC/SAE threads. If the two are forced together, either the bold or part threads will be ruined.

Bolts and nuts are also available in right- and left-hand threads. **Right-hand threads** must be turned clockwise to tighten. Less common **left-hand threads** must be rotated in a counterclockwise direction to tighten the fastener. Left-hand threads may be denoted by notches or the letter "L" stamped on them.

Bolt Strengths or Grades

Bolt strength indicates the amount of torque or tightening force that should be applied. Bolts are made from different materials having various degrees of hardness. Softer metal or harder metal can be used to make bolts. Bolts are made with different hardnesses and strengths for use in different situations.

Bolt grade markings are lines or numbers on the top of the head to identify bolt hardness and strength. The hardness or strength of metric bolts is indicated by using a property class indicator on the head of the bolt.

Bolt strength markings are given as lines. The number of lines on the head of the bolt is

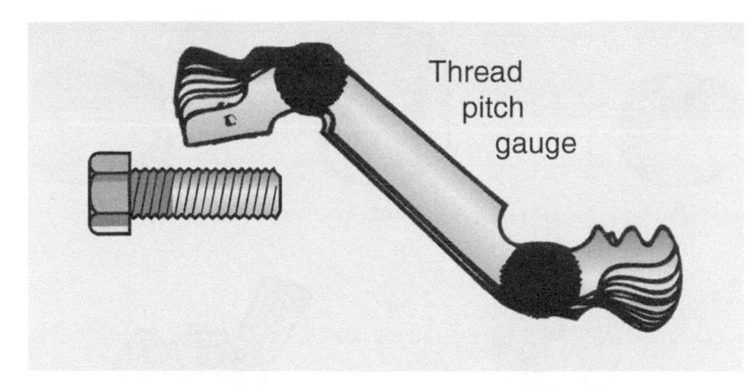

(A) Thread pitch gauge. The thread pitch gauge is fit against threads. Threads that match the gauge equal the pitch number printed on the gauge.

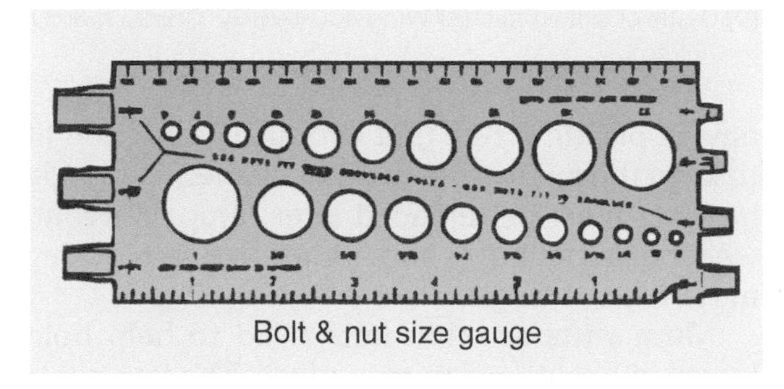

(B) Bolt and nut size gauge. Bolts and nuts can be fitted into a bolt and nut gauge to quickly tell their sizes.

Figure 6–3. Gauges can be used to tell thread, bolt, or nut sizes.

related to its strength. As the number of lines increases so does the strength.

Metric bolt strength markings are given as numbers. The higher the number is, the stronger the bolt. These markings apply to both bolts and nuts.

Tensile strength is the amount of pressure per square inch the bolt can withstand just before breaking when being pulled apart. The harder or stronger the bolt, the greater the tensile strength.

Torque

Torque is a measurement of the turning force applied when tightening a fastener. It is critical that bolts and nuts are tightened or torqued properly. Over-tightening will stretch and possibly break the bolt. Under-tightening could allow the bolt or nut to loosen and fall out.

Torque specifications are tightening values for the specific bolt or nut. They are given by the manufacturer. Discussed in the tool chapter, a torque wrench must be used to measure torque values.

If you cannot find the factory torque specification for a bolt, you can use a **general bolt torque chart.** It will give a general torque value for the size and grade of bolt. One is given in **Figure 6–4.** Normally, the bolt threads should be lubricated to get accurate results. Refer to the service or repair manual to see if the threads should be lubricated or dry.

A *tightening sequence,* or **torque pattern,** ensures that parts secured by several bolts are clamped down evenly. Generally, tighten fasteners in a crisscross pattern. This will pull the part down evenly, preventing warpage. It is commonly recommended on wheels, as shown in **Figure 6–5.**

Basically, tighten the fastener in steps. Begin at approximately half-torque, then continue to

Metric standard							SAE standard/foot pounds						
Grade of bolt		5D	.8G	10K	12K		Grade of bolt	SAE 1&2	SAE 5	SAE 6	SAE 8		
Min. tensile strength		71,160 PSI	113,800 PSI	142,200 PSI	170,679 PSI		Min. ten strength	64,000 PSI	105,000 PSI	133,000 PSI	150,000 PSI		
Grade markings on head		5D	8G	10K	12K	Size of socket on wrench opening	Markings on head					Size of socket or wrench opening	
Metric		Foot pounds				Metric	U.S. standard	Foot pounds				U.S. regular	
Bolt dia.	U.S. dec equiv.					Bolt head	Bolt dia.					Bolt head	Nut
6 mm	.2362	5	G	8	10	10 mm	1/4	5	7	10	10.5	3/8	7/16
8 mm	.3150	10	16	22	27	14 mm	5/16	9	14	19	22	1/2	9/16
10 mm	.3937	19	31	40	49	17 mm	3/8	15	25	34	37	9/16	5/8
12 mm	.4720	34	54	70	86	19 mm	7/16	24	40	55	60	5/8	3/4
14 mm	.5512	55	89	117	137	22 mm	1/2	37	60	85	92	3/4	13/16
16 mm	.6299	83	132	175	208	24 mm	9/16	53	88	120	132	7/8	7/8
18 mm	.709	111	182	236	283	27 mm	5/8	74	120	167	180	15/16	1.
22 mm	.8661	182	284	394	464	32 mm	3/4	120	200	280	296	1-1/8	1-1/8

Figure 6–4. This is a general bolt torque chart. It gives different values for each bolt tensile strength rating. These values apply to dry torque unless otherwise specified.

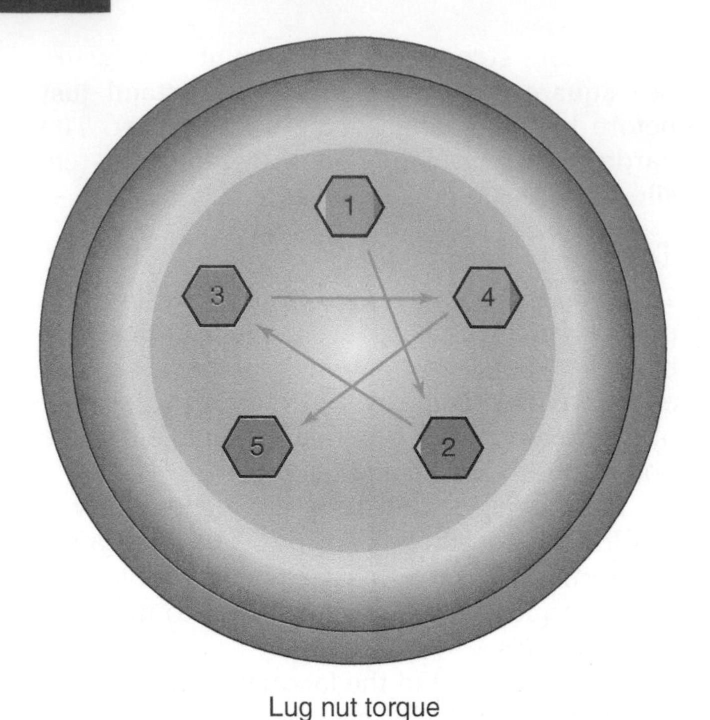

Figure 6–5. When tightening several bolts that hold one part, a wheel, for example, always use a crisscross pattern. This will prevent part warpage and damage.

three-fourths torque, and then full torque at least twice.

Be careful when tightening bolts and nuts with air wrenches. It is easy to stretch or break a bolt in an instant. The air wrench can spin the bolt or nut so fast that it can hammer the fastener past its yield point. This can strip threads or snap off the bolt.

NUTS

A **nut** uses internal (inside) threads and an odd shaped head that often fits a wrench. When tightened onto a bolt, a strong clamping force holds the parts together. Many different nuts are used by the automotive industry. Several are shown in **Figure 6–6.**

Castellated or **slotted nuts** are grooved on top so that a safety wire or cotter pin can be installed into a hole in the bolt. This helps prevent the nut from working loose. For example, castellated nuts are used with the studs that hold wheel bearings in position. Slotted nuts are also used on steering and suspension parts for safety.

Self-locking nuts produce a friction or force fit when threaded onto a bolt or stud. The top of the nut can be crimped inward. Some

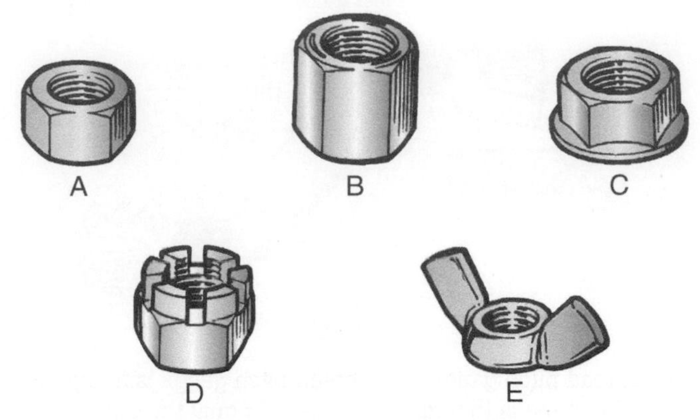

Figure 6–6. Nuts also come in various designs. Memorize their names. **(A)** Hex nut. **(B)** High or deep nut. **(C)** Flange nut. **(D)** Castle or slotted nut. **(E)** Wing nut. (Courtesy of Dorman Products)

have a plastic insert that produces a friction fit to keep the nut from loosening. Sometimes, locking nuts must be replaced after removal. Front-wheel drive spindles sometimes use self-locking nuts.

Jam nuts are thin nuts used to help hold larger, conventional nuts in place. The jam nut is tightened down against the other nut to prevent its loosening.

Wing nuts have two extended arms for turning the nut by hand. They are used when a part must be removed frequently for service or maintenance. Air cleaners sometimes use wing nuts. See **Figure 6–7.**

Acorn nuts are closed on one end for appearance and to keep water and debris off the threads. They can be used when they are visible and looks are important.

Special types of nuts are used to hold specific parts onto the vehicle. Sometimes a washer is formed onto the nut. Termed **body nuts,** the flange on the nut helps distribute the clamping force of the thin body panel or trim piece to prevent warpage. See **Figure 6–8.**

THREAD REPAIR

A collision repair technician must frequently repair damaged threads. A **tap** is a tool for cutting inside threads in holes. A tap is used to repair damaged threaded holes. It is rotated down into the threaded hole to recut the threads. A **die** cuts threads on the outside of bolts or studs. It too is rotated over the threads to clean them up.

Special **t-handles** fit over the tap or die for turning. You must hold the tool perfectly square to cut good threads. Oil the threads. Then rotate

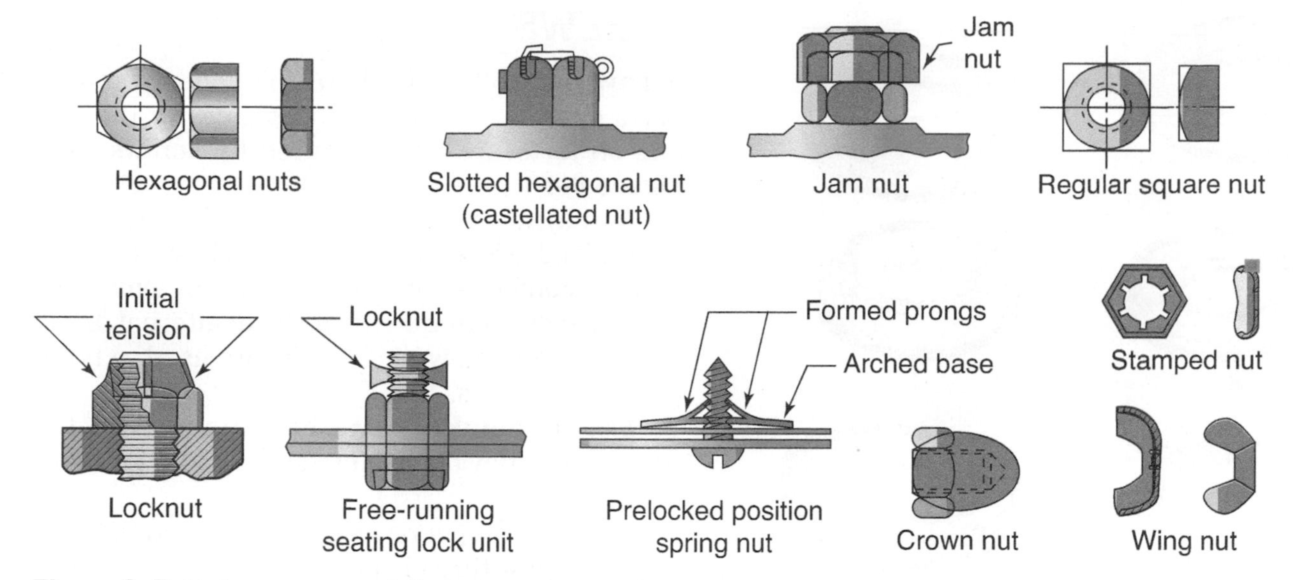

Figure 6–7. Body nuts are specially designed for specific holding applications.

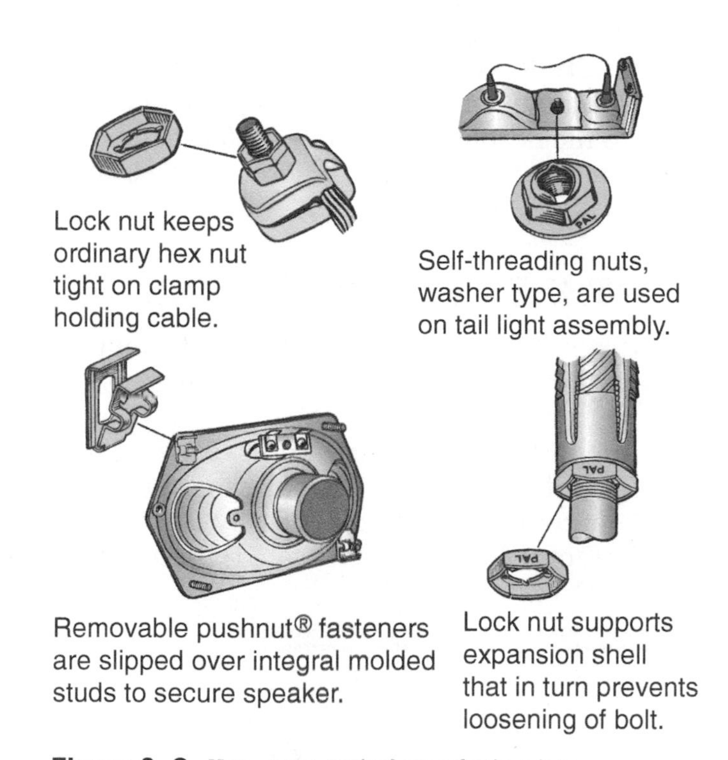

Lock nut keeps ordinary hex nut tight on clamp holding cable.
Self-threading nuts, washer type, are used on tail light assembly.
Removable pushnut® fasteners are slipped over integral molded studs to secure speaker.
Lock nut supports expansion shell that in turn prevents loosening of bolt.

Figure 6–8. Note some typical uses for jam juts.
(Courtesy of Palnut)

the tap or die about one-half of a turn and then back it out about one-fourth turn. This will clean metal shavings out and prevent tool breakage.

A **Helicoil®** or *thread insert* can be used to repair badly damaged internal threads. Basically, to use a thread insert, drill the hole oversize. Then tap the hole with new threads. Use the special tool to rotate the insert into the freshly threaded hole. This will allow you to use the original size bolt.

WASHERS

Washers are used under bolts, nuts, and other parts. They prevent damage to the surfaces of parts and provide better holding power. Several types are illustrated in **Figure 6–9.**

Flat washers are used to increase the clamping surface area. They prevent the smaller bolt head from pulling through the sheet metal or plastic.

A **wave washer** adds a spring action to keep parts from rattling and loosening.

Body or **fender washers** have a very large outside diameter for the size hole in them. They provide better holding power on thin metal and plastic parts.

Copper or **brass washers** are used to prevent fluid leakage, as on brake line fittings. **Spacer washers** come in specific thicknesses to allow for adjustment of parts. **Fiber washers** will prevent vibration or leakage but cannot be tightened to a great extent.

Finishing washers have a curved shape for a pleasing appearance. They are used on interior pieces.

Split lock washers are used under nuts to prevent loosening by vibration. The ends of these spring-hardened washers dig into both the nut and the part to prevent rotation.

Shakeproof or **teeth lock washers** have teeth or bent lugs that grip both the work and the nut. Several designs, shapes, and sizes are available. An external type has teeth on the outside and an internal type has teeth around the inside.

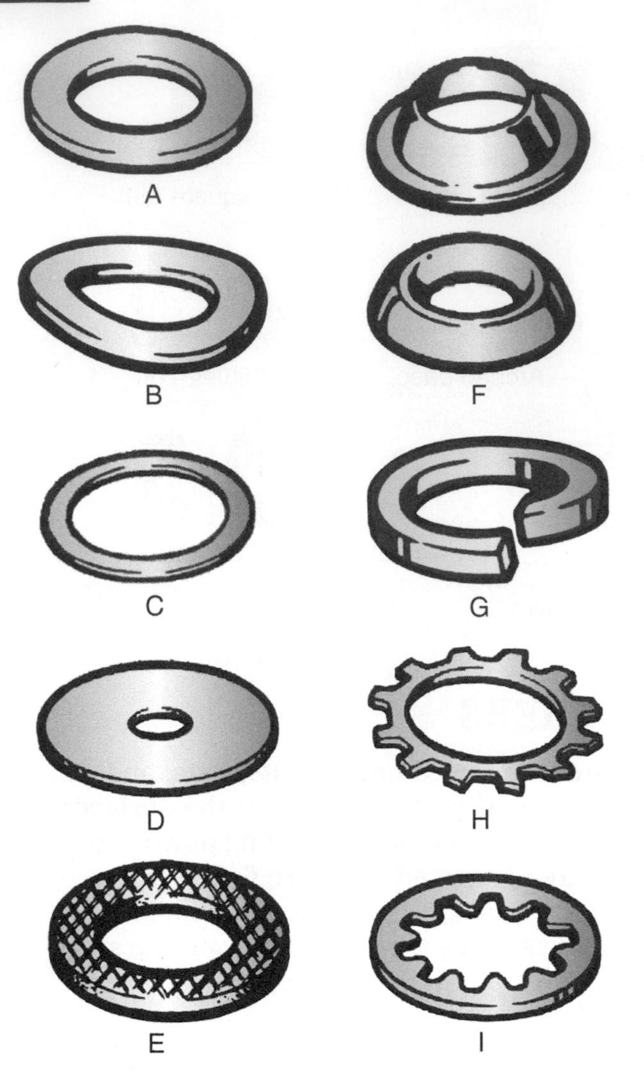

Figure 6–9. Know the washer types. **(A)** Plain flat washer. **(B)** Wave or spring washer. **(C)** Spacer washer. **(D)** Fender washer. **(E)** Fiber washer. **(F)** Finishing washer. **(G)** Split lock washer. **(H)** External lock washer. **(I)** Internal lock washer. (Courtesy of Dorman Products)

SCREWS

Screws are often used to hold nonstructural parts on a vehicle. Trim pieces, interior panels, and so forth are often secured by screws. See **Figure 6–10.**

Machine screws are threaded their full length and are relatively weak. They come in various configurations and will accept a nut.

Set screws frequently have an internal drive head for an Allen wrench. They are used to hold parts onto shafts.

Sheet metal screws have pointed or tapered tips. They thread into sheet metal for light holding tasks.

Self-tapping screws have a pointed tip that helps cut new threads in parts.

Trim screws have a washer attached to them. This improves appearance and helps keep the trim from shifting.

Headlight aiming screws have a special plastic adapter mounted on them. The adapter fits into the headlight assembly. Different design variations are needed for different makes and models of vehicles.

NONTHREADED FASTENERS

Nonthreaded fasteners, as implied, do not use threads. They include keys, snap rings, pins, clips, adhesives, etc.

Various **keys** and **pins** are used by equipment manufacturers to retain parts in alignment. It is important to be able to identify these keys and pins, order replacements, and replace them.

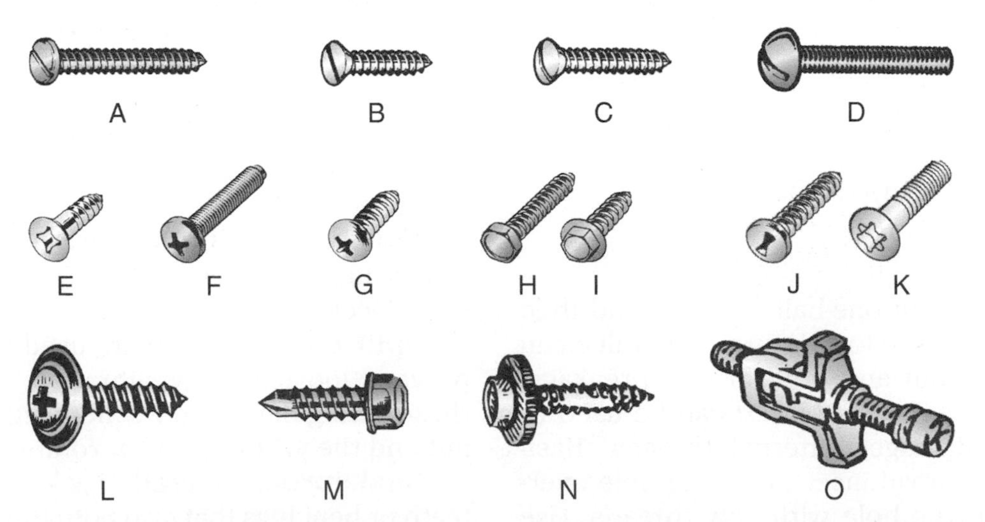

Figure 6–10. Study common screw names. **(A)** Pan head sheet metal screw. **(B)** Flat head sheet metal screw. **(C)** Oval head. **(D)** Slotted machine screw. **(E)** Phillips head screw. **(F)** Phillips machine screw. **(G)** Oval head sheet metal screw. **(H)** Hex or nutdriver screw. **(I)** Hex screw with flange or integral washer. **(J)** Clutch head. **(K)** Torx® head. **(L)** Trim screw. **(M)** Self-tapping screw. **(N)** Body screw. **(O)** Headlight aiming screw. (Courtesy of Dorman Products)

Square keys and **Woodruff keys** are used to prevent hand wheels, gears, cams, and pulleys from turning on their shafts. These keys are strong enough to carry heavy loads if they are fitted and seated properly. See **Figure 6–11.**

Round **taper pins** have a larger diameter on one end than the other. They are used to locate and position matching parts. They can also be used to secure small pulleys and gears to shafts. See **Figure 6–12.**

Dowel pins have the same general diameter their full length. They are used to position and align the parts of an assembly. One end of a dowel pin is chamfered, and it is usually 0.001 to 0.002 inch (0.025 to 0.05 mm) greater in diameter than the size of its hole. When replacing a dowel pin, be sure that it is the same size as the old one.

Cotter pins help prevent bolts and nuts from loosening, or they fit through pins to hold parts together. They are also used as stops and holders on shafts and rods. All cotter pins are used for safety and should NEVER be reused.

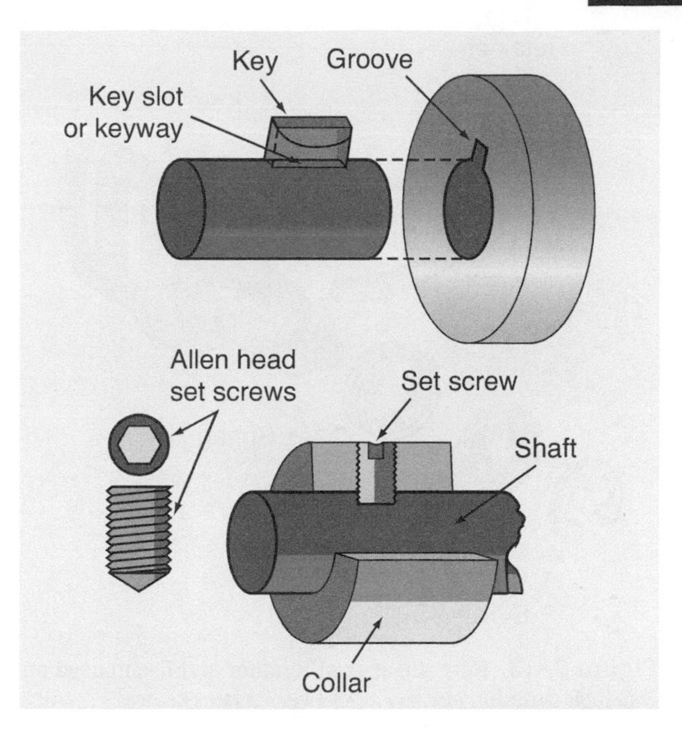

Figure 6–11. Keys and set screws are both used to align parts on shafts. **(A)** Key and keyway. **(B)** Set screw application.

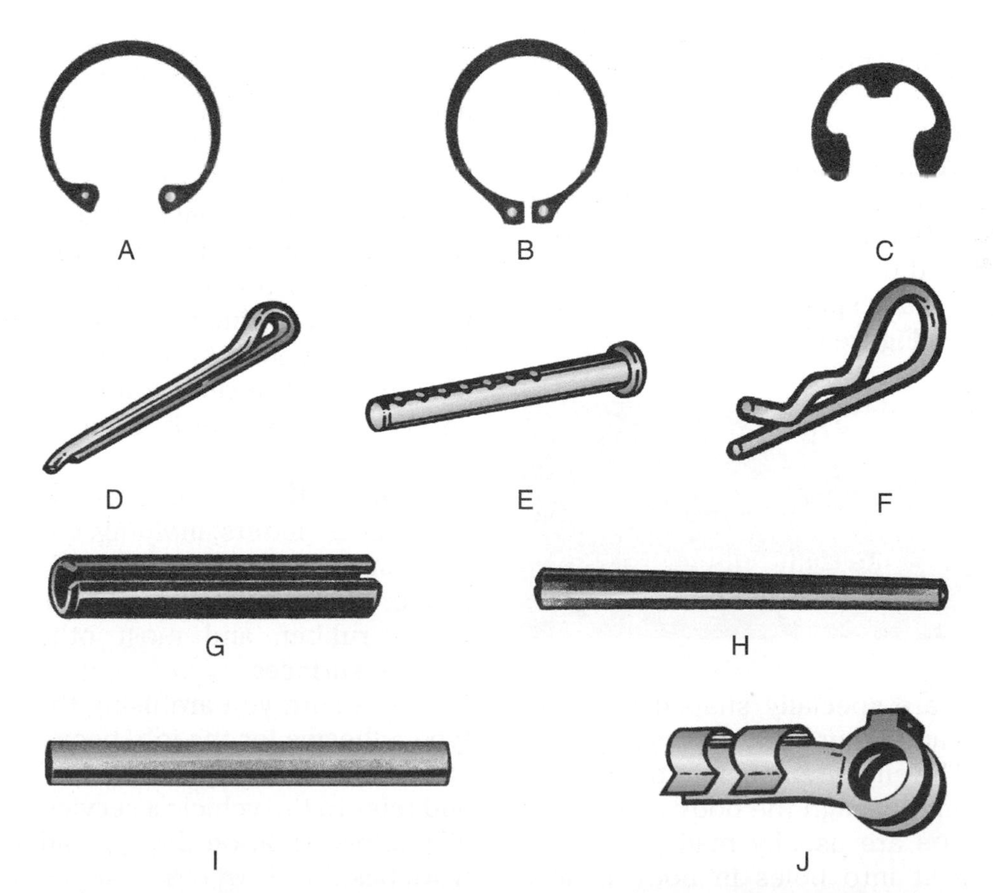

Figure 6–12. Know the nonthreaded fastener names. **(A)** Internal snap or retaining ring. **(B)** External snapring. **(C)** E-clip or snapring. **(D)** Cotter pin. **(E)** Clevis pin. **(F)** Hitch pin. **(G)** Split rollpin. **(H)** Taper pin. **(I)** Straight dowel pin. **(J)** Linkage clip. (Courtesy of Dorman Products)

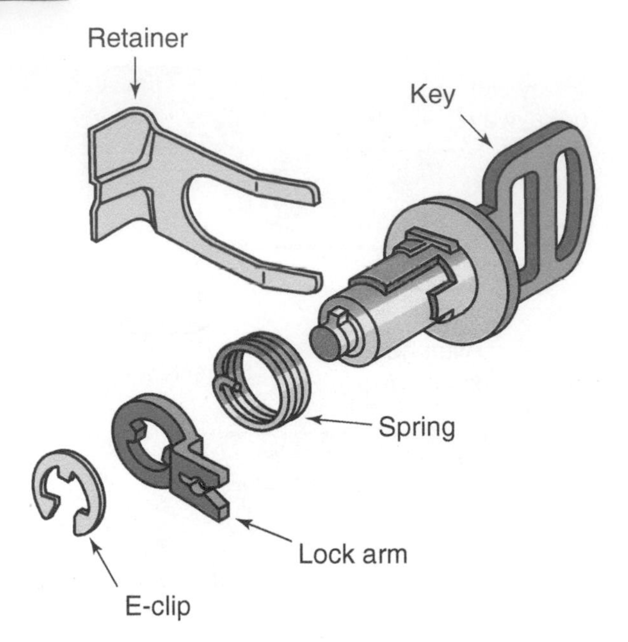

Figure 6–13. Note the special retainer and E-clip used on this lock cylinder. (Courtesy American Honda Motor Co., Inc.)

The cotter pin should fit into the hole with very little side play. If it is too long, cut off the extra length of cotter pin. Bend it over in a smooth curve. Sharply angled bends invite breakage. Bend the ends with needle nose pliers. Final bending of the prongs can be done with a soft-faced mallet.

Snap rings are nonthreaded fasteners that install into a groove machined into a part. They are used to hold parts on shafts. Special snap ring pliers are designed to flex and install or remove snap rings. They have special tips that will hold the snap ring. See **Figure 6–13.**

DANGER

Wear safety glasses when removing or installing snap rings. Being constructed of spring steel, they can shoot out with great force.

Body clips are specially shaped retainers for holding trim and other body pieces requiring little strength. The clip often fits into the back of the trim piece and through the body panel.

Push-in clips are usually made of plastic and they force fit into holes in body panels. Push-in clips are used to hold interior door trim panels, for example. They install easily, but can be difficult to remove. See **Figure 6–14.**

Pop rivets can be used to hold two pieces of sheet metal together. They can be inserted into a blind hole through two pieces of metal and then drawn up with a riveting tool or gun. This will lock the pieces together. There is no need to have access to the back of the rivets.

HOSE CLAMPS

Hose clamps are used to hold radiator hoses, heater hoses, and other hoses onto their fittings. See **Figure 6–15.**

ADHESIVES

Adhesives provide an alternate means of bonding parts together. The two types of adhesives most often used are epoxy and trim adhesive.

Epoxy is a two-part bonding agent that dries harder than adhesive. It comes in two separate containers, usually tubes. One contains the epoxy resin and the other contains a hardener. Epoxy does NOT shrink when it hardens and is waterproof and heat-resistant at moderate temperatures.

Read the instructions for the proper quantity to use. If both resin and hardener are NOT in proper proportion, the bond might fail. Some epoxy tubes automatically dispense the correct amount of resin and hardener.

Once mixed, the epoxy remains in a workable condition for only a brief time. Therefore, try to mix only as much as is required and use it as quickly as possible. Clamp the work while the glue cures, which can take several hours. Do NOT apply epoxy in low temperatures (below 50°F or 10°C), because it will NOT harden. Once an epoxy is applied, it is difficult to remove it from a surface.

Trim adhesive is used to install various trim pieces (letters, molding, emblems) onto the body surface. Trim adhesive dries to a pliable rubber-like consistency. It will bond plastics, metal, rubber, and most other materials to painted surfaces.

Make sure you are using the recommended type adhesive for the job, because performance characteristics vary. Read the label directions and refer to the vehicle's service manual for specific information on the type adhesive that will work best.

Make sure the surfaces on the part and body are properly cleaned. Mark the desired part alignment with masking tape if needed.

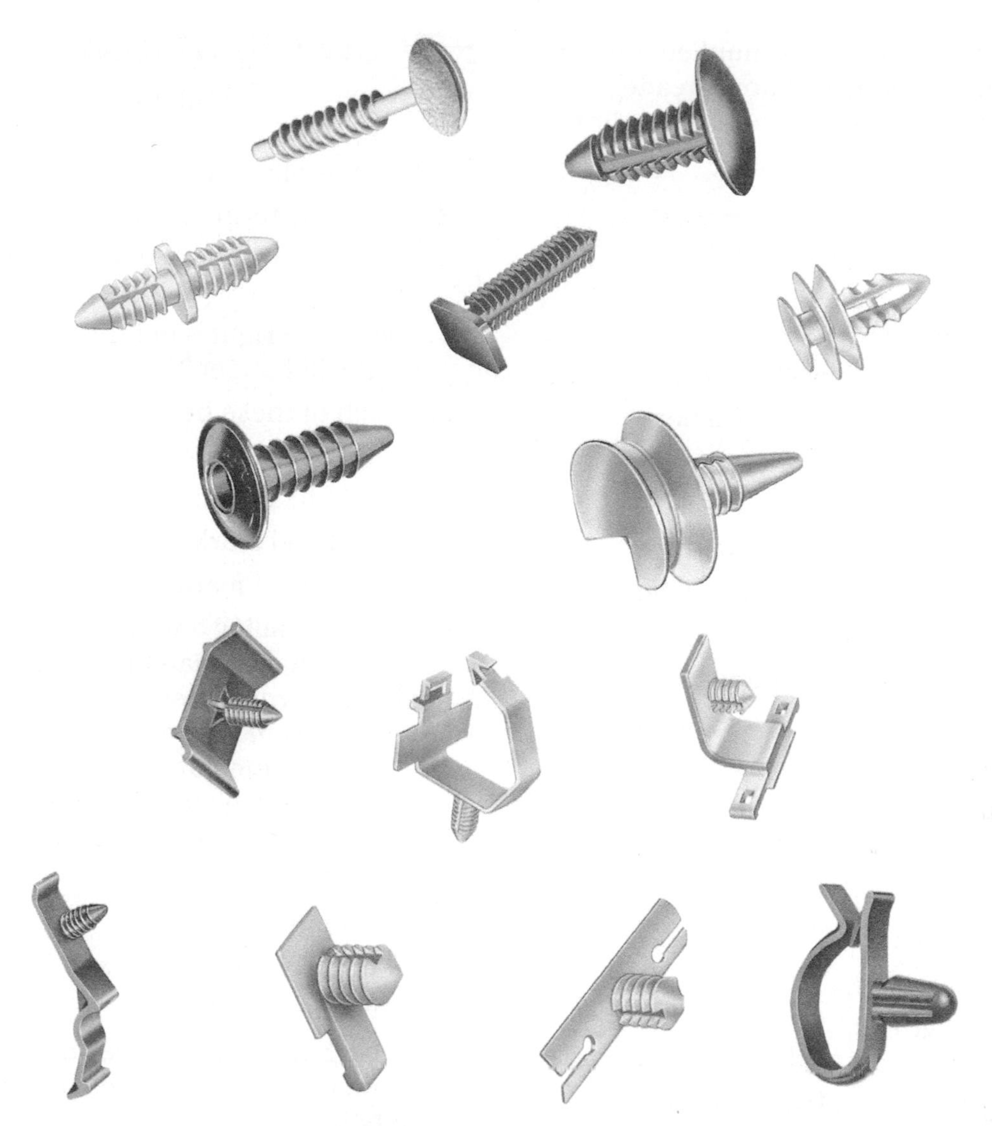

Figure 6–14. Here are a few of the special plastic retainers available. These types are often used in vehicle interiors. They quickly press into a hole. To remove them, you must carefully pry next to the retainer with a flat, forked trim tool. (Courtesy TRW Plastic Fasteners and Retainers Division, Westminster, MA and Roseville, MI)

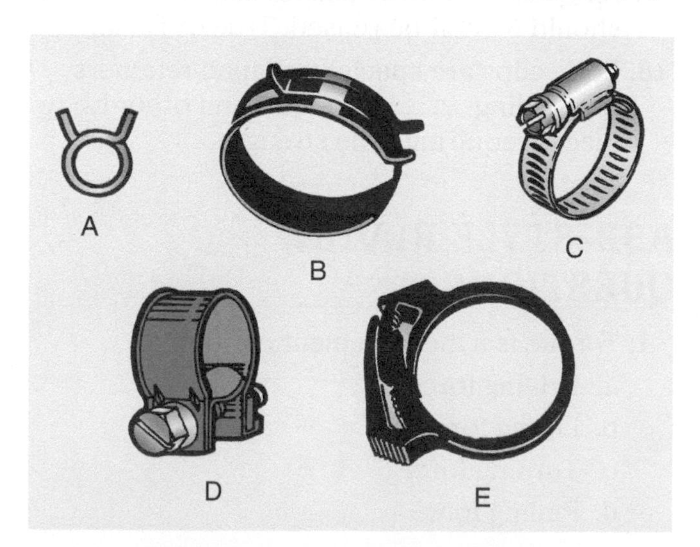

Figure 6–15. Note the hose clamp types. **(A)** Wire spring hose clamp. **(B)** Wire strap hose clamp. **(C)** Worm hose clamp. **(D)** Screw-nut hose clamp. **(E)** Plastic hose clamp. (Courtesy of Dorman Products)

Apply a moderate amount of adhesive to the part. When excessive adhesive squeezes out from under the part, extra cleanup will be required.

Carefully move the part straight into place on the body without smearing the adhesive. Press the part down tightly to compress the adhesive against the two surfaces. If needed, use masking tape to hold the part in place as the adhesive dries.

SUMMARY

- Fasteners make up the thousands of bolts, nuts, screws, clips, and adhesives that literally hold a vehicle together.
- Bolt strength indicates the amount of torque or tightening force that should be applied.

- Nonthreaded fasteners, as implied, do not use threads. Examples of nonthreaded fasteners are keys, snap rings, pins, clips, and adhesives.

TECHNICAL TERMS

fasteners
bolt
cap screw
bolt head
bolt length
bolt diameter
bolt size
bolt head size
thread pitch
thread pitch gauge
right-hand threads
left-hand threads
bolt strength
bolt grade markings
bolt strength markings
metric bolt strength markings
tensile strength
torque specifications
general bolt torque chart
torque pattern
nut
slotted nuts
self-locking nuts
jam nuts
wing nuts
acorn nuts
body nuts
tap
die
t-handles
Helicoil®
washers
flat washers
wave washers
body washers
fender washers
copper washers
brass washers
spacer washers
fiber washers
finishing washers
split lock washers
shakeproof lock washers
teeth lock washers
screws
machine screws
set screws
sheet metal screws
self-tapping screws
trim screws
headlight aiming screws
nonthreaded fasteners
keys
pins
square keys
Woodruff keys
taper pins
dowel pins
cotter pins
body clips
push-in clips
pop rivets
hose clamps
adhesives
epoxy
trim adhesive

REVIEW QUESTIONS

1. ______________ include the thousands of bolts, nuts, screws, clips, and adhesives that literally hold a vehicle together.
2. Define the term *cap screw.*
3. What is bolt thread pitch and how is it measured?
4. If you turn right-hand threads clockwise, what will happen?
5. Which of these bolts is strongest?
   a. Three head markings
   b. Two head markings
   c. No head markings
   d. One head marking
6. When installing a wheel on a vehicle, no service manual can be found for getting a factory torque specification.
   Technician A says to use an impact wrench on medium setting. *Technician B* says to use a general torque chart and a torque wrench. Who is correct?
   a. Technician A
   b. Technician B
   c. Both Technicians A and B
   d. Neither Technician
7. What general sequence should be used when tightening a series of bolts or nuts?
8. How do you use a thread repair insert?
9. All cotter pins are used for safety and should NEVER be reused. True or False?
10. Body clips are specially shaped retainers for holding ______________ and other body pieces requiring little strength.

ASE-STYLE REVIEW QUESTIONS

1. Torque is a measurement of:
   a. Driving force
   b. Lifting force
   c. Turning force
   d. Pulling force
2. A technician removes a nut with three dots on it. *Technician A* says that is has the

strength of grade 5. *Technician B* says that it has strength of grade 3. Who is correct?

a. Technician A
b. Technician B
c. Both Technicians A and B
d. Neither Technician

3. Which of the following types of washers is used to prevent loosening by vibration?

a. Flat
b. Fender
c. Finish
d. Split lock

4. When replacing a fastener, *Technician A* says that the same number of fasteners should always be used. *Technician B* says that stretched fasteners or fasteners with any signs of damage should be replaced. Who is correct?

a. Technician A
b. Technician B
c. Both Technicians A and B
d. Neither Technician

5. Which of the following is NOT a hose clamp type?

a. Orbital
b. Wire spring
c. Screw-nut
d. Worm

6. *Technician A* says that "one-time" fasteners must always be replaced following removal. *Technician B* says that cotter pins are to be used only once. Who is correct?

a. Technician A
b. Technician B
c. Both Technicians A and B
d. Neither Technician

7. *Technician A* says that an SAE is measured in millimeters. *Technician B* says that an SAE bolt is measured in inches. Who is correct?

a. Technician A
b. Technician B
c. Both Technicians A and B
d. Neither Technician

8. *Technician A* says that tensile strength is the amount of pressure per square inch that a bolt can withstand before breaking. *Technician B* says that tensile strength is the tightening value of the specific bolt or nut. Who is correct?

a. Technician A
b. Technician B
c. Both Technicians A and B
d. Neither Technician

9. *Technician A* says that a die is a tool that is used for cutting inside threads. *Technician B* says that a tap is a tool that is used for cutting inside threads. Who is correct?

a. Technician A
b. Technician B
c. Both Technicians A and B
d. Neither Technician

10. *Technician A* says that screws are often used to hold nonstructural parts on a vehicle. *Technician B* says that machine screws are threaded their full length and are relatively weak. Who is correct?

a. Technician A
b. Technician B
c. Both Technicians A and B
d. Neither Technician

ACTIVITIES

1. Inspect a car or truck. Write down the various types of fasteners you can locate. Create a chart listing their names and applications.
2. Read the directions on a few types of body adhesives. Write a short report on their use.
3. Visit a body supply house or hardware store. Inspect the various types of fasteners available.

CHAPTER

7 Body Shop Materials

OBJECTIVES

After studying this chapter, you should be able to:

- Select the right repair materials for the job.
- Explain the basic purpose of common body shop materials.
- Compare the use of similar shop materials.
- Summarize when to use different kinds of body filler and putty.
- Know how to select the right type of primer and paint.

INTRODUCTION

Collision repair materials include more than just refinishing or paint materials. They include the various fillers, primers, sealers, adhesives, sandpapers, and other compounds. It is critical that you understand their selection and use.

When consumers look at a vehicle's paint job, they often only see a shiny, bright color. They seldom understand all of the work involved in producing that long-lasting, tough, durable, high-gloss finish. There is hidden technology under the surface of the paint.

A professional collision repair and refinishing technician comprehends all of the "chemistry" and skill needed to do high-quality repairs.

REFINISHING MATERIALS

A car body is protected and beautified by a complete finishing system. All parts of the system work together to protect the vehicle. See **Figure 7–1.**

Refinishing materials is a general term referring to the products used to repaint the vehicle. Refinishing material chemistry has changed drastically. New paints last longer but require more skill and safety measures for proper application.

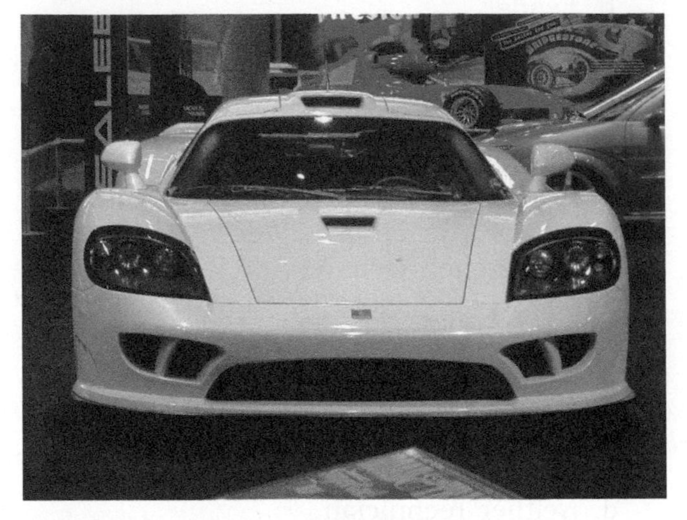

Figure 7–1. Many types of chemically advanced materials are used to repair collision damaged cars. The technology in today's refinishing materials results in a very beautiful yet "space-age tough" coating over the vehicle's body.

The **substrate** is the steel, aluminum, plastic, and composite materials used in the vehicle's construction. It will affect the selection of refinishing materials.

The vehicle's **paint** performs two basic functions—to beautify the body and to protect the metal from rust.

PRIMECOATS AND PAINTCOATS

A basic paint job on a car consists of several coats of two or more different materials. The most basic finish consists of:

1. Primer coats
2. Paintcoats

The *primer* has to improve adhesion of the paint. It is the first coat applied. Paint alone will not stick, or adhere. If you apply a paintcoat to bare substrate, the paint will peel, flake off, or look rough. This is why you must "sandwich" a primer between the substrate and the paint. Primer also prevents any chemicals from bleeding through and showing in the paint.

The term **colorcoat** refers to the paint applied over the primecoats. It is usually several light coats of one or more paints. The paintcoats are the "glamour coats," because they feature the eye-catching color, color effects, and gloss.

Basecoat-clearcoat paint systems use a colorcoat and a clearcoat over the primer. This is the most common paint system used today. The clear paint brings out the richness of the underlying color and also protects it.

PAINT TYPES

The general types of paint include:

1. Enamel/urethane
2. Waterbase/waterborne paint

As you will learn, there are variations within these categories. It is important that you know what type of finishes manufacturers use because there are slightly different methods required for refinishing them. Refer to **Figure 7–2.**

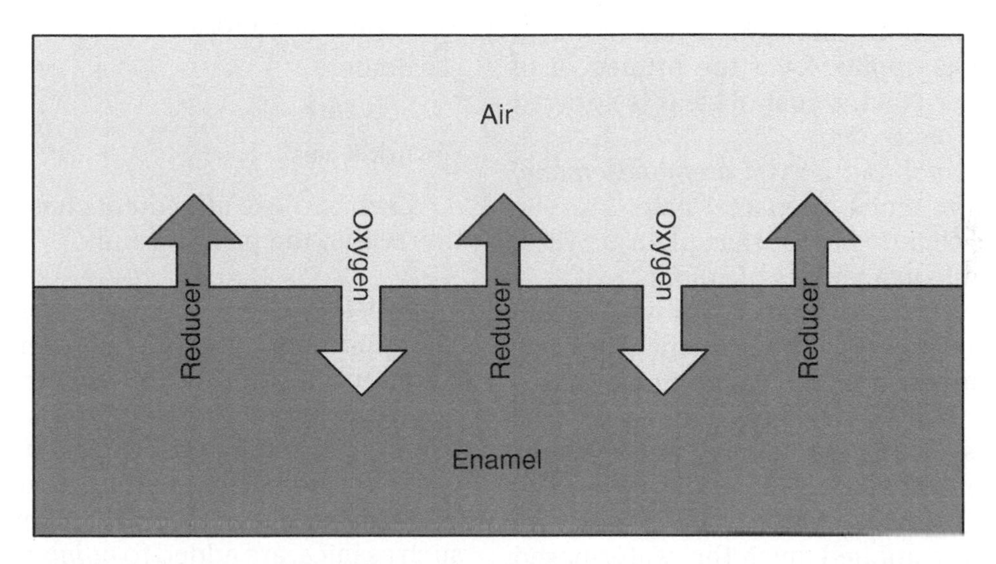

(A) Single-stage enamels dry by evaporation of the reducer (solvent) first then by oxidation (drying). Resin reacts with oxygen in the air to solidify the paint or primer. Heat speeds this action.

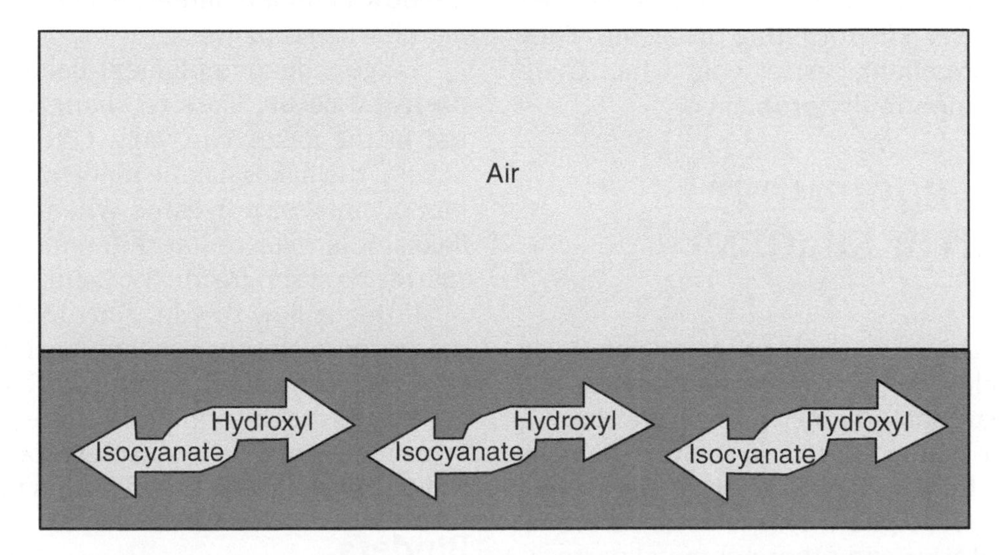

(B) Two-part urethane and polyurethane enamels cure by molecular cross-linking. The paint and a catalyst or hardener are mixed to cause this internal chemical reaction to make the paint or primer solidify. Heat also speeds this action.

Figure 7–2. Note how single-stage (one ingredient) and two-stage (two ingredient) paints, primers, and similar materials solidify and harden after being sprayed on as a liquid. (Courtesy of PPG Industries, Inc.)

Most **enamel** finishes used in collision repair are catalyzed (use a hardener) urethane enamels. Once applied, these materials, which can be color, clear, or primers, "dry" in a two-stage process.

First, some of the solvents used to thin or reduce the material must evaporate. Second, a chemical reaction occurs within the material and causes it to harden or "cure." This chemical change causes urethane enamel finishes to dry/cure with a gloss that does not require rubbing or polishing.

Two-stage paints consist of two distinct layers of paint: basecoat and clearcoat. *Basecoat-clearcoat enamel* is now the most common system used to repaint cars and trucks. First, a layer of color is applied over the primecoat of primer or sealer. Next, a coat of clear is sprayed over the color basecoat.

Acrylic enamel and *acrylic urethane enamel* are two specific types of enamel paint. Acrylic urethanes are slightly harder than plain acrylics. Each is available in a variety of colors.

Water-based/waterborne paints, as implied, use water to carry the pigment. They dry through evaporation of the water. Some manufacturers are using water-based paints on new vehicles. This is to help satisfy stricter emission regulations in some geographic areas. The basecoat of color is water-based. Then, an enamel paint is applied over the water-based paint to protect it from the elements.

Water-based/waterborne primers have been used for years as a fix for lifting problems. They serve as an excellent barrier coat when there are paint incompatibility problems.

ORIGINAL EQUIPMENT MANUFACTURER (OEM) FINISHES

The **OEM finishes** (factory paint jobs) on today's vehicles are "thermo-setting" high-solids basecoat-clearcoat enamels or water-based, low-emission paints. Common enamel finishes are baked in huge ovens to shorten the drying times and cure the paint. This is done before installing the interior and other nonmetal parts.

Vehicle manufacturers use several different types of finish materials, coating processes, and application processes. Each type of finish requires different planning and repair steps.

The most common types of OEM coating processes include:

1. Two-stage (basecoat/clearcoat)
2. Three-stage paint (tri-coat)
3. Multistage
4. Single-stage
5. Powder coat

These are explained fully in later chapters of this book.

CONTENTS OF PAINT

Paint's chemical content includes the following:

1. Pigments (colors)
2. Binders
3. Solvents
4. Additives

Each of these ingredients has a specific function within the paint formula.

Pigments

The **pigments** are fine powders that impart color, opacity, durability, and other characteristics to the primer or paint. They are a nonvolatile film-forming ingredient. The main purpose of the pigment is to hide everything under the paint.

Medium-size reflective pigment particles, such as mica, are added to *paints* to create a pearl effect. As you will learn later, *pearlescent colors* are now common and are sometimes difficult to match when repainting.

Large reflective pigment flakes are added to **metallic color.** The size, shape, color, and material in the flakes can vary. Often called "metal flakes," the flakes can be made of tiny but visible bits of metal or polyester. When light strikes the flakes, it is reflected at different angles like tiny "glittering stars" inside the paint.

If this is new to you, start looking at vehicle colors more closely. See if you can see the difference between a solid, a pearl, and a metallic color.

Solids are the nonliquid contents of the paint or primer. **High-solids materials** are needed to reduce air pollution or emissions when painting.

Binders

The **binder** is the ingredient in a color that holds the pigment particles together. It is the "backbone" or "film-former" of the paint. The binder helps the color stick to the surface. Various materials are used in the binder. The binder determines the type of paint—single-stage or base-clear.

Binder is usually modified with plasticizers and catalysts. They improve such properties as durability, adhesion, corrosion resistance, mar-resistance, and flexibility.

Solvents

The **solvent/reducer** is the liquid solution that carries the pigment and binder so it can be sprayed. *Reducers* are composed of one or several chemicals. They provide a transfer medium. Solvents are the volatile part of a paint. They are used to reduce (thin) a paint for spraying. Solvents give the paint its flow characteristics. They evaporate as the paint dries.

Remember! Thinning and reducing are needed to give the color the right "thickness" or **viscosity** to flow (spray) out smoothly onto the surface.

Some water-based paints come **premixed** (ready to spray) and they are NOT normally reduced. If required or directed, distilled water can be added to make a thinner, more liquid solution.

When using waterborne materials, the water used for equipment cleaning must be handled correctly.

1. It contains hazardous materials and should be disposed of as hazardous waste.
2. It must NOT be poured down the drain for disposal.
3. It must NOT be combined with other waste solvents such as reducers or thinners. Keep a separate container for storing hazardous water wastes.

Due to clean air regulations, some solvents are no longer being used. To meet clean air regulations, traditional solvents are being replaced by water or other solvents. Check all federal, state, and local ordinances.

Additives

Additives are ingredients added to modify the performance and characteristics of the paint (color). Additives are used to:

1. Speed up or slow down the drying process.
2. Lower the freezing point of a paint.
3. Prevent the paint from foaming when shaken.
4. Control settling of metallic and pigments.
5. Make the paint more flexible when dry.

DRYING AND CURING

Drying is the process of changing a coat of paint (color) or other material (clear) from a liquid to a solid state. Drying is due to evaporation of solvent, chemical reaction of the binding medium, or a combination of these causes.

The term *drying* is used with material that evaporates its solvent to harden. The term *curing* refers to a chemical action in the paint or other material itself that causes hardening.

Flash time is the first stage of drying when some of the solvents evaporate, which dulls the surface from a high gloss to a normal gloss.

A **retarder** is a slow-evaporating solvent or reducer used to retard, or slow, the drying process. A slow-drying solvent/reducer is often used in very warm weather. If a paint/clear dries too quickly, problems can result.

An **accelerator** is a fast-evaporating solvent or reducer for speeding the drying time. It is needed in very cold weather to make the paint or clear dry in a reasonable amount of time.

A general rule to follow in selecting the proper solvent or reducer is: the faster the shop drying conditions, the slower drying the solvent or reducer should be. In hot, dry weather, use a slow-drying solvent or reducer. In cold, wet weather, use a fast-drying solvent or reducer.

A "catalyst" is a substance that causes a chemical reaction. When mixed with another substance, it speeds the reaction but does not change itself. Catalysts are used with many types of materials—paints, clears, primers, putties, fillers, fiberglass, plastics. See **Figure 7–3.**

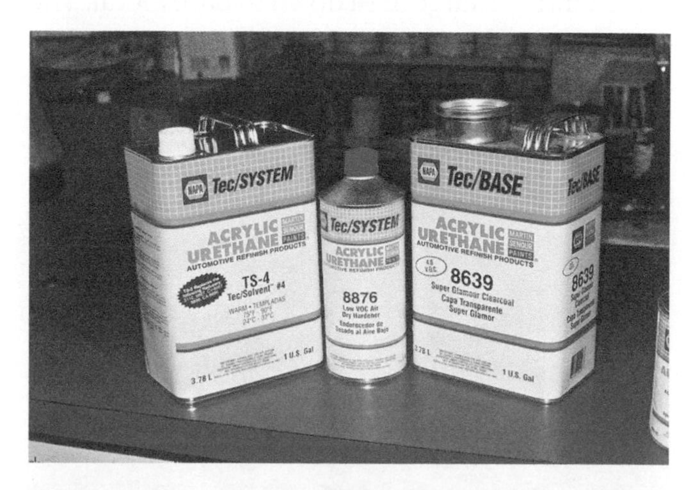

Figure 7–3. A catalyst, or hardener, is added to modern primers, colors, and clears to make them cure more quickly and efficiently. The solvent, the paint or primer, and the hardener must be mixed together in the correct amounts.

A **catalyst** or **hardener** is an additive used to make paint materials cure. The hardener speeds curing and makes the paint more durable.

The hardener is added to the paint right before it is sprayed. When an enamel catalyst is used, the paint can be wet sanded and compounded (polished) the next day. If you make a mistake (paint run, dirt in paint, etc.), you can fix the problem after the short curing time. The hardener will make the color or clear cure in just a few hours. Also, the vehicle can be released to the customer sooner with less chance of paint damage.

PRIMERS AND SEALERS

Primers come in many variations—primer, primer-sealer, primer-surfacer, primer-filler, etc. It is important to understand the functions of subcoating or primecoat materials. You must follow the manufacturer's instructions. Deviation from these directions will result in unsatisfactory work.

A plain primer is a thin undercoat designed to provide good adhesion for the paint. Primers can be used when the surface is very smooth and there is no potential problem with bleeding. If properly applied, some primers do not require sanding. See **Figure 7–4.**

Primers are usually two-component products because they provide better adhesion and corrosion resistance.

Self-Etching Primer

A **self-etching primer** has acid in it to prepare bare metal so that the primer will adhere properly. A self-etching primer is often used when you have sanded a large area down to bare metal. The self-etching primer will "bite" into the metal to bond securely. This will help prevent lifting and peeling. Some primer-sealers and primer-surfacers have etching materials in them.

Epoxy Primers

An **epoxy primer** is a two-part primer that cures fast and hard. Some material manufacturers recommend epoxy primer prior to the application of body fillers. Using an epoxy primer greatly increases body filler adhesion and corrosion resistance over bare metal. Epoxy primers most closely duplicate the OEM primers used for corrosion protection.

SEALERS

Bleeding or **bleedthrough** is a problem in which colors in the primecoat or old paint chemically seep into the new paint. This can discolor the new color.

A **sealer** is a midcoat between the paint (color) and the primer or old finish to prevent bleeding. Sealers differ from primer-sealers in that they cannot be used as a primer. Sealers are sprayed over a primer or primer-surfacer, or a sanded finish. Sealers do not normally need sanding, but some are sandable.

Sealers are sometimes used when a sharp color difference is visible after sanding. They are also used to prevent sand scratch swelling problems.

A **primer-sealer** is an undercoat that improves adhesion of the paint and also seals old painted surfaces that have been sanded. It will solve two potential problems (adhesion and bleed) with one application. See **Figure 7–5.**

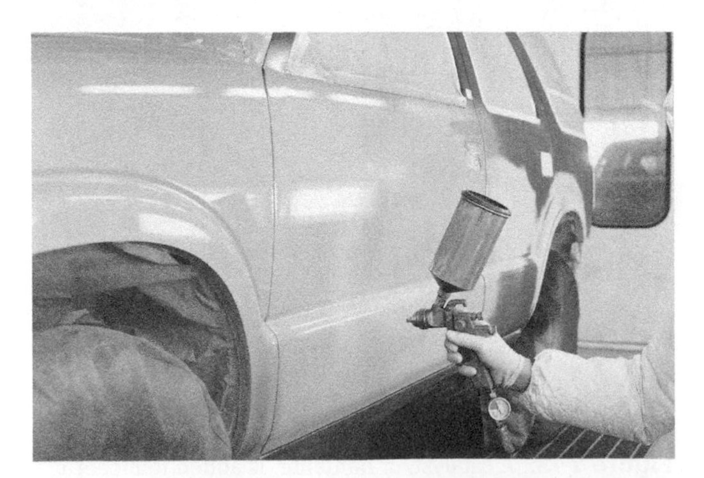

Figure 7–4. Primers are needed for the paint to bond to the substrate securely. There are many variations such as primer-sealer that increases adhesion and also blocks out any color or chemical differences of the old paint.

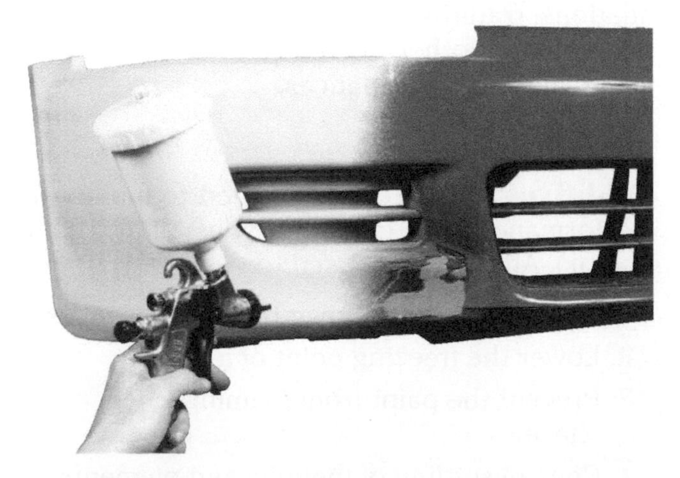

Figure 7–5. This primer-sealer is formulated for plastic parts. Plastic parts require different repair materials than metal body parts. (Courtesy of Urethane Supply Co.)

Primer-sealers provide the same protection as primers—adhesion and corrosion resistance. But they also have the ability to seal over a sanded old finish to provide uniform color holdout.

PRIMER-SURFACERS

A **primer-surfacer** is a high-solids primer that fills small imperfections and usually must be sanded. It is often used after a filler to help smooth the surface. Primer-surfacers are used to build up and level featheredged areas or rough surfaces and to provide a smooth base for paint. See **Figure 7–6.**

Strong adhesion is the first prerequisite of a primer. All automotive paint colors require the use of a primer or primer-surfacer as the first coat over bare substrate. A good primer-surfacer should be ready to sand in as short a period as 30 minutes.

A **primer-filler** is a very thick form of primer-surfacer. It is sometimes used when a very pitted or rough surface must be filled and smoothed quickly. It might be used on a solid, but pitted, body panel, for example.

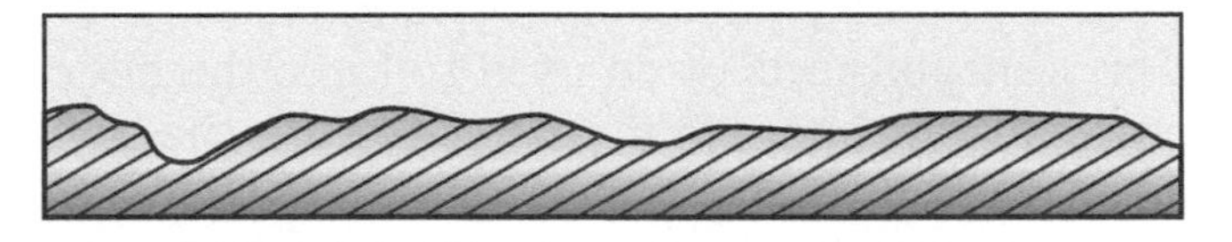

(A) This magnified cross-section shows that the surface is slightly rough from sanding. Some surface roughness or sand scratches are needed to make the spray coating adhere or stick to the car body.

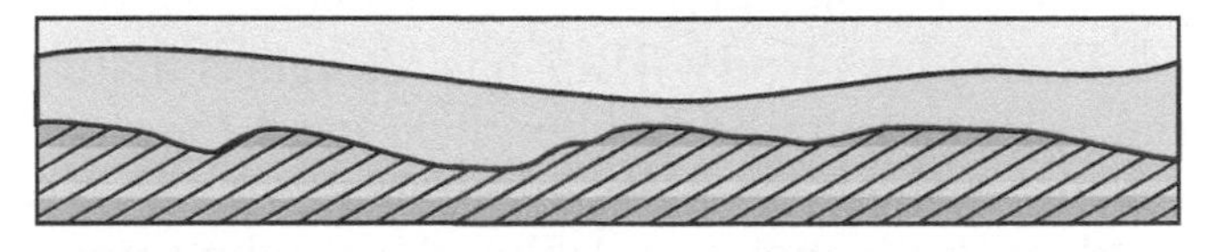

(B) A thick liquid primer-surfacer has been sprayed over the sanded surface. It has a high-solids content that flows and fills tiny scratches, sand marks, or imperfections in the vehicle body or body filler.

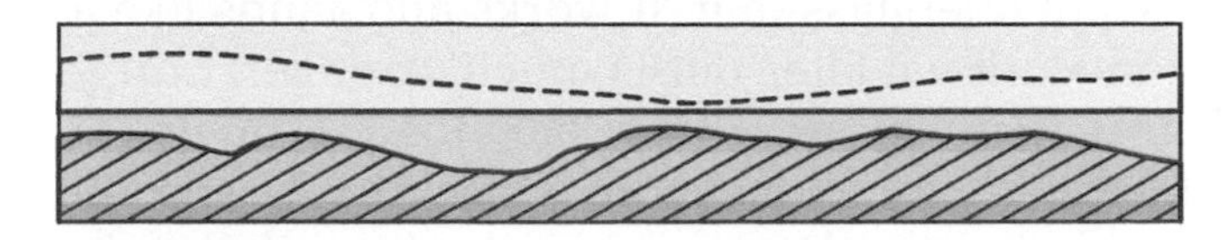

(C) Sanding the primer-surfacer will quickly level and smooth the surface. This readies the surface for a final coat of primer or primer-sealer and then for paintcoats (colorcoats and clearcoats).

Figure 7–6. The primer-surfacer is now the "workhorse" of the collision repair industry. (Courtesy of PPG Industries, Inc.)

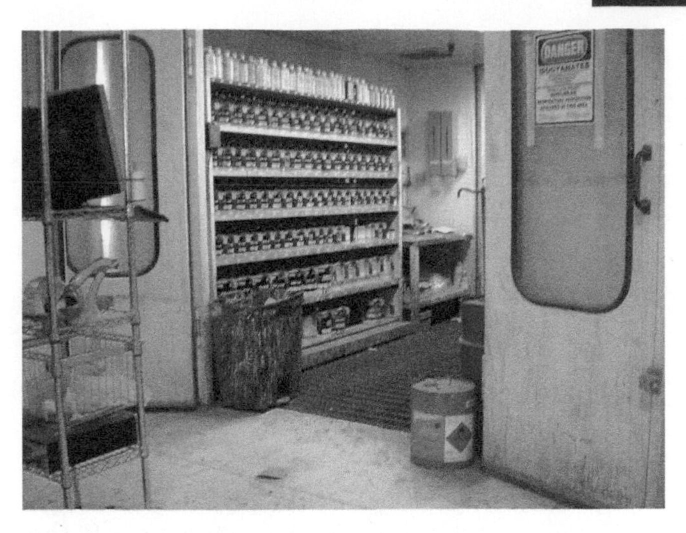

Figure 7–7. The mixing room contains all of the ingredients used by the shop's painter or refinish technician. The small room has extra ventilation to remove paint fumes while mixing paint or primer ingredients. Only mix and use paint materials from the same manufacturer or paint system.

USE A COMPLETE SYSTEM!

Remember! Always use a complete refinishing system. A **refinishing system** means all materials (primers, catalysts, reducers, colors, and clears) are compatible and manufactured by the same company. They are designed to work properly with each other. If you mix materials from different manufacturers, you can run into problems. The chemical contents of the different systems may not work well together. See **Figure 7–7.**

OTHER PAINT MATERIALS

A wax and grease remover is a fast-drying solvent often used to clean a vehicle. It will remove wax, oil, grease, and other debris that could contaminate and ruin the paint job.

A **flattener** is an agent added to paint to lower gloss or shine. It can be added to any color gloss paint to make it a semigloss or flat (dull) color. For example, some factory trim is painted semigloss or flat black. A flattening agent would be used in this instance. Flatteners can also be used where reflection off a high-gloss paint could affect driver visibility.

A **flex agent** is an additive that allows primers and colors to flex or bend without cracking. It is commonly added to materials being applied to plastic bumper covers, for example. Also called an **elastomer,** it is a manufactured compound with flexible and elastic properties that can be added to primers and paints.

Antichip coating, also called *gravel guard, Chip Guard,* or *vinyl coating,* is a rubberized material used along a vehicle's lower panels. It is designed to be flexible or rubbery to resist chips from rocks and other debris flying up off the tires. Antichip coatings are usually applied with a special spray gun.

Rubberized undercoat is a synthetic-based rubber material applied as a rust-preventive layer. It can be applied using a production gun or a spray can.

A **metal conditioner** is an acid used to etch bare sheet metal before priming. It is a chemical cleaner that removes rust from bare metal and helps prevent further rust.

A **conversion coating** is a special metal conditioner or primer used on galvanized steel, uncoated steel, and aluminum to prevent corrosion and aid adhesion. It is applied after acid etching or metal conditioning.

Corrosion is a chemical reaction of air, moisture, or corrosive materials on a metal surface. Corrosion of steel is usually referred to as *rust* or oxidation.

Paint stripper is a powerful chemical that dissolves paint for fast removal. If the paint has failed, you may have to use a chemical stripper. It is applied over the paint. After it soaks into and lifts the paint, a plastic scraper is used to remove the softened paint.

A **tack cloth** is used to remove dust and lint from the surface right before painting. It is a cheesecloth treated with nondrying varnish to make it tacky. A tack cloth must be wiped gently over the surface to keep the varnish from contaminating the paint.

BODY FILLERS

A **filler** is any material used to fill (level) a damaged area. There are several types of filler. You should understand their differences.

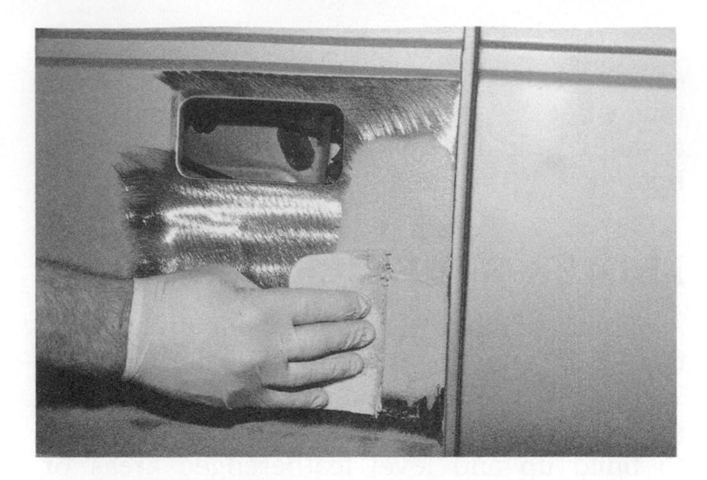

Figure 7–8. A body filler is a two-part material that is mixed together and then applied over small dents in metal body parts. The body filler will heat up and cure in a few minutes so it can be sanded.

Body filler is a heavy-bodied plastic material that cures very hard for filling small dents in metal. It is a compound of resin and plastic used to fill dents on vehicle bodies. This is shown in **Figure 7–8.**

Body fillers come canned and in plastic bottles. A dispenser is often used to force the filler onto a mixing board. A **mixing board** is the surface (metal or plastic) used for mixing the filler and its hardener.

Light body filler is formulated for easy sanding and fast repairs. It is used as a very thin top coat of filler for final leveling. It can be spread thinly over large surfaces for block or air-tool sanding the panel level.

Fiberglass body filler has fiberglass material added to the body filler. It is used for rust repair or where strength is important. It can be used on both metal and fiberglass substrates. Because fiberglass-reinforced filler is very difficult to sand, it is usually used under a conventional, lightweight plastic filler.

Short-hair fiberglass filler has tiny particles of fiberglass in it. It works and sands like a conventional filler but is much stronger. **Long-hair fiberglass filler** has long strands of fiberglass for even more strength. It is commonly used when you must repair holes in metal or fiberglass bodies.

Cream hardeners are used to cure body fillers. They usually come in a tube. Once the hardening cream is mixed in, the body filler will heat up and harden.

NOTE

The most common mistake is to use too *much hardener!* The body filler will set up or harden in a couple of minutes, before you have time to spread it on the body. Literally "tons" of body filler have been wasted because of hardener overuse. Using too much hardener can also cause problems with adhesion and pinholing.

GLAZING PUTTY/FINISHING FILLERS

Glazing putty is a material made for filling small holes or sand scratches. It is similar to body filler but it has more solid content. Putty is applied over the primecoat of primer-sealer or primer-surfacer to correct small surface imperfections. The purpose of glazing putties is to fill excessively rough surfaces or imperfections that cannot be filled with a primer-surfacer.

Spot putty is the same as glazing putty except it has even more solids. Spot putty is recommended for scratches or nicks up to 1/16 inch (1.5 mm) deep. It should NOT be used to fill large surface depressions. For larger depressions, use body filler or catalyzed putty.

Two-part putty comes with its own hardener for rapid curing. This is the main advantage of two-part putty. It dries much more quickly. Some two-part putties can be applied over paint to reduce sanding time.

To use two-part putty, follow label directions to mix the right amount of putty and hardener. Use a rubber or small plastic spreader to work the putty into any surface imperfections. Provide for a slight buildup of material over the imperfection. After adequate curing time, sand the putty down flush with the surrounding surface.

MASKING MATERIALS

Masking materials are used to cover and protect body parts from paint overspray. **Overspray** is unwanted paint spray mist floating around the spray gun. It can stick to glass and body parts, and takes considerable time to clean off.

Masking paper is special paper designed to cover body parts not to be painted. It comes in a roll. When mounted on a masking machine, masking tape is automatically applied to one edge of the paper, speeding your work. See **Figure 7–9.**

Masking plastic is used just like paper to cover and protect parts from overspray. It also comes in rolls and can cover large body areas more easily than paper. Masking plastic is used to cover areas of the vehicle away from the area being painted. Plastic should not be used right next to the area being sprayed. The plastic will not absorb the paint and can cause paint to drip down onto the body surface. See **Figure 7–10.**

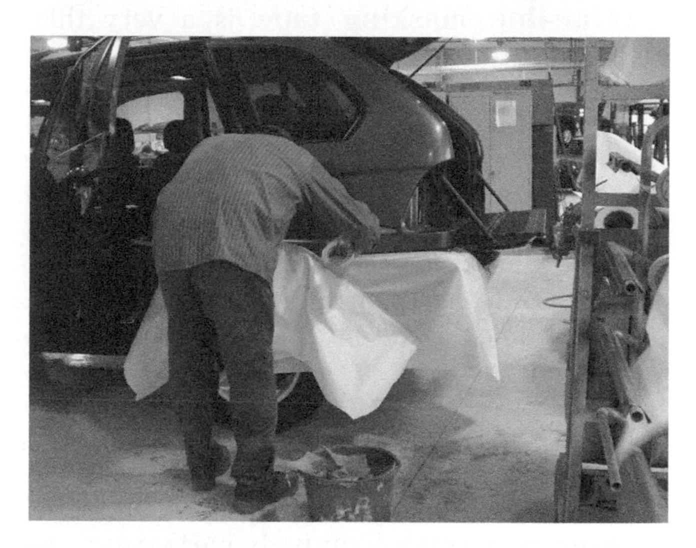

Figure 7–9. Masking materials protect undamaged surfaces on the vehicle from sanding, primer, and paint overspray. Masking paper is being placed around the lower area of the minivan. This will keep unwanted overspray off parts that are not to be painted.

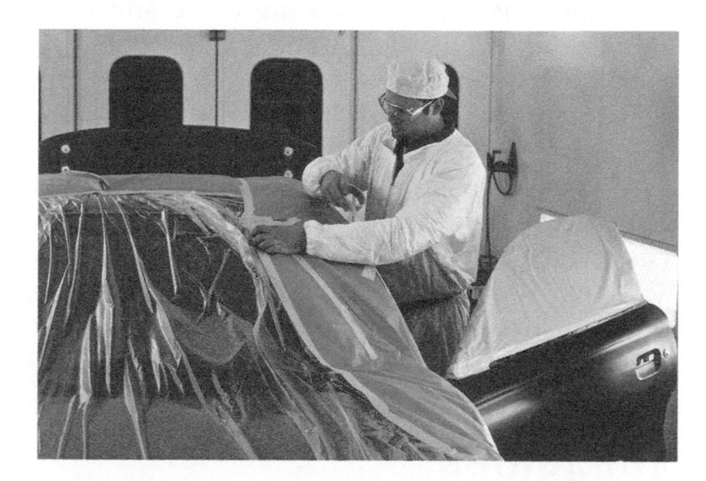

Figure 7–10. Large plastic sheets are sometimes used to mask large sections of a vehicle away from the area to be painted. Plastic can be draped over the body and held in place by a few pieces of tape. Plastic should not be used right next to a panel being painted, however. It will not absorb paint and may allow drips to fall onto the surface. Masking paper must be used right next to the area to be painted so it can absorb and hold overspray.

Wheel masks are preshaped plastic or cloth covers that fit over the vehicle's wheels and tires. Plastic wheel covers are disposable and should be used only once. Cloth covers are reused but should be cleaned off periodically. Preshaped plastic antenna, headlamp, and mirror covers are also available.

Masking tape is used to hold masking paper or plastic into position. It is a high-tack, easy-to-tear tape. It comes in rolls of varying widths, ½-inch (19 mm) being the most common. See Figure 7–10.

Fine-line masking tape is a very thin, smooth surface plastic masking tape. Also termed *flush masking tape,* it can be used to produce a better **paint part edge** (edge where old paint and new paint meet). When the fine-line tape is removed, the edge of the new paint will be straighter and smoother than if conventional masking tape were used.

Duct tape is a thick tape with a plastic body. It is sometimes used to protect parts from damage when grinding or sanding. Duct tape is thicker than masking tape and provides more protection for the surface under the tape.

Masking liquid, also called **masking coating,** is usually a water-based sprayable material for keeping overspray off body parts. Some are solvent-based. Masking liquid comes in a large, ready-to-spray container or drum. These materials are sprayed on and form a paint-proof coating over the vehicle.

Some masking coatings are tacky and used only during priming, and some when painting. They form a film that can be applied when the vehicle enters the shop. Others dry to a hard, dull finish.

These masking coatings can be removed when the vehicle is ready to return to the owner. They wash off with soap and water. Local regulations may require that liquid masking residue be captured in a floor drain trap, and not put into the sewer or storm drain system.

ABRASIVES

An **abrasive** is any material, such as sand, crushed steel grit, aluminum oxide, silicon carbide, or crushed slag, used for cleaning, sanding, smoothing, or material removal. Many types of abrasives are used by the collision repair and refinishing technician.

Grit refers to a measure of the size of particles on sandpaper or discs. A *coarse* sandpaper would have large grit. A *fine* sandpaper would have smaller grit.

Grit Ratings

A **grit numbering system** denotes how coarse or fine the abrasive is. For example, 16 grit would be one of the coarsest and 1500 grit would be one of the finest. The grit number is printed on the back of the paper or disc.

Very coarse grit of 16 to 60 is generally used for fast material removal. It will quickly remove paint and take it down to bare metal. This grit is commonly used on grinding discs and air files paper for rapid cutting of body fillers.

A **coarse grit** of 36 to 60 is basically used for rough sanding and smoothing operations. This coarseness might be used to get the general shape of a large body filler area.

Medium grit of 80 to 120 is often used for sanding body filler high spots and for sanding paint.

Fine grit of 150 to 180 is normally used to sand bare metal and for smoothing existing paint.

Very fine grit ranges from 220 to about 2000 and is used for numerous final smoothing operations. Larger grits of 220 to 320 are for sanding primer-surfacers and paint. Finer grits of 400 to 2000 are for colorcoat sanding and sanding before polishing or buffing. Very fine grits are usually wet sandpapers to keep the paper from becoming clogged or filled with paint.

Generally, start with the finest grit that is *practical.* A coarser grit will cut straighter but will create coarser scratches to fill.

GRINDING DISCS

Grinding discs are round, very coarse abrasives used for initial removal of paint, plastic, and metal (weld joints). Some are very thick and do not require a backing plate. Others are thinner and require a **disc backing plate** mounted on the grinder spindle. They are used for material removal operations. See **Figure 7–11.**

Grinding disc size is measured across the outside diameter. The most common grinding disc sizes are 7 and 9 inches (175 and 225 mm). The hole in the center of the disc must also match the shaft on the grinder or sander.

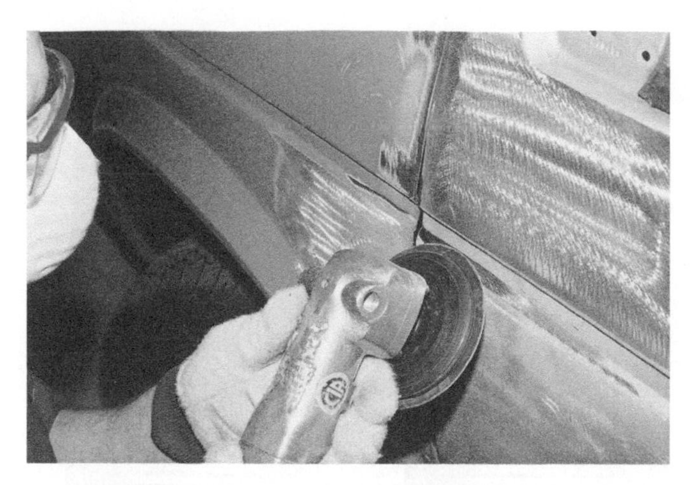

Figure 7–11. Various abrasives or grinding-sanding materials are used to remove the old paint and to sand the body filler and paint before refinishing. Here the body technician is using a very coarse grinding wheel to remove paint before application of the body filler.

SANDPAPERS

Sandpaper is a heavy paper coated with an abrasive grit. It is the most commonly used abrasive in collision repair. Sandpaper is used to remove paints and to smooth primers and fillers. There are many kinds, shapes, and grits of sandpaper. Each has its own advantage.

Sanding discs are round and are normally used on an air-powered orbital sander. They may use Velcro (hook and loop fibers) or a self-stick coating to hold the sandpaper onto the tool sanding pad.

Sanding sheets are square and can be cut to fit sanding blocks. Long sheets are also available for use on air files. See **Figure 7–12.**

Dry sandpaper is designed to be used without water. Its resin is usually an animal glue. This glue is not water resistant and will dissolve when wet, ruining the sandpaper.

Dry sandpaper is often used for coarse-to-medium-grit sanding tasks, like shaping and smoothing plastic filler. One example, 80-grit dry sandpaper is often used on plastic filler. It will quickly cut the filler down.

Wet sandpaper, as implied, can be used with water for flushing away sanding debris that would otherwise clog fine grits. Wet sandpaper comes in finer grits for final smoothing operations before and after painting. Wet sandpaper is available in grits from about 220 to 2000. See **Figure 7–13.**

Wet sandpaper is commonly used to block sand paint before compounding or buffing. Wet sanding will knock down any imperfections in the paint film. Buffing or compounding is then needed to make the paint shiny again.

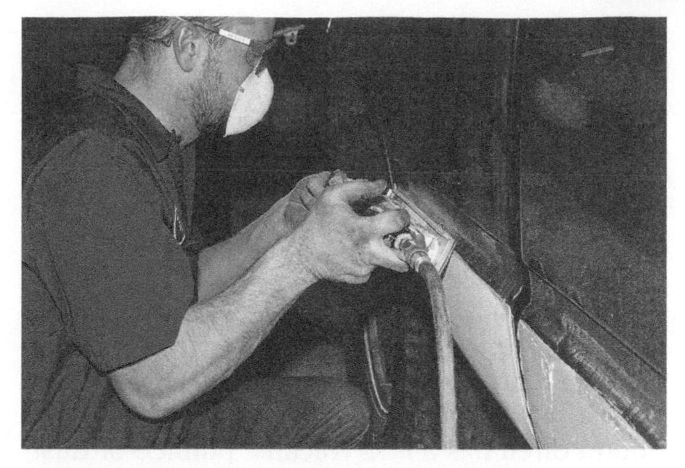

Figure 7-12. After application of the body filler, a medium-grit sandpaper is used to level, smooth, and shape the body filler to match the shape of the car's body panel.

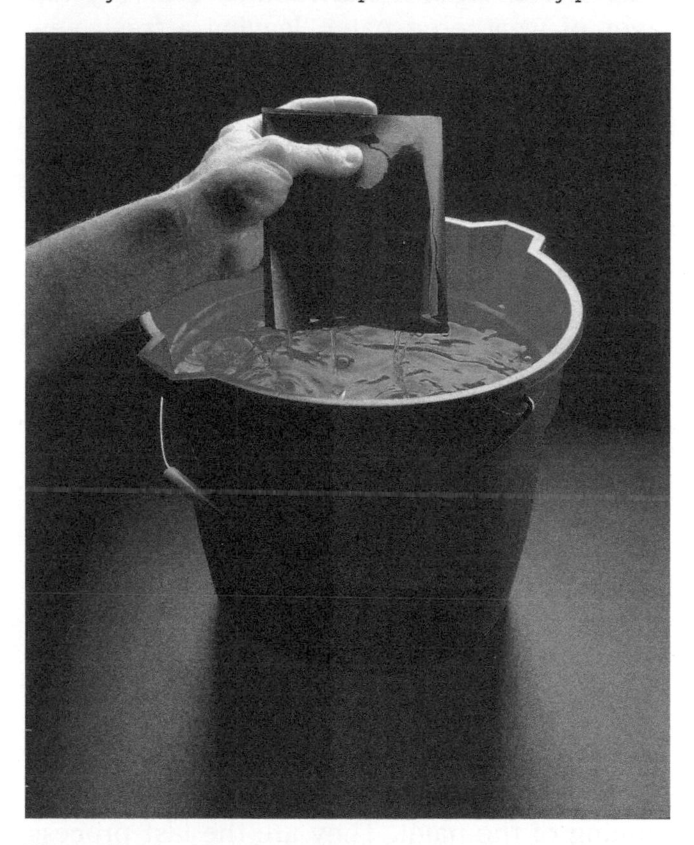

Figure 7-13. Very fine sandpaper and wet sandpaper are often used on a new paint surface to remove any imperfections. After the new paint has cured, it can be ultrafine wet or dry sanded and compounded or buffed to make the paint surface perfectly smooth and shiny. (Courtesy of Norton)

SCUFF PADS

Scuff pads are tough synthetic pads used to clean and lightly scratch the surface of paints and parts. Being like a sponge, they are handy for scuffing irregular surfaces, like on door jambs, around the inside of the hood and deck lids, and other obstructed areas. This will clean and lightly scuff these areas so the paint, primer, or sealer will stick.

COMPOUNDS

Compounding involves using an abrasive paste material to smooth and bring out the gloss of the applied paint. It can be applied by hand or with a polishing wheel on an air tool. A compound often has a fine volcanic pumice or dust-like grit in a water-soluble paste. When rubbed on a painted surface, a thin layer of paint or clear is removed. It will remove the very top layer of weathered paint, leaving a fresh new surface of paint.

A **hand compound** is designed to be applied by hand on a rag or cloth. **Machine compound** is formulated to be applied with an electric or air polisher. It will not cut as fast and will not break down with the extra friction and heat of machine application.

Rubbing compound is the coarsest type of hand compound. It will rapidly remove paint or clear but will leave visible scratch marks. Rubbing compound is designed for hand application, not machine application. It is often used on small areas to treat imperfections in the paint surface.

Polishing compound or *machine glaze* is a fine-grit compound designed for machine application. A polisher is used to carefully run the compound over the cured or dried paint or clear. Polishing compound is often used after a rubbing compound or after wet sanding. It will make the paint shiny and smooth. See **Figure 7–14.**

Hand glazes are for final smoothing and shining of the paint. They are the last process used to produce a professional finish. They are applied by hand using a circular motion, like a wax.

Buffing compounds come in other formulations as well. Read the label on the compound to learn about its use. See **Figure 7–15.**

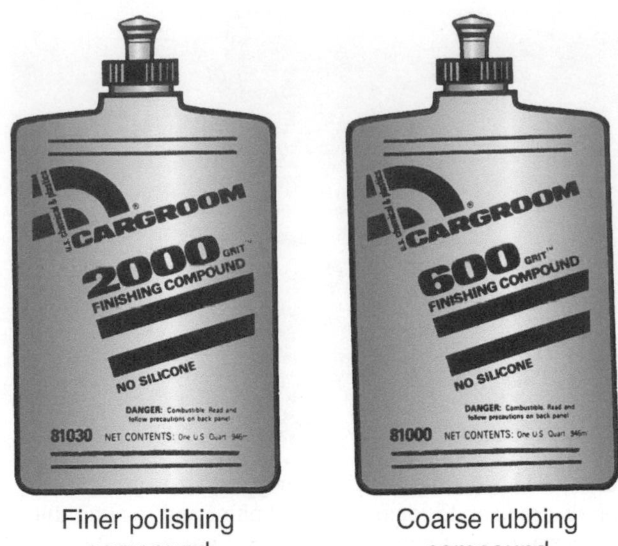

Figure 7-14. Compounds are used for final smoothing of painted surfaces. Some are coarser than others. Some are designed for hand application and others for machine use. Always read the label directions. (Courtesy of U.S. Chemicals and Plastics, Inc., Canton, Ohio)

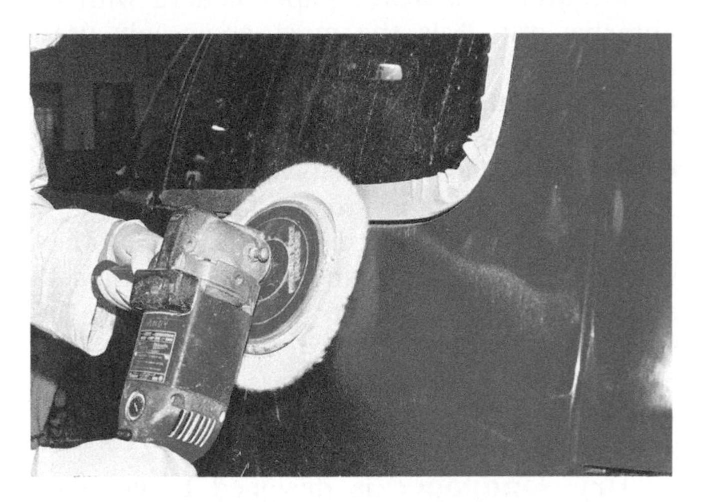

Figure 7-15. Here the detail technician is using a high-speed buffer to polish the paint surface. On new paint, it will increase smoothness and gloss. On old paint, it will remove the oxidized or dulled paint surface and uncover the bright, original color again.

ADHESIVES

Adhesives are special glues designed to bond parts to one another. Various types are available.

Weatherstrip adhesive is designed to hold rubber seals and similar parts in place. Weatherstrip adhesive dries to a hard rubber-type consistency. This makes it ideal for holding door seals, trunk seals, and other seals onto the body.

Plastic adhesive or **emblem adhesive** is designed to hold hard plastic and metal parts. It is used to install various types of emblems and trim pieces onto painted surfaces.

An **adhesive release agent** is a chemical that dissolves most types of adhesives. It is used when you want to remove a glued part without damaging it. The agent is sprayed onto the

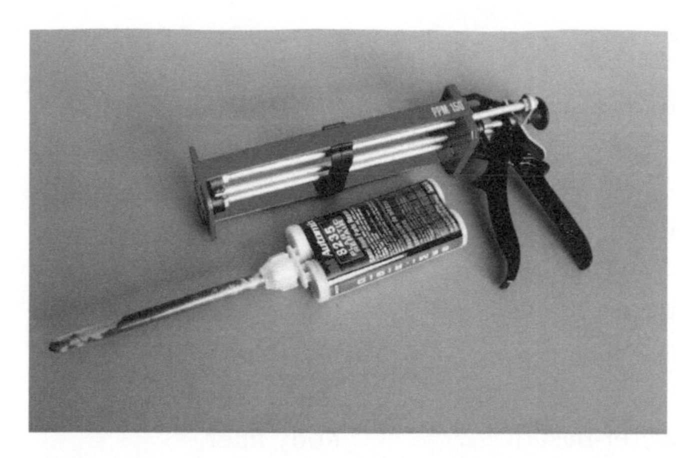

Figure 7-16. Numerous types of two-part epoxies are used to bond parts together during repairs. Make sure you use the type recommended by the vehicle manufacturer for the specific part being repaired. (Courtesy of Urethane Supply Co.)

adhesive. This softens the adhesive so the part can be lifted off easily.

EPOXIES

An *epoxy* is a two-part glue used to hold various parts together. The two ingredients are mixed together in equal parts. This makes the mixture cure through a chemical reaction. Always use the type of epoxy suggested by the vehicle manufacturer. See **Figure 7–16.**

SEALERS

Sealers are used to prevent water and air leaks between parts. They are flexible, which prevents cracking. Sealers come in several variations.

Seam sealers are designed to make a leakproof joint between body panels. They are often needed where two panels butt or overlap each other. Seam sealers come in different forms and each is applied differently. Read the directions.

Tube sealers are applied directly from the tube or by using a caulking gun. They squirt out like toothpaste and cure in a few hours.

Apply primer before applying seam sealer. Seam sealers are paintable but may need to be reprimed if product directions specify. Silicone sealers are NOT paintable and should NOT be used in auto body repair. Follow instructions on the product for finishing sealers.

Ribbon sealers come in strip form and are applied by hand. They are a thick sealer that must be worked onto the parts with your fingers.

HAZARDOUS MATERIALS

A **hazardous material** is any substance that can harm people or the environment. Product labels give important procedures for safe use of products to protect you and the environment. Follow all warnings given by product manufacturers. Most of the products used in a collision repair facility carry warnings and caution information that must be read and understood by all users.

Material safety data sheets (MSDS), available from all product manufacturers, detail chemical composition and precautionary information for all products that can present a health or safety hazard. Employers must know the general uses, protective equipment, accident or spill procedures, and other information for safe handling of hazardous materials. Training about hazardous materials must be given to employees as part of their job orientation. The best way to protect yourself when using paint and body materials is to be familiar with the correct application procedures. Follow all safety and health precautions found on MSDS and on product labels.

Right-to-know laws give essential information and stipulations for safely working with hazardous materials. The federal courts have decided that these regulations should apply to all companies, including the collision repair and refinishing professions. The general intent of the law is for employers to provide their employees with a safe working place as it relates to hazardous materials.

Types of Material Hazards

Irritants are materials that can affect your lungs, skin, and eyes. They can be found in solvents, reducers, polishes, body fillers, adhesives, and other materials. They could affect your health if they enter your lower respiratory system and if you have prolonged exposure to them.

Toxins are poisonous substances that can be divided into several categories. *Neurotoxins* affect your nervous system; they can be found in adhesives and thinners. *Liver toxins* damage your liver; they can be found in reducers and paints. *Reproductive toxins* can cause birth defects; they are found in gasoline and urethanes. *Blood toxins* can damage your red blood cells; they can be found in enamel clearcoats.

Corrosives can burn your skin and eyes. They are alkalines or acids. Examples are paint strippers, battery electrolyte, and some degreasers.

Carcinogens are substances that can cause cancer. They can be in some air-conditioning refrigerants, older brake and clutch dust, and in some body fillers.

Allergens can cause allergic reactions. They can be found in adhesives, hardeners, and other substances.

WASTE DISPOSAL AND RECYCLING

Many shops use "full-service" haulers to test and remove hazardous waste from the property. Besides hauling the hazardous waste away, the hauler will also take care of all the paperwork, deal with the various government agencies, and even advise the shop on how to recover disposal costs.

Some shops are now **recycling** materials (like paint solvent) so that it can be reused to clean spraying equipment. A solvent recycling machine is used to remove impurities from the solvent. These impurities are filtered out and stored in a plastic bag for proper disposal.

SUMMARY

- Collision repair materials include the various fillers, primers, sealers, adhesives, sandpapers, and other compounds common to collision repair facilities.
- The substrate is the metal, aluminum, plastic, or composite material used in the vehicle's construction. It will affect the selection of refinishing materials.
- There are two general types of paint: enamel and water-base (waterborne).
- A filler is any material used to fill (level) a damaged area.
- Masking materials, such as masking plastic, masking paper, masking tape, and duct tape are used to cover and protect body parts from paint overspray.
- Sealers are used to prevent water and air leaks between parts. They are applied in the form of seam sealers, tube sealers, and ribbon sealers.

TECHNICAL TERMS

refinishing materials
substrate
paint
colorcoat
basecoat-clearcoat
enamel
two-stage paints
water-based/waterborne paints
OEM finishes
pigments
metallic color
solids
high-solids materials
binder
solvent/reducer
viscosity
premixed
additives
flash time
retarder
accelerator
catalyst
hardener
self-etching primer
epoxy primer
bleeding
bleedthrough
sealer
primer-sealer
primer-surfacer
primer-filler
refinishing system
flattener
flex agent
elastomer
antichip coating
rubberized undercoat
metal conditioner
conversion coating
corrosion
rust
paint stripper
tack cloth
filler
body filler
mixing board
light body filler
fiberglass body filler
short-hair fiberglass filler
long-hair fiberglass filler
cream hardeners
glazing putty
spot putty
two-part putty
overspray
masking paper
masking plastic
wheel masks
masking tape
fine-line masking tape
paint part edge
duct tape
masking coating
abrasive
grit
grit numbering system
very coarse grit
coarse grit
medium grit
fine grit
very fine grit
grinding discs
disc backing plate

sandpaper
sanding discs
sanding sheets
dry sandpaper
wet sandpaper
scuff pads
hand compound
machine compound
rubbing compound
polishing compound
hand glazes
weatherstrip adhesive
emblem adhesive
adhesive release agent
epoxy
sealers
seam sealers
tube sealers
ribbon sealers
hazardous material
irritants
toxins
corrosives
carcinogens
allergens
recycling

REVIEW QUESTIONS

1. A _____________ is the steel, aluminum, composite, or plastic material used in the vehicle's construction.
2. What are two functions of a vehicle's paint or finish?
3. This refers to a factory paint job.
   a. Lacquer
   b. Enamel
   c. OEM paint
   d. ASE paint
4. Name the four ingredients in a color.
5. The term _____________ refers to a paint material that evaporates its solvent to harden. The term _____________ refers to a chemical action in the paint or other material itself that causes hardening.
6. What is a catalyst?
7. This is an undercoat that improves adhesion of the paint and seals painted surfaces that have been sanded.
   a. Primer
   b. Primer-sealer
   c. Primer-filler
   d. Primer-surfacer
8. A _____________ is a high-solids primer that fills small imperfections and usually must be sanded. It is often used after a filler to help smooth the surface.
9. What is corrosion?
10. What is masking liquid or masking coating?
11. In detail, explain the sandpaper grit numbering system and how it is used.

ASE-STYLE REVIEW QUESTIONS

1. *Technician A* says that an undercoat is another name for primer. *Technician B* says that an undercoat is "sandwiched" between the substrate and the paint. Who is correct?
   a. Technician A
   b. Technician B
   c. Both Technicians A and B
   d. Neither Technician
2. Which of the following is NOT a paint type?
   a. Enamel
   b. Urethane
   c. Water-base
   d. Bauxite
3. *Technician A* says that OEM stands for original equipment manufacturer. *Technician B* says that manufacturers use several different types of finish materials, coating processes, and application processes. Who is correct?
   a. Technician A
   b. Technician B
   c. Both Technicians A and B
   d. Neither Technician
4. Which of the following is NOT contained in paint?
   a. Solvents
   b. Binders
   c. Graphite
   d. Pigment
5. *Technician A* says that a primer-sealer is designed to fill small imperfections.

Technician B says that a primer-filler will fill small imperfections. Who is correct?

a. Technician A

b. Technician B

c. Both Technicians A and B

d. Neither Technician

6. *Technician A* says that it does not matter if you use different manufacturers' products when painting a vehicle. *Technician B* says that the same manufacturer's products should be used through the complete refinish process. Who is correct?

a. Technician A

b. Technician B

c. Both Technicians A and B

d. Neither Technician

7. Which of the following is the finest grit sandpaper?

a. 230

b. 24

c. 500

d. 1500

8. *Technician A* says that rubbing compound is coarser than polishing compound. *Technician B* says that following the use of polishing compound, a hand glaze is the last process used to produce a professional finish. Who is correct?

a. Technician A

b. Technician B

c. Both Technicians A and B

d. Neither Technician

9. *Technician A* says that epoxies are two-part glues used to hold various parts together. *Technician B* says that seam sealers are designed to make a leakproof joint between body panels. Who is correct?

a. Technician A

b. Technician B

c. Both Technicians A and B

d. Neither Technician

ACTIVITIES

1. Visit a "paint supply" house. Read the labels on several different kinds of products. Write a report on the hazards of using different body shop materials.

2. Check out different types of sandpaper. Inspect their grits and compare conventional and metric grit ratings. Mount different sandpapers on a piece of cardboard and explain each.

3. Apply different types of adhesive and epoxy to a piece of cardboard. Study how long it takes each to dry or cure. Write a report on your findings.

CHAPTER 8 Welding, Heating, and Cutting

OBJECTIVES

After studying this chapter, you should be able to:

- Describe when to use and when NOT to use certain welding processes for collision repair.
- Name the parts of a MIG welder.
- Summarize how to set up a MIG welder.
- Describe differences between MIG electrode wires.
- Explain the variables for making a quality MIG weld.
- Describe the various types of MIG welds and joints.
- Explain the resistance spot welding process.
- Explain the differences in welding aluminum compared to steel.
- Describe plasma arc cutting.

INTRODUCTION

This chapter introduces welding methods common to the collision repair industry. It defines technical terms and compares different types of welding found in a collision repair shop.

With major collision repair work, many of the panels on a vehicle must be replaced and welded into place. As you will learn, this requires considerable skill and care. The structural integrity of the vehicle is dependent upon how well you weld and install panels.

WHAT IS WELDING?

A **weld** is formed when separate pieces of material are fused together using heat. The heat must be high enough to cause melting. Pressure may be used to force the points together. See **Figure 8–1.**

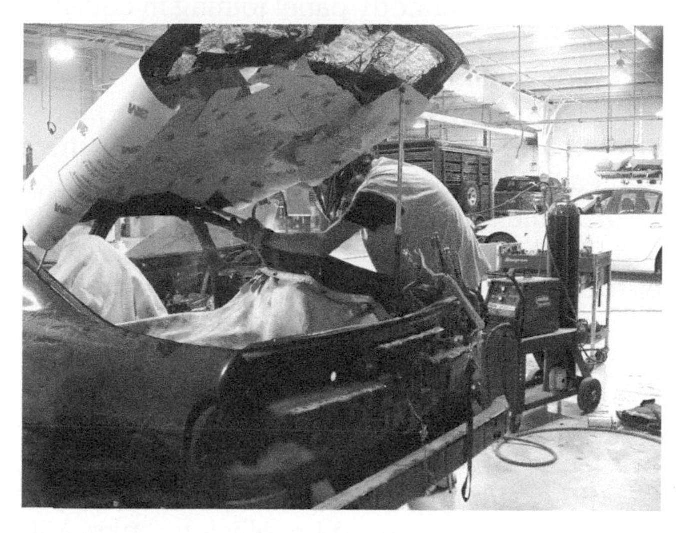

Figure 8–1. Welding is a vital aspect of fixing a badly damaged vehicle. Proper training and experience is needed to make quality welds safely.

The **base material** is the material to be welded, usually metal or plastic. Both can be welded in the collision repair industry.

Filler material from a wire or rod is added to the weld joint. The filler material makes the weld joint thicker and stronger.

WELD TERMINOLOGY

The **weld root** is the part of the joint where the wire electrode is directed. The **weld face** is the exposed surface of the weld on the side where you welded.

Visible **weld penetration** is indicated by the height of the exposed surface of the weld on the back side. Full weld penetration is needed to ensure maximum weld strength.

A **burn mark** on the back of a weld is an indication of good weld penetration. **Burn-through** results from penetrating too much into the lower base metal, which burns a hole through the back side of the metal.

Fillet weld parts include the following. The **weld legs** are the width and height of the weld bead. The **weld throat** refers to the depth of the triangular cross section of the weld.

Joint fit-up refers to holding workpieces tightly together, in alignment, to prepare for welding. It is critical to the replacement of body parts!

WELDING CATEGORIES

The four types of body panel joining in collision repair are fusion welding, pressure welding, adhesion bonding, and hybrid bonding.

Fusion welding is joining different pieces of metal together by melting and fusing them into each other. The pieces of metal are heated to their melting point, joined together (usually with a filler rod), and allowed to cool. Molecules of the metals combine. MIG, TIG, stick arc, and oxyacetylene welding are all fusion processes. Refer to **Figure 8–2.**

There are two general types of gas metal arc welding methods: **metal inert gas (MIG)** and **tungsten inert gas (TIG).**

MIG welding is a wire-feed fusion welding process commonly used in collision repair. MIG stands for "metal inert gas," even though some shielding gases used may be active. It is the accepted industry name for **gas metal arc welding (GMAW).**

MIG is sometimes called "wire-feed" because wire is automatically fed into the weld. MIG welding is the best method of structural welding on unibody vehicles.

Today's steels demand a technique that leaves a narrow heat-affected zone. Oxyacetylene and stick arc welding create too much heat, which will weaken or warp the steel.

TIG welding is generally used in engine rebuilding shops to repair cracks in aluminum cylinder heads and in reconstructing combustion chambers. It has very limited use in collision repair, yet it is growing.

Even though there is full fusion, stick arc welding is NOT recommended for repairs on thin gauge **high-strength steels (HSS).** The high heat used with stick arc welding weakens and warps the metal. Stick arc welding can be used on body-over-frame vehicles and thick low carbon steel frames, however.

Oxyacetylene welding is a form of fusion welding in which oxygen and acetylene are used

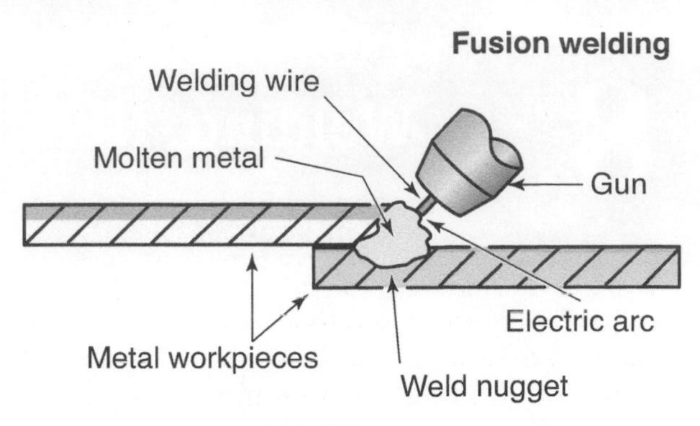

(A) Fusion welding uses an electric arc and metal filler wire to join metal. A welding wire is automatically fed out of the gun to form a strong weld nugget or bead.

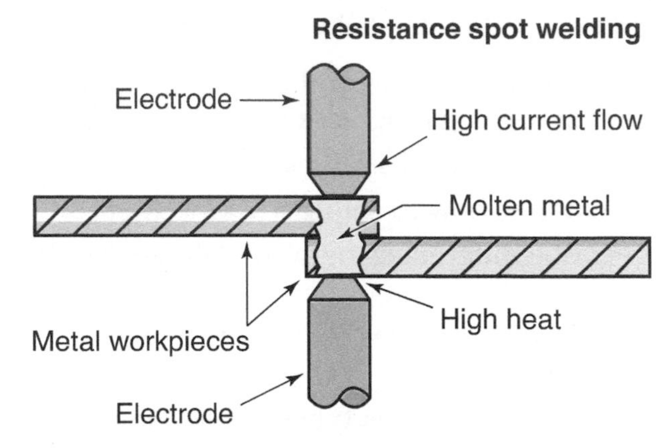

(B) Resistance spot welding uses an electric current and clamping force from electrodes to melt and join the panels without a filler wire. This is similar to the process used when manufacturing a vehicle.

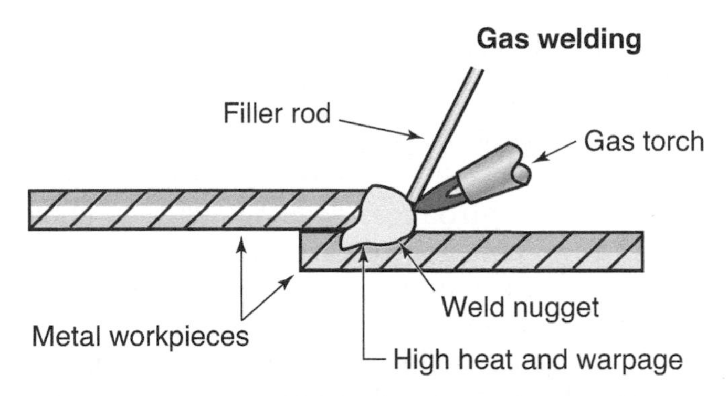

(C) Gas welding uses heat from an oxyacetylene torch and a filler metal to join the workpieces. Gas welding is seldom used in collision repair because of heat warpage of the metal body panels. Some manufacturers recommend gas brazing specific points on panels.

Figure 8–2. These are the three basic types of welding used in collision repair.

in combination. The two are mixed in a chamber, ignited at the torch tip, and used to join a welding filler rod with the base metal (see Figure 8–2C).

Oxyacetylene and shielded arc (stick) welding are also NOT recommended for most collision repair. They create too much heat for use with high-strength steels. However, they can still be used to repair some thick metals.

Squeeze-type resistance spot welding uses electric current through the base metal to form a small, round weld between the base metals. It is the only accepted form of pressure welding for collision repair. Resistance spot welding focuses the heat onto a small area. A series of pressure spot welds are sometimes used to secure replacement panels onto the body structure of wrecked cars or trucks. See Figure 8–2B.

HYBRID BONDING

Hybrid bonding refers to using more than one method to join structural body parts on a vehicle. Hybrid bonding is now being used during the manufacture of today's steel and aluminum unibody structures. See **Figure 8–3.**

Weld bonding uses adhesive and resistance spot welds to join steel or aluminum body panels together during vehicle manufacture. When on the vehicle assembly line, a weld-through structural adhesive is applied to the body flanges. Then spot welds are also used to fuse the body panels together.

A few manufacturers are using *friction stir welds* to assemble their vehicles. The panel flanges are clamped together and a small spinning wheel is forced against the panel. The friction from the spinning wheel generates enough heat to weld the panels together.

Rivet bonding uses adhesive and self-piercing metal rivets to join body panels on some aluminum unibody vehicles. At the factory, an epoxy adhesive is applied to flanges of the body panels. Then aluminum rivets are shot through the body panel flanges to join the aluminum panels together securely. The rivets pierce the top panel but expand and embed in the lower panel to join them.

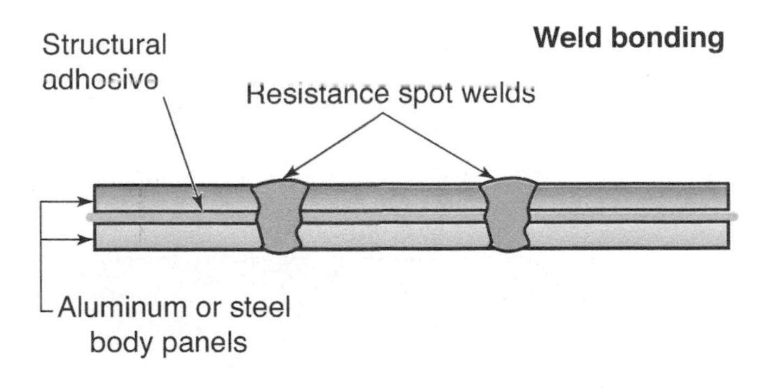

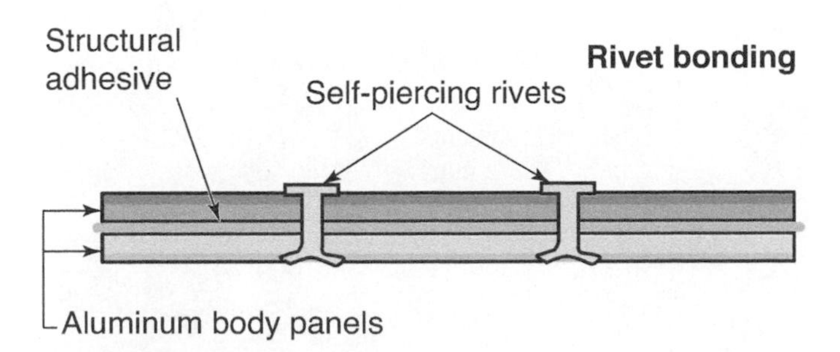

Figure 8–3. Auto manufacturers are now using hybrid methods of bonding structural panels together at the factory. Weld bonding uses both adhesive and resistance spot welds to hold steel or aluminum panels together. Rivet bonding uses structural adhesive and self-piercing rivets to join aluminum body panels.

MIG Welding Process

MIG welding uses a small diameter welding wire fed into the weld joint. The welding machine feeds the roll or wire out through the welding gun. A short arc is generated between the base metal and the wire. The resulting heat from the arc melts the welding filler wire and base metal to body panels. Look at **Figure 8–4.**

During the welding process, a **shielding gas** protects the weld from the atmosphere and prevents oxidation of the base metal. The type of gas used depends on the base metal to be welded, but C25 (argon/CO_2) is the most common.

MIG Welder Parts

The major parts of a MIG welder are:

1. Power supply—converts wall outlet AC to DC
2. Welding gun—feeds wire and gas into arc when trigger is pulled
3. Weld cable—large wires that connect welding gun to vehicle
4. Electrode wire—small welding wire fed down through center of gun
5. Wire feeder—mechanism for pushing wire through gun and into weld arc
6. Shielding gas—inert gas that surrounds and protects molten metal in weld
7. Regulator—pressure control device for setting gas pressure
8. Weld clamp—ground cable for connecting welder to vehicle

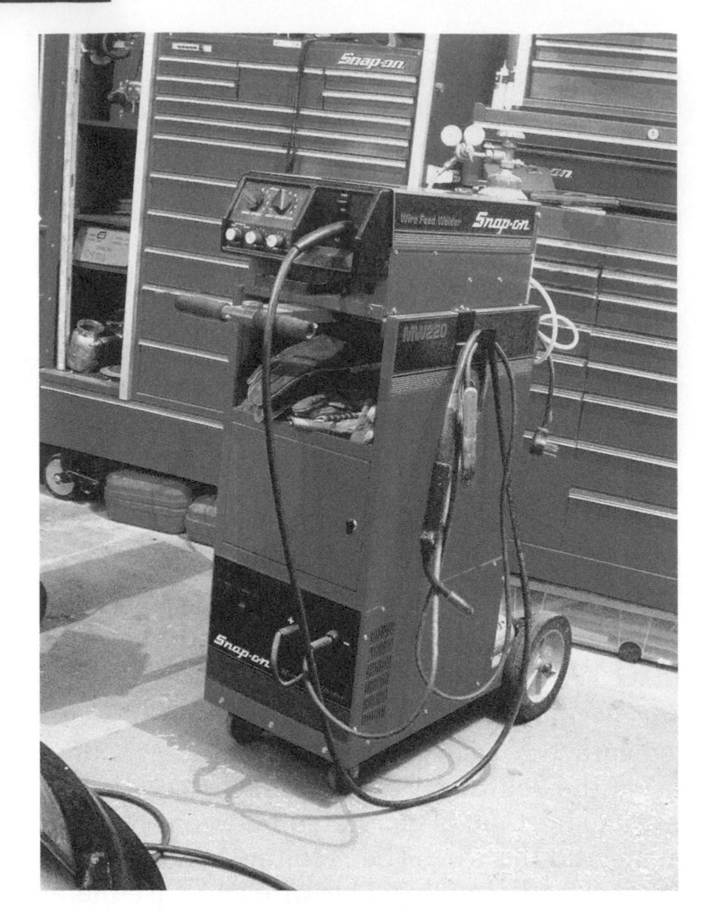

Figure 8–4. A MIG or metal inert gas welder, also called wire-feed welder, is the most commonly used welding machine in collision repair. It is easy to use and results in strong welds that match the strength of factory welds. (Courtesy of Snap-on Tools Corp.)

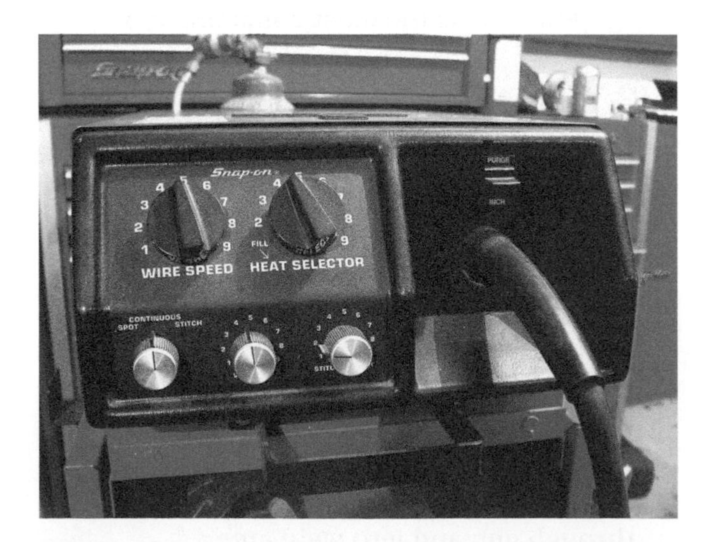

Figure 8–5. The major controls on a MIG are wire-feed speed and amperage setting. Both are primarily dependent upon the thickness of the metal to be welded.

A **welder amperage rating** gives the maximum current flow through the weld joint. The thickness of the metal being welded determines the amperage needed. See **Figure 8–5.**

Duty cycle is how many minutes the welder can safely operate at a given amperage level continuously over 10 minutes. The duty cycle rating is a percentage. A machine with 50 percent duty cycle can run 5 out of 10 minutes continuously (at rated amperage).

MIG Welding Gun

The **MIG welding gun,** also called a *torch,* delivers wire, current, and shielding gas to the weld site. It consists of a neck and handle, an on/off trigger, contact tip (or tube), and nozzle, **Figure 8–6.**

The **MIG contact tip,** or *tube,* transfers current to the welding wire as the wire travels through. It is usually made of copper or copper alloy. Its inside diameter must match the diameter

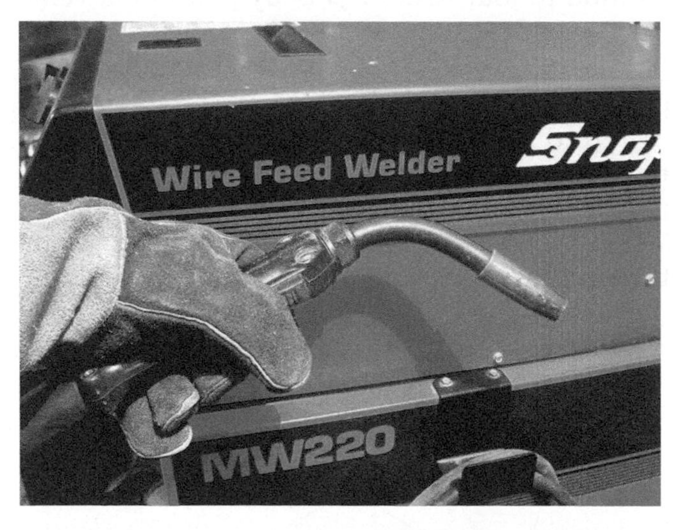

(A) A MIG welding gun will feed welding wire and inert gas through the head when the trigger is depressed.

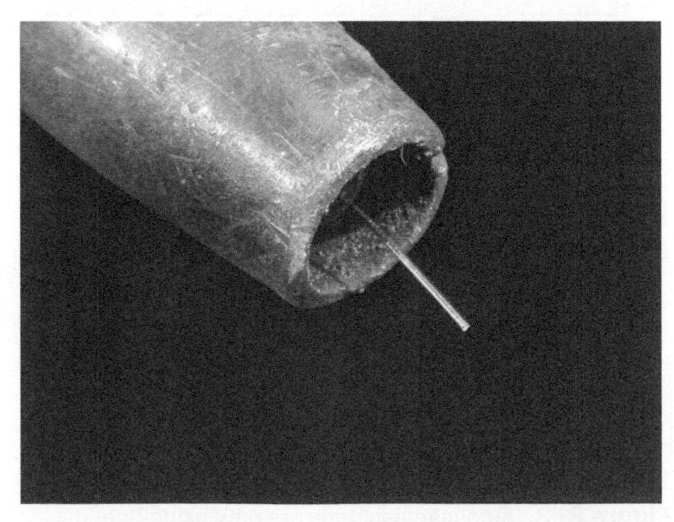

(B) Note how the wire feeds out of the welding gun tip. Inert gas is fed out around the wire tip to keep impurities in the air from contaminating the weld.

Figure 8–6. MIG welding gun feeds wire and inert gas to welding arc. (Courtesy Snap-on Tools Corp.)

of the electrode wire used. This is usually stamped on the tip in millimeters.

The *MIG nozzle* protects the contact tip and directs the shielding gas flow. It must be kept clean. A dirty nozzle can cause holes (porosity) in the weld.

Antispatter compound spray may help keep spatter from sticking to the nozzle. Spatter buildup still has to be cleaned off occasionally. Spattering tends to stick to the nozzle, especially when welding steel, causing porosity. If spatter builds up, it can create a "bridge" between the contact tip and nozzle and short out the welder.

MIG Shielding Gas

MIG shielding gas protects the weld area from oxygen, nitrogen, and hydrogen, which cause porosity in the weld. The gas also blows dirt and particles away. It is contained in a pressurized cylinder. See **Figure 8–7.**

The shielding gas cylinder has a flow meter/regulator that meters the gas out of the tank. In collision repair, most shops use C25 on their MIG welding machines. C25 is a mixture of argon gas and CO_2 gas for welding steel body panels. It contains 75 percent argon gas and 25 percent carbon dioxide gas to protect the weld from contamination.

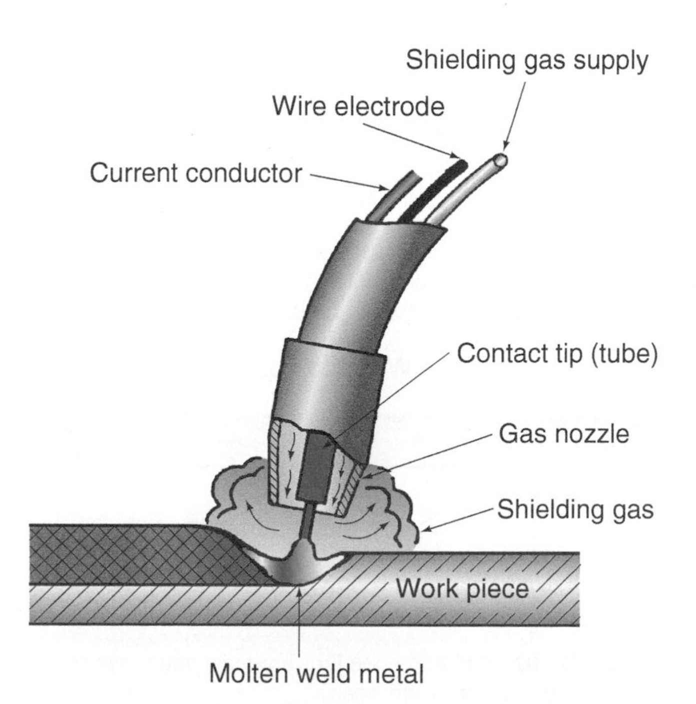

Figure 8–7. Note the MIG welder components and their relationships. (Courtesy of Lincoln Electric Co.)

When welding aluminum or stainless steel, straight argon gas is often recommended to protect the weld from contamination. If in doubt, check vehicle manufacturer recommendations for the type of welding gas and wire to use.

MIG Wire

MIG electrode wire comes in rolls that mount inside the MIG welder. See **Figure 8–8.** Rollers grasp and force the wire out to the gun whenever the gun trigger is pulled.

MIG Welding Variables

Many welders used for collision repair are 220 volt. There are also welders available that

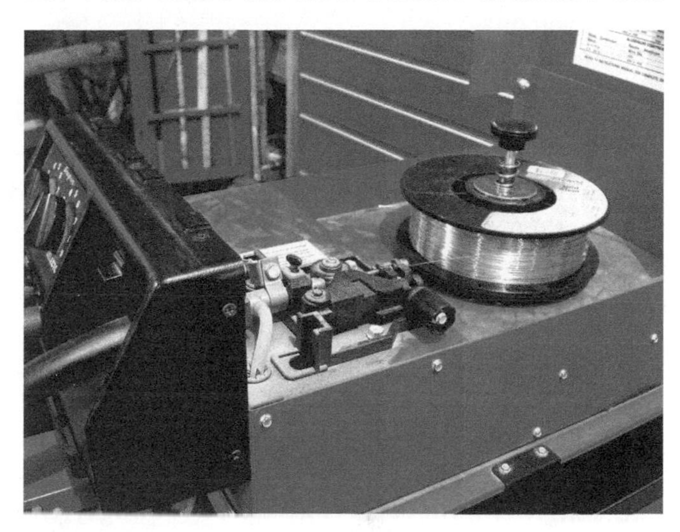

(A) A large roll of welding wire on top of the MIG welder is fed out through the welding hose and through the welding gun. The wire type must match the type of metal being welded.

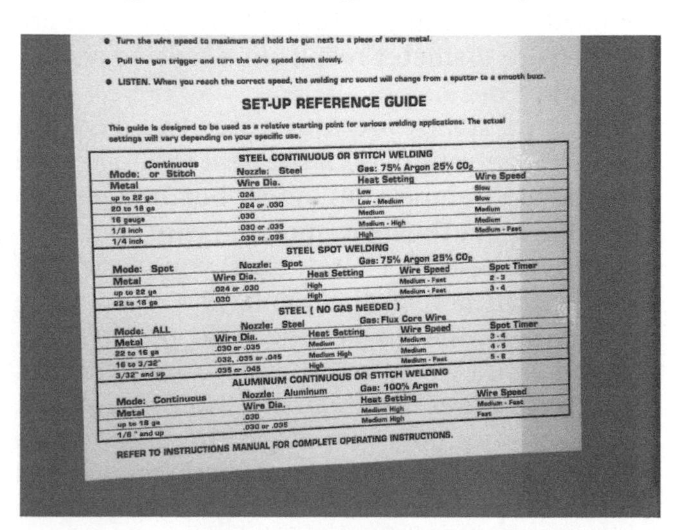

- Turn the wire speed to maximum and hold the gun next to a piece of scrap metal.
- Pull the gun trigger and turn the wire speed down slowly.
- LISTEN. When you reach the correct speed, the welding arc sound will change from a sputter to a smooth buzz.

SET-UP REFERENCE GUIDE

This guide is designed to be used as a relative starting point for various welding applications. The actual settings will vary depending on your specific use.

STEEL CONTINUOUS OR STITCH WELDING — Mode: Continuous or Stitch; Nozzle: Steel; Gas: 75% Argon 25% CO_2

Metal	Wire Dia.	Heat Setting	Wire Speed
up to 22 ga	.024	Low	Slow
20 to 18 ga	.024 or .030	Low - Medium	Slow
16 gauge	.030	Medium	Medium
1/8 inch	.030 or .035	Medium - High	Medium
1/4 inch	.030 or .035	High	Medium - Fast

STEEL SPOT WELDING — Mode: Spot; Nozzle: Spot; Gas: 75% Argon 25% CO_2

Metal	Wire Dia.	Heat Setting	Wire Speed	Spot Timer
up to 22 ga	.024 or .030	High	Medium - Fast	2 - 3
22 to 18 ga	.030	High	Medium - Fast	3 - 4

STEEL (NO GAS NEEDED) — Mode: ALL; Nozzle: Steel; Gas: Flux Core Wire

Metal	Wire Dia.	Heat Setting	Wire Speed	Spot Timer
22 to 16 ga	.030 or .035	Medium	Medium	3 - 4
16 to 3/32"	.032, .035 or .045	Medium High	Medium	4 - 5
3/32" and up	.035 or .045	High	Medium - Fast	5 - 6

ALUMINUM CONTINUOUS OR STITCH WELDING — Mode: Continuous; Nozzle: Aluminum; Gas: 100% Argon

Metal	Wire Dia.	Heat Setting	Wire Speed
up to 18 ga	.030	Medium High	Medium - Fast
1/8 " and up	.030 or .035	Medium High	Fast

REFER TO INSTRUCTIONS MANUAL FOR COMPLETE OPERATING INSTRUCTIONS.

(B) The chart on the MIG welder shows the setup information for different welding methods, different metal types, and different metal thicknesses.

Figure 8–8. Different size wire and kinds of inert gas can be installed on the MIG welder.

Welding variables to change	Desired changes							
	Penetration		Deposition rate		Bead size		Bead width	
	Increase	Decrease	Increase	Decrease	Increase	Decrease	Increase	Decrease
Current and wire feed speed	Increase	Decrease	Increase	Decrease	Increase	Decrease	No effect	No effect
Voltage	Decrease	Increase	No effect	No effect	Increase	Decrease	Increase	Decrease
Travel speed	Little effect	Little effect	No effect	No effect	Decrease	Increase	Increase	Decrease
Stickout	Decrease	Increase	Increase	Decrease	Increase	Decrease	Decrease	Increase
Wire diameter	Decrease	Increase	Decrease	Increase	No effect	No effect	No effect	No effect
Shielding gas percent CO_2	Increase	Decrease	No effect	No effect	No effect	No effect	Increase	Decrease
Gun angle	Backhand to 25°	Forehand	No effect	No effect	No effect	No effect	Backhand	Forehand

Figure 8–9. Study how to change variables to get better welding results.

use a standard 110-volt outlet. The higher voltage welders are more expensive but usually provide better welds. See **Figure 8–9.**

The **heat setting,** or **voltage,** determines the length of the arc. The more voltage, the longer the arc. The longer the arc, the wider and flatter the weld, since the weld wire melts off in larger drops. Too long an arc for the wire diameter used results in spattering. Too short an arc for the wire diameter results in a pulsing sound. See **Figure 8–10.**

To get a steady arc with a steady sound and correct penetration, both the heat (voltage) and wire speed (amperage) must be matched to each other. Set the heat, then the wire speed.

Travel speed is how fast you move the welding gun across the joint. The slower the travel speed, the deeper the weld penetration, the wider the weld, and the more bead height.

Travel direction refers to whether to push or pull the welding gun along the joint. **Push welding** means you aim or angle the gun ahead of the weld puddle. **Pull welding** means you aim or angle the gun back toward the weld puddle.

Electric **wire stick-out** is the length of unmelted wire that protrudes from the end of the MIG welding gun's contact tip during welding,

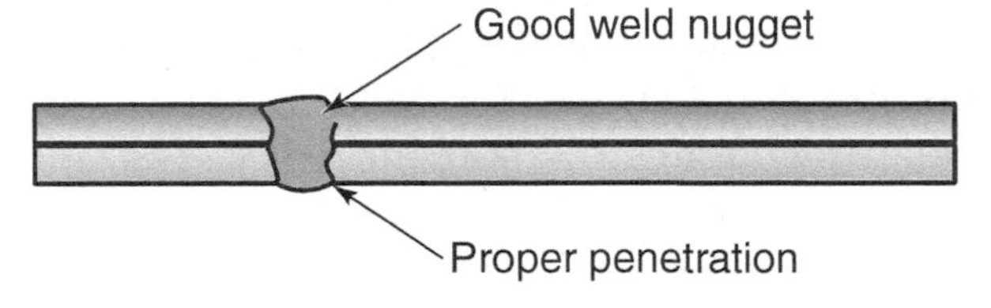

(A) A correct weld has full penetration and proper width and height. This weld would be very strong.

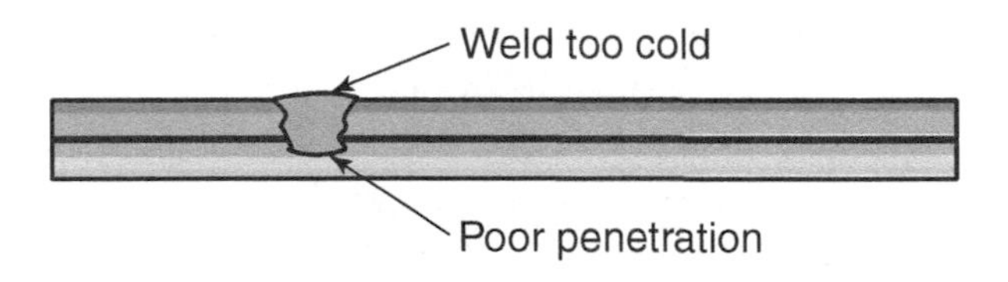

(B) Moving the gun too quickly would cause poor penetration. A bead would form only near the top of the base metals. This weld would break easily.

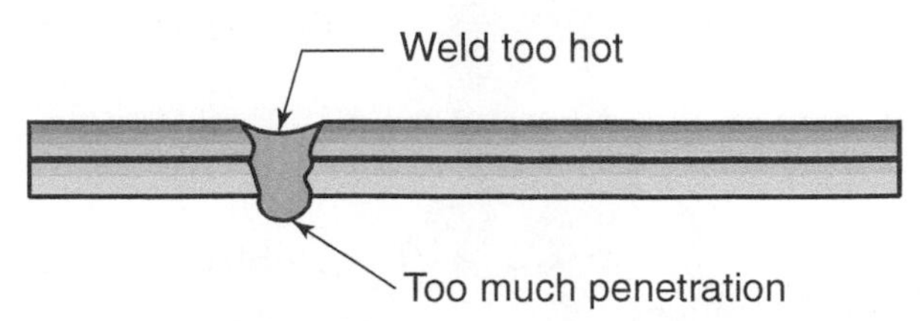

(C) If you move the gun too slowly too much heat will melt the bead down into the joint too much.

Figure 8–10. Welding speed, or how fast you move the welding gun, affects weld bead.

regardless of whether the tip sticks out of the nozzle or is recessed. Also called *tip-to-work distance* or *contact tip height,* wire stick-out should be kept between $\frac{1}{4}$ and $\frac{3}{8}$ inch (6–9 mm) for 0.023-inch (0.6 mm) wire. Wire stick-out should also be longer for larger diameter wires because of the higher heat (voltage) setting used.

Support the welding gun with the free hand, whenever possible, to control stick-out. Too much electrode stick-out lowers weld penetration. The wire becomes preheated and melts before penetrating deep enough into the weld.

Not enough electrode stick-out increases weld penetration, because the wire is too hot when contacting the workpiece.

Gun angle is the angle of the gun to the workpiece.

The angle of the gun to the workpiece varies, depending on the type of joint. For butt joints, hold the gun at 90 degrees. For "T" joints, hold the gun at 45 degrees. For lap joints, hold the gun at between 60 and 75 degrees. The thicker the workpiece, the greater the angle. The angle of direction of travel is always about 70 degrees from the workpiece, regardless of the type of joint. See **Figure 8–11.**

Straight polarity, or "DC straight," is when the electrode is negative. In DC straight, most of the heat is on the workpiece.

Reverse polarity, or "DC reverse," is when the electrode is positive and the workpiece is negative. In DC reverse, most of the heat is at the arc. Reverse polarity is commonly used for collision repair, because it provides the best fusion, leaving less weld on the surface to grind off. It

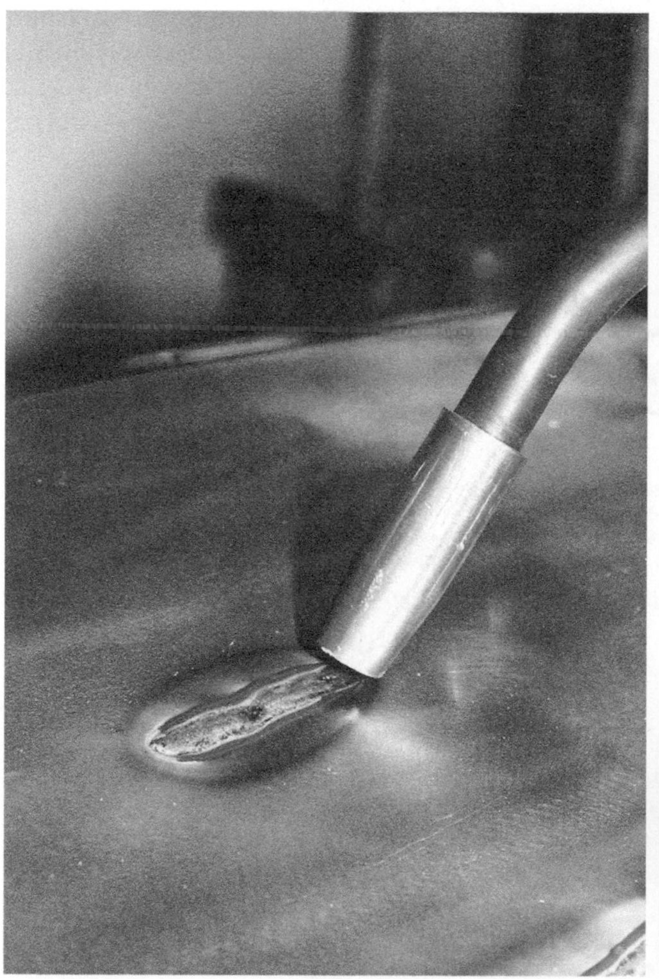

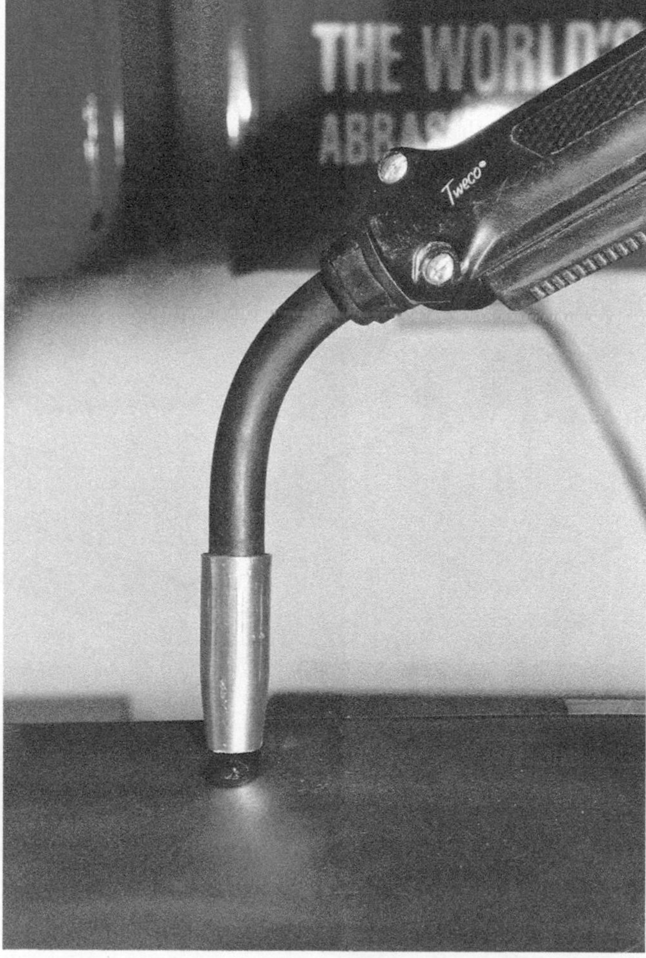

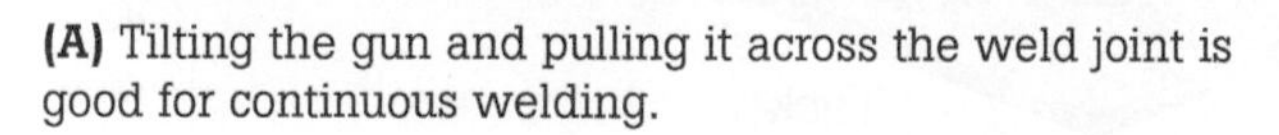

(A) Tilting the gun and pulling it across the weld joint is good for continuous welding.

(B) Holding the gun straight up when welding is often used when using plug welds to join structural panels.

Figure 8–11. The angle of the gun affects how the weld bead forms on metal. (Courtesy of Snap-on Tools Corp.)

also has a more stable arc and transfers less heat into the body panels.

MIG Weld Types

The types of MIG welds include tack, continuous, butt, fillet, and plug welds. You should understand each. See **Figure 8–12.**

A MIG **tack weld** is a short bead used for setup of a permanent weld. Tack welds help joint fit-up. They are usually placed about every 2 inches (51 mm) along a joint.

A **continuous weld** is a single weld bead along a joint. It could be a single pass weld. It could also be a series of short welds connected together to make one weld.

Skip welding produces a continuous weld by making short welds at different locations to prevent overheating. All of the small welds are finally joined to produce the continuous weld. This prevents heat buildup in one location on the part.

Stitch welding is a continuous weld in one location but with short pauses to prevent overheating. The operator can pause the machine manually to allow cooling. Some welders can also be programmed to pause automatically to prevent overheating (see Figure 8–12).

MIG **butt welds** are formed by fitting two edges of adjacent panels together and welding along the mating edges. They are often used to make two joints when sectioning frame rails, rocker panels, and door pillars. For butt welds, keep a gap between the two pieces the thickness of one piece. This helps weld penetration and prevents expansion and contraction problems. Also, hold the gun at 90 degrees to the joint.

An **insert,** or **backing strip,** made of the same metal as the base metal can be placed behind the weld. The backing helps proper fit-up and supports the weld.

A MIG **fillet weld** is a weld joining two surfaces with their edges or faces at about right angles to each other. The joint may be a lap joint or T-joint.

MIG **lap joints** are welds made on overlapping surfaces. They are commonly used on front and rear rails and floor pans. When welding a lap joint, the gun angle is kept between 60 and 75 degrees. If the lower piece is thicker than the top piece, angle more at the lower piece.

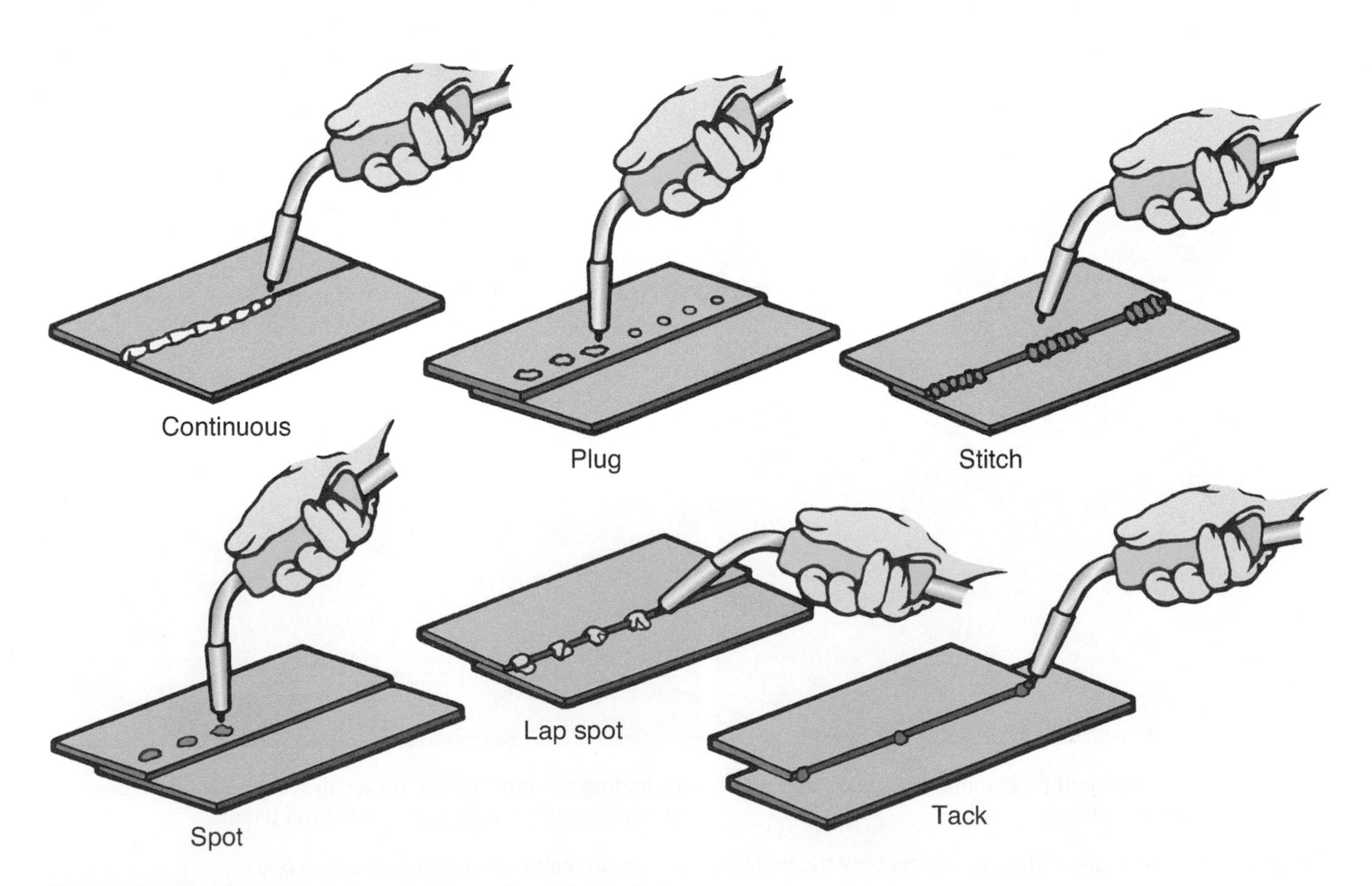

Figure 8–12. Study these six main types of welding techniques.

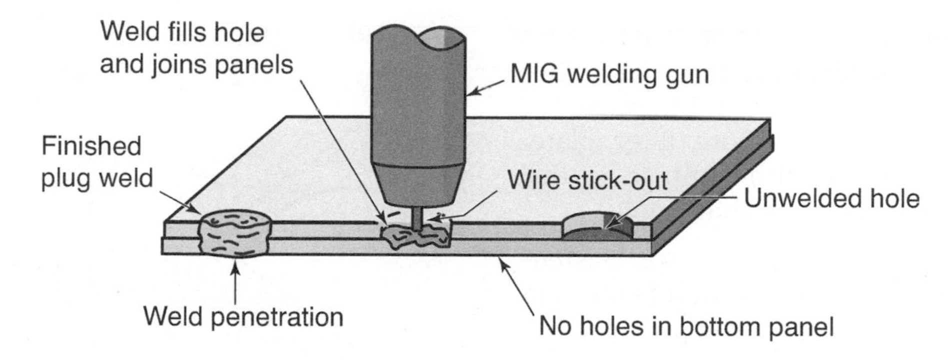

Figure 8–13. Plug welding is commonly used to replace factory welds when replacing structural panels on a vehicle. You must drill or stamp holes in the flange of a new panel and place it over the other body panel. Then the MIG welder is used to weld through a hole in the top panel to join it to the bottom panel. A series of plug welds are normally used to replace factory spot welds.

A MIG **plug weld** is made through a hole drilled in the top pieces. See **Figure 8–13.** It is started by drilling or punching holes in the top piece or pieces. The hole is filled with a weld nugget. Drill or punch the size holes recommended by the vehicle manufacturer in the top piece or pieces.

Start around the edge of the hole, then fill in the hole. A 5/16-inch (8 mm) hole works well for most collision repair, but refer to factory specs.

When plug welds are used to join three or more panels together, holes are punched or drilled in every piece except the bottom piece. The holes should be made progressively smaller from the top down. This will provide better fusion of each panel.

WELDING POSITIONS

Weld position refers to the orientation of the work pieces.

In **flat welding** the pieces are parallel to the bench or shop floor. Flat welding is the easiest because gravity pulls the puddle down into the joint. Flat is used whenever possible. It provides the best control. The weld bead does not flow away from the weld area.

In **horizontal welding** the pieces are turned sideways. Gravity tends to pull the puddle into the bottom piece. The gun can be pulled to the right or left. Pulling directs the heat at the puddle just laid, helping control penetration.

In **vertical welding** the pieces are turned upright. Gravity tends to pull the puddle down the joint. Welding in a vertical position works best when starting from the top and pulling the gun downward. The gun can be tipped downward slightly. A vertical up directs heat into the weld puddle, increasing penetration. Too much heat in the weld puddle makes it fluid, allowing gravity to pull it downward.

In **overhead welding** the piece is turned upside down. This is the most difficult type of weld position. Gravity tries to pull the puddle off the pieces and into the welder tip. Welding in an overhead position can be done by pulling the gun in either direction. Overhead welding takes the most skill because it is usually not as easy to control stick-out and gun angle.

Always make test welds on same type and thickness scrap metal in positions to be used before attempting to weld on the vehicle.

WELDING SAFETY

Use common sense while welding. The most important welding safety rules include:

1. Welding voltages and amperages can kill. Keep cables and connections in good shape.
2. Do NOT place the machine on a wet floor, or stand on a wet floor when welding. Keep the shop floor dry.
3. Arc rays are ultraviolet and can cause burns. Sparks or pieces of metal can also shoot out from the weld. Wear a welding helmet with face shield and filter plate.

A **welding filter lens,** sometimes called filter plate, is a shaded glass welding helmet insert for protecting your eyes from ultraviolet burns. They are graded with numbers from 4 to 12. The higher the number, the darker the filter. The American Welding Society (AWS) recommends grade 9 or 10 for MIG welding.

Note that there are **"self-darkening" filter lenses** available that instantly turn dark when the arc is struck. There is no need to move the face shield up and down. These filter plates work well but have one disadvantage in that their viewing window is somewhat small.

4. Wear a heavy shirt with long sleeves. Fasten the top button. Wear pants without cuffs and welding gloves. A leather apron provides good protection.
5. Breathing welding fumes can cause respiratory problems, especially when welding zinc-coated steel. Have adequate ventilation. Wear a respirator when welding.
6. Never have matches or a butane lighter in pockets. They can ignite or explode from the ultraviolet rays of welding.
7. To protect the glass and other areas from sparks, use a welding blanket.
8. Protect computers and other electronic parts while welding. They can be easily damaged. Do NOT allow cables to pass near computers or sensors. Remove the computer from the vehicle if welding within 12 inches (305 mm) of the computer.
9. Keep the current path short by placing the work clamp close to the weld location. Keep the power supply as far away from the vehicle as possible.

WELDING SURFACE PREPARATION

To prepare the surface for welding, you must first remove paint, undercoating, rust, dirt, oil, and grease. Use a plastic woven pad, grinder, sander, or wire brush. Apply weld-through primer to all bare metal mating surfaces.

The surfaces to be welded must be bare, clean metal. If they are NOT, contaminants will mix with the weld puddle and may result in a weak, defective weld.

HOLDING PARTS

Locking jaw pliers (Vise-Grip®), C-clamps, sheet metal screws, and special clamps are all necessary tools for welding. Clamping panels together correctly will require close attention to detail. See **Figure 8–14.**

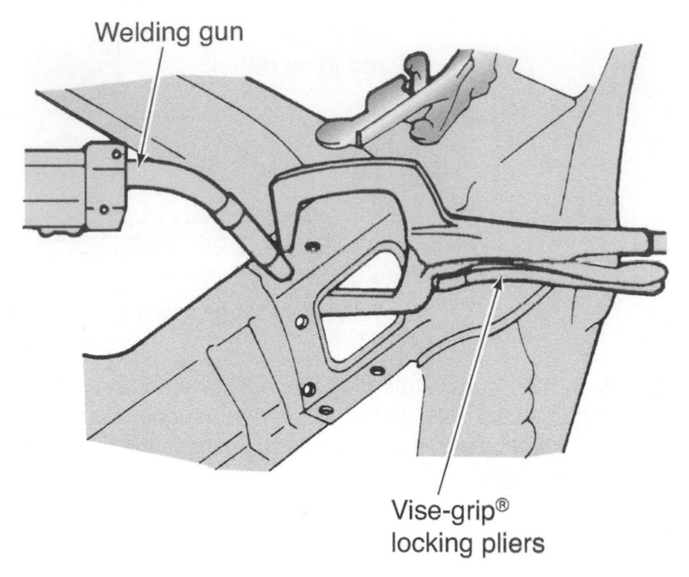

Figure 8–14. Fit-up involves making sure all areas of the panel fit together tightly and are in the proper locations. Clamping pliers are used to hold parts in contact while they are being welded. Try to position them close to the area to be welded.

Clamping both sides of a panel is not always possible. In these cases, a simple technique using self-tapping sheet metal screws or rivets can be employed.

When using the plug weld technique, the panels are held in place temporarily by setting a screw in every other hole. The empty holes are then plug welded. After the original holes are plug welded, the screws are removed and the remaining holes are then plug welded. See **Figure 8–15.**

WELD-THROUGH PRIMER

Weld-through primer is used for corrosion protection at weld zones. This primer must be sprayed onto clean surfaces. Most weld-through primers have poor adhesion qualities. Do NOT overuse them. Always follow directions closely. See **Figure 8–16.**

USING THE MIG WELDER

Before operating the MIG welder, be sure to:

1. Read the owner's manual carefully. Remember that when in doubt, follow equipment directions.
2. Use the proper power source, ideally on a separate circuit.
3. Use proper wire and shielding gas.

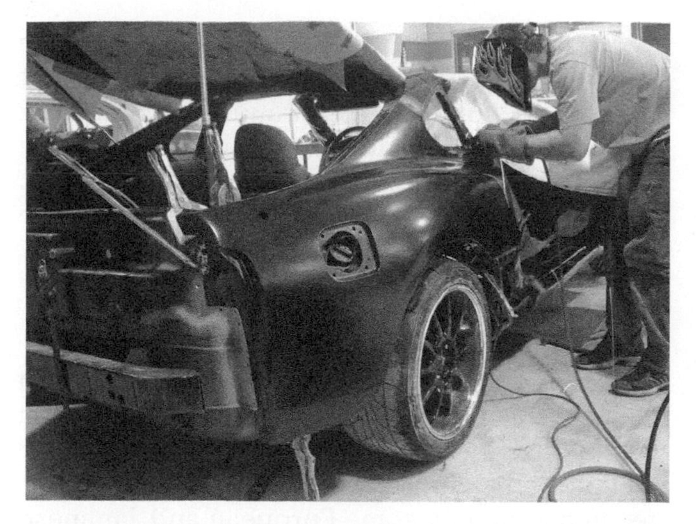

(A) After removal of a badly damaged panel, a new panel is fit into place and then welded on the vehicle.

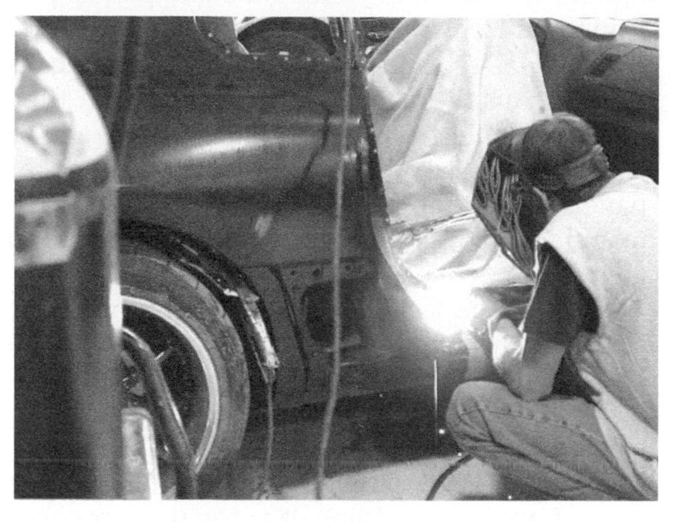

(B) High heat from the MIG welder joins the new body panel with the existing body structure.

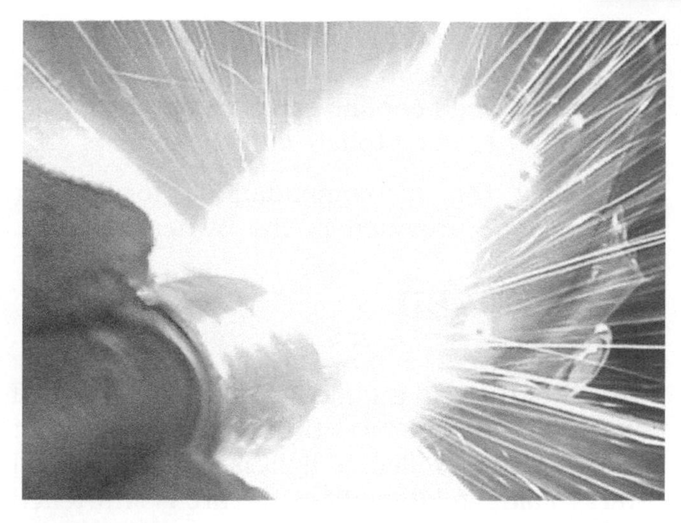

(C) Welding produces extreme heat and light that melts steel and makes it flow together in a weld bead.

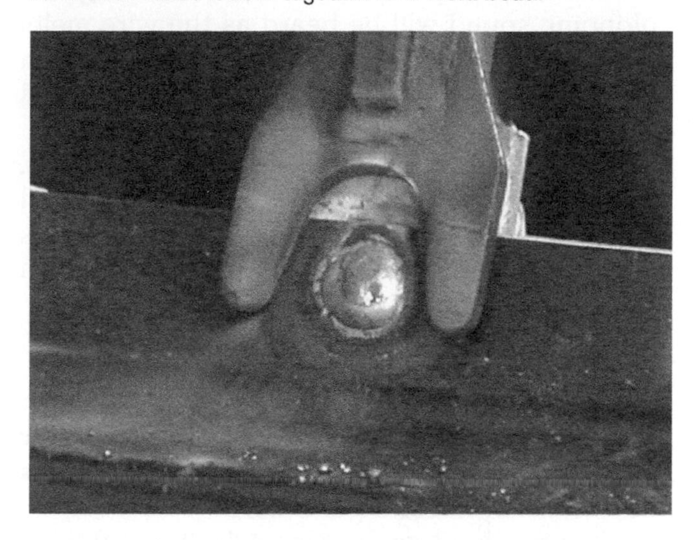

(D) Plug welds, like this one, are commonly used to secure the new structural panel to the vehicle during major collision repairs.

Figure 8–15. Most of today's structural body panels must be welded during replacement.

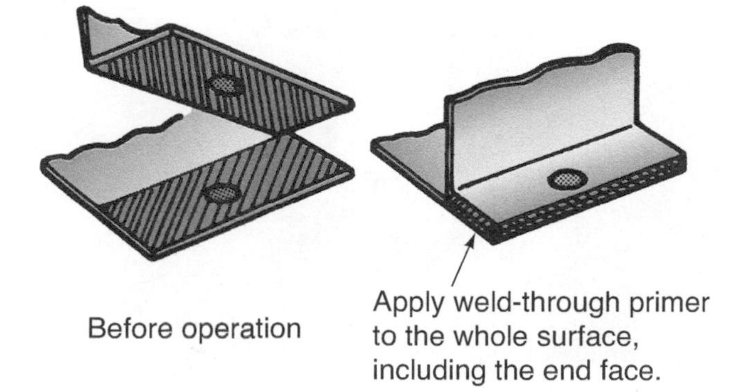
Before operation
Apply weld-through primer to the whole surface, including the end face.

Figure 8–16. Weld-through primer should be applied to bare metal before welding. It can be applied with a spray can or brush. Use only a light coat. This will restore proper rust protection to bare metal.

4. Set all drive rollers, cable liners, and tensions to manufacturer's specifications.
5. Set the welder to the proper voltage and speed suggested for the thickness of the metal.
6. Adjust the shielding gas flow rate to the recommended settings.
7. Cover upholstery and glass to prevent spark damage. Sparks can be lessened by making sure the welding area is clean, reducing the voltage setting, and making sure the wire stick-out distance is correct.

8. Allow the weld to cool naturally. Do NOT use water or compressed air to cool the weld. Forced cooling can cause cracking. If the weld can be touched, it is cool enough.

Follow the recommendations for welder maintenance provided in the owner's manual.

WIRE SPEED

MIG **wire speed** is how fast the rollers feed the wire into the weld puddle. An even, high-pitched buzzing sound indicates the correct wire-to-heat ratio. A steady, reflected light is desirable; it will start to fade in intensity as the arc is shortened and wire speed is increased.

If the wire speed is too slow, a hissing and plopping sound will be heard as the wire melts away from the puddle and deposits the molten glob. There will be a much brighter reflected light.

Too much wire speed will choke the arc. More wire is being deposited than the head and puddle can absorb. The result is the wire melts into tiny balls of molten metal that fly away from the weld, creating a strobe light arc effect.

SHIELDING GAS FLOW RATE

MIG **gas flow rate** is a measurement of how fast gas flows over the weld puddle. Precise gas flow is essential for a good weld.

If the flow of gas is too high, it will flow in eddies and reduce the shielding effect. If there is NOT enough gas, the shielding effect will also be reduced. Adjustment is made in accordance with the distance between the nozzle and the base metal, the welding current, travel speed, and welding environment (nearby air currents). The standard flow rate is 25 cubic feet per hour (0.75 cubic meter per hour).

HEAT BUILDUP PREVENTION

As mentioned previously, too much heat when welding or heating distorts and weakens the metal. Always make sure you do not allow excess heat to transfer into any area of a panel. Use stitch or skip welding methods described earlier.

Stitch and skip welding will prevent costly and time-consuming panel warpage. Another method of preventing heat buildup is heat sink compound.

Heat sink compound is a paste that can be applied to parts to absorb heat and prevent warpage. It comes in a can and can be applied and reused. The heat sink compound is sticky and can be placed on the panel next to the weld. Heat will flow into the compound and out of the metal to prevent heat damage.

RESISTANCE SPOT WELDING

Squeeze-type resistance spot welding has two electrode arms that apply pressure and electric current to the metals being joined. No filler metal or shielding agent is needed. This type is recommended by some European and Japanese vehicle manufacturers. It can be used to replace factory spot welds on some panels and components.

Squeeze-type resistance spot welding is primarily used for cosmetic panels when they are accessible from both sides. It is used for some structural parts like pillars and rocker panels only when recommended by the vehicle manufacturer. This process cannot be used on aluminum.

Resistance spot welding is not new, but there are some recent equipment developments. Modern spot welders for the shop are generally easier to use and more effective for making strong welds. Refer to **Figure 8–17.**

Squeeze-type resistance spot welding is a type of pressure welding. It is the main process

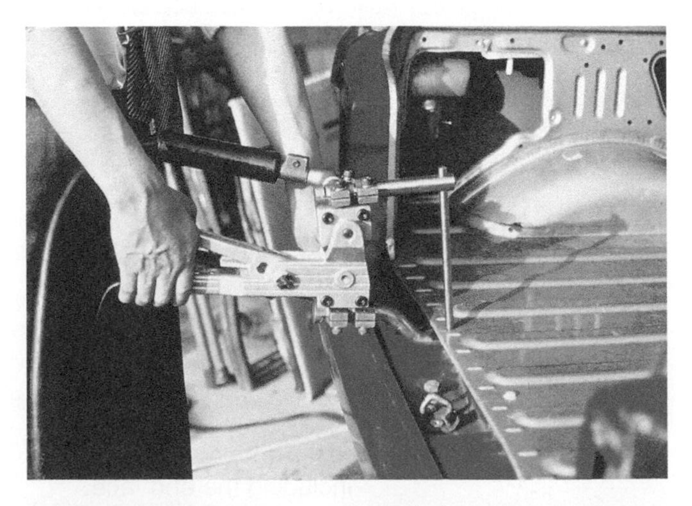

Figure 8–17. This technician is using a resistance spot welder to install a floor panel. Panels are clamped together by large electrodes. When current passes through electrodes and panels, a spot weld is formed to secure the panels together. (Courtesy of Data Welder)

used in the factory. Over 99 percent of factory welds are resistance spot welds. Factory spot welds are usually done by robots. Extremely high current and pressures are used.

Many manufacturers recommend both MIG plug welds and resistance spot welding for replacing factory spot welds. They recommend resistance spot welding for repairs on body panels and some structural areas, including radiator core supports, pillars, rocker panels, exposed pinch weld areas on window and door openings and roofs.

At least one vehicle manufacturer recommends removing the galvanized coating from outside the joint before resistance spot welding. Unless otherwise directed, do NOT remove the galvanized coating. This removes corrosion protection.

Resistance Spot Welder Settings

Basic resistance spot welding parts include:

1. Transformer with controls—converts AC into regulated DC.
2. **Arm sets**—hold welding tips and conduct current to tips.
3. **Electrode tips**—allow current flow through spot weld.

Three separate transformer controls are needed for quality welds, including a pressure multiplier, current adjuster, and a timer. These three settings depend on each other for good resistance spot welds. There are also computer-controlled spot welders available that automatically adjust settings depending on the thickness of material dialed in. See **Figure 8–18.**

Use a hand-held electrode shaper to maintain spot weld tips. A shaper that attaches to a drill is also available. A file can be used, but is NOT as accurate. The ridges left by filing need to be polished with emery cloth or the tips will NOT make full contact with the workpiece.

The spot welder tips must be aligned in a straight line as seen from the front and side. If the tips come together at an angle, the weld will be weak. If the tips do NOT come together at all, the weld area will be offset, resulting in no weld. Always check tip alignment before welding and between groups of welds.

The electrode tips also need to be tightly fastened to the arm sets. They tend to loosen during use, affecting current flow and tip alignment.

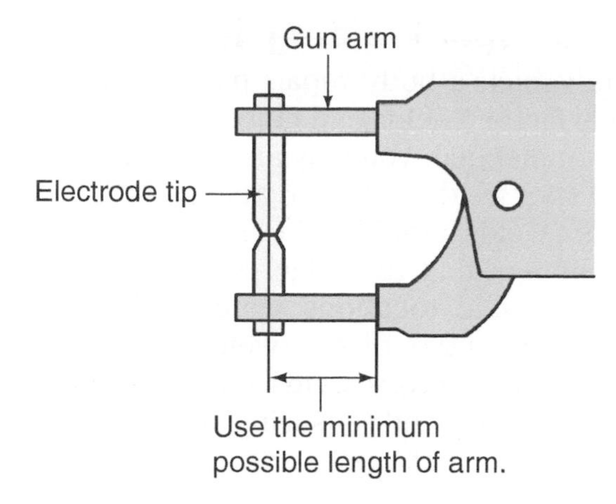

(A) Use the shortest arm lengths that will work.

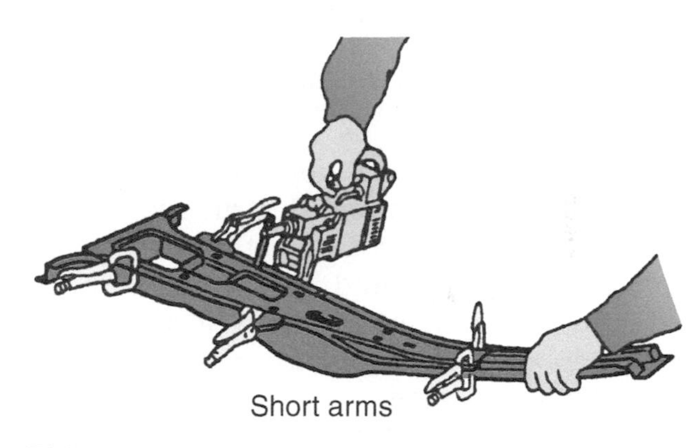

(B) Short arms will reach many weld areas. (Courtesy of Nissan North America, Inc.)

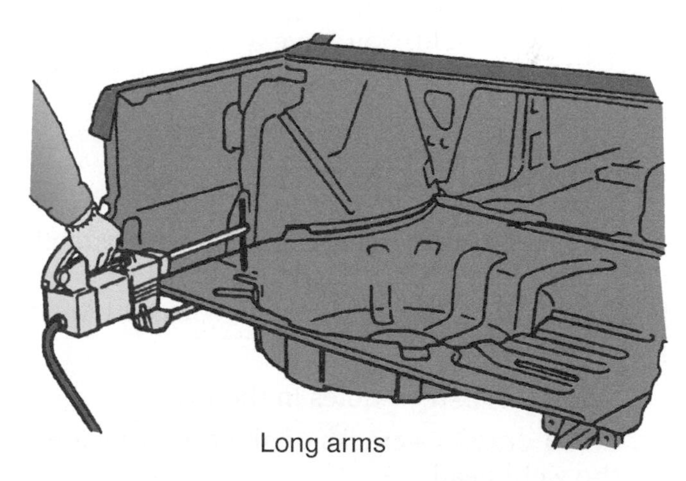

(C) A longer arm length might be needed on very large panels. (Courtesy of Nissan North America, Inc.)

Figure 8–18. Spot weld arm length affects clamping pressure.

When servicing welder parts, follow the instructions in the operating manual. It will give directions for the specific make and model of welder.

Resistance Spot Welding Techniques

Check the vehicle's body repair manual to find the original factory welds and number of replacements recommended. You may also compare the number of spot welds on the original panel.

The spot welds should be in the center of the flange without riding the edge. Make sure the original spot weld locations were NOT used. Check that the pitch of the welds is a little shorter than the factory welds. Make sure the spots are evenly spaced (ensuring strength).

Spot weld current, time, and pressure settings are adjusted for:

1. Type of metal
2. Metal thickness
3. Length of arm sets
4. Distance electrode tips are from the metal edge

There are two basic types of weld inspection: visual inspection and destructive testing.

Visual weld inspection is the most practical method on a repaired vehicle because the weld is not taken apart. Visual weld inspection involves looking at the weld for flaws, proper size, and proper shape.

Destructive testing forces the weld apart to measure weld strength. Force is applied until the metal or weld breaks.

Basically, you have a good weld if metal tears off with weld. You have a bad weld if two pieces break cleanly at the weld with no metal tear-out.

WELD PROBLEMS

A welding problem causes a weak or cosmetically poor joint that reduces quality. The chart in **Figure 8–19** lists weld problems and their possible causes.

1. **Weld porosity**—holes in the weld
2. **Weld cracks**—cracks on the top or inside the weld bead
3. **Weld distortion**—uneven weld bead
4. **Weld spatter**—drops of electrode on and around weld bead
5. **Weld undercut**—groove melted along either side of weld and left unfilled
6. **Weld overlap**—excess weld metal mounted on top and either side of weld bead
7. *Too little penetration*—weld bead sitting on top of base metal
8. *Too much penetration*—burn-through beneath lower base metal

WELDING ALUMINUM

Several vehicles now have body, frame, and chassis parts made of aluminum. Whole bodies made of aluminum are now available. As a result, the information needed for welding aluminum is growing.

Aluminum is light and relatively strong. It is naturally corrosion resistant. Aluminum forms its own corrosion barrier of aluminum oxide when exposed to air. A disadvantage of aluminum is its high cost.

There are some major differences to keep in mind when working with aluminum as opposed to steel, particularly when it comes to welding. Pure aluminum is lightweight and useful more for its ability to be formed than for its strength. When used on vehicles, it is alloyed with other elements and heat-treated for additional strength.

Concerning welding, pound for pound, aluminum is the best conductor of electricity. It conducts heat three times faster than steel. Aluminum becomes stronger, NOT brittle, in extreme cold. It is also easily recyclable. Aluminum conducts heat faster than steel, and also spreads heat faster. Therefore, it requires special attention when welding.

Aluminum looks similar to magnesium which, if welded, could start a flash fire. To make sure the part is aluminum, brush the part with a stainless steel brush. Aluminum turns shiny. Magnesium turns dull gray.

DANGER

If the part is found to be magnesium, do NOT try to weld it. It can start to burn with tremendous heat.

When welding aluminum, be sure to protect wire harnesses and electronics from potential damage from spreading heat. Aluminum takes more voltage and amperage for the same thickness of material.

Defect	Defect condition	Remarks	Probable causes
Pores/pits (porosity)	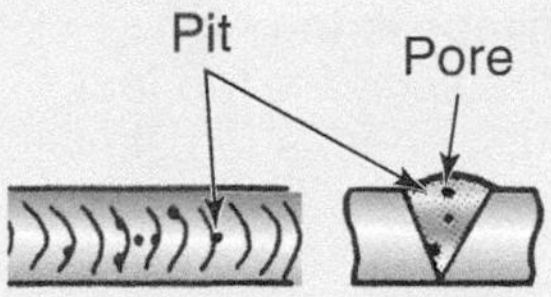 Pit Pore	Holes form when gas is trapped in the weld metal.	Rust or dirt on the base metal. Rust or moisture adhering to the wire. Improper shielding action (the nozzle is blocked or the gas flow volume is low). Weld is cooling off too fast. Arc length is too long. Wrong wire used. Gas is sealed improperly. Weld joint surface is not clean. Electrode contamination.
Undercut	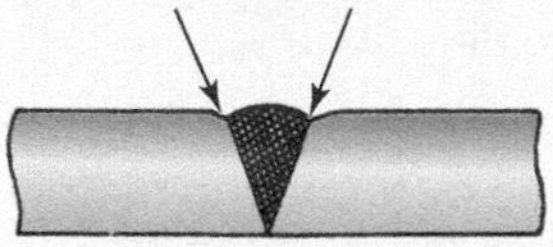	The overmelted base metal creates grooves or an indentation. The base metal's section is made smaller and, therefore, the weld zone's strength is severely lowered.	Arc length is too long. Improper gun angle. Welding speed is too fast. Current is too high. Torch feed is too fast. Torch angle is tilted.
Improper fusion	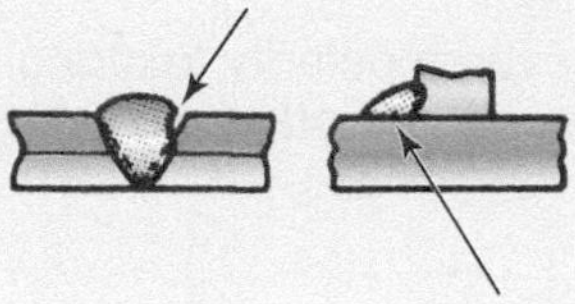	An absence of fusion between weld metal and base metal or between deposited metals.	Improper torch feed operation. Voltage is too low. Weld area is not clean. Improper gun angle.
Overlap	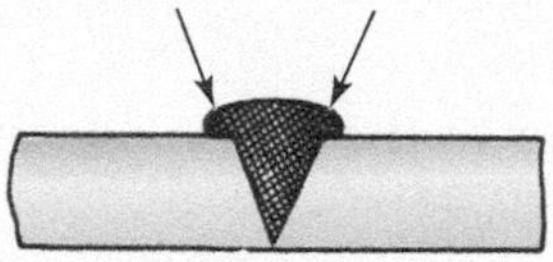	Apt to occur in a fillet weld rather than a butt weld. Causes stress concentration and results in premature corrosion.	Welding speed is too slow. Arc length is too short. Torch feed is too slow. Current is too low.
Insufficient penetration	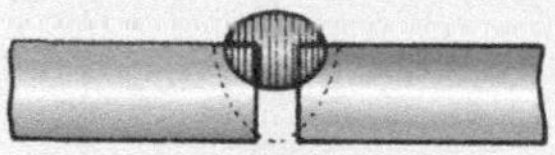	Insufficient deposition made under the panel.	Welding current is too low. Arc length is too long. The end of the wire is not aligned with the butted portion of the panels. Groove face is too small. Gun speed is too fast. Improper electrode extension.
Excess weld spatter	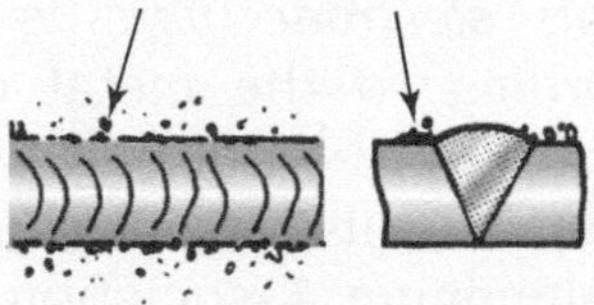	Shows up as speckles and bumps along either side of the weld bead.	Arc length is too long. Rust on the base metal. Gun angle is too severe. Worn tube or drive rolls. Wire spool too tight. Voltage is too high. Wire speed too slow.
Spatter (short throat)	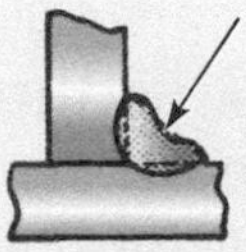	Prone to occur most often in fillet welds.	Current is too high. Wrong wire used.
Waviness of bead	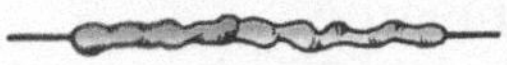	Uneven bead pattern usually caused by torch mishandling.	Wavering hands. Electrode extension too long.

Figure 8–19. Study weld problems and causes carefully.

Defect	Defect condition	Remarks	Probable causes
Cracks		Usually occur on the top surface only.	Stains on welded surface (paint, oil, rust, etc.). Voltage is too high. Wire speed is too fast. Gun speed is too slow.
Bead not uniform		Weld bead is misshapen and uneven rather than streamlined and even.	Contact tip hole is worn or deformed and wire is oscillating as it comes out of the tip. Gun is not held steady during welding.
Burn-through		Holes in the weld bead.	Welding current is too high. Gap between the metal is too wide. Gun speed is too slow. Gun-to-base metal distance is too short. Reverse polarity to straight polarity (gun negative, work positive).

Figure 8–19. (*Continued*).

Use the following guidelines when MIG welding aluminum:

1. Use aluminum wire and 100 percent argon shielding gas.
2. Set the wire speed faster than with steel.
3. Hold the gun closer to vertical when welding aluminum. Tilt it only about 5 to 10 degrees.
4. Use only the forward welding method with aluminum. Always push—never pull. When making a vertical weld, start at the bottom and work up.
5. Set the tension of the wire drive roller lower to prevent twisting.
6. Use about 50 percent more shielding gas with aluminum.
7. Because there tends to be more spatter with aluminum, use an antispatter compound to control buildup at the end of the nozzle and contact tip.
8. Shop squeeze-type resistance spot welders do NOT have enough amperage for aluminum. Do NOT use "shop-type" resistance spot welders on aluminum.
9. Always use skip and stitch welding techniques to prevent heat warping. Set wire speed slightly faster. Hold the gun closer to the vertical, compared to steel.
10. Use only the push method when welding aluminum. Pushing helps take away any remaining aluminum oxide which must be cleaned off before welding. When vertical welding aluminum, always start at the bottom and work up.
11. When welding aluminum, there will be more spatter, but the spatter will NOT stick to the nozzle as with steel.

Aluminum electrode wire is classified by series according to the metal or metals the aluminum is alloyed with, and whether or not the aluminum is heat-treated. The series are set up by the Aluminum Association, not the AWS. The number does NOT indicate the strength of the electrode.

Heat crayons or **thermal paint** can be used to determine the temperature of the aluminum or other metal being heated. They will melt at a specific temperature and warn you to prevent overheating.

As in **Figure 8–20,** the crayon or paint is applied next to the aluminum area to be heated. The mark will begin to melt when the crayon's or paint's melting point is almost reached. The melting will let you know that you are about to reach the melting point of the aluminum.

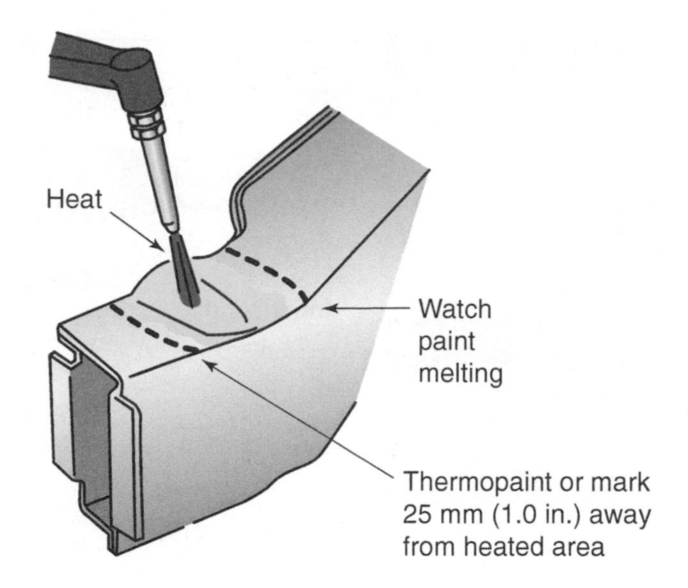

Figure 8–20. Thermal paint or crayon can be used to prevent overheating. Because aluminum does not change color when heated, it is easy to overheat it and blow holes in parts. Thermal paint or crayon will melt when the melting point of aluminum is almost reached. (Courtesy of American Honda Motor Co., Inc.)

Oxyacetylene Welding

Even though oxyacetylene welding is no longer used for collision repair, it can still be used for cleaning and heating on unibody vehicles. Therefore, oxyacetylene welding basics should be understood.

A typical **oxyacetylene welding outfit,** shown in **Figure 8–21,** consists of the following:

1. **Cylinders**—steel tanks that hold the oxygen and the acetylene.
2. **Regulators**—diaphragm valves that reduce pressure coming from the tanks to the hoses.
3. **Hoses**—lines from the regulators to the torch.
4. **Torch**—mixes oxygen and acetylene in the proper proportions and produces a flame capable of melting steel.

Each regulator has a cylinder pressure gauge and a working pressure gauge. The gauges show the settings of the regulators. Working **oxygen pressure** ranges from 5 to 100 psi (0.35 to 7 kg/cm^2). Working **acetylene pressure** ranges from 1 to 12 psi (0.07 to 0.84 kg/cm^2).

There are two main types of torches: welding and cutting. A **welding torch** has two valves for adjusting gas flow. A **cutting torch** has a third oxygen valve and a lever or trigger for increased oxygen flow. The heat of the flame, combined with the blast of oxygen, will rapidly cut thick steel. See **Figure 8–22.**

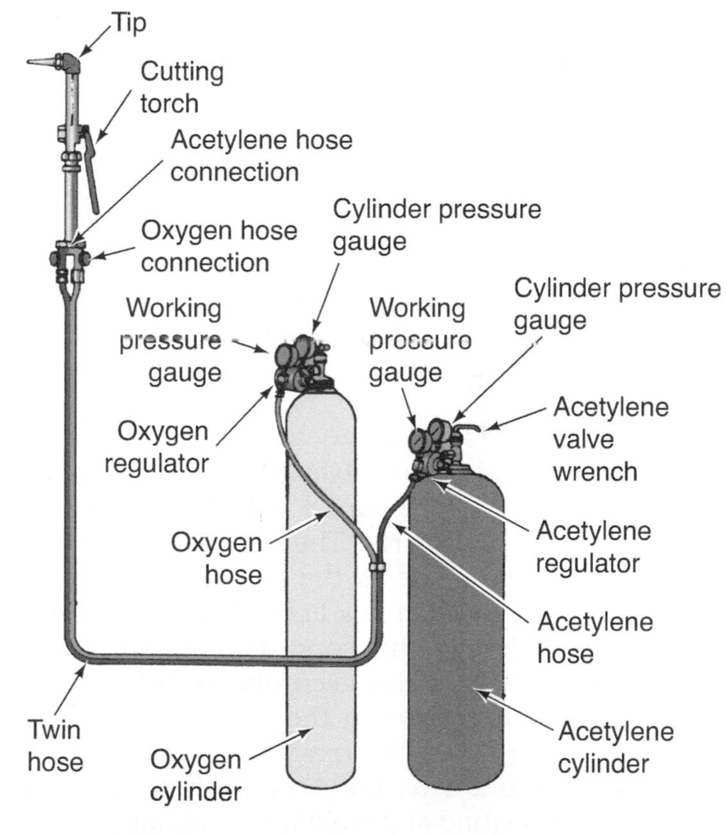

Figure 8–21. Study the parts of an oxyacetylene outfit. One tank holds acetylene and the other oxygen. Regulators control the amount of gas pressure going to the welding torch. Valves on the torch allow to further control gas mixture and flow to produce good flame.

All oxyacetylene welding should be done with a number 4, 5, or 6 tinted filter lens. A **spark lighter** is a necessity for producing a spark and igniting an oxyacetylene torch.

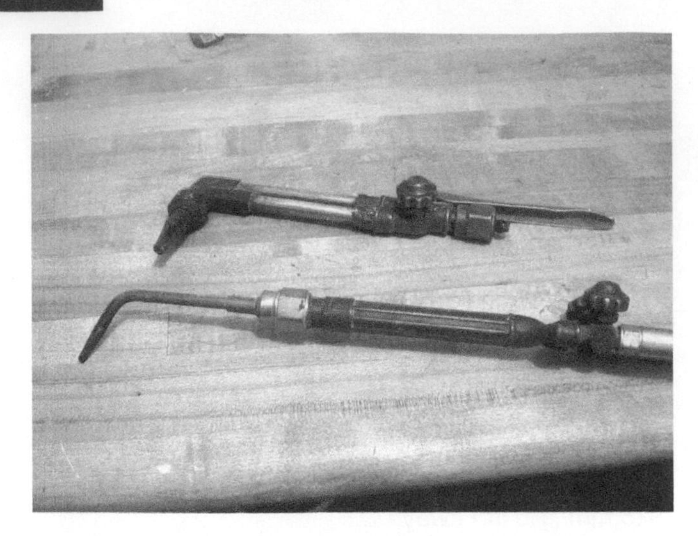

Figure 8–22. Compare a welding torch and a cutting torch. A cutting torch has three control valves and a trigger for controlling high gas flow from the tip.

Flames and Adjustment

When acetylene and oxygen are mixed and burned, the condition of the flame varies depending on the ratio of oxygen and acetylene used.

Shown in **Figure 8–23,** there are three types of flames:

A **neutral flame** or standard flame is produced by mixing acetylene and oxygen in a 1-to-1 ratio. A neutral flame has a brilliant white core surrounded by a clear blue outer flame.

A **carburizing flame,** also called a reducing flame, is obtained by mixing slightly more acetylene than oxygen. Figure 8–23B shows that this flame has three parts. The core and the outer flame are the same as the neutral flame. However, between them is a light-colored acetylene cone enveloping the core. The length of the acetylene cone varies according to the amount of surplus acetylene in the gas mixture. For a carburizing flame, the oxygen-acetylene mixing ratio is about 1 to 1.4. A carburizing flame is used for heating and welding aluminum, nickel, and other alloys.

An **oxidizing flame** is obtained by mixing slightly more oxygen than acetylene. It resembles the neutral flame in appearance, but the inner core is shorter and its color is a little more violet. The outer flame is shorter and fuzzy at the end. Ordinarily, this flame oxidizes melted metal, so it is NOT used in the welding of mild steel.

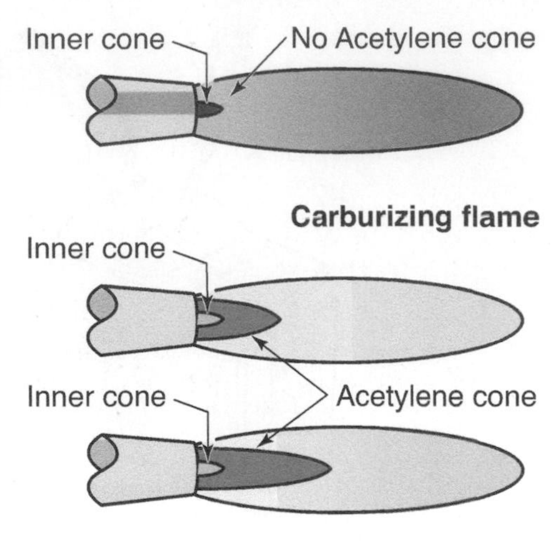

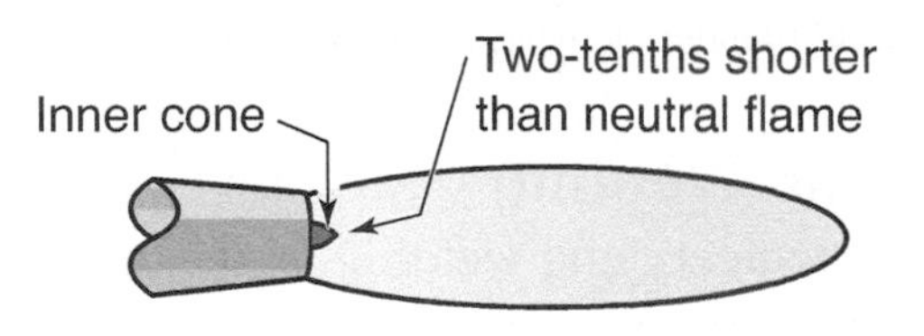

Figure 8–23. Note the types of oxyacetylene flames.

Oxyacetylene Torch Flame Adjustment

When using an oxyacetylene welding torch, proceed as follows:

1. Attach the appropriate size tip to the end of the torch. Use the standard size tip for mild steel. Keep in mind that each torch manufacturer has a different system for measuring the size of the tip orifice.
2. Set the oxygen and acetylene regulators to the proper pressure.
3. Open the acetylene hand valve about half a turn and ignite the gas. Continue to open the hand valve until the black smoke disappears and a reddish yellow flame appears. Slowly open the oxygen hand valve until a blue flame with a yellowish white cone appears. Further open the oxygen hand valve until the center cone becomes sharp and well defined. This is a neutral flame and is used for welding mild steel.
4. If acetylene is added to the flame or oxygen is removed from the flame, a carburizing

flame will result. If oxygen is added to the flame or acetylene is removed from the flame, an oxidizing flame will result.

Brazing

Brazing is like soldering at relatively low temperatures around 800°F (427°C). An adhesion bond is made by melting a filler metal and allowing it to spread into the pores of the workpiece. The natural flow of the filler material into the joint is called capillary attraction. In brazing, the filler metal does NOT fuse with the workpiece.

Braze welding is classified as either soft or hard brazing, depending on the temperature at which the brazing material melts. **Soft brazing** or **soldering** is done with brazing materials that melt at temperatures BELOW 900°F (468°C). **Hard brazing** is done with brazing materials that melt at temperatures ABOVE 900°F (468°C).

Brazing is applied only for sealing purposes. This is a method of welding whereby a filler rod, whose melting point is lower than that of the base metal, is melted without melting the base metal. Brass brazing is frequently applied to automotive bodies.

Shutting Down Oxyacetylene Equipment

Always turn off the oxyacetylene torch when it is not in use. Never lay down a lit torch. Turn the torch off when it is not being held in your hand. Do this by first closing the acetylene hand valve, then the oxygen hand valve. Shutting off the acetylene valve first will immediately extinguish the flame. If the oxygen is shut off first, the acetylene will continue to burn, throwing off a great deal of smoke and soot.

Close the main valves on the tops of the cylinders when finished. Then crack open the torch valves to bleed the hoses of pressure. Finally, close the torch valves to ready it for the next use.

PLASMA ARC CUTTING

Plasma arc cutting creates an intensely hot air stream over a very small area that melts and removes metal. Extremely clean cuts are possible with plasma arc cutting. Because of the tight focus of the heat, there is no warpage, even when cutting thin sheet metal. See **Figure 8–24.**

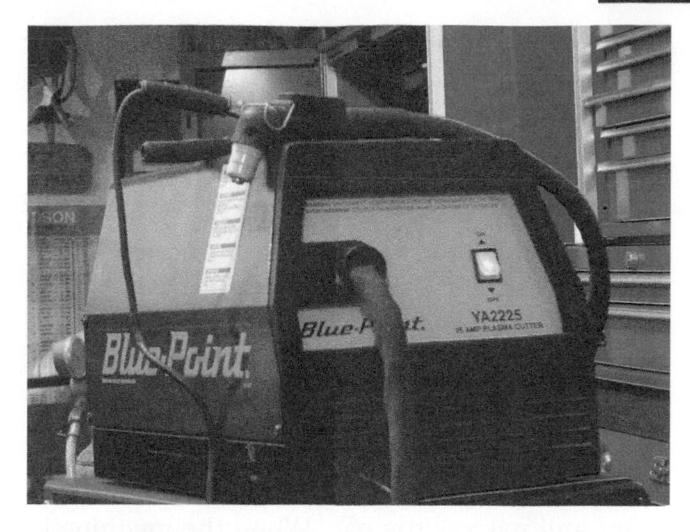

(A) The plasma arc welder is designed to rapidly cut metal using electric arc.

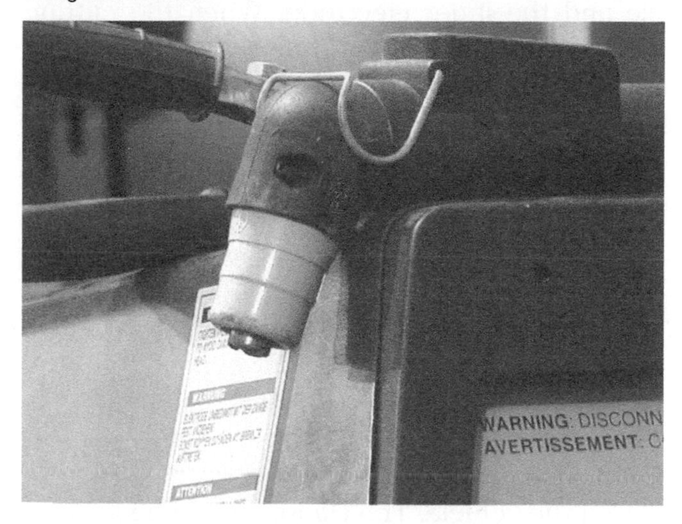

(B) The plasma arc cutting tip directs compress air over the cutting arc to rapidly melt and remove molten metal.

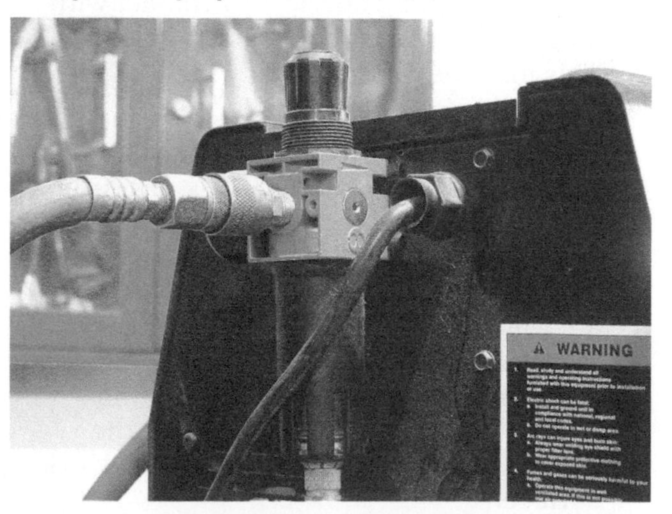

(C) Note how the shop air hose connects to the pressure regulator-filter on the back of the plasma arc cutting machine.

Figure 8–24. Study the major parts of the plasma arc cutting machine. (Courtesy of Snap-on Tools Corp.)

Plasma arc cutting is replacing oxyacetylene as the best way to cut metals. It cuts damaged metal effectively and quickly but will NOT destroy the properties of the base metal. The old method of flame cutting just does not work that well anymore.

In plasma arc cutting, compressed air is often used for both shielding and cutting. As a shielding gas, air covers the outside area of the torch nozzle, cooling the area so the torch does not overheat.

Air also becomes the cutting gas. It swirls around the electrode as it heads toward the nozzle opening. The swirling action helps to constrict and narrow the gas. When the machine is turned on, a pilot arc is formed between the nozzle and the inner electrode. When the cutting gas reaches this pilot arc, it is super-heated—up to 60,000°F (3,298°C). Look at **Figure 8–25.**

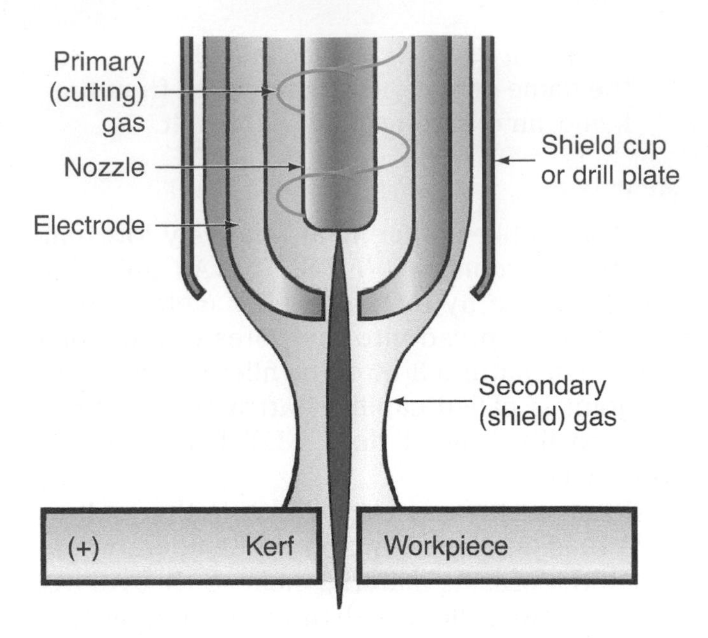

Figure 8–25. Study plasma arc cutting process.

Operating a Plasma Arc Cutter

To operate a typical plasma arc cutter, proceed as follows:

1. Connect the unit to a clean, dry source of compressed air with a minimum line pressure of 60 psi at the air connection.
2. Connect the torch and ground clamp to the unit. After plugging the machine in, connect the ground clamp to a clean metal surface on the vehicle. The clamp should be as close as possible to the area to be cut.
3. Move the cutting nozzle into contact with an electrically conductive part of the work. This must be done to satisfy the work safety circuit.
4. Hold the plasma torch so that the cutting nozzle is perpendicular to the work surface. Push the plasma torch down. This will force the cutting nozzle down until it comes in contact with the electrode. Then the plasma arc will start. Release downward force on the torch to let the cutting nozzle return to its normal position. While keeping the cutting nozzle in light contact with the work, drag the gun lightly across the work surface.
5. Move the plasma torch in the direction the metal is to be cut. The speed of the cut will depend on the thickness of the metal. If the torch is moved too fast, it will not cut all the way through. If moved too slowly, it will put too much heat into the workpiece and might also extinguish the plasma arc.

SUMMARY

- A weld is formed when separate pieces of material are fused together through the application of heat. The heat must be high enough to cause the melting of the pieces to be joined.
- Metal inert gas (MIG) welding is a wire-feed fusion welding process commonly used in collision repair. Tungsten inert gas (TIG) is generally used in automotive engine rebuilding shops to repair cracks in aluminum cylinder heads and in reconstructing combustion chambers but has very limited applications in collision repair.
- The major parts of a MIG welder are power supply, welding gun, weld cable, electrode wire, wire feeder, shielding gas, regulator, and wire clamp.
- The types of MIG welds are tack, continuous, butt, fillet, and plug welds.
- Plasma arc cutting creates an intensely hot air stream over a very small area, which melts and removes metal. It is replacing oxyacetylene torches as the best way to cut metals.

TECHNICAL TERMS

weld
base material
filler material
weld root
weld face
weld penetration
burn mark
burn-through
weld legs
weld throat
joint fit-up
fusion welding
metal inert gas (MIG)
tungsten inert gas (TIG)
gas metal arc welding (GMAW)
high-strength steels (HSS)
oxyacetylene welding
squeeze-type resistance spot welding
hybrid bonding
weld bonding
rivet bonding
shielding gas
welder amperage rating
duty cycle
MIG welding gun
MIG contact tip
antispatter compound
heat setting
voltage
travel speed
travel direction
push welding
pull welding
wire stick-out
gun angle
straight polarity
reverse polarity
tack weld
continuous weld
skip welding
stitch welding
butt welds
insert
backing strip
fillet weld
lap joints
plug weld
flat welding
horizontal welding
vertical welding
overhead welding
welding filter lens
self-darkening filter lenses
weld-through primer
wire speed
gas flow rate
heat sink compound
arm sets
electrode tips
visual weld inspection
destructive testing
weld porosity
weld cracks
weld distortion
weld spatter
weld undercut
weld overlap
heat crayons
thermal paint
oxyacetylene welding outfit
cylinders
regulators
hoses
torch
oxygen pressure
acetylene pressure
welding torch
cutting torch
spark lighter
neutral flame
carburizing flame
oxidizing flame
brazing
soft brazing
soldering
hard brazing
plasma arc cutting

REVIEW QUESTIONS

1. Explain the difference between a welding base material and a filler material.
2. Define the term "weld penetration." How can you tell if it is correct?
3. List ten advantages of MIG welding.
4. This term refers to metals NOT containing iron.
   a. Nonalloy
   b. Alloy
   c. Nonferrous
   d. Ferrous
5. The ______________ protects the contact tip and directs the shielding gas flow.
6. This type of welding gas combines with the weld to contribute to weld quality.
   a. Inert gas
   b. Active gas
   c. Biodegradable gas
   d. Butane gas
7. Explain the effects of the voltage setting on a MIG welder.
8. ______________ is how fast you move the gun across the joint.
9. How does moving more slowly or quickly affect the answer in question 8?
10. Explain the difference between push and pull welding.
11. What is the difference between skip and stitch welding?
12. This is the most difficult welding position.
    a. Horizontal
    b. Vertical
    c. Flat
    d. Overhead

13. A ____________ primer is used to add zinc antirust protection to weld zones.
14. List and explain eight welding problems.

ASE-STYLE REVIEW QUESTIONS

1. A technician is practicing welding on an old panel. A loud hissing and popping sound is produced. This is normally caused by:
   a. Wire speed or feed too fast
   b. Wire speed or feed too slow
   c. Poor cable ground
   d. Wrong wire size

2. When metal inert gas (MIG) welding, the wire melts into tiny balls of molten metal that fly away from the weld. A strobe light effect is produced. What could cause this welding problem?
   a. Wire speed or feed too fast
   b. Wire speed or feed too slow
   c. Poor cable ground
   d. Wrong wire size

3. *Technician A* says that if the flow of gas is too high, it will reduce the shielding effect. *Technician B* says that if there is NOT enough gas, the shielding effect will be reduced. Who is correct?
   a. Technician A
   b. Technician B
   c. Both Technicians A and B
   d. Neither Technician

4. *Technician A* says that you should use stitch or skip welding methods to reduce heat buildup. *Technician B* says that heat sink compound will reduce the chance of panel warpage when welding. Who is correct?
   a. Technician A
   b. Technician B
   c. Both Technicians A and B
   d. Neither Technician

5. When welding aluminum, which of the following should you use to monitor heat buildup?
   a. Heat crayons
   b. Thermometer
   c. Pyrometer
   d. None of the above

6. *Technician A* says that magnesium parts should not be welded because they can begin to burn violently. *Technician B* says that magnesium is a metal that may start to burn during welding. Who is correct?
   a. Technician A
   b. Technician B
   c. Both Technicians A and B
   d. Neither Technician

7. *Technician A* says that oxyacetylene is still the most common method of welding structural panels. *Technician B* says that it should NOT be used for cleaning and heating on unibody vehicles. Who is correct?
   a. Technician A
   b. Technician B
   c. Both Technicians A and B
   d. Neither Technician

8. Which of the following processes often uses compressed air for both shielding and cutting?
   a. Oxyacetylene
   b. MIG
   c. TIG
   d. Plasma arc

ACTIVITIES

1. Visit your guidance counselor. Ask about welding courses offered in your area. Give a report to the class about your findings.
2. Practice destructive tests of welds. Make MIG and spot welds on scrap metal. Tear them apart with a hammer and chisel. Visually inspect the welds and write a report on your findings.
3. Visit a body shop. While wearing all protective gear and a helmet with an approved lens, observe experienced collision repair welders working. Write a report on what you have learned.

CHAPTER 9 Vehicle Construction

OBJECTIVES

After studying this chapter, you should be able to:

- Define the most important parts of a vehicle.
- Explain body design and frame variations.
- Compare unibody and body-over-frame construction.
- Identify the major structural parts, sections, and assemblies of body-over-frame vehicles.
- Identify the major structural parts, sections, and assemblies of unibody vehicles.
- Summarize how to classify vehicles by body, engine, and drivetrain configurations.

INTRODUCTION

Vehicle construction refers to how a vehicle is made. If you know how a vehicle is "put together" or constructed, you will be prepared to repair it properly when damaged. You must be able to identify the basic parts of a vehicle and compare design variations. This will give you the vocabulary to fully grasp information in later text chapters. So study carefully! See **Figure 9–1.**

As you will learn, the modern motor vehicle is no longer a simple "buggy with an engine." The present-day motor vehicle is a maze of interacting mechanical-electrical systems. In fact, over 15,000 parts are used in a typical vehicle. Damage to one part can affect the operation of another seemingly unrelated part. As a result, you must understand the whole vehicle and its systems to safely and effectively repair collision damaged vehicles.

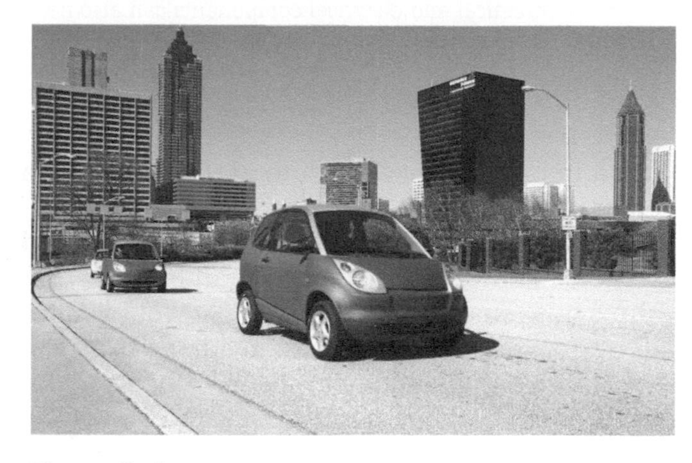

Figure 9–1. Vehicle manufacturers now use many exotic materials in the design and construction of their vehicles. This makes the job of auto body repair technician even more challenging. (Courtesy of Georgia Power)

During a collision, severe damage often occurs to the vehicle's unibody or frame structure. Depending upon the type of construction, varying methods must be used to repair the damage properly. This chapter gives you essential information that will help you understand later chapters.

CRASH TESTING

Automobile manufacturers are challenged by having to design vehicles that are light, *aerodynamic* (have low wind resistance), and are yet strong and safe.

Computer-simulated crash testing helps to determine how well a new vehicle might survive a collision. Computer-simulated testing is used before building a prototype, or first real vehicle, to find weak or faulty structural areas before investing in mass production.

It is critical that the passenger compartment is strong enough to help prevent injury to the driver and passengers. It is also important that the front and rear sections collapse

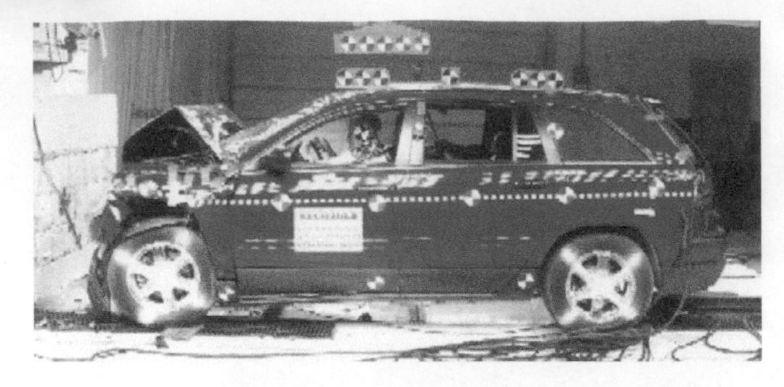

Figure 9–2. During a collision, severe structural damage often occurs to the unibody or frame near the area of impact. Mechanical and electrical components can also be damaged. (Courtesy of DaimlerChrysler Corporation)

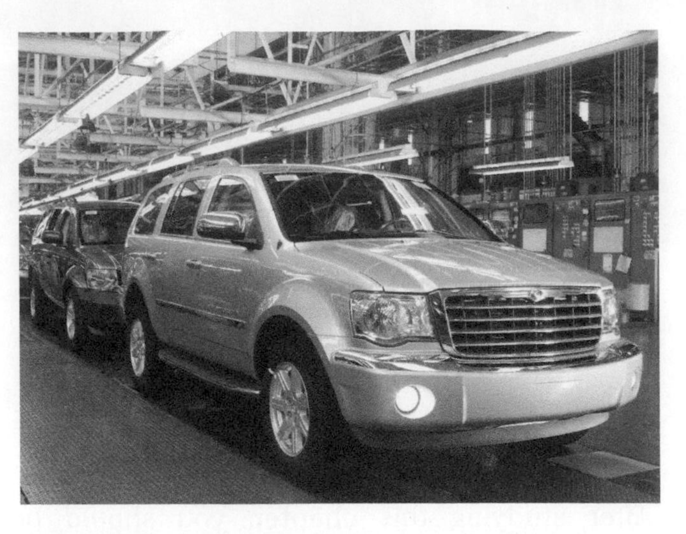

Figure 9–3. To properly repair a damaged vehicle, you must know how it is constructed. Here you can see vehicles coming off the assembly line at the factory. (Courtesy of DaimlerChrysler Corporation)

upon impact to absorb some of the energy of a collision.

Certified crash tests are done using a real vehicle and sensor-equipped dummies that show how much impact the people would suffer during a collision. Computer readings from the sensors in the dummies give feedback about each crash test for body structure evaluation.

Crush zones are built into the frame or body to collapse and absorb some of the energy of a collision. The front and rear of the vehicle collapses while the passenger compartment tends to retain its shape. This helps reduce the amount of force transmitted to the occupants. See **Figure 9–2.**

VEHICLE CLASSIFICATIONS

Vehicle classification relates to the construction, size, shape, number of doors, type of roof, and other criteria of a motor vehicle. To communicate properly in collision repair, you must understand these basic terms.

VEHICLE CONSTRUCTION

There are three main types of vehicle construction: body-over-frame, unibody, and space frame. Each has its own unique repair challenges. See **Figure 9–3.**

Parts and Components

The term *part* or **component** generally refers to the smallest units on a vehicle. An **assembly** is several parts that fit together to make up a more complex unit. For example, a car bumper assembly might be made up of several parts—bumper frame, bumper cover, bumper brackets, and so on.

A **panel** is a general term that refers to a large removable body part. For example, a quarter panel is a large body section forming the rear side of the body over and behind the rear wheels. A rocker panel would be a body part along the bottom of a door opening.

Similarly, the term **pan** referes to a floor-related component, for example, front floor pan, rear floor pan. In auto body, the names of parts usually refer to the location and purpose of the part. This makes it relatively easy to remember automotive part names.

Chassis

The **chassis** basically includes everything under the body—suspension system, brake system, wheels and tires, steering system. It consists of the mechanical systems that support and power the car.

Full Frames

Body-over-frame vehicles have separate body and chassis parts bolted to the frame. The engine and other major assemblies are mounted on the frame. This type of frame consists of two side rails connected by a series of cross-members. See **Figure 9–4.**

Most full frames are wide at the rear and narrow at the front. The narrow front construction

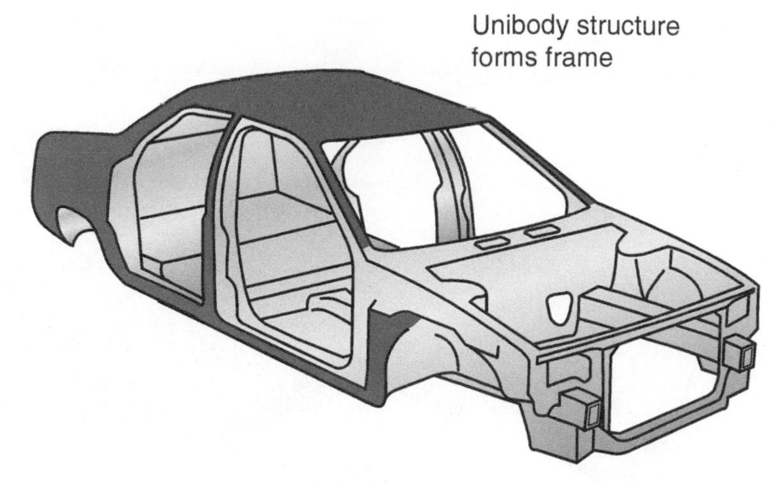
Unibody structure
forms frame

(A) Unibody construction welds major body panels together to form the frame for attaching the engine, drivetrain, suspension, and other parts. This type of construction is commonly used on cars.

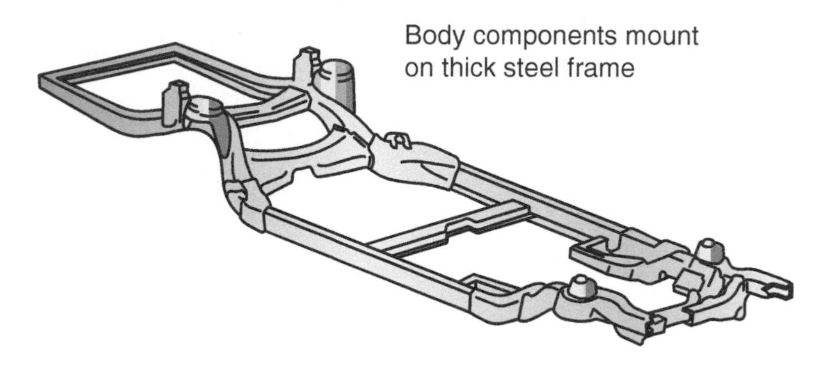
Body components mount
on thick steel frame

(B) With body-over-frame construction, a thick gauge steel frame provides the foundation for holding other parts. This type of construction is commonly used on large trucks and SUVs.

Figure 9–4. Two very different methods are used to construct modern vehicles: unibody and body-over-frame construction.

enables the front wheel to make a sharper turn. A wide frame at the rear provides better support of the body.

Other characteristics of a separate frame are:

1. A full-frame vehicle is heavier.
2. High amounts of energy are absorbed by the frame during a collision.
3. Suspension and drivetrain parts can be quickly assembled on the frame.
4. The heavy frame is made of thick sheet metal approximately ⅛ inch (3 mm) thick.

The **frame rails** are the long steel members that extend along the sides of the vehicle. The **torque boxes** are the structural parts of the frame designed to allow some twisting to absorb road shock and collision impact. The **frame horn** is the very front of the frame rails where the bumper attaches.

Crossmembers are thick metal stampings that extend sideways across the frame rails. They are often used to support the engine, suspension, and other chassis parts. **Spring hangers** are sometimes formed on the frame to hold the suspension system springs. **Rubber body insulators** are used between the frame and body to reduce noise and vibration.

Although unibody construction is the trend, body-over-frame construction is still being used. Full- or partial-frame construction is used on some full-size vehicles, most full-size pickup trucks, and some small pickups.

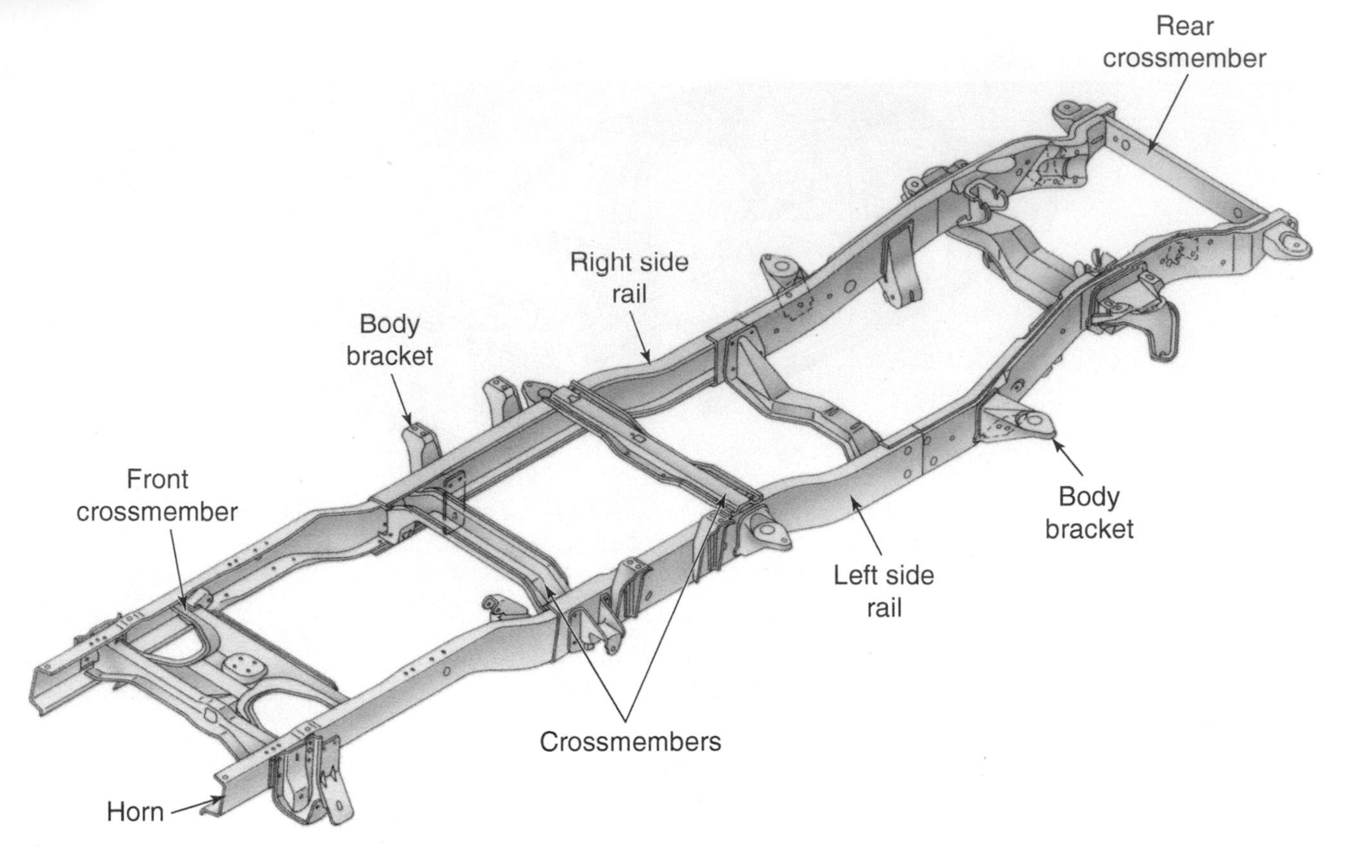

Figure 9–5. Study the parts of a full frame. (Courtesy of DaimlerChrysler Corp.)

The **frame** is an independent, separate part because it is not welded to any of the major units of the body shell. The strong side rails are normally made of U-shaped channel- or box-shaped sections. Various brackets, braces, and openings are provided for the parts of the chassis.

A **perimeter frame,** as its name implies, has the frame rail near the outside, or perimeter, of the vehicle. It is the most common type of full frame. It utilizes full-length side rails with torque boxes in the four corners of the center section. A perimeter frame has good side impact strength. See **Figure 9–5.**

A **ladder frame** has long frame rails with a series of straight crossmembers formed in several locations. It is a seldom used modification of the perimeter frame.

A **partial frame** is a cross between a solid frame and a unibody. **Sub-frame assemblies** are used at the front and rear while the unibody supports the middle area of the vehicle. The sub-frame is used to support the suspension and drivetrain.

Unibody Construction

Unibody construction uses body parts that are welded and bolted together to form an integral vehicle. No separate heavy-gauge steel frame under the body is needed. In unibody designs, heavy-gauge, cold-rolled steels have been replaced with lighter, thinner, high-strength steel alloys or aluminum alloy. See **Figure 9–6.**

The concept of unibody construction first proved successful in the aircraft industry, where lightweight, high-strength fuselages were needed. Adapted to the auto industry, unitized construction eliminated the need for a separate, rigid frame. The strength and rigidity of the vehicle was integrated into the body shell. See **Figure 9–7.**

The body shell is formed by welding sheet metal into a box- or egg-like configuration. Strength is achieved through shape and design of the individual parts instead of their mass and weight. The entire inner structure works together for structural integrity.

The eggshell concept is an ideal model for understanding the principle of unibody design.

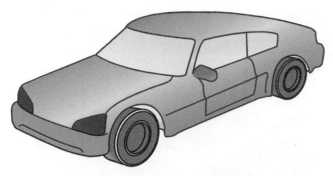

(A) The outer body provides an attractive painted covering for the vehicle.

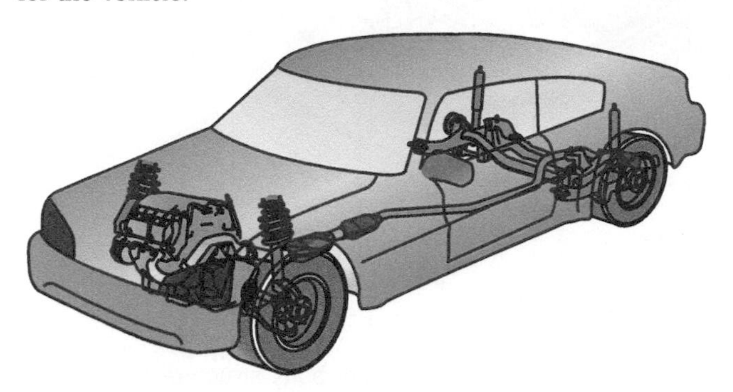

(B) This phantom view shows how internal parts fit inside the unibody vehicle.

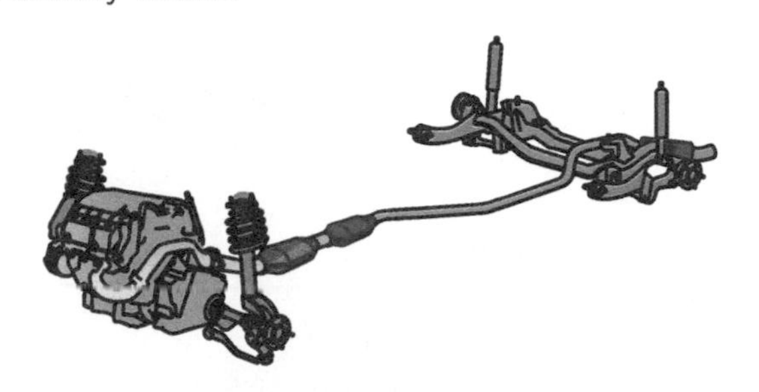

(C) The powertrain or drivetrain fastens to the unibody at the frame rails and other reinforced body points.

Figure 9–6. These photos show the major construction of a unibody vehicle.

Even when pressing hard on an eggshell, it is comparatively difficult to destroy its thin structure. All the force applied by your finger is not concentrated in one place but is dispersed over the shell surface. In engineering, this concept is called a **stressed hull structure.**

Space Frame

Similar to a unibody, a **space frame** vehicle has a metal body structure covered with an outer skin of plastic or composite panels. It is a relatively new type of vehicle construction. Quite often, the roof and quarter panels are not welded to the structure as they are with traditional unibodies. Exterior body panels are attached with mechanical fasteners or adhesives. See **Figure 9–8.**

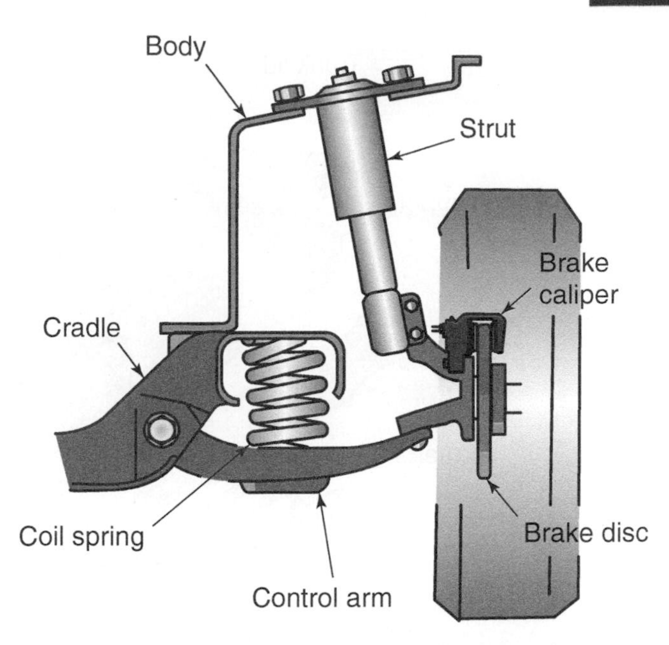

Figure 9–7. The suspension and braking systems bolt directly to the body on a vehicle with unitized construction.

After a collision, a space frame is more likely to have hidden damage because of the ability of plastic panels to hide more severe damage. Rust protection is also important since the plastic body panels may look good but the hidden metal frame structure may become deteriorated.

Basically, unibody vehicles are made up of numerous simple parts. Single-layer stamped steel panels, channels, and boxed or closed steel sections form the unibody.

Support members are often bolted to the bottom of the unibody to hold the engine, transmission, and suspension in alignment. They are needed in high-stress areas to reduce body flex.

JOINING PARTS

Stationary parts, like the floor, roof, and quarter panels, are permanently welded or adhesive bonded into place. **Hinged parts,** like doors, hood, and deck lids, will swing up and open.

Fastened parts are held together with various fasteners (bolts, nuts, clips, etc.). Many parts, like the fenders, hood, and grille, bolt into place. These bolted-on parts also add to the strength of the vehicle.

Welded parts are permanently joined by melting the material so that it flows together and bonds when cooled. Both metal and plastic parts can be welded.

Press-fit or **snap-fit parts** use clips or an interference fit to hold parts together. This assembly method is becoming more common to

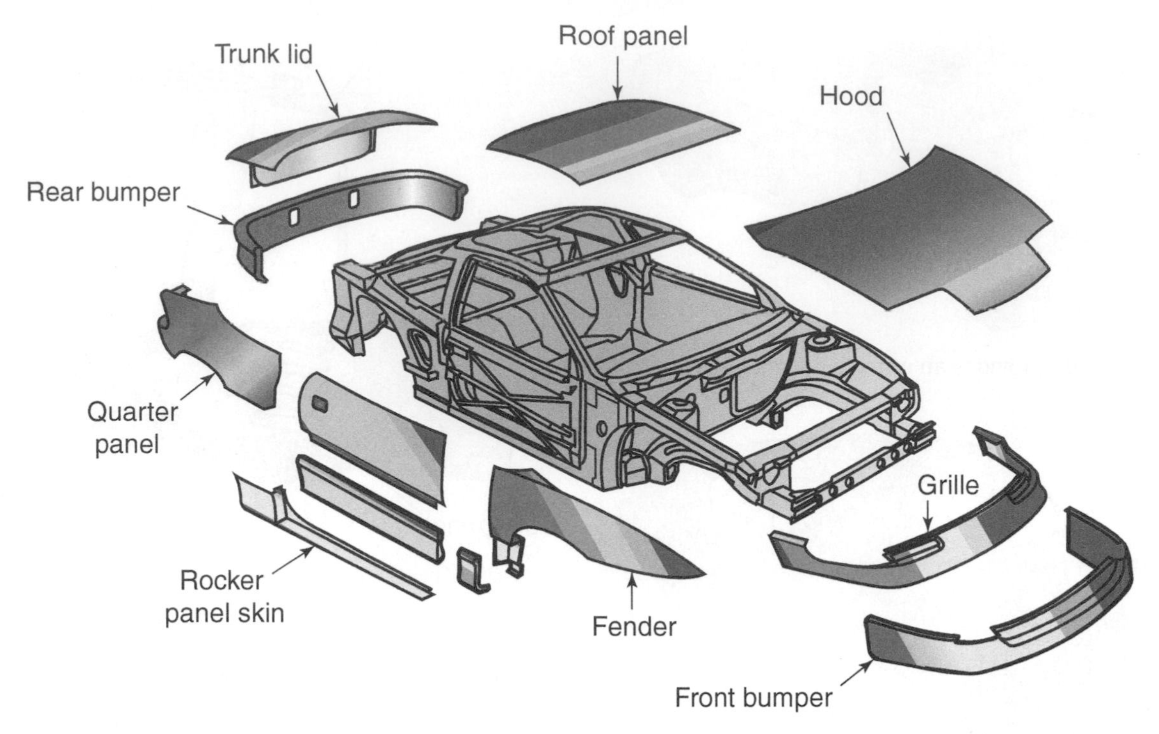

Figure 9–8. Note the space frame construction. Composite (plastic) panels fasten to a metal inner body structure. Composite panels can be made flexible to resist door dings and small dents.

reduce manufacturing costs. Grilles, bumper covers, inner door trim, and other nonstructural parts may use clips to snap into place.

Adhesive-bonded parts use a high-strength epoxy or special glue to hold the parts together. Both metal and plastic parts can be adhesive joined. **Structural adhesive** can also be used to bond parts together. See **Figure 9–9.**

A **composite unibody** is made of plastics and other materials, like carbon fiber, to form the vehicle. The frame is made totally of plastics or other composite materials, keeping metal parts to a minimum. This cuts weight while increasing strength, rigidity, performance, and fuel economy. Although this type of vehicle is not being mass produced, several manufacturers are experimenting with composite unibody construction.

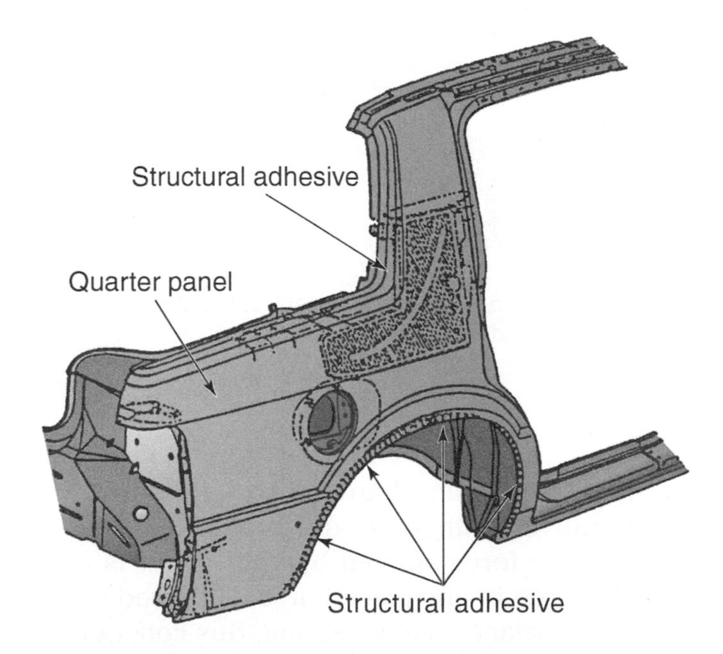

Figure 9–9. Structural adhesives are commonly used to help hold parts securely together. Adhesive helps make body structure quieter and stronger. (Courtesy of DaimlerChrysler Corp.)

MAJOR BODY SECTIONS

For simplicity and to help communication in collision repair, a vehicle is commonly divided into **three body sections**—front, center, and rear. It is important to understand how these sections are constructed to properly repair them. Study **Figure 9–10.**

The **front section,** also called **nose** *section,* includes everything between the front bumper and the fire wall. The bumper, grille, frame rails, front suspension parts, and, usually, the engine are a few of the items included in the front section of a vehicle.

The nickname "front clip" or "doghouse" is used to refer to the front body section. Front

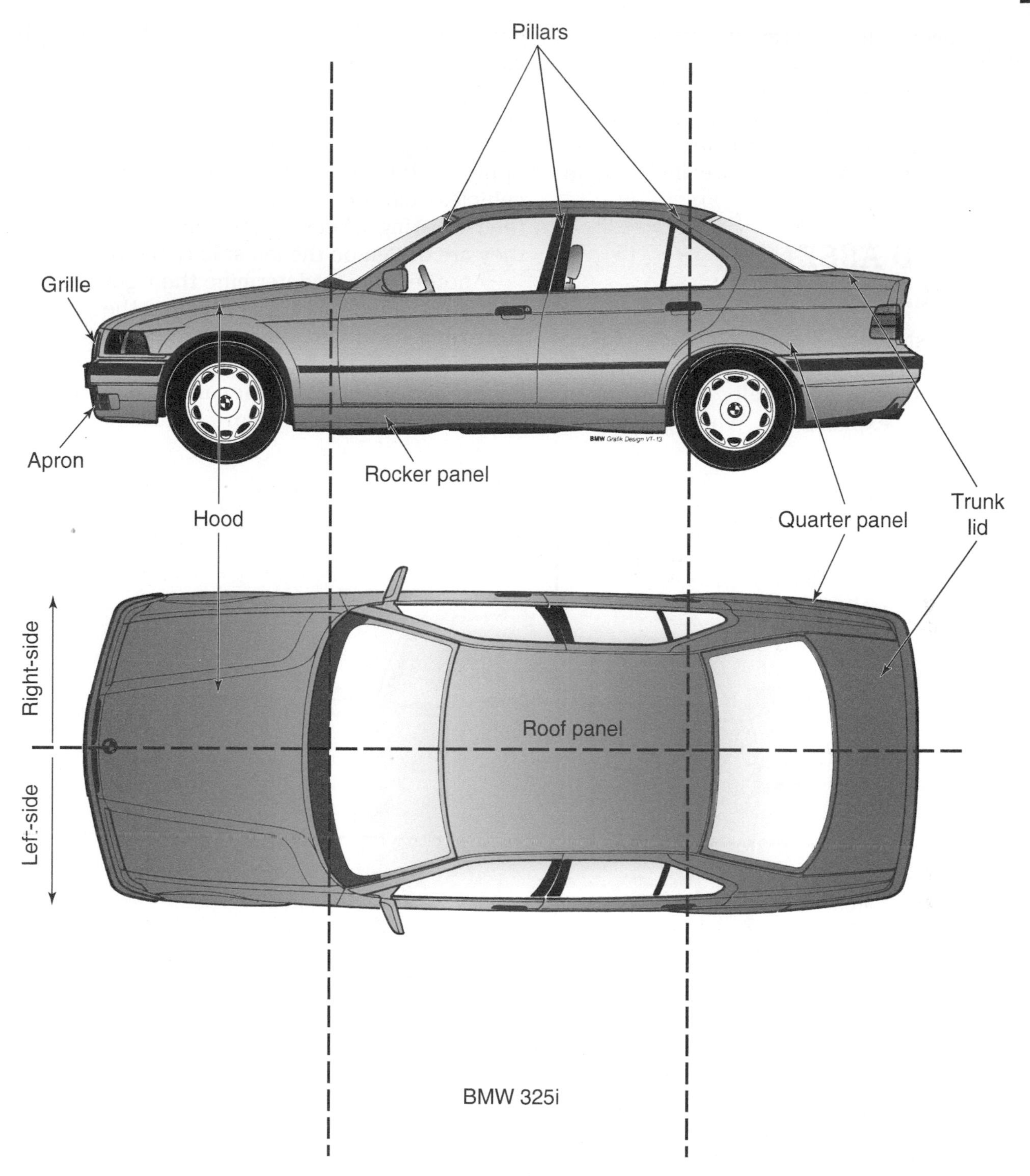

Figure 9–10. The vehicle is divided into three major sections for better communication. Study the parts included in each section. (Courtesy of BMW of North America)

sections are often purchased in one piece from an **automotive recycler** or "salvage yard." The empty engine compartment forms the "doghouse."

The **center section** or *midsection* typically includes the body parts that form the passenger compartment. A few parts in this section include the floor pan, roof panel, cowl, doors, door pillars, glass, and related parts. A slang name for the center section is the "greenhouse" because it is surrounded by glass.

The **rear section,** *tail section,* or *rear clip,* commonly consists of the rear quarter panels, trunk or rear floor pan, rear frame rails, trunk or deck lid, rear bumper, and related parts. Also called the "cathouse," it is often sectioned or cut off of a salvaged vehicle to repair severe rear impact damage.

When discussing collision repair, repair personnel often refer to these sections of the vehicle. It simplifies communication because everyone knows which parts are included in each section.

PANEL AND ASSEMBLY NOMENCLATURE

A *panel* is a stamped steel or molded plastic sheet that forms a body part. Various panels are used in a vehicle. Usually, the name of the panel is self-explanatory. When panels are joined with other components, the result is called an *assembly*.

The **vehicle left side** is the steering wheel side on vehicles built for American roads. The **vehicle right side** is the passenger side or side opposite the steering wheel. Remember that vehicles built for other countries will often have their steering wheel on the right side because they are driven on the left side of the road.

Another way to determine the right and left sides of a vehicle is to stand behind the vehicle. Your right hand would be on the right side and left hand would be on the left side of the vehicle. Panels and parts are often called out as left or right side, as shown in **Figure 9–11.**

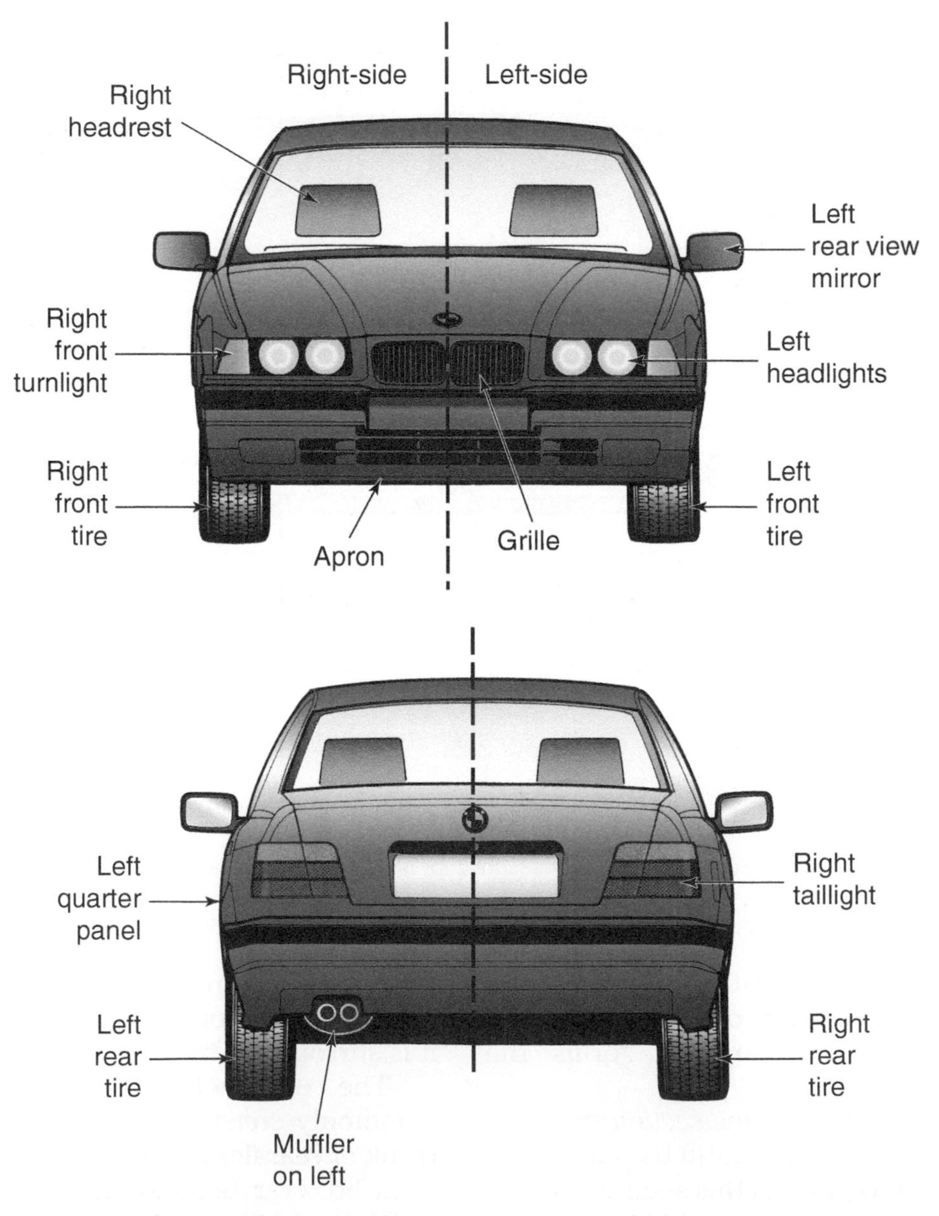

Figure 9–11. Note the names of parts in the front and rear sections of the vehicle. (Courtesy of BMW of North America)

FRONT SECTION PARTS

The *frame rails* are the box frame members extending out near the bottom of the front section. They are usually the strongest part of a unibody.

The **cowl** is near the rear of the front section, right in front of the windshield. This includes the top cowl panel and side cowl panels.

The **front fender aprons** are inner panels that surround the wheels and tires to keep out road debris. They often bolt or weld to the frame rails and cowl.

The **shock towers** or **strut towers** are reinforced body areas for holding the upper parts of the suspension system. The coil springs, and strut or shock absorbers fit up into the shock towers. They are normally formed as part of the inner fender apron. See **Figure 9–12.**

The **radiator core support** is the framework around the front of the body structure for holding the cooling system radiator and related parts. It often fastens to the frame rails and inner fender aprons.

The **hood** is a hinged panel for accessing the engine compartment (front-engine vehicle) or trunk area (rear-engine vehicle). See **Figure 9–13. Hood hinges,** bolted to the hood and cowl panel, allow the hood to swing open. The hood is normally made of two or more panels welded or bonded together to prevent flexing and vibration.

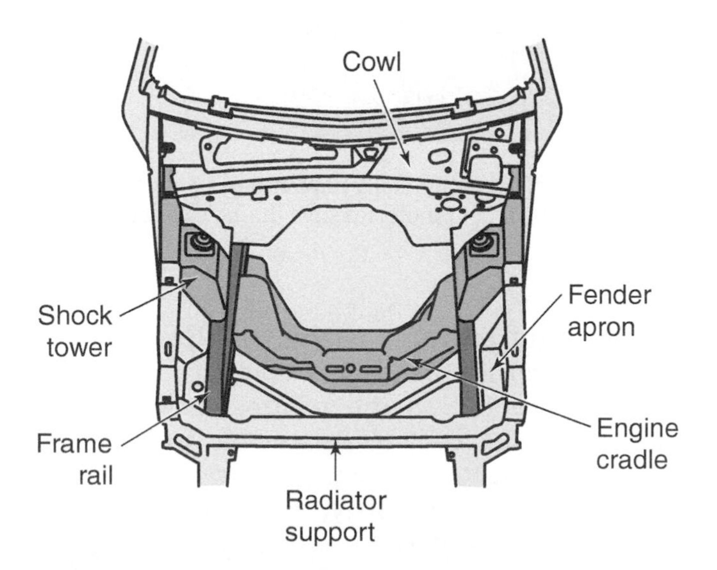

Figure 9–12. This top view of unibody construction shows how structural members are added to support the engine, suspension, and other mechanical systems.

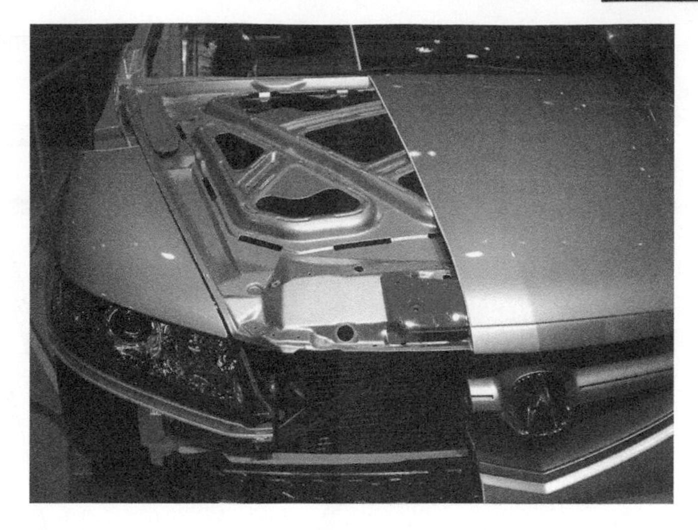

Figure 9–13. A cutaway of a hood panel shows how inner structural panels are used to reduce flex and vibration.

The **dash panel,** sometimes termed **fire wall** or **front bulkhead,** is the panel dividing the front section and the center passenger compartment section. It normally welds in place.

The **front fenders** extend from the front doors to the front bumper. They cover the front suspension and inner aprons. They normally bolt into place around their perimeter.

The **bumper assembly** bolts to the front frame horns or rails to absorb minor impacts.

CENTER SECTION PARTS

The **floor pan** is the main structural section in the bottom of the passenger compartment.

With front-wheel drive vehicles, the floor pan can be relatively flat. With rear-wheel drive vehicles, a **tunnel** is formed in the floor pan for the transmission and drive shaft. The drive shaft needs room to extend back to the rear axle assembly.

Pillars are vertical body members that hold the roof panel in place and protect in case of a rollover accident. See **Figure 9–14.**

The **front pillars** extend up next to the edges of the windshield. They must be strong to protect the passengers. Also termed **A-pillars,** they are steel box members that extend down from the roof panel to the main body section.

Center pillars or **B-pillars** are the roof supports between the front and rear doors on four-door vehicles. They help strengthen the roof and provide a mounting point for the rear door hinges.

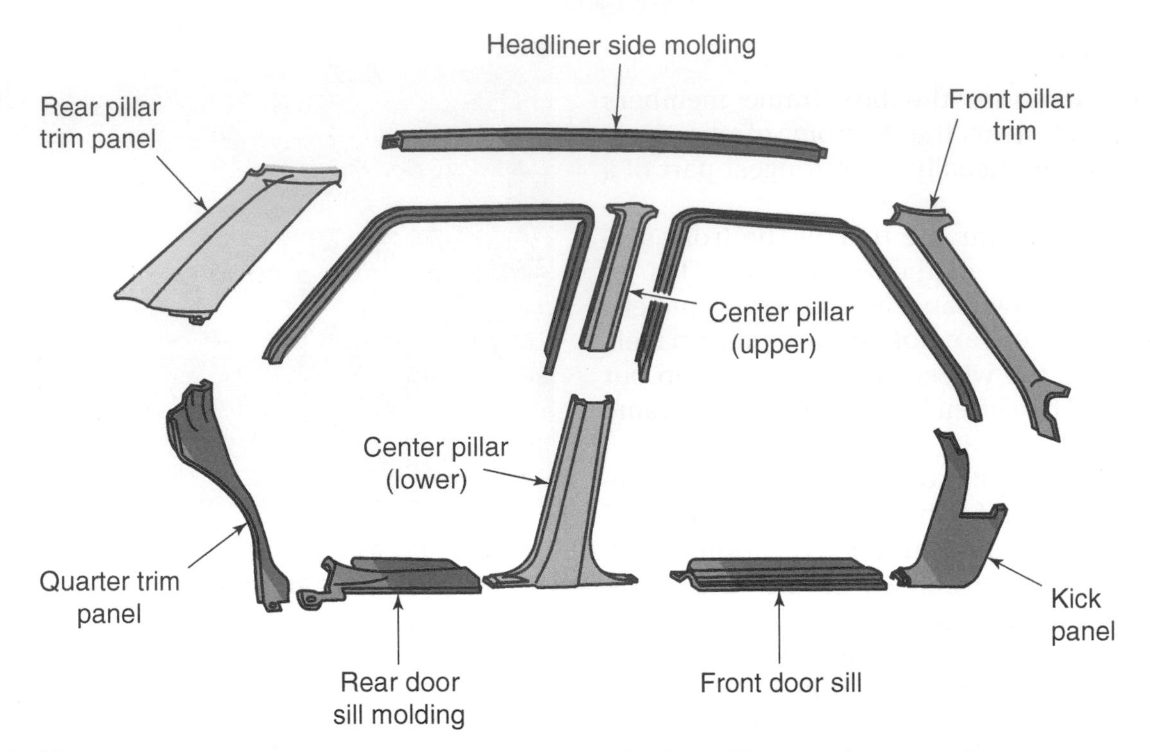

Figure 9–14. Pillars hold the roof in place and provide openings for doors. They must be extremely strong to protect the driver and passengers of a vehicle.

Rear pillars extend up from the quarter panels to hold the rear of the roof and rear window glass. Also called **C-pillars,** their shape can vary with body style.

Rocker panels or **door sills** are strong beams that fit at the bottom of the door openings. They normally are welded to the floor pan and to the pillars, kick panels, or quarter panels. The **kick panels** are small panels between the front pillars and rocker panels.

The **rear shelf** or **package tray** is a thin panel behind the rear seat and in front of the back glass. It often has openings for the rear speakers. The **rear bulkhead panel** separates the passenger compartment from the rear trunk area.

The *doors* are complex assemblies made up of an outer skin, inner door frame, door panel, window regulator, glass, and related parts. **Door hinges** bolt between the pillars and door frame. The **window regulator** is a gear mechanism that allows you to raise and lower the door glass.

Side impact beams are metal bars or corrugated panels that bolt or weld inside the door assemblies to protect the passengers. They prevent the door from opening upon impact and help protect the passenger area, as shown in **Figure 9–15.**

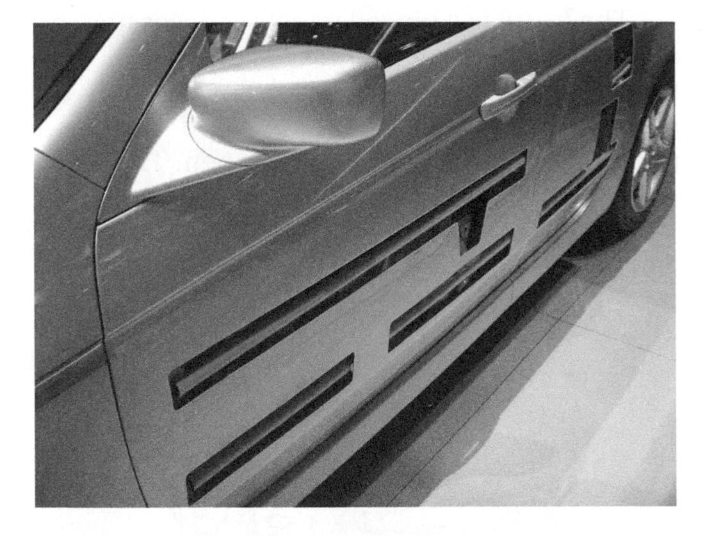

Figure 9–15. Doors normally have strong steel beams under the door skin to protect people during side impact collisions.

The **roof panel** is a large multipiece panel that fits over the passenger compartment. It is normally welded to the pillars. Sometimes it includes a sun roof or removable top pieces, termed T-tops.

The **dash assembly,** sometimes termed **instrument panel,** is the assembly including the soft dash pad, instrument cluster, radio, heater and A/C controls, vents, and similar parts.

REAR SECTION PARTS

The **trunk floor panel** is a stamped steel part that forms the bottom of the rear storage compartment. Quite often, the spare tire fits down into this stamped panel. It often welds to the rear rails, inner wheel houses, and lower rear panel.

The **deck lid,** or **trunk lid,** is a hinged panel over the rear storage compartment. A **rear hatch** is a larger panel and glass assembly hinged for more access to the rear of the vehicle. See **Figure 9–16.**

The **quarter panels** are the large, side body sections that extend from the side doors back to the rear bumper. They are welded in place and form a vital part of the rear body structure.

The **lower rear panel** fits between the trunk compartment and the rear bumper between the quarter panels.

Rear shock towers hold the top of the rear suspension. The **inner wheel housings** surround the rear wheels.

GASKETS AND SEALS

Various **gaskets** and **rubber seals** are used to prevent air and water leakage between body parts. Seals or **weatherstripping** are often used around doors and the rear deck lid. The rubber seal is partially compressed when the door or lid is closed to form a leakproof connection. Another example, a rubber gasket often seals the stationary glass where it fits into the body.

ANTICORROSION MATERIALS

Anticorrosion materials are used to prevent rusting of metal parts. Various types of anticorrosion materials are available. For example, **undercoating** is often a thick tar or synthetic rubber-based material sprayed onto the underbody of the vehicle. After performing repairs, you must restore all corrosion protection. See **Figure 9–17.**

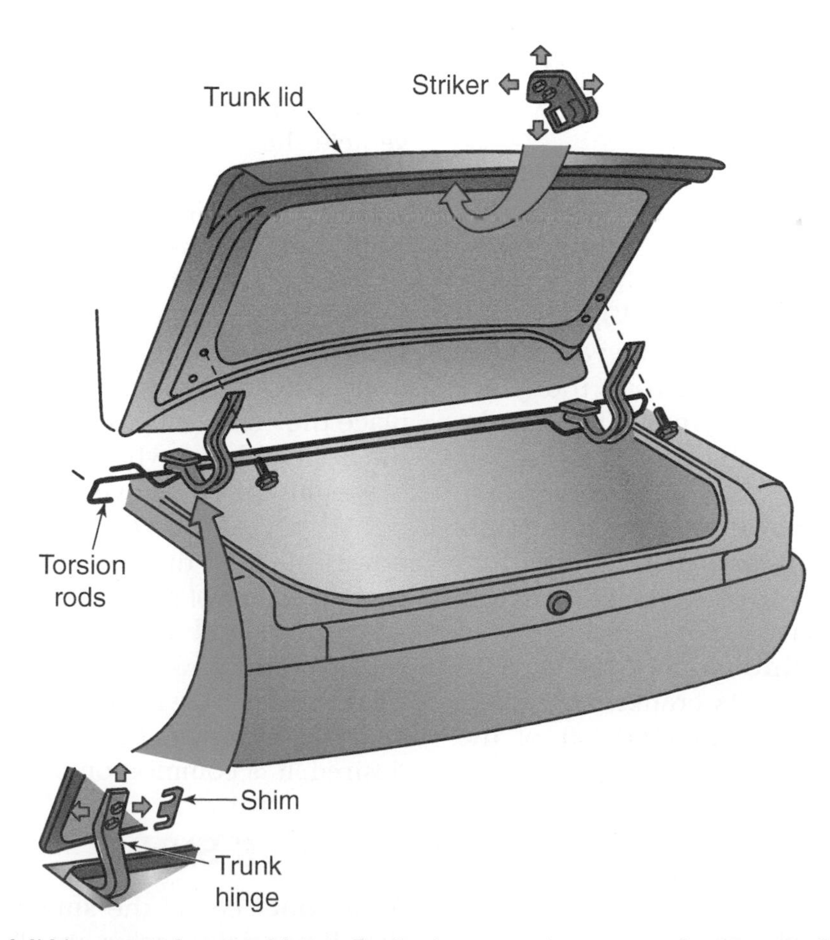

Figure 9–16. The deck lid is mounted on two hinges. Torsion bars or springs are used to keep the lid open when needed. The striker engages the latch to keep the lid closed.

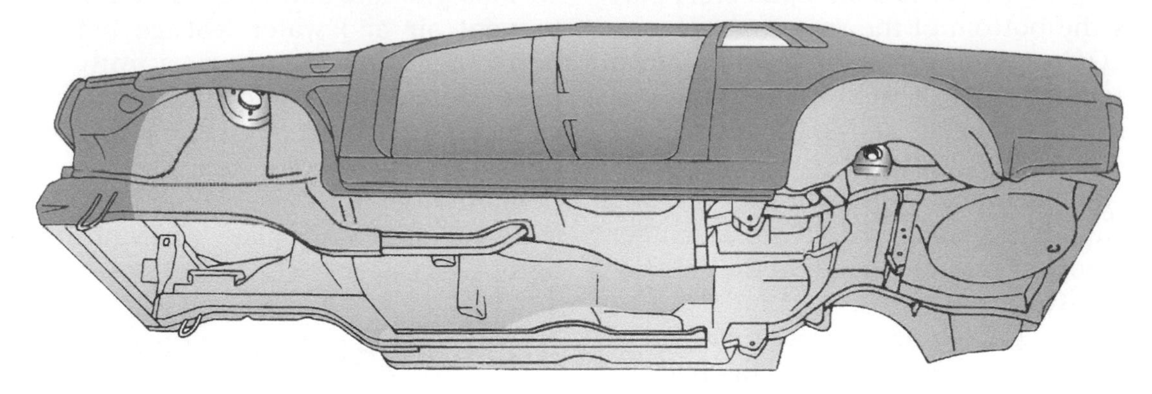

Figure 9–17. Anticorrosion materials are applied to body panels to keep them from rusting due to exposure to road salt, water, and other debris. (Courtesy of Nissan North America, Inc.)

SOUND-DEADENING MATERIALS

Sound-deadening materials are used to help quiet the passenger compartment. They are insulation materials that prevent engine and road noise from entering the passenger area.

ENGINE LOCATIONS, DRIVELINES

There are four basic drivetrain designs: front-wheel drive (FWD), rear-wheel drive (RWD), rear-engine, rear-wheel drive (RRW), and mid-engine, rear-wheel drive (MRD). The vast majority of unibody vehicles on the road today are FWD with the engine in the front. These variations affect vehicle construction and repair methods.

A **longitudinal engine** mounts the crankshaft centerline front-to-rear when viewed from the top. Front-engine, RWD vehicles use this type of engine mounting.

A **transverse engine** mounts sideways in the engine compartment. Its crankshaft centerline extends toward the right and left of the body. Both front-engine and rear-engine vehicles use this configuration.

A **front-engine, front-wheel drive (FWD)** vehicle has both the engine and transaxle in the front. Constant velocity (CV) axles extend out from the transaxle to power the front drive wheels. This is one of the most common configurations.

A **front-engine, rear-wheel drive (RWD)** vehicle has the engine in the front and the drive axle in the rear. The transmission is often right behind the engine and a drive shaft transfers power back to the rear axle. A few vehicles have the engine in the front and the transmission in the rear, however.

A **rear-engine, rear-wheel drive (RRD)** vehicle has the engine in the back and a transaxle transfers power to the rear drive wheels. Traction upon acceleration and cornering is good because the weight of the engine and transaxle are over the rear drive wheels.

A **mid-engine, rear-wheel drive (MRD)** vehicle has the engine located right behind the front seat, or centrally located. This helps to place the center of gravity in the middle so that the front and rear wheels hold the same amount of weight. This improves cornering ability.

All-wheel drive uses two differentials to power all four drive wheels. This is used on several makes of passenger vehicles.

Four-wheel drive systems use a transfer case to send power to two differentials and all wheels. The transfer case can be engaged and disengaged to select two- or four-wheel drive as desired. It is common on off-road vehicles.

VEHICLE SIZES

A **compact car** is the smallest body classification. It normally uses a small, 4-cylinder engine, is very lightweight, and gets the highest gas mileage.

An **intermediate car** is medium in size. It can use a 4-, 6-, or 8-cylinder engine and has average weight and physical dimensions. It usually has unibody construction, but a few vehicles have body-over-frame construction.

A **full-size car** is the largest classification. It is large, heavy, and often uses a high performance V8 engine. Full-size cars can have either unibody or body-over-frame construction.

ROOF DESIGNS

A **sedan** refers to a body design with a center pillar that supports the roof. Sedans come in both 2- and 4-door versions.

A **hardtop** does not have a center pillar to support the roof. The roof must be reinforced to provide enough strength. A hardtop is also available in both 2- and 4-door versions.

A **hatchback** has a large third door at the back. This design is commonly found on small compact cars so that more rear storage space is available.

A **convertible** uses a retractable canvas roof with a steel tube framework. The top folds down into an area behind the seat. Some convertibles use a removable hardtop.

A **station wagon** extends the roof straight back to the rear of the body. A rear hatch or window and **tailgate** open to allow access to the large storage area.

VANS AND TRUCKS

A **van** has a large box-shaped body to increase interior volume or space. A full-size van normally is front-engine, RWD. A **minivan** is smaller and often uses front-engine, FWD with unibody construction.

A **pickup truck** normally has a separate cab and bed. A front-engine, RWD is typical.

SUMMARY

- Vehicle classification relates to the construction, size, shape, number of doors, type of roof, and other criteria of a motor vehicle.
- There are three main types of vehicle frame construction: body-over-frame, unibody, and space frame. Each has its own unique repair challenges.
- A vehicle is commonly divided into three body sections:
  1. Front, or nose, section
  2. Center section, or midsection
  3. Rear section, tail section, or rear clip
- The three vehicle sizes are compact, intermediate, and full size.

TECHNICAL TERMS

certified crash tests
crush zones
vehicle classification
component
assembly
panel
pan
chassis
body-over-frame
frame rails
torque boxes
frame horn
crossmembers
spring hangers
rubber body insulators
frame
perimeter frame
ladder frame
partial frame
sub-frame assemblies
unibody
stressed hull structure
space frame
support members
stationary parts
hinged parts
fastened parts
welded parts
snap-fit parts
adhesive-bonded parts
structural adhesive
composite unibody
three body sections
front section
automotive recycler
center section
rear section
vehicle left side
vehicle right side
cowl
front fender aprons
shock towers
strut towers
radiator core support
hood
hood hinges
dash panel
fire wall
front bulkhead
front fenders
bumper assembly
floor pan
tunnel
pillars
front pillars
A-pillars
center pillars
B-pillars
rear pillars
C-pillars
rocker panels
door sills

kick panels
rear shelf
package tray
rear bulkhead panel
door hinges
window regulator
side impact beams
roof panel
dash assembly
instrument panel
trunk floor panel
deck lid
trunk lid
rear hatch
quarter panels
lower rear panel
rear shock towers
inner wheel housings
gaskets
rubber seals
weatherstripping
anticorrosion materials
undercoating
sound-deadening materials
longitudinal engine
transverse engine
front-engine, front-wheel drive (FWD)
front-engine, rear-wheel drive (RWD)
rear-engine, rear-wheel drive (RRD)
mid-engine, rear-wheel drive (MRD)
all-wheel drive
four-wheel drive
compact car
intermediate car
full-size car
sedan
hardtop
hatchback
convertible
station wagon
tailgate
van
minivan
pickup truck

REVIEW QUESTIONS

1. How many parts are used in a typical vehicle?
   a. 1,000
   b. 10,000
   c. 15,000
   d. 50,000
2. ______________ are built into the frame or unibody to collapse and absorb collision energy.
3. What are three main types of vehicle construction?
4. Describe some characteristics of a separate frame.
5. ______________ are used between the frame and body to reduce noise and vibration.
6. What is a perimeter frame?
7. Explain how the concept of unibody construction was first developed.
8. What is a space frame?
9. A vehicle has been hit in the front. The front section must be replaced. *Technician A* says to call automotive recyclers or salvage yards to find a front clip. *Technician B* says to order new parts to ensure a good repair. Who is correct?
   a. Technician A
   b. Technician B
   c. Both Technicians A and B
   d. Neither Technician
10. Describe the term "doghouse."
11. How do you tell the right and left side of a vehicle?
12. This is the area at the rear of the front section, right in front of the windshield.
   a. Kick panel
   b. Crossmember
   c. Side panel
   d. Cowl
13. What is the difference between FWD and RWD vehicles regarding the floor pan?
14. This part helps strengthen the roof and provide a mounting point for the rear door hinges.
   a. A-pillar
   b. B-pillar
   c. C-pillar
   d. D-pillar
15. The ______________ are the large, side body sections that extend from the side doors back to the rear bumper. They are welded in place and form a vital part of the rear body structure.

ASE-STYLE REVIEW QUESTIONS

1. *Technician A* says that the "right side" of the vehicle is determined as if you were sitting in the driver seat. *Technician B* says that the "right side" of the vehicle is determined as if

you were standing in front of the vehicle looking back. Who is correct?

a. Technician A
b. Technician B
c. Both Technicians A and B
d. Neither Technician

2. *Technician A* says that the body-over-frame construction of a vehicle has separate body and chassis parts bolted to the frame. *Technician B* says that unibody construction uses body parts that are welded and bolted together to form an integral vehicle. Who is correct?

a. Technician A
b. Technician B
c. Both Technicians A and B
d. Neither Technician

3. *Technician A* says that space frame construction uses a perimeter frame to strengthen the body. *Technician B* says that space frame construction has a metal body structure covered with an outer skin of plastic or composite panels. Who is correct?

a. Technician A
b. Technician B
c. Both Technicians A and B
d. Neither Technician

4. Which of the following methods of joining parts is not used on a unibody construction vehicle?

a. Bolts
b. Welding
c. Pop rivets
d. Adhesive bonding

5. *Technician A* says that unibody parts can be single layer, hat channel, box, or other shapes. *Technician B* says that unibody parts can be flat steel, box, or open hat channel shapes. Who is correct?

a. Technician A
b. Technician B
c. Both Technicians A and B
d. Neither Technician

6. *Technician A* says that a space frame vehicle is less safe because it has plastic body parts. *Technician B* says that unibody construction uses heavier steel welded together to make it stronger because there is no real frame. Who is correct?

a. Technician A
b. Technician B
c. Both Technicians A and B
d. Neither Technician

7. *Technician A* says that a unibody-constructed vehicle is divided into four sections (front, driver, passenger, and rear). *Technician B* says that a unibody-constructed vehicle is divided into three sections (front, center, and rear). Who is correct?

a. Technician A
b. Technician B
c. Both Technicians A and B
d. Neither Technician

8. *Technician A* says that a good paint is all that is needed to protect the vehicle from corrosion following a collision repair. *Technician B* says that gaskets and seals are used to prevent air and water leakage. Who is correct?

a. Technician A
b. Technician B
c. Both Technicians A and B
d. Neither Technician

9. All-wheel drive:

a. Can be engaged and disengaged to select four- or two-wheel drive
b. Uses a transfer case
c. Is used on large trucks for more traction
d. Has all four wheels engaged at all times

10. *Technician A* says that a hardtop is a body design that does not have a center pillar that supports the roof. *Technician B* says that a sedan is a body design that does not have a center pillar that supports the roof. Who is correct?

a. Technician A
b. Technician B
c. Both Technicians A and B
d. Neither Technician

ACTIVITIES

1. Have a class discussion comparing the advantages and disadvantages of conventional frame versus unibody construction.
2. Examine a vehicle in the shop. See how many parts you can identify. Study how the vehicle is constructed.
3. Discuss front- and rear-wheel drive vehicles. What are the advantages and disadvantages of each?
4. Name the makes and models of vehicles that use steel, aluminum, and plastic or composite construction. Discuss each.

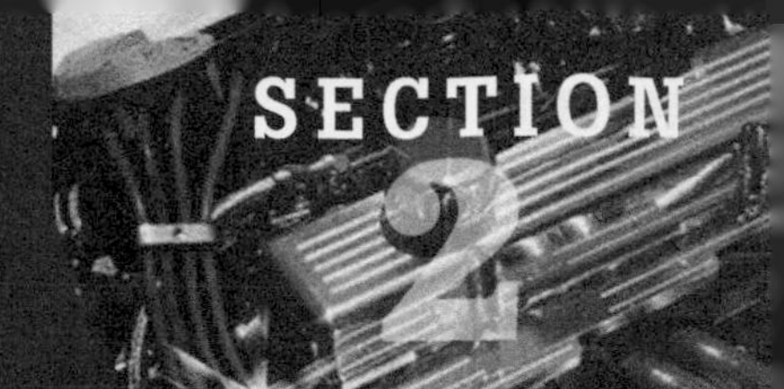

CHAPTER

10 Metal Straightening Fundamentals

OBJECTIVES

After reading this chapter, you should be able to:

- Describe different types of metals used in vehicle construction.
- Summarize the deformation effects of impacts on steel.
- Use a hammer and dolly to straighten.
- Explain how to straighten with spoons.
- List the steps for shrinking metal.
- Summarize paintless dent removal.
- Prepare a surface for filler.
- Properly mix filler and hardener.
- Correctly apply and shape filler.
- List common mistakes made when using filler and spot putty.

INTRODUCTION

This chapter introduces you to basic metalworking (straightening) methods. It explains how to analyze minor damage to sheet metal before showing you how to repair the damage. Good metalworking skills are critical to your success as a collision repair technician.

An untrained person can spend more time shaping and sculpting body filler than properly reworking the damaged metal. Not only does this waste valuable shop time, but the quality of the repair also suffers. An improperly straightened panel will have tension that can cause the filler to crack, lose adhesion, or fall off. This, of course, does nothing to build customer satisfaction.

To do quality sheet metal repairs, you must first know how to return the sheet metal to its original shape. Then, you can use a thin layer of filler to smooth the surface above the panel. This chapter will help you develop these essential skills.

SHEET METAL

There are two types of sheet metal used in automobile construction—hot-rolled and cold-rolled.

Hot-rolled sheet metal is made by rolling at temperatures exceeding 1,472°F (792°C). It has a standard manufacturing thickness range of $\frac{1}{16}$ to $\frac{5}{16}$ in. (1.6 to 7.9 mm). It is often used for comparatively thick parts such as frames and crossmembers.

Cold-rolled sheet metal is hot-rolled sheet metal that has been acid rinsed, cold rolled thin, then **annealed** (reheated and then cooled in a controlled manner to strengthen the metal and prevent it from becoming brittle). It has a dependable thickness accuracy, surface quality, and better workability than hot-rolled steel. Most unibodies are made from cold-rolled steel.

Low-carbon or **mild steel (MS)** has a low level of carbon and is relatively soft and easy to work. Much of the sheet metal used in vehicles today is low-carbon or mild steel. It can be safely welded, heat shrunk, and cold worked without seriously affecting its strength. Mild steel has a yield strength of up to 30,000 psi (2,100 kg/cm^2).

Because MS is easily deformed and relatively heavy, vehicle manufacturers have begun using high-strength steels in load-carrying parts of the vehicle.

High-strength steel (HSS) is stronger than low-carbon or mild steel because of a heat treatment. Most new vehicles contain HSS in their structural components. It has a yield strength of up to 60,000 psi (4,200 kg/cm^2). HSS experiences an increase in stress, exceeding this yield strength, when deformed during a collision.

The same properties that give strength offer some unique challenges. When HSS is deformed on impact, it is more difficult to restore than MS.

STEEL STRENGTH

When flat sheet steel is formed into a shape for a panel or a part, it takes on certain properties that harden it.

For example, a roof panel is relatively flat. If hit lightly in the center, the panel will usually bend and then pop back to its original shape. However, if you hit a panel with a curved shape, the panel will hardly move. Although both are the same steel, the one that has been changed the most will be stronger and more resistant to bending.

The same is true for panels whose shape has been changed during a collision. The structure of the metal in the affected areas has changed, causing the metal to become harder and more resistant to corrective forces. See **Figure 10–1.**

To repair collision damage, a technician should understand what property changes have taken place in the metal.

Deformation refers to the new, undesired bent shape the metal takes after a collision or impact. There are various ways to measure the strength of a metal. All relate to the metal's ability to resist deformation.

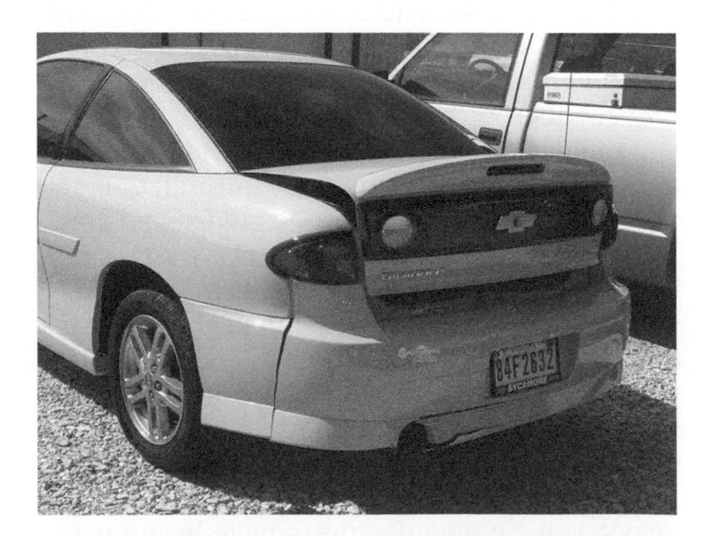

Figure 10–1. Before starting work to repair a vehicle, evaluate the damage. Would it be cheaper to purchase a new or used panel, or should you straighten the panel?

1. *Tensile strength* is the property of a material that resists forces applied to pull it apart. **Tension** includes both yield stress and ultimate strength. **Yield stress** is the amount of strain needed to permanently deform a test specimen. **Ultimate strength** is a measure of the load that breaks a specimen. The tensile strength of a metal can be determined by a tensile testing machine.
2. **Compressive strength** is the property of a material to resist being crushed.
3. **Shear strength** is a measure of how well a material can withstand forces acting to cut or slice it apart.
4. *Torsional strength* is the property of a material that withstands a twisting force.

Strength is expressed in pounds per square inch (psi) or kilograms per centimeter squared (kg/cm^2).

Even though most types of steel look alike, there are differences in their chemical makeup and crystalline structure. These invisible differences can affect strength and sensitivity to heat. There is a variety of HSS. All have unique properties that dictate the way in which they can be repaired.

PHYSICAL STRUCTURE OF STEEL

Steel, just like all matter, is composed of atoms. These very small particles of matter are arranged to form grains that can only be seen with a microscope. Grains are formed into patterns called the grain structure.

The **grain structure** in a piece of steel determines how much it can be bent or shaped. To change the shape of flat sheet steel, you must change the shape and position of all the individual grains that are located in the area of the creases, folds, or curves.

In MSs, the individual grains can withstand a considerable amount of change and movement before splitting or breaking. To demonstrate this, bend a piece of automotive sheet steel (part of a fender) back and forth several times. Notice that in the bend, the metal will become very hot. The heat is generated by the internal friction created as the individual grains move against each other.

EFFECT OF IMPACT FORCES

The grain pattern of a metal will determine how it reacts to force. Sheet metal's resistance to change has three properties: elastic deformation, plastic deformation, and work hardening. All of these properties are related to the yield point.

Yield point is the amount of force that a piece of metal can resist without tearing or breaking.

Elastic deformation is the ability of metal to stretch and return to its original shape. For example, take a piece of sheet metal and gently bend it to form a slight arc. When released, it will spring back to its original shape.

Spring-back is the tendency for metal to return to its original shape after deformation. It will occur in any area that is still relatively smooth. Many such areas will spring back to shape if they are released by relieving the distortion in the buckled areas.

Plastic deformation is the ability of metal to be bent or formed into different shapes. When metal is bent beyond its elastic limit, it will have a tendency to spring back. However, it will NOT spring back all the way to its original shape. This is because the grain structure has been changed.

Plasticity is important to the collision repair technician because both stretching and permanent deformation take place in various areas of most damaged panels.

WORK HARDENING

Work hardening is the limit of plastic deformation that causes the metal to become hard where it has been bent. For example, if a welding rod is bent back and forth several times, a fold or buckle will appear at the point of the bend. The plastic deformation has been so great that the metal will be very hard and stiff at the bend.

KINDS OF DAMAGE

A part is **kinked** when:

1. It has a sharp bend of a small radius, usually more than 90 degrees over a short distance. See **Figure 10–2.**

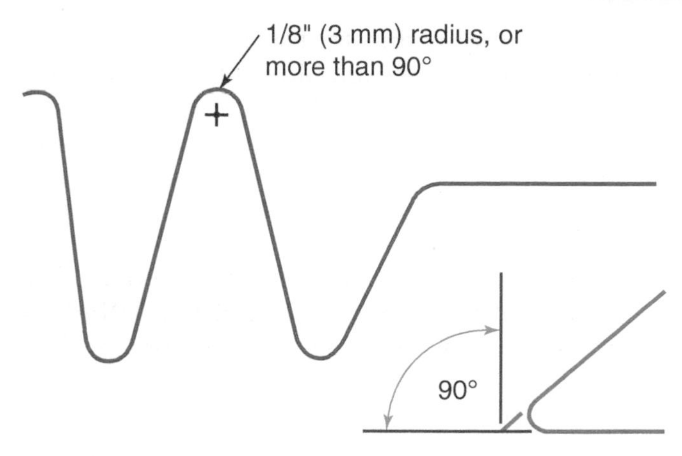

Figure 10–2. The radius of the bend determines whether you have a kink or a bend. A kink generally results when metal is folded more than 90 degrees. A bend in sheet metal can be easily repaired but not a sharp kink that has deformed the metal badly.

2. After straightening, there is a visible crack or tear in the metal or there is permanent deformation that cannot be straightened to its precollision shape without the use of excessive heat.

A part is **bent** when:

1. The change in the shape of the part between the damaged and undamaged areas is smooth and continuous.
2. Straightening the part by pulling restores its shape to precollision condition without any areas of permanent deformation.

USING BODY HAMMERS

The body hammer is often used to remove small dents in sheet metal parts. The body hammer is designed to strike the sheet metal and rebound off the surface.

A **high spot** or *bump* is an area that sticks up higher than the surrounding surface. A **low spot** or *dent* is just the opposite; it is recessed below the surrounding surface. Minor low and high spots in sheet metal can often be fixed with a body hammer.

The term **raising** means to work a dent outward or away from the body. The term **lowering** means to work a high spot or bump down or into the body.

The secret of metal straightening is to hit the right spot at the right time, with the right amount of force. When using a body hammer, swing in a circular motion at your wrist. Do not swing the hammer with your whole arm and shoulder. Hit the part squarely and let the hammer rebound off the metal. Space each blow ⅜ to ½ inch (9.5 to 12.7 mm) apart until the damaged metal is level.

The face of the hammer must fit the contour of the panel. Use a flat face on flat or low-crown panels. Use a convex-shaped or high-crown face when bumping inside curves.

Heavy body hammers should be used for roughing out the damage. **Finishing** or **dinging hammers** should be used for final shaping. The secret to finish hammering is light taps. It is also important to hit squarely. Hitting with the edge of the hammer will put additional nicks in the metal.

STRAIGHTENING WITH DOLLIES

In the rough-out phase, a heavy steel dolly is sometimes used as an impact tool. Dollies are often used as striking tools on the back panels. Sometimes you can reach into obstructed areas with a steel dolly more easily than with a hammer. You can strike the back side of the dented panel with the dolly to raise low areas and to unroll buckles.

The contour of the dolly must fit the contour of the back side of the damaged area. This will make the blows from the dolly force the metal back into its original contour. If the wrong surface hits the panel (sharp edge of the dolly, for example), you will cause further damage to the panel.

Start out with light blows from the dolly while watching the front of the panel. Make sure you are hitting exactly where needed. Gradually increase the force of your blows to raise the damage. It is normally better to use several moderate blows than to use a few hard blows. Numerous well-placed blows with the dolly will let you better control how you work the metal back into shape.

HAMMER-ON-DOLLY

Hammer-on-dolly is a method used to exert a powerful but concentrated smoothing force to a small area on a damaged panel. The dolly is held against the back of the damage and the hammer hits the metal right over the top of the dolly. This exerts a pinching force on the metal between the dolly and the hammer head. A small area of damaged metal is crushed and flattened between the faces of the dolly and hammer. See **Figure 10–3.**

Hammer-on-dolly straightening requires you to repeatedly move the point of hammer impact and dolly slightly. Each blow should overlap the next. By repeatedly moving hammer-on-dolly blows, you can steadily work out minor damage over a large area. Generally, try to work out the damage methodically. Start at the outside and gradually work toward the center of the damage. See **Figure 10–4.**

A proper hammer-on-dolly blow will make a slight high-pitched "ping" sound. The force of the blow goes into the panel and then into the dolly. Hitting the dolly makes the pinging sound. If you accidentally miss the spot backed by the dolly, a more dull or dead sound is produced as only the panel is hit. If you miss the dolly with a hammer tap, a small unwanted dent is often produced in the panel.

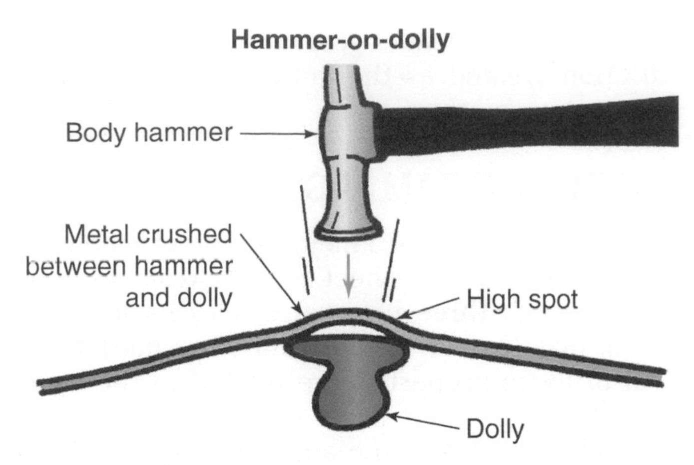

Figure 10–3. With the hammer-on-dolly method, place the dolly right behind the damage and hit the metal right over the dolly to straighten the metal in the small area between the tools.

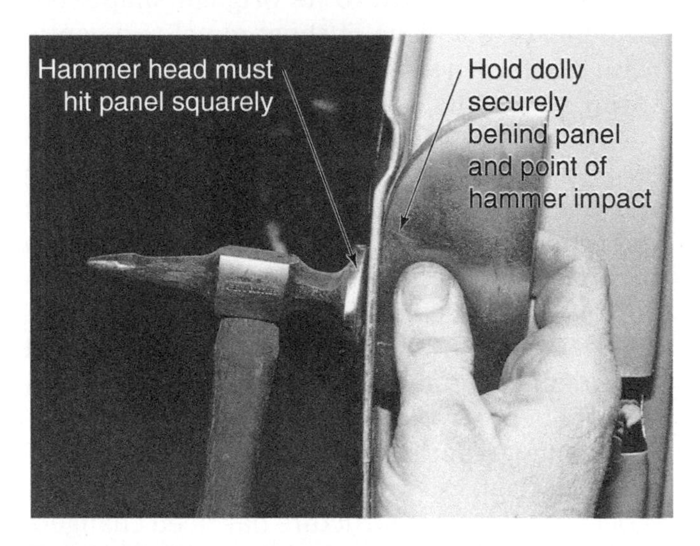

Figure 10–4. A dolly is normally held behind the area to be straightened to support the sheet metal when being hit by the body hammer. Here the technician is using the flat surface off the dolly to straighten the flat area of the door skin lip. (Courtesy of Snap-on Tools Corp.)

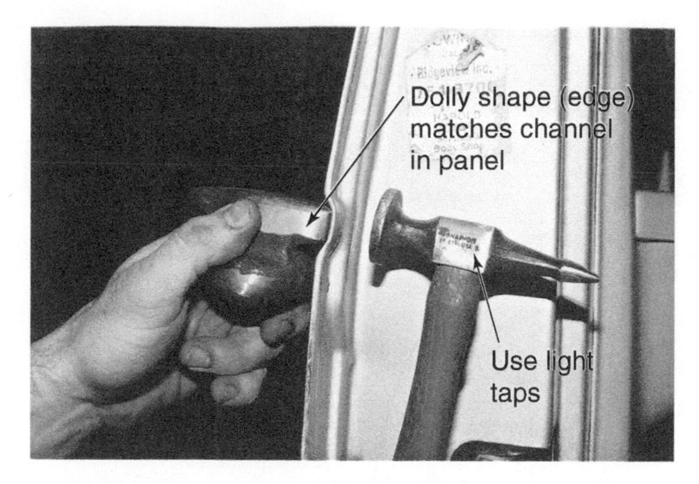
Dolly shape (edge) matches channel in panel
Use light taps

Figure 10–5. The shape or contour of the dolly and hammer head must mimic or be the same as the repair area. Note how the dolly edge was selected with the same shape as the channel in the door panel. Carefully placed hammer blows have reshaped the badly damaged door skin at the channel area. (Courtesy of Snap-on Tools Corp.)

With hammer-on-dolly, the shapes of the dolly and hammer head must match the desired shape of the panel. If the area to be straightened is flat, the dolly surface and hammer head must be flat. If the panel is curved, the dolly and hammer head must also be curved to match the panel's shape. When you bump or hit the damage with the hammer, the metal is flattened against the dolly and a tiny area is formed into the shape of the hammer head and dolly face. Look at **Figure 10–5.**

Never use a flat surface on a dolly to try to straighten a curved panel. You will damage the panel further.

Always start out with light hammer blows. A common mistake is to use excessively hard or poorly aimed hammer blows, which dent, stretch, and damage the panel. By starting light and working up to stronger blows, you can better control the movement of the metal to avoid unwanted dents. Carefully observe the results of each blow to make sure you are slowly reshaping the metal as desired.

Hold the dolly securely against the back of the panel. Hit the area lightly so that the hammer bounces back. Light hammer-on-dolly blows are used to smooth small, shallow dents and bulges. Hard hammer-on-dolly blows can be used to stretch the metal.

To lower a bulge, place the dolly against the back side of the panel directly behind the bulge and use a hammer from the front side. There will be a slight rebound as your hammer hits the dolly. The dolly will then hit the back side of the panel. As the force of the dolly pressing against the panel is increased, the flattening action will also increase.

With hard blows using hammer-on-dolly, the metal is smashed between the hammer and dolly. This tends to crush the metal thinner and make it stretch out to fill a slightly larger surface area. All blows that are designed to stretch should be hard and accurate. Remember that an inaccurate hard blow can damage the panel.

Keep in mind that light hammer blows are for straightening, not stretching. In other words, when using the hammer-on-dolly technique for stretching, hit hard and do not miss!

Hammer-on-dolly is used only if there is access to the back side of the panel.

Remember! You can control the effects of hammer-on-dolly straightening by:

1. Using a hammer with a different shaped head
2. Using a different shaped dolly face
3. Altering how hard you hit the metal
4. Changing how hard you push the dolly against the back of the panel

HAMMER-OFF-DOLLY

Hammer-off-dolly is used to raise low spots and lower high spots simultaneously. The hammer hits the panel slightly to one side of where the dolly is being held. It is often used to rough out or shape large areas of damage during initial straightening. In this procedure, hold the dolly under the lowest area on the back of the panel. Then hit any high area right next to the dolly with your hammer. Hammer off to one side of the dolly, not directly on top of the dolly. Look at **Figure 10–6.**

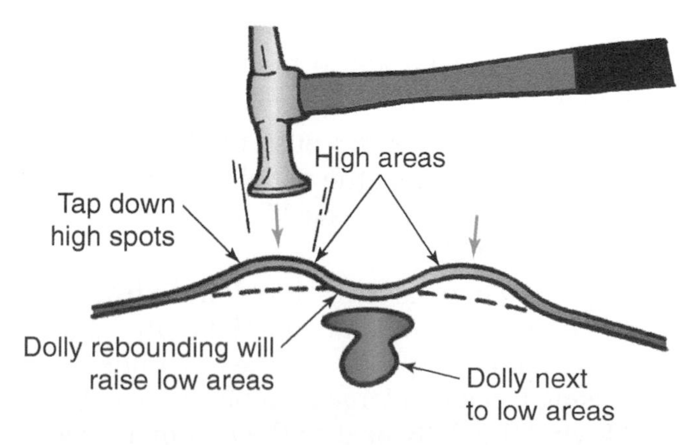

Figure 10–6. With the hammer-off-dolly method, place the dolly next to the area to be hit. Then strike the high spots next to the dolly.

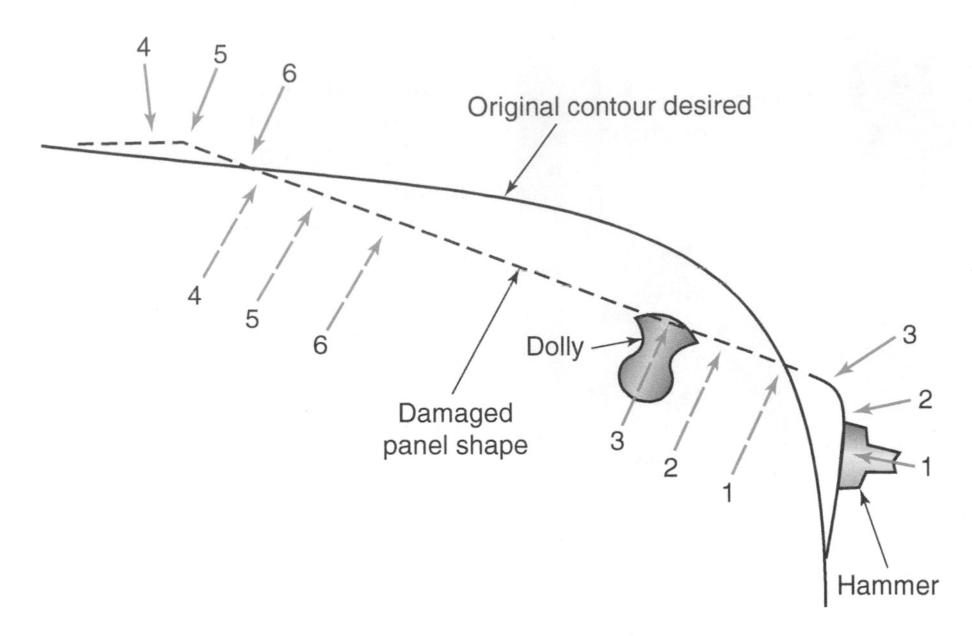

Figure 10–7. Note the steps for removing damage from a curved shape using a hammer and dolly. First, start at one end of the damage, on the right. Then work the damage on the other side. Roll out the damage toward the middle. Filler would then be needed to give the area its final contour.

Generally, use the hammer and dolly to roll out the damage in reverse order than it was formed. Generally, the damage must be rolled out working toward the center. Start at the outer perimeter off the damage and work to the middle of the damage. See **Figure 10–7.**

For example, if the panel has a large buckle, you could use the hammer-off-dolly method. Place the dolly on the low spot at the back of the panel. Then hit a high spot with your hammer. This will lower the high spot and raise the low spot without stretching the metal. The hammer blow will push the high spot down and the rebound of the dolly will force the low spot up.

Remember! You can control hammer-off-dolly straightening by:

1. Altering how hard you hit the panel. Start out with light blows and then increase their force if needed to lower high spots in the panel.
2. Changing how hard to push the dolly against the back of the panel. Pushing harder tends to increase lifting action to raise low spots.
3. Adjusting how far away the dolly is from the hammer blows. Moving the dolly father away tends to spread out the lowering-raising force to a large area on the panel. Moving the dolly next to the hammer blow tends to concentrate the lowering-raising force more.

STRAIGHTENING WITH SPOONS

Spoons can be used to pry out damage, struck with a hammer to drive out damage, and as a dolly in hard-to-reach areas. Some are even designed to be used in place of a body hammer.

Spring hammering is a method of bumping damage with a hammer and a dinging spoon. The dinging spoon is lightweight and has a low crown. Hold the spoon firmly against a ridge or crease. Hit the spoon with a bumping hammer to work the high spot down. See **Figure 10–8.** Always keep firm pressure on the spoon when spring hammering. It must never be allowed to bounce.

The force of the blow on the spoon is distributed over a large area of the ridge. Begin at the ends of the ridge and work toward the high point, alternating from side to side.

Spoons can be used to back up the hammer or in combination with a slapper spoon. With a long body spoon, you can often reach into restricted places. Pressure can be applied to tension areas with the spoon, while high areas are bumped down. See **Figure 10–9** and **Figure 10–10.**

Spoons can also be used to pry up metal or to drive out deep dents. In **Figure 10–11,** note how a double-end spoon is being used to pry out a dent in a door panel. The door is supported on blocks of wood to provide clearance for the panel. Use care not to stretch the metal by prying it out too much. Once the dent is roughed out, a body hammer can be used to finish the area.

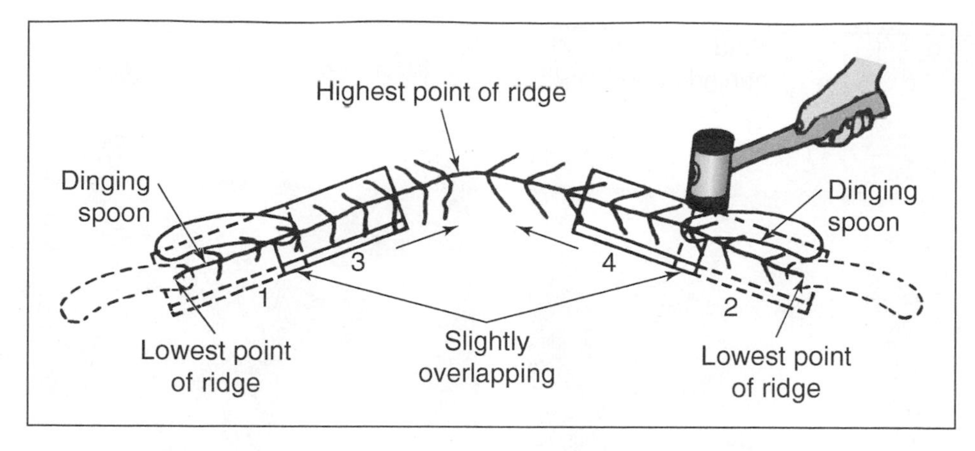

Figure 10–8. A large dinging spoon can be used to lower a ridge formed in a damaged panel. Start at the outer ends of the ridge and work your way to the center.

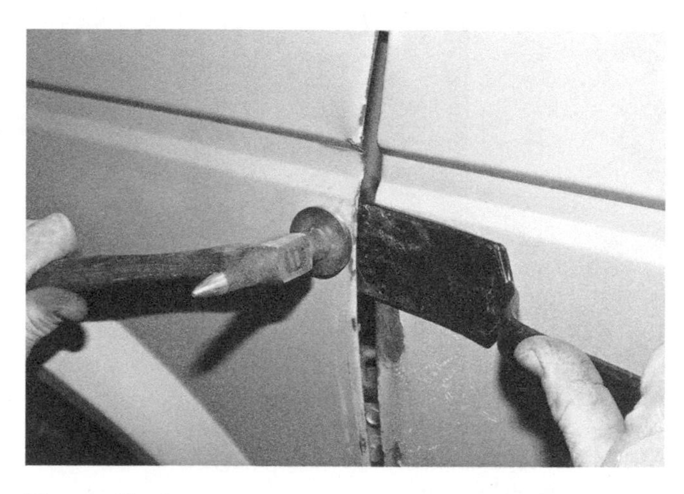

Figure 10–9. A spoon is being used as a prybar and dolly. It has been forced between the front fender and the door to back up damage on the edge of the fender. The backs of fenders are often forced into the fronts of doors during frontal collision.

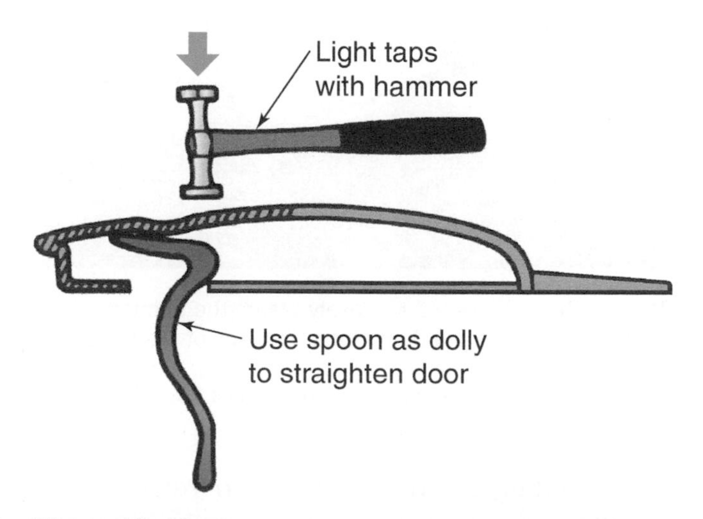

Figure 10–10. Use a curved spoon to reach in behind a damaged panel to serve as a dolly. Tap on the outside of the panel with a hammer while pressing the spoon in from the back.

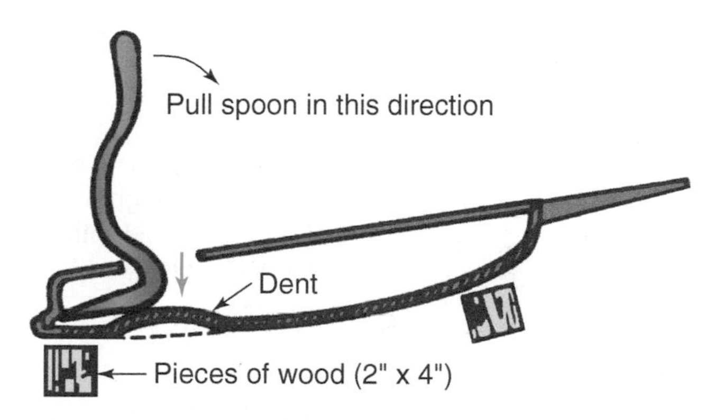

Figure 10–11. You can also use a curved spoon to pry out dents in panels, a door panel in this example. Pieces of wood can also be used to raise a door or panel off the work surface.

STRAIGHTENING WITH PICKS

Picking hammers, pry picks, a dolly edge, and a scratch awl can be used to pick or push up metal. When picking up a small dent, it is better to use several light blows. See **Figure 10–12.** After an area has been raised, use a file to identify any remaining low spots.

Picks can be used to pry up metal in areas that cannot be reached with a dolly or spoon. A vehicle door is a good example. See **Figure 10–13.** A pick can sometimes be inserted through a drainage hole. This eliminates the need to remove the inside door trim or to drill holes in the outer panel for pulling the dent.

When picks are used to remove small dents without having to repaint the panel, it is termed **paintless dent removal.** This method only works with very small dents that do not damage the finish (paint). See **Figure 10–14.**

When prying with a pick, be careful not to stretch the metal by exerting too much pressure. Start with the point of impact or the lowest

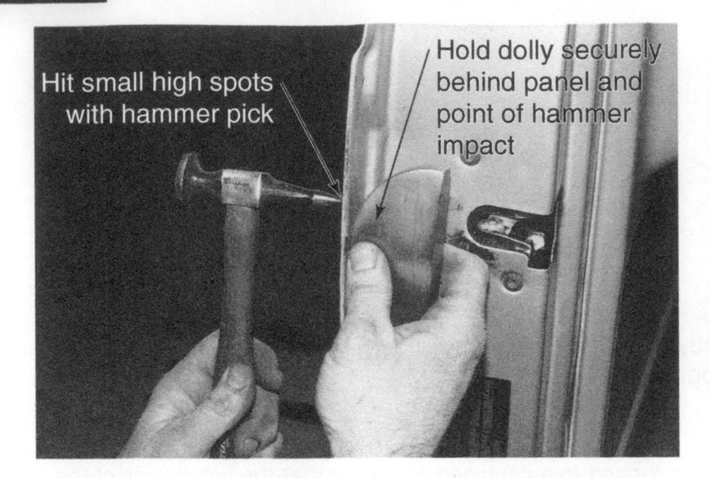

Figure 10–12. The pick end of a body hammer is being used to carefully lower tiny high spots remaining in the repair area of a door panel. The dolly-off method is being used to avoid hammer rebound.

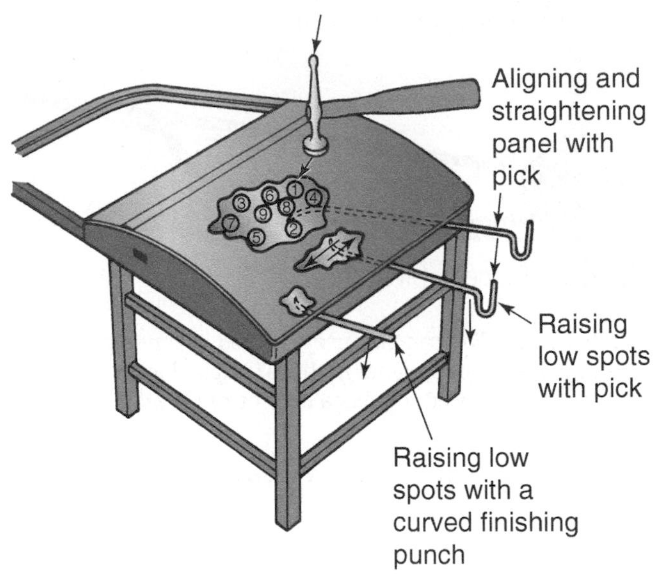

Figure 10–13. Pry picks are often used to remove small dents and other hard-to-reach areas. Pry on dents with a pick while applying light taps from the hammer on the other side. Picks will fit through small openings in the side of a door or other part.

point. Slowly pry up the damaged area. On the larger areas, use a flat blade pick rather than a pointed one. Tap down pressure areas, while prying up low tension areas.

PULLING DAMAGED AREAS

Dents can be pulled out with a number of tools: suction cups, pull rods, and dent pullers. Pulling is often needed because access to the inside of many panels is blocked by reinforcements and other parts. With a puller, you can repair a simple dent in a minimal amount of time. Refer to **Figure 10–15.**

First, study the damage to determine the point and angle of the impact. Then you can find where pulling force is needed to remove the damage.

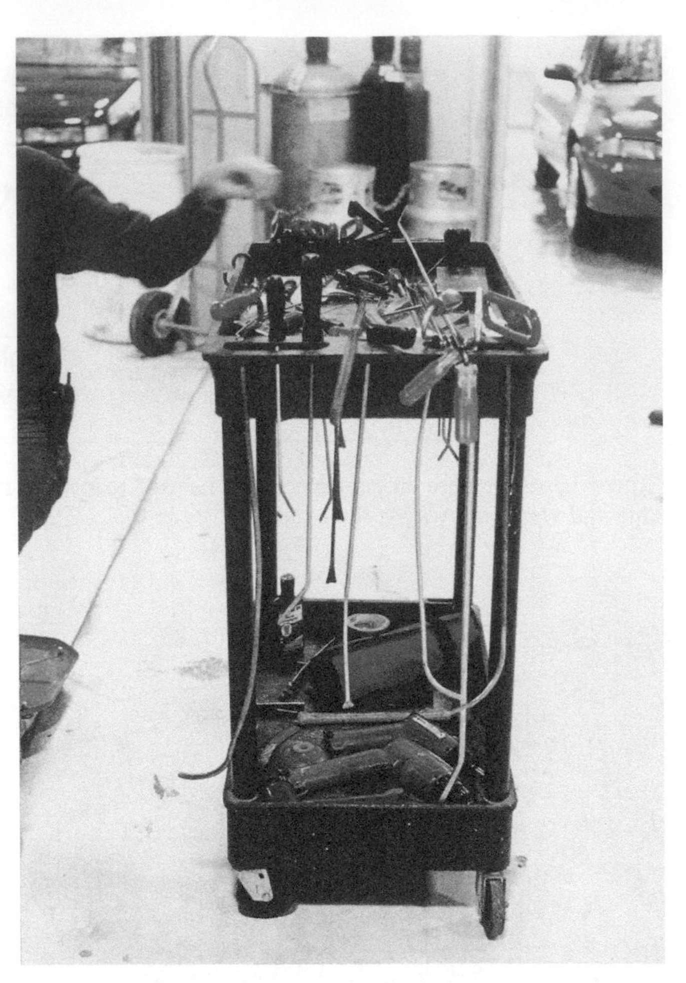

(A) The cart contains many specialized tools of the paintless dent removal technician.

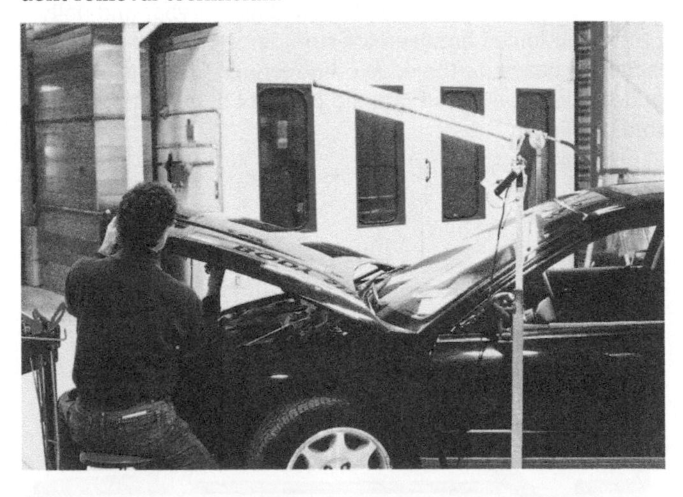

(B) Bright light is needed to closely watch the painted surface as you work out dents from the back of the panel.

Figure 10–14. Paintless dent removal takes special skill and patience. (continued)

Straightening with Suction Cup

A *suction cup* can be used to straighten shallow dents. Wet the area and install the cup. If hand

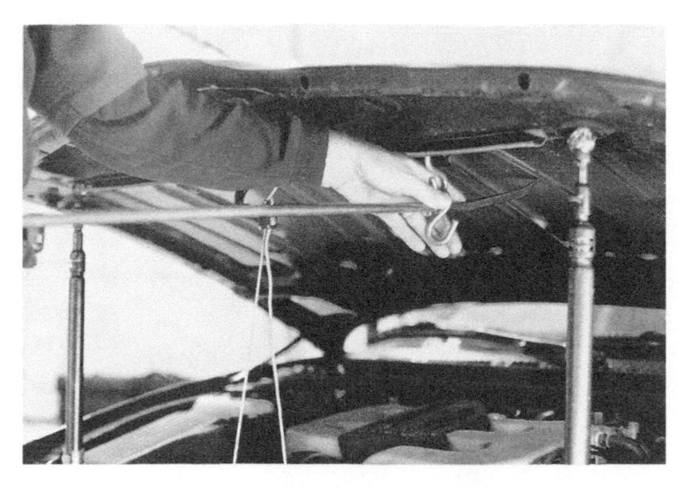

(C) Special bracing is being used to hold the long prybar or pick to lift the dent from the bottom of the hood panel.

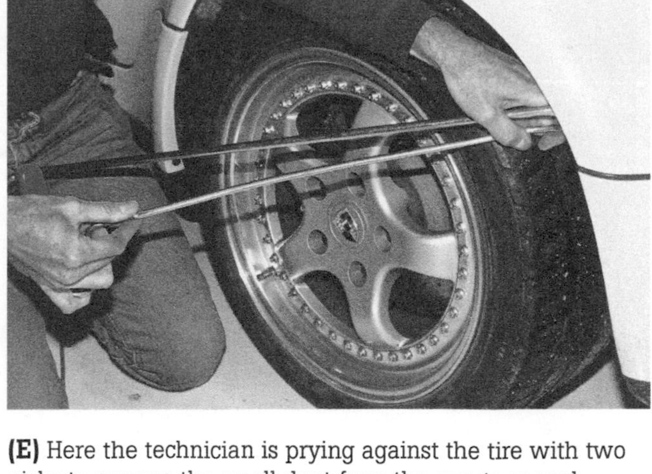

(E) Here the technician is prying against the tire with two picks to remove the small dent from the quarter panel without repainting it.

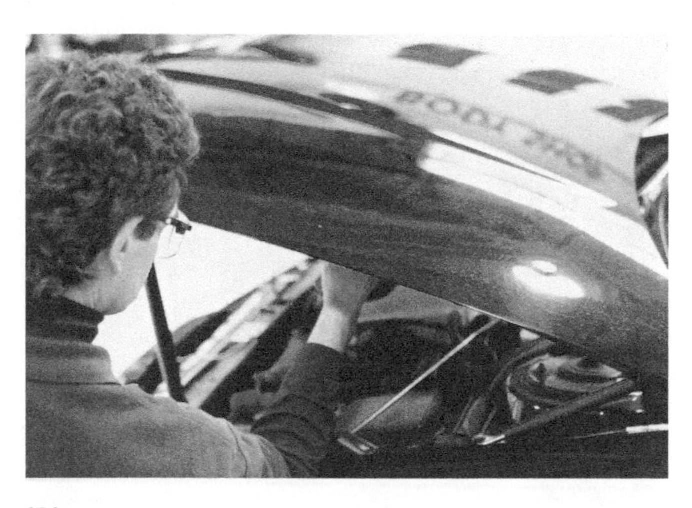

(D) The technician is closely watching the small dent as he pushes it out from the bottom of the hood.

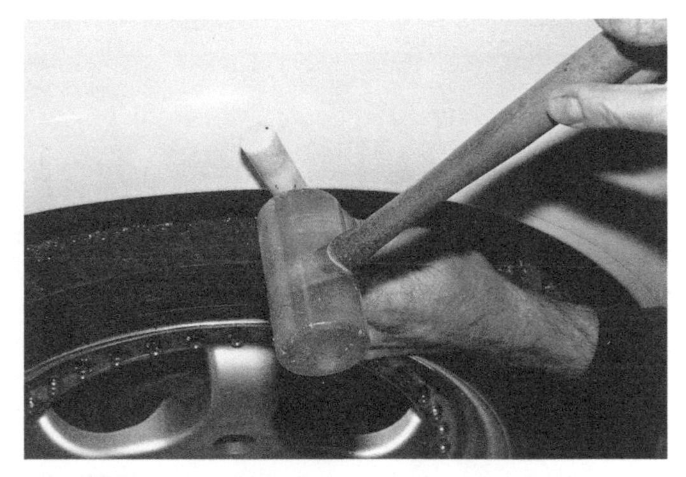

(F) To finally straighten the surface, a plastic rod is being tapped on with a plastic hammer to flatten the surface without damaging the paint.

Figure 10–14. (***Continued***)

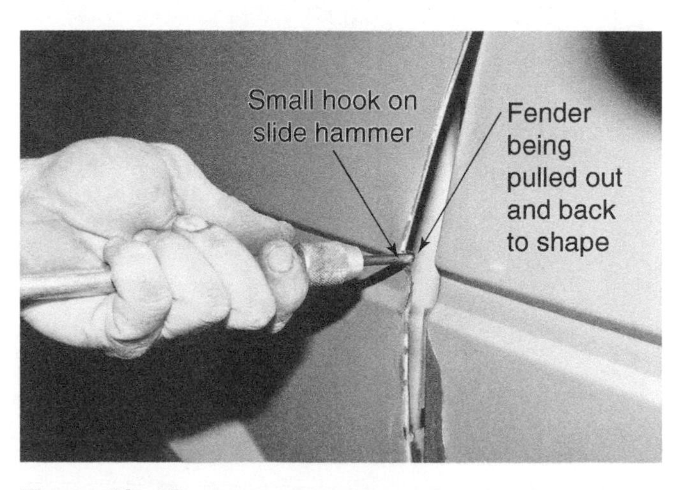

Figure 10–15. Slide hammers can be fitted with various ends, like this hook, for pulling on the edges of panels. Slide hammer blows have straightened this fender lip next to the channel or body contour.

held, pull straight out on the cup's handle. If mounted on a slide hammer, use a quick blow to pop the dent out.

A **vacuum suction cup** uses a remote power source (separate vacuum pump or air compressor airflow) to produce negative pressure (vacuum) in the cup. This increases the pulling power because the cup will be forced against the panel tightly. Larger, deeper dents can be straightened with a vacuum suction cup.

Straightening with Studs

A **stud spot welder** joins "pull rods" on the surface of a panel so that you do not have to drill holes. It is one way to straighten dents. Straightening with spot-welded studs avoids drilling or punching through the metal and undercoating, which can lead to rust. Refer to **Figure 10–16.**

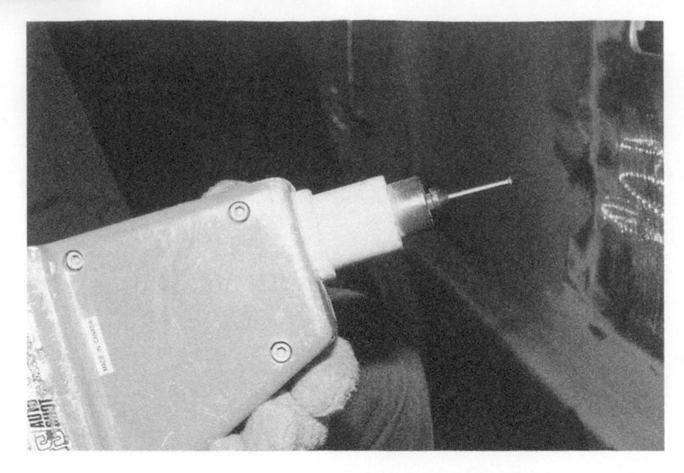

(A) This dent pulling equipment uses a special spot welder that welds studs onto the panel to be straightened. Fit a nail or stud into the tip of the welding gun as shown.

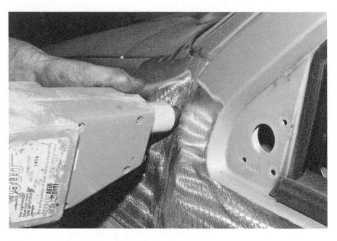

(B) Hold the stud welder against the panel and pull the trigger to weld the stud onto the surface of the panel.

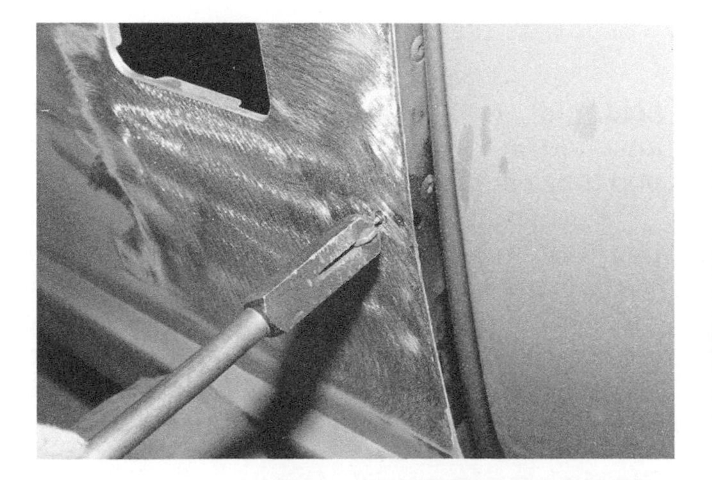

(C) Attach a slide hammer to the end of the welded-on stud.

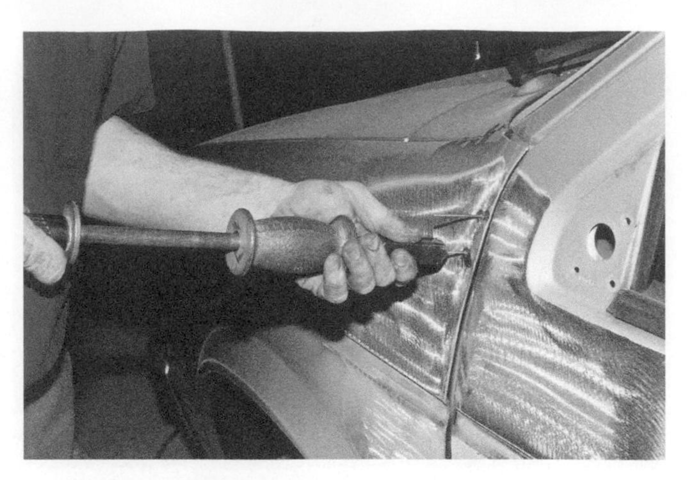

(D) Use slide hammer blows and a body hammer to work the dented metal outward.

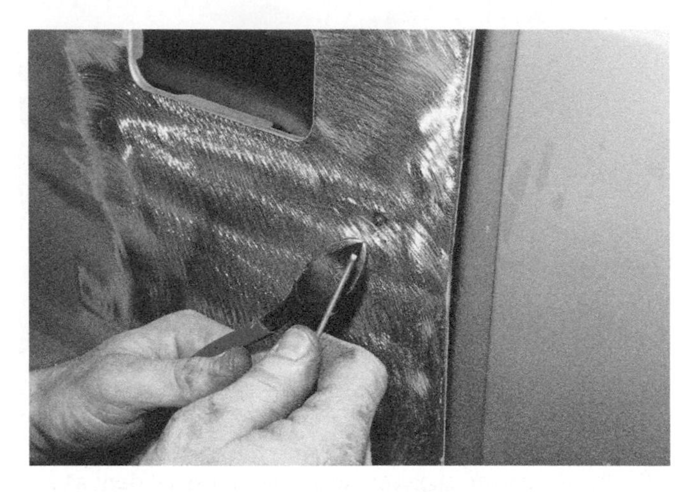

(E) After pulling out the dent, cut off the welded studs with side cut pliers.

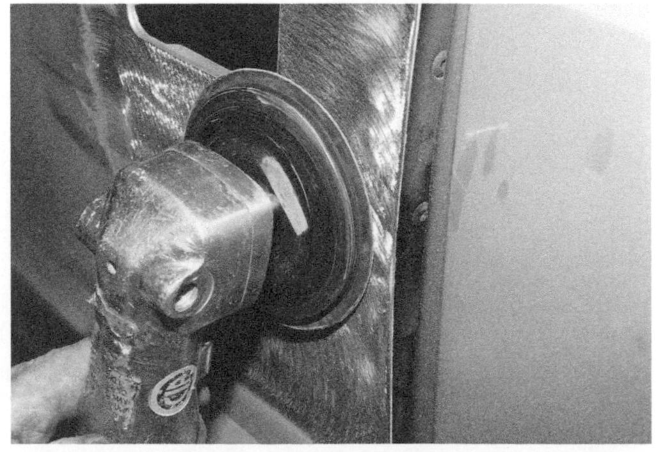

(F) Grind the stud weld nuggets flush with the panel.

Figure 10–16. Never drill holes in panels that will be repaired. Holes must be welded shut and this can lead to rusting since rust protection is burned off by welding.

To use a stud welding gun, remove paint in the damaged area. Install a stud into the gun. Press the gun against the dented area. Pull the trigger to weld the pin onto the surface of the panel. Weld enough pins onto the area to remove the damage.

Next, attach a slide hammer to each of the pins and pull out the damage in steps. You could also use a pulling chain on a frame rack if needed. After bringing the surface of the dent almost out to the desired level, grind off the studs. This will allow you to remove the dent without drilling holes in the panel. See **Figure 10–17.**

SHRINKING METAL

Shrinking metal removes strain or tension on a damaged, stretched sheet metal area. During impact, the metal can be stretched. When pulled or hammered straight, the area can still have tension or strain on it. This is because the stretched metal no longer fits in the same area. The metal will tend to pop in and out when you try to finally straighten it. You would have to use heat to shrink the metal back to its original dimensions.

If a strained area is filled with body filler, road vibrations can cause the panel to make a popping or flapping noise. After prolonged movement of the strained area, the filler can crack or fall off. Eventually, you will be required to spend extra time correcting the work that should have been done properly in the first place.

Principles of Shrinking

A steel bar will expand (lengthen) when heated and contract (shorten) when cooled. If heated while butted against a solid object at both ends, it cannot lengthen and will bulge out in the middle or hottest area. Then when cooled, the length of the bar will decrease. This is the principle of shrinking metal.

The processes involved in shrinking a steel bar also apply to the shrinking of a warped area in a piece of sheet metal. A small spot in the center of the warped area is heated to a dull red. When the temperature rises, the heated area swells and attempts to expand outward toward the edges of the heated circle. Since the surrounding area is cool and hard, the panel cannot expand. As a result, a strong compression load is generated.

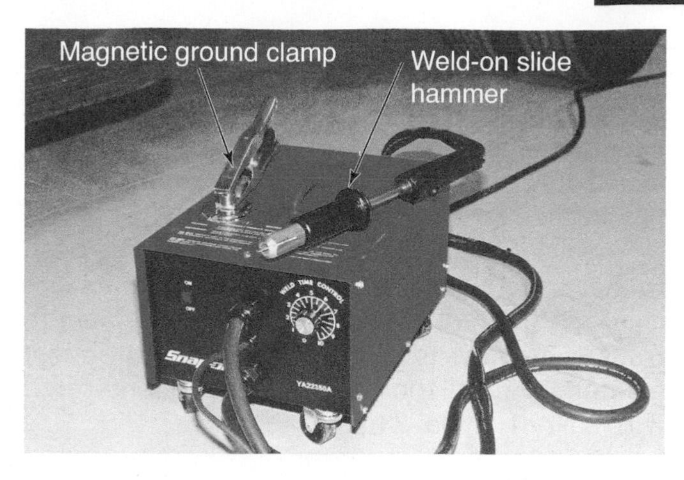

(A) The slide hammer has a tip that welds itself to the body panel. The ground cable has a magnet that allows for easy attachment to the bare metal on the panel.

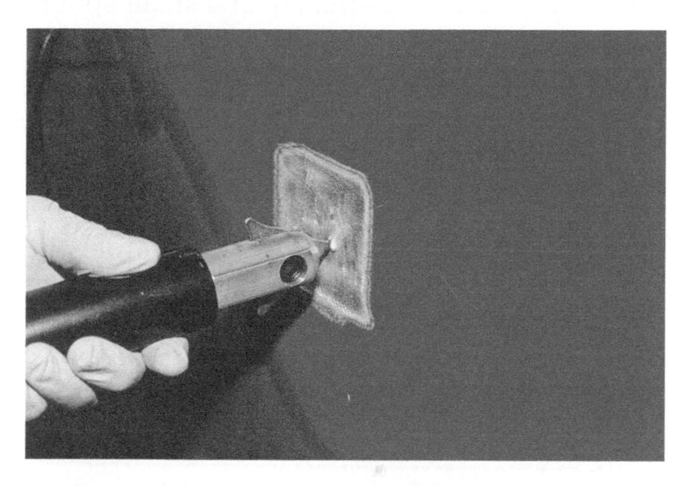

(B) Hold the slide hammer head against the panel and press the trigger. This will weld the metal tip of the tool to the metal panel.

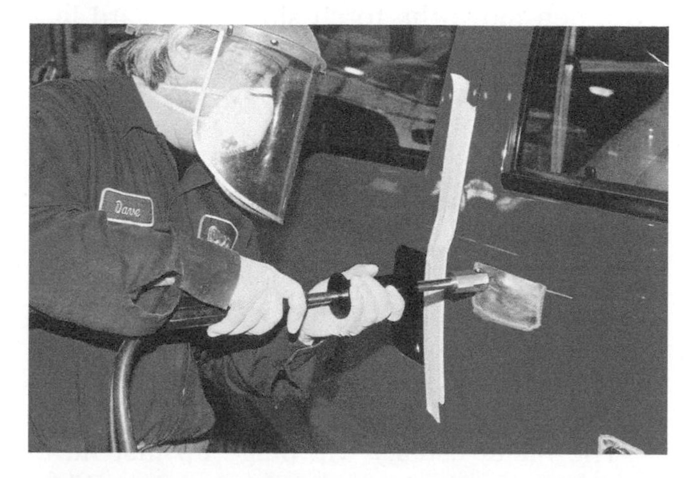

(C) Pull on the tool while sliding the hammer handle back and forth. To remove the tool from the panel, twist or rotate the tool to break the spot weld.

Figure 10–17. Study the use of this type of weld-on dent pulling equipment. (Courtesy of Snap-on Tools Corp.)

If heating continues, the stretching of the metal is centered in the dull red-hot portion, pressing it out. This causes it to thicken, thus relieving the compression load. If the red-hot area is suddenly cooled, the steel will contract and the surface area will shrink.

A variety of welding equipment can be used to heat metal for shrinking. Attachments are available for spot and MIG welding equipment to transform them into shrinking tools; the most commonly used tool is the oxyacetylene torch with a No. 1 or No. 2 tip.

Torch Shrinking

Torch shrinking uses the heat of an oxyacetylene torch to release tension in the panel. To shrink an area with a torch, heat a small spot in the bulge to a cherry red. Shrink in the highest spot of the stretched area, then in the next highest spot, until the area has been shrunk back to its proper position.

The size of the area to be heated, or the "hot spot," is determined by the amount of excess metal. The larger the area, the harder the heat is to control. An average-sized area to heat is usually about the size of a quarter. Smaller areas should be used on flat panels because they tend to warp easily. The area should never be larger than the size of the hammer face being used.

Use a neutral flame and a small tip to heat the panel. Bring the point of the cone straight down to within ⅛ inch (3 mm) of the metal. Hold the torch steady until the metal starts to turn red. Then move the torch slowly outward in a circular motion until the area is cherry red.

! WARNING !

Do not heat the metal past a cherry red. It will start to melt, and a hole may be burned through the metal. Also, remember that aluminum will not change color or turn red when heated.

The metal usually will bulge up instead of down because the top of it is heated first. When it starts to bulge, the rest of the metal in the area follows. When the area has been heated, tap around it to drive the molecules of metal closer together. You may have to support the panel with a dolly to prevent the metal from collapsing. Push the dolly *lightly* under the metal. When the redness disappears, use a hammer and dolly to level the area around the shrink.

! WARNING !

Never use hard, hammer-on-dolly blows to level the area when shrinking. This will restretch the metal.

Once the redness has disappeared and the area has been smoothed, cool the area with a wet rag or sponge. This will cause metal contraction. A slight amount of distortion could result. Straighten any warpage before heating the next spot.

Remember! It is easy to overshrink. When this occurs, the metal in the area last heated is usually collapsed or pulled flat. Sometimes the metal surrounding the heated area can even be pulled out of the proper contour. To fix overshrinking use hard, hammer-on-dolly blows to stretch the affected area.

Shrinking a Gouge

A **gouge** is caused by a focused impact that forces a sharp dent or crease into a panel. A gouge causes the metal to be stretched. Gouges must be shrunk to their original size to properly repair the damage. Simply picking up the low area would distort the panel. Filling the gouge with filler without restoring the panel's original contour will leave tension in the panel that could cause the filler to crack or pop off.

IDENTIFYING STRETCHED METAL

Stretched metal has been forced thinner in thickness and larger in surface area by impact. When metal is severely damaged in a collision, it is often stretched in the badly buckled areas. These same areas are also sometimes stretched slightly during the straightening process. Most of the stretched metal will be found along ridges, channels, and buckles in the direct damage area. When there are stretched areas of metal, it is impossible to correctly straighten the area back to its original contour. The stretched areas can be compared to a bulge on a tire. There is no place for the area to fit within the correct panel contour.

When an area is stretched, the grains of metal are moved farther away from each other. The metal is thinned and work-hardened. Shrinking is needed to bring the molecules back to their original position and to restore the metal to its proper contour and thickness.

Before shrinking, dolly the damaged area back as close to its original shape as possible. Then you can accurately determine whether or not there is stretched metal in the damaged area. It will usually pop in and out if stretched. If it is stretched, you must shrink the metal.

FILING THE REPAIR AREA

When the area has been straightened smooth as possible, use a body file to locate any remaining high and low spots. File across the damaged area to the undamaged metal on the opposite side. This will keep the filing action on the correct plane with the good part of the panel. Look at **Figure 10–18.**

Push the file forward by its handle for the cutting stroke. Control file downward pressure and direction by holding the front of the file. Use as long a stroke as possible.

The scratch pattern created by the file on the metal identifies any high and low spots. You can then further work the metal into shape before using body filler.

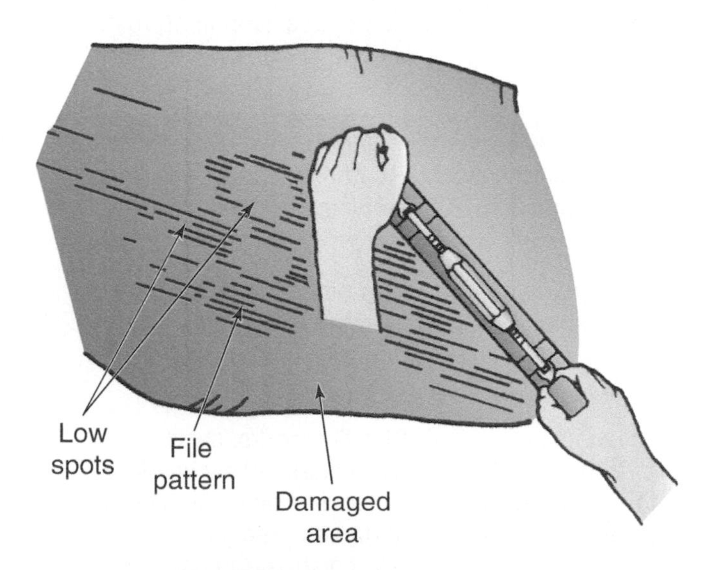

Figure 10–18. Filing will help you locate high and low spots that need further work. Low spots will NOT have file marks.

WORKING ALUMINUM

Aluminum is used for some automotive panels, such as hoods and deck lids. The repair of aluminum requires much more care than working steel panels. Aluminum is much softer than steel, yet it is more difficult to shape once it becomes work-hardened. It also melts at a lower temperature and distorts readily when heated.

Because aluminum is soft, it responds very readily to the hammer-on-dolly method. If hammered too hard or too much, the panel will stretch. Use several light strokes rather than a few heavy blows.

Aluminum does not readily bend back to its original shape after being buckled by an impact. Therefore, it does not respond well to the hammer-off-dolly method. Be careful not to create additional damage when attempting to lower ridges with hammer and dolly blows.

Raising small dents with a picking hammer or pry bar is an excellent way to repair aluminum panels. However, do not raise the panel too far and stretch the soft aluminum.

Spring hammering with a hammer and spoon is an excellent way to unlock stress in high-pressure areas of aluminum. The spoon distributes the force of the blow over a wider area.

Because aluminum is soft, reduce hand pressure on the body file. Use a file with rounded edges to avoid scratching and gouging the metal.

Sand carefully on aluminum. A coarse grit grinding disc will quickly burn through aluminum. The heat from grinding can also warp the panel. A No. 80 grit open coat disc can be used, but sand carefully to remove only paint and primer, not the aluminum. Make two or three passes, then quench the area with a wet rag to cool the metal in the panel.

Featheredging of aluminum should be done with a dual-action sander. Use No. 80 or No. 100 grit paper and a soft, flexible backing pad.

Heat shrink stretched aluminum slowly to avoid distorting the panel. Do not heat the spot over 1,200°F (584°C). Use a thermal crayon or paint to monitor heating. Mark the part with the crayon when it is still cold. When the stated temperature has been reached, the crayon or paint mark will liquefy.

Unlike steel, aluminum does not turn red as it is heated. Instead, it turns ash gray just before it melts. Thus, a lack of caution will result in a melted panel. Also, quench or cool the heated area very slowly to avoid distortion.

USING BODY FILLER

After the damaged metal has been bumped, pulled, pried, and dinged, the application of body filler is next.

Body fillers are designed to cover up minor surface irregularities that remain after metal straightening. Keep in mind that the quality of the repair and finish is adversely affected by the wrong choice of filler. The chart in **Figure 10–19** shows various types of filler and their uses.

Preparing Surface for Filler

One of the most important steps in applying body fillers is surface preparation. Begin by washing the repair area with soap and water to remove dirt and grime. Then clean the area with wax and grease remover to eliminate wax, road tar, and grease. Use a cleaner that will remove the **silicones** often present in automotive waxes.

Mask any trim, parts, or adjacent panels that could be damaged by grinding, sanding, and filling. Use masking tape or duct tape to protect them.

Grind the area to remove the paint 3 to 4 inches (75 to 100 mm) around the area to be filled. Remember! Never apply body filler over

Comparing Body Fillers			
Filler	**Composition**	**Characteristics**	**Application**
Conventional fillers			
Lightweight fillers	Microsphere glass bubbles; fine grain talc; polyester resins	Spreads easily; nonshrinking; homogeneous; no settling	Dings, dents, and gouges in metal panels
Premium fillers	Microspheres; talc; polyester resins; special chemical additives	Sands fast and easy; spreads creamy and moist; spreads smooth without pinholes; dries tack-free; will not sag	Dings, dents, and gouges in metal panels
Fiberglass-reinforced fillers			
Short strand	Small fiberglass strands; polyester resins	Waterproof; stronger than regular fillers	Fills small rustouts and holes. Used with fiberglass cloth to bridge larger rustouts
Long strand	Long fiberglass strands; polyester resins	Waterproof; stronger than short strand fiberglass fillers; bridges small holes without matte or cloth	Cracked or shattered fiberglass. Repairing rustouts, holes, and tears
Specialty fillers			
Aluminum filler	Aluminum flakes and powders; polyester resins	Waterproof; spreads smoothly; high level of quality and durability	Restoring classic and exotic vehicles
Finishing filler/ polyester putty	High-resin content; fine talc particles; microsphere glass bubbles	Ultra-smooth and creamy; tack-free; nonshrinking; eliminates need for air dry type glazing putty	Fills pinholes and sand scratches in metal, filler, fiberglass, and old finishes
Sprayable filler/ polyester primer-surfacer	High-viscosity polyester resins; talc particles; liquid hardener	Virtually nonshrinking; prevents bleed-through; eliminates primer/glazing/ primer procedure	Fills file marks, sand scratches, mildly cracked or crazed paint films, and pinholes. Seals fillers and old finishes against bleed-through

Figure 10–19. This chart shows general composition, characteristics, and applications for various types of body fillers.

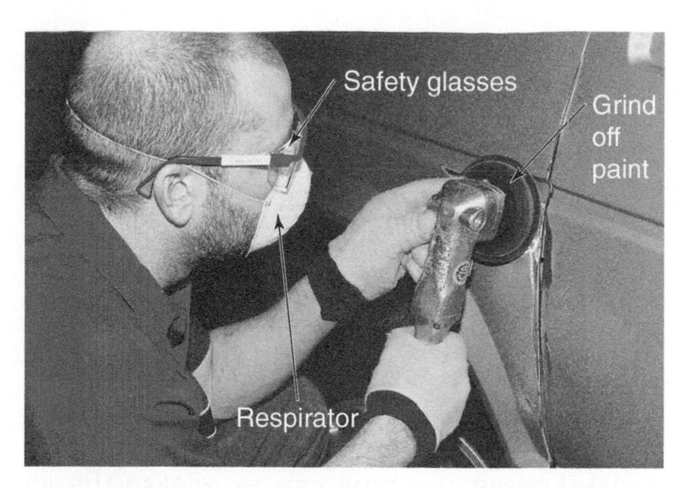

Figure 10–20. Before applying filler, grind the area to remove all paint. Coarse (36 or 40 grit) grind marks will help the filler bond to the metal. Mask the trim or adjacent panels so you do not accidentally damage surfaces not being repaired and repainted. Use compressed air to blow off dust from the repair area.

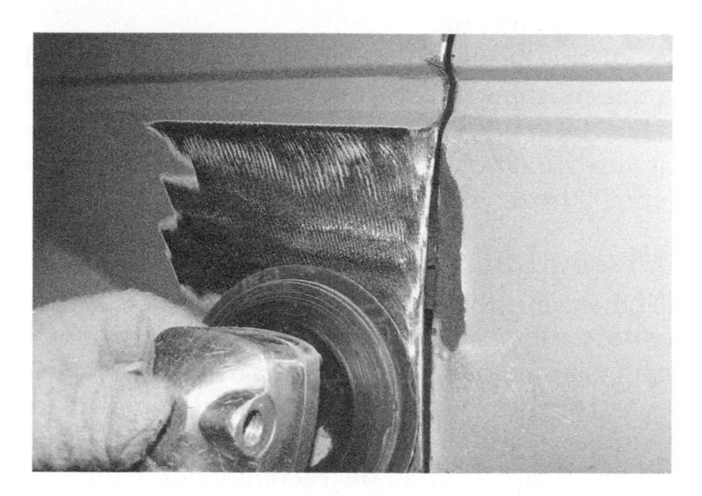

Figure 10–21. Grind methodically to just remove paint and scuff the metal. Do not grind too long in one location or you can thin the metal or even grind a hole in it. Start at the top. Grind straight across the panel and then drop down so that grind marks overlap each other. You want to texture the steel so that the filler will bond to the panel securely.

paint! Apply filler only to bare metal. Filler will NOT bond properly to paint, causing problems. See **Figure 10–20.**

Use a No. 40 grit grinding disc to remove the paint. Grinding also etches the metal to provide better adhesion. Grind only enough to remove the finish. Do not grind too much or you will thin and weaken the metal. See **Figure 10–21** to **Figure 10–23.**

If you are applying filler over a metal patch, do not hammer down the excess weld bead. Grind it level with the surface. Hammering a weld down distorts the metal, creates stress, and increases the area to be filled.

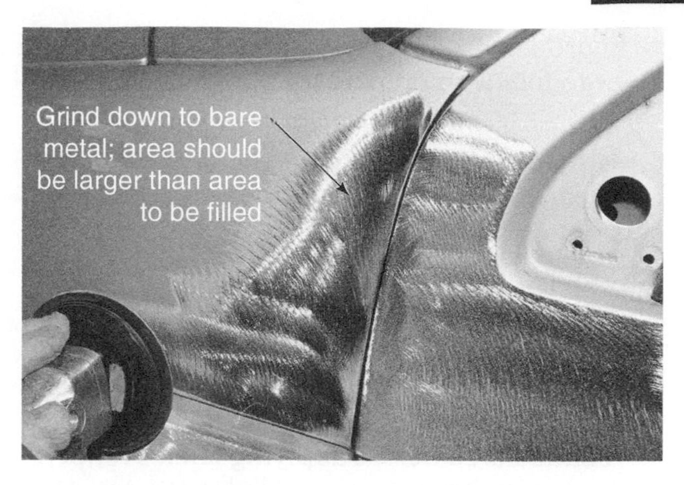

Figure 10–22. Grind an area slightly larger than the damaged area. This will give you enough area to feather out the body filler flush with the undamaged area of the panel.

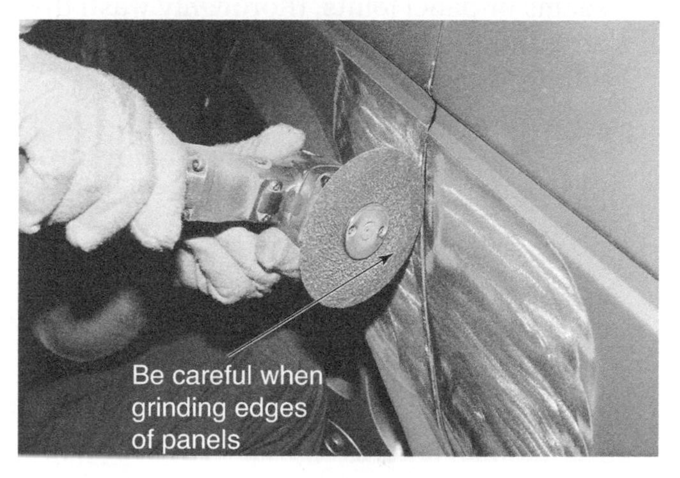

Figure 10–23. Here the technician is grinding the edges of the door and fender to straighten the edges. Wear eye protection and gloves to prevent injury.

After removing the finish from the repair area, blow away the sanding dust with compressed air and wipe the surface with a tack rag to remove any remaining dust particles.

Note that some paint and vehicle manufacturers recommend applying primer to bare metal (usually aluminum) before applying a filler. Filler may not bond as well to bare aluminum as it will to an epoxy-type primer. Refer to the paint or vehicle manufacturer's instructions.

PREPARING SURFACE FOR FILLER

Surface Preparation Problems

Surface preparation involves the many steps needed to clean, straighten, and smooth the surface before refinishing. Many problems are linked to improper surface preparation. Below is a list of rules to follow to prepare for applying filler.

1. Before applying filler, sand or grind the surface to the bare metal, making sure all rust, spots of paints, weld scale, etc. are removed.
2. After sanding or grinding, blow off the area with a high-pressure air gun. Wipe the area with a clean cloth to remove any fine dust or moisture that may be left on the surface.
3. Make sure no solvents are used to clean the sanded area before applying filler. Trapped vapors will result, causing pinholing and poor adhesion.
4. If body filler is to be applied to brazed seams or panel joints, thoroughly wash the area and thoroughly blow out the seam or joint with an air blow gun.
5. Avoid applying filler over seams or joints that were pop riveted. Too much movement takes place, which will cause the filler to crack.
6. For best results, the filler, shop, and parts should all be above 65°F (18°C).
7. With high humidity conditions, use a heat lamp to warm and dry the area to be prepared. This will eliminate moisture accumulation between the bare metal and filler, which will cause poor adhesion.

Mixing Filler

Mix the can of filler to a uniform and smooth consistency. It must be free of lumps and not wet on top. Fillers can be shaken on a paint shaker for several minutes.

Proper *filler mixing* is needed to prevent these problems:

1. The filler in the upper portion of the can will be too thin. This results in runs and sags when applying filler.
2. The filler can cure slowly or not at all.
3. The filler can have a gummy, soft condition when sanded. It can have a very tacky surface after curing that will clog your sandpaper.
4. The filler can cause poor featheredging. It will tear off the metal and form a small lip at its outer edge.
5. The filler can blister and lift when coated with primers and refinishing materials.
6. The filler in the bottom of the can will be too thick. When you use the bottom, the filler will be very coarse and grainy.
7. The filler will have pinholing, or small air holes will form in the filler.
8. The filler will cause poor color holdout when the area is coated with primers and refinishing materials.

Mixing the Hardener

Mixing hardener is done by squeezing the tube back and forth with your fingers to mix the material. Loosen the tube cap to release the air. Knead (squeeze) the tube thoroughly to ensure a smooth, pastelike consistency. The hardener should be like toothpaste when squeezed out.

If you do NOT mix the hardener in the tube, the result can be the same problems listed for poor filler mixing.

If the hardener is kneaded thoroughly and remains thin and watery, you have **defective (bad) hardener.** It should not be used because it has broken down chemically. Hardener can spoil if frozen or if stored too long.

Mixing Filler and Hardener

Numerous problems can occur from improper **catalyzing** (mixing) of *hardener* (filler catalyst) and filler. Before catalyzing, make sure the materials (filler and hardener) to be used are compatible. They should be manufactured by the same company and be recommended for use with each other. See **Figure 10–24.**

The following tips will help eliminate problems relating to mixing filler and its catalyst.

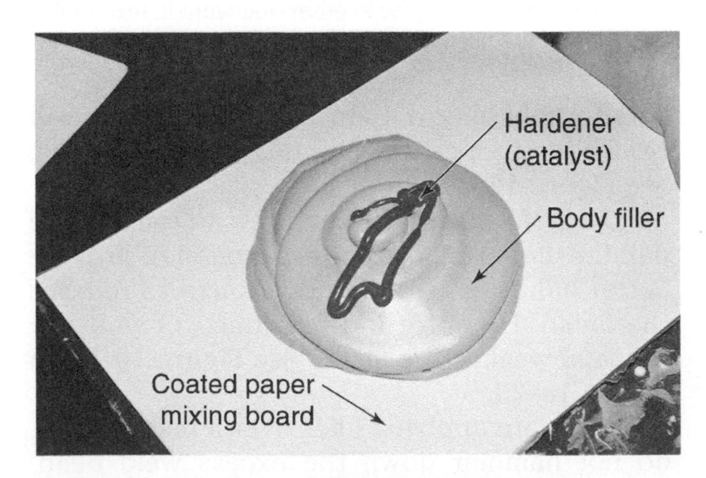

Figure 10–24. Always add the amount of hardener recommended by the manufacturer of the product. Generally, for a "baseball-size" amount of body filler, use about a 6-inch bead of hardener, as shown.

Open the can of filler without bending its lid. Remove the desired amount of filler. Use a clean putty knife or spreader.

Place the filler on a smooth, clean filler mixing board. A **filler mixing board** is a clean, nonporous surface for mixing filler and hardener. You can use sheet metal, glass, or hard plastic.

! WARNING !

Cardboard should NOT be used as a filler mixing board. It is porous and contains waxes for waterproofing. These waxes will be dissolved in the mixed filler and cause poor bonding. Cardboard also absorbs some of the chemicals in the filler and hardener, changing the filler's curing quality slightly. Cardboard fibers can also stick in the filler and ruin the finish. Mixing boards with a handle are also available.

Add hardener according to the proportion indicated on the product label. Too little hardener will result in a soft, gummy filler that will not adhere properly to the metal. It will also not sand or featheredge cleanly. See **Figure 10–25.** Too much hardener will produce excessive gases, resulting in pinholing and hardening before you have time to apply the filler. Look at **Figure 10–26.**

A general rule is this: for each golf ball sized "glob" of filler, use a 1-inch (25 mm) bead of hardener. If the filler is as big as a baseball, use about a 6-inch (152 mm) bead of hardener. However, always refer to the manufacturer's instructions for exact mixing directions.

Filler over-catalyzation results when you use too much hardener for the amount of filler. This must be avoided when adding hardener to the filler. In addition to paint color bleed-through

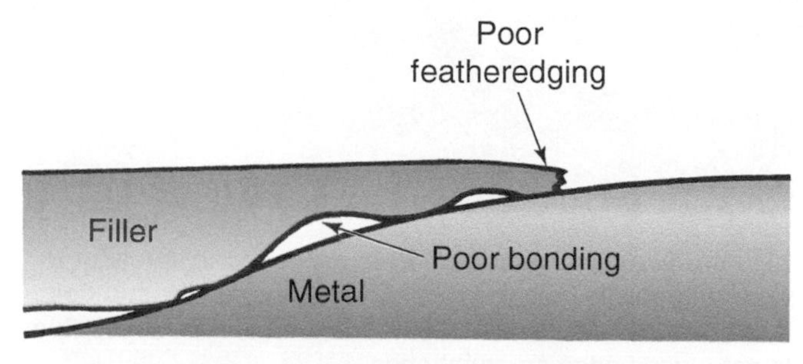

Figure 10–25. If you do not use enough hardener, the filler will not bond to the panel properly and will not featheredge or sand properly.

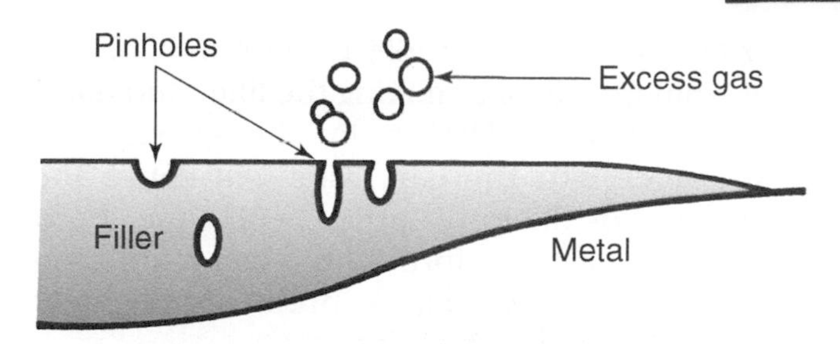

Figure 10–26. A common mistake is to use too much hardener. This will cause excess gas and pinholes in the hardened filler. The filler will also harden on your mixing board before you have time to apply it to the vehicle.

and pinholing, a reverse curing action may occur, causing poor adhesion and poor sanding properties.

Filler under-catalyzation is caused by not using enough hardener in the filler. It will result in the filler not curing properly, resulting in tacky surfaces and poor adhesion properties.

With a clean putty knife or spreader, use a scraping motion (back and forth) to mix the filler and hardener together thoroughly and achieve a uniform color. Scrape filler off both sides of the spreader and mix it in. Every few back-and-forth strokes, scrape the filler into the center of your mixing board by circling inward. Look at **Figure 10–27.**

If the filler and hardener are not thoroughly mixed to a uniform color, soft spots will form in the cured filler. The result is an uneven cure, poor adhesion, lifting, and blistering.

Reinstall the cover on the can of filler right away. This will keep out dust and dirt. It will also help prevent liquids in the filler from evaporating.

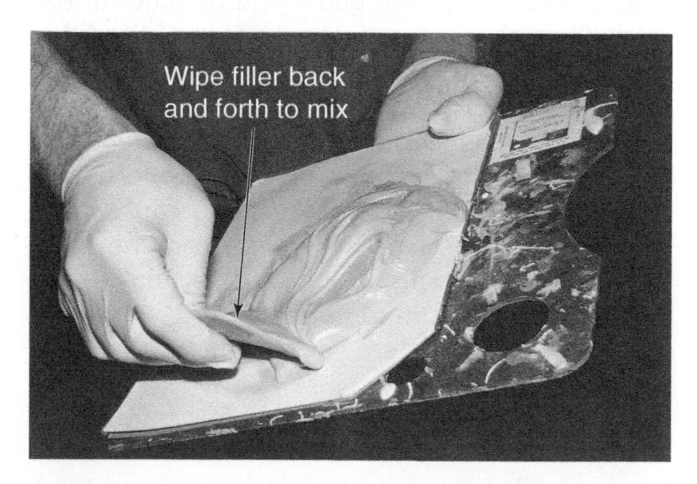

Figure 10–27. Do not stir body filler and hardener because this can force air bubbles into the material. Scrape the filler back and forth across the board in different directions until mixed to the same color. This handy mixing board uses tear-off sheets of coated paper so you do not have to clean your mixing board after use.

Always use clean tools when removing the filler from the can and mixing the filler and hardener together. Do NOT redip the spreader or mixed filler into the can. This will cause the whole can of filler to harden with time. Hard lumps of filler might form in the can and/or applied filler. This will cause problems the next time you try to use the filler.

Use different spreaders to mix and apply the filler. A small amount of unmixed filler will always remain on the mixing spreader. If any is applied, you will have soft spots in the cured filler. The paint finish may peel.

Applying the Filler

Apply the mixed filler as soon as you have finished mixing. First, apply a thin coat of filler to the repair area. Press firmly to force filler into the sand scratches and holes. This will strengthen the bond. Refer to **Figure 10–28.**

Work the filler patch in two directions (left to right, then top to bottom). This will greatly reduce pinholing. Buildup layers should NOT be more than ⅛ inch (3 mm) thick. See **Figure 10–29.**

Spread the filler approximately 3 inches (75 mm) beyond the repaired area. This will ensure better adhesion, and allow you to featheredge the patch.

When this layer cures and has been sanded, apply more coats to build up the repair area to a proper contour. Allow each application to cure before sanding and applying the next coat of filler.

Build up the final layer of filler slightly above the panel surface. Make the filler slightly thicker than needed. This will allow you to sand off the waxy film that forms on the surface of the filler. You will also be able to sand the filler down smooth on an equal plane with the existing panel.

Always use a clean plastic *spreader* or *spatula* to apply filler. Chunks of old filler could fall into the new soft filler. This can cause large pockets to be gouged as you spread the filler. Also, for your final coating of filler, make sure the spreader has a smooth edge. If worn and nicked, used spreaders will not make a smooth layer of filler.

If needed, you can use your fingers to bend the spreader to match the shape of the contour. Use a smaller spreader on small repair areas. A larger spreader will fill large areas more easily.

Avoid using filler in cold temperatures. When the filler, shop, or panel are cold, the filler will NOT cure properly. It will have a tacky surface and poor sanding properties. Large pinholes

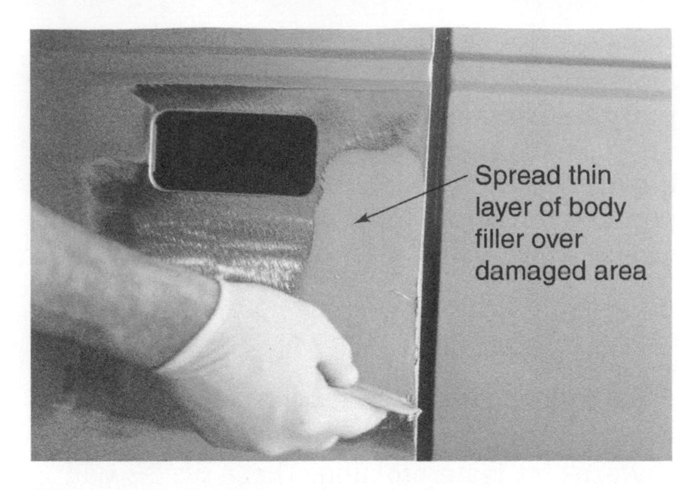

(A) Spread the material one way (horizontally) and then the other way (bottom to top). This will help level the filler and fill low areas on the panel.

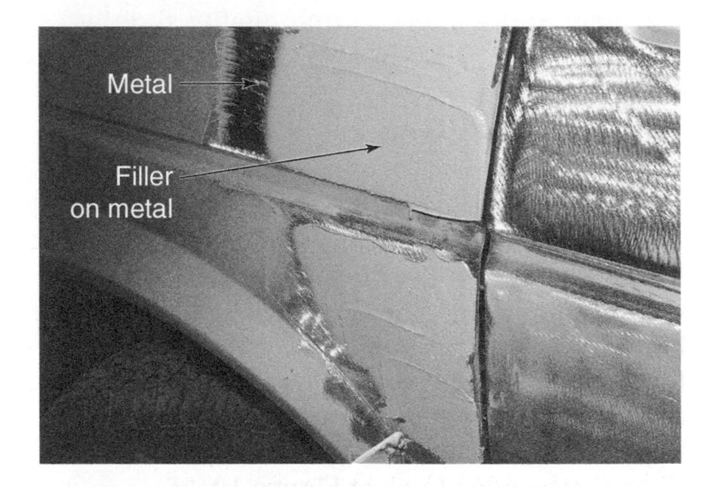

(B) Wipe the body filler on the low spots of the panel. Avoid going over paint with the body filler. Work carefully but quickly so the filler does not start to cure.

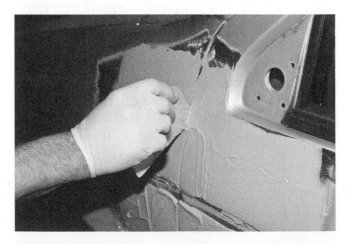

(C) Here the technician is using the edge of the spreader to remove the filler from the gap between the fender and door. If not removed while still soft, it would be almost impossible to get a good edge on panel ends.

Figure 10–28. After blowing off the panel, use a clean spreader to wipe the filler across the repair area.

could also form. Filler should be stored at room temperature (65° to 70°F or 18° to 21°C). Use a heat lamp to warm cold surfaces if needed.

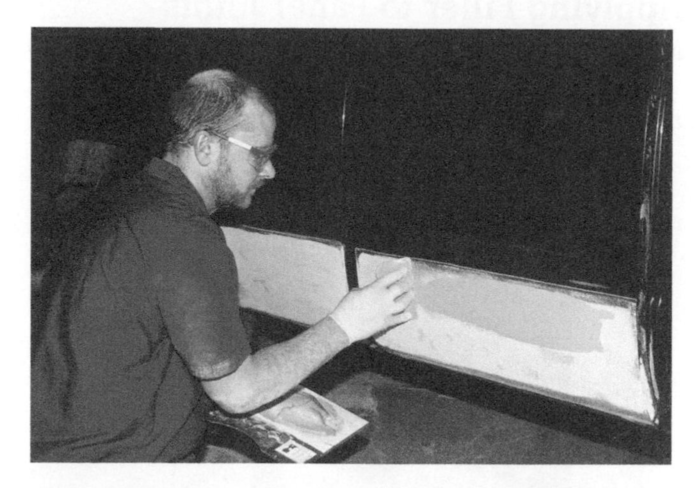

Figure 10–29. After initial sanding, a second coat of body filler is often needed to fill any remaining low spots.

In winter, moisture can form on metal surfaces when a cold vehicle is brought inside. In summer, condensation could form on the metal. Again, use a heat lamp to dry damp surfaces before applying filler. If the repair area is not first warmed to remove moisture, poor adhesion, poor featheredging, pinholing, and lifting could result.

Make sure all holes, gaps, joints, cracks, etc. are welded. Holes left under filler allow moisture to accumulate between the metal and filler, eventually resulting in bond failure.

Shaping Filler

Allow the filler to cure to a semihard consistency. This usually takes 15 to 20 minutes. Scratch the filler with your fingernail. If the scratch leaves a white mark, the filler is ready to be filed. See **Figure 10–30.**

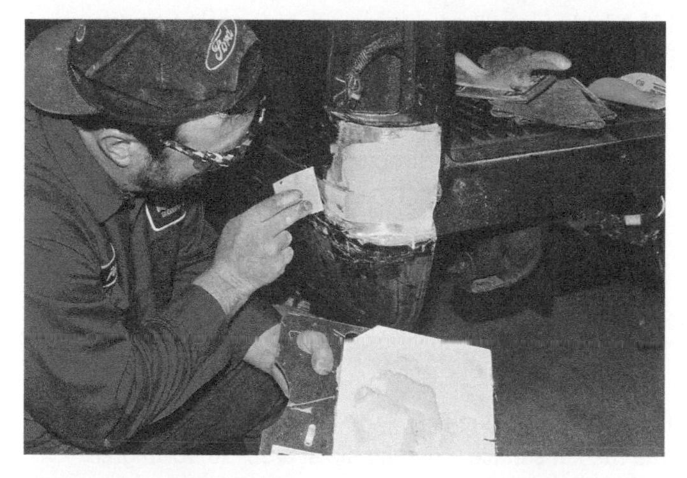

(A) After metal straightening, a small spreader is being used to apply body filler to restore the basic shape of body contour.

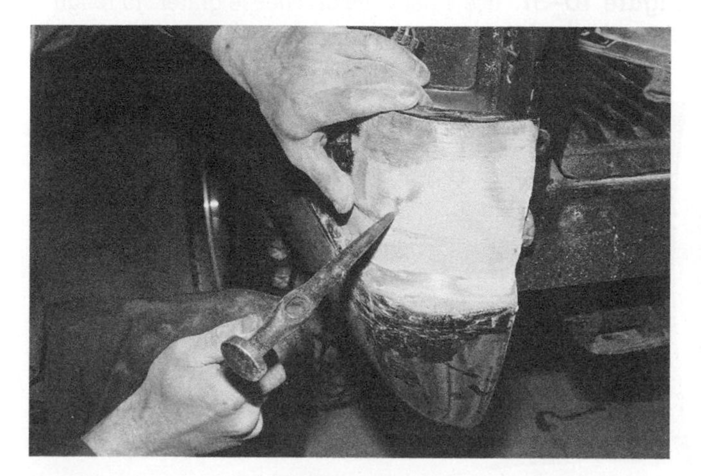

(B) After initial sanding, high spots must be picked down with a body hammer to just below the filler.

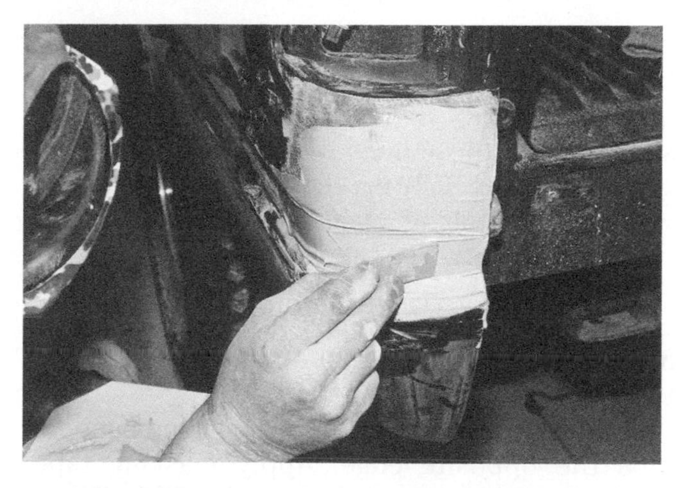

(C) After cutting the spreader to the desired width for body contour, more body filler is applied and sculpted onto the panel.

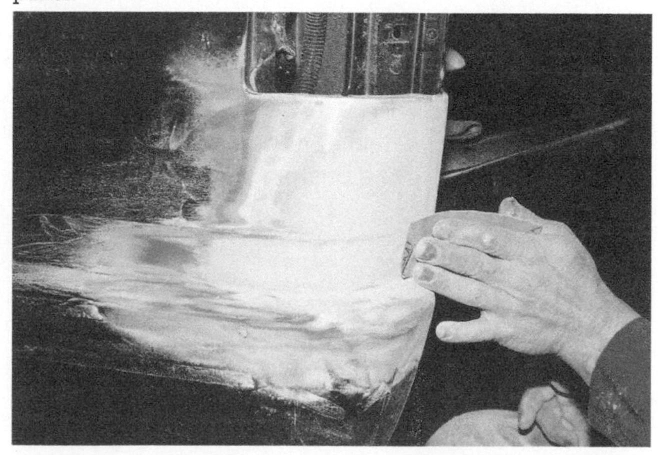

(D) Sanding blocks and hand sanding are needed to restore the original shape to the panel. Only finger sand when the shape of the fingers match the desired shape of the contour.

Figure 10–30. Here the technician is using body filler on a complex, irregular-shaped area of the body panel.

Filler filing involves using a coarse "cheese grater" or body file to rough shape the semihard filler. You will knock off the high spots and rough edges. Since the filler is only partially hard, the body file will quickly remove excess filler. It will force the semisoft filler through the large holes in the file face.

If you do NOT rough shape the filler with a grater, you will waste time and sandpaper. Sandpaper will become loaded quickly. It will also create unwanted dust. See **Figure 10–31.**

To use the body file, hold it at a 30- to 40-degree angle. Pull it lightly across the semihard filler. See **Figure 10–32.** Work the file in several directions. Stop filing when the filler is slightly above the desired level. This will be sufficient for sanding out the file marks and for feathering the edges. If the filler is undercut, additional filler must be applied. See **Figure 10–33.**

Applying Filler to Body Lines

Many vehicles have sharp body lines in doors, quarter panels, hoods, etc. Maintaining the sharpness of these lines when doing filler work is difficult, especially in recessed areas. The best way to get straight, clean lines is to file each plane, angle, or corner separately.

Apply masking tape along one edge. Then apply filler to the adjacent surface. Before the filler sets up, pull the tape off. This will remove the excess filler from the body line.

After the first application is dry and sanded, tape the opposite edge. Apply masking tape along the body line and over the filler. Then, coat the adjacent surface with filler. When the tape is removed and the filler sanded, the result is a straight, even line or corner.

Applying Filler to Panel Joints

Many panels have joints that are factory finished with a *seam sealer* to allow the panel to flex and move. Often, both halves of the joint suffer

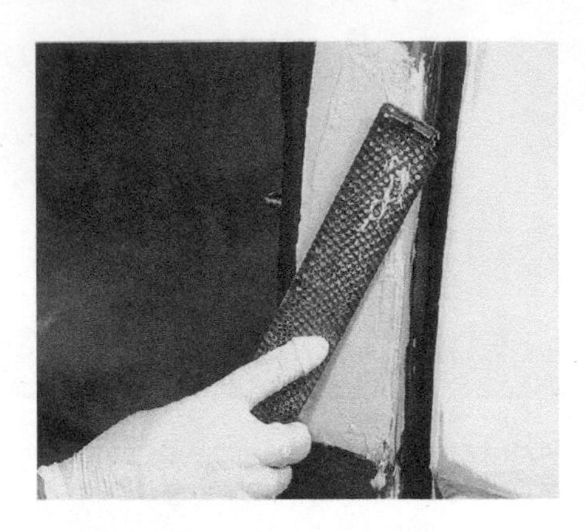

(A) A body file will quickly remove high spots from the filler. It is faster than sanding and does not produce dust.

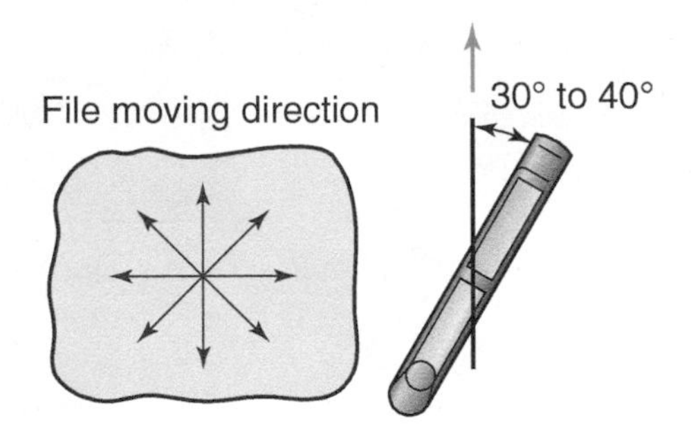

(B) Hold the body file flat and move it in all directions to true the flat surface. Hold the file at a 30- to 40-degree angle.

Figure 10–31. Use a body file or "cheese grater" to rough shape filler when it is partially cured.

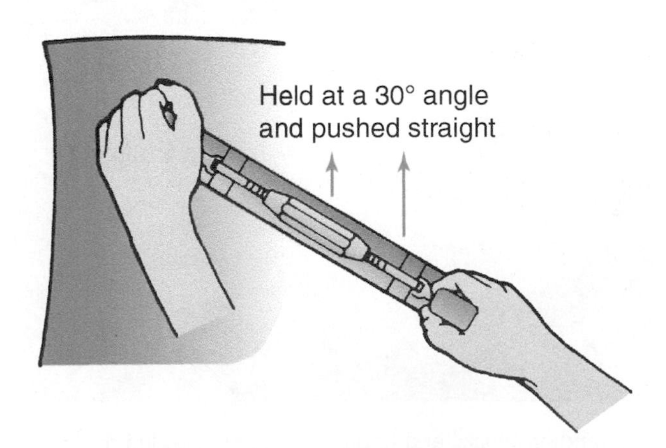

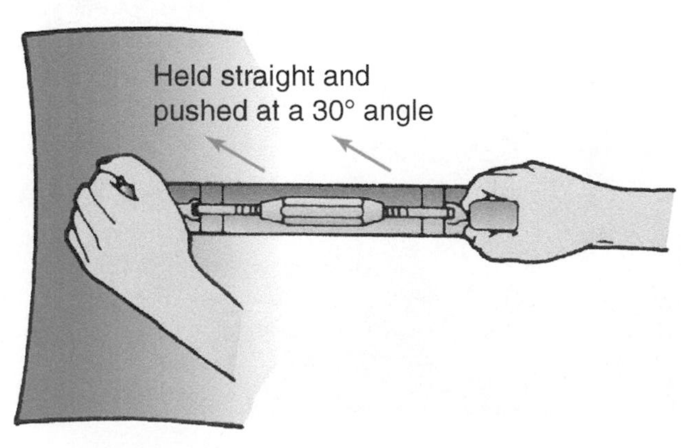

Figure 10–32. Shown are two methods for filing or board sanding of filler. (Left) Push the file or sanding board sideways while holding it at a 30-degree angle. (Right) Hold the tool straight and push it sideways at a 30-degree angle. Always put equal pressure on both ends of the file or sanding board.

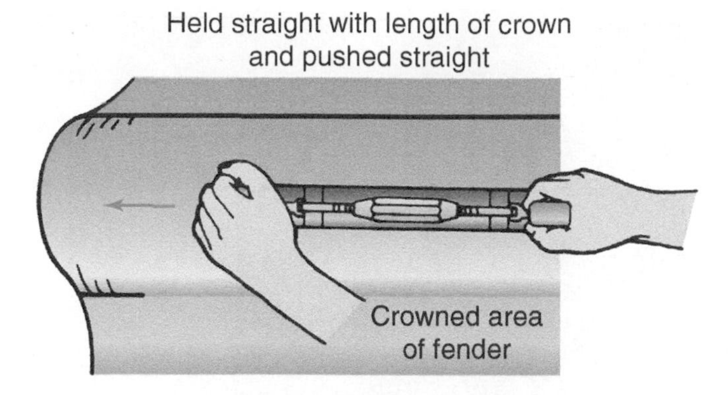

and

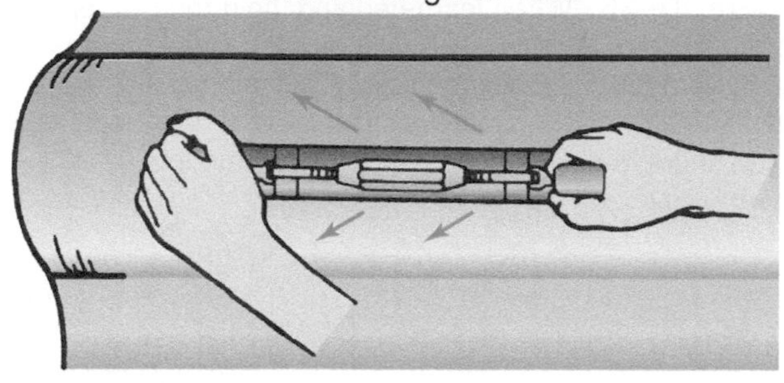

Figure 10–33. Note two methods for filing or sanding a crowned or curved surface. (Top) Push straight along the crown to true the top of the crown. (Bottom) Angle and push the tool off to the side to shape and true the curves on the sides of the crown. Twist the tool with your wrists to match the curved shape.

damage and require filling. Never make the mistake of covering the seam sealer with body filler. The filler will crack over the body flex joint.

Sanding the Filler

After filing, sand out all file marks and begin to shape the filler more accurately. Use a No. 36 or No. 40 grit disc on a sanding board or block first. An air file can also be used on large flat areas. Do not try to sand out all imperfections in the first coat of filler. Only sand the first coat to get the general shape of the repair.

A common mistake is oversanding the first layer of filler below the desired level. Two or more coats of plastic filler are normally needed to get a good, smooth surface.

After sanding the first layer of filler to shape, blow off the area and apply a second layer of plastic filler. Work the filler in two directions to fill any imperfections or holes in the repair.

After this layer cures, sand it to shape with No. 36 to No. 40 grit sandpaper. Follow this with No. 80 grit sandpaper until all large scratches are removed.

DANGER

Do not breathe the dust created when sanding filler. Wear the proper dust respirator to keep the plastic dust out of your lungs.

Finally, smooth the filler with No. 180 grit sandpaper. A sanding block or air file can again be used, as well as a long sanding board. A DA disc orbital sander will work fine on smaller areas.

Be careful not to oversand. **Filler oversanding** results in the filled area being below the desired level, which makes it necessary to apply more filler.

Filler undersanding leaves the filled area high or thicker than the surrounding panel. A hump would be formed at the filled area. See **Figure 10–34.**

After final sanding, blow with an air gun and wipe with a tack cloth. This removes any fine sanding dust that might be hiding surface

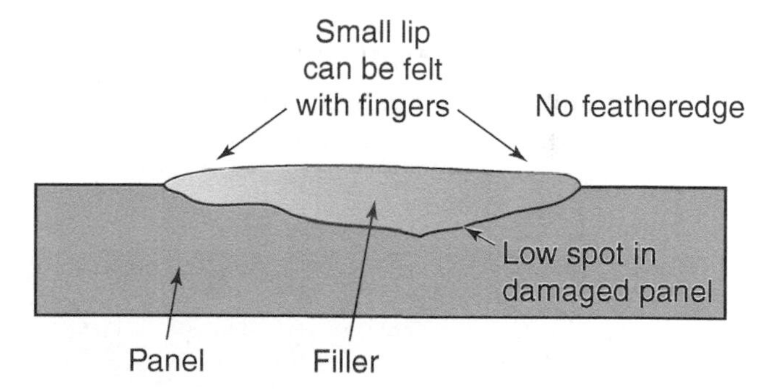

(A) The filler has not been featheredged properly. You want to be able to feel a small lip at the edge of the filler.

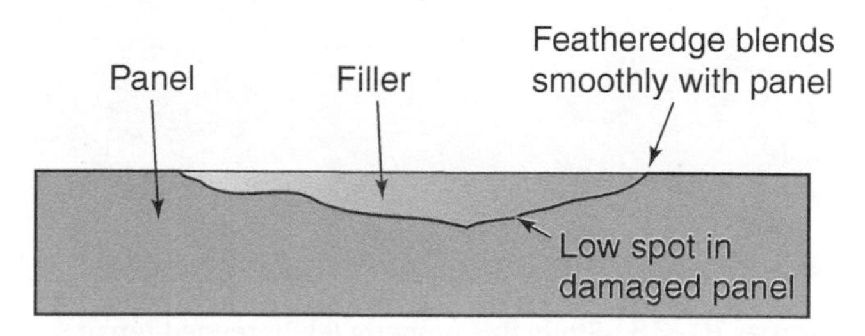

(B) This filler has a good featheredge and blends smoothly into the panel.

Figure 10–34. Compare incorrect and correct body filler featheredge.

pinholes. It also exposes holes lying just below the surface. These holes and remaining sand scratches must be filled.

Run your hand or straightedge over the surface to check for evenness. Do not trust "eyeballing" for accuracy. Paint does NOT hide imperfections; it highlights them. Do not be satisfied until the repaired surface is perfectly smooth.

Remember! If you can feel the slightest bump, paint will make it show up much more. The dull surface of filler and sanded paint does not visibly show surface imperfections.

Featheredging

Featheredging involves sanding the repair area until the filler and old paint blend smoothly into each other. You must use fine sandpaper, 180 grit or finer. Sand until you remove any small lip where different materials on the surface meet. Look at **Figure 10–35.**

Featheredging is commonly done with a DA sander. When sanding, hold the sander flat on the surface. Avoid tilting the sander to remove material more quickly. This will sand a small hole into the filler. By holding the sander flat, you will plane off the filler smoothly. Refer to **Figure 10–36.**

On large areas with filler, use an air file or large sanding board with 180 grit sandpaper. The large sandpaper surface area will help you quickly straighten door panels, fenders, and other large, relatively flat panels.

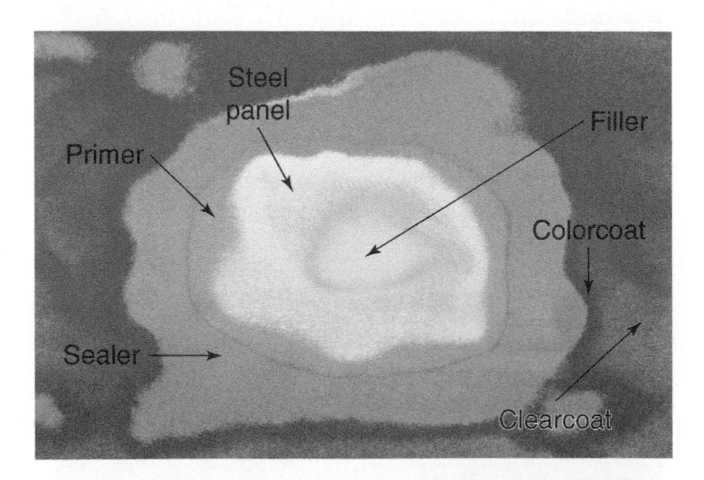

Figure 10–35. Study this properly featheredged repair area. Note the small amount of filler inside the dent in the center area. Note wide lines around the borders of primer, colorcoat, and clearcoat. If the line between different materials is sharp or thin, the area is not featheredged properly.

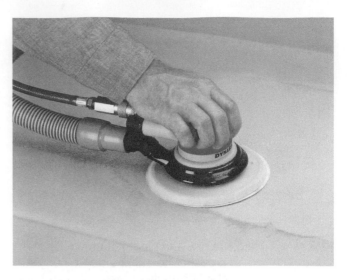

Figure 10–36. When featheredging, hold the sander flat on the surface. Sand the body filler until it is flush with the surrounding undamaged area. A common mistake is oversanding, trying to remove small surface imperfections. If you find a low spot, apply more filler to the low area. Then resand.

Priming

Priming is done after filling to cover any bare metal as well as the filler. After using filler, primer-surfacer is often sprayed on the repair area. Since primer-surfacer can be thick, it will help fill small sand scratches in the filler and paint.

For the best and quickest results when applying primer-surfacer, spray two or three coats with a five to fifteen minute flash time between coats. You will actually save time by following flash recommendations versus spraying coats wet on wet.

It is difficult to tell when a thick coat of primer-surfacer is truly dry. The surface will appear dry while there is still a lot of solvent trapped below the surface. The lower layer of primer-surfacer is still trying to dry and shrink.

On the other extreme, thin dry coats of primer-surfacer can cause loss of adhesion, not only to the substrate, but also to the topcoat color. Always spray wet coats of primer-surfacer. Wait an hour or more before sanding the primer-surfacer.

If the primer-surfacer is sanded before all of the solvent has evaporated, the material in the scratches will continue to shrink down in the scratches. They will show up in the final finishing color topcoats as sanding scratches.

Finishing Fillers (Putties)

Once the primer is dry, small pinholes and scratches can be filled with *spot putty* or *glazing putty* as shown in **Figure 10–37.** If you are using a one-part putty, apply it directly to your spreader. If using a polyester (two-component) putty, mix the putty and hardener according to the manufacturer's instructions.

Place a small amount of putty onto a clean rubber squeegee. Apply a thin coat over the primer. Use single strokes and a fast scraping motion. Use a minimum number of strokes when applying lacquer-based putties. They dry very fast. Repeated passes of the spreader may pull the putty away from the primer.

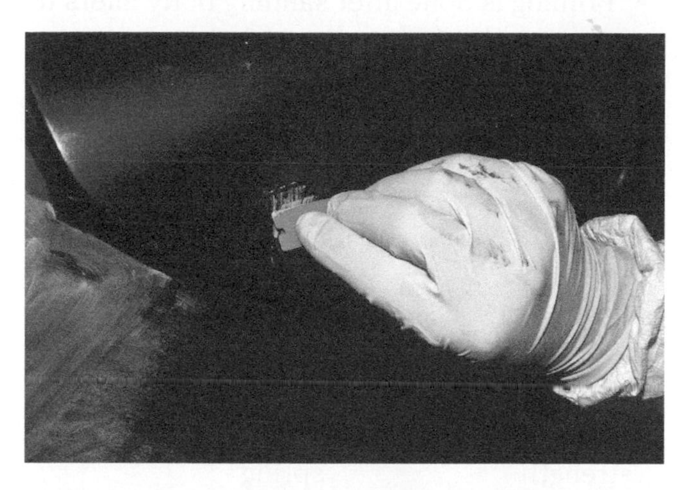

(A) Here the technician is using a tiny spreader to apply two-part body putty to a small chip in the paint.

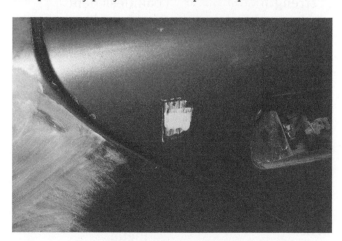

(B) It will be very easy to sand and featheredge the chip to be level with the existing paint.

Figure 10–37. Two-part spot putty is being used to fill small chips in paint.

WARNING

A common mistake is to use spot putty as a filler. Spot putty is NOT as strong as filler. Use spot putty only to fill small imperfections in the primer. Do NOT apply it to bare metal or painted surfaces. Most spot putties are designed to be applied over primer.

Allow the putty to dry completely before sanding smooth with No. 240 grit sandpaper. Sanding the putty too quickly results in sand scratches in the finish.

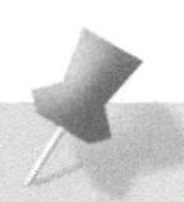

NOTE

Excessive use of glazing putties is usually an indication of a lack of skill and training. They should be used only on small pinholes and other small surface problems in the primer.

Sanding Guide Coat

A **guide coat** is often used to check for high and low spots on your repair area. A guide coat is a thin layer of a different color primer or a special powder applied to the repair area. By watching what happens to the guide coat with light sanding, you can find low and high spots. See **Figure 10–38.**

If the second color primer or guide coat powder does not sand off, you have found a low spot. If either sands off too quickly, you have found a high spot. Both situations require further work before painting.

Ideally, the second color primer or dry guide coat powder should all sand off at the same time. This shows that the surface is flat and ready for sealer, colorcoat, and other operations.

Final check all areas to be refinished. Look around edges carefully to find any remaining surface imperfections. You want to find any surface problems now or before painting.

Make sure you hand sand the edges on the repair panels to prepare them for painting.

Many technicians like to wet sand repair areas as a final check of the repair. When the

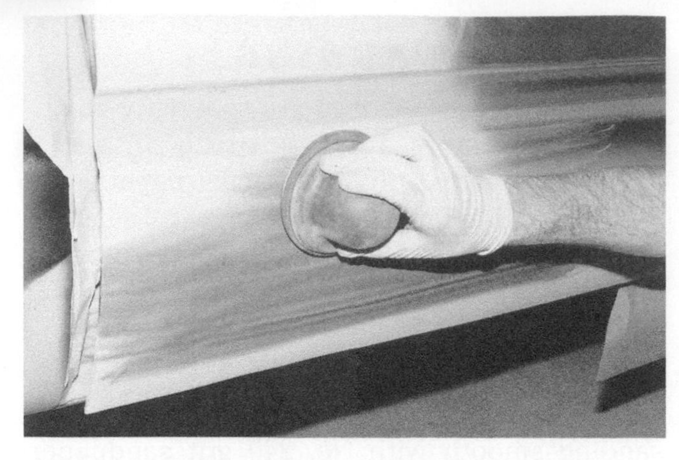

(A) Work the sponge applicator down into the powder. Wipe the powder over the entire area of repair. You can also mist a different color primer over the repair area as a guide coat when final sanding.

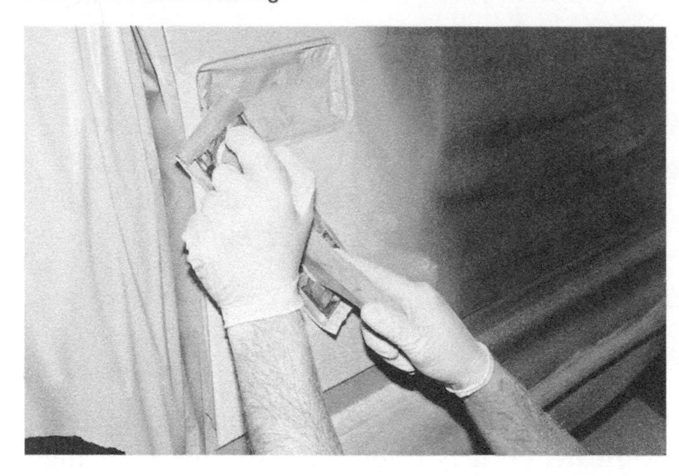

(B) If the powder or primer does not sand off in a small area, that area is still too low and would look like a dent when painted. If the powder sands off too quickly, that area is high and must be sanded level.

Figure 10–38. After spraying on primer, check that the surface is level and smooth. Dry guide powder or a different color primer can be used when checking the repair surface for problems.

surface is wet, it is much easier to notice minor imperfections in the surface. Wet sanding also produces a very smooth surface.

SUMMARY

- The two types of sheet metal used in auto body work are hot-rolled and cold-rolled. Hot-rolled sheet metal is used for comparatively thick parts such as frames and crossmembers. Cold-rolled sheet metal is used for most unibodies.
- The various tools used to straighten metals include body hammers, spoons, dollies, suction cups, slide hammers, and spot-welded studs.
- Shrinking metal removes strain or tension on a damaged, stretched sheet metal area.
- Aluminum is used for a variety of automotive panels such as hoods and deck lids. It is much softer than steel, yet it is more difficult to shape once it becomes work-hardened. It also melts at a lower temperature and distorts readily when heated.
- Body fillers are designed to fill minor surface irregularities that remain after straightening.
- Featheredging involves sanding the repair area until the filler and the finish (old paint) blend smoothly into each other.
- Priming is done after sanding body fillers to prepare the surface for refinishing.

TECHNICAL TERMS

annealed
mild steel (MS)
deformation
tension
yield stress
ultimate strength
compressive strength
shear strength
grain structure
yield point
elastic deformation
spring-back
plastic deformation
work hardening
kinked
bent
high spot
low spot
raising
lowering
finishing hammers
dinging hammers
hammer-on-dolly
hammer-off-dolly
spoons
spring hammering
paintless dent removal
vacuum suction cup
stud spot welder
shrinking metal
torch shrinking
gouge
stretched metal
silicones
defective (bad) hardener
catalyzing

filler mixing board
filler over-catalyzation
filler under-catalyzation
filler filing
filler oversanding
filler undersanding
featheredging
guide coat

REVIEW QUESTIONS

1. What is the difference between mild steel and high-strength steel?
2. Which of these terms refers to a measure of how well a material resists a twisting force?
   a. Tensile strength
   b. Torsional strength
   c. Yield stress
   d. Compression strength
3. ____________ ____________ is the ability of metal to stretch and return to its original shape.
4. ____________ ____________ is the limit of plastic deformation that causes the metal to become hard where it has been bent.
5. When is a part kinked?
6. When is a part bent?
7. Explain the difference between a high spot and a low spot on a panel.
8. The term ____________ means to work a dent outward or away from the body. The term ____________ means to work a high spot or bump down or into the body.
9. Describe the difference between hammer-on- and hammer-off-dollying.
10. A vacuum suction cup uses a remote power source (separate vacuum pump or air compressor airflow) to produce negative pressure (vacuum) in the cup. True or false?
11. What is the main advantage of using a stud/nail welder over a screw-in puller?
12. When should you shrink metal?
13. How do you torch shrink metal?
14. Aluminum turns "cherry red" when heated near its melting point. True or false?
15. ____________ ____________ are designed to cover up minor surface irregularities that remain after metal straightening.
16. List seven rules for applying body filler.
17. This is done to mix a tube of hardener.
    a. Knurling
    b. Shaking
    c. Spreading
    d. Kneading
18. Why should cardboard not be used as a mixing board for filler?
19. Explain how you should file filler.
20. ____________ ____________ results in the filled area being below the desired level, which makes it necessary to apply more filler.

ASE-STYLE REVIEW QUESTIONS

1. Which of the following types of steel is used in unibody structural components?
   a. Hot-rolled steel
   b. Mild steel
   c. High-strength steel
   d. Mild-strength steel

2. *Technician A* says that the secret of metal straightening is to hit the right spot at the right time, with the right amount of force. *Technician B* says that damage should be removed in the opposite direction from how it occurred. Who is correct?
   a. Technician A
   b. Technician B
   c. Both Technicians A and B
   d. Neither Technician

3. A technician is removing a small dent from a panel with a body hammer. However, the repair is going slowly because small nicks are forming where the hammer strikes the panel. Which of the following could be the problem?
   a. Not using dolly
   b. Dolly too large
   c. Not hitting squarely with hammer
   d. Hammer has serrated face

4. *Technician A* says that the contour of the dolly must fit the contour of the backside of the damaged area. *Technician B* says that the dolly contour should be the opposite of the panel to quickly drive out damage. Who is correct?
   a. Technician A
   b. Technician B
   c. Both Technicians A and B
   d. Neither Technician

5. Which of the following metalworking methods should be used to smooth small, shallow dents and bulges because it concentrates force in a small area?
   a. Hammer-off-dolly
   b. Hammer-on-dolly
   c. Hammer stretching
   d. Hammer shrinking

6. Which of the following metalworking techniques is used to raise low spots and lower high spots simultaneously?
   a. Hammer-off-dolly
   b. Hammer-on-dolly
   c. Hammer stretching
   d. Hammer shrinking

7. *Technician A* says that you should never punch or drill holes in panels. *Technician B* says that this is acceptable when the panel is going to be replaced? Who is correct?
   a. Technician A
   b. Technician B
   c. Both Technicians A and B
   d. Neither Technician

8. Filler has been applied to a panel and numerous pinholes are found in the material. Which of the following is the most common cause for this problem?
   a. Improper surface prep
   b. Undermixing
   c. Not enough hardener
   d. Too much hardener

9. Which of the following grits of sandpaper should be used when featheredging body filler?
   a. 36
   b. 80
   c. 180
   d. 600

10. Which of the following can be used to check for high and low spots when final sanding a repair area on a compound curve?
   a. Guide coat
   b. Straightedge
   c. Template
   d. Inspection

ACTIVITIES

1. Obtain a damaged panel (fender, hood, door, or lid). Use a hammer to place a small dent in a flat area of the panel. Use the information in this chapter to grind, fill, and smooth the dent using filler.
2. Featheredge, prime, and spot putty the area filled in activity number 1.
3. Read the mixing instructions on several brands of filler. Make a report on your findings. What differences in mixing hardener and filler did you find?

CHAPTER

11 Plastics and Composite Repair

OBJECTIVES

After studying this chapter, you should be able to:

- List typical plastics and composite applications in vehicle construction.
- Identify automotive plastics through the use of international symbols (ISO codes) and by making a trial-and-error weld.
- Describe the basic differences between welding metal and welding plastic.
- Outline the basics of hot-air and airless welding.
- Repair interior and unreinforced hard plastics.
- Perform two-part adhesive repairs.
- Repair RRIM and other reinforced plastics.

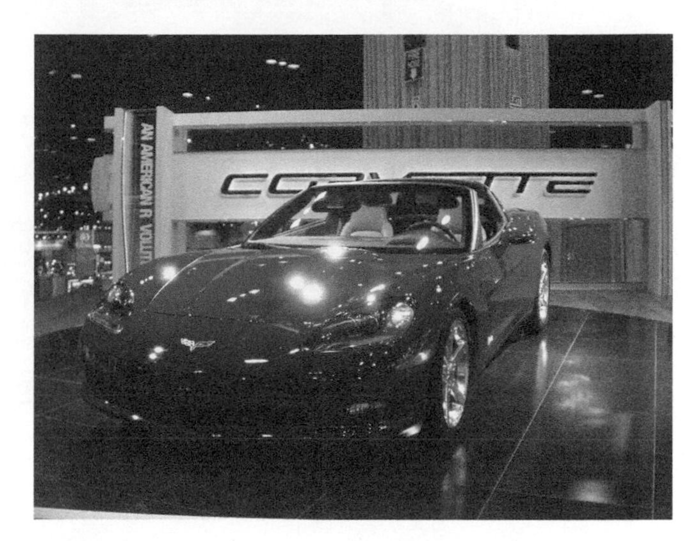

Figure 11–1. Plastics and composites are now very common in modern vehicles. This car uses a composite plastic skin over a full perimeter steel or optional aluminum frame. This improves corrosion resistance and reduces weight for better fuel economy and higher performance. (Courtesy of General Motors Corporation)

INTRODUCTION

The terms **composites** and **plastics** refer to a wide range of materials synthetically compounded from crude oil, coal, natural gas, and other substances. Unlike metals, they do not occur in nature and must be manufactured. Plastics have become an important part of today's vehicles. Today, more and more plastic is being used in automobile manufacturing. Look at **Figure 11–1.**

Plastic parts include bumper covers, fender extensions, fascias, fender aprons, grille openings, stone shields, instrument panels, trim panels, fuel lines, and engine parts. See **Figure 11–2.** Fuel saving and weight reduction programs by auto makers have made plastic parts more common.

TYPES OF AUTO PLASTICS

Two general types of plastics are used in automotive construction: thermoplastics and thermosetting plastics. See **Figure 11–3.**

Thermoplastics can be repeatedly softened and reshaped by heating, with no change in their chemical makeup. They soften or melt when heated and harden when cooled. Thermoplastics are weldable with a plastic welder.

Thermosetting plastics undergo a chemical change by the action of heating, a catalyst, or ultraviolet light. They are hardened into a permanent shape that CANNOT be altered by reapplying heat or catalysts. Thermosets are NOT weldable, but they can be repaired with flexible parts repair materials.

The table in **Figure 11–4** on page 172 shows some of the more common plastics with their full chemical name, common name, and their locations on a vehicle.

Composite plastics, or "hybrids," are blends of different plastics and other ingredients designed to achieve specific performance characteristics.

Note: A standard symbol is stamped on the side under each resin part to show the type of material used.

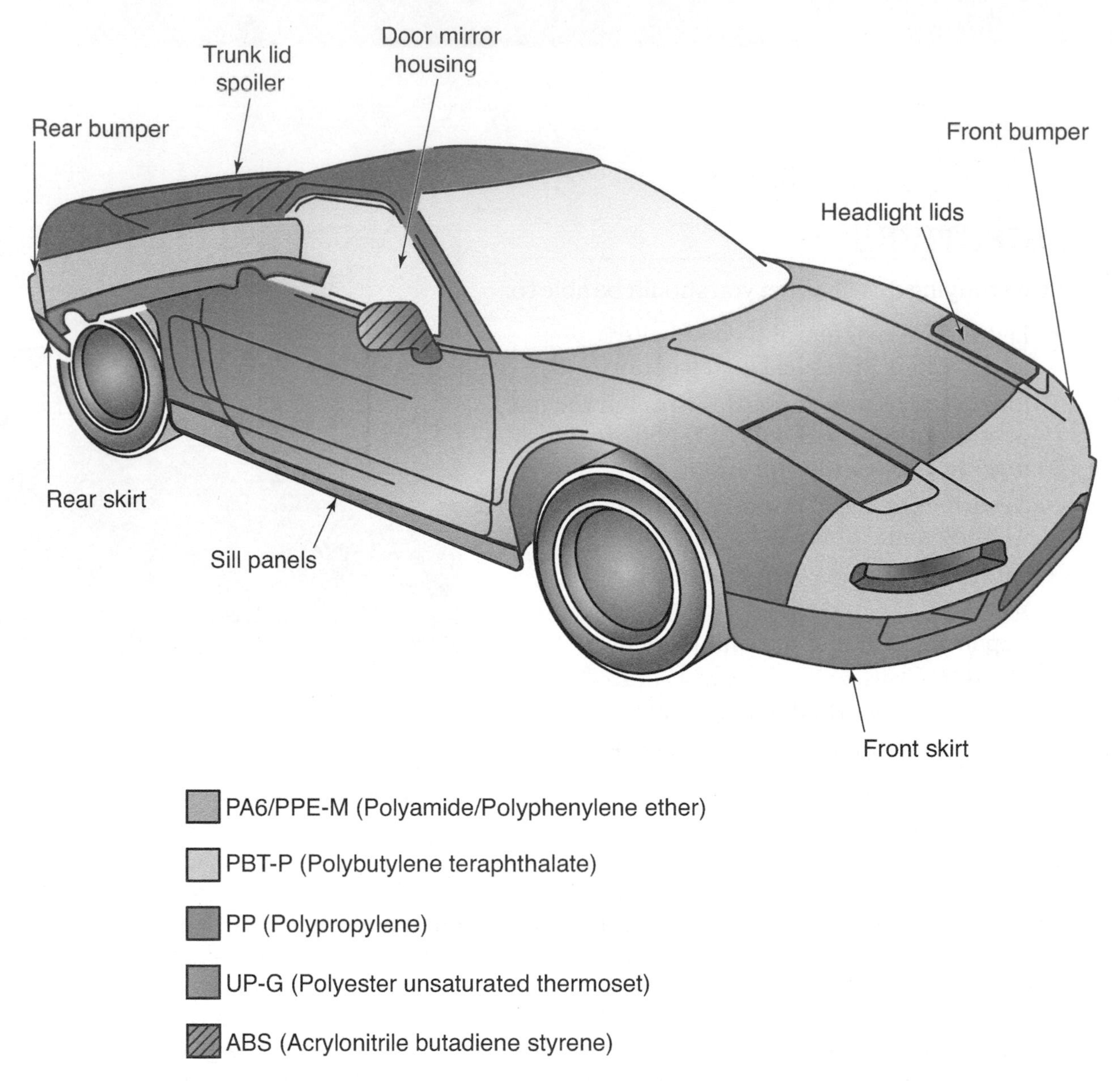

Figure 11–2. Note the types of composite parts used on this aluminum body vehicle.

PLASTICS SAFETY

Working with plastics, fiberglass, and composites requires you to think about safety at all times. The resin and related ingredients can irritate your skin, lungs, eyes, and stomach lining. The curing agent or hardener can produce harmful vapors.

Read and understand the following safety points before using any of these types of products:

1. Read all label instructions and warnings carefully.
2. When cutting, sanding, or grinding plastics, dust control is important.
3. Wear rubber gloves when working with fiberglass resin or hardener. Long sleeves, buttoned collar, and cuffs are helpful in preventing sanding dust from getting on your skin. Disposable paint suits will keep dust away from clothes.

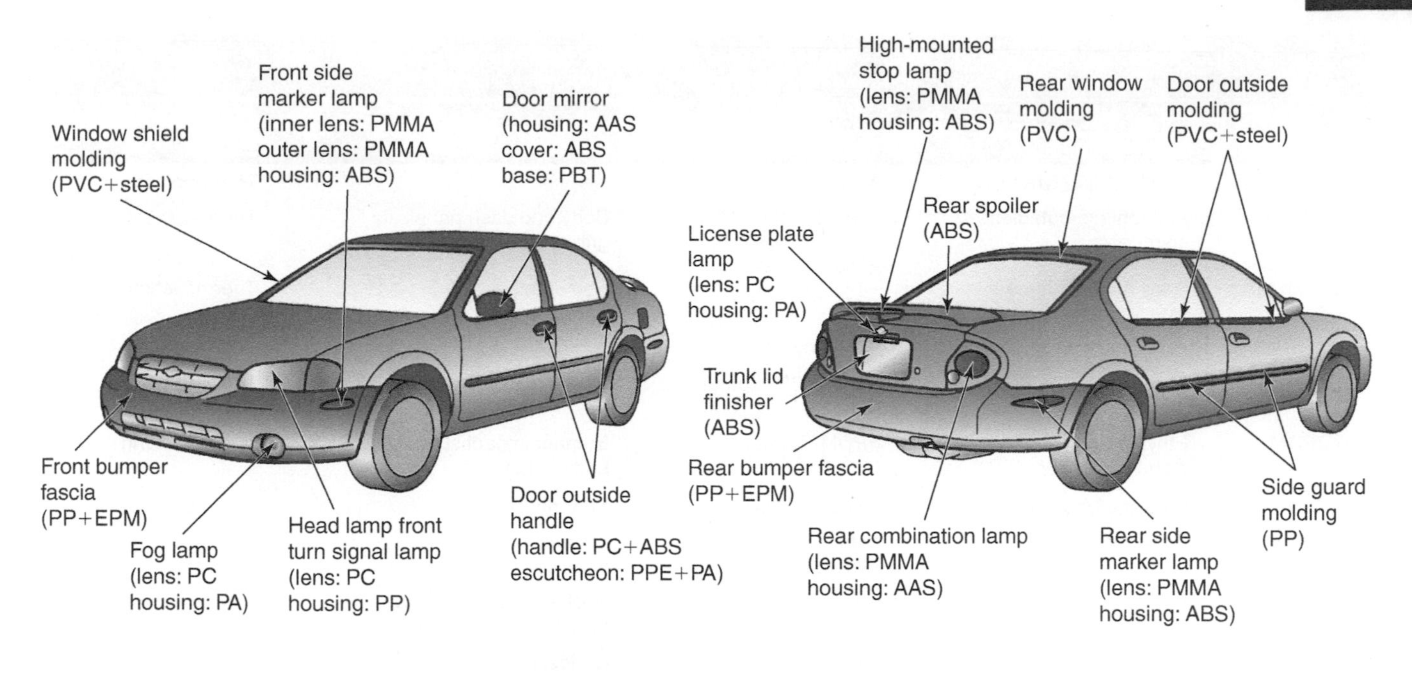

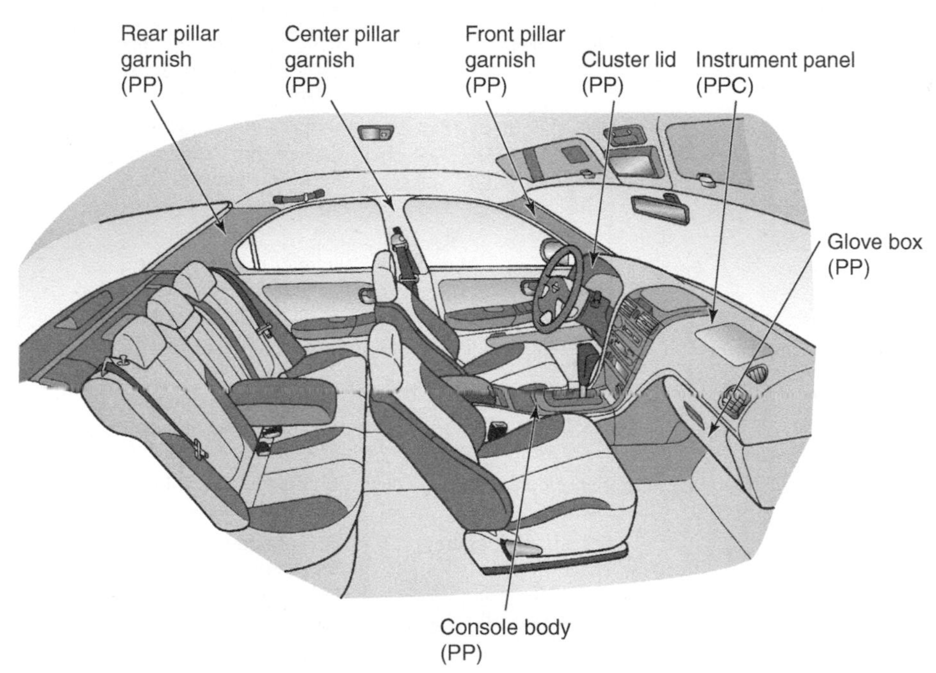

Figure 11–3. Study the location of different kinds of composites (plastics) on a typical vehicle. (Courtesy of Nissan North America)

4. A protective skin cream should be used on any exposed areas of the body.
5. If the resin or hardener comes in contact with your skin, wash with borax soap and water or alcohol.
6. Safety glasses are always a necessity.
7. Always work in a well-ventilated area.
8. Wear a respirator to avoid inhaling sanding dust and resin vapors.
9. Some shop chemicals can react with certain plastics. Keep brake fluid, solvents, and gasoline off exposed plastics. Use only manufacturer-approved solvents to clean plastics.
10. PVC-type plastics produce a poison gas when burned. Keep them away from excess heat and flames.

PLASTIC IDENTIFICATION

There are several ways to identify an unknown plastic. One way to identify a plastic is by **international symbols,** or **ISO codes,** which are molded into plastic parts. The symbol or abbreviation is formed in an oval on the back of

Symbol, Chemical Name, Trade Name, and Design Applications of Commonly Used Automotive Plastics				
Symbol	Chemical name	Trade name	Design applications	Thermosetting or thermoplastic
AAS	Acrylonitrile-styrene	Acrylic Rubber	—	Thermoplastic
ABS	Acrylonitrile-butadiene-styrene	ABS, Cycolac, Abson, Kralastic, Lustran, Absafil, Dylel	Body and dash panels, grilles, headlamp doors	Thermoplastic
ABS/MAT	Hard ABS reinforced with fiberglass	—	Body panels	Thermosetting
ABS/PVC	ABS/Polyvinyl chloride	ABS Vinyl	—	Thermoplastic
EP	Epoxy	Epon, EPO, Epotuf, Araldite	Fiberglass body panels	Thermosetting
EPDM	Ethylene-propylene-diene-monomer	EPDM, Nordel	Bumper impact strips, body panels	Thermosetting
EVA	Ethylene/Vinyl Acetate	Elvax, Microthane	Soft trim parts	Thermosetting
PA	Polyamide	Nylon, Capron, Zytel, Rilsan, Minlon, Vydyne	Exterior trim panels	Thermosetting
PBT	Polybutylene	Bexloy "M"	Rocker cover moldings, fascias	Thermosetting
PC	Polycarbonate	Lexan, Merlon	Grilles, instrument panels, lenses	Thermoplastic
PPO	Polyphenylene oxide	Noryl, Olefo	Chromed plastic parts, grilles, headlamp doors, bezels, ornaments	Thermosetting
PE	Polyethylene	Dylan, Fortiflex, Marlex, Alathon, Hi-fax, Hosalen, Paxon	Inner fender panels, interior trim panels, valances, spoilers	Thermoplastic
PF	Phenol-Formaldehyde resin	Bakelite, Genal, Resinox	Ashtrays	Thermosetting
PP	Polypropylene	Profax, Olefo, Marlex, Olemer, Aydel, Dypro	Interior moldings and panels, inner fenders, radiator shrouds, bumper covers	Thermoplastic
PS	Polystyrene	Lustrex, Dylene, Styron, Fostacryl, Duraton	—	Thermoplastic
PUR	Polyurethane	Castethane, Bayflex	Bumper covers, front and rear body panels, filler panels	Thermosetting
TEO	Ethylene/Propylene	Thermoplastic, Rubber	Bumper fascia, valance panels, air dams	Thermoplastic
TPUR	Polyurethane	Pellethane, Estane, Roylar, Texin	Bumper covers, gravel deflectors, filler panels, soft bezels	Thermoplastic
PVC	Polyvinyl chloride	Geon, Vinylete, Pliovic	Interior trim, soft filler panels	Thermoplastic
RIM	"Reaction injection molded" polyurethane	—	Bumper covers	Thermosetting
RRIM	Reinforced RIM-polyurethane	—	Exterior body panels	Thermosetting
SAN	Styrene-acrylonitrite	Lustran, Tyril, Fostacryl	Interior trim panels	Thermosetting
SMC	Sheet Molded Compound	—	Body panels	Thermosetting
TPR	Thermoplastic rubber	—	Valance panels	Thermosetting
UP	Polyester	SMC, Premi-glas, BMC, Selection Vibrin-mat	Fiberglass body panels	Thermosetting

Figure 11–4. This chart lists symbols, chemical names, trade names, applications, and types of commonly used automotive plastics.

the part. One problem is that you usually have to remove the part to read the symbol.

If the part is NOT identified by a symbol, the **body repair manual** will give information about plastic types used on the vehicle.

A **floating test** can be used to help determine the type of plastic. Cut a piece of plastic off the part to be repaired. Drop the sliver of plastic into a container of water. Watch to see if the piece of plastic sinks or floats in the water.

If the plastic floats in the water, it is thermoplastic. You would then know that you can repair the part with either welding or an adhesive. If the plastic piece sinks in the water, it is thermoset plastic and must be repaired with an adhesive.

A reliable means of identifying an unknown plastic is to make a trial-and-error weld on a hidden or damaged area of the part. Try several different filler rods until one sticks. Most suppliers offer only a few types of plastic filler rods; the range of possibilities is not that great. The rods are color coded. Once you find a rod that works, the base material is identified.

Some technicians like to cut a sliver off the damaged part and use it as a welding rod. Cut the piece from a location on the part that cannot be seen after installation. Try using this piece as a welding rod. If the plastic fails to weld, you should use an appropriate adhesive to repair the plastic damage.

PLASTIC PART REMOVAL

There are various types of fasteners used to secure plastic parts to the vehicle. These fasteners include screws, clips, or adhesive. Refer to the vehicle's service manual for directions about part removal. See **Figure 11–5.**

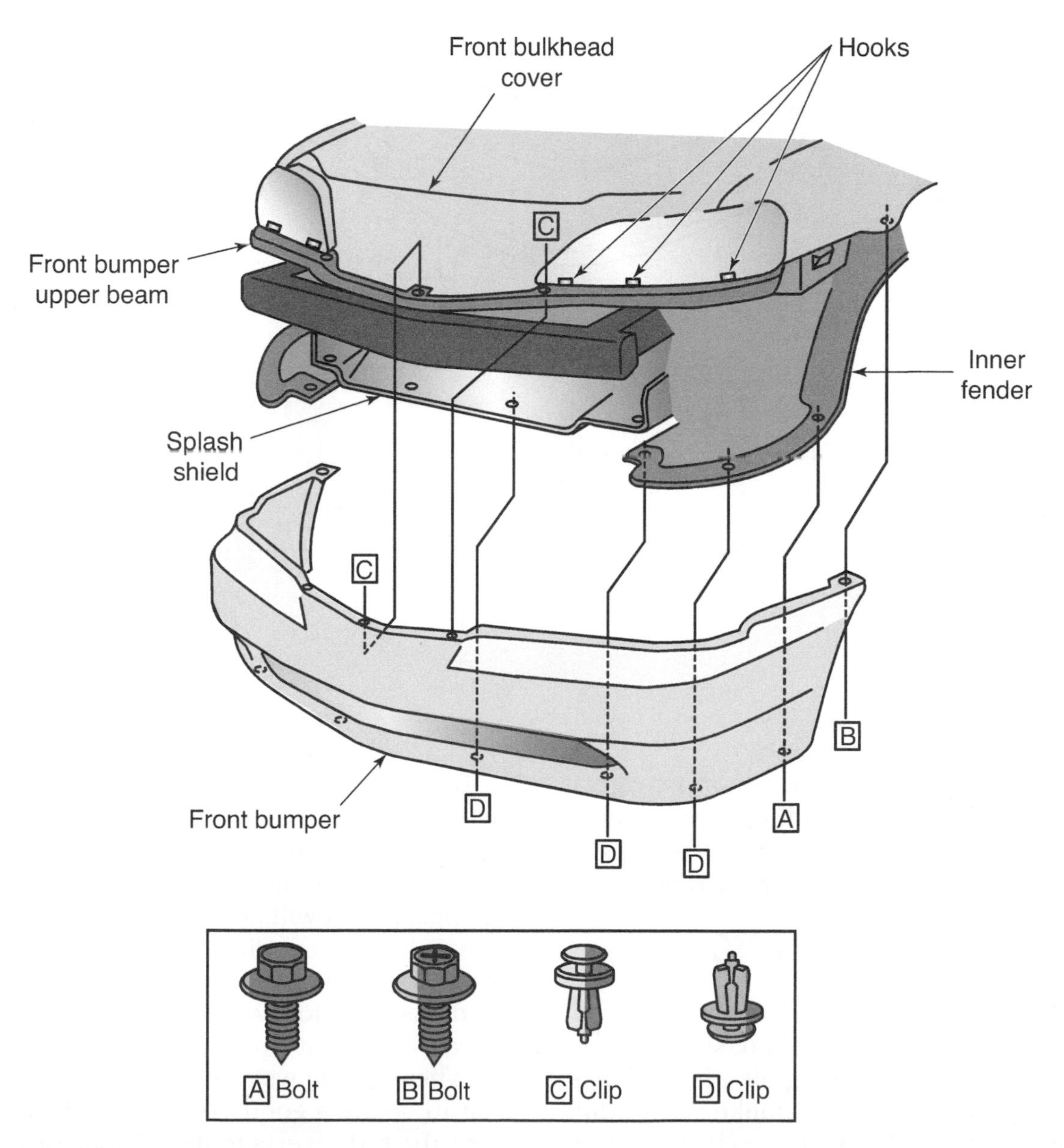

(A) Note how this front bumper is held on a unibody.

Figure 11–5. Various methods are used to secure plastic parts to a vehicle.

(continued)

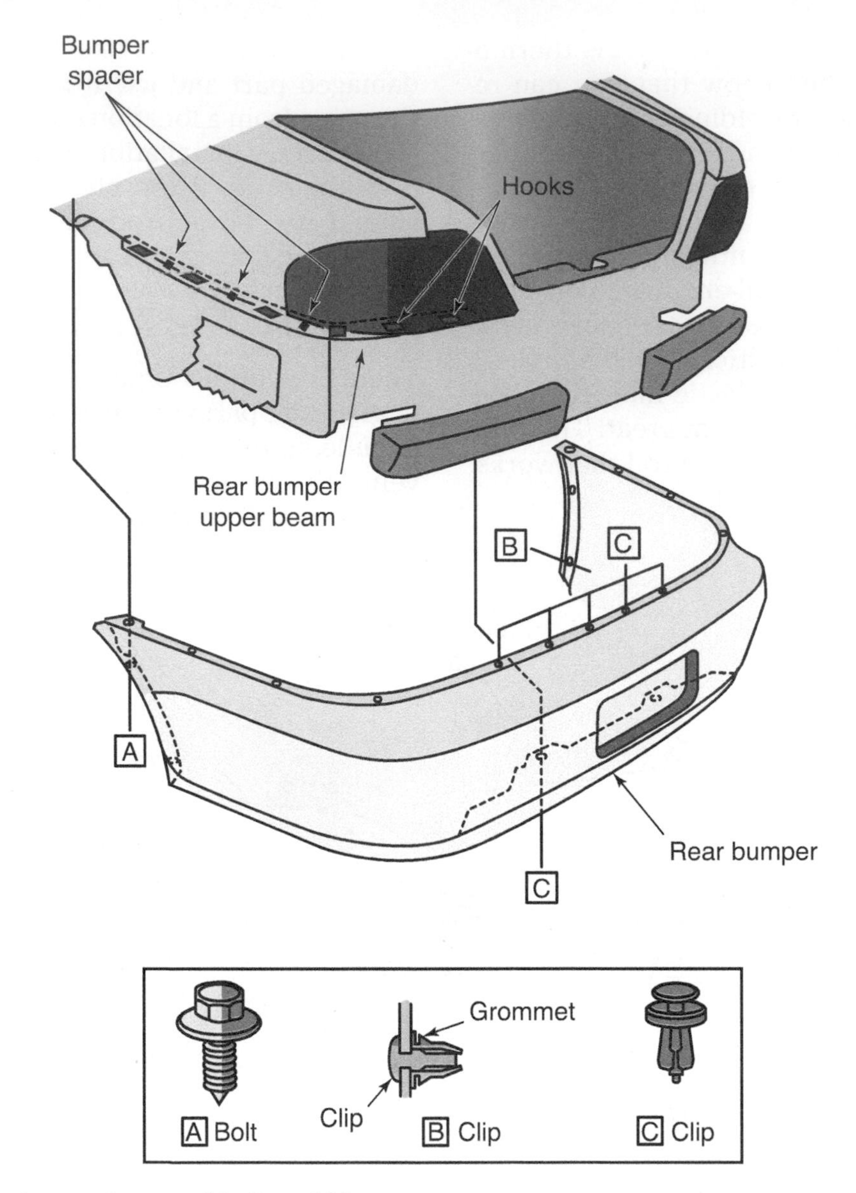

(B) Study how the rear bumper is secured to the vehicle.

Figure 11–5. (***Continued***)

If the plastic part has only minor damage, it can often be repaired by welding or, more commonly, by using a two-part plastic repair adhesive. By repairing the part, you save time.

PRINCIPLES OF PLASTIC WELDING

Plastic welding uses heat and sometimes a plastic filler rod to join or repair plastic parts. The welding of plastics is not unlike the welding of metals. Both methods use a heat source, welding rod, and similar techniques (butt joints, lap joints, etc.). See **Figure 11–6.**

Because a plastic rod does not become completely molten, a plastic weld might appear incomplete. The outer surface of the rod becomes molten while the inner core remains semisolid. The plastic rod will not look completely melted, except for molten flow on either side of the bead. Even though a strong and permanent bond has been formed, you may think you have a weak, cold-joint weld.

When plastic welding, force the rod into the joint to create a good bond. When heat is taken away, the rod reverts to its original form. A combination of heat and pressure is used when welding plastic. Normally, apply pressure on the welding rod with one hand while applying heat with the tool. Use a constant fanning motion with hot air from the welding torch.

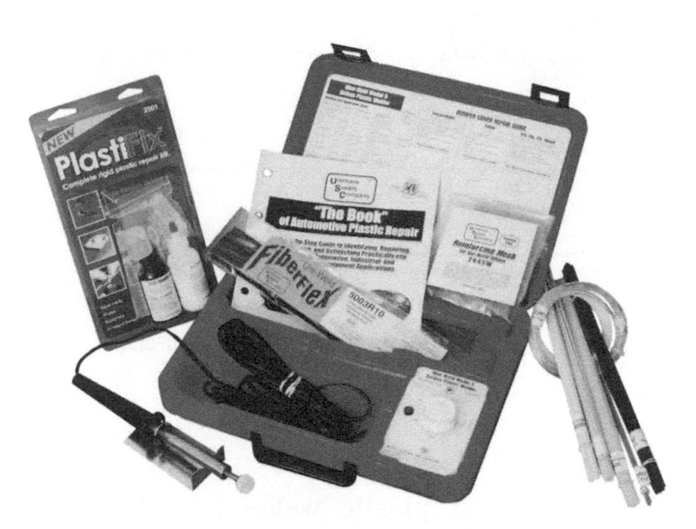

Figure 11–6. This is a typical plastic welder. Note the different types of plastic welding rods provided. The type of rod used must match the type of plastic part. (Courtesy of Urethane Supply Co.)

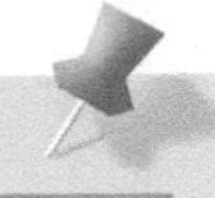

NOTE

Too much pressure on the rod tends to stretch the bead. Too much heat will char, melt, or distort the plastic. Competent plastic welding takes practice.

HOT-AIR PLASTIC WELDING

Hot-air plastic welding uses a tool with an electric heating element to produce hot air (450° to 650°F or 230° to 340°C), which blows through a nozzle and onto the plastic. The air supply comes from either the shop's air compressor or a self-contained portable compressor that comes with the welding unit.

Most hot-air welders use a tip working pressure of around 3 psi (0.21 kg/cm^2). Air pressure regulators reduce the air pressure first to around 50 psi, and then to the working pressure of about 3 psi (0.21 kg/cm^2). A typical hot-air welder is illustrated in **Figure 11–7.**

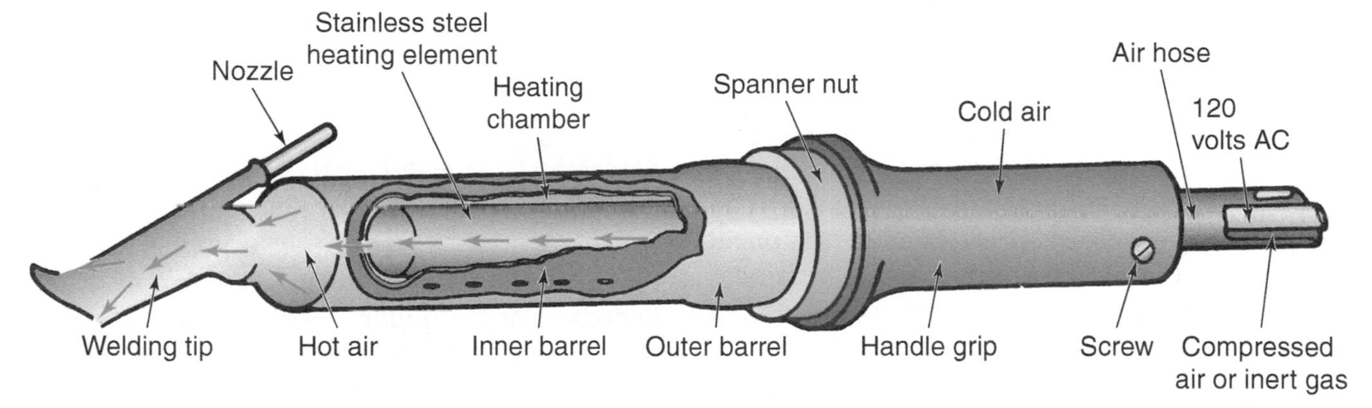

(A) Study the parts of the plastic welder.

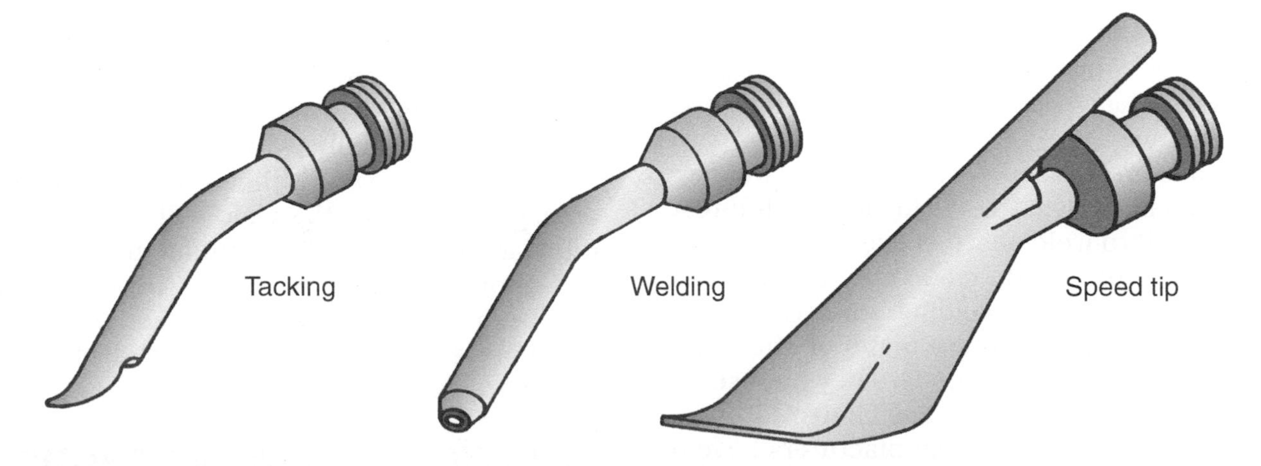

(B) Note the types of plastic welding tips. (Courtesy of Seelye, Inc.)

Figure 11–7. Close-up of a typical plastic welder.

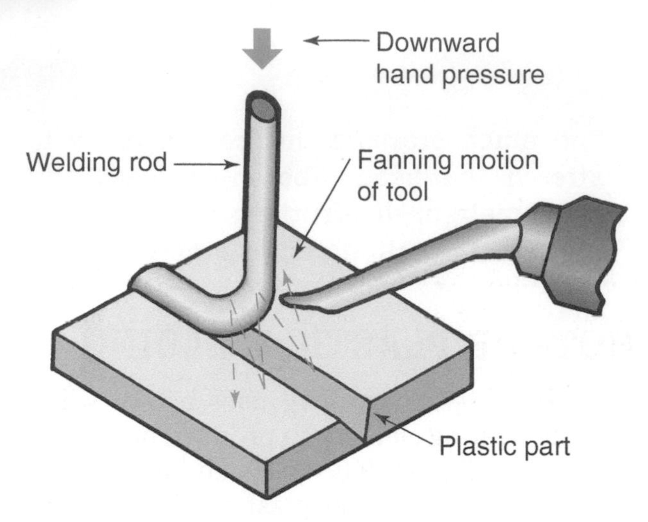

Figure 11–8. When welding plastic, you must use the proper combination of heat and pressure. Hand pressure is needed to force the plastic rod down into the weld joint. Fan the welder over the joint to heat the rod and base material properly.

The hot-air torch is used in conjunction with the welding rod, which is normally $\frac{3}{16}$ inch (5 mm) in diameter. The plastic welding rod must be made of the same material as the plastic being repaired. This will ensure proper strength, hardness, and flexibility of the repair. See **Figure 11–8.**

One of the problems with hot-air welding is that the plastic welding rod is often thicker than the panel to be welded. This can cause the panel to overheat before the rod has melted. Using a smaller diameter rod with the hot-air welder can often correct such warpage problems.

Three types of welding tips are available for use with most hot-air plastic welding torches. They are:

Tacking tips—shaped to tack weld broken sections of plastic together before welding. If necessary, tack welds can be easily pulled apart for realigning.

Round tips—used to make short welds, to weld small holes, to weld in hard-to-reach places, and to weld sharp corners.

Speed tips—hold, feed, and automatically preheat the plastic welding rod. This design feeds the rod into the base material, thus allowing for faster welding speeds. They are used for long, fairly straight welds. See **Figure 11–9.**

Some hot-air welder manufacturers have developed specialized welding tips and rods to meet specific needs. Check the product catalog for more information.

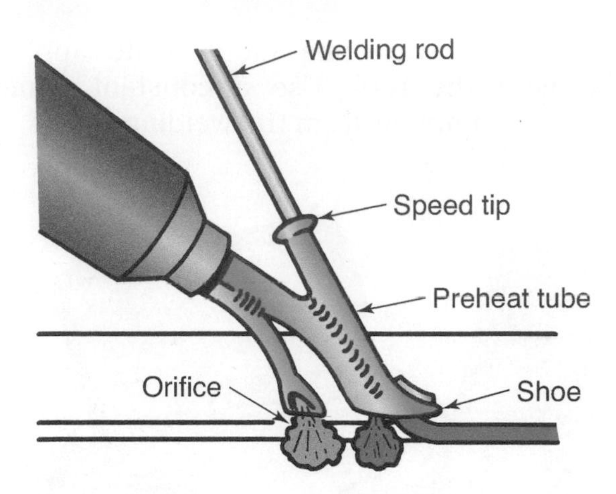

Figure 11–9. Note the construction of a high-speed plastic welding tip.

Using Hot-Air Plastic Welders

No two hot-air plastic welders work exactly alike. For specific instructions, always refer to the owner's manual and other material provided by the hot-air welder manufacturer.

Some manufacturers advise against using their welder on plastic thinner than $\frac{1}{8}$-inch (3.2 mm) because of distortion. It is sometimes acceptable to weld thin plastics if they are supported from underneath while welding.

AIRLESS PLASTIC WELDING

Airless plastic welding uses an electric heating element to melt a smaller $\frac{1}{8}$-inch (3 mm) diameter rod with no external air supply. It has become very popular. Airless welding with a smaller rod helps eliminate two troublesome problems: panel warpage and excess rod buildup. See **Figure 11–10.**

When setting up an airless welder, set the temperature dial at the appropriate setting. This will depend upon the specific plastic being worked on. It will normally take about 3 minutes for the welder to fully warm up.

Make sure the rod is the same material as the damaged plastic or the weld will be unsuccessful. Many airless welder manufacturers provide rod application charts. When the correct rod has been chosen, it is good practice to run a small piece through the welder to clean out the tip before beginning.

PLASTIC WELDING METHODS

The basic methods for hot-air and airless welding are very similar. To make a good plastic weld

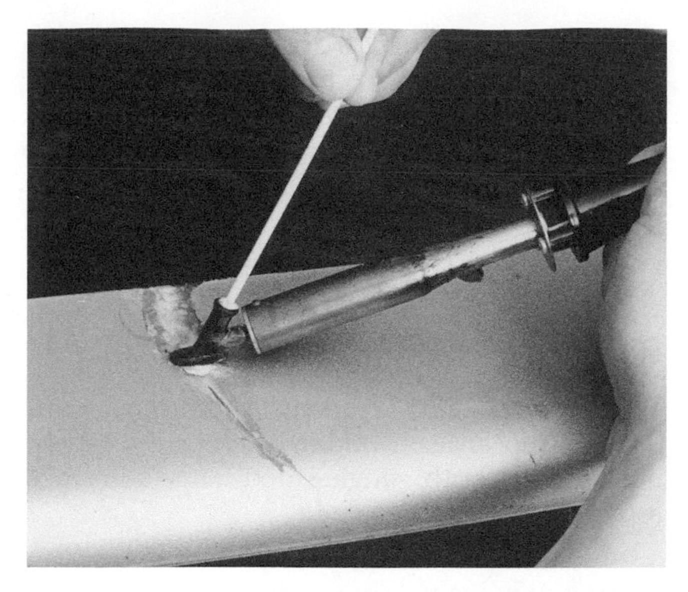

Figure 11–10. Practice is needed to make good plastic welds. Welding both sides of the part is the best method when possible. Using too much heat or not enough heat is a common problem when plastic welding. (Courtesy of Urethane Supply Co.)

with either procedure, keep the following factors in mind:

1. Plastic welding rods are frequently color coded to indicate their material. Unfortunately, the **rod color coding** is not uniform among manufacturers. It is important to use the reference information provided. If the rod is not compatible with the base material, the weld will NOT hold.
2. Too much heat will char, melt, or distort the plastic. Too little heat will not provide weld penetration between the base material and the rod.
3. Too much pressure stretches and distorts the weld.
4. The angle between the rod and base material must be correct. If it is too shallow, a proper weld will NOT be achieved.
5. Use the correct welding speed. If the torch movement is too fast, it will NOT permit a good weld. If the tool is moved too slowly, it can char the plastic.

PLASTIC TACK WELDING

On long tears where backup is difficult, small *tack welds* can be made to hold the two sides in place before doing the permanent weld. For larger areas, a patch can be made from a piece of plastic and tacked in place.

WELDING A PLASTIC V-GROOVE

Prepare the rod for welding by cutting the end at approximately a 60-degree angle. When starting a weld, hold the nozzle about ¼ to ½ inch (6 to 12 mm) above and parallel to the base material. Hold the rod at a right angle to the work. Position the cut end of the rod at the beginning of the weld.

Direct the hot air from the tip alternately at the rod and the base material. Concentrate the heat more on the rod when starting to weld. Keep the rod lined up and press it into the seam. Light pressure is sufficient.

Once the rod begins to stick to the plastic, start to move the torch and use the heat to control the flow. After you start your weld, direct more of the heat into the base material. Be careful not to melt or char the plastic. As the welding continues, a small bead should form along the entire weld joint.

As you plastic weld and use up the rod, you must regrip the rod. Unless it is done carefully, you will lift the rod away from the weld. This will allow air to be trapped under the weld, weakening it. To prevent this, you must develop the skill of continuously applying pressure on the rod while repositioning your fingers. This can be done by applying pressure with your third and fourth fingers while moving the thumb and first finger up the rod.

At the end of a weld, maintain pressure on the rod as the heat is removed. Hold the rod still for a few seconds to make sure it has cooled and does not pull loose. Then carefully cut the rod with a sharp knife or clippers.

Do NOT attempt to pull the rod from the joint after making the weld. About 15 minutes cooling time is needed for rigid plastic and 30 minutes for thermoplastics.

Smooth the weld area by grinding with No. 36 grit sandpaper. Excess plastic can be removed with a sharp knife before grinding. When grinding, do NOT overheat the weld area because it will soften. Use water to cool the plastic while grinding, if needed.

After rough grinding, check the weld visually for defects. Any voids or cracks are unacceptable. Bending should NOT produce any cracks. A good plastic weld is as strong as the part itself!

The weld area can be finish sanded using No. 220 grit sandpaper followed by a No. 320 grit. Either a belt or orbital sander may be used, plus hand sanding as required. If refinishing is to be done, follow the procedure designed specifically for plastics.

PLASTIC SPEED WELDING

Plastic speed welding uses a specially designed tip to produce a more uniform weld and at a high rate of speed. You must preheat both the rod and base material. The rod is preheated as it passes through a tube in the speed tip. The base material is preheated by a stream of hot air passing through a vent in the tip.

A pointed shoe on the end of the tip applies pressure to the rod. You do not have to apply pressure to the rod. The shoe smoothes out the rod, creating a more uniform appearance in the finished weld. On panel work, speed welding is commonly used.

With speed plastic welding, the conventional two-hand method is replaced by a faster and more uniform one-hand operation. Once started, the rod is fed automatically into the preheat tube as the welding torch is pulled along the joint. Speed tips are designed to provide the constant balance of heat and pressure. The average welding speed is about 40 inches per minute (1,000 mm per minute).

CONTROLLING SPEED WELDING RATE

The angle between the torch and base material determines the **speed welding rate.** For this reason, hold the torch at a 90-degree angle when starting the weld. Hold the torch at a 45-degree angle after you begin welding.

If the welding rate is too fast, bring the torch back to the 90-degree angle temporarily to slow it down. Then gradually move to the desired angle for proper welding speed.

Remember, once started, speed welding must be maintained at a fairly constant rate. The torch cannot be held still. To stop welding before the rod is used up, bring the torch back past the 90-degree angle and cut off the rod at the end of the shoe.

A good speed weld in a V-groove will have a slightly higher crown and more uniformity than the normal hand weld. It should appear smooth and shiny, with a slight bead on each side. For best results and faster welding speed, clean the shoe on the speed tip with a wire brush to remove any residue that might create drag on the rod.

AIRLESS MELT-FLOW PLASTIC WELDING

Melt-flow plastic welding is the most commonly used airless welding method. It can be utilized for both single-sided and two-sided repairs.

A typical melt-flow procedure is as follows:

1. With the welding rod in the preheat tube, place the flat shoe part of the tip in the V-groove.
2. Hold it in place until the rod begins to melt and flow out around the shoe.
3. A small amount of force is needed to feed the rod through the preheat tube. The rod will NOT feed itself. Care should be used not to feed it too fast.
4. Move the shoe slowly. Crisscross the groove until it is filled with melted plastic.
5. Work the melted plastic well into the base material, especially toward the top of the V-groove.
6. Complete a weld length of about 1 inch (25 mm) at a time. This will allow smoothing of the weld before the plastic cools.

PLASTIC STITCH-TAMP WELDING

Plastic stitch-tamp welding involves melt-flow fusion followed by using the pointed end of the welding tip to help bond the plastic rod and base plastic together. It is primarily used on hard plastics, like ABS and nylon, to ensure a good base-rod mix.

After completing the weld using the melt-flow procedure, remove the rod. Turn the shoe over and slowly move the pointed end of the tip into the weld area to bond the rod and base material together. Stitch-tamp the entire length of the weld. After stitch-tamping, use the flat shoe part of the tip to smooth out the weld area.

SINGLE-SIDED PLASTIC WELDS

Single-sided plastic welds are used when the part cannot be removed from the vehicle. To make a single-sided weld, proceed as follows:

1. Set the temperature dial on the welder for the plastic being welded. Allow it to warm up to the proper temperature.
2. Clean the part by washing with soap and water, followed by a good plastic cleaner.
3. Align the break using aluminum body tape.
4. V-groove the damaged area 75 percent of the way through the base material. Angle or bevel back the torn edges of the damage at least ¼ inch (6 mm) on each side of the damaged area. Use a die grinder or similar tool.
5. Clean the preheat tube, and insert the rod. Begin the weld by placing the shoe over the V-groove and feeding the rod through. Move the tip slowly for good melt-in and heat penetration.
6. When the entire V-groove has been filled, turn the shoe over and use the tip to stitch-tamp the rod and base material together into a good mix along the length of the weld.
7. Resmooth the weld area using the flat shoe part of the tip, again working slowly. Then cool with a damp sponge or cloth.
8. Shape the excess weld buildup to a smooth contour, using a razor blade and/or abrasive paper.

TWO-SIDED PLASTIC WELDS

A **two-sided plastic weld** is the strongest type of weld because you weld both sides of the part. When making a two-sided weld, be sure to do the following:

1. Allow the welder to heat up. Then clean the preheat tube.
2. Clean the part with soap and water and plastic cleaner.
3. Align the front of the break with aluminum body tape, smoothing it out with a stiff squeegee or spreader.
4. V-groove 50 percent of the way through the back side of the panel.
5. Weld the back side of the panel using the melt-flow method. Move slowly enough to achieve good melt-in.
6. When finished, smooth the weld with the shoe.
7. Quick-cool the weld with a damp sponge or cloth.
8. Remove the tape from the front of the piece. V-groove deep enough that the first weld is penetrated by the second V-groove.
9. Weld the seam, filling the groove completely.
10. Use a razor blade or slow speed grinder to reshape the contour.

REPAIRING VINYL DENTS

Vinyl is a soft, flexible, thin plastic material often applied over a foam filler. Vinyl over foam construction is commonly used on interior parts for safety. Common vinyl parts are the dash pads, armrests, inner door trim, seat covers, and exterior roof covering. Dash pads or padded instrument panels are expensive and time consuming to replace. Therefore, they are perfect candidates for repair. See **Figure 11–11.**

Most *dash pads* are made of vinyl-clad urethane foam to protect people during a collision. Surface dents in foam dash pads, armrests, and other padded interior parts are common in

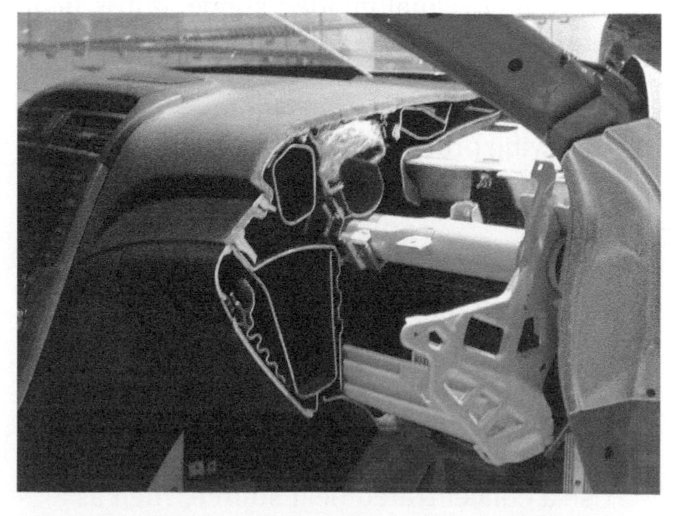

Figure 11–11. Study the construction of a typical dash pad. Note the steel reinforcing bar behind the dash panel.

collision repair. These dents can often be repaired by applying heat as follows:

1. Soak the dent with a damp sponge or cloth for about half a minute. Leave the dented area moist.
2. Using a heat gun, heat the area around the dent. Hold the gun 10 to 12 inches (250 to 300 mm) from the surface. Keep it moving in a circular motion at all times, working from the outside inward.
3. Heat the area to around 130°F (54°C). Do NOT overheat the vinyl or it will blister. Keep heating it until the area is too hot to touch. If available, use a digital thermometer to meter the surface temperature.
4. Wearing gloves, massage the pad. Force the material toward the center of the dent. The area may have to be reheated and massaged more than once. In some cases, heat alone may repair the damage.
5. When the dent has been removed, cool the area quickly with a damp sponge or cloth.
6. Apply vinyl treatment or preservative to the part.

HEAT RESHAPING PLASTIC PARTS

Many bent, stretched, or deformed plastic parts, such as flexible bumper covers and vinyl-clad foam interior parts, can often be straightened with heat. This is because of **"plastic memory,"** which means the piece wants to keep or return to its original molded shape. If it is bent or deformed slightly, it will return to its original shape if heat is applied.

To reshape a distorted bumper cover, use the following procedure:

1. Thoroughly wash the cover with soap and water.
2. Clean with plastic cleaner. Make sure to remove all road tar, oil, grease, and undercoating.
3. Dampen the repair area with a water-soaked rag or sponge.
4. Apply heat directly to the distorted area. Use a concentrated heat source, such as a heat lamp or high-temperature heat gun. When the opposite side of the cover becomes uncomfortable to the touch, it has been heated enough.
5. Use a paint paddle, squeegee, or wood block to help reshape the piece if necessary.
6. Quick-cool the area by applying cold water with a sponge or rag.

! WARNING !

Do not overheat textured vinyl or you will damage the vinyl surface.

PLASTIC BUMPER TAB REPLACEMENT

When a bumper cover has been torn away from its mounting screws, the mounting tabs will often be broken or torn away. Mounting tabs must be repaired with a two-sided weld to provide enough weld strength.

If the material is a thermoplastic, either the hot-air or airless method may be used. If the piece is a thermosetting plastic, airless welding must be used. If welded properly, the repaired piece will be as strong as the original, undamaged part.

The following is the procedure for rebuilding a mounting tab that has been torn off:

1. Begin by cleaning the piece as described before.
2. Bevel back the torn edges of the mounting tab at least ¼ inch (6 mm) on both sides.
3. Rough up the plastic and wipe dust free.
4. Use aluminum body tape to build a form in the shape of the missing tab. Turn the tape edges up to form the thickness of the new tab.
5. Set the temperature dial on the welder for the type of plastic being repaired. Allow the unit to warm up.
6. Begin the weld. Push the rod slowly through the preheat tube. Slightly overfill the form, working the melted plastic into the base material.
7. Smooth and shape the weld. Quick-cool the weld area.
8. Remove the tape. V-groove along the tear line on the other side about halfway through the piece.

9. Weld the groove and quick-cool. Finish the weld to the desired contour using a slow-speed grinder with a No. 60 or 80 grit disc.

PLASTIC ADHESIVE REPAIR SYSTEMS

A **plastic adhesive repair system** is a high-strength glue or epoxy used to repair damage to plastic parts. The minor damage to the part is cleaned, ground out, and sanded. Then the adhesive is applied to the damaged area. A spreader is used to work the adhesive down into the damage. The repair is then sanded to shape it, much like plastic body filler.

Adhesive repair of plastics is often preferable to plastic welding, especially on more severe damage. If applied properly, adhesives produce a stronger repair that takes little more time than welding. Refer to the vehicle service manual and material instructions to make sure you are using the right kind of adhesive and correct repair procedures.

Adhesive repair systems are of two types: cyanoacrylate (CA) and two-part. Two-part is the most commonly used.

Cyanoacrylates (CAs) are one-part, fast curing adhesives used to help repair rigid and flexible plastics. They are used as a filler or to tack parts together before applying the final repair material. CAs are sometimes known as "super glues." They can be a valuable tool for the repair of plastic parts. CAs set up very quickly.

Although one-part, an activating agent can be used to accelerate the bonding process of a CA. Care must be used NOT to apply too much activating agent. If too much is used, the product foams, causing a weaker bond.

CAs do NOT work equally well on all plastics. There is no hard and fast rule. When CAs are used, be sure to use products from reliable suppliers and follow the manufacturer's guidelines for using them.

Two-part adhesive systems consist of a base resin and a hardener (catalyst). The resin comes in one container and the hardener in another. When mixed, the adhesive cures into a plastic material similar to the base material in the part. Two-part adhesive systems are an acceptable alternative to welding for many plastic repairs.

Not all plastics can be welded, while adhesives can be used in all but a few instances. If adhesive repair is chosen, you must first identify the type of plastic. A good way to do this is through a plastic flexibility test.

To do a plastic flexibility test, use your hands to flex and bend the part and compare it to samples of plastic. Compare the flexibilities. Use the repair material that most closely matches the characteristics of the part's base material.

USE THE CORRECT ADHESIVE!

WARNING

When working with an adhesive system, use the manufacturer's categories to decide on a repair product and procedure. There are many plastic and repair material variations. The vehicle manufacturer's repair manual is the most accurate source of information. The service manual will recommend products and procedures for the exact type of plastic in the part.

It is important to keep in mind that there are differences between manufacturers' repair materials. When using plastic repair adhesives, remember that:

1. Mixing product lines is NOT acceptable. Choose a product line and use it for the entire repair.
2. Most product lines have two or more adhesives designed for different types of plastic.
3. The product line usually includes an adhesion promoter, a filler product, and a flexible coating agent. Use each as directed.
4. Some product lines are formulated for a specific base material. For instance, one manufacturer offers individual products for use with each type of plastic (TPO, urethanes, or Xenoy, for example), regardless of plastic flexibility.

A product line might use a single flexible filler for all plastics, or there might be two or more flexible fillers designed for different types of plastic.

TWO-PART PLASTIC ADHESIVE REPAIRS

Regardless of which manufacturer's products are used, two-part adhesive repairs share the common preparation steps:

1. Clean the part. First, use soap and water and then a plastic cleaner. See **Figure 11–12.**
2. Make sure both the part and the repair material are at room temperature for proper curing and adhesion.
3. Mix the two parts of the adhesive thoroughly and in the proper proportions.
4. Apply the material within the time guidelines given in the product literature. Use heat if indicated by the manufacturer. See **Figure 11–13.**
5. Follow the cure time guidelines given in the product literature. Regulated heat can speed curing.
6. Support the part adequately during the cure time to ensure that the damaged area does NOT move before the adhesive cures. This would weaken the repair.
7. Follow the product literature for guidelines on when to reinforce a repair.

An **adhesion promoter** is a chemical that treats the surface of the plastic so the repair material will bond properly. Some plastics (TPO, PP, and E/P, for example) require an adhesion promoter. There is a simple test to perform that indicates whether or not the plastic will require an adhesion promoter. Lightly sand a hidden spot on the piece, using a high-speed grinder and No. 36 grit paper.

If the material gives off dust, it can be repaired with a standard structural adhesive system. If the material melts and smears or has a greasy or waxy look, then you must use an adhesion promoter. Many plastic fillers and adhesives contain an adhesion promoter. Check their labels.

Here is a typical way to use a two-part epoxy adhesive to repair a flexible bumper cover:

1. Clean the entire cover with soap and water. Wipe or blow-dry. Then clean the surface with a good plastic cleaner. See **Figure 11–14.**
2. V-groove the damaged area. Then grind about a 1½-inch (38 mm) taper around the damage for good adhesion and repair strength.

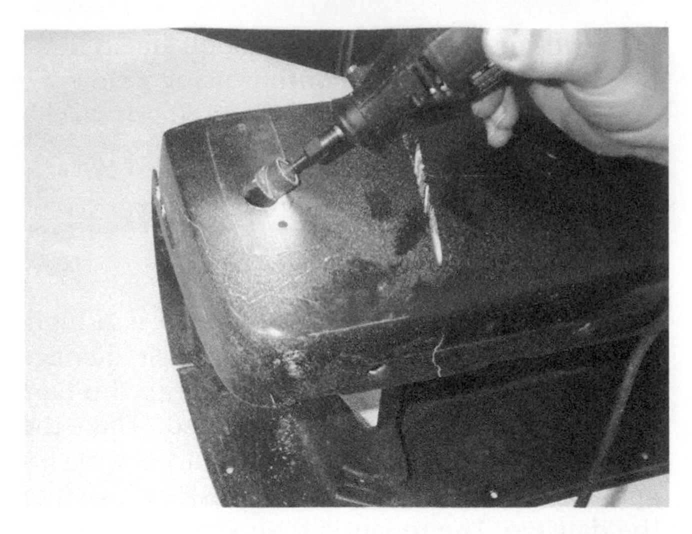

(A) Grind and chamfer the hole or damage to be repaired.

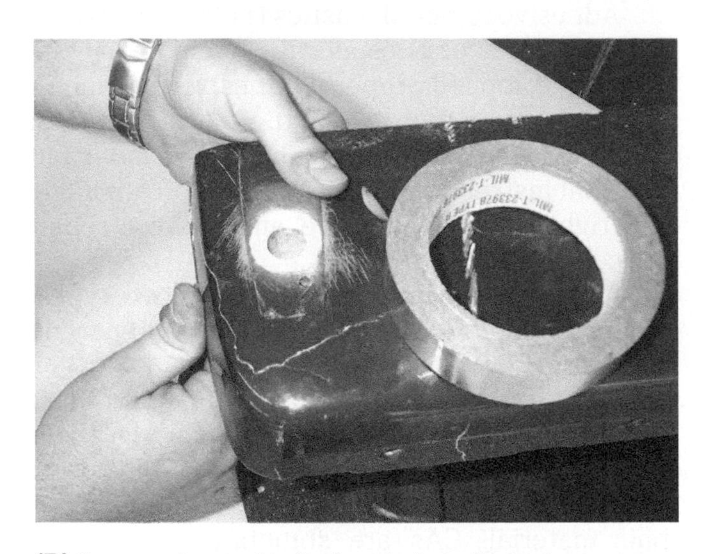

(B) Tape can be used to back up hole in the part.

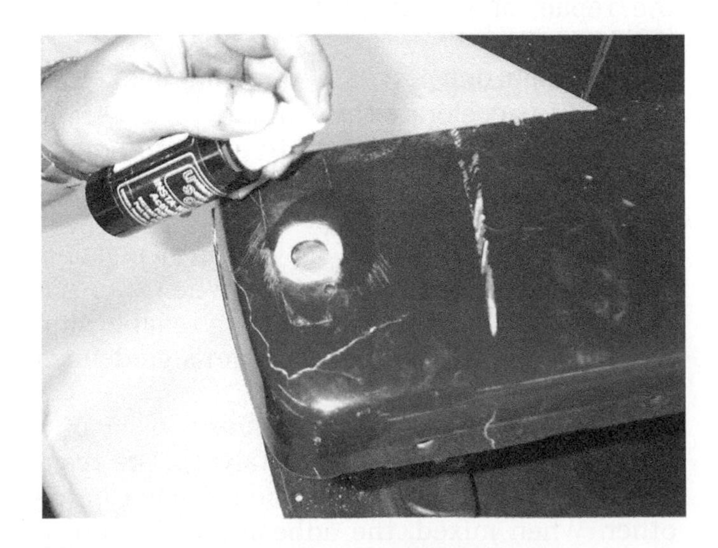

(C) Apply primer to the sanded area to be repaired.

Figure 11–12. Preparation of the plastic part to be repaired is critical. (Courtesy of Urethane Supply Co.)

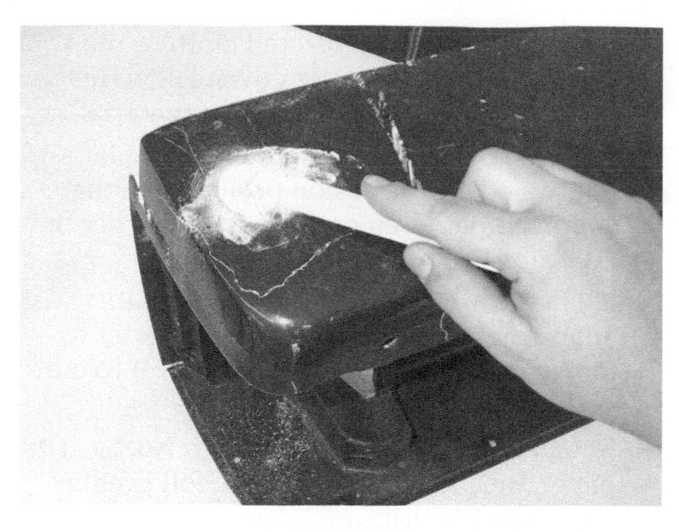

(A) After mixing, the technician is using a wood spreader to apply repair material to the hole.

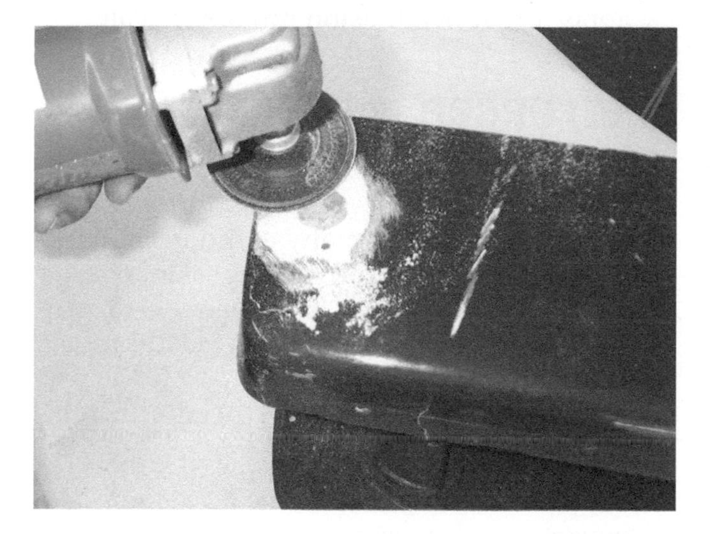

(B) Grind the repair material and reapply, if needed.

Figure 11–13. Applying repair material to the plastic part. (Courtesy of Urethane Supply Co.)

3. Use a sander with No. 180 grit paper to featheredge the paint around the damaged area. Then blow off the dust. Depending on the extent of the damage, the back side might need reinforcement. To do this, use steps 4 through 6.
4. To reinforce the repair area, sand and clean the back side of the cover with plastic cleaner. Then, if needed, apply a coat of adhesion promoter.
5. Dispense equal amounts of both parts of the flexible epoxy adhesive. Mix them to a uniform color. Apply the material to a piece of fiberglass cloth using a plastic squeegee. See **Figure 11–15.**

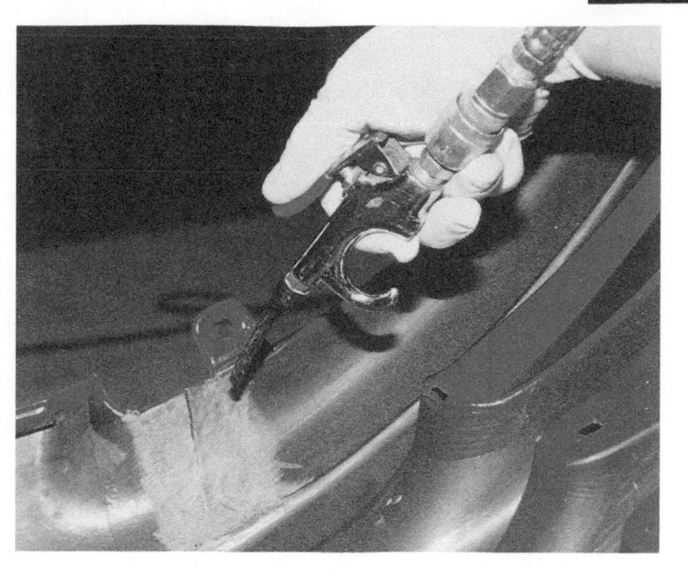

(A) First, clean the area to be repaired with soap and water. Then wipe the area with silicone and wax remover before blow-drying.

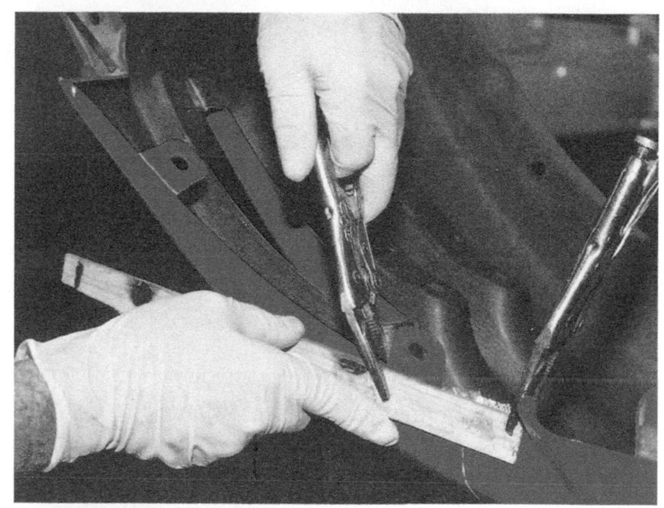

(B) If needed, clamp a wood stirring stick to the bumper to hold the tear in alignment.

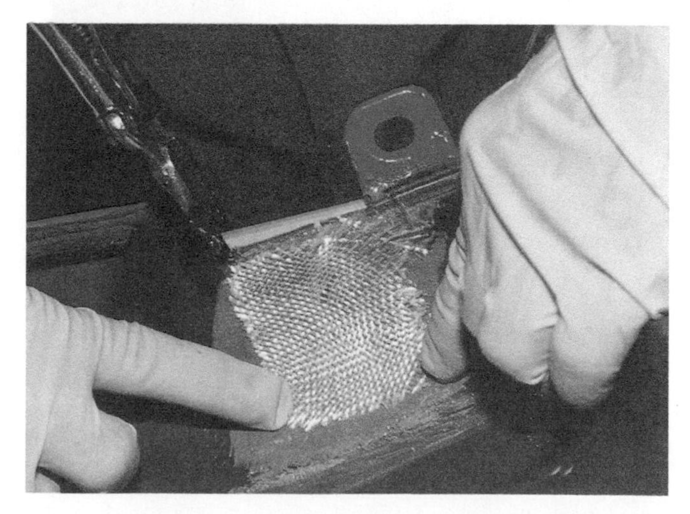

(C) Cut and fit the fiberglass cloth over the tear in the bumper.

Figure 11–14. Note the methods to prepare a large tear in a plastic bumper cover for repair.

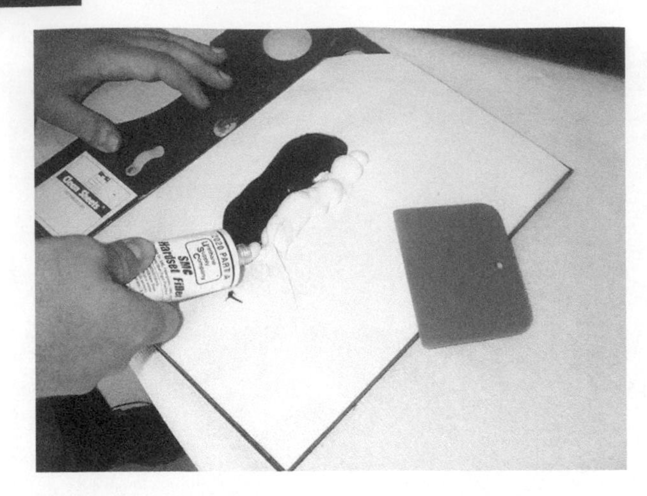

(A) Mix the correct type of flexible repair material in the mixing board.

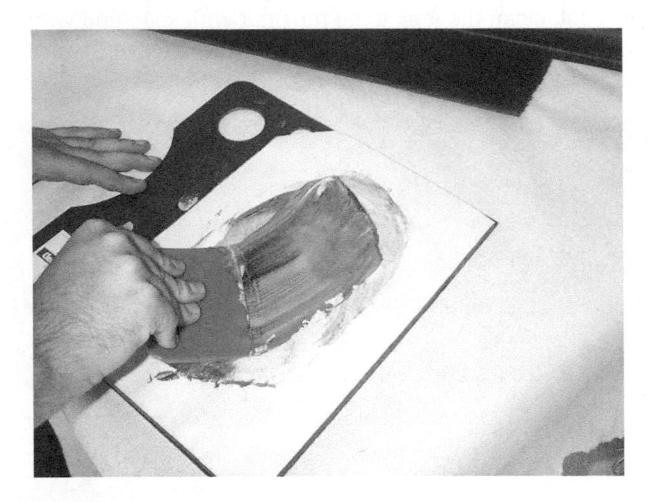

(B) Wipe, do not stir, the repair material to avoid air bubbles in the material.

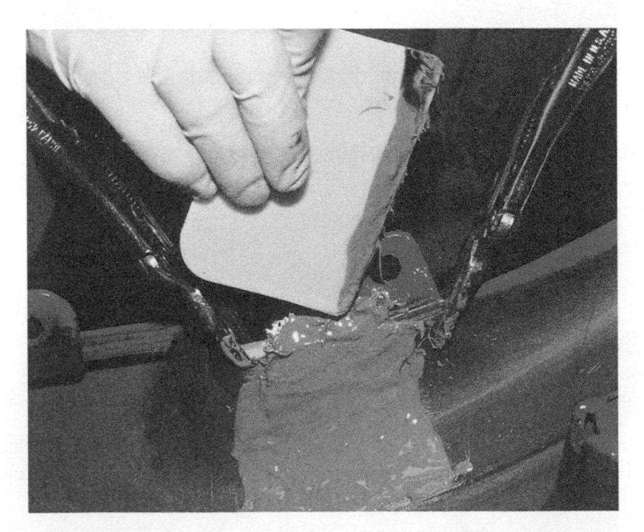

(C) Apply repair material to the bumper and then to the fiberglass cloth.

Figure 11–15. Study the major steps for repair of the back side of a large tear in the bumper. (A and B, Courtesy of Urethane Supply Co.)

6. Attach the plastic-saturated cloth to the back side of the bumper cover. Fill in the weave with additional adhesive material.
7. With the back side reinforcement in place, apply a coat of adhesion promoter to the sanded repair area on the front side. Let the adhesion promoter dry completely.
8. Fill in the area with adhesive material. Shape the adhesive with your spreader to match the shape of the part. Allow it to cure properly. See **Figure 11–16.**
9. Rough grind the repair area with No. 80 grit paper, then sand with 180 grit, followed by smoother 240 grit.
10. If additional adhesive material is needed to fill in a low spot or pinholes, be sure to apply a coat of adhesion promoter again.

REINFORCED PLASTIC REPAIRS

Reinforced plastic—including *reinforced reaction injection molded (RRIM) polyurethane*—parts are being used in many unibody vehicles. They provide a durable plastic skin over a steel unibody. The table in **Figure 11–17** provides an overview of reinforced plastic repair materials.

The damage that generally occurs in reinforced plastic panels includes:

- One-sided damage, such as a scratch or gouge
- Punctures and fractures
- Panel separation, where the panel pulls away from the metal space frame
- Severe damage, which requires full or partial panel replacement
- Minor bends and distortions of the space frame, which can be repaired by pulling and straightening
- Severe kinks and bends to the space frame, which require replacement of that piece along factory seams or by sectioning

Remember! Combinations of these types of damage often occur on a single vehicle. Depending on the location and amount of damage, there are four different types of repairs. These are:

1. Single-sided repair
2. Two-sided repair

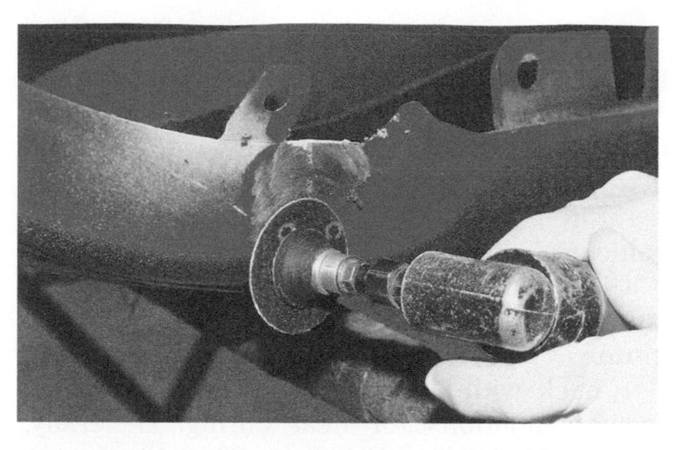

(A) Grind the area around the split or crack to remove the paint and scuff the surface.

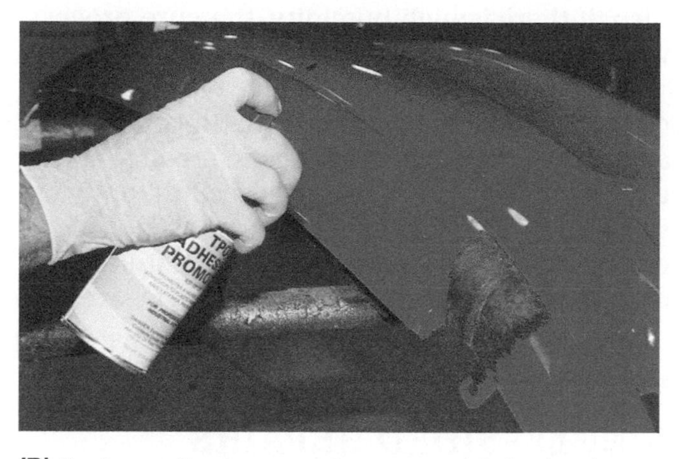

(B) Apply an adhesion promoter or a special plastic primer to the repair area.

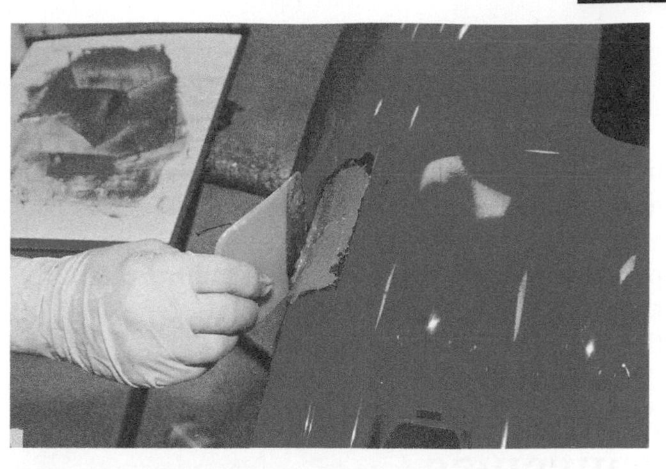

(C) Mix and apply the flexible repair material to the front damage on the bumper.

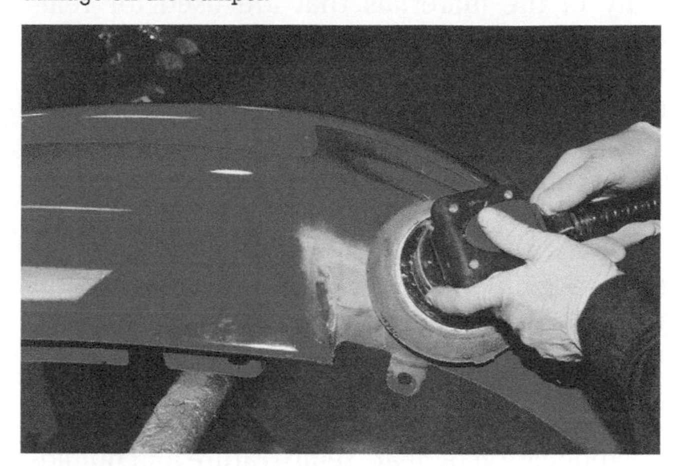

(D) Grind and sand the repair material to featheredge it into the existing surface contour on the bumper. You can then prime and paint the bumper cover.

Figure 11–16. Once the rear repair has cured, you can apply repair material to the front of the bumper cover.

Reinforced Plastic Repair Material Selection Chart					
	Applicable repair product				
Type of repair	Panel adhesive	Patching adhesive	Structural filler	Cosmetic filler	Glass fiber reinforcement
Panel replacement	X				
Panel sectioning	X		X_1	X_1	X
One-sided repairs				X_1	
Two-sided repairs	X_2	X_2	X	X	X

Notes: 1. Some panel adhesives can also be used as structural and cosmetic fillers, depending on sanding characteristics.
2. Panel adhesives can also be used as patching adhesives, but not vice versa.

Figure 11-17. Study the reinforced plastic repair chart. It gives recommended repairs and materials.

3. Panel sectioning
4. Full panel replacement

To select a repair method, a thorough examination of the vehicle is required. Examine all affected reinforced plastic panels. First, check the entire panel for signs of damage. Also check all panel seams for adhesive bond failure. Examine the back of the panel to determine the extent of the damage.

REINFORCED PLASTIC ADHESIVES

Many of the materials that are used for reinforced plastic repair are two-part adhesive products. Two-part adhesive means a base material and a hardener must be mixed to cure the adhesive. Each must be mixed together in the proper ratio. Both parts must be thoroughly mixed together before use.

Work life or **open time** is the time when it is still possible to disturb the adhesive and still have the adhesive set up for a good bond. This work life time will be provided by the manufacturer. The cure time of some adhesives used in reinforced plastic repair can be shortened with the application of heat. Temperature and humidity can affect work life and cure time.

After mixing, remember that each product has a work life or open time. If you move or disturb the adhesive as it starts to harden, you will adversely affect its durability.

REINFORCED PLASTIC FILLERS AND GLASS CLOTH

Two filler products are specifically formulated for use on reinforced plastic. They are cosmetic filler and structural filler.

Cosmetic filler is typically a two-part epoxy or polyester filler used to cover up minor imperfections. Do NOT use fillers designed for sheet metal on reinforced plastic.

Structural filler is used to fill the larger gaps in the panel structure while maintaining strength. Structural fillers add to the structural rigidity of the part.

All two-part products will shrink to some degree. The use of heat will help to speed the drying time and will eliminate some of the shrinkage.

Check with the product manufacturer for temperatures and dry times. If the product is NOT properly heated to a full cure, shrinkage will occur as the product cures with time. The "rule of thumb" is to heat the material to a surface temperature higher than any temperatures that the vehicle will be subject to when it is on the road. If it is a black vehicle sitting in the sun in midsummer, this could be about 170°F (77°C) or more.

Check with the product manufacturer for recommendations for heat curing. Generally, 200° to 250°F (93° to 121°C) for 20 to 40 minutes should do it. Remember that at lower temperatures, the product will have to be heated longer. Also, if there is high humidity, the cure process will take longer.

There are several different types of glass cloth available. Rovings and mattings are NOT appropriate for reinforced plastic repair. Choose unidirectional cloth, woven glass cloth, or nylon screening. The cloth weave must be loose enough to allow the adhesive to fully saturate the cloth, leaving no air space around the weave.

REINFORCED PLASTIC, SINGLE-SIDED REPAIRS

Single-sided damage is surface damage that does NOT penetrate or fracture the rear of the panel. Damage might pass all the way through a panel, but no pieces of the panel have broken away. If the break is clean and all of the reinforcing fibers have stayed in place, then a single-sided repair would be adequate.

For a single-sided repair, you must bevel deep to penetrate the fibers in the panel. The broken fibers must come into contact with the adhesive.

The following is a typical single-sided repair procedure for reinforced plastic:

1. Clean the repair area with soap and water.
2. Clean again using mild wax and grease remover.
3. Remove any paint from the surrounding area by sanding with No. 80 grit sandpaper.
4. Scuff sand the area surrounding the damage.
5. Bevel the damage to provide an adequate area for bonding.

6. Mix two-part filler according to the manufacturer's instructions.
7. Apply the filler and cure as recommended.

Once the filler has been sanded, apply additional coats as required and resand. The product manufacturer will provide grit recommendations.

TWO-SIDED REPAIRS OF REINFORCED PLASTIC

A two-sided repair is normally needed on damage that passes all of the way through the panel. This would include damage to the reinforcing fibers.

A *backing strip* or **backing patch** is bonded to the rear of the repair area to restore the reinforced plastic's strength. The patch also forms a foundation for forming the exterior surface to match the original contour of the panel.

To make a two-sided repair in a reinforced plastic panel, proceed as follows:

1. Clean the surface surrounding the damage with a good wax and grease remover. Use a No. 36 grinding disc to remove all paint and primer at least 3 inches (75 mm) beyond the repair area.
2. Grind, file, or use a hacksaw to remove all cracked or splintered material away from the hole on both the inside and outside of the repair area.
3. Remove any dirt, sound deadener, and the like from the inner surface of the repair area. Clean with reducer, lacquer thinner, or a similar solvent.
4. Scuff around the hole with No. 80 grit paper to provide a good bonding surface.
5. Bevel the inside and outside edge of the repair area about 30 degrees to permit better patch adhesion.
6. Clean the repair area thoroughly.
7. Cut several pieces of fiberglass cloth large enough to cover the hole and the scuffed area. The exact number of pieces will depend on the thickness of the original panel.
8. Prepare a mixture of resin and hardener. Follow the label recommendations.
9. Using a small paintbrush, saturate at least two layers of the fiberglass cloth with the activated resin mix.
10. Apply the material to the inside or back surface of the repair area. Make sure the cloth fully contacts the scuffed area surrounding the hole.
11. Saturate three more layers of cloth with the mix. Apply it to the outside surface. These layers must also contact the inner layers and the scuffed outside repair area.
12. With all of the layers of cloth in place, form a saucer-like depression in them. This is needed to increase the depth of the repair material. Use a squeegee to work out any air bubbles.
13. Clean all tools with a lacquer thinner immediately after use.
14. Let the saturated cloth patch become tacky. An infrared heat lamp can be used to speed up the process. If one is used, keep it 12 to 15 inches (300 to 375 mm) away from the surface. Do NOT overheat the repair area because too much heat will cause distortion.
15. With No. 50 grit paper, disc sand the patch slightly below the contour of the panel.
16. Prepare more resin and hardener mix. Use a plastic spreader to fill the depression in the repair area. You need a sufficient layer of material for grinding down smooth and flush.
17. Allow the patch to harden. Again, a heat lamp can be used to speed the curing process.
18. When the patch is fully hardened, sand the excess material down to the basic contour. Use No. 80 grit paper and a sanding block. Finish sand with No. 120 or finer grit paper.

There are several ways to hold the patch in place from the front side of the panel. One method is to use a pull rod. Drill a hole in the middle of the patch. Insert the end of the rod. Position the patch, and pull it snug with the pull rod. Apply heat using a heat gun on the front, or have someone else apply the heat to the back of the patch.

This same two-sided repair can be made by attaching sheet metal to the back side of the panel with sheet metal screws. Sand the sheet metal and both sides of the part to provide good adhesion. Before fastening the sheet metal, apply resin and hardener mix to both sides of the rim of the hole. Follow the procedures described earlier for the remainder of the repair.

When the inner side of the hole is NOT accessible, apply a fiberglass patch to the outer side only. After the usual cleaning and sanding operations, apply several additional layers of fiberglass cloth to the outer side of the hole. Before it dries, make a saucer-like depression in the cloth to provide greater depth for the repair material.

REPAIRING RRIM

Reinforced reaction injection molded (RRIM) polyurethane is a two-part polyurethane composite plastic. Part A is the isocyanate. Part B contains the reinforced fibers, resins, and a catalyst. The two parts are first mixed in a special mixing chamber, then injected into a mold. RRIM parts are becoming more common in fenders and bumper covers.

Since RRIM is a thermosetting plastic, heat (100° to 140°F or 37° to 59°C) is applied to the mold to cure the material. The molded product is made to be stiff yet flexible. It can absorb minor impacts without damage. This makes RRIM an ideal material for exposed areas.

Gouges and punctures can be repaired using a structural adhesive. If the damage is a puncture that extends through the panel, a backing patch is required. To make a typical backing patch repair, proceed as follows:

1. Clean the damaged area thoroughly using the plastic cleaner recommended by the manufacturer and a clean cloth. Wipe dry.
2. Remove any paint film in and around the damage with an orbital sander and No. 180 grit disc.
3. Using a No. 50 grit disc, enlarge the damaged area, tapering out the damage for about 1 inch (25 mm). Wipe or blow away any loose particles.
4. Clean the back side of the damaged area with the plastic cleaner.
5. Use a No. 50 grit disc to scuff sand the area. Extend the area to about 1½ inches (38 mm) beyond the damage. Align the front of the panel with body tape, if necessary.
6. Cut a piece of fiberglass cloth to cover the damaged area and the part of the panel that has been scuff sanded.
7. Mix the adhesive according to the manufacturer's recommendations. Apply a layer of adhesive to the back side of the panel about ⅛ inch (3 mm) thick.
8. Place the fiberglass patch into position on the adhesive. Cover it with a sheet of waxed paper. Use a roller to force the adhesive into the fibers of the patch.
9. Remove the waxed paper and add another layer of adhesive. Work out the adhesive to just beyond the edges of the patch. Allow the adhesive to cure, following the manufacturer's recommendation.
10. Now move to the front side of the panel. Apply a layer of adhesive, completely covering the damaged area. Build it up to slightly higher than the surrounding contour. Allow it to cure.
11. Apply heat to help speed the cure of the patch.
12. Contour the adhesive to the adjoining surface by block sanding using No. 220 grit paper.
13. Finish by feathering with an orbital sander and a No. 320 disc.

SPRAYING VINYL PAINTS

Vinyl repair paints are usually ready for spraying as packaged. Since application properties cannot be controlled with thinners or other additives, air pressure is an important factor.

When applying vinyl paints by siphon feed guns, the normal air pressure range is between 40 and 50 psi (2.8 and 3.5 kg/cm^2) at the gun. With pressure systems, the air pressure is reduced to 30 to 40 psi (2.1 to 2.8 kg/cm^2). Overspray can be controlled by decreasing the air pressure.

There is no retardant for vinyl paints. If blushing occurs, allow the initial coat to set up and reapply the color in a much lighter coat.

Vinyl and soft ABS plastics should be thoroughly cleansed with vinyl cleaner and allowed to dry. Then treat the surface with vinyl prep. **Vinyl prep** is a chemical solution that opens the pores of the vinyl material. Wipe off the vinyl prep right after it is applied. The surfaces are then ready for color and/or clearcoating.

Figure 11–18 shows a few tips for installing a large, flexible bumper.

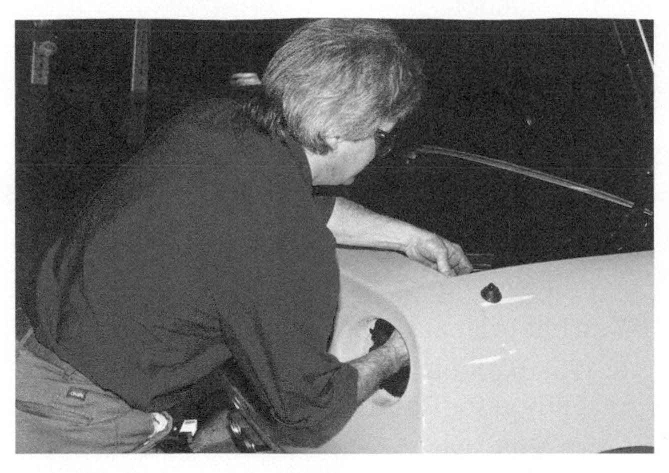

(A) Fit the part onto the vehicle and hand start a couple of fasteners but do not tighten them.

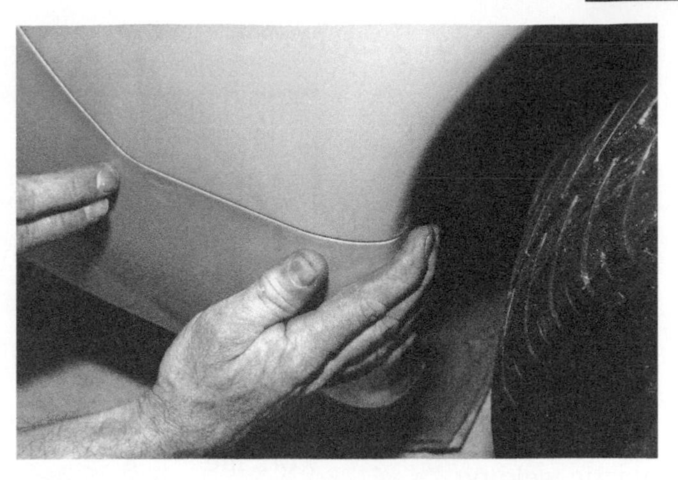

(C) When the parts have been aligned, you can then tighten the fasteners to keep the parts in alignment.

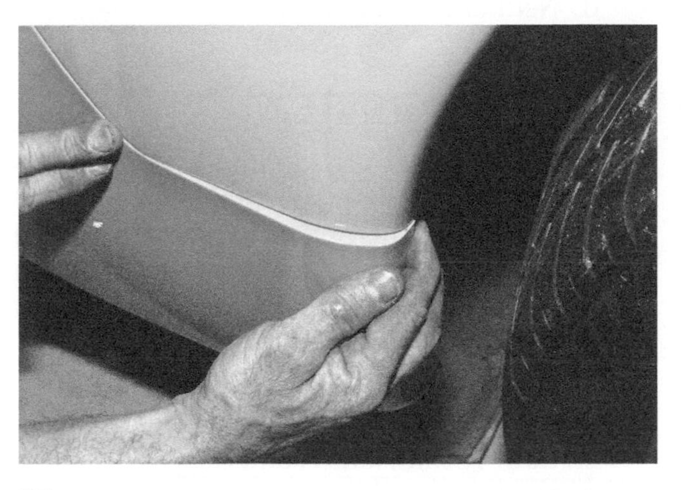

(B) Align all surfaces on the flexible plastic part with the other body panels.

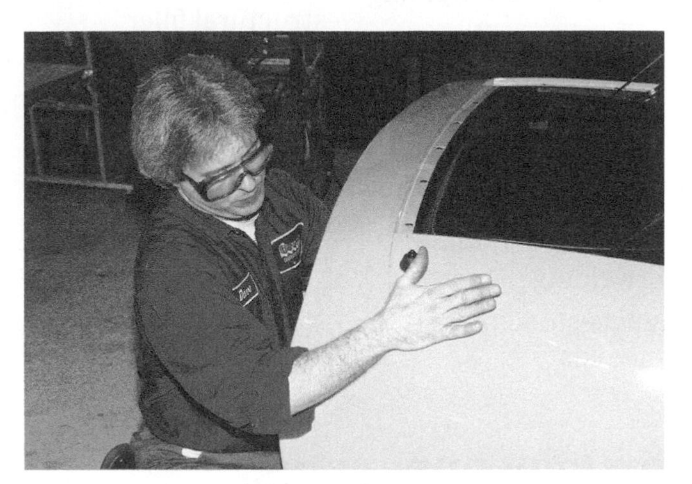

(D) Sight down all surfaces on the flexible part and push the part into perfect alignment as you tighten each fastener on the inside of the panels.

Figure 11–18. Note the basic steps for installing a flexible plastic part, a rear bumper cover.

SUMMARY

- Plastics and composites are terms that refer to a wide range of materials synthetically compounded from crude oil, coal, natural gas, and other substances. Bumpers, fender extensions, fascias, fender aprons, grille openings, stone shields, instrument panels, trim panels, fuel lines, and engine parts can be constructed of these materials.
- Two general types of plastics are used in automotive construction: thermoplastics and thermosetting plastics. Thermoplastics can be repeatedly softened and reshaped by heating with no change in their chemical makeup; thermosetting plastics undergo a chemical change and are hardened into a permanent shape that CANNOT be altered by reapplying heat or catalysts.
- One way to identify a plastic is by international symbols, or ISO codes, which are molded into plastic parts. If there is no ISO code, refer to the body repair manual for information.
- Plastic welding uses heat and sometimes a plastic filler rod to join or repair plastic parts. The types of plastic welding include hot air and airless.

TECHNICAL TERMS

composites
plastics
thermoplastics
thermosetting plastics
composite plastics
international symbols
ISO codes
body repair manual
floating test
plastic welding
hot-air plastic welding
airless plastic welding
rod color coding
plastic speed welding
speed welding rate
melt-flow plastic welding
plastic stitch-tamp welding
single-sided plastic welds
two-sided plastic weld
vinyl
plastic memory
plastic adhesive repair system
cyanoacrylates (CAs)
two-part adhesive systems
adhesion promoter
work life
open time
cosmetic filler
structural filler
single-sided damage
backing patch
reinforced reaction injection molded (RRIM) polyurethane
vinyl prep

REVIEW QUESTIONS

1. Define the term "plastics."
2. In speed welding, the hot-air torch is held at a ______________-degree angle to the base material to start the weld.
   a. 45
   b. 90
   c. 30
   d. 120
3. Explain the difference between a thermoplastic and a thermosetting plastic.
4. When *Technician A* grinds the base material, it melts and smears, so an adhesion promoter is used to make the repair. Under the same circumstances, *Technician B* says that an adhesion promoter is NOT needed. Who is correct?
   a. Technician A
   b. Technician B
   c. Both Technicians A and B
   d. Neither Technician
5. A ______________ ______________ is a curved body repair part made by applying plastic repair material over a part and then removing the cured material.
6. The ______________ and ______________ ______________ are used to help the factory hold panels in place while the adhesive cures.
7. What is a backing strip or patch?
8. Which of the following is the correct repair method for RRIM?
   a. Adhesive
   b. Welding
   c. Both a and b
   d. Neither a nor b

ASE-STYLE REVIEW

1. *Technician A* says to identify a plastic by international symbols, or ISO codes, molded into plastic parts. *Technician B* says that the body repair manual will give information about plastic types used on the vehicle. Who is correct?
   a. Technician A
   b. Technician B
   c. Both Technicians A and B
   d. Neither Technician
2. *Technician A* says that one of the ways to identify plastic is by international symbols, which are molded into plastic parts. *Technician B* says that all plastic parts are repaired in the same manner and identification is not necessary. Who is correct?
   a. Technician A
   b. Technician B
   c. Both Technicians A and B
   d. Neither Technician
3. When plastic welding, *Technician A* forces the rod into the joint with slight pressure. *Technician B* uses test welds to help select the correct plastic welding rod. Who is correct?
   a. Technician A
   b. Technician B
   c. Both Technicians A and B
   d. Neither Technician

4. Which of the following is the preferred method of repairing plastic damage?
   a. Hot-air welding
   b. Airless welding
   c. Reshaping
   d. Adhesive repair

5. *Technician A* says that not all plastics can be welded, while adhesives can be used in all but a few instances. *Technician B* says that plastic welding can be used on all plastic with better success. Who is correct?
   a. Technician A
   b. Technician B
   c. Both Technicians A and B
   d. Neither Technician

6. *Technician A* says that if the plastic material GIVES OFF DUST when ground, it can be repaired with a standard structural adhesive system. *Technician B* states that if the material MELTS and smears or has a greasy or waxy look when ground, then you must use an adhesion promoter. Who is correct?
   a. Technician A
   b. Technician B
   c. Both Technicians A and B
   d. Neither Technician

7. Which of the following types of repair can be used when reinforced plastic damage does NOT break away large pieces of the panel?
   a. Single-sided repair
   b. Double-sided repair
   c. Spot putty repair
   d. Epoxy repair

8. When performing a two-sided repair of reinforced plastic, which of the following should be used on the rear of the panel?
   a. Heat lamp
   b. Duct tape
   c. Baking patch
   d. Nothing

9. *Technician A* says that when using the single-side weld method, the weld should penetrate 75 percent of the base material. *Technician B* says that when using the two-sided weld method, a second weld should fuse with weld for the other side. Who is correct?
   a. Technician A
   b. Technician B
   c. Both Technicians A and B
   d. Neither Technician

10. When repairing reinforced plastic parts, *Technician A* says that full panel replacement is always needed. *Technician B* says that complete inspection of the panel is necessary to find all the damage. Who is correct?
    a. Technician A
    b. Technician B
    c. Both Technicians A and B
    d. Neither Technician

ACTIVITIES

1. Inspect plastic body parts. Try to find an identification code on the back of each part. Make a report on the type of plastic used for different parts.
2. Make a one-side repair on a plastic part. Summarize the repair in a report. Describe the type of plastic, damage, and steps for repairing the part.
3. Visit a body shop. Talk to technicians about new methods of repairing plastics. Report your findings to the class.

CHAPTER

12 Replacing Hoods, Bumpers, Fenders, Grilles, and Lids

OBJECTIVES

After studying this chapter, you should be able to:

- Remove and install fenders.
- List the various methods for adjusting mechanically fastened panels.
- Perform hood-to-hinge, hood height, and hood latch adjustments.
- Remove, install, and adjust deck lids.
- Remove, install, and adjust bumpers.
- Replace grilles and other bolt-on body parts.

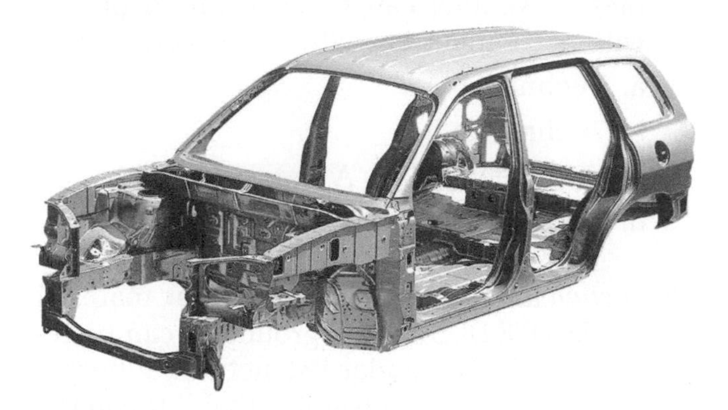

Figure 12–1. Even with the unibody designs, vehicles still have many bolt-on parts and panels. It is important that you know how to properly remove and replace them. (Courtesy of Hyundai Motor Co.)

INTRODUCTION

A collision damaged vehicle can require a variety of repair operations. Repair steps will depend on the nature and location of the damage. Panels with minor damage can often be straightened and filled with body filler. Minor bulges, dents, and creases can be fixed using the techniques discussed in earlier chapters. However, quite often the damage is too great and parts must be replaced.

This chapter covers replacement procedures for hoods, fenders, bumpers, deck lids, and similar bolt-on parts. As **Figure 12–1** shows, many major parts bolt on to the vehicle.

You must know how to properly remove, install, and adjust these parts. As explained in this chapter, some parts can be removed, installed, and aligned without too much difficulty. However, when replacing several adjoining parts (front end parts, for example), you must use specific procedures to get all parts to align properly with the rest of the vehicle.

HOW ARE PARTS FASTENED?

The methods of fastening parts to cars and trucks has changed in the past few years. Many parts that were held with bolts and screws in the past now snap into place. Plastic retainers now hold these parts onto the vehicle. This is done to save time during vehicle manufacturing.

Fastener variations can make repair more challenging. See **Figure 12–2.** Parts can be held by screws, bolts, nuts, metal or plastic clips, adhesives, and other methods. To efficiently replace parts, you must carefully study part construction. Inspect parts closely to find out how they are held on the vehicle. This will let you make logical decisions about which parts to remove first, second, and so on, and the methods needed.

Keep this in mind! On-the-job experience is the only way to become competent and fast at body part *removal and replacement (R and R).* Sometimes you must remove one part at a time. In other instances, it is better to remove several parts as an assembly.

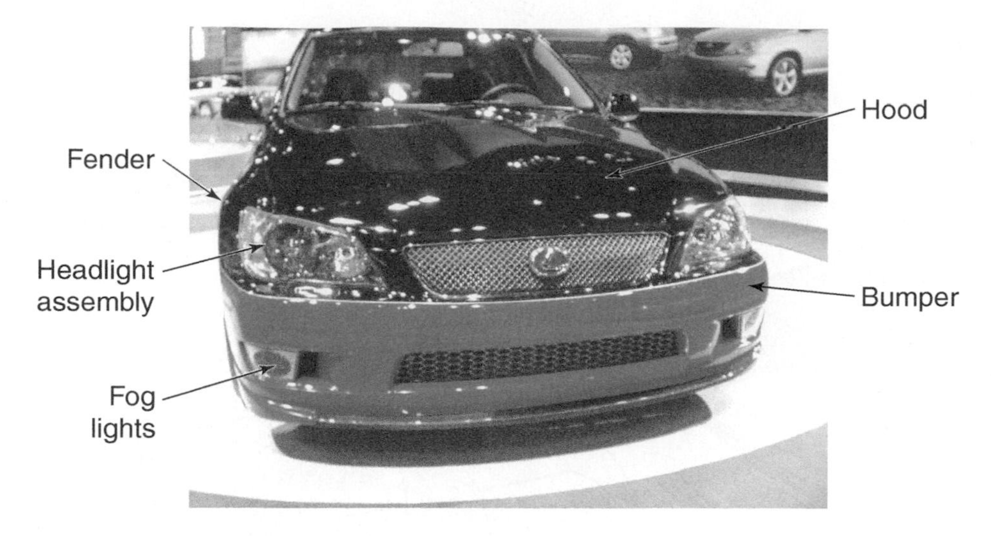

Figure 12–2. Note some of the parts that bolt onto this unibody vehicle.

REFER TO ESTIMATE

When starting work, refer to the estimate to get guidance on where to begin. The estimator will have determined which parts need repair and which should be replaced. Use this information and shop manuals to remove and replace parts efficiently.

The estimate is an important reference tool for doing repairs. It must be followed. The estimator has determined which parts must be repaired.

The estimate is also used to order new parts. You may want to make sure all ordered parts have arrived. Compare new parts on hand with the parts list. If anything is missing, have the parts person order. This will save time and prevent your stall from being tied up waiting for parts.

WHERE TO START

Generally, start removing large, external parts first. For example, if the front end has damage, you must remove the hood first. This will give you more room to access rear fender bolts. This will also allow more light into the front for finding and removing hidden bolts in the frontal area. Use this kind of logic to remove parts efficiently.

If in doubt about how to remove a part, refer to the vehicle's service manual. Factory service manuals normally have a body repair section. The *body repair section* of the manual explains and illustrates how parts are serviced. The manual will give step-by-step instructions for the specific make and model vehicle. It will give bolt locations, torque values, removal sequences, and other important information.

As one example of a repair variation, look at **Figure 12–3.** The rear quarter panels on this vehicle bolt in place. Most vehicles have welded quarter panels. This one also has aluminum body panels that must be repaired differently than steel.

HOOD REMOVAL AND REPLACEMENT

The *hood* provides an external cover over the front of the vehicle. It is one of the largest, heaviest panels on a vehicle. In a front-engine vehicle, it provides access to the engine compartment. With a rear-engine car, it serves as a trunk lid.

Before removing the hood, analyze part conditions. Open and close the hood. Check for binding and bent hinges. If applicable, inspect hood alignment with the fenders and cowl. This will help you determine what must be done during repairs.

To remove a hood, first disconnect any wires and hoses. Wires often connect to an underhood light. Hoses might run to the hood for the windshield washer system. Refer to **Figure 12–4.**

Next, remove the hood hinge bolts. If the hood is not badly damaged and will be reused, mark hood hinge alignment. To mark the hood, make alignment marks around the sides of the hood hinge where it contacts the hood. You may

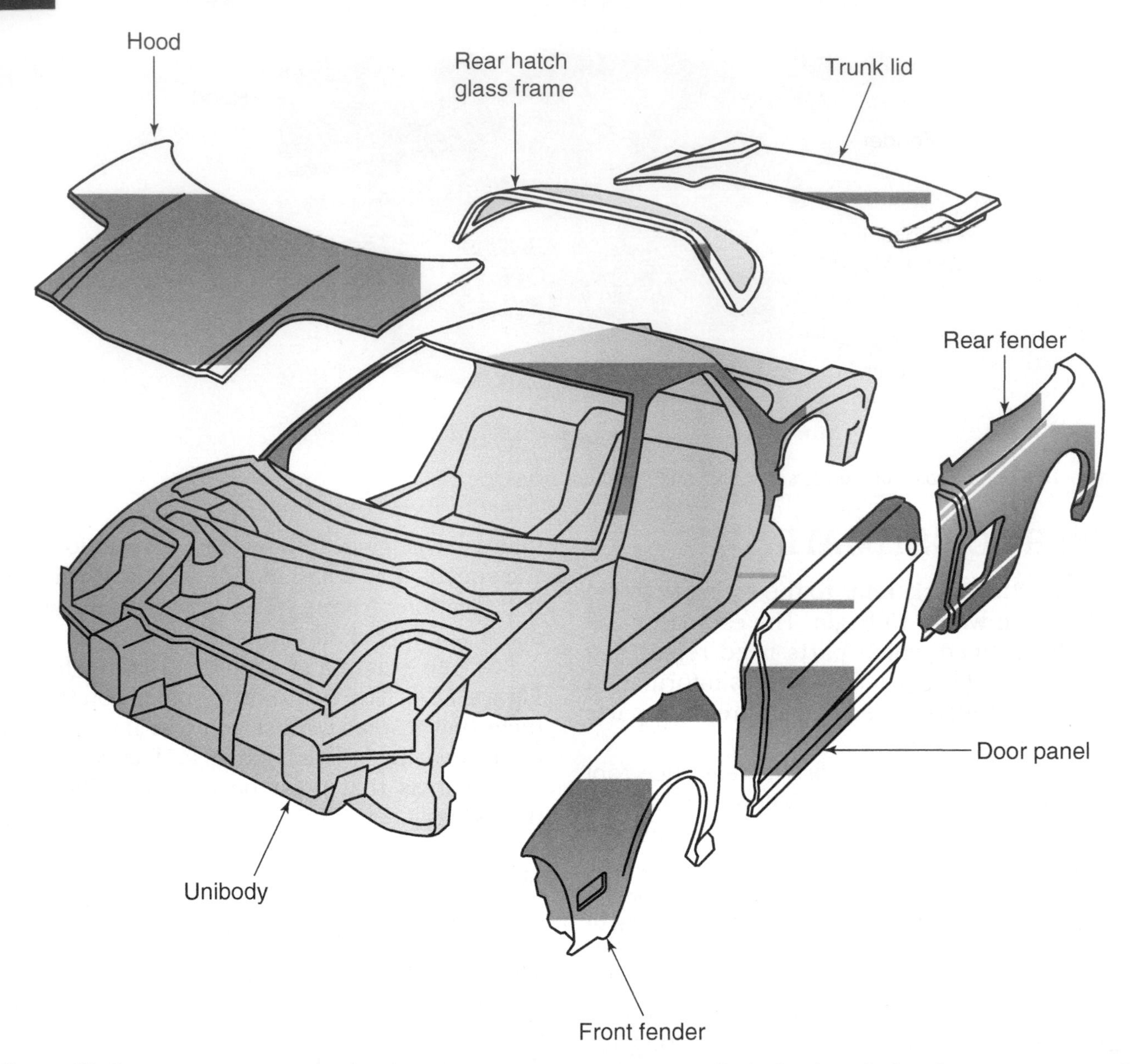

Figure 12–3. The hood, deck lid, fenders, and doors commonly bold onto a unibody. A unique design, the rear quarter panels also bolt on in this rear-engine, high-performance, aluminum-bodied vehicle.

also want to mark the hinge where it mounts on the body. You can then use these marks to rough adjust the hinges and hood during reinstallation.

To prevent part damage, have someone help you hold the hood. Place your shoulder under the hood while holding the bottom edge of the hood with one hand. This will keep the hood from sliding down and hitting the cowl or fenders. Use your shoulder to support the weight of the hood. With your free hand, remove the hood bolts. Your helper should do the same. Do not let the weight of the hood rest on the bolts as you loosen them.

Note the location of any **hood hinge spacers** that help adjust the hood. If there is no major damage, you may need to reinstall the spacers in the same locations. Place the hood out of the way, where it will not fall over.

Hood Hinge Removal and Replacement

Hood hinges allow the hood to open and close while staying in alignment. They must hold considerable weight while keeping the hood open. They are often damaged in a frontal impact.

If they are badly bent, you will have to replace the hood hinges. If the hood is equipped with large coil springs, you may also have to install the old springs on the new hinges. A **hood hinge spring tool** should be used to stretch the spring off and on. It is a hooked tool that will easily pry the end of the spring off of and onto its mount.

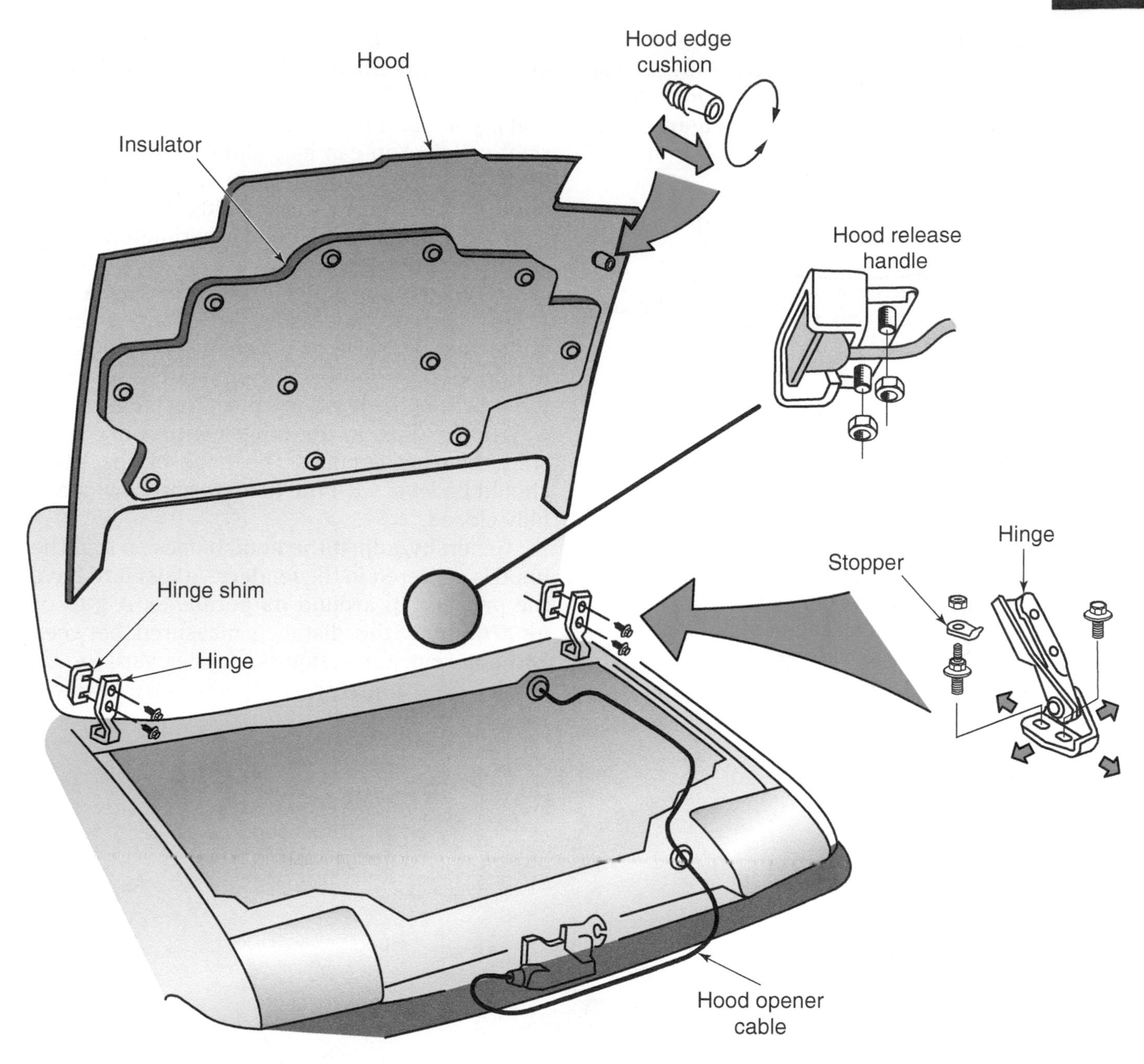

Figure 12–4. Study the parts of a typical hood assembly and cable hood release mechanism.

If necessary, unbolt the hinges from the inner fender panels. Again, mark their alignment if the panels are not damaged. Install the new hinges. Snug the bolts down; do not tighten them. You will have to adjust the hood and hinges later.

Hood Adjustment

Install the hood in reverse order of its removal. Again, have someone help you hold the hood while installing its bolts. Snug down but do not tighten the hood bolts. You will need to adjust the hood before tightening the bolts fully. A misaligned hood is shown in **Figure 12–5.**

! WARNING !

After installing the hood, close the hood slowly. If it is not centered, it could hit and dent the fenders. It may be a good idea to place tape over the fender edges to protect them.

Hood adjustments are made at the hinges, at the adjustable stops, and at the hood latch. You can adjust the hood up or down and forward or rearward. This allows you to align the hood with the fenders and cowl vertically and horizontally. The holes in the hinges are slotted. This allows the hinges to be raised or lowered at the cowl or fender and the hood to be moved forward or rearward at the hinges. See **Figure 12–6.**

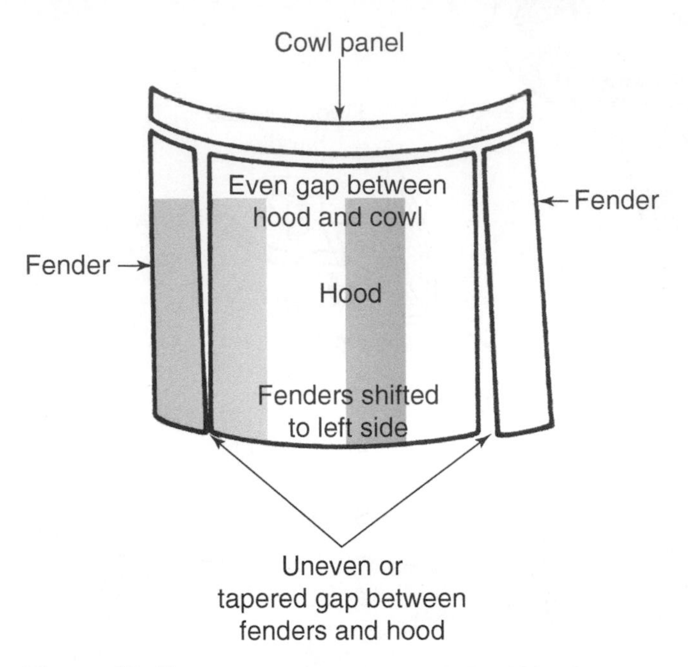

Figure 12–5. The gap around the hood should be the same. The problems may be due to fenders being out of alignment.

Hood hinge adjustments control the general position of the hood in the fenders and the rear hood height. By loosening the hood-to-hinge bolts, you can move the front end of the hood right or left. You can also slide the hood to the front or back. Tighten them down when the hood is centered in the opening. You want an equal gap around the hood's perimeter. There should be enough of a gap at the back edge to clear the cowl panel. Refer to **Figure 12–7A.**

By partially loosening the hinge-to-body bolts, you can raise or lower the rear height of the hood. Do not loosen the bolts too much or the weight of the hood will push the hinge all the way down. Tap on the hinges with a mallet to shift them as needed. The back of the hood should be level with the fenders and cowl when fully closed.

Generally, adjust the hood hinges so that the hood is centered in the fenders. Adjust it to have the proper gap around its perimeter. A **gap** or **clearance** is the distance measured between two adjacent parts, hood-to-fender gap, for example. Then adjust the hinges to raise or lower the back of the hood.

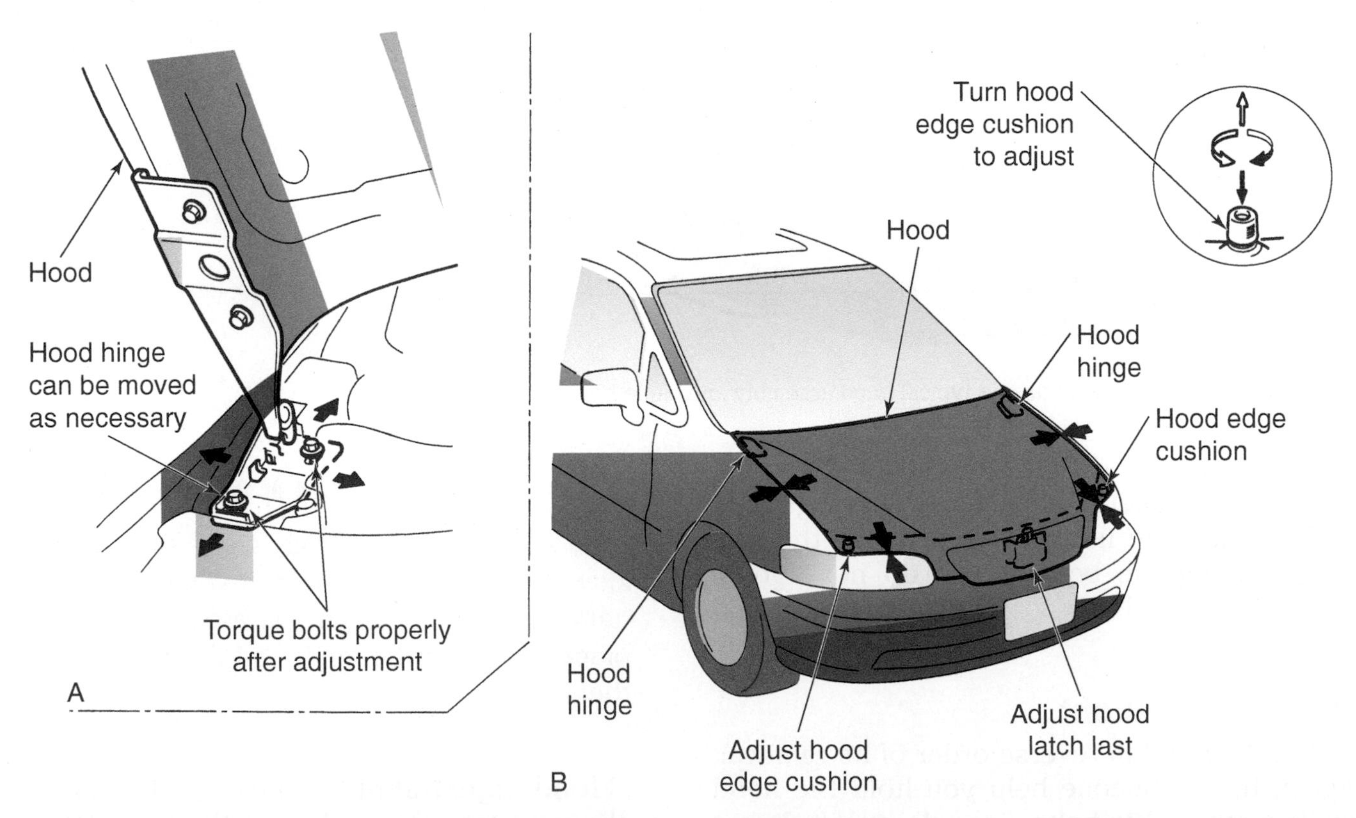

Figure 12–6. (A) When adjusting hood alignment, loosen the hinge-to-body bolts slightly. This will let you shift the hinge mounting in the elongated holes right-left and fore-aft. To avoid paint damage, slowly lower the hood while checking its alignment. Tighten the hinge bolts when the hood is aligned with the cowl and fenders. **(B)** Hood edge cushions must be adjusted so the height of the hood is even with the fenders. You may want to remove the latch during hood adjustment. (Courtesy of American Isuzu Motors, Inc.)

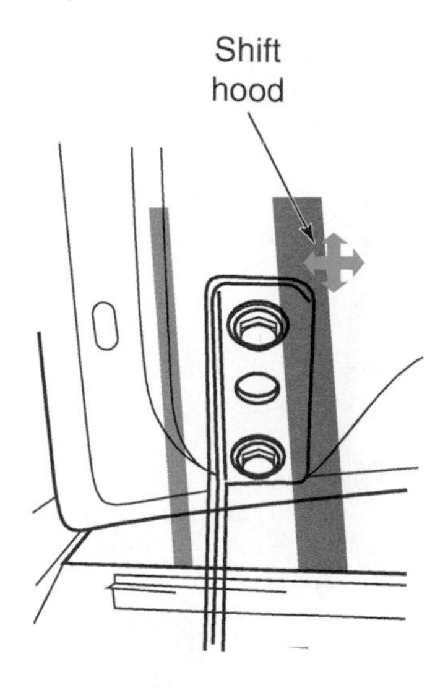

(A) With the hood-to-hinge bolts loose, shift the hood as needed to position it on the body. Align the hood straight on the body and obtain the correct clearance at the back of the hood.

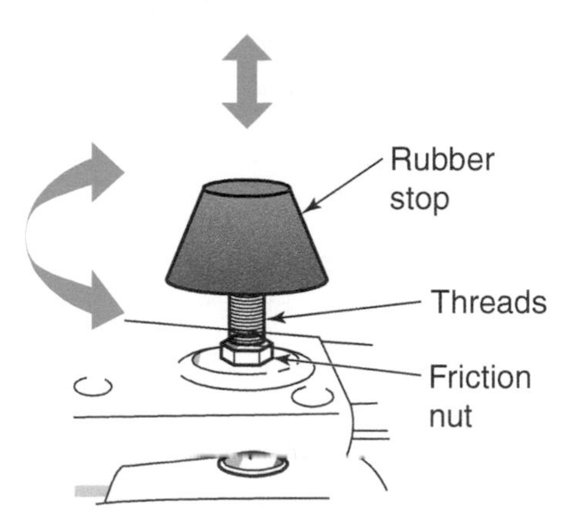

(B) Turn the bumpers up or down to make the front of the hood level with the fender and other parts.

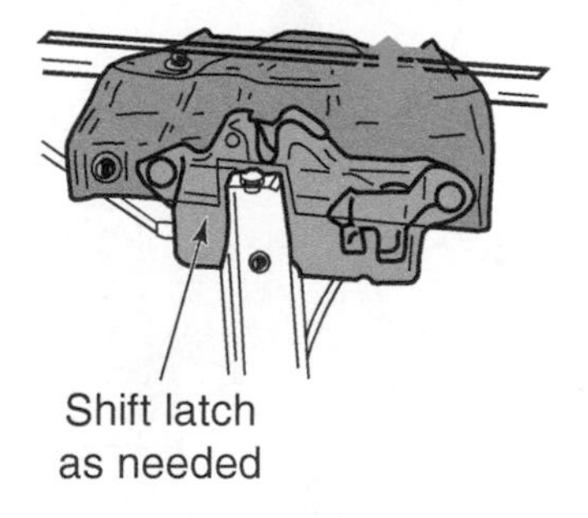

(C) Close the hood slowly. It should not shift sideways when the striker engages the latch. Center the latch in the striker and adjust the latch up or down to pull the hood lightly down against the bumpers.

Figure 12–7. Study the basic methods of adjusting a hood. (Courtesy of DaimlerChrysler Corporation)

The **hood stop adjustment** controls the height of the front of the hood. It is usually made of rubber bumpers mounted on threaded studs. By loosening the locknut, you can rotate to raise or lower the stops and hood. Adjust the hood stops so that the hood is even with the front of the fenders and fascia. Tighten the locknuts after adjustment. See **Figure 12–7B.**

Hood Latch Removal, Replacement, and Adjustment

The **hood latch mechanism** keeps the hood closed and releases the hood when activated. Some hood latches are opened by moving a lever behind the grille. Most have a cable release that runs into the passenger compartment. All have slots for adjustment. See **Figure 12–7C.**

A **cable hood release,** as shown in **Figure 12–8,** consists of the following:

- The **hood release handle** can be pulled to slide a cable running out to the hood latch. It is normally mounted on the lower left side of the passenger compartment.
- The **hood release cable** is a steel cable that slides inside a plastic housing. One end fastens to the release handle and the other to the hood latch.
- The **hood latch** has metal arms that grasp and hold the hood striker. The spring-loaded arms lock over the hood striker when the hood is closed. When the cable release is pulled, the arms release the striker so the hood can open.
- The **hood striker** bolts to the hood and engages the hood latch when closed.

Before removing a hood latch, scribe mark its location if necessary. Remove its bolts and disconnect any cable. Slots in the latch mount provide up and down and side to side adjustment.

Hood latch adjustment controls how well the hood striker engages the latch mechanism. Basically, with the hood centered and set at the right height, adjust the latch for proper closing.

Slowly lower the hood while watching to see if the striker centers itself in the latch. The hood should not pivot right or left when it engages the latch. If the hood moves to one side when closed, shift the latch right or left as needed.

The latch should also produce a slight downward compression of the rubber stops. This keeps the hood from bouncing up and down. If you must slam the hood down to engage the latch, raise the latch. If the hood will move up and down when latched, lower the latch. See **Figure 12–9.**

After adjustment, tighten the latch bolts. Make sure the latch releases the hood properly.

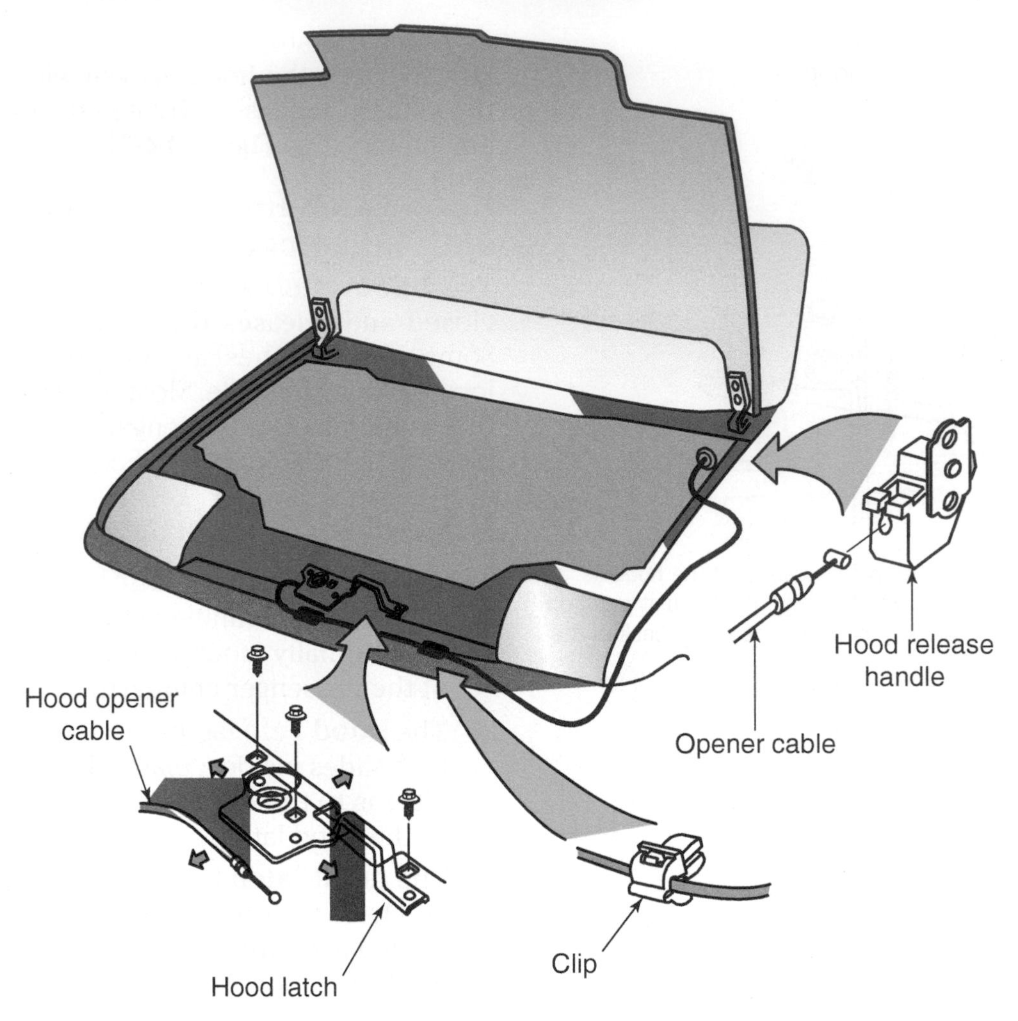

Figure 12–8. Study the parts and adjustment of the hood release mechanism.

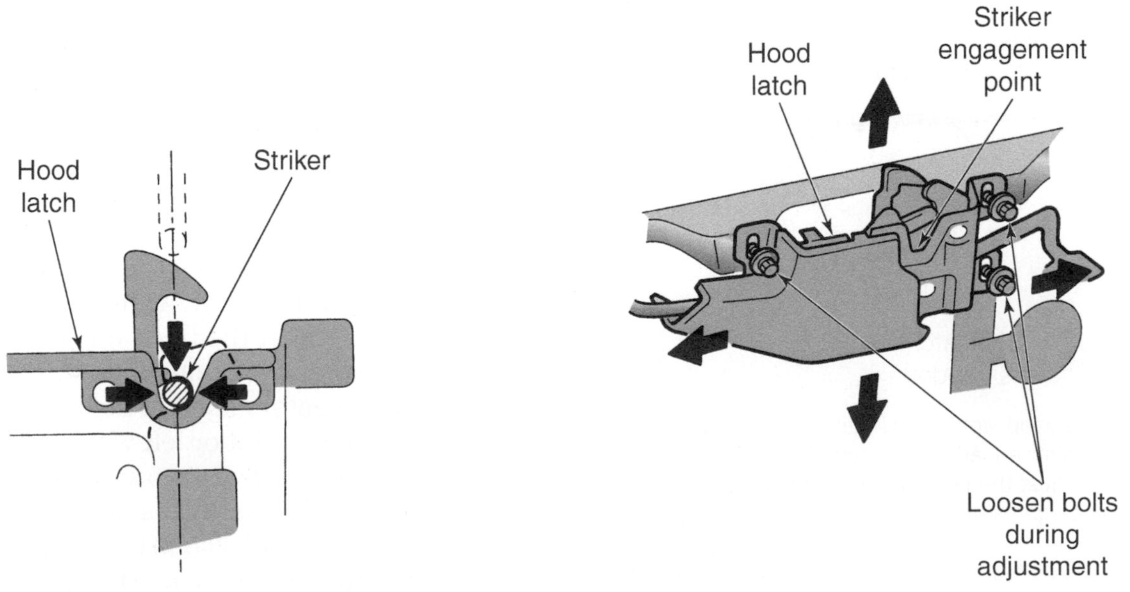

(A) With the hood alignment and height adjusted, adjust the latch. Move the latch until the striker is centered in the latch as shown.

(B) The latch should be positioned so that it places a slight downward pull on the hood when it is fully engaged with the striker.

Figure 12–9. Study how to adjust hood latch. (Courtesy of American Isuzu Motors, Inc.)

Always check the vehicle's service manual for specific hood adjustment procedures.

BUMPER REMOVAL, REPLACEMENT, AND ADJUSTMENT

New vehicle **bumpers** are designed to withstand minor impact without damage. They protect other parts from light impact with sheer mass and bulk.

Bumper designs are light, yet strong. Many use an outer covering of flexible plastic with a heavy steel or aluminum inner bumper. Some have a plastic honeycomb or foam structure behind their flexible cover. Many have a large one-piece cover over the lower front half of the vehicle nose.

To remove a bumper, first disconnect the wiring going to any lights. Procedures vary, so you may need to refer to a service manual. Some bolts can be hidden behind parking lights, inner fender panels, etc. See **Figure 12–10.**

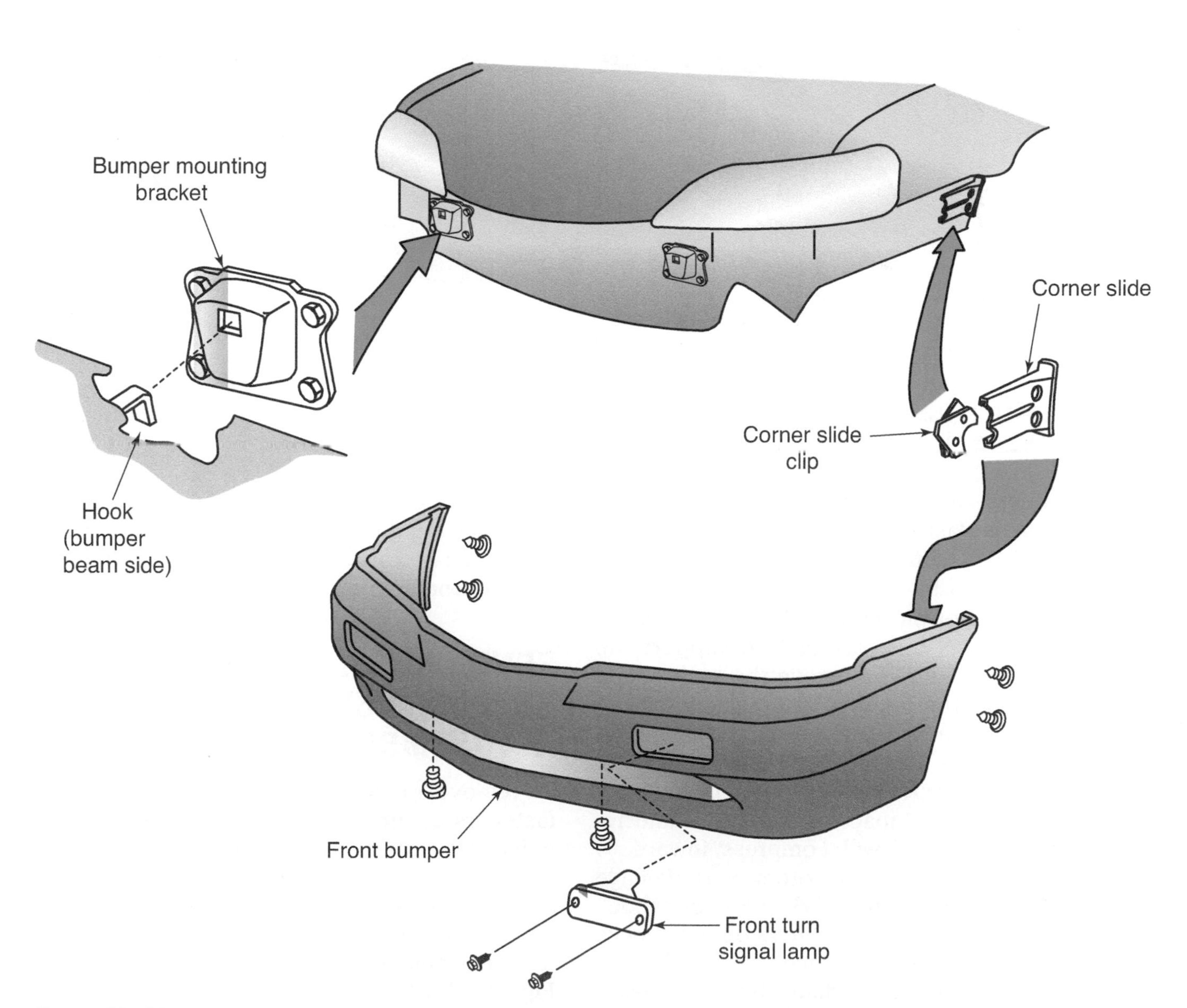

Figure 12–10. Various methods are used to secure the front bumper to a vehicle. Removal of the lights and molding will often give access to mounting hardware for removal of the bumper. Also note screws and bolts that come in from the bottom and rear of the bumper.

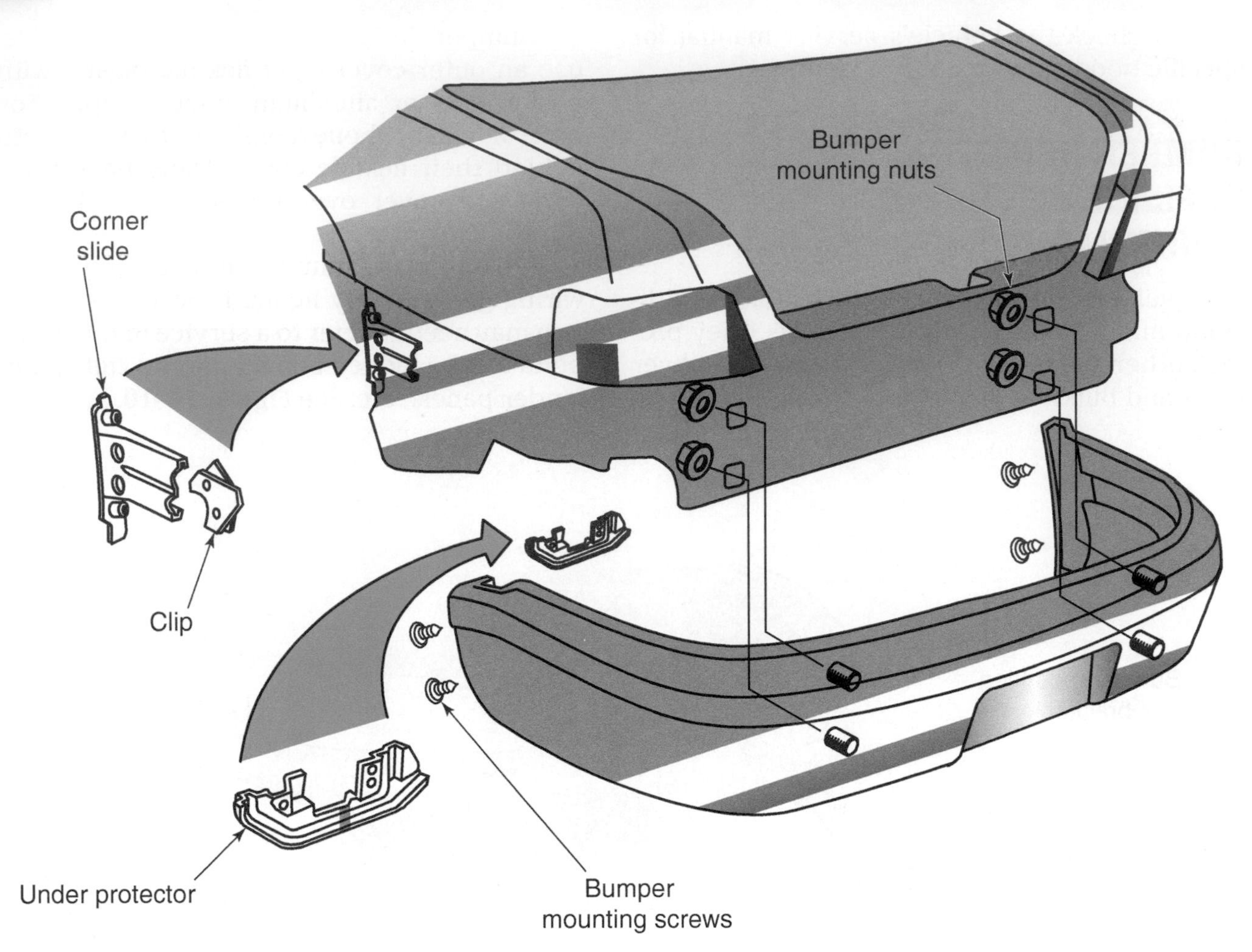

Figure 12–11. Replacement of the rear bumper is similar to that of the front bumper. Always remember to disconnect all wires so they are not damaged when you lift the bumper off.

Bumpers can be heavy and clumsy. Before removing the last mounting bolts, support the bumper. Get a helper or use a floor jack. If the bumpers are to be repaired or reused, place a block of wood or piece of thick foam rubber on the jack saddle. Raise the jack to support the weight of the bumper. Remove the bolts. Then you can work the bumper and jack away from the vehicle. These general procedures also apply to the rear bumper. See **Figure 12–11.**

Bumper shock absorbers are used to absorb some of the impact of a collision and reduce damage. They will compress inward to help prevent bumper and other part damage during a low-speed impact. When bumper shock absorbers are used, bolts or nuts on the shocks often hold the bumper in place.

With major front end damage, sometimes it is best to remove the large assemblies, like the front clip or bumper-spoiler assembly. This will let you gain access to hard-to-reach parts on the assembly more easily. This may allow you to service damaged bumper, lights, brackets, and other front end parts in less time. **Figure 12–12** shows an assortment of clips that may be needed when replacing fastened parts.

FENDER REMOVAL, REPLACEMENT, AND ADJUSTMENT

To remove a fender, find and remove all of the fasteners securing it to the vehicle. Also remove any wires going to fender-mounted lights. Fenders are usually bolted to the radiator core support, inner fender panels, and cowl. Bolts are often hidden behind the doors, inner fender panels, and under the vehicle. Refer to **Figure 12–13.**

With all of the bolts removed, carefully lift the fender off. Transfer any needed parts (trim, body clips, etc.) from the old fender over to the new fender.

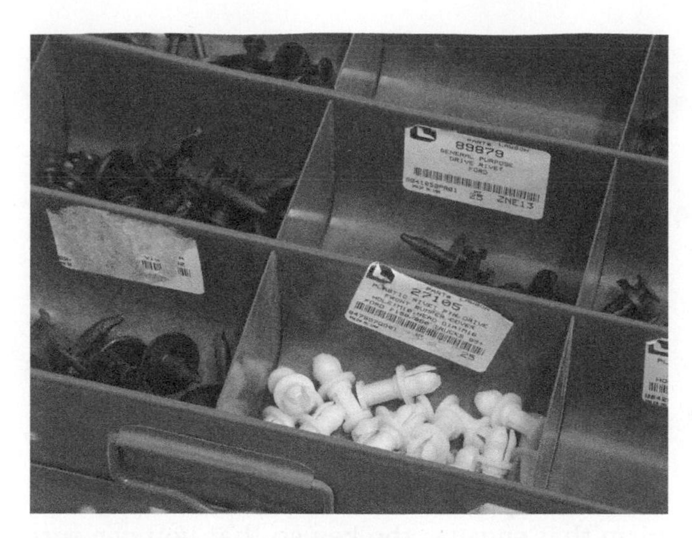

Figure 12–12. Various methods are used to secure the front bumper to a vehicle. Removal of the lights and molding will often give access to mounting hardware for removal of the bumper. Also note screws and bolts that come in from the bottom and rear of the bumper. (Courtesy of American Honda Motor Co., Inc.)

Install the replacement fender in reverse order of the removal. If the doors or cowl are undamaged, place masking or duct tape over their edges. This will protect their finish from scratches when installing the fender.

When installing the fenders, hand start the fender bolts. Do not tighten them. Leave the bolts loose enough that you can adjust the fender. Shift the fender on its bolts so that it aligns with other body parts properly. Shift the fender forward or backward until the fender, door, and cowl have the correct spacing or gap. Also adjust the fender in and out so that it is flush with the door and parallel with the hood. Tighten the fender bolts after you have the fender in alignment.

Fender shimming is an adjustment method that uses spacers under the bolts that attach the fender to the cowl or inner fender panel. By changing shim thicknesses, you can move the position of the fender for proper alignment.

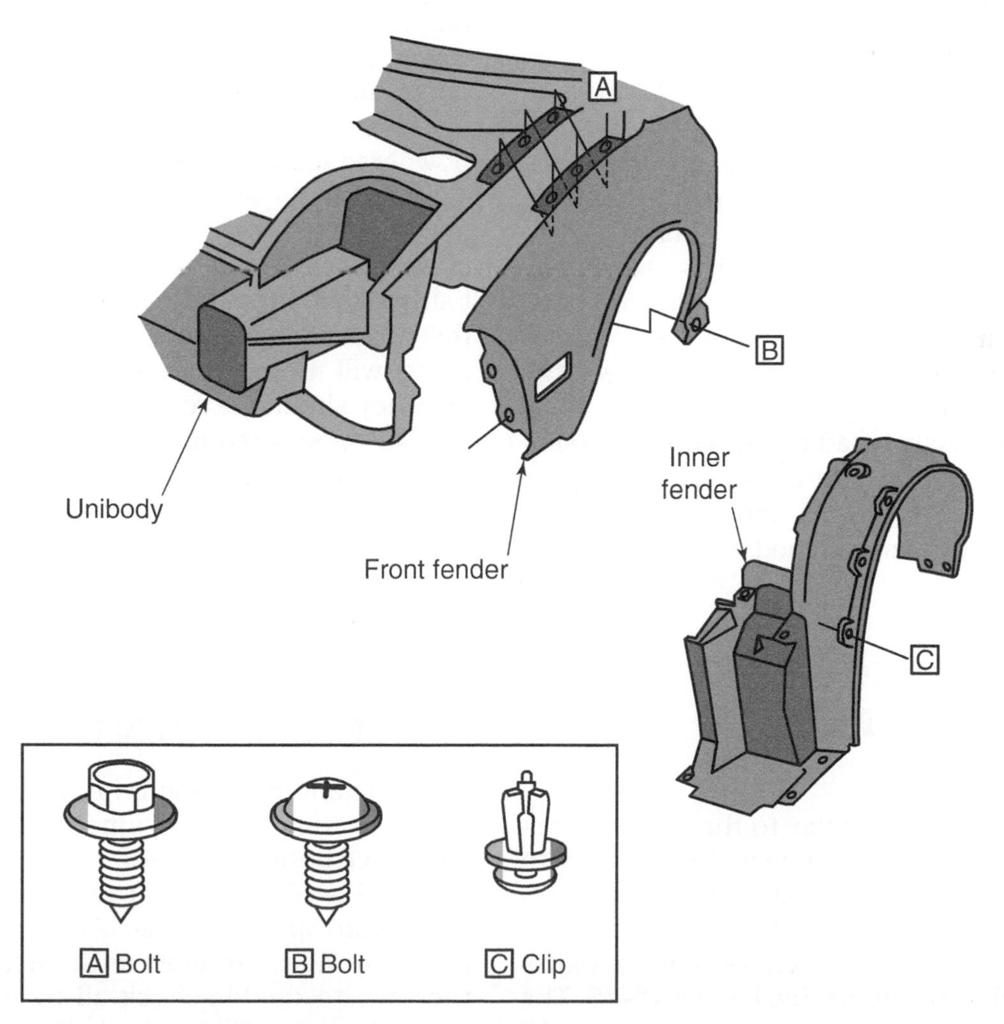

Figure 12–13. Fender bolts are located around the outside of the fender. Some are hidden behind the inner fender panel or at the rear behind the front door around the cowl.

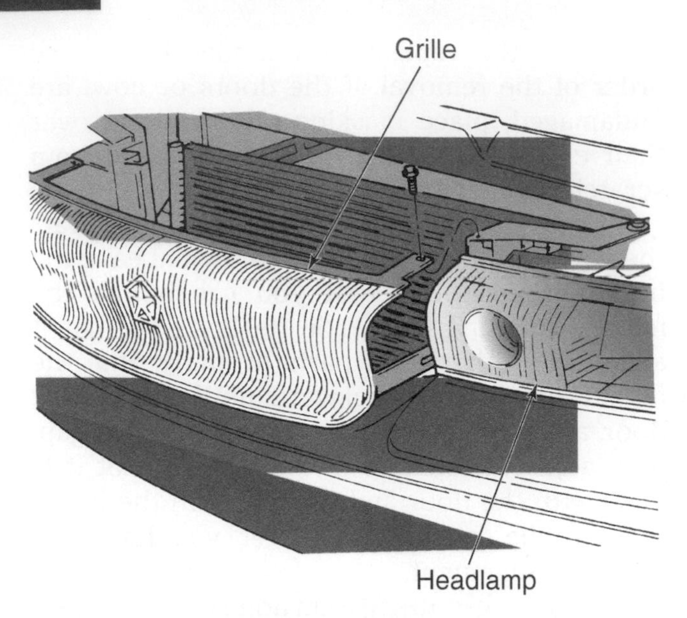

Figure 12–14. Most new grilles are made of plastic. Small clips and screws hold the grille in place. (Courtesy of DaimlerChrysler Corporation)

GRILLE REMOVAL AND REPLACEMENT

Grilles are often held in place with small screws, rivits, and clips. You might have to remove a cover to access grille fasteners (see **Figure 12–14**). An air ratchet is handy for reaching down and unscrewing grille bolts. When installing a grille, make sure all clips are undamaged and installed. Since most grilles are plastic, be careful not to overtighten any bolts or screws. You could crack the grille. Select the correct rivet size.

Some grilles can be adjusted. They have slotted or oversized holes in them. By leaving the bolts loose, you can shift and align the grille with other parts. Once aligned, tighten the grille fasteners slowly.

DECK LID REMOVAL, REPLACEMENT, AND ADJUSTMENT

The deck lid is very similar to the hood in construction. Two hinges connect the deck lid to the rear body panel. The trailing edge is secured by a locking latch.

Deck lid or hatch door removal and replacement is similar to a hood. See **Figure 12–15.** The deck lid must be evenly spaced between the adjacent panels. Slotted holes in the hinges and/or caged plates in the deck lid allow it to be moved. To adjust the deck lid forward or rearward, slightly loosen the bolts on both hinges. Close and adjust the deck lid as required. Then raise the lid and tighten the bolts.

Weatherstripping is a rubber seal that prevents leakage at the joint between the movable part (lid, hatch, door) and the body. To prevent air and water leaks, the deck lid must contact the weatherstripping evenly when closed. The latch must be adjusted so that it holds the lid or hatch closed against the weatherstripping.

Lock cylinders contain a tumbler mechanism that engages the key so that you can turn the key and disengage the latch. When you insert your key into a door or lid, it engages the lock cylinder. The lock cylinder then transfers motion to the latch.

The lock cylinder on door and deck lids is usually held on the panel with a retainer. A sealing gasket may also seal out water and dust. To remove a lock cylinder, pry the retainer sideways. This will free the lock cylinder. Sometimes, lock cylinders are held by small screws. If necessary, lubricate a lock cylinder with dry powdered graphite.

Lid struts are usually spring-loaded, gas-filled units that hold the lid open and cause it to close more slowly. The struts often engage small ball sockets mounted on the body. The ends of the struts snap-fit over the ball sockets. Bad lid struts will no longer support the weight of the lid. They should be replaced.

Lid torsion rods are spring steel rods used to help lift the weight of the lid. They extend horizontally across the body and engage a stationary bracket. Some torsion rod brackets have adjustment slots. You can change tension on the torsion rods by moving them in these slots. Refer to **Figure 12–16.**

PANEL ALIGNMENT

After installing all new body panels, you must check overall panel alignment. Make sure that clearance between panels is equal. As shown in **Figure 12–17,** the gap around all panels must be within specifications. Also check that all panel surfaces are even with each other. Take the time to double-check all panels to ensure good alignment. This is a sign of a professional technician.

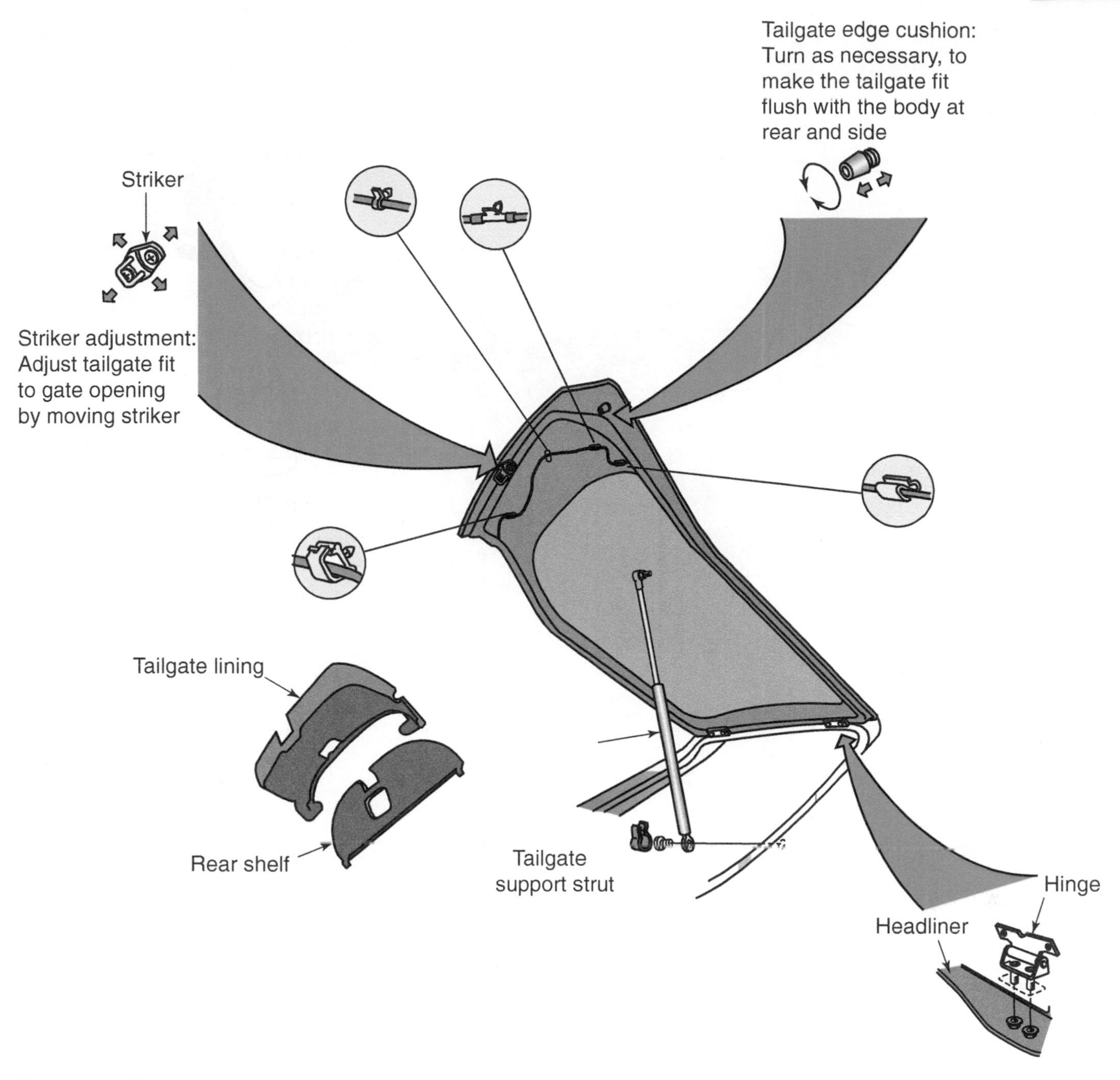
Tailgate edge cushion: Turn as necessary, to make the tailgate fit flush with the body at rear and side
Striker
Striker adjustment: Adjust tailgate fit to gate opening by moving striker
Tailgate lining
Rear shelf
Tailgate support strut
Hinge
Headliner

Figure 12–15. Study the parts of a rear hatch lid.

TRUCK BED REMOVAL AND REPLACEMENT

Truck beds are usually bolted to the frame. To remove the bed, simply remove the bolts that extend up through brackets on the frame. Keep track of bolt lengths and rubber mounting cushion locations. They must be reinstalled in their original locations. See **Figure 12–18.**

Truck tailgates mount on two hinges. A steel cable often limits how far down the tailgate will open. See **Figure 12–19.** Latches in the sides of the tailgate engage strikers on the body. The handle on the outside of the tailgate moves small linkage rods that run out to the latches.

WARNING

Truck tailgates are surprisingly heavy. Ask someone to help you when removing or installing one.

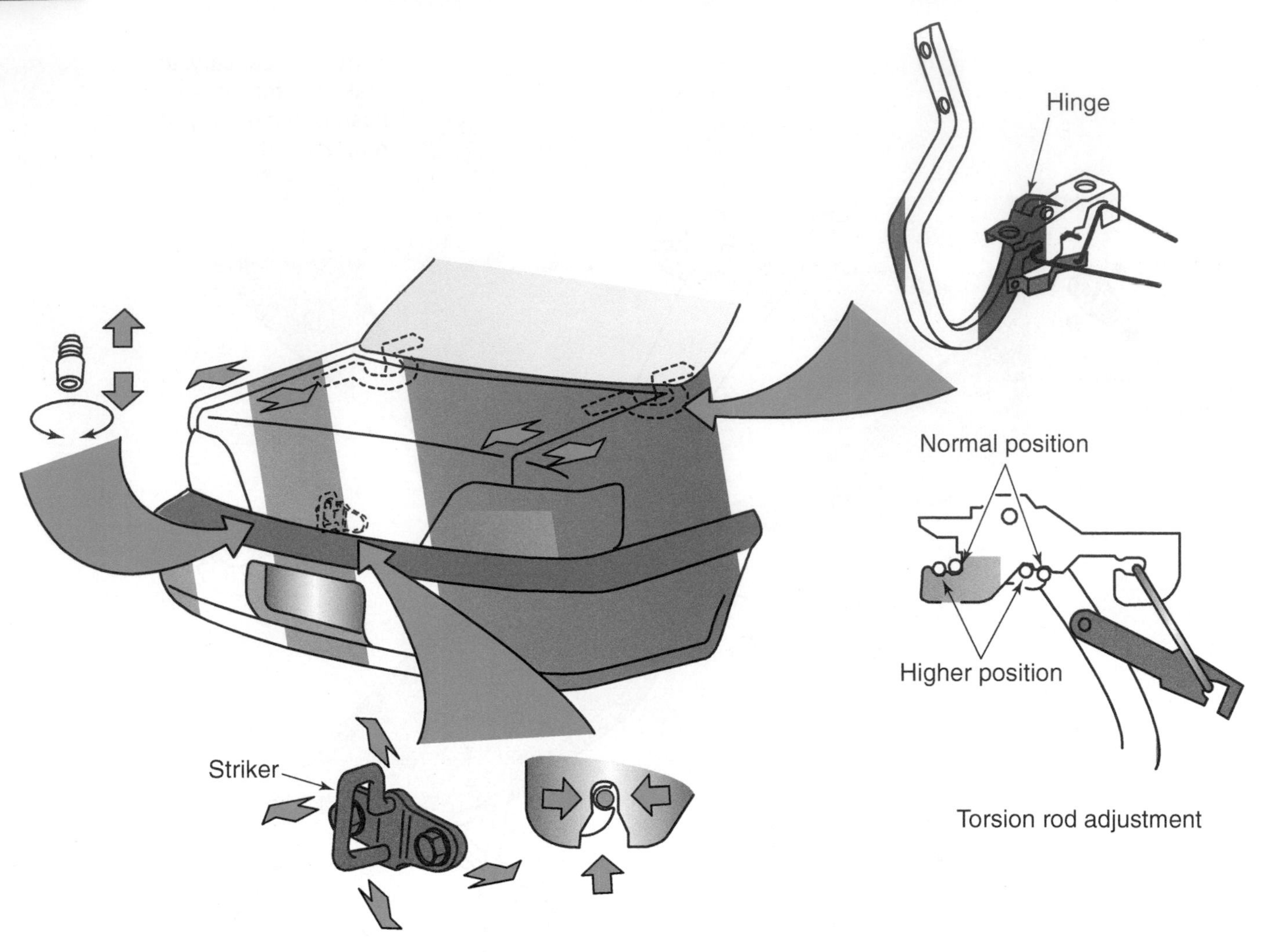

Figure 12–16. Deck lids can also be held open by torsion rods. Some can be adjusted by moving the location of the rod in a mount.

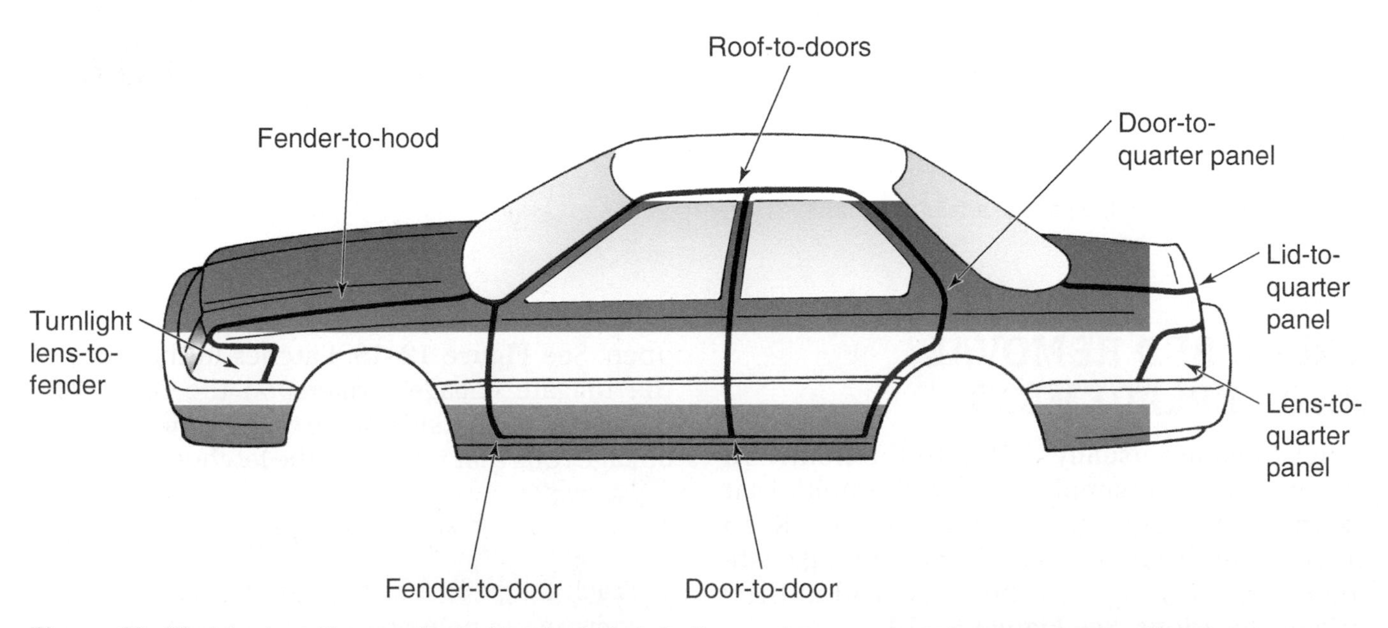

Figure 12–17. After installing panels, double-check their fit. You want even gaps or clearances among all parts. (Courtesy of Honda Motor Co.)

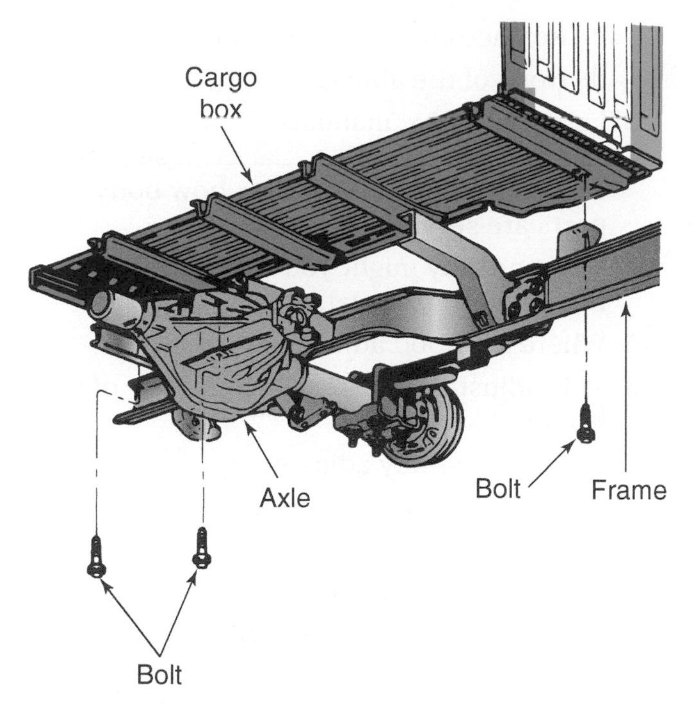

Figure 12–18. Truck beds normally bolt to the full frame. After removing all bolts, wires, and other parts, the bed can be lifted off the frame. (Courtesy of DaimlerChrysler Corporation)

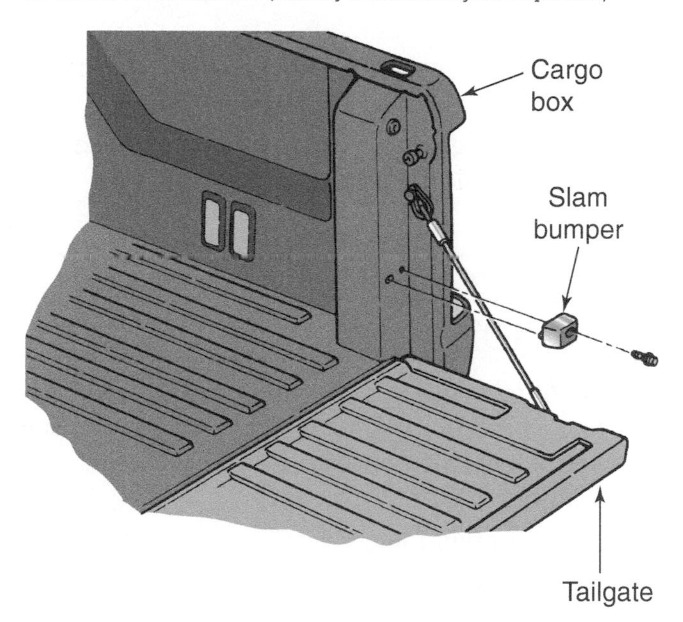

Figure 12–19. A truck tailgate is serviced like other hinged parts. It must align properly when closed and engage strikers properly. (Courtesy of DaimlerChrysler Corporation)

INSTALLING SOUND-DEADENING PADS

Sound-deadening pads are often bonded to the inside surface of trunk cavities and doors to reduce noise, vibration, and harshness. Sound-deadening material is made of a plastic or asphalt-based material. It prevents the thin sheet metal panels from acting like large metal sounding drums to quiet the passenger compartment. The original factory material is bonded and, sometimes, heat formed to the surface.

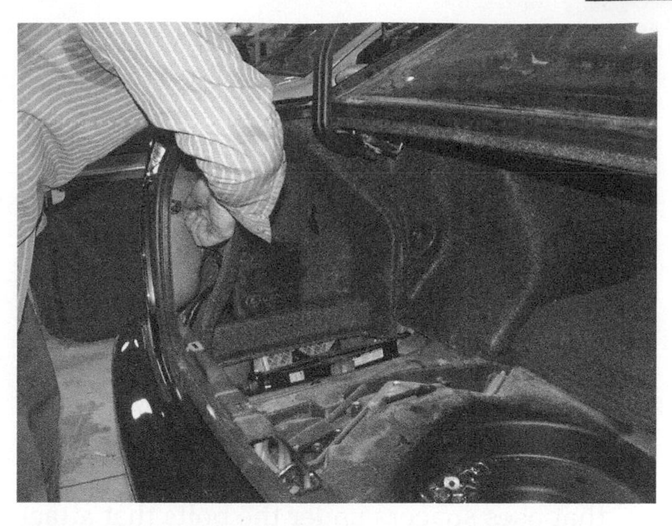

Figure 12–20. The technician is reinstalling sound-deadening panels and trim in the truck after major repair. (Courtesy of Riverdale Body Shop)

During collision repair, sound-deadening pads must be replaced to match precollision performance. After repair, the area must be properly refinished to provide rust protection before the sound-deadening material is applied.

Some pads are available as factory service parts. Be sure to check the factory body repair manual for details. If a factory pad is not available, the sound-deadening qualities must be restored with a suitable replacement product. These should be available from several sources. See **Figure 12–20.**

One sound-deadening product is available with an adhesive on the back. Cut it to size and shape. Peel off the backing, and apply. The sheets can be heated with a heat gun to make them flexible to conform to the contour of the sheet metal.

SUMMARY

- When starting work, refer to the estimate to get guidance on where to begin. The estimator will have determined which parts need repair and which should be replaced. Use this information to begin removal and replacement (R and R).
- Hood hinges allow the hood to open and close while staying in alignment. They must hold considerable weight while keeping the

hood open. They are often damaged in a frontal impact.

- A cable hood release consists of the hood release handle, hood release cable, hood latch, and the hood striker.
- Bumpers today are designed to be light, yet strong. Many use an outer covering of flexible plastic with a heavy steel or aluminum inner bumper. Some have a plastic honeycomb structure behind their flexible cover. The trend is also to a large one-piece cover over the lower front half of the vehicle nose.
- Fender shimming is an adjustment method that uses spacers under the bolts that attach the fender to the cowl or inner fender panel. By changing shim thicknesses, you can move the position of the fender for proper alignment.
- After installing all new body panels, you must check overall panel alignment. Make sure that clearance between panels is equal and that the gap around all parts is within specifications.

TECHNICAL TERMS

hood hinge spacers
hood hinges
hood hinge spring tool
hood adjustments
gap
clearance
hood stop adjustment
hood latch mechanism
cable hood release
hood release handle
hood release cable
hood latch
hood striker
hood latch adjustment
bumpers
bumper shock absorbers
fender shimming
weatherstripping
lock cylinders
lid struts
lid torsion rods
sound-deadening pads

REVIEW QUESTIONS

1. List five ways parts can be held together.
2. A vehicle has a damaged fender. The estimate says to "R and R" the fender. This means you should:
   a. Remove and repair the fender.
   b. Remove and replace the fender.
   c. Replace and realign fender.
   d. None of the above.
3. Factory service manuals often have a ____________ ____________ section that explains and illustrates how body parts are serviced.
4. How and why might you want to mark a hood before removal?
5. Where are hood adjustments made?
6. This adjustment controls the height of the front of the hood.
   a. Hinge-to-body adjustment
   b. Hinge-to-hood adjustment
   c. Hood stop adjustment
   d. None of the above
7. Describe the parts of a cable hood release.
8. Fender ____________ is an adjustment method that uses spacers under the bolts that attach the fender to the cowl or inner fender panel.
9. What is the purpose of weatherstripping?
10. Bad lid ____________ ____________ will no longer support the weight of the lid. They should be replaced.

ASE-STYLE REVIEW QUESTIONS

1. *Technician A* says that most quarter panels are welded in place. *Technician B* says that some quarter panels are held in place with fasteners. Who is correct?
   a. Technician A
   b. Technician B
   c. Both Technicians A and B
   d. Neither Technician

2. A vehicle has minor front end damage. Before removing the hood, *Technician A* says to open and close the hood to analyze part conditions. *Technician B* says to mark hood hinge alignment. Who is correct?
   a. Technician A
   b. Technician B
   c. Both Technicians A and B
   d. Neither Technician

3. Which of the following fasteners should be removed for hood replacement if hood hinges and fender aprons are not damaged?

a. Hinge-to-apron

b. Hinge-to-cowl

c. Hinge-to-hood

d. Hinge-to-firewall

4. During hood adjustment, the hood pivots sideways when closed. This is normally caused by:

a. Damaged hood hinges

b. Damaged hinge springs

c. Misaligned hinges

d. Misaligned latch

5. When installing a new fender, *Technician A* says to tighten the fender bolts and adjust the hood to the fender. *Technician B* says to leave the fender bolts loose so the fender can be adjusted to the hood. Who is correct?

a. Technician A

b. Technician B

c. Both Technicians A and B

d. Neither Technician

6. *Technician A* says that sound-deadening ma terial is combustible and must be removed from any area to be welded or flame cut. *Technician B* says that these materials are fireproof. Who is correct?

a. Technician A

b. Technician B

c. Both Technicians A and B

d. Neither Technician

7. A vehicle that has suffered a hard hit to the front requires fender apron replacement and straightening of the cowl. Which of the following operations would not be necessary?

a. Get help to remove hood.

b. Mark hood hinge alignment.

c. Read dimensions manual on vehicle.

d. Pull aprons before removal.

8. A rear trunk lid has torsion bars. *Technician A* says that you must always replace the torsion bars to change opening tension. *Technician B* says that sometimes torsion bar tension can be adjusted. Who is correct?

a. Technician A

b. Technician B

c. Both Technicians A and B

d. Neither Technician

9. *Technician A* says that the hood should not be adjusted to compress the rubber hood stops. *Technician B* says to close the hood briskly after replacement to seat it in the opening. Who is correct?

a. Technician A

b. Technician B

c. Both Technicians A and B

d. Neither Technician

10. *Technician A* says that fender and hood adjustments must be made simultaneously to achieve a satisfactory result. *Technician B* says to adjust the fenders first and then the hood. Who is correct?

a. Technician A

b. Technician B

c. Both Technicians A and B

d. Neither Technician

ACTIVITIES

1. Inspect several cars. Determine if their bolt-on panels are adjusted properly. Is the gap between panels or components equal all the way around all panels? Make a report of your findings.

2. Using a service manual, summarize the procedures for removing a hood and fender from three different makes of cars. Write a report on how these procedures vary.

3. After getting instructor permission, loosen the bolts on a hood latch and hood. Move the hood and latch out of alignment. Adjust the hood and latch.

CHAPTER

13 Servicing Doors, Glass, and Leaks

OBJECTIVES

After studying this chapter, you should be able to:

- R and R a door and adjust it.
- Replace both welded and adhesive-bonded door skins.
- Replace an SMC door skin.
- R and R and adjust a door regulator.
- R and I (remove and install) a windshield.
- R and I other stationary glass.
- Find and fix air and water leaks.
- Describe gasket, full cutout, and partial cutout glass replacement procedures.
- Describe the basics of vent window and tailgate door glass service.

INTRODUCTION

Doors are the most used—and abused—parts of a vehicle. They are opened and closed thousands and thousands of times over the life of a vehicle. They must do this while still being strong enough to stay closed and protect the driver and passengers from injury during a collision. Doors must also seal out water and wind noise to keep the interior dry and quiet. Look at **Figure 13–1.**

Glass also plays an important role in the safety and appearance of a vehicle. Glass adds to structural integrity and visibility. Windshields, door glass, stationary glass, and related parts must all be serviced properly to keep the vehicle safe to drive.

DOORS

Vehicle doors allow entry into and exit from the passenger compartment. They are designed to be strong assemblies that provide easy access while being dependable structural units of the vehicle. It is important that you understand door construction and service because doors are commonly damaged in collisions.

DOOR CONSTRUCTION

There are two basic door designs: framed doors and hardtop doors. **Framed doors** surround the sides and top of the door glass with a metal frame, helping keep the window glass aligned. The door frame seals against the door opening. **Hardtop doors** have the glass extending up out of the door without a frame around it. The glass itself must seal against the weatherstripping in the door opening.

Illustrated in **Figure 13–2,** the basic parts of a door include the following:

1. **Door frame**—the main steel frame of the door. Other parts (hinges, glass, handle, etc.) mount on the door frame.
2. **Door skin**—the outer panel over the door frame. It can be made of steel, aluminum, composite, or plastic.
3. *Door glass*—must allow good visibility out of the door.
4. **Door glass channel**—serves as a guide for the glass to move up and down. It is a U-shaped channel lined with a low friction material, felt for example.
5. **Door regulator**—a gear and arm mechanism for moving the glass. When you turn the window handle or press the window button, the regulator moves the glass up or down.
6. **Door latch**—engages the **door striker** on the vehicle body to hold the door closed.
7. *Inner and outer door handles*—use linkage rods to transfer motion to the door latch,

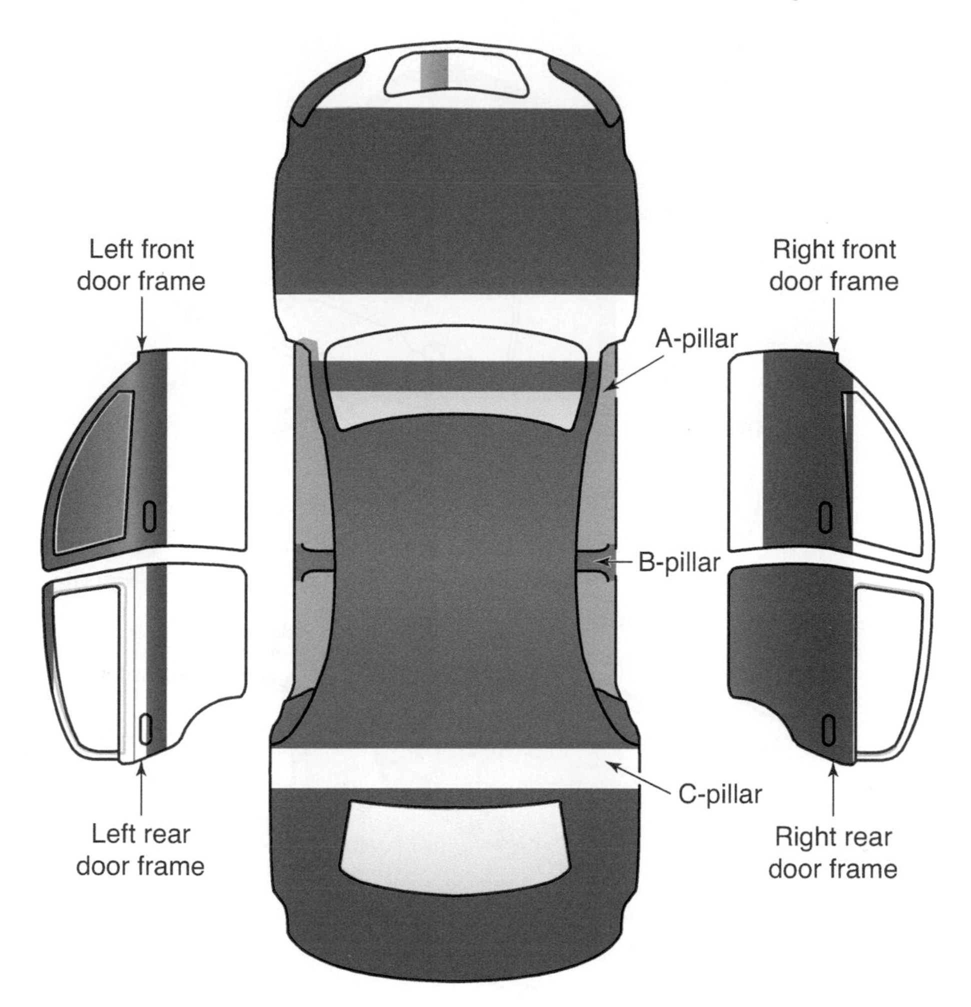

Figure 13–1. The top disassembled view of this vehicle shows doors and large glass areas. Doors are structurally very important to the integrity of the passenger compartment during a side impact collision.

allowing you to activate the latch to open the door.

8. **Door trim panel**—an attractive cover over the inner door frame. Various parts (inner handle, window buttons, speakers) can mount in the inner trim panel.
9. A plastic or paper **door dust cover** fits between the inner trim panel and door frame to keep out wind noise.
10. **Door weatherstripping** fits around the door or door opening to seal the door-to-body joint. When the door is closed, the weatherstripping is partially compressed to prevent air and water leaks.
11. *Rearview mirror* can often mount on the outside of the door frame. A remote mirror knob may provide mirror adjustment on the inner trim panel.

DOOR ADJUSTMENTS

Doors must be accurately adjusted so that they close easily, do not rattle, and do not leak. The door hinges must be adjusted to hold the door in the center of its opening when closed. The door striker must be adjusted to engage the latch smoothly. This section will describe various door adjustments.

Adjusting Door Hinges

Doors must fit their openings and align with the adjacent body panels.

When the doors on a four-door sedan need adjusting, start at the rear door. Since the quarter panel cannot be moved, the rear door must be adjusted to it. Once the rear door is adjusted, the front door can then be adjusted to fit the rear door. Then, the front fender can be adjusted to fit the front door.

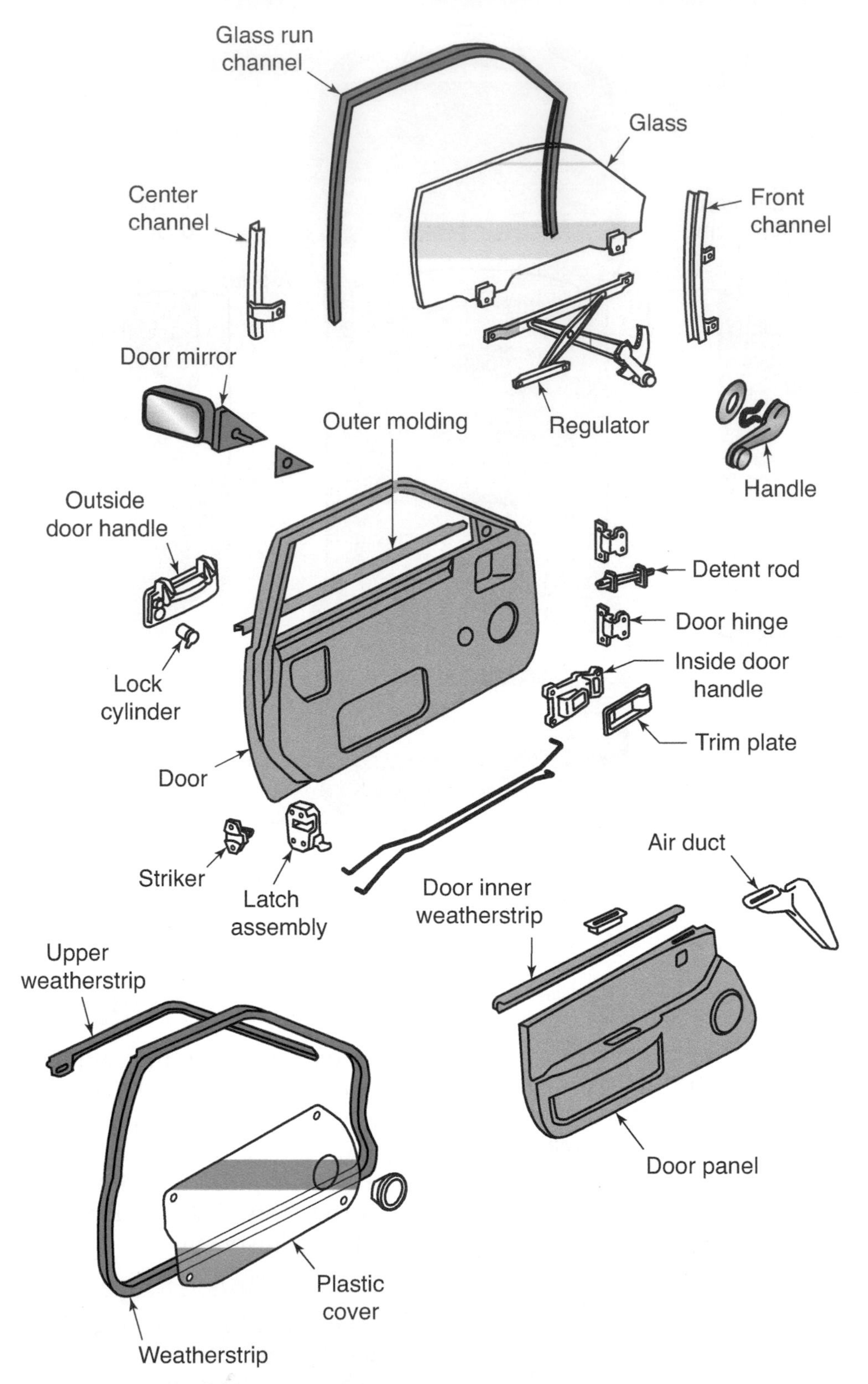

Figure 13–2. Know the parts of a typical door assembly.

On hardtop models, the windows can be adjusted to fit the weatherstripping. Hardtop windows are usually adjusted starting with the front edge of the glass and working toward the back. The front window is then adjusted to it. The rear door window is adjusted to the front window rear edge and the opening for the rear door assembly.

Doors are attached to the body with hinges. The bolted hinge can be adjusted forward, rearward, up, and down easily. The use of shims

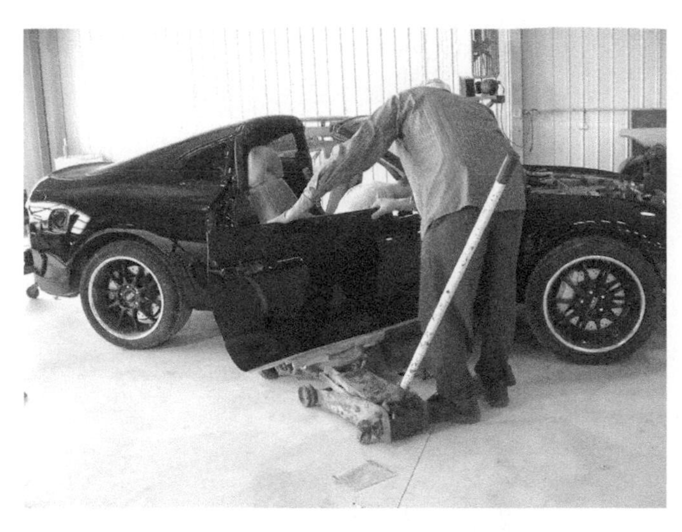

Figure 13–3. When working on a door, use a holding tool to keep the door in alignment while removing or installing hinge bolts. This door tool fits over the saddle of the floor jack.

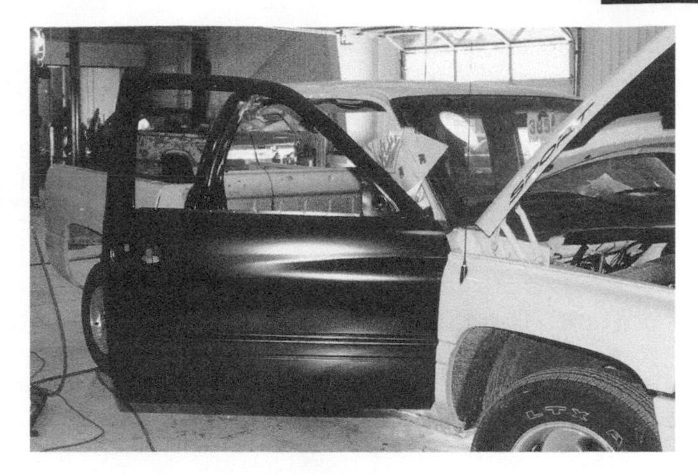

Figure 13–4. After door installation, be careful the first time you close the door. Make sure the edges do not hit the fender or other body parts.

behind the hinge also allows the hinge to be moved as desired.

To adjust a door in its opening, follow these steps:

1. Determine which hinge bolts must be loosened to move the door in the desired direction.
2. Use a jack and wooden block or door holding tool to support the weight of the door. The wooden block or tool on the jack will prevent the jack saddle from chipping the paint on the door edge. See **Figure 13–3.**

WARNING

Do not slam the door after adjusting it. You could damage the latch or striker if they are no longer in alignment.

3. Loosen the hinge-to-body bolts just enough to permit movement of the door.
4. Move the door as needed to align it. Tighten the hinge bolts and check the fit to be sure there is no binding or interference with the adjacent panel.
5. Repeat the operation until the desired fit is obtained. Then check the striker pin alignment for proper door closing. See **Figure 13–4.**
6. Loosen the door striker and move it up or down as needed. If the door tends to move up, move the striker down. If the door tends to drop when engaging the striker, shift the striker upward. See **Figure 13–5.**
7. The door and glass must also be checked to ensure proper alignment to the roof rail and vertical weatherstripping.

When door adjustments are necessary, it may be helpful to remove the striker plate.

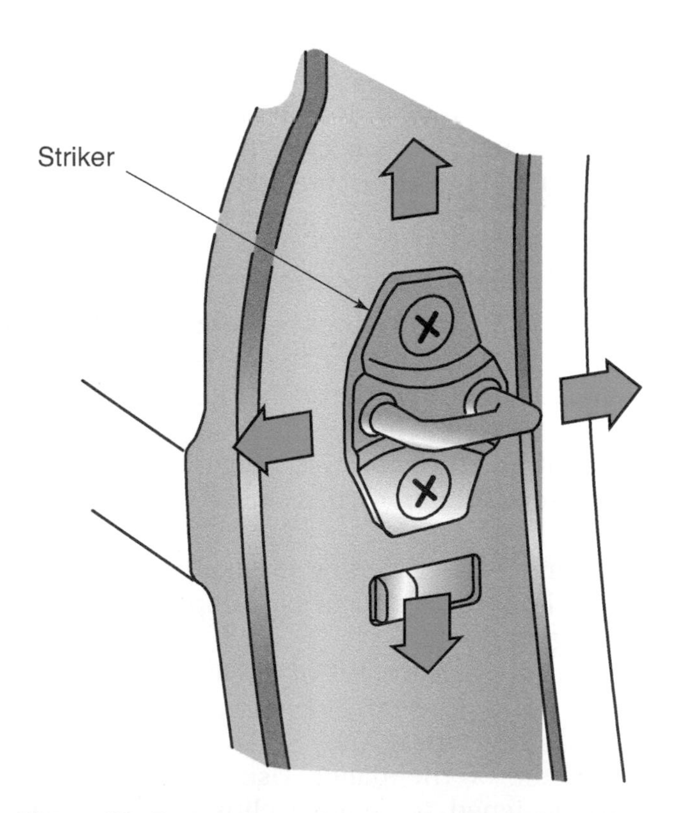

Figure 13–5. The door striker should be loosened and adjusted to hold the door tight against the weatherstripping. If the door tends to move up or down when engaging the striker, raise or lower it.

Doing so allows the door to be centered in the opening more easily.

You might have to loosen the fender at the rear bottom edge to reach the bolts. If the hinge pins are worn out, replace the hinges. This will remove clearance in the hinges and also readjust the door.

In-and-out adjustments are also very important. The door must be aligned in and out to fit the body panels. To adjust the door in or out, loosen the hinge-to-door bolts. Shift the door as needed and then tighten the hinge bolts.

If the top of the door is moved out, it will also move the opposite bottom corner in. If the bottom of the door is moved in on the hinge, it will move the opposite corner out.

The key is to move the door in or out equally on both hinges. Then it will only affect the front of the door because the amount of adjustment decreases toward the back. The center door post, striker pin, and lock will determine the position of the rear of the door. The front edge of the door should always be slightly in from the fender. This will help prevent wind noise from entering the gap between the door and fender.

Some hinges are welded to both the door and body. Obviously, no adjustments can be made to the welded door hinge. If only slightly out of alignment, you can spring or bend the hinge mounts to adjust welded hinges.

Door Inner Trim Panel R and R

To work on parts inside the door, you must remove the inner door trim panel and related parts. Remove any screws that hold on the armrest and other trim pieces. You may have to pop out small decorative plugs over some of the screws. Refer to the service manual if in doubt.

Remove the window crank handle. It can be held on by a screw or by a clip from behind. See **Figure 13–6.**

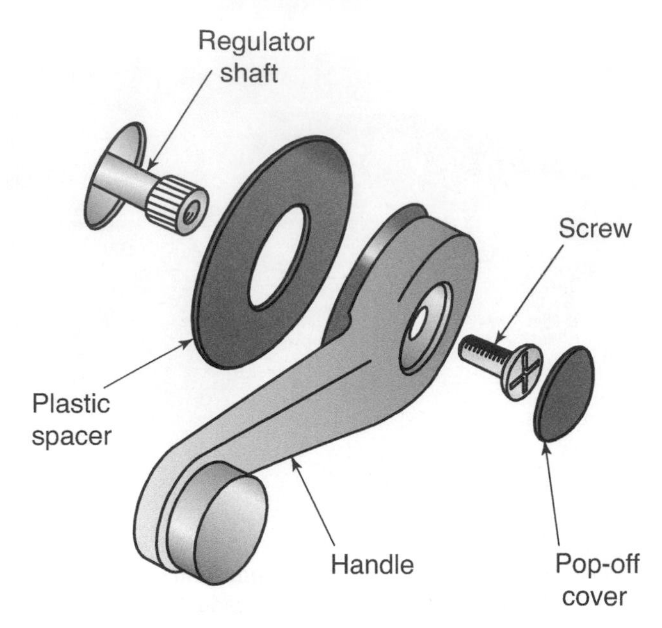

(A) A small screw under a plastic bezel holds this window crank.

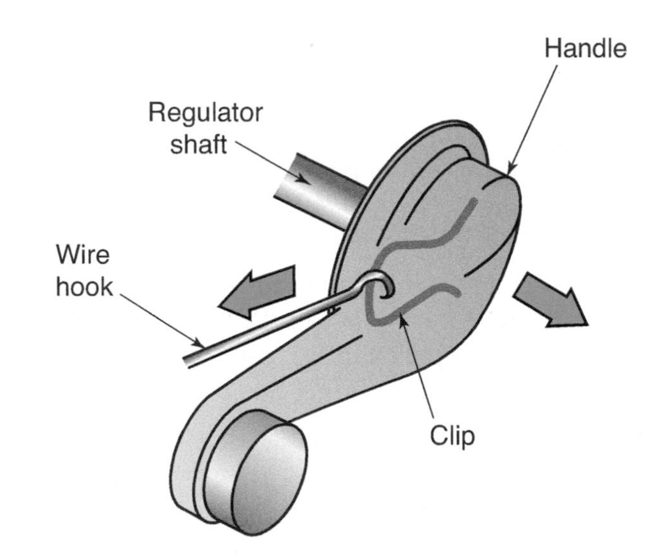

(B) A spring clip holds this window crank. A hook, fork tool, or shop rag can be used to pop the clip out of its groove.

Figure 13–6. Note two common methods of holding window crank handles in place.

With all screws out of the door inner trim panel, you will usually have to pop out a series of plastic clips. They install around the perimeter of the panel. Use a **forked trim tool** designed to remove clips in trim parts. Slide it between the door and panel. Then pry out the plastic clips without damaging the panel.

As you lift off the door inner trim panel, disconnect any wires going to the panel. Feed the wires through the panel. See **Figure 13–7.**

With the door panel off, peel back the paper or plastic water shield over the door. Pull slowly so you do not damage it. You now have access to the bolts and nuts securing the window regulator. See **Figure 13–8.**

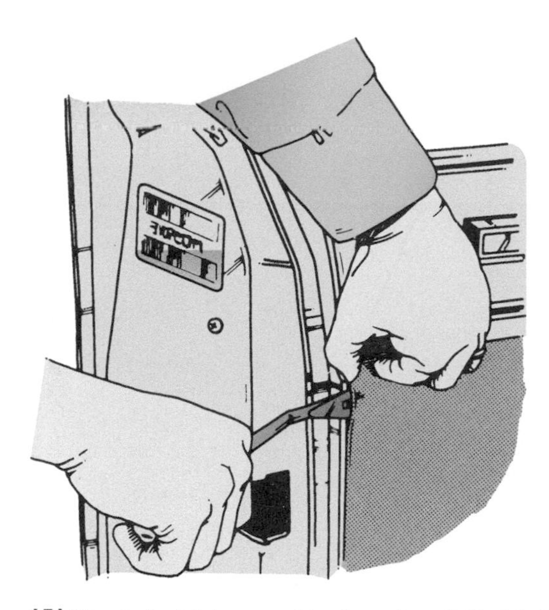

(A) The forked trim panel tool can be slid behind the inner door panel to pop out plastic clips without damage to the panel. Make sure the forked tool surrounds the plastic clip when prying.

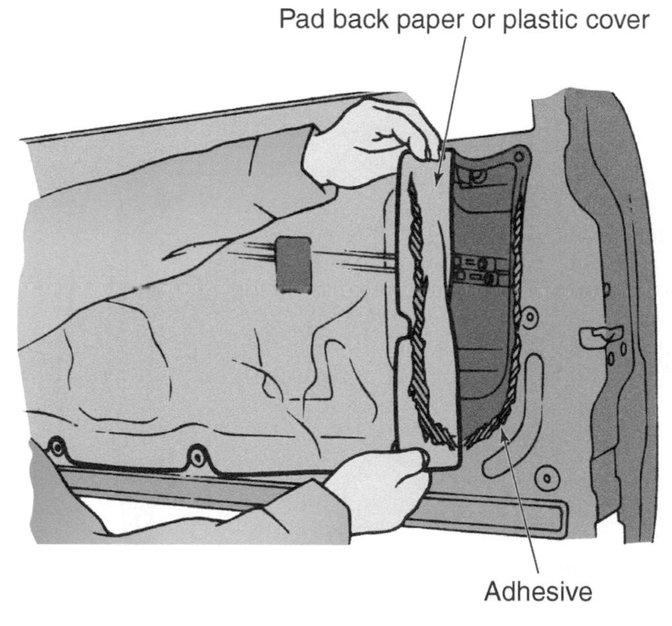

(B) To prevent tearing, slowly pull back the paper or plastic moisture shield behind the door panel. It must be reused.

Figure 13–7. Carefully remove clip inner door panel. (Courtesy of DaimlerChrysler Corporation)

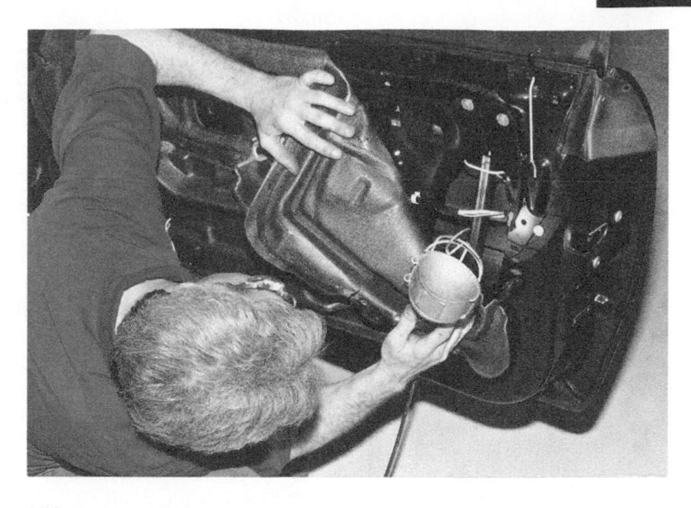

(A) A drop light is needed to see inside of the door.

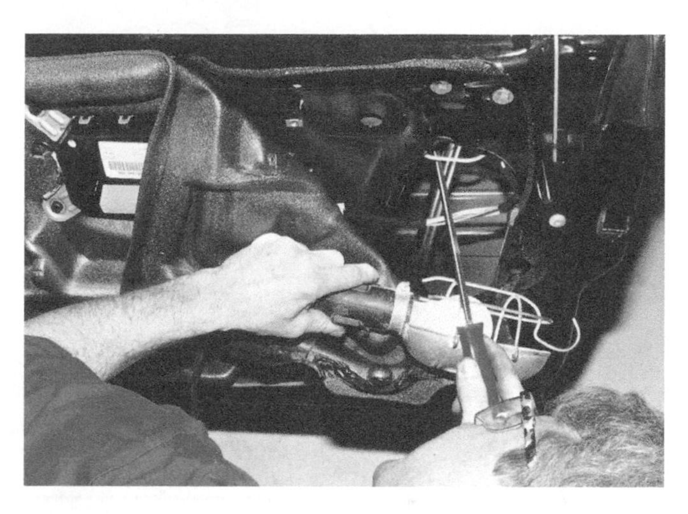

(B) Here a long screwdriver is being used to pop off the small spring clip that secures the door latch release rod.

Figure 13–8. Working inside a door can be challenging because of the restricted area.

When replacing a door inner trim panel, check that all plastic clips are fully in the panel. They can slide out of position and not align with the holes in the door. Bond the paper or plastic water shield back into place. Then feed any wires through the panel.

Fit the panel over the top lip on the door and down into position. Starting at one end, use your hand to pop each clip into the door. Lean down and check that each clip is started in its hole. Then use your hand to pop each clip into place. Install the other parts in reverse order of removal.

Window Glass and Regulator R and I, Adjustment

Small nuts and bolts or rivets secure the window regulator and glass guides or tracks in position. Usually, the glass bolts to the upper arms of the regulator. On a few older vehicles, the glass may be held on with special adhesive or epoxy.

To remove the glass, unbolt it from the regulator or drill out the rivets. You must then remove any parts that prevent you from sliding the glass out of the door. This can vary, so refer to the manual if needed. Look at **Figure 13–9.**

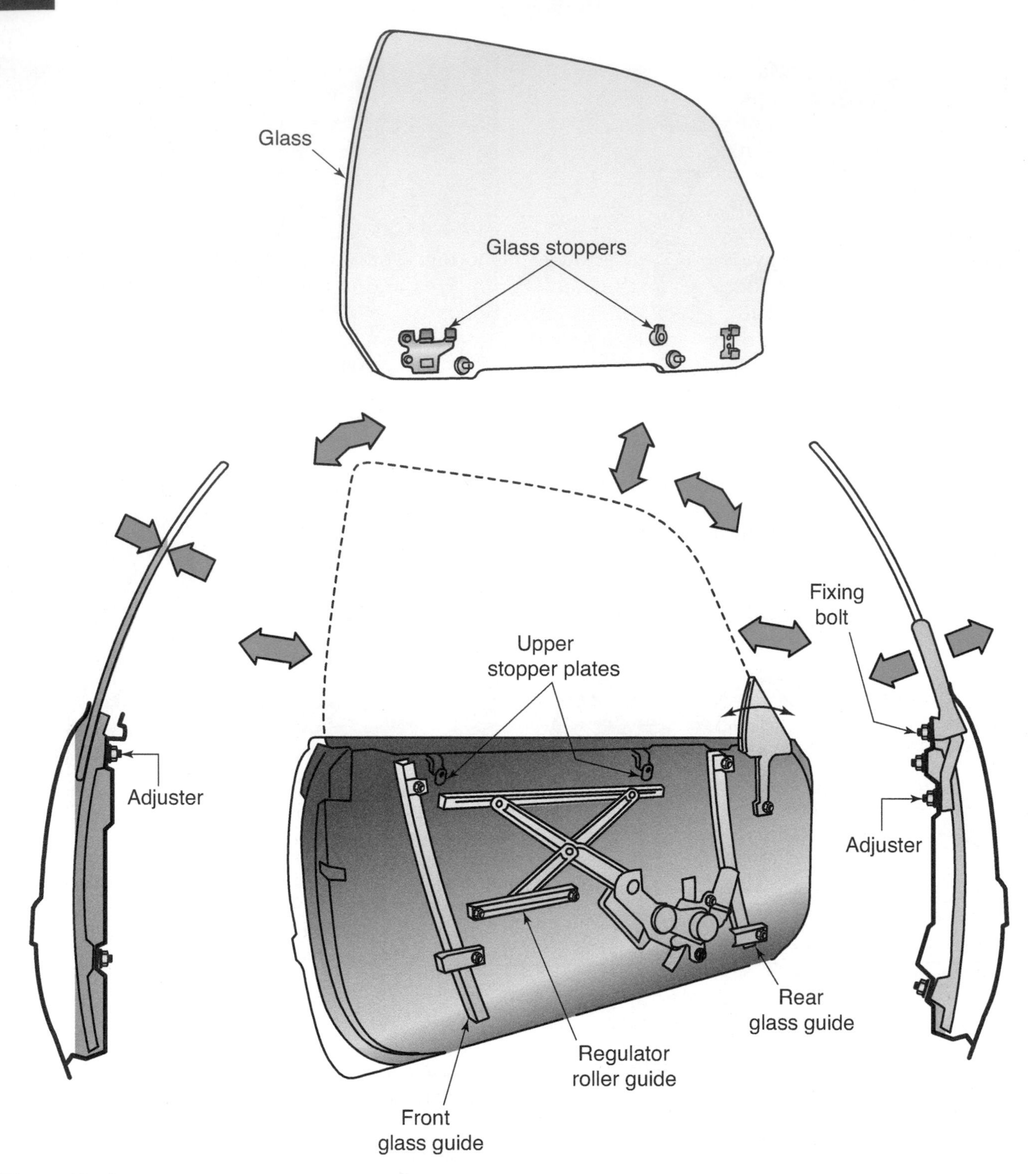

Figure 13–9. Study the internal part of a door. Note the adjustment points for window glass.

If the glass was broken, use a vacuum cleaner to remove all broken glass from inside the door. Install the new glass and bolt it to the regulator. Make sure you use all rubber, plastic, and metal washers.

! WARNING !

Do not slam the door before adjusting the glass. With a hardtop door, the glass can hit and break on the top of the door opening.

To adjust the glass and regulator, roll the window all the way up. Make sure it is centered in the frame or door opening. If necessary, loosen the regulator mounting fasteners. Shift the regulator and glass as needed. Turning the window crank one way or the other may help shift the regulator. When the glass is properly positioned, tighten the regulator fasteners.

Stops may also be provided to limit upward travel of the glass. Adjust the stops so they limit upward glass travel. Double-check the door glass adjustment with the door closed. Inspect where the glass contacts the inner door channel or weatherstripping. It must fully seal the door opening.

If needed, lubricate high friction points on the regulator. Lubricate the large gear and the arms where they rub together. The window glass should slide up and down easily without binding.

Door Lock and Latch R and R

Door lock assemblies usually consist of the outside door handle, linkage rods, the door lock mechanism, and the door latch. Various types of exterior door handles are available. With a push-button-type handle, the button contacts the lock lever on the latch to open the door. However, most exterior door handles operate through one or more rods.

Door handles can be replaced by raising the window and removing the interior trim, panel, and water shield to gain access to the inside of the door. Exterior door handles are often held on with screws or bolts. A short screwdriver or small, ¼-inch drive socket is often needed to remove an outside door handle.

Inside door lock mechanisms are generally the pull handle type. The mechanisms are connected to the lock by one or more lock cylinder rods. Clips or bushings are used to secure the rods in place.

The door lock mechanism usually mounts through a hole in the door. A spring clip often fits over the inside of the lock to hold it in place. An arm on the lock transfers motion through a rod to the door latch.

To remove the lock, place a drop light inside the door. While looking through one of the large openings in the inside of the door, pop off the small clip holding the lock rod. Then pry the clip off the lock. You can use a screwdriver or pliers depending upon the amount of space around the lock. Slide the lock and washer off the outside of the door.

Electric door locks often use electric solenoids to move the linkage to the door locks. When you turn the key or press a door lock button, current flows to the solenoids in the doors. The solenoids convert the electrical energy into motion. The solenoid motion moves the lock linkages and latches. This locks or unlocks the doors.

In **Figure 13–10,** note the solenoid-operated door lock mechanism.

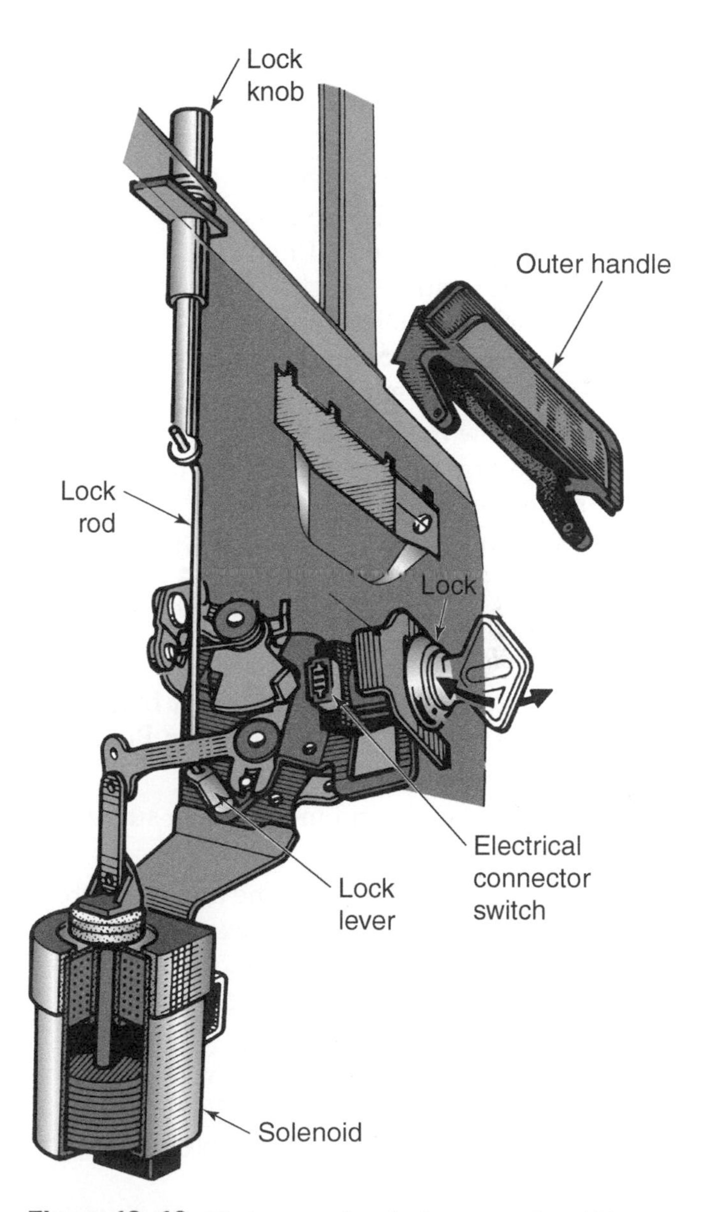

Figure 13–10. Most power door locks use a solenoid to move lock mechanisms and latches. The switch on the lock electrically energizes the solenoid. The solenoid then converts electrical energy into motion. (Courtesy of DaimlerChrysler Corporation)

Door Skin Replacement

Like other damaged panels, a door skin can be straightened or replaced. The decision is based on the amount of door frame damage.

The door skin wraps around—and is flanged around—the door frame. The door skin is secured to the frame either by welding or with adhesives. Typical replacement procedures are needed for both types of skins.

Replacing Welded Door Skins

A **welded door skin** has spot welds that hold the skin onto its frame. To replace a welded door skin, follow manufacturer recommended procedures and these basic steps:

1. Remove the trim panel and disconnect the negative side of the battery to isolate all power door accessories.
2. Before removing the door, check to see if the hinges are sprung. Check the alignment of the door with respect to its opening. If the door frame is bent, do not try to replace the door skin. Straighten the door frame or obtain a replacement door.
3. Inspect how the skin is fastened to the door. Determine how much interior hardware must be removed.
4. To prevent loss, place all removed parts and hardware inside the vehicle or in a parts tray.
5. If it only has minor damage, straighten and/or align the inner door frame.
6. Remove the door glass to prevent breakage or pitting while repairing the door. Place it inside the vehicle for protection.
7. Remove the door and move it to a suitable work area.
8. Apply tape to the door frame and measure the distance between the lower line of the tape and the edge of the skin. Also measure the distance between the edge of the skin and the door frame.
9. Remove the paint from the spot welds in the **skin hem** (folded door edge). Using a drill and spot weld cutter or hole saw, remove the spot welds.
10. Use a plasma arc cutter or grinder to remove the welded portion of the skin from the door frame.
11. Grind off the edge of the door skin hem flange, as illustrated in **Figure 13–11A.**

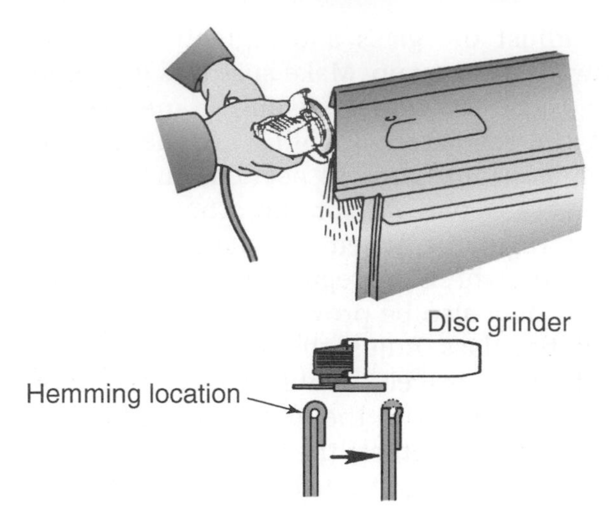

(A) Grind off the door skin hem flange as shown.

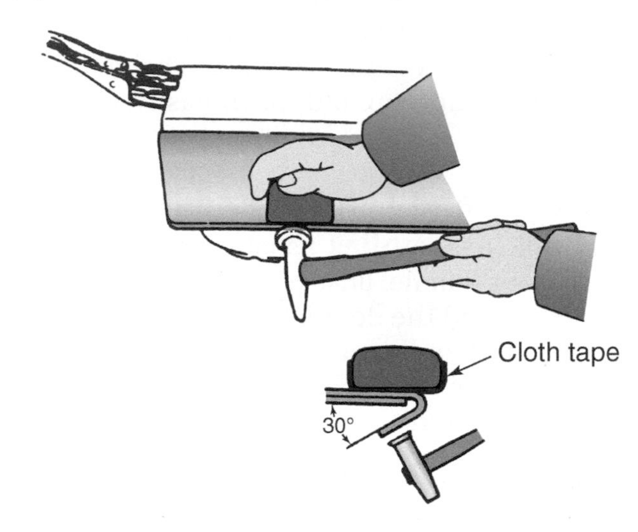

(B) Use a hammer and dolly to straighten and fit the hem flange.

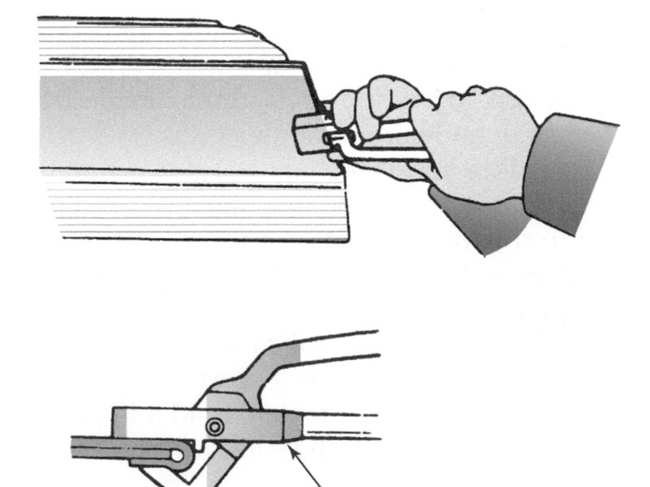

(C) Use flanging pliers to force the new door skin down over the door frame.

Figure 13–11. Follow the major steps for replacing a welded door skin.

Grind off just enough metal that the skin can be separated from the flange. Do not grind into the frame. Also, do not use a cutting torch or power chisel to separate the panels. The frame can be distorted or be accidentally cut.

12. Separate the reinforcing strip on the top of the skin, if applicable.
13. Using a hammer and chisel, start to separate the skin from the frame. Use a pair of tin snips to cut around any spot welds that could not be cut or ground out.
14. When the skin moves freely, remove it. Use clamping pliers to remove what remains of the hem flange. Any remaining spot welds, braze, and rust should be ground or blasted off.
15. With the skin removed, examine the frame for damage. Repair any remaining inner door damage at this time. If necessary, remove damage to the inner flange with a hammer and dolly.
16. Apply weld-through primer to bare metal mating surfaces. Cover other bare metal with an antirust primer or other rust protection material.
17. Prepare the new skin for installation. Using a drill or hole punch, make holes for plug welds. Remove the paint from the weld and braze locations with a sander. Apply weld-through primer to the bare metal mating surfaces.
18. Some door skins have a silencer pad that must be attached to the skin. To do this, clean the skin with alcohol, then heat it and the silencer pad with a heat lamp. Finally, glue the pad to the skin.
19. Apply body sealer to the back side of the new skin. Apply the sealer evenly, ⅜ inch (9 mm) from the flange, in a ⅛-inch (3 mm) bead.
20. Using clamping pliers, attach the new skin to the door and align it properly. Weld where required.
21. Use a hammer and dolly to flange the hem. See **Figure 13–11B.** Cover the dolly face with masking tape to avoid marring the skin. Bend the hem flange gradually in three steps. Be careful not to bend or throw the skin out of alignment.
22. After working the flange within 30 degrees of the frame, use a flanging tool to finish the hem flange, as shown in **Figure 13–11C.** Check alignment of the door in the opening.
23. Weld the plug or spot weld locations of the glass opening. Then tack weld the hem flange.
24. Drill holes into the new door skin to accommodate moldings, trim, and so forth. Make sure all edges are cut in prior to installing any parts.
25. Install all door parts. Prepare the door surfaces for refinishing.
26. Place the door on the vehicle. Align the door with the adjacent panels. Check for proper operation.

Sealing Door Seams

Remember that all joints and seams must be protected from rust. Use an appropriate seam sealer to keep water and contaminants out of the door and provide long-term protection.

Allow seam sealer to dry properly before painting. Drying time depends on the type of sealer, its thickness, and the temperature and humidity in the area. Normally, the lower the temperature, the longer the necessary dry time. Also, the higher the humidity, the longer the dry time.

Replacing Adhesive-Bonded Door Skins

An **adhesive-bonded door skin** is bonded, not welded, to the door frame. It requires different replacement methods:

1. After removing all hardware, trim material, and the glass, remove the door from the vehicle.
2. Use a grinder to grind the edge of the door. This will make it possible to safely separate and remove the damaged skin.
3. Peel off the remaining hem flange using a chisel.
4. Use sandpaper or a blaster to remove any rust from areas that are too tight for a grinder. Then sand or grind all areas where the door skin meets the door frame.
5. If necessary, straighten the door frame.
6. Thoroughly clean the edge of the door frame, inside and out, with a good adhesive cleaner.

7. Check the fit of the replacement door skin.
8. Prime both sides of the door frame with adhesive primer.
9. Cut the tip of the adhesive nozzle to provide a ⅛-inch (3 mm) bead of adhesive.
10. Apply the adhesive in a continuous bead. The adhesive can be applied to the inside of the door skin creases or to the door skin side of the door frame.
11. Carefully position the door skin on the frame.
12. Flange the door skin in the usual manner. Be sure to wipe away any excess adhesive along the flange. Check door alignment in the opening before the adhesive cures.
13. Seal the crimped seam with seam sealer.
14. To protect against rust, apply an antirust compound to the inside of the door.
15. Bond or tack weld the tabs at the top edge of the door skin. Use the method that best suits the design of the door. This step may not be needed on certain vehicle makes.
16. Paint and reassemble the door.

Replacing SMC (Composite) Door Skins

Sheet molded compound, or **SMC,** door skin panels are similar to fiberglass. Some doors are made completely of SMC, except for steel door intrusion beams and the steel lock and hinge reinforcements.

To replace an SMC door skin, proceed as follows:

1. Cut away the center of the skin. Air shears work well because cut depth is easily controlled. If you use a saw, be careful not to hit or cut internal door parts.
2. To remove the remaining door skin, heat the bonding areas with a heat gun. Then apply pressure with a prybar or chisel to remove the rest of the material. Be careful not to damage the door flange.
3. Sand the door frame flange to remove all remaining adhesive. Clean the bonding areas of the replacement skin with soap and water. Allow them to dry. Sand the bonding areas to expose the SMC fibers. Wipe dry with a clean cloth.
4. Apply a bead of two-part adhesive to the door frame flange, as shown in **Figure 13–12.**

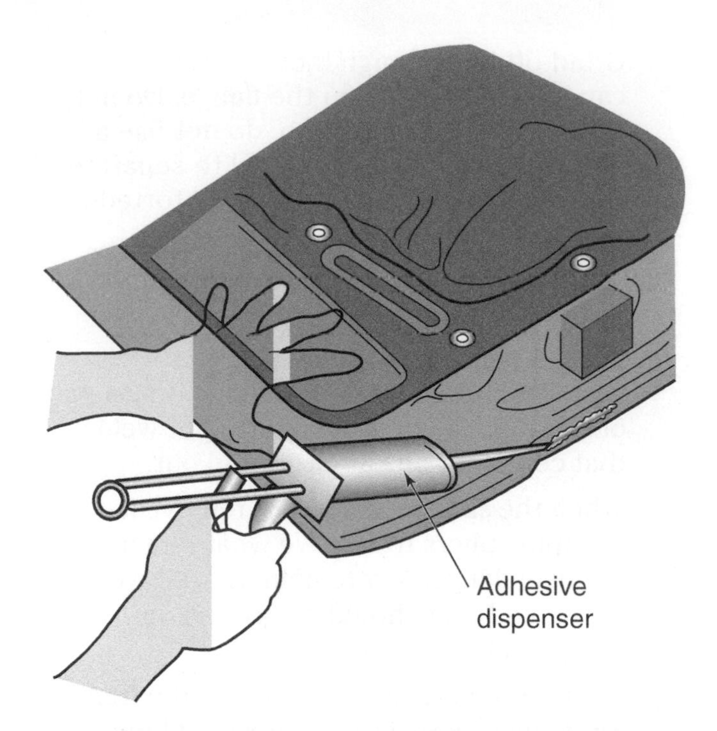

Figure 13–12. Installing an adhesive-bonded door skin is similar to installing a welded-on skin. However, you must use a special two-part adhesive to bond the skin onto the frame.

5. Set the skin on the door frame and lightly clamp it. Do not squeeze too tight. You want to leave adhesive between the skin and frame. Check door alignment in the opening before the adhesive cures.

To complete the job, allow the adhesive to cure, paint the door, and then reassemble and mount it on the vehicle.

Door Reinforcements

All the doors of unibody vehicles have inner metal reinforcements at various locations. There are some other door frame reinforcements, such as at the hinge locations and the door lock plate. Door intrusion beams are normally used inside side doors.

A **door intrusion beam** is welded or bolted to the metal support brackets on the door frame to increase door strength. Methods of strengthening doors are given in **Figure 13–13.**

GLASS

Vehicle glass allows the passengers clear visibility out of the passenger compartment and also protects them from wind, rain, and road debris. Glass is often broken during a collision and must be serviced. Passenger-side air bag deployment

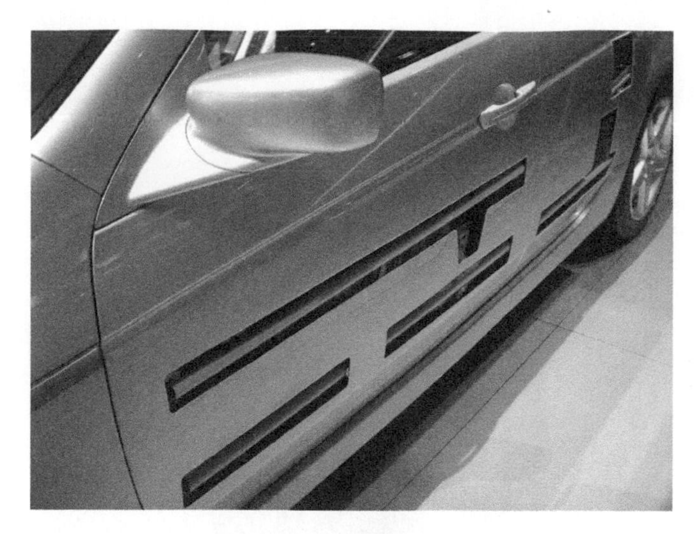

Figure 13–13. The cutaway shows intrusion beams behind the door skin to protect the driver and passengers from side impact or "T-bone" collision. Door intrusion beams are made of high-strength steel and should be replaced if bent or damaged.

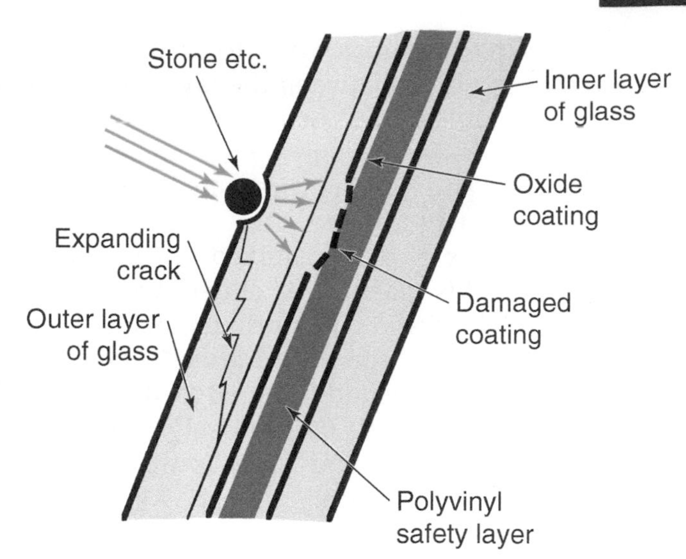

Figure 13–14. Study what happens when laminated glass is broken.

can break the windshield. Side air bag deployment can sometimes shatter door glass.

Windshields

Today's vehicles are built with a lot of glass that affords greater visibility for driving. Frequently, this glass is broken during a collision or by flying gravel or vandalism. Glass may also need to be removed from areas of damage before the damage can be straightened.

Glass also plays an important role in aerodynamics styling. Air drag is reduced by fitting the glass accurately to the sheet metal and eliminating trim. This approach reduces wind noise and provides a more sleek, uncluttered appearance.

Stationary glass panels in modern unibody vehicles also play an important role in the strength of the body structure. The stationary glass is an integral part of the upper body structure. It provides lateral bracing to help prevent roof collapse during a rollover. For this reason, when stationary glass is replaced, it must be installed in the same manner as it was by the manufacturer.

If the glass is installed incorrectly, you could be putting a vehicle back on the road that is not structurally sound. It is important for you to be familiar with the various techniques used to remove and install glass properly.

Types of Glass

For years, the glass used in most vehicles was either laminated or tempered. Both are considered safety glass because of their construction. Today, other types of glass are also found in vehicles.

Laminated plate glass consists of two thin sheets of glass with a layer of clear plastic between them. It is used for windshields. When this type of glass is broken, the plastic material will tend to hold the shattered pieces in place and prevent them from causing injury. See **Figure 13–14.**

Tempered glass is a single piece of heat-treated glass that shatters into small pieces when broken. However, it has more impact resistance than regular glass. It is used for side and rear window glass but never for windshields.

Both laminated and tempered glass can be tinted. **Tinted glass** contains a shaded vinyl material to filter out most of the sun's glare. This is helpful in reducing eye strain and prevents fading of the interior. Some windshields are shaded to reduce the sun's glare by means of a dark tinted band or section across the top. Tinted glass is usually recommended if the vehicle is to be equipped with air conditioning.

Glass can also be tinted by adding small quantities of metal powder to the other normal ingredients of glass to give it a particular color.

Glass can also be fitted with a defrosting circuit or antenna. **Self-defrosting glass** has a conducting grid or invisible layer that carries electric current to heat the glass. A grid type is common in rear windows. Windshields use a transparent conducting medium.

A **window antenna wire** for radio reception is placed either between the layers of laminated glass (windshield) or printed on the surface of the glass (rear window). Some glass has antenna wires and heating wires side by side.

Anti-lacerative glass has one or more additional layers of plastic affixed to the inside of the glass. This glass gives added protection against shattering and cuts during impact.

Modular or **encapsulated glass** has a plastic trim molding attached to its edge. It also fits the contours of a vehicle more closely than glass used in the past. Modular glass is the newest glass used in unibody applications.

Windshield Service

Replacement of the windshield involves two different methods: gasket installation or adhesive installation. The adhesive installation is further divided into two methods: the full cutout and the partial cutout method.

WARNING

When replacing glass, be aware of the following:

1. If you fail to restore the original structural integrity of a vehicle during repair, it could be violating federal law.
2. Butyl tape alone CANNOT be used to completely replace urethane, because it has no structural bonding properties. It only holds the windshield in place and prevents leaks. NEVER use butyl tape ALONE to install a windshield.

A **windshield gasket** is a rubber molding shaped to fit the windshield, body, and trim. The gasket installation method is common in older vehicles but still finds use in present day vehicles. The gasket is grooved to accept the glass, a sheet metal flange, and sometimes the exterior reveal molding. See **Figure 13–15A.** The gasket locking strip must be removed before the glass can be removed from the opening.

The **adhesive installation,** as the name implies, uses an adhesive material to secure the glass in place. See **Figure 13–15B.** The use of adhesives permits the windshield to be mounted flush with the roof panel, decreasing wind drag and noise. Rubber stops and spacers separate the glass from the metal.

Reveal molding is metal or plastic trim that fits around the vehicle's glass to cover the gap between the body and any glass adhesive. Depending upon the molding design, it can be held in place with small clips, adhesive, or a friction fit.

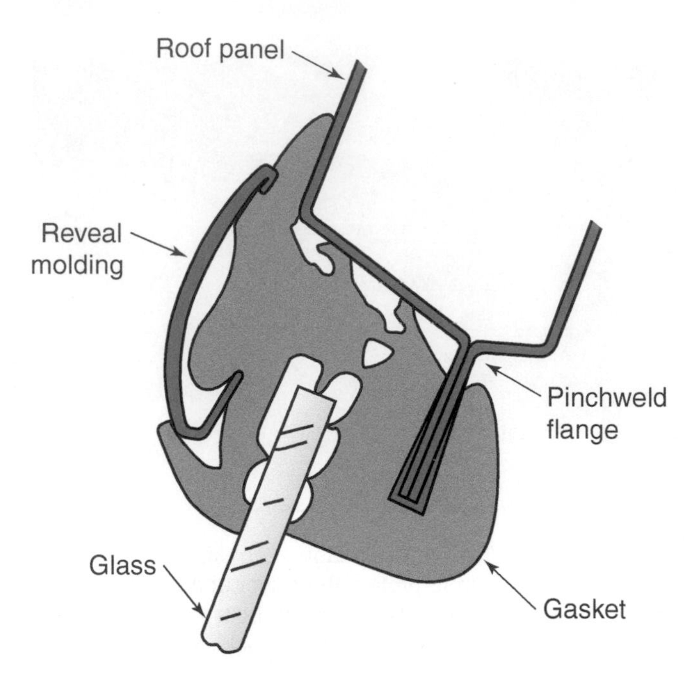

(A) The rubber gasket is shaped to fit around the glass and the body structure. Note this cross section of a windshield gasket.

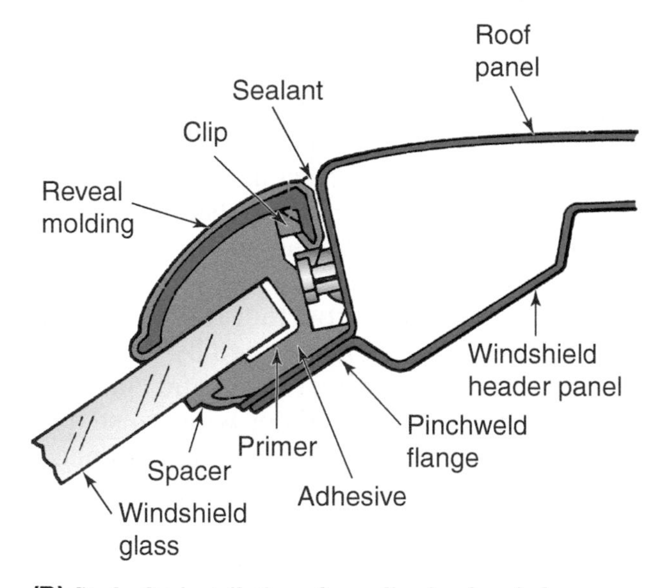

(B) Study the installation of an adhesive-bonded windshield. Metal or plastic trim covers the edge of the glass and adhesive. Note this cross section of an adhesive-bonded windshield.

Figure 13–15. Some windshields are held in place with a gasket or rubber seal; others use an adhesive material.

The **partial cutout method** of windshield replacement uses some of the original adhesive. The old adhesive must be in good condition and of sufficient thickness. It serves as a base for the new adhesive.

When the original adhesive is defective or requires complete removal, the **full cutout method** of windshield replacement is used.

Broken Glass

It is important to clean up pieces of broken glass from the seats, carpet, and air ducts before returning the vehicle to the customer. Vacuum the interior and blow out around the glass mounting area and vent ducts. Vacuum up as much glass as possible. Then, blow out glass from the heater and behind the dashboard with low pressure compressed air.

DANGER

If you fail to clean up broken glass properly, someone could be cut and injured. Also, if you fail to clean out dash ducts, glass can blow into people's eyes when the heater or A/C blower is turned on. Wear gloves and a full face shield!

Windshield Gasket Method

Before removing the windshield, remove the interior and exterior moldings. Any garnish moldings on the interior face of the windshield are secured in place by screws or retaining clips. All of the garnish moldings should be removed first. If necessary, the rearview mirror should be removed as well.

WARNING

The instructions in this text are for general purposes. Always refer to the service manual for the exact make and model vehicle. It will give the detailed instructions and specifications needed.

On the exterior of the vehicle, remove the reveal moldings. The reveal molding is usually secured by retaining clips attached to the body opening. A projection on the clip engages the flange on the reveal molding.

To replace a windshield using a gasket, proceed as follows:

1. Place protective covers over adjacent panels. Put on safety glasses and gloves.
2. Be sure all moldings, trim, and hardware are removed. Remove the windshield wiper arms.
3. If the glass has a built-in antenna wire, disconnect the antenna leads. The wires are usually at the lower center of the windshield. Tape the leads to the glass.
4. Locate the locking strip on the outside of the gasket. Pry up the tab and remove the locking strip to open the gasket all the way around the windshield.
5. Use a putty knife to pry the gasket away from the pinchweld inside and outside of the vehicle.
6. With an assistant in the passenger compartment, push the windshield and gasket out of the body opening. If the glass was not cracked and is to be reused, exert even pressure on the glass so it will not break.
7. Clean the windshield opening with solvent to remove any dirt or residual sealer.
8. Place the glass on a cloth-covered bench or table to protect it. If the glass was removed for body repairs, leave the gasket intact.
9. If the glass was removed because it was broken, remove the gasket from the glass. Install the gasket on the replacement glass.
10. Cracks that develop in the outer edge of the glass are sometimes caused by low or high spots or poor spot welds in the pinchweld flange. Examine the body pinchweld and correct any problems.
11. Install setting blocks and spacers.
12. Carefully install the glass on the blocks to verify fit. Center the windshield. Check the gap between the glass and the pinchweld. The gap should be uniform around the entire pinchweld.
13. After the windshield is lined up, apply several strips of masking tape. Apply the tape from the glass to the vehicle body.
14. Slit each piece of tape at the end of the glass. Then lift the new windshield out and set it aside. To permanently install the

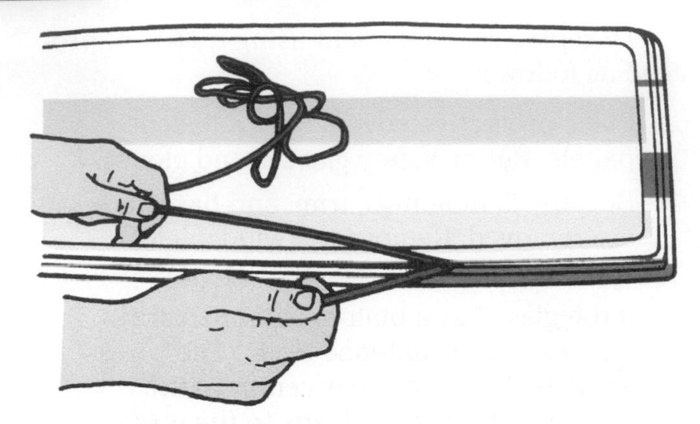

Figure 13–16. When installing windshield with a large rubber gasket, install a piece of cloth cord inside the gasket. Then, when you pull the cord, it will force the edge of the rubber gasket over the lip of the body.

windshield, you will line up the tape on the body with the tape on the glass.

15. Insert a cloth cord in the pinchweld groove of the gasket. Start at the top of the glass so the cord ends meet in the lower center of the glass. Tape the ends of the cord to the inside of the glass. See **Figure 13–16.**
16. Squirt a soapy solution in the pinchweld groove for easier installation.
17. Apply waterproof sealer to the base of the gasket.
18. With an assistant, install the glass and gasket assembly in the body opening. Use your masking tape to align the glass. Slip the bottom groove over the pinchweld.
19. Slowly pull the cord ends so that the gasket slips over the pinchweld flange. Work the bottom section of the glass in first, then the sides, and finally the top. The glass might crack if the cord is pulled from only one end.
20. Dispense a small bead of waterproof sealer around the body side of the gasket.
21. Remove excess sealer with solvent.
22. Install the reveal and garnish moldings.
23. Check the windshield for water leaks using a low-pressure stream of water.
24. Place a soapy solution in the locking strip groove. Replace the locking strip by spreading the groove. Feed the strip into the opening. The soapy solution lubricates the groove and makes it easier to slide the strip through.

Windshield Full Cutout Method

When using the full cutout method, first remove the windshield according to the following procedure:

1. Protect both the interior and the exterior of the vehicle from damage. Cover the front seat and instrument panel. Also cover the painted surfaces next to the windshield area.
2. Remove the rearview mirror. Take off the wipers, antenna, moldings, and any other parts that might get in the way. Remove the cowl vent panel if it makes it easier to reach around the edge of the windshield.
3. Using a hook tool, lift the molding at the bottom of the windshield. Once it can be securely grasped, pull it out from around the windshield. Do this carefully so the molding is not damaged.
4. With a utility knife, score the exposed urethane all the way around the outside of the windshield. Cut as close to the glass as you can. This makes it easier to insert the vibrating power knife.
5. Using a power knife, cut through the adhesive next to the glass. Cut as close to the glass as possible.

   Pneumatic windshield cutters use shop air pressure and a vibrating action to help cut the adhesive around glass. They have a variety of blade designs available for use on different windshields. Many have blades with depth stops to prevent pinchweld damage. With some designs, you may have to use two or more blades to remove some windshields.

   Electric adhesive cutters use either 12- or 120-volt power supplies to produce a vibrating action to assist in cutting the adhesive around glass. They operate similar to pneumatic windshield cutters. Some power cutters are used on the outside of the vehicle. Others are designed to be used from inside the passenger compartment. See **Figure 13–17.**

   Piano wire (fine steel wire) can also be used to cut the adhesive. Use a 3- to 4-foot length of the lightest gauge wire that can be purchased. The cutting procedure with piano wire is a two-person job. After pushing the wire through to the interior, you and

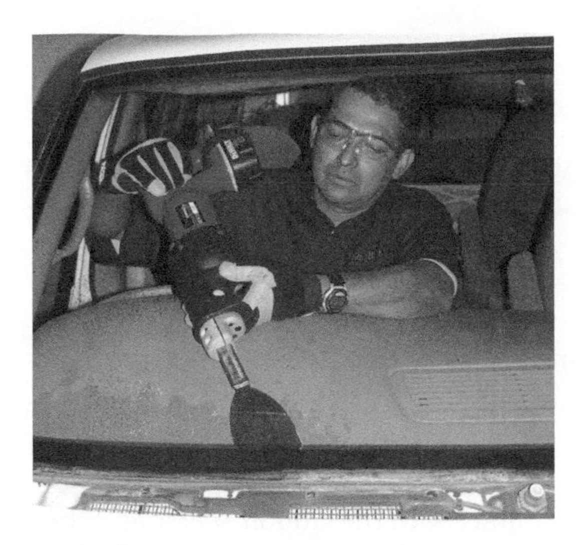

Figure 13–17. Here the technician is using a power knife to cut out the adhesive for windshield removal. (Courtesy of Equalizer Industries)

your helper must pull the wire around the windshield to cut the windshield free.

When removing a piece of modular or encapsulated glass, especially one that is undamaged, most auto-makers recommend using the vibrating power knife to remove the glass instead of piano wire.

6. Carefully lift out the glass.

To prepare for the installation of the windshield, proceed in the following manner:

1. Cut out the remaining urethane adhesive from the pinchweld with a razor knife. Be careful not to cut or damage the headliner. Make sure no loose pieces of old adhesive are left. If the windshield had been replaced before with butyl tape or other unknown materials, it is especially important to remove this material thoroughly.
2. Check for corrosion in the pinchweld area. If there is corrosion, remove it with a wire brush, then sand if needed. Use a grit recommended by the adhesive manufacturer.
3. Dry set the new windshield. Check for at least ¼ inch (6 mm) of clearance around the windshield. Adjust the setting blocks as needed to get proper alignment. After the windshield is lined up, apply several strips of masking tape. Bridge from the windshield to the body. See **Figure 13–18.**
4. Slit the pieces of tape at the edge of the glass. Lift the windshield out and set it aside. When you set the new windshield on the adhesive, line up the tape on the vehicle with the tape on the windshield to get it positioned.

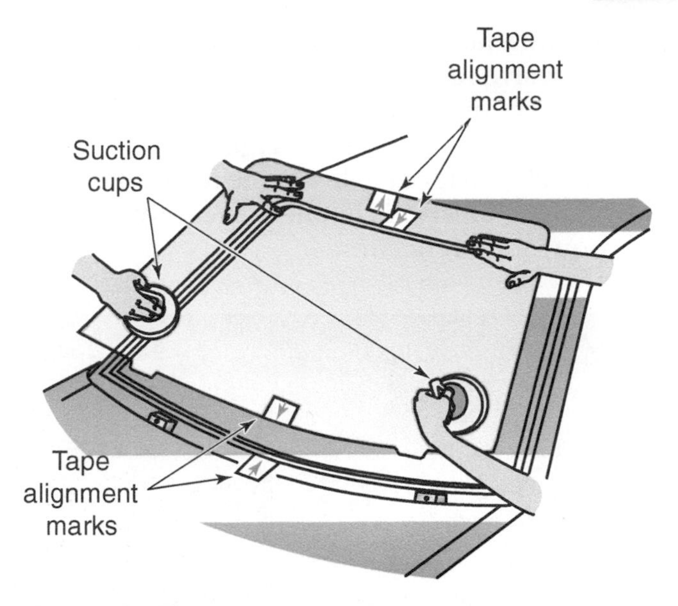

Figure 13–18. Ask someone to help when you are lowering a window straight down onto the adhesive bead. Suction cups will help hold the glass.

5. Use a urethane adhesive cleaner on a lint-free dry cloth to wipe the pinchweld area. This removes any loose urethane. Let the cleaner dry.
6. Use a urethane primer in the pinchweld area. Do not use a liquid butyl primer or a ribbon sealer primer. Apply the primer to all bare metal in the pinchweld area.
7. Clean the windshield edge with a recommended solvent. Wipe dry with a clean, lint-free cloth.
8. Place a ½-inch (12 mm) coat of urethane primer on the inside contact surface of the windshield. Apply it all the way around. Let it dry for the required time.
9. Install square ribbon sealer to the inside edge of the pinchweld. For shallow pinchwelds, use 5⁄16 × 5⁄16 inch (8 × 8 mm). For deeper pinchwelds, use ⅜ × ⅛ inch (9 × 9 mm). Square ribbon sealer provides better support than round sealer. It also does not squeeze into the space needed for the urethane.

WARNING

Using an adhesive other than urethane can result in the shop and you being held liable. If the vehicle is involved in another collision and the glass reacts differently than the original installation, you and the shop could be sued.

10. Apply a fast-curing, high-strength urethane adhesive following the manufacturer's instructions. Apply it directly behind the pinchweld, as shown in **Figure 13–19.** Hold the dispenser at a 45-degree angle. If too much adhesive is applied, excessive squeeze-out occurs.

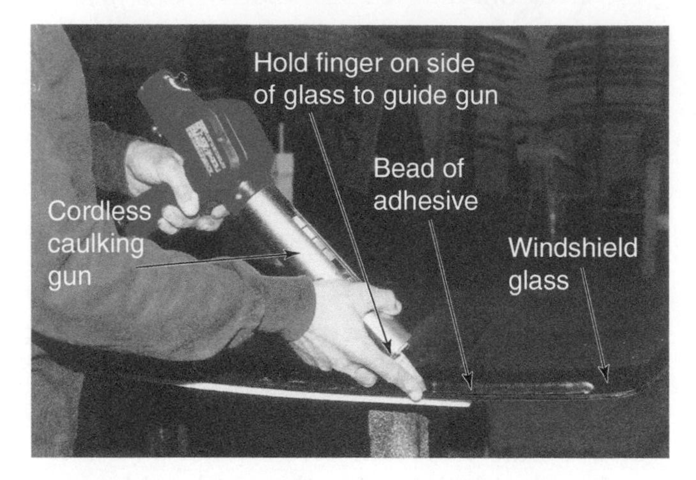

(A) The technician is using a dispenser to apply a continuous bead of adhesive to the flange of the windshield.

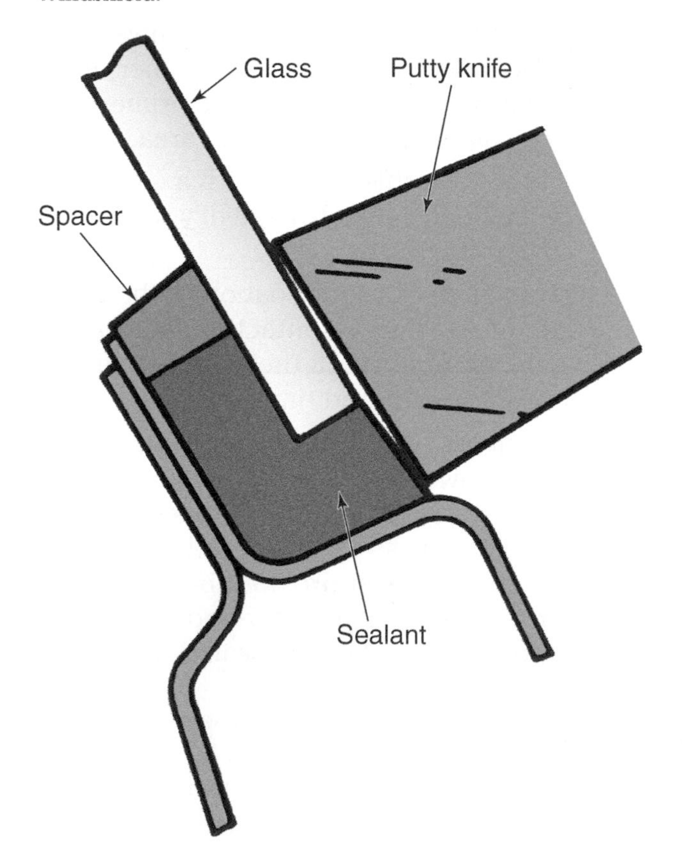

(B) Use a plastic spreader or putty knife to level off and remove excess adhesive.

Figure 13–19. Apply adhesive slowly in a uniform bead of the recommended size.

! WARNING !

The adhesive must be strong enough to deflect a top-mounted air bag without allowing the windshield to be blown out.

The final step is to install the windshield. This is done as follows:

1. Set the windshield into place. Line up the pieces of masking tape on the glass and body. Press firmly so the glass makes contact with the ribbon sealer and the urethane adhesive.
2. Look for squeeze-out along the edge of the windshield. Use a paddle to spread it evenly. Smooth the surface and remove any excess adhesive. Fill all spaces between the glass and the metal.
   Remember! At least ¼ inch (6 mm) of the windshield surface must be bonded to the vehicle body.
3. Install the moldings. Clean up the area with a liquid adhesive cleaner.
4. Attach the cowl vent panel, wiper, antenna, and other parts.

The ribbon sealer will hold the windshield in place while the urethane adhesive cures. The urethane adhesive will reach its maximum strength in 4 or 5 days. Follow the manufacturer's recommendations for curing times. Curing times are affected by temperature and humidity.

Partial Cutout Method

The partial cutout method is recommended only under ideal curing conditions. Most of the steps are the same as in the full cutout method. One difference is that it is not necessary to remove all the old adhesive. The old adhesive left on the pinchweld serves as the base for the new adhesive.

Other Glass R and I

The removal and installation of rear and many stationary side windows follow the above methods closely. Procedures vary slightly for different vehicle makes. However, many of the operations are similar.

When working on small side windows, use duct or masking tape to secure the window while working. When inside the passenger compartment

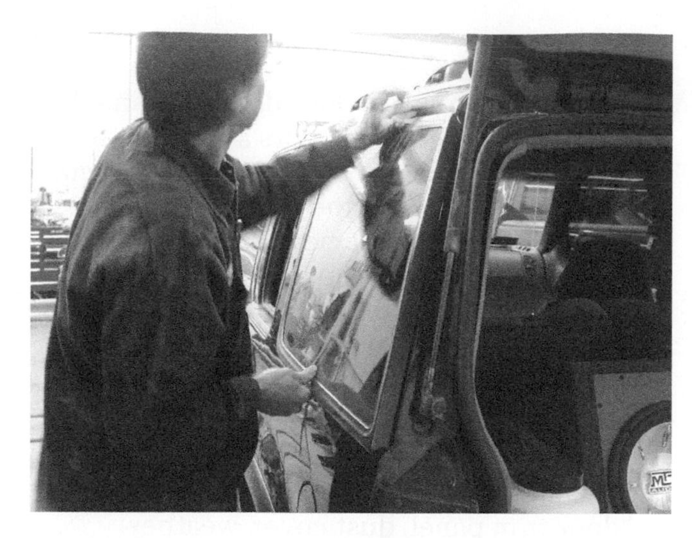

Figure 13–20. Service of stationary side glass is very similar to methods just discussed. Here the technician is fitting rear glass back into the opening. Adhesive and small screws secure the glass to the vehicle.

working, it is easy for the glass to fall out and break on the shop floor. See **Figure 13–20.**

AIR AND WATER LEAKS

Air leaks will result in a complaint of wind noise in the passenger compartment. They often result from improperly adjusted doors, window glass, or damaged weatherstripping.

Water leaks will result in a complaint of water leaking into the passenger compartment or trunk. The most common causes of water leaks are poor seal around the windshield, window glass, sun roof, doors, or lids.

Improper door adjustment is the most common cause for both air and water leaks. The doors must provide a good seal between the weatherstripping and the body openings. The weatherstripping should be compressed sufficiently in the opening to prevent water, dust, and drafts from entering the vehicle. Door hinges wear and allow the doors to drop down, out of alignment.

To find body leaks, you can use several methods:

To conduct a **water hose test,** have someone squirt water onto the possible leakage areas while you watch for leaks inside the vehicle. Direct the water to flow over gaps in parts that might be leaking. Dripping water will result around any gap or leak in parts.

To conduct an **air hose leak test,** place a soapy water solution on possible leakage points and use low pressure air on the inside of the vehicle. When you find a leak, bubble will form in the soapy water.

An **air leak tape test** involves covering potential leaks with masking tape and driving the vehicle. If covering an area stops wind noise, you have found the air leak.

An **electronic leak detector** uses a signal generator tool and signal detector tool to find leaks. One person sits in the vehicle with the detector. Another person moves the generator tool around possible leakage points. The detector will make an audible "beep" if the signal passes through a body opening. This shows you the location of leakage points.

After finding the leak, you must adjust the door or lid, replace the weatherstripping, or seal the glass to fix the leak. You must use common sense and the procedures given in this and other chapters to stop the air or water leakage.

REARVIEW MIRROR SERVICE

Both exterior and interior rearview mirrors require repair or replacement after collision damage. See **Figure 13–21.**

External rearview mirrors normally bolt to the outside of the driver and passenger doors. Screws on the outside or inside of the door secure the mirrors. A gasket normally fits between the mirror and door surface. See **Figure 13–22.**

If only the mirror is broken on external mirrors, you can sometimes replace the mirror glass. Heat the mirror with a heat gun to soften the adhesive. Then pry off the broken pieces of mirror. Bond the new mirror into its housing with an approved adhesive.

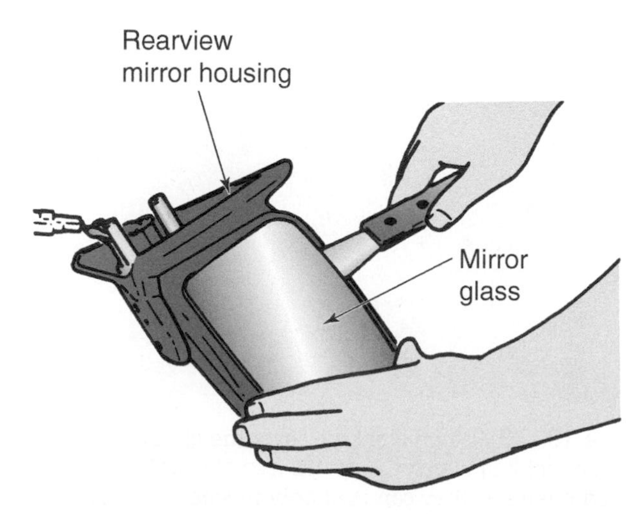

Figure 13–21. Pry off the old mirror.

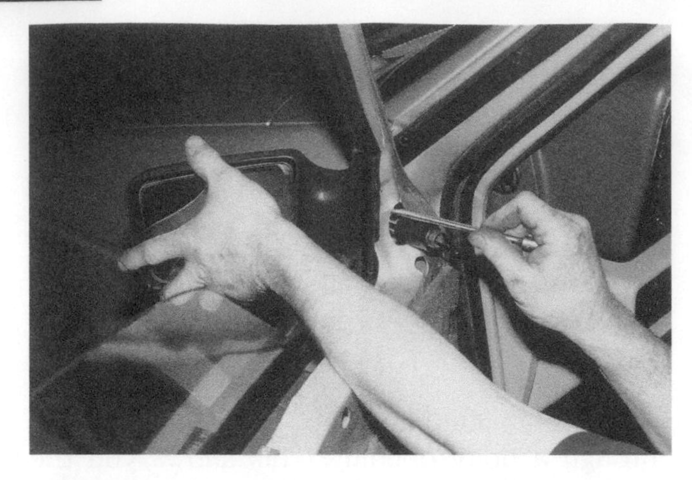

Figure 13–22. Here the technician is using a long extension and ¼-inch drive socket to remount the outside rearview mirror.

Some interior rearview mirrors attach to the windshield with a special adhesive. You must clean the glass with a recommended cleaner. Spray on a clear primer agent. Then, apply a small bead of adhesive. Hold the mirror mounting pad stationary on the windshield for a few minutes until the adhesive cures.

PROTECT GLASS WHEN WELDING

Glass can be pitted and easily damaged when welding and grinding. If hot bits of molten metal fall on the glass, they will burn small pits into the glass. This is an expensive, time-consuming mistake. Always cover all glass with a welding blanket or remove the glass when welding or grinding, as shown in **Figure 13–23.**

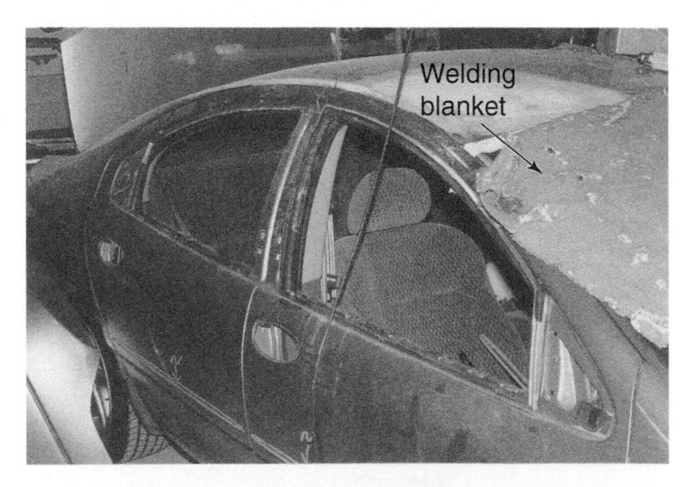

Figure 13–23. When welding, cover the glass and protect it with a welding blanket. If sparks from the welding bead land on the glass, they can melt or burn small indentations in the glass, requiring glass replacement.

SUMMARY

- There are two basic door designs: framed and hardtop. Framed doors surround the sides and top of the door glass with a metal frame, helping keep the window glass aligned. The door frame seals against the door opening. Hardtop doors have the glass extending up out of the door without a frame around it. The glass itself must seal against the weatherstripping in the door opening.
- The basic parts of a door include the door frame, door skin, door glass, door glass channel, regulator, door latch, handles, door trim panel, dust cover, weatherstripping, and rearview mirror.
- Air leaks will result from improperly adjusted doors, window glass, or damaged weatherstripping. The most common causes of water leaks are poor seal around the windshield, window glass, sun roof, doors, or lids.

TECHNICAL TERMS

framed doors
hardtop doors
door frame
door skin
door glass channel
door regulator
door latch
door striker
door trim panel
door dust cover
door weatherstripping
forked trim tool
door lock assemblies
welded door skin
skin hem
adhesive-bonded door skin
sheet molded compound
SMC
door intrusion beam
laminated plate glass
tempered glass
tinted glass
self-defrosting glass
window antenna wire
anti-lacerative glass
modular glass
encapsulated glass
windshield gasket
adhesive installation
reveal molding
partial cutout method
full cutout method
pneumatic windshield cutters
electric adhesive cutters
piano wire
air leaks
water leaks
water hose test
air hose leak test
air leak tape test
electronic leak detector

REVIEW QUESTIONS

1. ______________ are the most used—and abused—parts of a vehicle.
2. Explain the difference between a frame door and a hardtop door.
3. List and describe the 11 major parts of a door.
4. The driver's door is sagging badly and will not close easily. *Technician A* says to check for worn hinges. *Technician B* says to loosen and adjust the hinges. Who is correct?
   a. Technician A
   b. Technician B
   c. Both Technicians A and B
   d. Neither Technician
5. This should be used when removing interior door trim panels.
   a. Pneumatic knife
   b. Electric knife
   c. Forked tool
   d. Slide hammer
6. What can happen if you slam a hardtop door after adjusting a door?
7. This can cause exterior door handle problems.
   a. Worn bushings
   b. Bent or incorrectly adjusted lock cylinder rods
   c. No lubrication on handle, linkage, or latch
   d. All of the above
   e. None of the above
8. Summarize the five major steps in replacing an SMC door skin.
9. This type of glass shatters into tiny pieces when broken.
   a. Laminated glass
   b. Tempered glass
   c. Modular glass
   d. Encapsulated glass
10. What is the difference between the partial and full cutout methods of windshield replacement?

ASE-STYLE REVIEW QUESTIONS

1. *Technician A* says to adjust the door in its opening and then the striker. *Technician B* says to adjust the striker first to make sure it engages the latch. Who is correct?
   a. Technician A
   b. Technician B
   c. Both Technicians A and B
   d. Neither Technician
2. When adjusting the doors on a four-door vehicle, which of the following should be adjusted first?
   a. Front fenders
   b. Front doors
   c. Rear doors
   d. Strikers
3. *Technician A* says that door strikers never need adjustment. *Technician B* says that on some vehicles, a special wrench must be used to loosen and tighten the hinge bolts. Who is correct?
   a. Technician A
   b. Technician B
   c. Both Technicians A and B
   d. Neither Technician
4. A door on a two-door hardtop has been centered in its opening. However, the door still moves down slightly when the striker engages the latch. Which of the following should be done?
   a. Readjust door
   b. Move door hinges up
   c. Move striker down
   d. Move striker up
5. A door is going to be removed for outer skin replacement. The door frame is not damaged. Which of the following tasks should NOT be done?
   a. Remove hinge bolts
   b. Place jack under door
   c. Remove striker
   d. Mark hinges

6. *Technician A* says that you cannot adjust a door with welded door hinges. *Technician B* says that you can spring or bend the hinge mounts to adjust welded hinges. Who is correct?

a. Technician A

b. Technician B

c. Both Technicians A and B

d. Neither Technician

7. Which of the following is used to hold most door locks in doors?

a. Adhesive

b. Bolts

c. Nuts

d. Spring clips

8. A door on a vehicle is centered in its opening but the bottom is sticking out farther than the fender and rocker panel. *Technician A* says to move the upper hinge inward. *Technician B* says to move the lower hinge inward. Who is correct?

a. Technician A

b. Technician B

c. Both Technicians A and B

d. Neither Technician

9. A vehicle has an air leak somewhere around the rear door. *Technician A* says to cover the areas of potential leakage with masking tape to help locate the air leak. *Technician B* says to have an assistant use an electronic air leak detector around the back door. Who is correct?

a. Technician A

b. Technician B

c. Both Technicians A and B

d. Neither Technician

10. *Technician A* says to remove door glass during door skin replacement to gain access to the regulator. *Technician B* says that door glass removal is seldom needed during welded door skin replacement. Who is correct?

a. Technician A

b. Technician B

c. Both Technicians A and B

d. Neither Technician

ACTIVITIES

1. Inspect a vehicle to check for proper alignment of doors and lids. Can you find any misaligned parts? Compare the alignment of doors and panels on different vehicles. Write a summary or make a large poster of your findings.

2. After getting permission from your instructor, use service manual/textbook procedures to correctly remove, install, and adjust a hood latch.

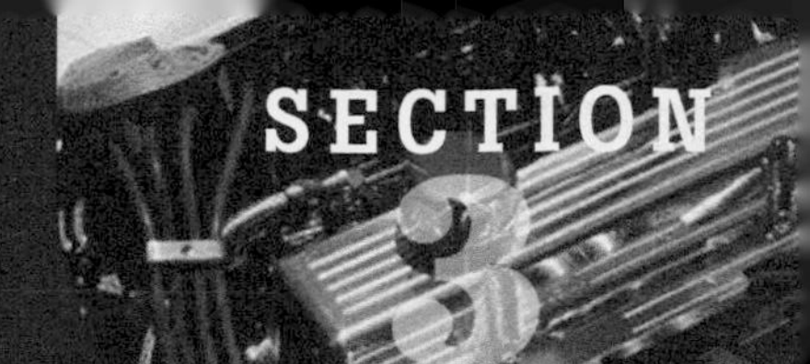

CHAPTER 14 Vehicle Surface Preparation

OBJECTIVES

After studying this chapter, you should be able to:

- Prepare a vehicle for painting/refinishing.
- Properly clean a vehicle using soap, water, air pressure, and a wax-grease remover.
- Evaluate the condition of the vehicle's paint.
- Describe methods for removing the damaged paint if needed.
- Properly prepare and treat bare metal surfaces.
- Correctly sand and featheredge surfaces.
- Apply an undercoat.
- Mask a vehicle properly.

INTRODUCTION

Vehicle preparation involves all of the final steps prior to painting/refinishing, including cleaning, sanding, stripping, masking, priming, and other related tasks.

Keep in mind that it is foolish to apply any kind of finish to a surface that is NOT properly prepared. The paint work will look bad or not hold up. Thorough vehicle preparation pays off in material savings, job quality, and customer satisfaction.

As you will learn, even if the original finish is in good condition, it should be lightly sanded or scuffed after washing to remove "dead film" and to block or smooth out small imperfections. If the paint surface is in poor condition, the paint should be removed down to the bare metal. In this way, a good foundation for the new finish is achieved.

VEHICLE CLEANING

Initial washing involves a complete cleaning of the vehicle to remove mud, dirt, and other foreign matter. Washing should be done before bringing the vehicle into the shop. This will prevent road debris from entering the shop area. Look at **Figure 14–1.**

Wet the whole vehicle with a water hose. Concentrate water flow onto trim pieces, around windows, and other areas that can trap and hold debris. Dirt also collects in door jambs, around the trunk and hood openings, and in wheel wells.

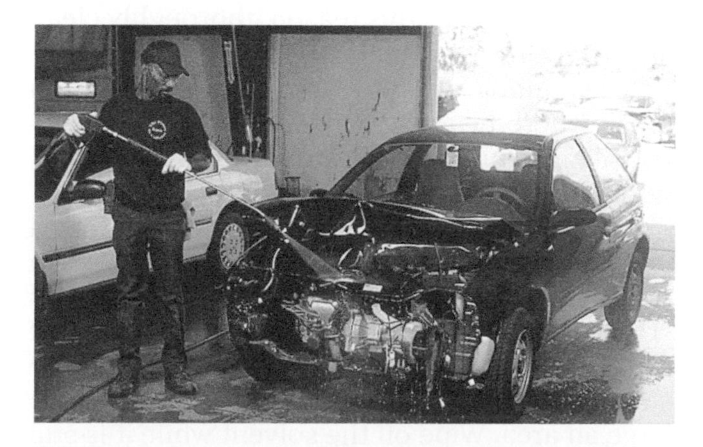

Figure 14–1. Thoroughly wash the vehicle with soap and water before starting work. All dirt and debris must be removed before starting repairs. Some shops also like to use a pressure washer, as shown.

WARNING

Failure to remove foreign matter from the vehicle can allow it to blow or fall into the wet paint when spraying. This avoidable problem is very frustrating and a waste of time!

Scrub all surfaces thoroughly with a detergent and water. A sponge works well. Wash the top first, then the front, rear, and sides. Rinse the vehicle thoroughly and let it dry completely. Remember that all adjacent panels must be as clean as the area to be refinished.

DANGER

Never use gasoline as a cleaning solvent. A tremendous fire could result. Gasoline is also a poor wax-removing solvent and can itself deposit contaminating substances on the surface.

WARNING

Do NOT use paint reducers for cleaning. They can be absorbed into the paint film. Blistering or lifting of the new paint can result.

Using Wax and Grease Remover

Paint or other finish will NOT adhere to a waxy or oily surface. For this reason, thoroughly clean all surfaces to be painted with a wax and grease or prepainting cleaning agent. Concentrate on areas where heavy wax buildup can be a problem. This would include around trim, moldings, door handles, and radio antennae.

To apply a prepaint surface cleaner, fold a clean, dry cloth. Soak it with the solvent. Then clean the painted surface. While the surface is still wet, fold a second clean cloth and dry off the wet solvent. Work small areas and wet the surface liberally. Never attempt to clean too large an area. Wipe off the solvent while it is still wet or before it dries.

Some technicians like to use one hand to wipe on the cleaning agent and the other to dry the same area. By using both hands and two rags, you can more easily wipe off the solvent while it is still wet and remove all surface debris.

If you fail to remove contaminants (especially tar and grease) from the surface before final sanding, this debris can be embedded in the filler or primer. Problems can then result when you are spraying on the paint.

Many shops like to use wax and grease remover before sanding and again right before painting. This ensures that all contaminants have been removed from the vehicle's surface before painting/refinishing.

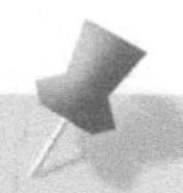

NOTE

Most paint techs now use lint-free disposable clothe wipes for the paint wipedown. Laundering or washing used rags might not remove all oil, wax, or silicone residue. Disposable wipes are now preferred to avoid a lint and debris problem.

To remove any last trace of moisture and dirt from seals and moldings, use compressed air at low pressure. Use a blow gun to blow out behind any area that could hold moisture.

SURFACE EVALUATION

There are several characteristics of the finish that may affect the refinishing procedures. These finish characteristics include the type of the existing finish and the condition of existing finish.

You should make a visual inspection of the condition and appearance of the finish. During the inspection, answer these questions:

1. Has the finish been damaged because of age?
2. Has the finish been damaged because of weathering?
3. Does the finish have environmental damage?
4. Has the finish faded?
5. Will the gloss of the finish cause problems with matching?
6. How much texture or orange peel does the finish have?
7. Which conditions must be repaired prior to refinishing?

Both the customer and appraiser should be informed of any additional work that will be required prior to refinishing.

There are several factors that may affect the aging and durability of an automotive finish. The life span of a finish can be affected by its exposure to acid rain, industrial fallout, ultraviolet (UV) radiation, and hard water.

If a vehicle has been exposed to these elements, the damage may have to be repaired before refinishing. The finish may have to be removed before refinishing.

A *visual inspection* of the finish should include looking for:

1. Fading, dulling, whitening, or similar changes in gloss
2. Cracking or checking (tiny spots are in paint film)
3. Blistering (paint film is lifting or bubbling)
4. Spotting (paint is discolored)
5. Cratering (deep cavities are formed in paint film)
6. Other paint problems

Surface evaluation is a close inspection of the paint to determine its conditions. Once the vehicle has been cleaned, inspect the paint surface carefully.

Look for any signs of **paint film breakdown,** including checking, cracking, or blistering. Pay particular attention to the gloss level; low gloss often indicates surface irregularities. See **Figure 14–2.**

To do a **paint adhesion check,** sand through a small area of the old finish and featheredge it. If the featheredge does NOT break or crumble, the paint may be properly adhered. If you cannot featheredge the paint, it must be removed before repainting.

Preexisting Damage

Preexisting damage includes paint cracking, scratches in paint, acid rain damage, and industrial fallout damage. If there is preexisting damage, the vehicle's owner should be contacted and the situation explained. It is then the decision of the vehicle owner whether to authorize additional repairs. Some types of preexisting damage may have to be repaired before the new finish can be applied or match the existing finish.

Acid rain is caused by the release of various chemicals into the atmosphere. It results

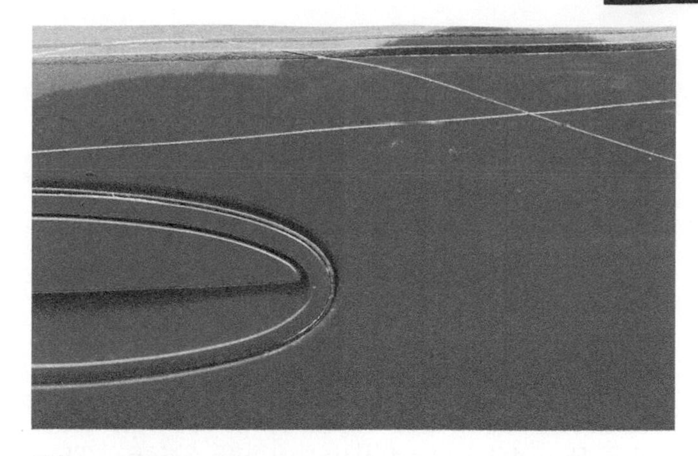

(A) This paint is scratched and would require heavy sanding to featheredge the paint.

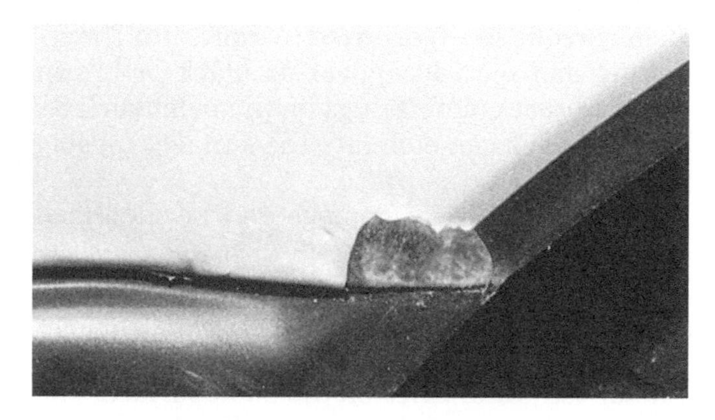

(B) This paint is suffering from body rust. The area should be sand or plastic bead blasted and then sanded.

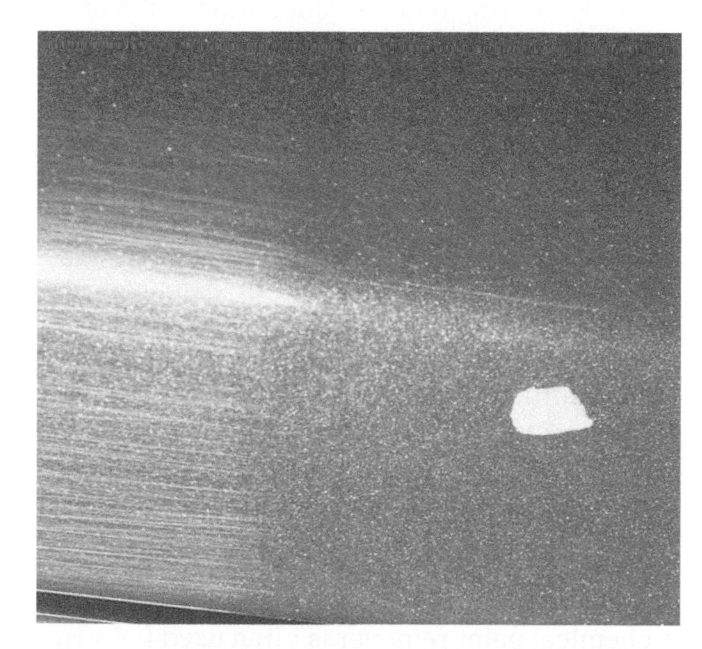

(C) This paint has a flake in it, possibly indicating a lack of paint adhesion. The panel may have to be completely stripped of paint.

Figure 14–2. If your evaluation finds serious problems with the vehicle's finish, you may have to strip the paint off completely.

when these chemicals are absorbed by rain water and form acids. When it rains or snows, these acids settle on the paint surface. They can become stronger as the water evaporates.

Acid rain damage may cause craters to be etched into the paint film, changes in pigment colors, and fading or dulling.

Acid rain damage can be identified with a magnifying glass while feeling the surface for depressions.

Industrial fallout is when metallic particles are released into the atmosphere from steel mills, foundries, and railroad operations. This is another source of paint damage. The metallic particles fall onto the vehicle's surface. They then corrode when exposed to moisture. The resulting damage will appear as black or brown spots or rust-colored rings on the paint surface. The particles can etch into the surface, causing a coarse or sandy surface.

Industrial fallout damage can be identified by feel or wiping a terry cloth towel over the surface. The metallic particles will catch on the cloth and can be easily seen.

Hard water spotting damage forms when rain or tap water dries on the paint surface. The water evaporates, leaving hard minerals on the paint surface. Hard water spotting leaves a round white ring on the paint surface. It is often repairable because the mineral deposits are on top of the paint film.

UV radiation damage results from excessive exposure of the paint film to the sun's radiation. Exposure to UV radiation can cause discoloration, cracking, checking, dulling, or yellowing.

When paint is badly aged or damaged, the finish should be completely removed. There are three common ways of stripping paint from metal surfaces: chemical stripping, abrasive blasting, and sanding or grinding.

CHEMICAL STRIPPING

Chemical stripping uses a chemical action to dissolve and remove paint down to bare metal. A chemical paint remover is often used for stripping large areas of paint. Chemical stripping is effective in those places where a power sander cannot reach.

Before applying paint remover, mask off the area to ensure that the remover does NOT dissolve any paint NOT meant to be stripped. Use two or three thicknesses of masking paper to give adequate protection. Cover any crevices to prevent the paint remover from seeping to the bottom of a panel.

DANGER

Paint remover (stripper) should be applied following the manufacturer's instructions. Pay attention to warnings regarding ventilation and smoking. Also wear protective clothing such as rubber gloves, long sleeve shirts, and goggles. If paint remover comes in contact with your skin or eyes, it can cause serious chemical burns.

WARNING

Some paint removers can harm body filler beneath the paint. The chemical residue can be difficult to remove completely. If the chemical residue is NOT cleaned properly, it can cause paint adhesion problems.

Before applying the paint remover, slightly sand the surface of the paint to be stripped. This will help the chemical stripper penetrate and dissolve the paint more quickly.

To apply paint remover, brush on a heavy coat in one direction only, to the entire area being treated. Use a soft bristle brush. Do NOT brush the material out. Allow the paint remover to stand and soak until the finish is softened.

Although paint remover is quickly effective on most paints, some surfaces can prove stubborn. More than one application of remover may be needed.

Caution should be taken when removing the loosened paint coatings. Some paint removers are designed to be neutralized by water. Others are more easily removed with a squeegee or scraper. See **Figure 14–3.**

Be sure to rinse off any residue that remains by using a cleaning solvent and abrasive pad. Follow immediately by wiping with a clean rag. This rinsing operation is essential. Many paint removers contain wax. If left on the surface, the residue will prevent the paint from adhering, drying, and hardening properly.

After chemical stripping, you will sometimes have to remove small patches of remaining

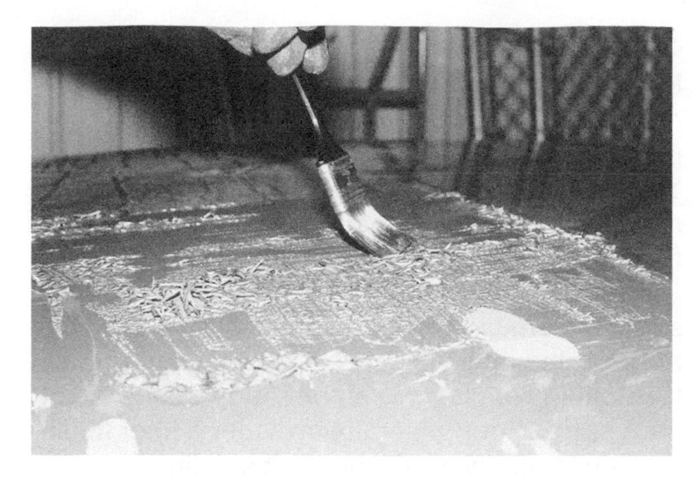

(A) Apply chemical stripper with a paint brush while wearing protective gloves and goggles.

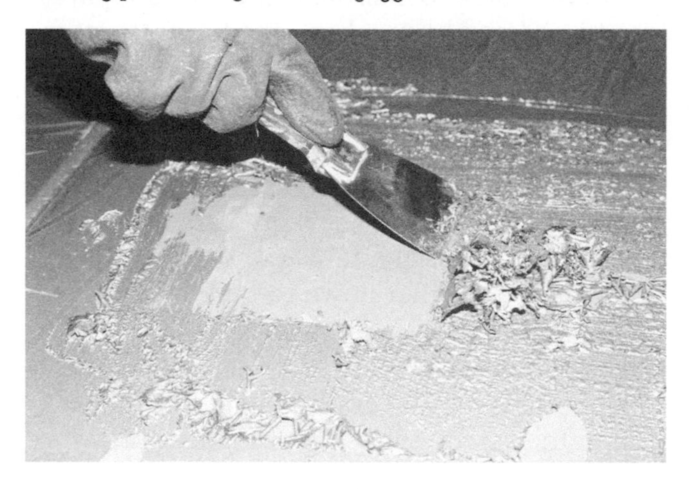

(B) Use a scraper to remove softened paint before sanding.

Figure 14–3. Here a technician is using a chemical paint stripper.

semisoftened paint. For fast removal, use a scuffing disc mounted on a grinder. Scuffing wheels will work well in restricted areas.

BLASTING PAINT

Abrasive blasting involves using air pressure, a blasting gun, and an abrasive (plastic beads or other medium) to remove paint. Blasting leaves a clean, dry surface that is ideal for refinishing. Specialty shops have large blasters that can remove all of the paint from a vehicle in a few hours. Collision repair shops often have smaller blasters for removing paint from smaller areas. Look at **Figure 14–4.**

Blasting will quickly reveal hidden rust that can result in scaling and other problems after refinishing. In addition, blasting makes hard-to-reach areas accessible. This method also saves time when compared with sanding/grinding or chemical stripping.

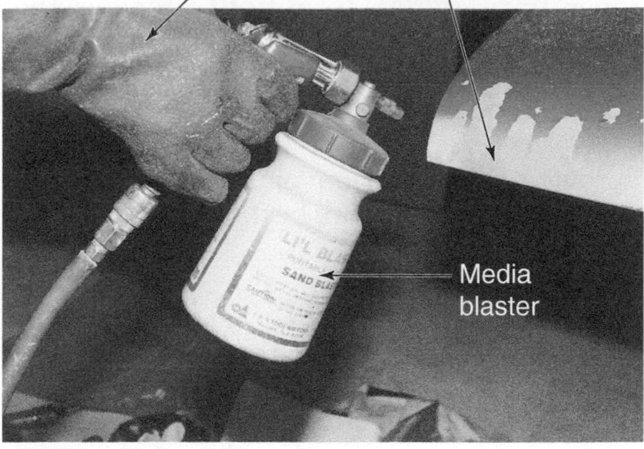

Figure 14–4. Blasting is good on small rust areas. It will remove rust from pits without thinning the metal. Blasting with soft media or plastic beads is better on larger areas.

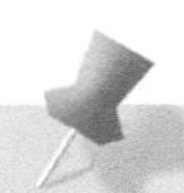

NOTE

Sandblasting can warp thin sheet steel, aluminum, plastic, and other substrates. Sand or hard media blasting is NOT recommended on large flat panels that could warp.

Plastic stripping media, however, will remove paint from almost any surface without damage. Methods of using a plastic stripping medium are similar to the conventional sandblasting methods.

REMOVING PAINT

Machine grinding is suitable for removing the finish from small flat areas and gently curved areas. Start with a No. 40 grit paper on a soft backing pad. Hold the face of the pad at a slight angle to the surface. Work back and forth evenly over the area to remove the bulk of the finish down to the metal. Follow this with a No. 80 grit paper and then No. 180 grit paper. Go over the entire area to be repaired.

! WARNING !

When using the grinder, care must be taken to prevent gouging, scarring, or heat warping the metal.

BARE METAL TREATMENT

Proper **bare metal treatment** prepares the metal for primer. It can also inhibit erosion. Several metal treatment systems are available that ensure a good bond.

Self-etching primers etch the bare metal to improve paint adhesion and rust resistance. Self-etching primers work best on lightly sanded surfaces.

PREPARING METAL REPLACEMENT PARTS

Many manufacturers and parts suppliers prime replacement panels. The function of this **new part primer coat** is to protect the metal against rust. It does not necessarily provide a firm basis for a paint system. Although most primers do have this dual function, the supplier should always be consulted.

Clean the new part with wax and grease remover. Then examine the part for scratches and other imperfections. Sand any imperfections until smooth but do NOT remove the coating completely. Scuff sand the entire panel. Then apply primer before painting. If in doubt about the coating, check with the manufacturer of the part for the recommended finishing procedure.

Clean e-coated replacement panels with a wax and grease remover. Wipe them with liberal amounts of solvent, changing rags frequently. Then treat the panels with a metal conditioner.

SANDING/FEATHEREDGING

One of the most important parts of surface preparation is *sanding*. Sanding prepares the surface for painting in several ways:

1. Chipped paint can be sanded to taper the sharp edges. Otherwise, the chip would show up as ridges under the new finish.
2. Cracking, peeling paint, and minor surface rust can be removed by sanding before applying a fresh paint. If they are NOT removed, these conditions will continue to deteriorate and will eventually ruin the new finish.
3. Primed areas must be sanded smooth and level.
4. The entire surface to be refinished must be scuff sanded to improve adhesion of the new finish. Scuff sanding also removes any trace of contaminants on the existing finish.

Selecting Sandpaper

Because **coated abrasives** (sandpapers) are often used to prepare the vehicle surface for painting, using the correct abrasive is critical. You must select the proper sandpaper for optimum productivity, cost efficiency, and best finish.

Open coat sandpaper is good for sanding softer materials, such as old paint, body filler, plastic, and aluminum. Open coat can prevent premature loading or clogging of the sandpaper. **Closed coat sandpaper** generally provides a finer finish and is commonly used when wet sanding.

Mentioned in earlier chapters, **grit sizes** vary from coarse to microfine grades. Sandpaper grits are ordered by number—the lower the number, the coarser the grit. Refer to **Figure 14–5.**

Here are some general uses for different sandpaper grits:

1. Roughing sandpaper or very coarse sandpapers (No. 24 to 60 grit) are used for very fast material removal of paint, primer, and old body filler down to bare metal.
2. Smoothing sandpaper or medium-grit sandpapers (No. 80 to 240 grit) are used to smooth, level, and featheredge body filler into the surrounding repair area.
3. Finish sandpaper or fine sandpapers (No. 280 to 600 grit) are used for final primer, primer-surfacer, and color or paint sanding before painting.
4. Finesse sandpaper or very fine sandpapers (No. 600 to 2000 grit) are used for removing minor flaws in new paint before buffing with an abrasive compound to restore the gloss in the paint. Finesse or very fine sandpapers can be wet or dry sandpaper.

Generally, select the finest grit paper that will do the job. Fine paper may remove material more slowly, but it will leave a smoother surface.

A common mistake is to use too coarse a sandpaper. Coarser paper will sand more quickly, but it will leave deep sanding marks that can show up in the new paint job. Finer paper would have to be used to sand the surface down to remove these scratches.

Power Grinding and Sanding

Power grinding is done to quickly remove large amounts of paint and other materials. An air grinder is one of the fastest methods to remove material.

Abrasive Grading Scales for Sandpaper

	CAMI (U.S. Std) (See Note 1)	FEPA (P-Scale) (See Note 2)	Finishing Scale	Average Grit Particle Size		Auto Body Use
				Microns	Inches	
FINISHING (Fine)	1200					Finish sanding before buffing or polishing. Wet or dry paper.
	1000	P2000		9.6	0.00042	
	800	P1500		12.3	0.00051	
		P1200	A16	15.8	0.00060	
	600			16.0	0.00062	
		P1000		18.3	0.00071	Finish sanding of paint runs or other imperfection in new paint. Wet or dry paper.
	500			19.7	0.00077	
		P800	A25	21.8	0.00085	
	400		A30	23.6	0.00092	
		P600	A35	25.8	0.00100	Finish sanding before priming and painting. Wet or dry paper.
	360			28.8	0.00112	
		P500		30.2	0.00018	
		P400	A45	35.0	0.00137	
	320			36.0	0.00140	
		P360		40.5	0.00158	
	280			44.0	0.00172	
SMOOTHING (Medium)		P320	A60	46.2	0.00180	Final sanding of good paint. Wet or dry paper.
		P280		52.5	0.00204	
	240		A65	53.5	0.00209	
		P240	A75	58.6	0.00228	
		P220	A90	65.0	0.00254	
	220			66.0	0.00257	Final sanding of body filler and paint. Dry paper.
	180	P180	A110	78.0	0.00304	
	150		A130	93.0	0.00363	
		P150		97.0	0.00378	Initial smoothing and final leveling of body filler. Dry paper.
	120			116.0	0.00452	
		P120	A160	127.0	0.00495	
	100			141.0	0.00550	
		P100	A200	156.0	0.00608	
	80			192.0	0.00749	
ROUGHING (Coarse)		P80		197.0	0.00768	Rough sanding of body filler and plastics. Dry paper.
		P60		260.0	0.01014	
	60			268.0	0.01045	
		P50		326.0	0.01271	
	50			351.0	0.01369	
		P40		412.0	0.01601	Coarse grinding and sanding to remove paint. Dry paper.
	40			428.0	0.01669	
		P36		524.0	0.02044	
	36			535.0	0.02087	
		P30		622.0	0.02426	
	30			638.0	0.02488	
	24			715.0	0.02789	
		P24		740.0	0.02886	

NOTES:

1. CAMI = Coated Abrasives Manufacturers Institute (North America) (Allows a wide tolerance range of particle sizes within the definition of a particular grit)
2. FEPA = Federation of European Producers Association (More consistent sized grit particles than CAMI)

Figure 14–5. Study the uses of different sandpaper grits. You must know which coarseness of sandpaper to use for each task. Study grits within each main category: roughing, smoothing, and finish sanding.

Power sanding normally uses an air sander to begin smoothing operations. Often, a dual-action sander is used to level surface imperfections.

DANGER

Always wear the proper dust mask when sanding. The dust can be harmful if inhaled.

When power sanding, replace the sandpaper when paint begins to cake or "ball up" on the paper. This paint buildup can scratch or gouge the surface and reduce the sanding action of the disc. Slowing down sander speed will also help prevent paint buildup and prolong sandpaper life. See **Figure 14–6.**

Types of Sanding

There are several types of sanding that a painter must master. Most are done during the surface preparation stage but are performed after priming.

Remember, the smoother the surface, the easier the refinishing work.

Bare metal sanding is done to smooth rough metal surfaces. If the metal work has been done properly, little sanding of bare metal should be required. But once in a while the metal is very rough from grinding or welding. In such cases, power sand it with No. 80 grit sandpaper to level out burrs, nibs, and deep scratches.

Paint sanding is needed when the finish is rough or in poor shape and to level and smooth primed areas. Since the primer is primarily intended to fill low spots and scratches, thorough sanding must be done to leave material in the low spots and cut away the high spots. Block sanding is highly recommended for this purpose.

Sanding Methods

Sanding can be done with a sanding block or by using power equipment. Most heavy sanding—such as removal of the old finish—is done by power sanders. Delicate final sanding operations are usually done by hand with a sanding block. Hand and power sanding can also be done wet (with water) or dry (without water). Sandpapers are available in dry or wet-or-dry types.

Block sanding is a simple back-and-forth action with the sandpaper mounted on a blocking tool. It is often used on flat surfaces. Block sanding helps level the surface or make it flat.

Use the following general steps when block sanding:

1. Use sandpaper that fits the sanding block. If needed, cut the sheet of sandpaper to fit the block. Fit the sandpaper under the ends of the block.
2. Hold the block flat against the surface. Apply even, moderate pressure along the length of the block. Sand back and forth with long, straight strokes. See **Figure 14–7.**
3. Do NOT sand in a circular motion. This will create sand scratches that might be visible under the finish. To achieve the best results, always sand in the same direction as the body lines on the vehicle.

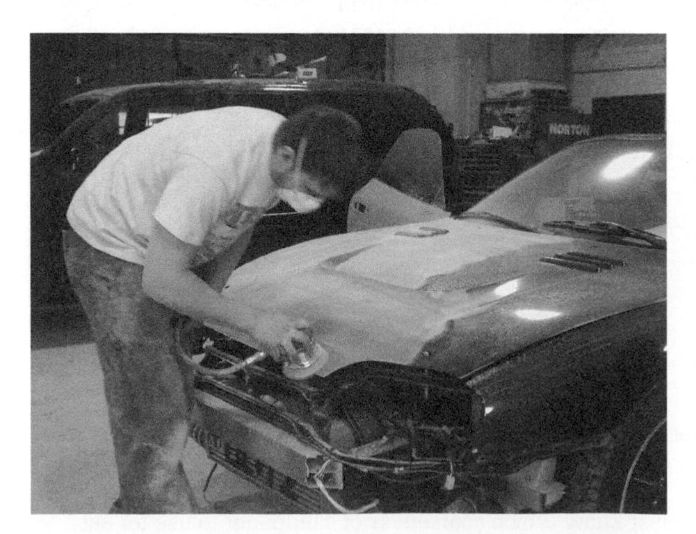

Figure 14–6. Most initial sanding is done with a DA for fast yet accurate paint removal or featheredging.

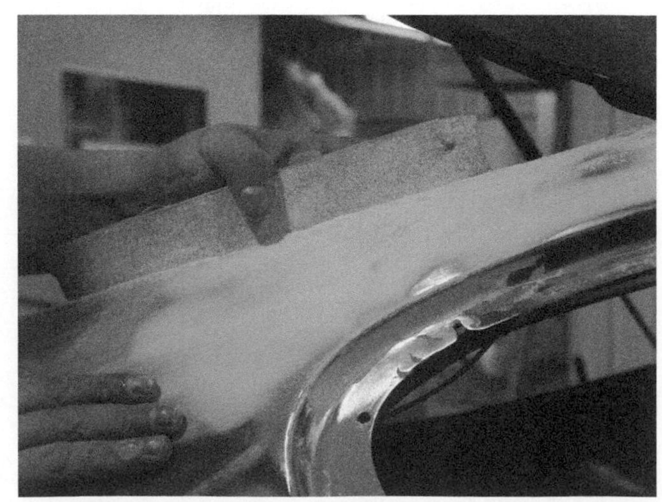

Figure 14–7. Dry block sanding works well when using smoothing sandpapers. Block sanding will quickly level body filler and feather it accurately. Never sand flat surfaces by hand or with your fingers without using a block.

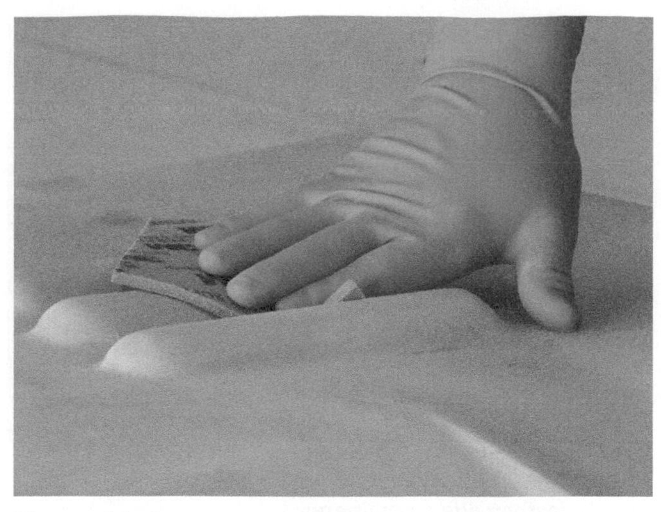

Figure 14–8. A soft, flexible block or sanding sponge should be used on very curved surfaces. The soft block will flex to match the surface profile. Here the technician is sponge sanding the louvers in a custom fiberglass hood.

4. To sand convex or concave panels, use a flexible backing pad. See **Figure 14–8.** You can also use the side of your hand to hand sand concave (curved inward) surfaces. You can use the palm of your hand to hand sand convex (curved outward) surfaces. You must hold your hand to match the shape of the surface.

WARNING

Never try to sand a flat surface while holding the sandpaper in your hand. An irregular surface will result.

5. Carefully find and sand scratches using a finer grit paper.
6. When block sanding primer or filler, make certain to sand the area until it feels smooth and level. Rub your hand or a clean cloth over the surface to check for rough spots.

Remember! If you can feel the slightest bump or dip in the surface, it will show up after painting. A surface will look smooth when sanded dull or when in primer. However, a shiny, reflective paint will exaggerate or magnify any surface roughness.

Block sanding can be done wet or dry. **Dry sanding** is often done with coarser nonwaterproof sandpaper, without using water. It is commonly done to remove material quickly. The majority of two-component primer-surfacers can be sanded dry.

Wet sanding is done with finer waterproof sandpaper, using water to flush away sanded particles. Some primers are wet sanded. Clearcoats are sanded with sandpaper as fine as No. 2,000 grit. Wet sanding reduces the problem of paper clogging.

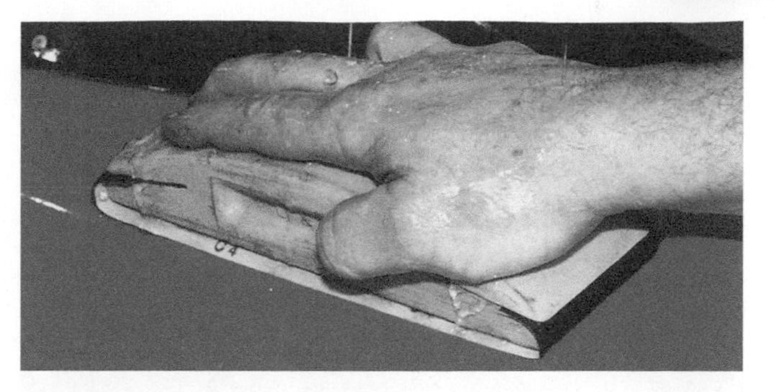

Figure 14–9. When wet sanding, water is applied to the body surface to carry away particles and to avoid clogging of finer paper grits. Again, use a sanding block to support the sandpaper on larger flat or slightly curved surfaces.

Wax and silicone can penetrate beneath the surface. Because this contamination is NOT easily detected, you might want to add wax and grease remover or soap to the water when wet sanding. Look at **Figure 14–9.**

Scuff Pads

Scuff padding is done with a nylon pad on hard-to-reach areas to clean and scuff the surface. Scuff padding is often done inside door jambs, around hood and trunk openings, and other restricted areas. Since the scuff pad is flexible, it will scuff irregular surfaces easily.

Paint scuffing is needed to make sure the new paint bonds properly. If you paint over a smooth, hard surface, the new paint will not have anything to bond to and it will peel off. Paint scuffing can be done with fine sandpaper or a scuff pad, wet or dry.

When scuff pad sanding, you can place the pad over a sanding block on flat surfaces. You can also use your hand to hold and shape the pad on curved or restricted areas. See **Figure 14–10.**

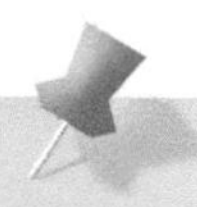

NOTE

Scuff pad coarseness ratings can vary. Refer to manufacturer data to obtain the coarseness rating needed.

Abrasive grinding discs are used for jobs such as grinding off rust and removing paint. They are available in many grit sizes and in diameters of 3 to 9 inches (76 to 229 mm). The

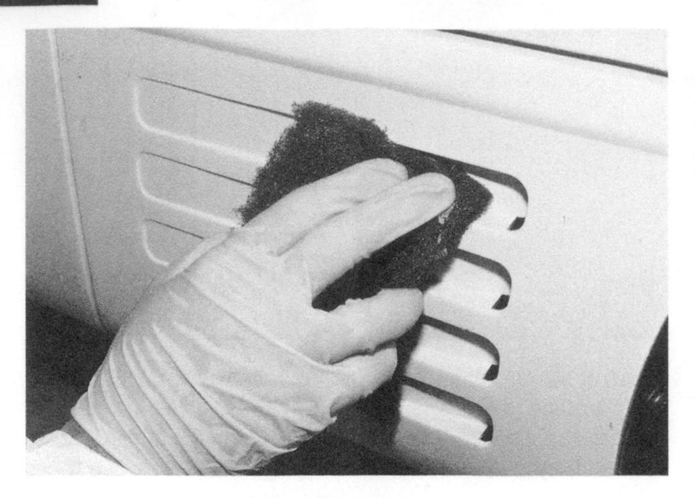

Figure 14–10. A scuff pad is needed to rough up and dull all existing painted surfaces that are hard to reach. The technician is scuffing inside the fender louvers so new paint will bond or adhere properly to existing paint. All gloss or shine must be removed from all surfaces to be painted or the new paint could peel or flake off.

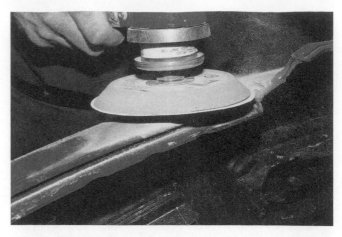

Figure 14–11. Here a repair area is being DA sanded to quickly featheredge a repair area.

grinding disc is first assembled to the backing plate and then the disc/plate assembly is attached to the grinder.

FEATHEREDGING

If a new coat of paint is applied over a broken area of the old finish, the broken film will be very noticeable through the paint. The broken areas must be featheredged. **Featheredged** means the sharp edge of the broken paint film is gradually tapered down by sanding. Then the bare metal areas are filled with a primer and the entire area is sanded smooth and level.

Hand featheredging with a sanding block is usually a two-step procedure:

1. Cut down the edges of the broken areas with a coarse No. 80 grit paper and follow with No. 220 grit.
2. Complete the taper of the featheredge with either a No. 320 or No. 400 grit paper and water. This will produce a finely tapered edge and eliminate coarse paper scratches.

When *featheredging* with an air sander, use a dual-action sander with a flexible backing pad. Use a No. 80 grit for the rough cut, followed by a No. 180.

Start by positioning the sanding disc flat against the work surface. Using the outer edge, or approximately 1 inch (25 mm) of the sanding disc, cut away the rough paint edges. Do NOT hold the sander at an angle greater than 10 degrees from the surface or it will cut a deep gouge in the paint. Refer to **Figure 14–11.**

After initially leveling the rough paint edges, lay the sander flat on the panel. Finish tapering the paint layers by moving the sander back and forth in a crosscutting pattern. Start over the chipped area and work in an outward direction. Stop frequently and run your hand over the sanded area to feel for rough edges. When the surface feels smooth where the old paint and primer meet, featheredging is complete.

! WARNING !

A common mistake when using a DA is to tilt the sander to remove small surface imperfections. This will cause an indentation in the surface that will show up after painting. Normally, hold the sander flat on the surface to avoid this problem.

PRIMING SYSTEMS

Primers and sealer spray coats form the foundation for an attractive, durable topcoat of paint. If the primer is NOT correct, the paint appearance will suffer, possibly cracking or peeling.

Most surfaces must be primed and sealed before refinishing for several reasons:

1. To fill scratches
2. To provide a good base for the paint
3. To promote adhesion of the paint to the substrate
4. To provide rust resistance

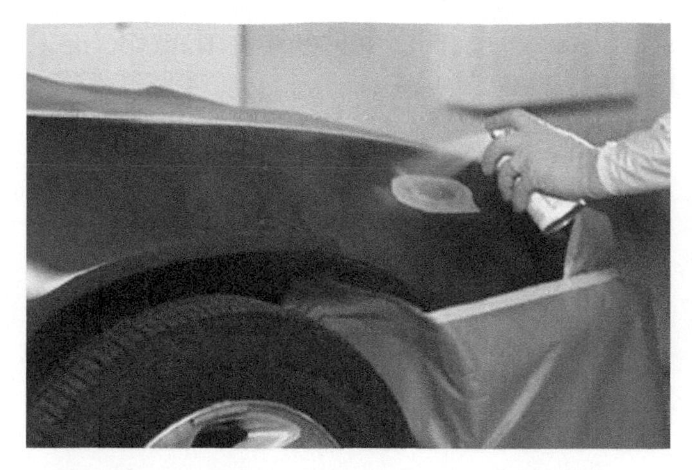

Figure 14–12. Spray primer over repair areas before final sanding. After drying or curing, sand the primer with finishing or fine sandpaper to final check the surface for imperfections.

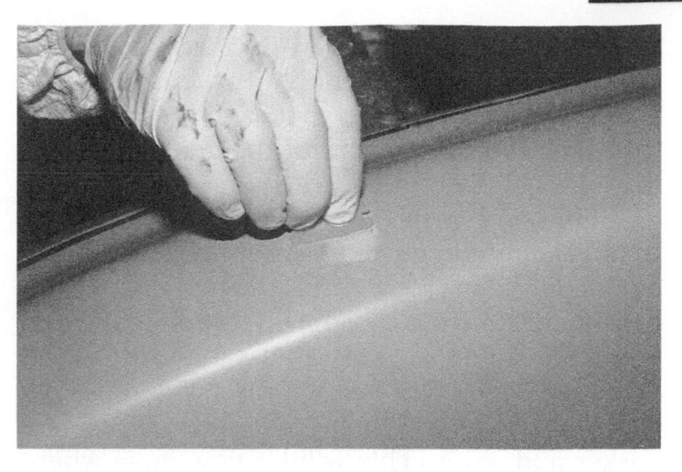

Figure 14–13. Two-part spot puttying is a quick way to fill small pin holes in the paint or primecoat, or primer-surfacer. Then only a small area must be sanded and feathered.

Primer-surfacers are used to provide both priming and filling in one step. *Primer-sealers* are applied to prevent solvents in the paint from being absorbed into the porous primer-surfacer. These three primecoats—*primer,* primer-surfacer, and primer-sealer—can be used together, by themself, or in various combinations of each product. This will depend on the surface condition and size of the job.

Sealers are used to improve adhesion between the old and new finishes. To provide good adhesion, use a sealer over an old lacquer finish when the new finish is to be enamel. Under other conditions, a sealer is desirable but NOT absolutely necessary.

Apply the first coat of primer and allow it to flash dry. Follow the recommendations on the label for flash time. Then apply two or three more medium wet coats for additional film buildup. Again, allow flash time between each coat. When making a spot repair, extend the additional coats several inches out from the first coat. See **Figure 14–12.**

Allow the primercoat to dry thoroughly. After the primercoat is dry, block sand the area until it is smooth. For best results, use No. 320 grit sandpaper. If very fine scratches still appear, another coat of primercoat might be all that is required to fill them.

USING SPOT PUTTY

As discussed earlier in the book, during vehicle prep you may find small scratches or pits that require additional filling with glazing putty. Glazing or spot putty is used to fill small scratches and pinholes after priming.

Two-part (two-component) putties come with two ingredients that must be mixed to start the curing process. They include polyester putties (finishing fillers) and polyester primer-fillers. Both products must be mixed with hardener and can be applied to filler, bare metal, or painted surfaces.

Because today's two-component putties harden chemically, they cure quickly and can be primed and refinished without the worry of sand scratch swelling.

To apply the two-part spot putty, mix the two ingredients properly on a clean mixing board. Then use a rubber or plastic squeegee to apply the material to the small scratch or surface imperfection. See **Figure 14–13.**

Allow the two-part putty to air dry or cure until it is hard. Refer to the instructions for drying/curing times. Test with a fingernail for hardness before sanding. If it is sanded too soon, the two-part putty will continue to shrink, leaving part of the surface imperfection unfilled. Once it hardens, dry sand the putty with No. 80 to 180 grit sandpaper. You can also wet sand the putty with No. 220 grit sandpaper.

After sanding the area, clean the surface and then reprime. If the putty has been wet sanded, make sure to dry the surface thoroughly before applying primer.

USING A GUIDE COAT

A *guide coat* is a very thin coat of powder or primer that assists in pointing out minor high and low spots in the existing surface. A guide coat is applied by spraying or dusting a very light coat of a different color material over the repair area. Sanding reveals the high spots and the low spots by contrasting the colors of the guide coat and the material under it.

Some new primer-surfacers are formulated to have a built-in guide coat feature. After being sprayed over the repair area, the primer-surfacer has a darker, semigloss film on its surface. When you block sand the repair area, sanded areas will become lighter and less glossy, while any low spots that are not being sanded will remain darker and shiny. This will let you know where more material is needed to level the repair area. See **Figure 14–14.**

A **surface high spot** shows up when sanding quickly cuts through the guide coat. A **surface low spot** shows up when sanding will NOT remove the guide coat.

When the surface is flat and ready for painting, the guide coat will sand off evenly or at the same time. Minor surface irregularities can be corrected by applying coats of primer and resanding. Two-component spot putty can be applied to fill deeper low spots and pits.

Light sanding or *scuffing* should be done on all areas where the old finish is in good condition. The purpose is to partially reduce the paint gloss to improve adhesion. Use a dual-action sander, or use a sanding block. Never use a rotary disc grinder or sander.

It is a good idea to carefully inspect the vehicle surfaces after sanding and scuffing. If you can see any shiny area on the old paint, sand or scuff that area. This will ensure that the new finish adheres properly.

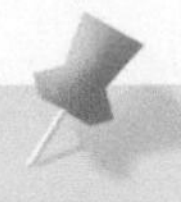

NOTE

Some primer-surfacers have a built-in guide coat. Sanding lightens the prime-coat, while unsanded areas stay a shade darker.

MASKING

Masking keeps paint mist from contacting areas other than those to be refinished or painted. It is a very important step in the vehicle preparation process. Masking has become even more important because of two-component-type paints. Once these paints dry, the overspray CANNOT be removed with a thinner or other solvent. It must be removed with a rubbing compound or by other time-consuming means. See **Figure 14–15.**

Using Masking Paper and Tape

Masking paper is a roll of paper designed to cover parts of a vehicle. Automotive masking paper comes in various widths—from 3 to 36 inches (75 to 915 mm). It is heat resistant so that it can be used safely in heated booths. It also has good wet strength, freedom from loose fibers, and resistance to solvent penetration. See **Figure 14–16.**

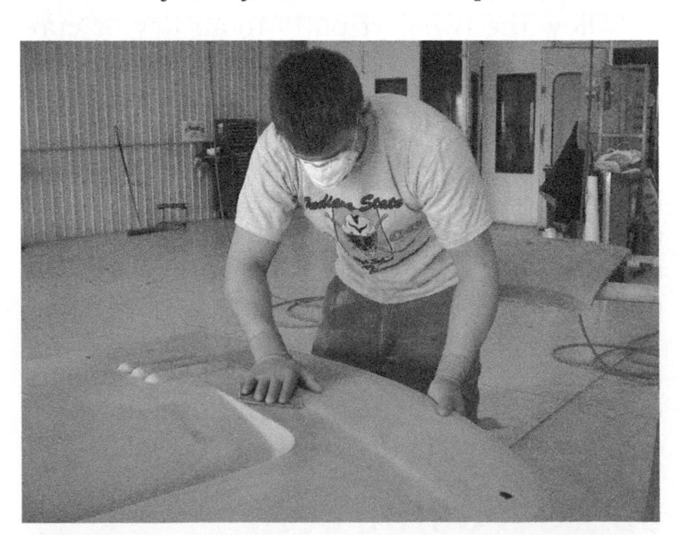

Figure 14–14. A sanding sponge is handy when sanding along sharply curved body lines. Here the technician is using a sanding sponge on the custom hood body line by flexing the sponge to match the shape of the body line.

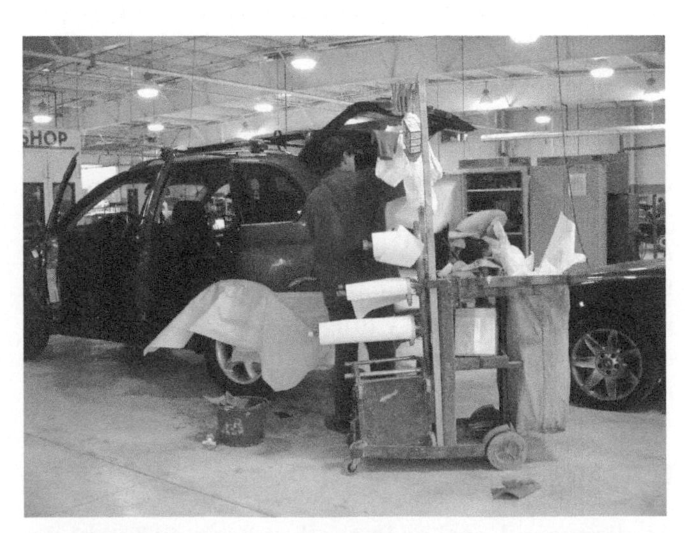

Figure 14–15. The masking paper dispenser is a time saver. This unit has different widths of paper and masking tape on it.

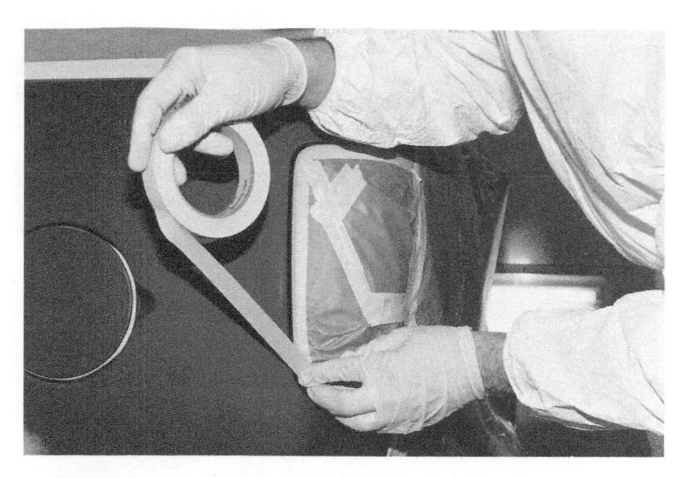

Figure 14–16. When using masking tape, pull lightly on the tape with one hand without stretching the tape. Moving the hand up or down will control the direction of the tape application. The other hand is used to press the tape down securely on the surface. Note the use of masking paper over the taillight assembly.

! WARNING !

Never use newspaper for masking a vehicle since it does NOT meet any of these requirements. Newspaper also contains printing inks that are soluble in some paint solvents. These inks can be transferred to the underlying finish or bleed into the new paint, causing staining.

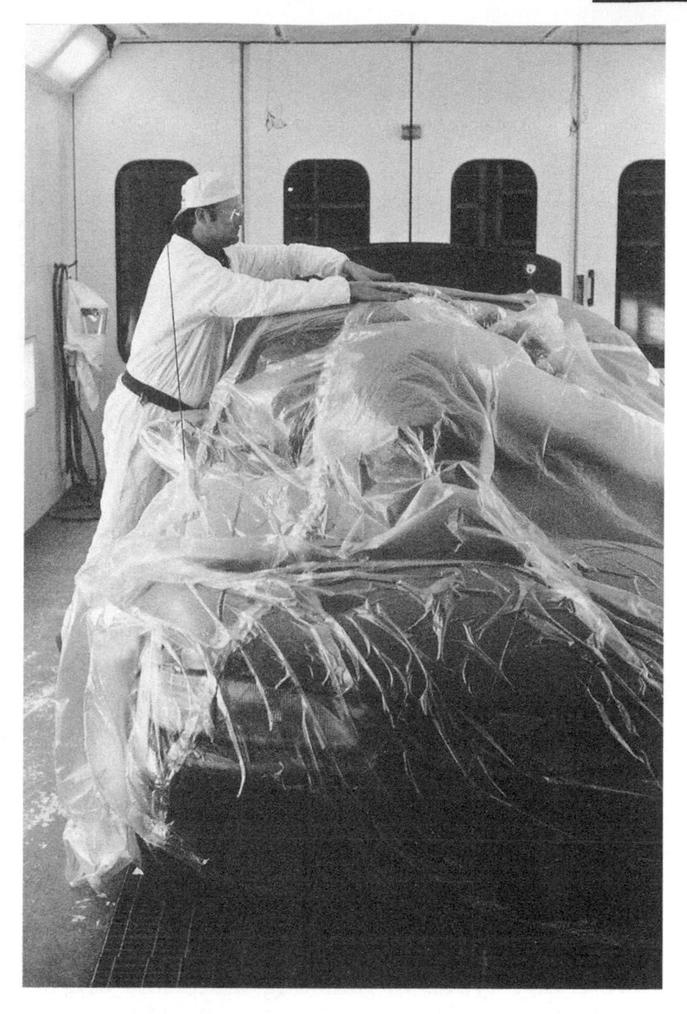

Figure 14–17. Masking plastic is used to cover areas away from the panel or panels to be painted. It should not be used right next to the area to be sprayed.

Masking plastic comes in large sheets for covering large areas of the vehicle. Masking plastic should be used away from the area to be painted. You do not want the paint spray to hit the plastic, because paint can drip off the plastic and onto the paint surface. Refer to **Figure 14–17.**

Masking foam or **masking rope** is a self-stick foam rubber cord designed for quickly and easily masking behind doors, hoods, gas cap lids, and other panels to block overspray.

Masking tape is very sticky paper tape designed to cover small parts and also to hold the masking paper in place. Automotive masking tape comes in various widths—from ¼ to 2 inches (6.4 to 50 mm). Larger width tapes are used only occasionally.

Refinishing masking tape should NOT be confused with tape bought in hardware or house paint stores for home use. This kind of tape will NOT hold up to the demanding requirements of automotive refinishing.

A **masking paper dispenser** applies tape to one edge of the paper as the paper is pulled out. This saves time when masking any vehicle. The average size vehicle can take two rolls of tape to be completely masked. The use of masking paper and tape dispensing equipment makes it easy to tear off the exact amount needed.

Fine-line masking tape is a very thin, smooth surface plastic masking tape. Also termed *flush masking tape,* it can be used to produce a better *paint part edge* (edge where old paint and new paint meet). When the fine line tape is removed, the edge of the new paint will be straighter and smoother than if conventional masking tape were used. See **Figure 14–18.**

Masking Covers

Masking covers are specially shaped cloth or plastic covers for masking specific parts. There are several types of masking covers available. They can save time when masking.

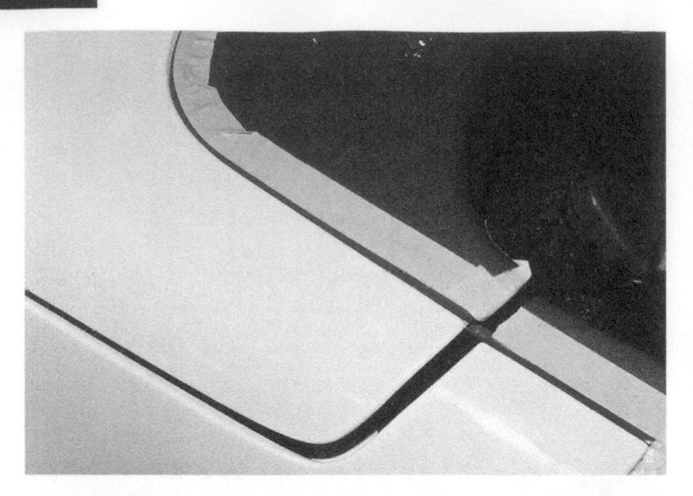

Figure 14–18. Note how a technician has applied fine line masking tape first and has then gone over it with conventional masking tape. This will let you have better control of fine line tape application for more accurate masking. Always check sharply curved masked areas for leaks. When the tape is curved, it can lift up and allow overspray to go under the tape.

One is the *tire cover* that eliminates the need for masking off the tire. Others include a body cover and a frame cover. Covers are also available in a variety of sizes and shapes to mask headlights, taillights, antennas, mirrors, etc.

Masking Procedures

Before any types of masking materials are applied, the vehicle must be completely cleaned and all dust blown away. Masking tape will NOT stick to surfaces that are NOT clean and dry. It is important that the tape is pressed down firmly and adheres to the surface. Otherwise, paint will creep under it.

There are no clear ground rules on when to mask and when to remove parts. This would include parts like trim, moldings, door handles, etc. The decision to remove or mask depends upon the design of the vehicle, and the expectations of the customer. If a part can be removed easily, this is better than trying to mask around the part. Also, if you cannot sand and clean right up to the part, the part should be removed. If it will be difficult to mask the piece, you might save time removing the part from the vehicle. Each part will require an individual decision. See **Figure 14–19.**

Removal of trim and moldings is more often necessary when using a base/clear system than with a single-stage finish. The film buildup can be greater with base/clears. This additional thickness makes the paint edge more likely to crack or chip.

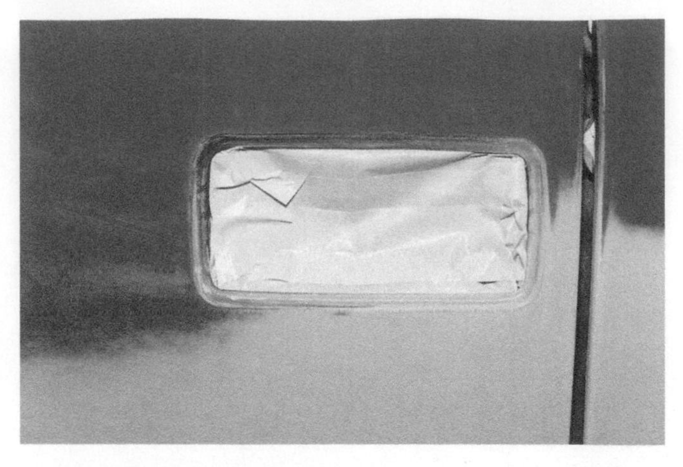

(A) This door handle has been removed and its hole masked closed. This is the best way to paint a door because the paint will deposit under the door handle.

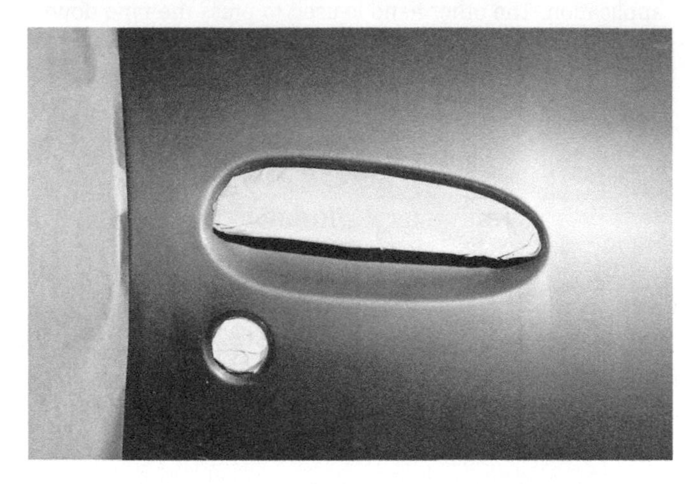

(B) Higher costs prevented the technician from removing this door handle and lock before painting. The handle and lock had to be carefully masked.

Figure 14–19. Note two different ways of masking. When practical, part removal allows for a superior paint job.

It is wise to completely clean and detail the vehicle before masking and again after the refinishing job is completed. This is because masking over a dirty vehicle can cause a "dirty paint job!"

If the painting environment is cold and damp, the masking tape may NOT stick to the glass or trim parts. Condensation on them can prevent the tape from sticking properly. Wipe the parts off before masking them. When masking door jambs, be sure to cover both the door lock assembly and the striker bolt. They can become filled and clogged with paint if not masked.

Although masking tape is elastic, do not stretch the tape when making a straight line. Use fine line tape to cover tightly curved surfaces.

When applying masking tape, hold and peel the tape with one hand. Use your other hand to guide and secure the tape to the vehicle. This provides tight edges for good adherence. This also allows you to change directions and go around corners.

To cut the tape easily, quickly tear upward against your thumbnail. This permits a clean cut of the tape without stretching.

WARNING

Be careful that the masking tape does NOT overlap any area to be painted. After painting, you can remove paint from parts but you cannot add missing paint to the body. Loop or overlap the inner tape edge to follow curves. The tape will stretch to conform to the curves. Difficult areas such as wheels can be masked using this process, but more often covers are used to save time.

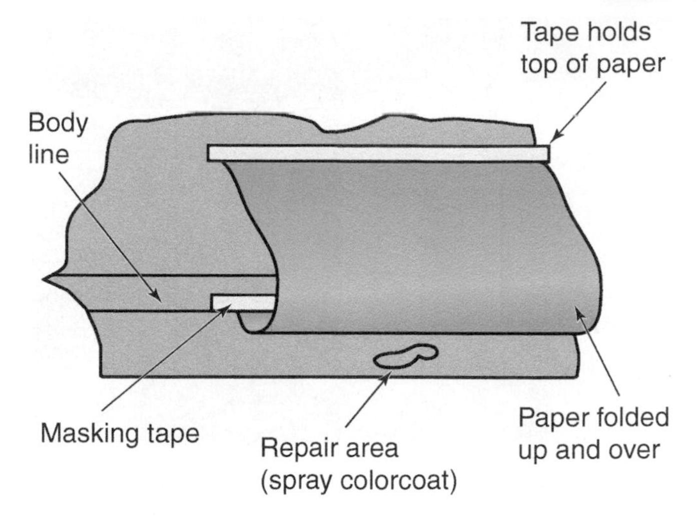

Figure 14–20. Reverse masking will help blend a repair area. Overspray will hit the folded-over paper and blend more smoothly into the old paint.

Before masking glass areas, remove accessories such as wiper blades. The wiper shafts can be protected in the same manner as radio antennas and door handles. Use tape or special covers.

Overspray results when you do not seal the area NOT to be painted and paint/clear gets on an uncovered surface. You would have to then take the time to use solvent or compound to remove the overspray problem.

Fine line tape can be used to protect existing pinstripes from overspray. Also use fine line tape for precise color separation in two-color painting and for creating vivid, clean stripes. Its added flexibility makes painting of curved lines easier, with less reworking.

Double masking uses two layers of masking paper to prevent bleed-through or finish-dulling from solvents. It is needed when spraying horizontal surfaces (hood, trunk, etc.) next to other horizontal surfaces. Overspray will tend to soak through the adjacent masked area and onto the old paint.

Reverse masking or back taping requires you to fold the masking paper back and over the masking tape. See **Figure 14–20.** It is often used during spot repairs to help blend the painted area and make it less noticeable. This also helps prevent bleed-through. The paper is taped on the inside and allowed to bellow slightly, which keeps it lifted a bit from the surface.

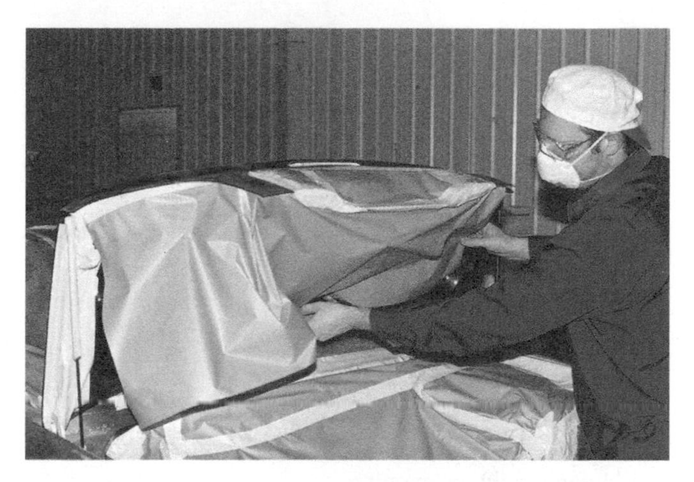

Figure 14–21. This technician is masking the trunk area of a vehicle so he can paint the trunk lid and rear of the vehicle.

Before painting them, the most difficult areas to mask can be door, hood, and trunk openings. You must carefully apply masking tape and paper to from a large unsupported mask to keep overspray out of the openings. Note how this was done to a trunk in **Figure 14–21.**

Figure 14–22 shows how to mask a wheel opening.

Masking foam is being applied to the bottom of a hood in **Figure 14–23A.** This will keep overspray from going down into the gap between the hood and the fender. It will produce a soft edge of spray next to the self-stick foam rope.

Figure 14–23B shows masking foam applied to the back of a gas cap cover. This, too, will quickly mask the gap between the parts to prevent a dull mist of overspray from depositing behind parts.

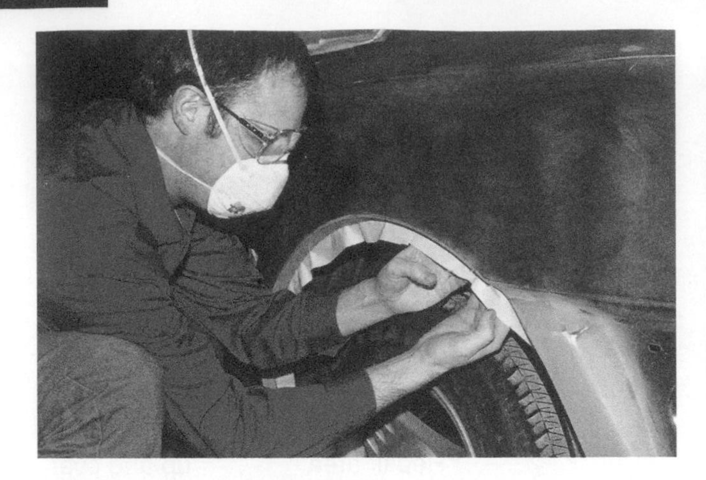

(A) First, apply wide masking tape to the inner edge of the wheel opening.

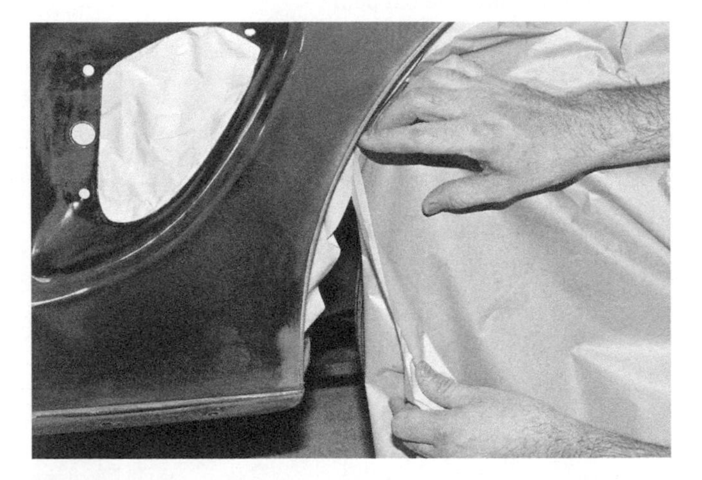

(B) Apply masking paper and tape to the masking tape already on the wheel opening.

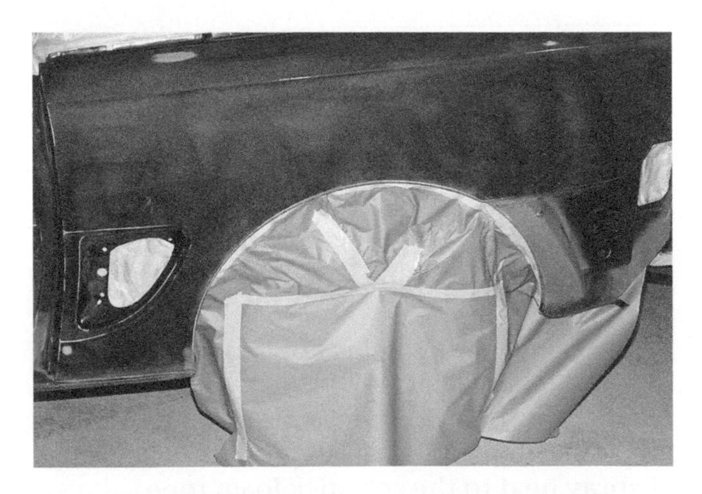

(C) Apply more tape and paper, as needed, to cover the wheel and tire. This will let you paint the panel edges properly.

Figure 14–22. Note how this wheel opening has been masked.

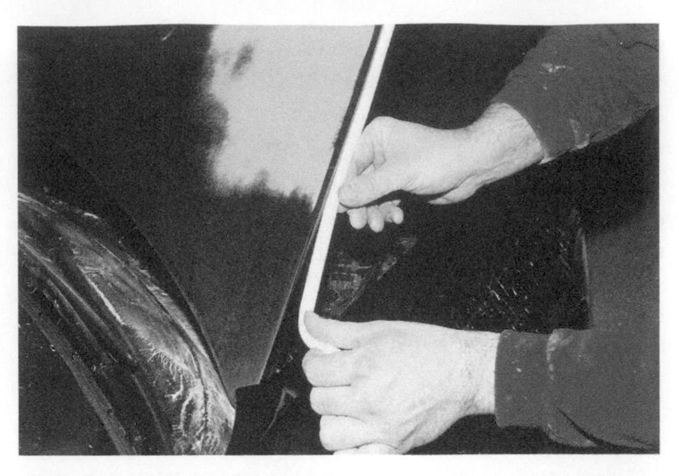

(A) The technician is applying self-stick foam rope or cord to the bottom of the hood lip. When the hood is closed, the rope will mask and prevent paint from entering the gap between the hood and the fender.

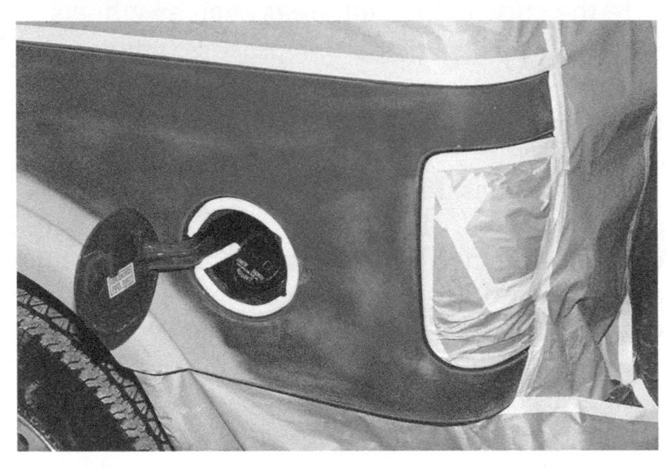

(B) Masking rope has been applied behind the gas cap door to keep overspray off surfaces under and behind the small door.

Figure 14–23. Note the convenience of masking rope when backmasking panel openings.

Liquid Masking Material

Liquid masking material seals off the vehicle to protect undamaged panels and parts from overspray. Liquid masking is used on areas where masking is necessary but difficult to apply, including wheel wells, headlights, grille, underbody chassis, and even the engine compartment.

Masking liquid, also called masking coating, is usually a water-based sprayable material for keeping overspray off body parts. Some are solvent-based. Masking liquid comes in a large, ready-to-spray container or drum. These materials are sprayed on and form a paint-proof coating over the vehicle.

Some masking coatings are tacky. They form a film that can be applied when the vehicle enters the shop. Others dry to a hard, dull finish.

Masking coatings can be removed when the vehicle is ready to return to the owner. It washes off with soap and water. Local regulations may require that liquid masking residue be captured in a floor drain trap, and not put into the sewer system.

To mask a vehicle using the liquid masking system, proceed as follows:

1. Partially mask the area to be painted by going around it with masking paper. Fold the paper over onto the area to be painted. Secure the paper with masking tape.
2. Apply the liquid masking material. Use a heavy, single overlapping coat. Apply the material to all surfaces not to be painted. This would include bumpers, grilles, doors, windshields, body panels, wheels, wheel wells, door jambs, and even the entire engine compartment. See **Figure 14–24.**

   An airless spray system is generally recommended for applying the masking material.
3. Fold the masking paper back over the liquid masking material. Wipe away any material from the area to be painted with a damp sponge. Allow the surface to dry.
4. Prepare the surface. Then apply primer and paint according to the manufacturer's instructions.

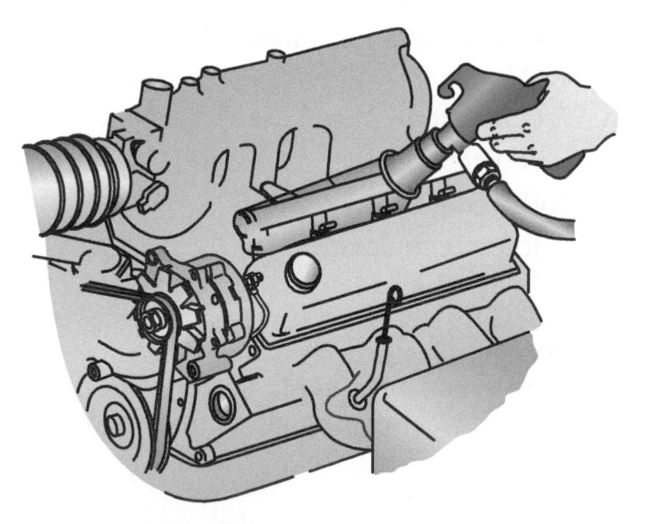

Figure 14–24. Spray liquid mask onto areas NOT to be painted. After painting, masking liquid and overspray can be washed off with soap and water. Here the windshield is being washed to remove masking liquid. (Courtesy of 3M Automotive Trades Division)

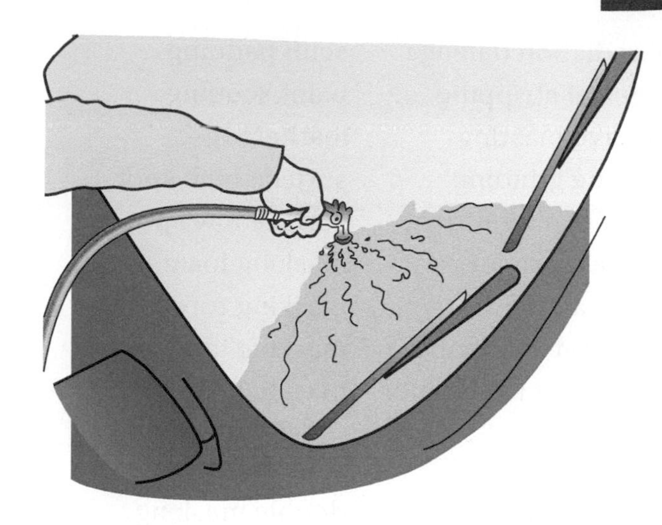

Figure 14–25. After the paint has hardened sufficiently, wash off the liquid masking material.

5. Allow the paint to dry, then unmask the vehicle. Liquid masking may be used in both air dry or bake conditions.
6. After the paint is cured, wash off the dried liquid masking material with a garden hose or pressure washer. See **Figure 14–25.**

SUMMARY

- Vehicle preparation involves all of the final steps prior to painting, including cleaning, sanding, stripping, masking, priming, and other related tasks.
- Open coat sandpaper is good for sanding softer materials such as paint, body filler, plastic, and aluminum. Closed coat sandpaper generally provides a finer finish and is commonly used in wet sanding.
- Masking keeps paint mist from contacting areas other than those to be refinished or painted. Some masking materials include masking paper and tape, masking foam, plastic sheeting, cloth, plastic covers, and liquid masking material.

TECHNICAL TERMS

vehicle preparation
initial washing
surface evaluation
paint film breakdown
paint adhesion check
preexisting damage
acid rain
industrial fallout
hard water spotting damage

UV radiation damage
chemical stripping
abrasive blasting
machine grinding
bare metal treatment
new part primer coat
coated abrasives
open coat sandpaper
closed coat sandpaper
grit sizes
power grinding
power sanding
bare metal sanding
paint sanding
block sanding
dry sanding
scuff padding
paint scuffing
featheredged
surface high spot
surface low spot
masking foam
masking rope
masking tape
masking paper dispenser
masking covers
double masking
reverse masking
liquid masking material

REVIEW QUESTIONS

1. *Technician A* uses a circular motion when block sanding. *Technician B* block sands in a back-and-forth direction. Who is correct?
   a. Technician A
   b. Technician B
   c. Both Technicians A and B
   d. Neither Technician
2. Paint film breakdown will show up as ____________, ____________, or ____________.
3. How do you do a paint adhesion check?
4. ____________ are used to provide both priming and filling in one step.
5. Which of the following statements concerning masking is INCORRECT?
   a. Newspaper works well and saves money as paint masking paper.
   b. Removal of trim, as opposed to masking, is preferred in some instances.
   c. Masking tape will NOT stick to surfaces that are NOT clean and dry.
   d. Using plastic covers on tires eliminates the need for masking them.
6. List four ways of masking the parts of a vehicle.
7. Name three common ways of stripping paint from metal surfaces.
8. Define the term "abrasive blasting."
9. Why is plastic bead blasting often preferred over sandblasting?
10. ____________ ____________ etch the bare metal to improve paint adhesion and rust resistance, while providing the priming and filling properties of primer-surfacer.
11. Explain four ways that sanding prepares the surface for painting.
12. Describe four general uses for different sandpaper grits.
13. How do you use a guide coat?

ASE-STYLE REVIEW QUESTIONS

1. *Technician A* says to wipe the vehicle down with wax and grease remover during vehicle prep. *Technician B* says to wipe the wax and grease remover off while it is still wet. Who is correct?
   a. Technician A
   b. Technician B
   c. Both Technicians A and B
   d. Neither Technician
2. When inspecting a vehicle before repairs, *Technician A* says to check for environmental damage. *Technician B* says to check the entire repair area for imperfections. Who is correct?
   a. Technician A
   b. Technician B
   c. Both Technicians A and B
   d. Neither Technician
3. *Technician A* says that some paint removers can damage plastic body panels. *Technician B* says that sand blasting is better than plastic media blasting on aluminum. Who is correct?
   a. Technician A
   b. Technician B
   c. Both Technicians A and B
   d. Neither Technician

4. When sanding off old paint down to the metal, which of the following grits of abrasive should be used?

a. 24 grit

b. 40 grit

c. 100 grit

d. 400 grit

5. *Technician A* says to use the finest sandpaper possible for adequate material removal. *Technician B* says that this would be too slow. Who is correct?

a. Technician A

b. Technician B

c. Both Technicians A and B

d. Neither Technician

6. Which of the following should a technician use to final sand a curved body surface?

a. Sanding board

b. Hard rubber block

c. Soft, flexible sanding block or pad

d. Air file

7. Which of the following is often used to final check the repair area for low and high spots?

a. Straightedge

b. Micrometer

c. Guide coat

d. Color coat

8. Which sandpaper grit would be used to dry sand and featheredge a repair area?

a. 36 or 40 grit

b. 40 or 80 grit

c. 80 or 120 grit

d. 180 or 240 grit

9. A technician finds very small flaws in the sanded repair area. Which product would help level these areas the most?

a. Primer

b. Primer-seal

c. Primer-filler

d. Primer-putty

10. *Technician A* says to only use masking paper away from the area to be painted. *Technician B* says to use masking plastic right next to the area to be painted. Who is correct?

a. Technician A

b. Technician B

c. Both Technicians A and B

d. Neither Technician

ACTIVITIES

1. Visit a body shop. Ask the owner to let you watch a worker prepare a vehicle for painting.

2. Make a chart showing the steps for preparing a vehicle for painting.

CHAPTER

15 Shop and Equipment Preparation

OBJECTIVES

After studying this chapter, you should be able to:

- Describe the recommended maintenance program for a spray booth.
- Explain the importance of proper material atomization, viscosity, and temperature.
- Measure the viscosity of material using a Zahn cup.
- Describe the advantages of a captive spray gun system.
- Operate and maintain a spray gun.
- Complete a spray pattern test.
- Explain the use of electronic or computerized mixing scales.
- Adjust a spray gun to prepare for refinishing a vehicle.

INTRODUCTION

To complete a professional painting/refinishing job, your shop and equipment must be in perfect condition! A dirty spray booth, a poorly maintained spray gun, contaminated air supply, and other avoidable situations will all ruin your work. Sloppy shop conditions will usually result in a sloppy paint job.

There are a number of shop and equipment variables that affect the refinishing operation. These variables include the spraying environment, as well as the spraying equipment and their adjustments. ALL are important. You must pay close attention to these variables because they can affect the quality of your work. See **Figure 15–1.**

Remember! A professional painting technician will spend more time maintaining the shop and equipment than on any other single task. Spraying the vehicle takes only a very short amount of time by comparison.

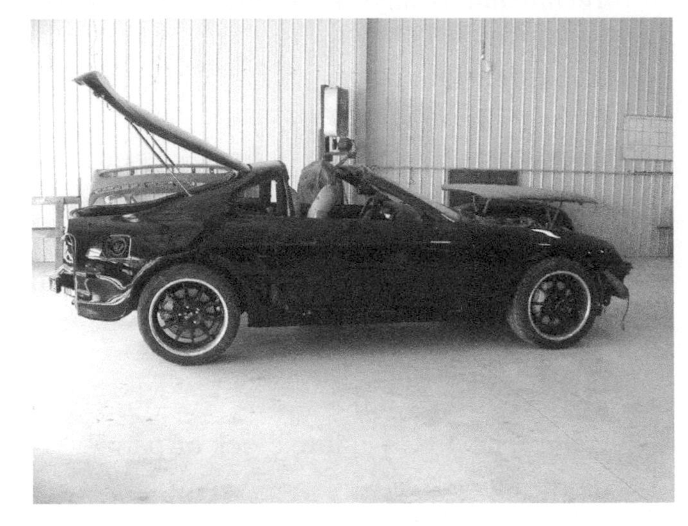

Figure 15–1. The cleanliness of your prep area, spray booth, and shop in general affects the quality of the finished product. Always keep all areas clean and organized.

PAINTING ENVIRONMENT

A painting technician must have a suitable work environment. Automotive refinishing materials must be kept free of dust and dirt during spraying and while drying. In fact, today's clearcoat finishes will magnify any dust, dirt, or other flaws in the finish.

The proper **painting environment** must address these variables:

1. Cleanliness—to keep dirt out of paint
2. Temperature/humidity—to provide proper paint curing or drying conditions
3. Light—to properly light vehicle and paint as it is applied
4. Compressed air/pressure—to send clean air, at the right pressure, to the spray gun

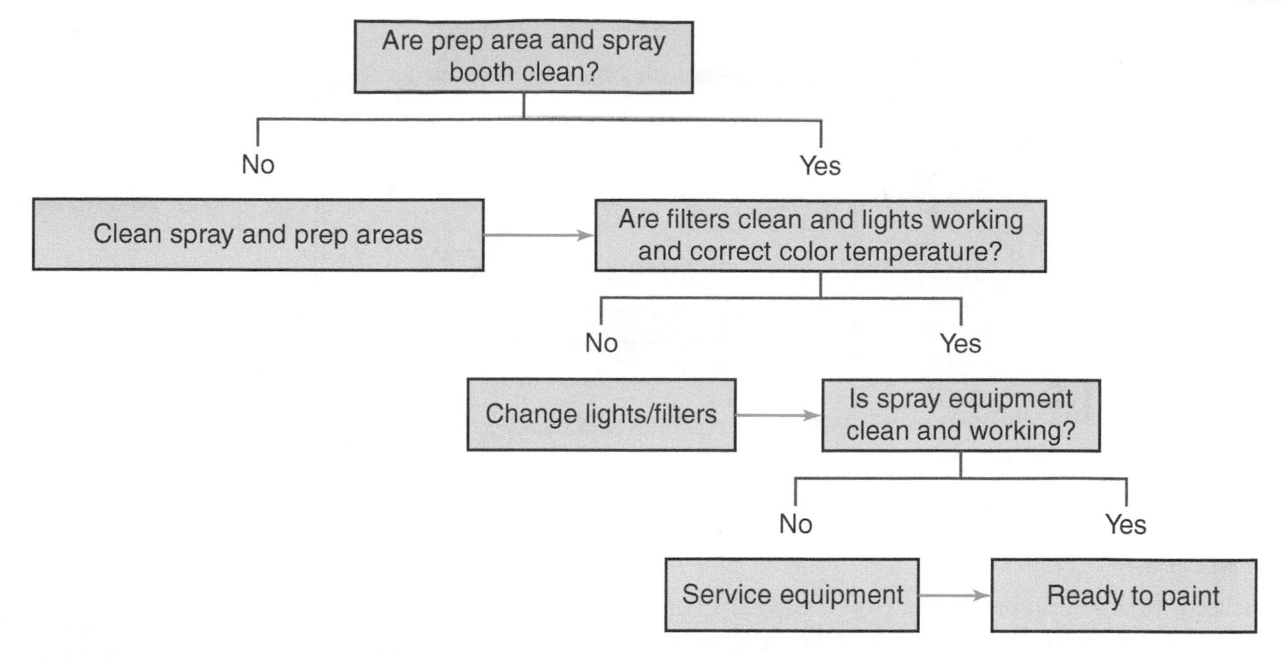

Figure 15–2. This chart shows the major steps for preparing equipment and the painting area.

There are many ways of keeping dirt from becoming a problem in a finish. During body repairs, dirt can be controlled by:

1. Using a dustless, or vacuum, sanding system
2. Cleaning the vehicle before bringing it into the shop
3. Having the paint prep area separate from the body repair area
4. Using prep stations
5. Maintaining the compressed air system's filters and water traps

Before beginning a refinish operation, you must *prep* (prepare) the equipment and painting area. As diagrammed in **Figure 15–2,** you should:

1. Clean the spray booth.
2. Check the spray booth filters for clogging and replace them if needed.
3. Replace any burned-out bulbs.
4. Drain any moisture from the compressed air system. Check filters and dryers.

PREPARING SPRAY BOOTH

Improper booth cleanliness may result in foreign matter entering the fresh finish. See **Figure 15–3.** This can require you to sand out the debris and redo the area. You will waste time and materials if you try to paint a vehicle in a dirty environment.

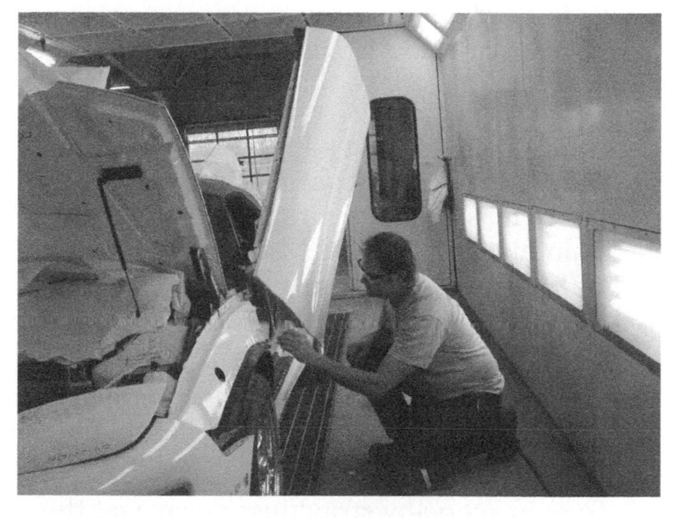

Figure 15–3. The spray booth provides controlled, clean conditions for painting. The paint technician is preparing a custom car for paint work.

The *spray booth* must provide the technician with:

1. A clean environment (see **Figure 15–4**).
2. Constant temperature. The materials, vehicle, and airflow should be at room temperature during spraying.
3. Daylight-corrected lighting.
4. Proper air movement for removing hazardous fumes and overspray, and for correct drying and curing of the paint film.

Before pulling the vehicle into the booth, make sure the area is perfectly clean and

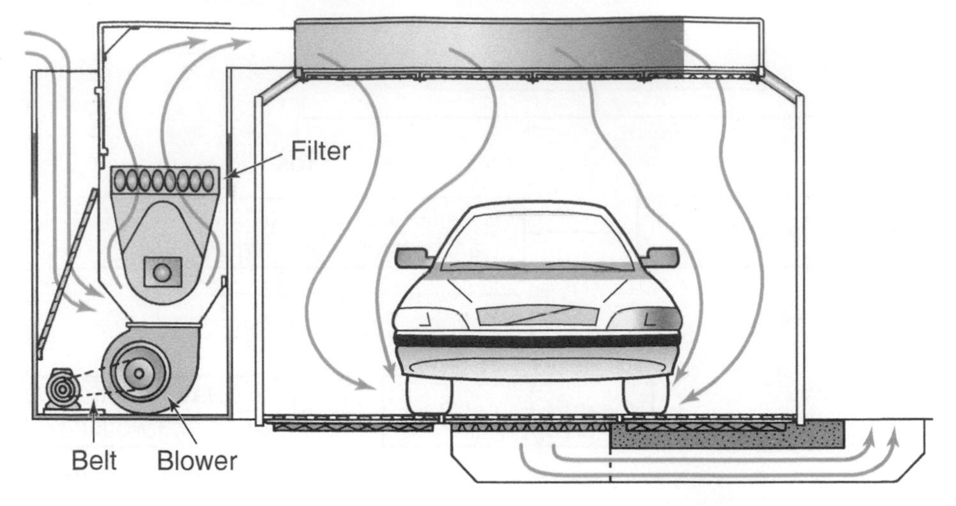

Figure 15–4. Airflow through the booth and filters helps keep any dirt from entering wet paint.

organized. Routine maintenance is necessary for proper spray booth performance. A regular program of cleaning, filter replacement, examining seals and lighting is important for the spray booth to operate properly.

Daily spray booth cleaning includes these tasks:

1. Remove all masking paper, empty cans, and other nonessential items. Clean up scrap, masking paper, rags, and so forth. Maintain and clean ALL equipment used in the booth.
2. Vacuum the booth. The collected material should be stored in a fireproof container. Keep the booth free of dirt and overspray at ALL times. Floors and walls should be cleaned after every job.
3. To help keep any stray dust down, wet the spray booth floor before spraying.
4. Drain oil and water filters and traps (see **Figure 15–5**).
5. Clean the air hoses by wiping them with a damp rag or tack cloth. Clean ALL air hoses several times a day. Accumulations of dirt and dust on their outer surfaces might drop off onto the freshly painted surfaces.
6. Inspect filters and replace them if necessary.

The continuous flow of air through the booth will eventually load the filters with dirt and overspray. These filters should be inspected and replaced at the recommended intervals. When they are replaced, the filters recommended by the booth manufacturer should be used. See **Figure 15–6.** Several types of filtration systems are available. See **Figure 15–7.**

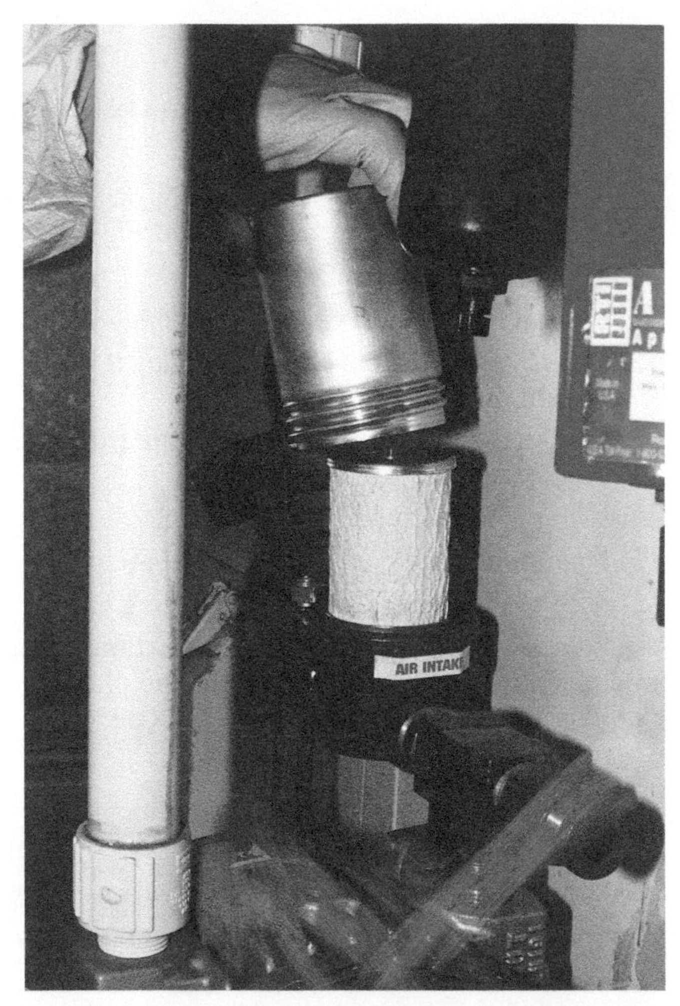

Figure 15–5. Filters should be checked and changed periodically. This is an air supply filter for a spray booth that keeps moisture and oil out of your "paint job."

Monitor the manometer readings daily and know what a normal reading should be. The **manometer** indicates when the intake filters are overloaded. Some booths have a pressure switch that shuts off the air supply and exhaust fan when the intake filter is clogged.

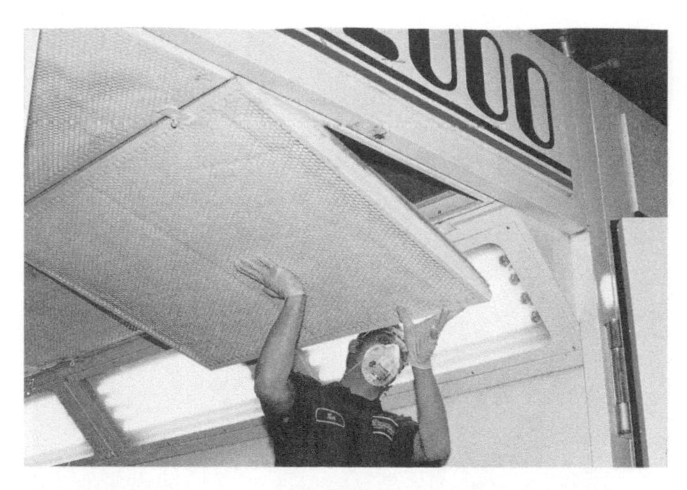

Figure 15–6. Here the technician is changing large air filters in the ceiling of the paint booth.

> **DANGER**
>
> Clogged booth filters are a fire hazard because they could ignite under certain conditions.

Weekly spray booth cleaning includes the following:

1. Vacuum the top of the spray booth and blow off exterior glass and walls.
2. Secure access doors and blow off interior walls and ceiling with the fan running.
3. Clean the light fixtures. Periodically check the lighting inside the booth and replace weak or burned-out bulbs. Improper lighting can lead to poor finishes.

To do a *monthly spray booth cleaning:*

1. Inspect the spray booth for air leaks and caulk and reseal when necessary.
2. Inspect and clean sprinkler heads. Replace plastic bags over sprinkler heads.

Annual spray booth cleaning includes these tasks:

1. Clean the plenum chamber and fan blade. Pay special attention to corners at the base of the chamber. Paint dust accumulation in this area creates a flammable situation.
2. Oil the plenum and fan blade.
3. Inspect the exhaust stack for paint buildup in the damper area. Excessive buildup here will prevent dampers (butterflies) from opening and closing properly.

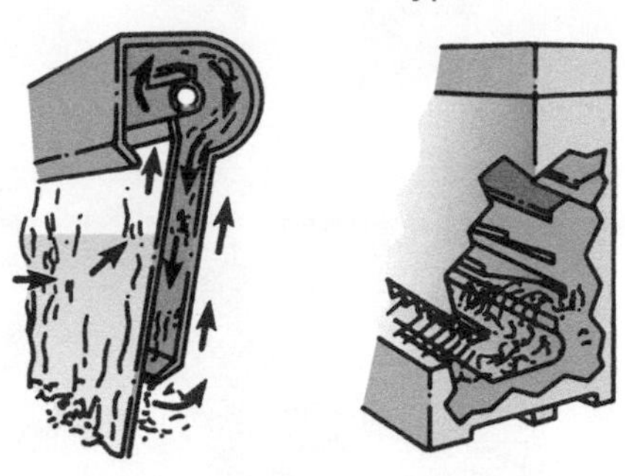

(A) Wet filtration.

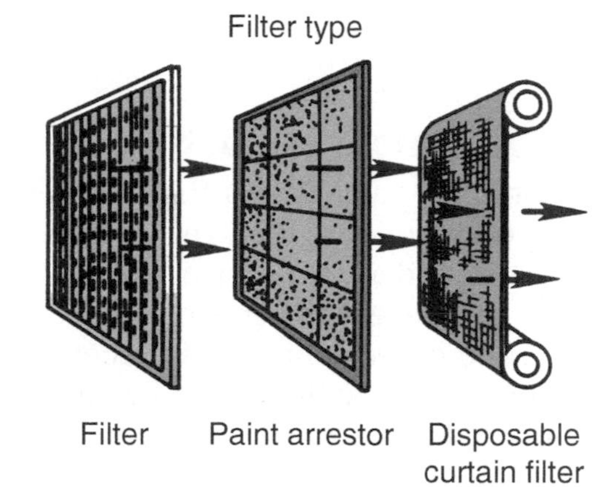

(B) Dry filtration.

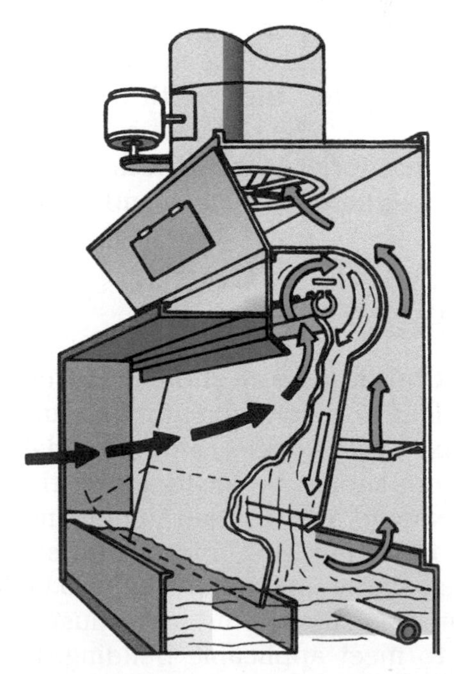

(C) A combination of water spray and centrifugal separation.

Figure 15–7. Different methods of spray booth filtration.

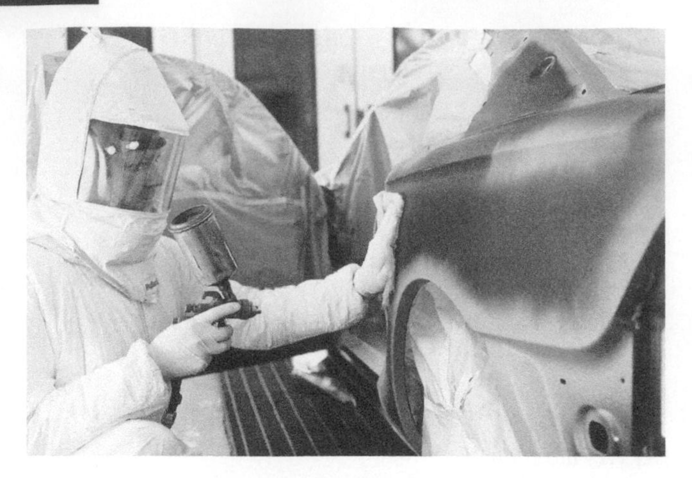

Figure 15–8. A tack rag should be used to wipe dust off the body while also blowing surfaces off with air from a spray gun or nozzle to lift and remove any debris that could harm your paint finish.

Prep with Vehicle in Booth

After driving the vehicle into the spray booth, close the booth doors tightly. Turn on the air filtration system and allow it to run a few minutes. Then **tack rag** the entire vehicle to remove any loose dust and other debris on surfaces. This is needed before proceeding with the refinishing operation. See **Figure 15–8.**

The booth doors must be kept tightly closed during spraying. If it becomes necessary to open a door, be sure the exhaust fan and air supply are turned off. In fact, many spray booths are equipped with door switches that automatically shut off the exhaust fan.

Personal cleanliness cannot be overemphasized. Never enter the booth wearing dirty clothes or shoes. The dirt can easily be transferred to the vehicle and into the finish. All clothing and gloves should be clean and lint-free.

MIXING AND STORAGE AREA PREP

The **paint mixing room** should provide a safe, clean, well-lit area for a painting technician to store, mix, and reduce paint materials. The mixing room should be located near the spray booth. It should also contain the mixing equipment if an intermix (in-shop mixing) system is used. The paint mixing room may also include a technician prep area. This area must be constructed to meet applicable building, fire, and electrical codes. The paint mixing area must be kept clean to reduce the amount of dust and dirt that can be introduced to the paint and painter.

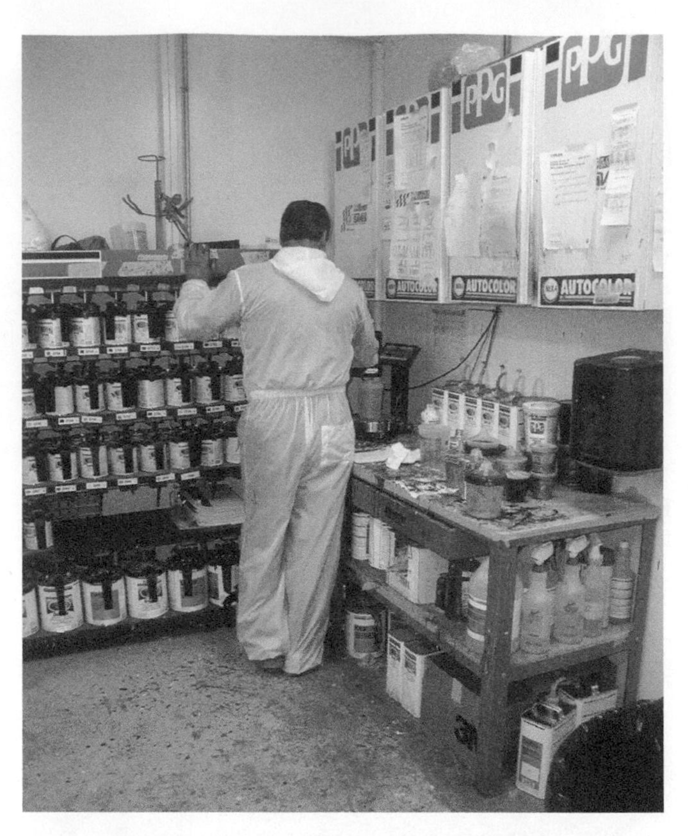

Figure 15–9. The paint mixing room is a ventilated area for mixing paint, preparing spray guns, coveralls, and other materials.

A **painter prep area** is a shop area that provides:

1. A clean area for a technician to dress
2. Clean storage for painting suits
3. A place to clean and store personal safety equipment
4. A good location to have emergency eye wash and first aid equipment

Dirt can enter the material as it is being mixed, so a clean, well-lit mixing area is required. Federal and local laws will dictate the type of mixing area the shop must have. In many cases, this means an enclosed space with its own ventilation system and explosion-proof lighting. See **Figure 15–9.**

The mixing area must have adequate ventilation and fire protection (per federal, state, and local codes). It must also have proper mixing and measuring equipment such as paint shakers, paddle agitators, churning knives, paint mixing sticks, mixing cans, and other equipment.

PREPARING SPRAY EQUIPMENT

If spray equipment is NOT adjusted, handled, and cleaned properly, it will apply a defective coating to the surface. The most common

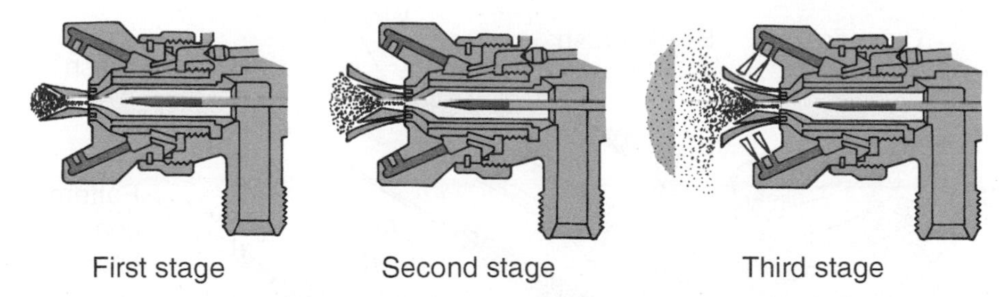

Figure 15–10. Note the three stages of atomization shown by this cutaway view of a spray gun.

problems and suggested remedies are given in the equipment service manuals. These variables can affect the appearance of the color and the outcome of the refinishing operation. When preparing the spray equipment, you must:

1. Clean the spray equipment.
2. Set up the spray equipment with the proper fluid needle, fluid nozzle, and air cap for the material to be sprayed.
3. Adjust the temperature in the spray booth if necessary.
4. Adjust the air pressure.
5. Make a test spray pattern.

Compressed Air System Preparation

The compressed air system can be a source of problems for the technician. *Air supply system problems* can introduce dirt, moisture, and oil into the air supply. From there, this contamination can get into the paint. To avoid air supply problems:

1. Check and replace oil and water filters and traps on a regular basis.
2. Drain moisture from the system daily. Draining the system in the morning allows more moisture to be removed because the air is cool and moisture has condensed.

Atomization Is Important!

A thorough understanding of atomization is the key to using a spray gun correctly. **Atomization** breaks primer, paint, or clear into a spray of tiny, uniform droplets. When properly applied to the vehicle's surface, these droplets flow together to create an even film thickness with a mirrorlike gloss. Proper atomization is essential when working with today's basecoat-clearcoat finishes.

Illustrated in **Figure 15–10,** atomization takes place in three basic stages.

In the first stage, the material passes through the fluid tip and is surrounded by air streaming from the annular ring. This turbulence begins the breakup of the material.

The second stage of atomization occurs when the material stream is hit with jets of air from the containment holes. These air jets keep the stream from getting out of control and aid in the breakup of the material.

In the third phase of atomization, the material is struck by jets of air from the air cap horns. These jets hit the material from opposite sides, causing it to form into a fan-shaped spray.

In **Figure 15–11,** note the common types of spray guns.

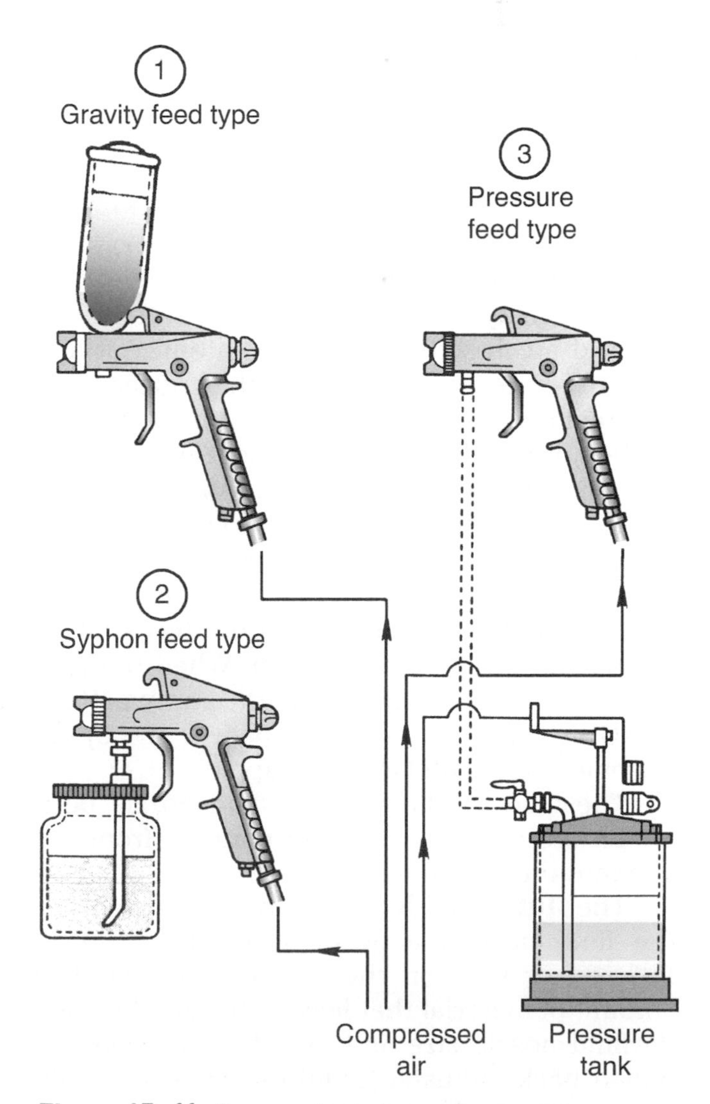

Figure 15–11. Compare basic types of spray guns.

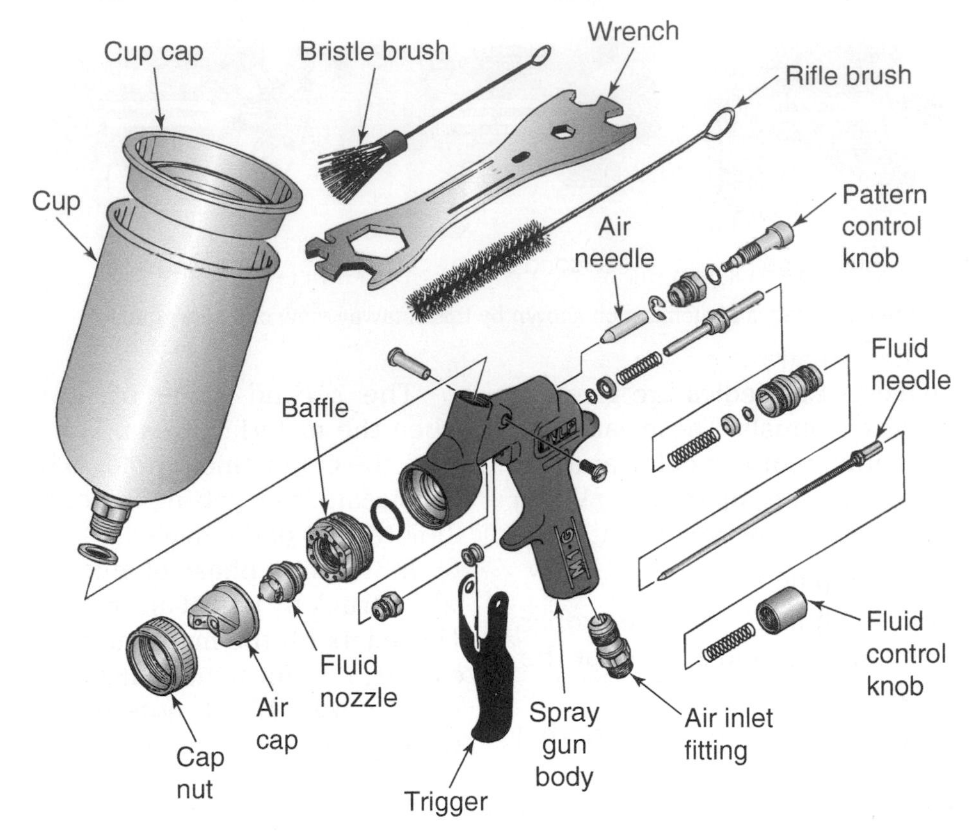

Figure 15–12. Study the basic parts of a typical gravity feed spray gun. The parts of other spray gun designs are similar. (Courtesy of ITW Automotive Refinishing, 1-800-445-3988)

Spray Gun Parts Review

The principal components of a typical spray gun are illustrated in **Figure 15–12.**

The **spray gun air cap** directs the compressed air into the material to atomize it and form the spray pattern. Each of the orifices has a different function. See **Figure 15–13.** The **center orifice** located at the fluid nozzle creates a vacuum for the discharge of the paint, primer, clear, etc. The **side orifices** determine the spray pattern by means of air pressure. The *auxiliary orifices* promote atomization of the paint.

Airflow through the two side orifices forms the shape of the spray pattern. When the **pattern control knob** is closed, the spray pattern is ROUND. As the knob is opened, the spray becomes more OBLONG in shape.

The fluid needle and the fluid nozzle both meter and direct the flow of material from the gun into the air stream.

The **fluid nozzle** forms an internal seat for the fluid needle, allowing the **fluid needle** to open or shut off the flow of material. The amount of material that leaves the gun depends on fluid nozzle size and how far the needle is pulled back (adjusted). Fluid nozzles are available in a variety of sizes to properly handle paints of various types and viscosities.

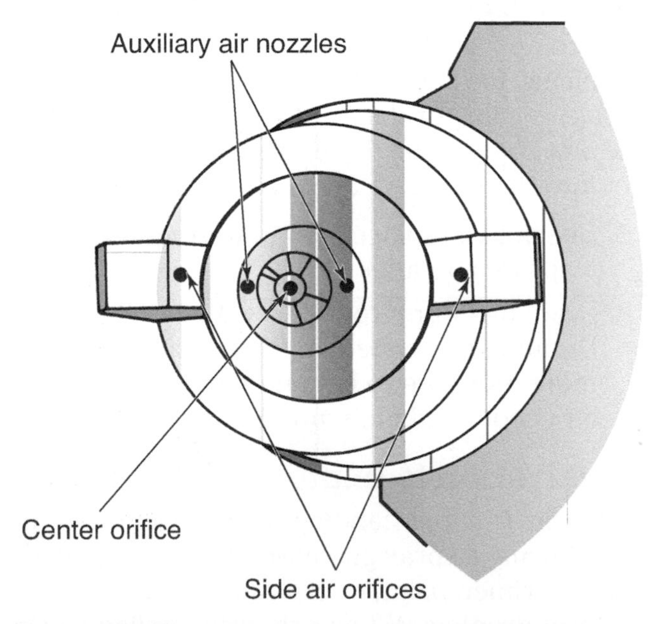

Figure 15–13. The center orifice, located at the fluid nozzle, creates a vacuum for the discharge of paint, primer, clear, etc. The side orifices determine the spray pattern by means of air pressure. Auxiliary orifices help atomize paint. (Courtesy of PPG Industries, Inc.)

The **fluid control knob** changes the distance the fluid needle moves away from its seat in the nozzle when the trigger is pulled. This controls flow.

Like the fluid valve, the air valve is opened by the trigger. The distance the air valve opens is regulated by a screw adjustment. When the trigger is pulled partway, the air valve opens. When it is pulled a little farther, the fluid nozzle opens.

Note how the pressure feed spraying system is hooked up:

1. Connect the regulated air hose from the air control device on the tank to the air inlet on the gun.
2. Connect the mainline air hose from the regulator to the air regulator inlet on the tank.
3. Connect the fluid hose from the fluid outlet on the tank to the fluid inlet on the gun.

Paint pressure tanks are available in sizes from 2 quarts to 10 gallons (2–38 liters). They are available in single, dual, and nonregulated models.

MIXING PAINT AND SOLVENT

When preparing for spraying, you must reduce the primer, paint, or clear to the proper viscosity. Directions on the can or product information sheet will explain reducing procedures.

When mixing and using paint and solvents or other additives, you must measure and mix their contents accurately. This is essential to doing high-quality paint work. You must be able to properly mix reducers, hardeners, and other additives into the paint. If you do NOT, serious paint problems will result.

Mixing instructions are normally given on the product information sheet or can. This may be a percentage or parts of one ingredient compared to the other.

A **percentage reduction** means that each material must be added in certain proportions or parts. For instance, if a paint requires 50 percent reduction, this means that one part reducer (solvent) must be mixed with two parts of paint.

Mixing by parts means that for a specific volume of paint or other material, a specific amount of another material must be added. If you are mixing a gallon of paint, for example, and directions call for 25 percent reduction, you would add 1 quart of reducer. There are 4 quarts in a gallon, and you want one part or 25 percent reducer for each four parts of paint.

Proportional numbers denote the amount of each material needed. The first number is usually the parts of paint needed. The second number might be used to denote the amount of hardener or other additives required. The third number is usually the solvent (reducer).

For example, the number 4:1:1 might mean to add four parts of color, one part hardener, and one part solvent. For a gallon of color, you would add 1 quart of hardener and 1 quart of solvent. This can vary, so always refer to the exact directions on the paint can.

A **mixing chart** converts a percentage into how many parts of each material must be mixed. Study the percentages and parts of each material that must be mixed.

Using Mixing Sticks

Graduated **mixing sticks** have scale markings that allow you to easily mix paint, primer, clear, solvent, and additives in the correct proportions. They are provided by the paint system manufacturer. Several are needed to provide mixing guides for each type of paint. Look at **Figure 15–14.**

Each mixing stick will have a ratio or percentage printed at the top. Measurement marks and numbers are placed along the tool for pouring out the correct quantity of each material quickly. Select the mixing stick with the correct ratio and type of material to be sprayed.

Obtain a can, pail, or container with straight sides. Tapered sides on the container would upset your measurements. It should be big enough to hold ALL paint, hardener, solvent, etc. needed for the job. A gallon or larger container saves mixing time for an overall or complete refinishing job. If you are only doing a small area and 1 cup will do, mix the materials in the spray gun cup. If you are using a pressure tank spray gun, measure and mix the materials in the tank.

For this example, let us say that the mixing stick is for a mixing ratio of 4:1:1 for color, hardener, and solvent.

1. Place the correct paint mixing stick for the type of material into the container.
2. Pour the amount of paint or primer you might use into the bucket. Stop pouring when the paint is even with any of the numbers on the left of the stick. This might be 1 through 7, for example, depending on the quantity of paint needed.

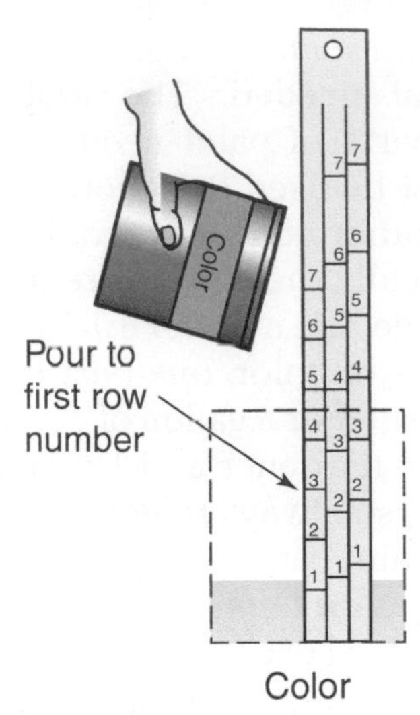

(A) Depending on information on top of the mixing stick, you usually pour in color primer first. Pour in the amount of material needed for the job. Stop when you reach any of the numbers on the left column of the mixing stick.

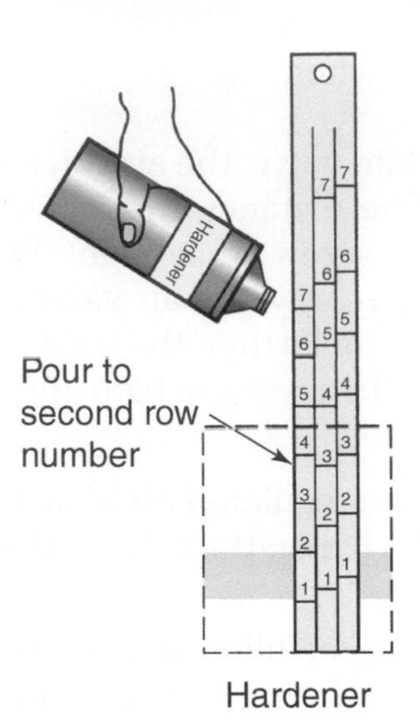

(B) If used, pour hardener or catalyst in next. Pour material into the container until it is even with the same number on the mixing stick, but in the next column. If the paint was even with the number 3, pour in hardener to number 3 on the next, or center, column on the stick.

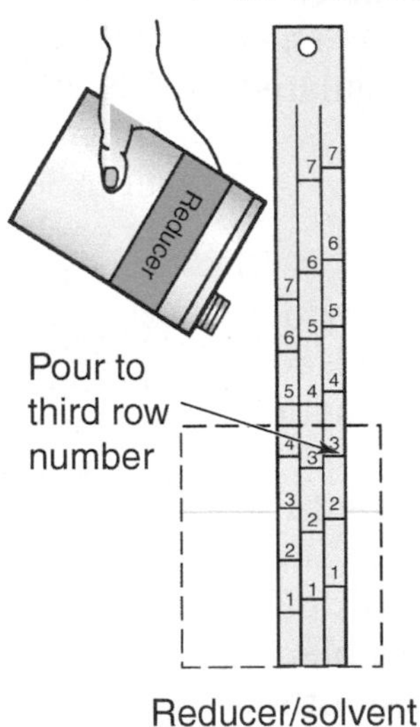

(C) Pour in solvent until the liquid is even with 3 on the right-hand column of the stick. Pour all materials slowly so that you do not add too much. Stir the materials with a metal stick.

Figure 15–14. Study the basic steps for using a mixing stick. (Courtesy of BASF)

For more paint, you might fill to lines 6 or 7. For a spot repair, you might only need to make the material even with lines 2 or 3, for example. Make sure the paint is perfectly even with any of the numbers on the mixing stick. If color is listed on the left, the paint should be even with any number column in that column.

3. Pour in hardener until it is even with the same number (from step 2) in the next column on the stick. If the material already in the container aligns with 3, pour in hardener until it aligns with 3 but in the second column.
4. Pour in the final ingredient (usually solvent) until it aligns with the same number in the last column on the mixing stick. This is demonstrated in Figure 15–14.

After adding the correct amounts of each material, mix them thoroughly with your metal mixing stick. You can then fill your spray paint gun with properly mixed paint.

When filling your spray gun, always use a paint strainer over the cup. The **paint strainer**

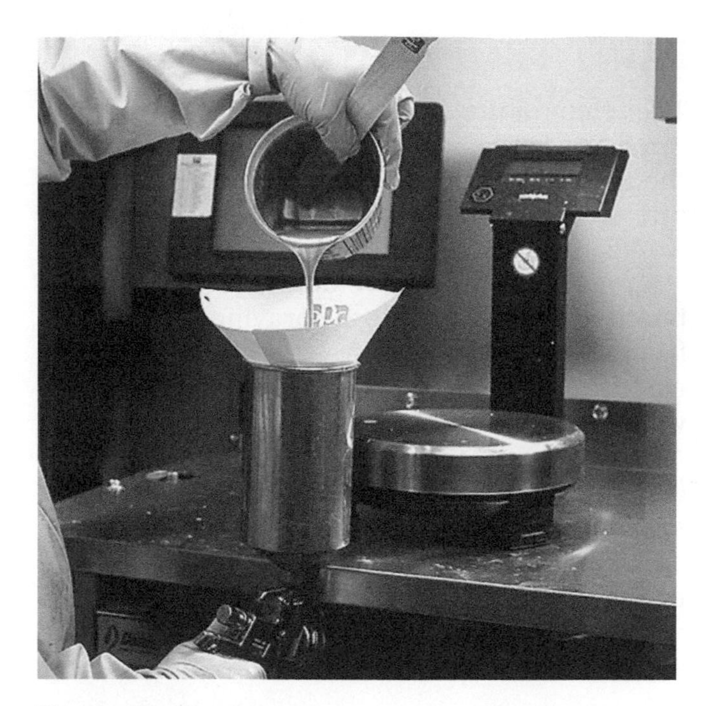

Figure 15–15. Always use a strainer when mixing paint ingredients. It will keep debris out of the paint materials and result in better paint work. (Courtesy of PPG Industries, Inc.)

is a paper funnel-mesh strainer that keeps debris out of the spray gun. It should be used when anything is poured into your spray gun cup! Contaminants can accidentally get into new materials. Dirt and dust can also fall off the top of containers when you are pouring! Refer to **Figure 15–15.**

VISCOSITY

Viscosity refers to the thickness or ability to resist flow of the paint, primer, or clear. Using an incorrect viscosity paint will result in various finish defects. The material must be thoroughly mixed and properly thinned or reduced.

Viscosity can be measured by means of a **viscosity cup.** This is another very accurate method of ensuring proper material thickness. The flow characteristics of liquids relate directly to the degree of internal friction. Therefore, anything that influences the internal friction (such as solvents or temperature change) will influence flow. Similarly, paint flow affects how well the paint will atomize and "flow out" on the vehicle surface.

The two types of paint viscosity measuring cups are the *Ford cup* and the **Zahn cup.** The Zahn-type cup is inexpensive and more common.

The paint manufacturer will give a recommended viscosity value in **viscosity cup seconds.** It will vary between 17 and 30 seconds depending on the type of paint and type of cup used. Refer to the paint specifications on the can for an exact value.

If the material DRAINS TOO QUICKLY out of the viscosity cup, you have added too much solvent. More paint will be needed. If the cup DRAINS TOO SLOWLY, you have not added enough solvent. Remix until the paint passes the viscosity cup test.

If the material is TOO THICK, your paint will develop orange peel or a rough film. If paint is TOO THIN, excess solvent can cause the paint to have poor hiding and other problems.

Make sure you use the reducer designed for the shop temperature and conditions. The amount of reduction should be the same regardless of temperature.

Various finishes are manufactured to spray at specific viscosities. It is very important to follow the label directions for each type of material being mixed.

Using a Zahn Viscosity Cup

The Zahn cup is cylindrical and has an orifice at the bottom. To determine viscosity with a Zahn cup, proceed as follows:

1. Prepare the paint to be tested. Mix, strain, and reduce as directed by the manufacturer.
2. Fill the cup by submerging it in the paint (see **Figure 15–16**).
3. After removing the cup, release the flow of the paint and trigger the stopwatch. Keep your eyes on the flow, NOT on the watch.
4. When the solid stream of paint "breaks" (indicating air passing through orifice), stop the watch. A stopwatch is ideal for measuring paint viscosity with a viscosity cup. Most painting technicians prefer a digital stopwatch because it is easily read.

The result is expressed in seconds. Manufacturers recommend specific viscosities for their various types of paint.

Using a Graduated Mixing Cup

A **graduated mixing cup** is a clear plastic cup with paint ratio markings for mixing spray materials. Its markings are similar to the paint mixing sticks explained earlier. You must add each paint ingredient until the material is equal to the

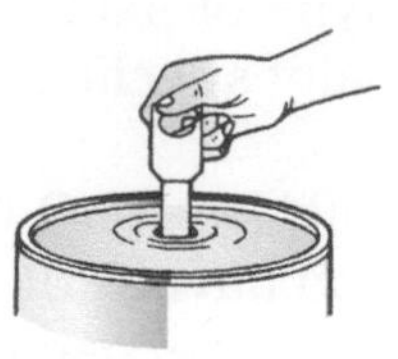

(A) Dip the cup into the paint until it is full.

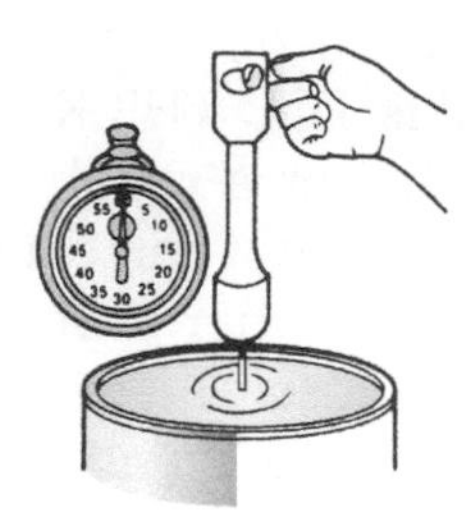

(B) Remove the cup, and as it clears the surface of the paint, begin timing the flow of paint from the small hole in the bottom of the cup.

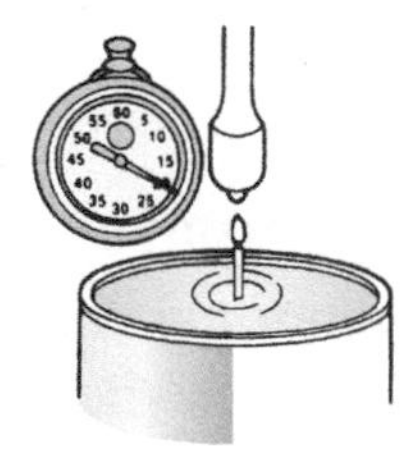

(C) Stop the timer when the stream of paint breaks.

Figure 15–16. Using a Zahn cup. (Courtesy of BASF)

correct marking on the side of the cup. Ounce markings are also provided for adding each ingredient.

Using a Computerized Mixing Scale

A **computerized mixing scale,** or electronic scale, is programmed to automatically indicate how much of each paint ingredient to use by weight. After selecting the needed paint formula on the keypad, the computerized scale will prompt you to add a specific amount of each ingredient. As you pour each material into a cup on the scale, the scale readout will go to zero or beep when the right amount has been dispensed. When zero is reached, you have added the right amount of paint material for that paint code. The scale will then prompt you to add the next ingredient until the proper mixture is achieved.

Electronic scales are commonly used in large collision repair facilities that mix their own paint.

PAINT TEMPERATURE

The temperature at which paint is sprayed and dried has a great influence on the smoothness of the finish. This involves not only the temperature of the shop, but the temperature of the work surface as well.

You should pull the vehicle into the shop and booth long enough before spraying that its surfaces can warm up. Never spray warm paint on a cold surface or cool paint on a hot surface. This will upset the flow characteristics of the paint.

Appropriate reducers should also be used for warm and cold weather applications. For example, a **hot weather solvent** (reducer) is designed to slow solvent evaporation to prevent problems. A **cold weather solvent** is designed to speed solvent evaporation so the paint flows and dries in a reasonable amount of time.

CAPTIVE SPRAY GUN SYSTEM

Because different materials require different setups, many shops use a captive spray gun system. In a **captive spray gun system,** individual guns are set up and used for applying each type of material. Each would be clean, adjusted, and ready for use. You would have separate spray guns for each type of material, as follows:

1. For applying primers
2. For applying sealers
3. For applying basecoats
4. For applying clearcoats

Having a gun adjusted for applying each material saves time. Also, your work will be better because you will know how each gun setting will apply its own material.

Adjusting the Spray

Proper spray gun operation is critical to refinishing. Spray guns are precision engineered tools. They must be treated as such.

A **good spray pattern** should deposit an even, oval-shaped mist of liquid on the body surfaces being repaired and painted. The paint should go on smoothly in a medium-to-wet coat, without sagging or running.

A good pattern depends on the proper mixture of air and paint droplets. Adjusting the spray gun is much like fine-tuning an engine fuel system for the proper mixture of air and fuel.

There are three basic adjustments that will give the proper spray pattern, degree of wetness, and air pressure: air pressure, pattern control, and fluid control.

To adjust a typical paint spray gun:

1. Adjust the air pressure. If this is set at the dryer-regulator (or transformer), you must account for pressure loss through the hose and fittings. Due to friction, as air passes from the dryer-regulator to the gun, pressure will be lost. The air pressure at the dryer-regulator and at the gun varies depending on the length and diameter of the hose.

   A **gun-mounted pressure gauge** or gun-mounted gauge-regulator is the best method to measure and adjust spray gun air pressure. Install the gauge or regulator between the hose coupler and the gun. This will let you set actual pressure at the gun.

   The optimum spraying pressure is the lowest needed to obtain proper atomization, flow rate, and pattern width. *High spray gun pressure* results in excessive paint loss through overspray and poor flow due to high solvent evaporation before the paint reaches the surface. *Low spray gun pressure* produces poor drying characteristics due to high solvent retention and makes the paint film prone to bubbling and sagging.

   Proper spray gun air pressure varies with the kind of material sprayed and type of gun. Many low volatile organic compound (VOC) regulations require 10 psi (0.7 kg/cm^2) or less at the air cap. Always follow the spray gun manufacturer's air pressure recommendations for the type of material to be sprayed.

2. Set the size of the spray pattern using the **pattern control knob.** Turn the pattern control knob all the way in to create a small, round pattern. Back the knob out to produce a wide pattern.

3. Use the **fluid control knob** to adjust the amount of fluid leaving the spray gun. As shown in **Figure 15–17,** regulate the volume of paint according to the selected pattern size. Back the fluid knob out to increase the paint flow. Screw the knob inward to decrease the flow.

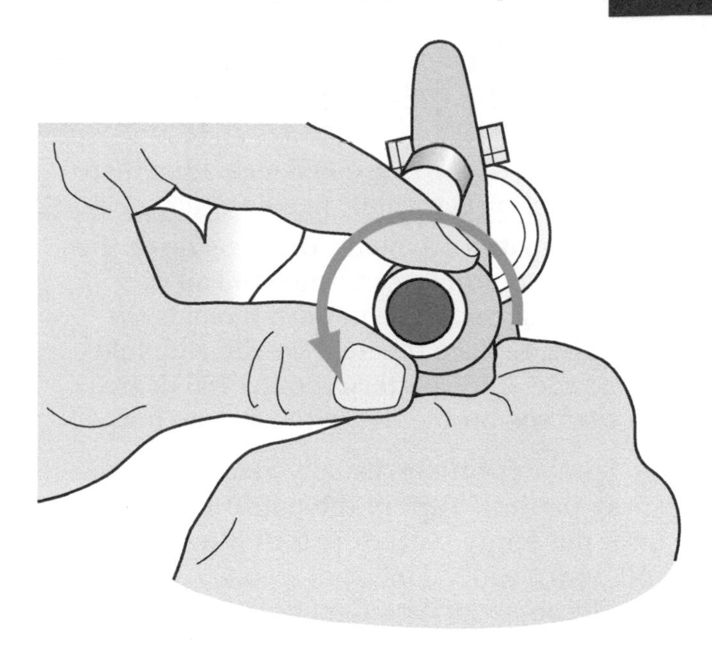

Figure 15–17. The fluid control knob on the spray gun controls the volume of color, primer, or clear leaving the gun.

Spray Pattern Test

A **spray pattern test** checks the operation of the spray gun on a piece of paper. Before attempting to paint the vehicle, it is very important to test the spray pattern.

Hold the gun 2 to 6 inches (50 to 150 mm) away from the paper. Hold the gun 4 to 6 inches (100 to 150 mm) away when spraying clears. Pull the trigger all the way back and release it immediately. This burst of paint should leave a long, slender pattern on the test paper. See **Figure 15–18.**

A spray pattern test that is:

1. Heavy in the middle could mean too little air flow.
2. Divided in the middle indicates too much air flow.

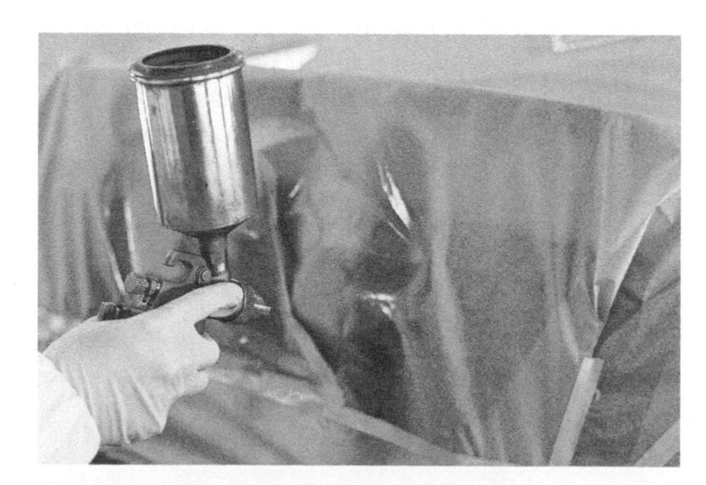

Figure 15–18. After filling the spray gun with material, always check the spray pattern and spray gun operation. You want to find and correct any problems before spraying the vehicle.

3. Too much paint at top or bottom might be caused by a restriction at the fluid needle or air cap horn.
4. Leaning to one side could mean that there is a restriction at the fluid needle or air cap horn.
5. If the pattern is heavy on one side or the top or bottom, try turning the air cap 180 degrees. If the pattern remains the same, replace the fluid needle and fluid nozzle. If the pattern rotates 180 degrees, then the problem is in the air cap horns.

Spraying primer usually requires a smaller spray pattern. Turn in the pattern control knob until the spray pattern is 6 to 8 inches (150 to 200 mm) wide. For spot repair, the pattern should be about 5 to 6 inches (125 to 150 mm) from top to bottom.

If the paint droplets are coarse and large, close the fluid control knob about one-half turn or increase the air pressure 5 psi (0.35 kg/cm^2). If the spray is too fine or too dry, either open the fluid control knob about one-half turn or decrease the air pressure 5 psi (0.35 kg/cm^2).

Next, test the spray pattern for uniformity of paint distribution. Loosen the air cap retaining ring and rotate the air cap so that the horns are straight up and down. In this position, you will get a horizontal spray pattern instead of a vertical one.

Spray again on your test paper. However, hold down the trigger until the paint begins to run. This is known as flooding the pattern. Inspect the lengths of the runs. If ALL adjustments are correct, the runs will be almost equal in length. See **Figure 15–19A.**

The uneven runs in the split pattern shown in **Figure 15–19B** are a result of setting the spray pattern too wide or the air pressure too low. Turn the pattern control knob in one-half turn or raise the air pressure 5 pounds (0.35 kg/cm^2). Alternate between these two adjustments until the runs are even in length.

If the runs are longer in the middle than on the edges, too much material is being discharged. Turn in the fluid control knob until the runs are even in length. See **Figure 15–19C.**

DANGER

Always wear a suitable air respirator when doing any spraying.

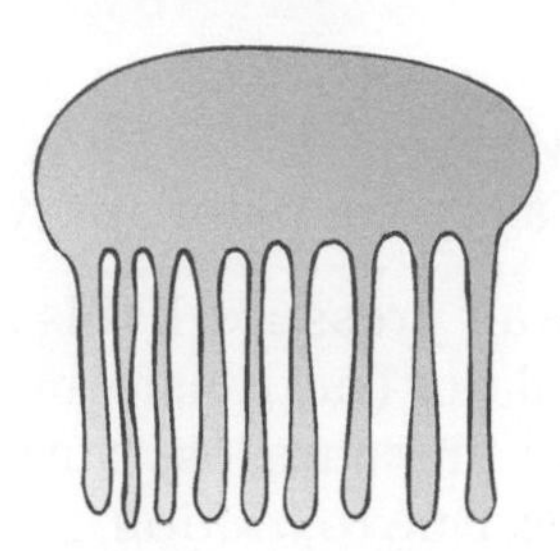

(A) Balanced pattern

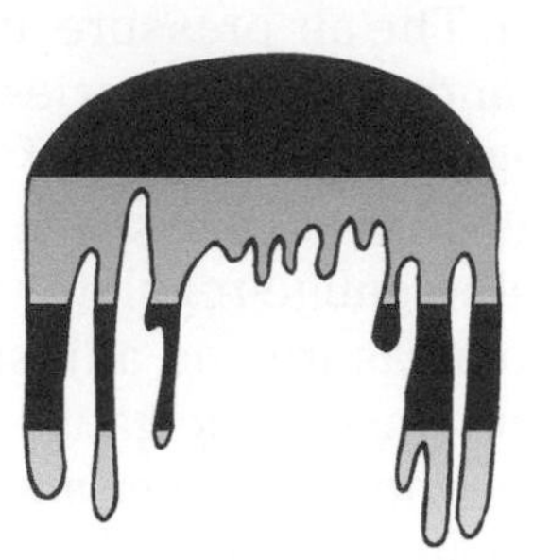

(B) Split pattern

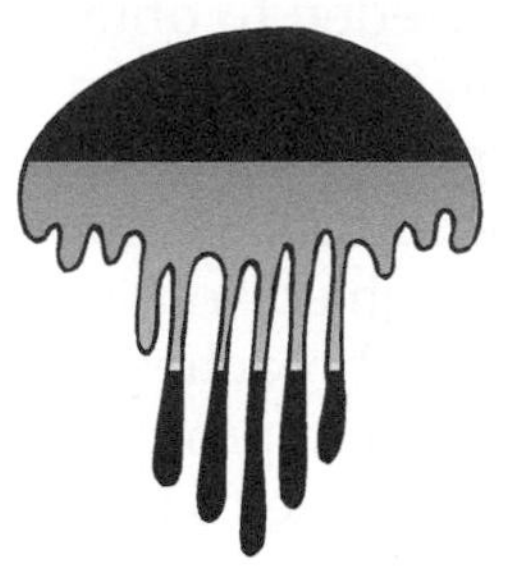

(C) Heavy center pattern

Figure 15–19. With the cap turned sideways on the gun, test spray further. Spray a heavy coat of paint onto the test paper to flood the pattern. Inspect the length of the runs. If all adjustments are correct, the runs will be almost equal in length.

SUMMARY

- A painter must have a suitable painting environment. The following variables must be addressed: cleanliness, temperature/humidity, light, and compressed air/pressure.
- Atomization breaks paint into a spray of tiny, uniform droplets. When properly applied, these droplets flow together to create an even film thickness with a mirrorlike gloss. Proper atomization is essential when working with today's basecoat-clearcoat finishes.
- Paint viscosity refers to the paint's thickness or ability to resist flow. It can be measured by means of a Ford cup or a Zahn cup. The Zahn cup is the more common, and less expensive, cup used.

- In a captive spray gun system, individual guns are set up and used for applying each type of material. This system saves time and improves work quality because each gun will already be at the correct setting when needed.

TECHNICAL TERMS

painting environment
manometer
tack rag
paint mixing room
painter prep area
atomization
spray gun air cap
center orifice
side orifices
pattern control knob
fluid nozzle
fluid needle
fluid control knob
percentage reduction
mixing by parts
mixing chart
mixing sticks
paint strainer
viscosity
viscosity cup
Zahn cup
viscosity cup seconds
graduated mixing cup
computerized mixing scale
hot weather solvent
cold weather solvent
captive spray gun system
good spray pattern
gun-mounted pressure gauge
pattern control knob
fluid control knob
spray pattern test

REVIEW QUESTIONS

1. Clearcoat finishes will magnify any dust, dirt, or other flaws in the finish. True or false?
2. List four functions of a spray booth.
3. Daily spray booth cleaning requires you to do ALL of the following EXCEPT:
   a. Remove ALL nonessential items.
   b. Vacuum the floor.
   c. Check blower belt tension.
   d. All of the above.
   e. None of the above.
4. After pulling the vehicle into the spray booth, ______________ the entire vehicle to remove any loose dust and other debris.
5. Name some expendable materials that should always be kept on hand.
6. To avoid air supply problems, do ALL of the following EXCEPT:
   a. Check and replace oil and water filters on a regular basis.
   b. Drain moisture from the system daily.
   c. Replace deteriorated air hoses because they can introduce dirt into the system.
   d. All of the above.
   e. None of the above.
7. ______________ breaks the material into a spray mist of tiny, uniform droplets.
8. A spray gun has too much paint being applied on one side during a pattern test. *Technician A* says to check for a clogged side orifice in the cap. *Technician B* says to check for proper fluid needle adjustment. Who is correct?
   a. Technician A
   b. Technician B
   c. Both Technicians A and B
   d. Neither Technician
9. If the label on a can of material says to reduce 100 percent, what would you do?
10. Paint mixing sticks have scale markings that allow you to easily mix ______________, ______________, and ______________ in the correct proportions.
11. In your own words, how do you use paint mixing sticks?
12. If the liquid material drains too quickly out of the viscosity cup, you have added too much color and not enough reducer. True or false?
13. What is a captive spray gun system?
14. Summarize the three steps for adjusting a spray gun.

ASE-STYLE REVIEW QUESTIONS

1. *Technician A* says that you will usually spend more time maintaining the shop and the equipment than on any other single task. *Technician B* says that you will spend more time painting. Who is correct?
   a. Technician A
   b. Technician B
   c. Both Technicians A and B
   d. Neither Technician

2. *Technician A* says that the spray booth should be self-cleaning because of the airflow through the system filters. *Technician B* says that booth cleaning is a daily process. Who is correct?

a. Technician A
b. Technician B
c. Both Technicians A and B
d. Neither Technician

3. *Technician A* says to use a tack rag to clean the vehicle once in the paint booth. *Technician B* says you should also blow off the vehicle. Who is correct?

a. Technician A
b. Technician B
c. Both Technicians A and B
d. Neither Technician

4. A spray gun spray pattern is too small. *Technician A* says to turn the fluid control knob in for more flow. *Technician B* says to turn the airflow control knob out for more flow. Who is correct?

a. Technician A
b. Technician B
c. Both Technicians A and B
d. Neither Technician

5. What does the mixture ratio 4:1:1 mean?

a. Add 4 quarts of hardener and 1 quart of solvent to a gallon of paint.
b. Add 4 parts of solvent and 1 part of hardener to a gallon of paint.
c. Add 1 pint of hardener and 1 pint of solvent to a gallon of paint.
d. Add 1 quart of hardener and 1 quart of solvent to a gallon of paint.

6. Which of the following should be used when filling a spray gun with paint?

a. Strainer
b. Funnel
c. Mixing stick
d. Zahn cup

7. *Technician A* says that paint temperature affects finish smoothness. *Technician B* says that solvent speed also affects finish smoothness. Who is correct?

a. Technician A
b. Technician B
c. Both Technicians A and B
d. Neither Technician

8. *Technician A* says that a pressure gauge-regulator between the spray gun and hose will help obtain more accurate gun pressure setting. *Technician B* says that using the pressure gauge-regulator on the wall is better. Who is correct?

a. Technician A
b. Technician B
c. Both Technicians A and B
d. Neither Technician

9. How far away should you hold an HVLP spray gun during a pattern test?

a. 2–4 inches
b. 4–6 inches
c. 6–8 inches
d. 12–14 inches

10. To check spray pattern uniformity, *Technician A* rotates the air cap so that the horns are straight up. *Technician B* floods the pattern with excess paint. Who is correct?

a. Technician A
b. Technician B
c. Both Technicians A and B
d. Neither Technician

ACTIVITIES

1. Inspect the condition of your spray booth. Is it ready for use? Make a report on its condition.

2. Make a wall chart showing how to use one type of paint mixing stick. Place callouts and steps on the chart for display in the classroom.

3. Make a spray pattern test of a spray gun. Try adjusting the gun knobs to make good and poor spray patterns.

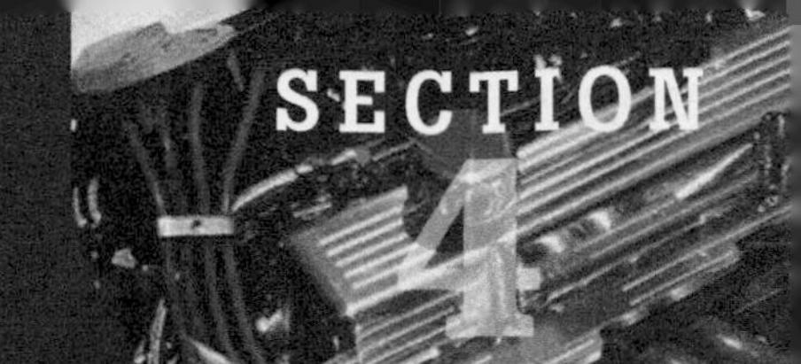

CHAPTER 16 Painting Fundamentals

OBJECTIVES

After studying this chapter, you should be able to:

- Explain the difference between spot refinishing, panel refinishing, and overall refinishing.
- Properly use a spray gun.
- Summarize the different kinds of spray coats.
- Outline general colorcoat/clearcoat application procedures.
- Explain the key points to keep in mind when applying multistage finishes.
- List general rules for painting/refinishing a vehicle.

INTRODUCTION

From the customer's standpoint, the paint is the most important aspect of a body repair job. The topcoat of paint is what the customer sees and evaluates. As a painting technician, you must therefore take special pride in producing a beautiful finish. To do this, you must understand the priming and painting materials and how they are applied.

With today's high-solid, low-VOC paints and high-efficiency spray guns, refinishing procedures have changed. The industry is now using high-volume, low-pressure (HVLP) spray equipment to reduce paint waste and emissions. These changes have made painting and refinishing even more challenging.

PREPARATION REVIEW

All body straightening should be done and the vehicle should be ready for painting/refinishing. Carefully pull the vehicle into a clean paint booth and center it. See **Figure 16–1.**

Make sure the air circulation system of the spray booth is turned on and working properly. See **Figure 16–2.** To prevent airborne contamination, close the booth door and allow the air circulation system to purge the booth of airborne debris. See **Figure 16–3** and **Figure 16–4.**

Check all masking tape and paper one last time. Make sure none of the tape has pulled up or paper has been torn. Inspect all edges and paper closely for openings that could allow overspray leaks. If needed, install wheel cover

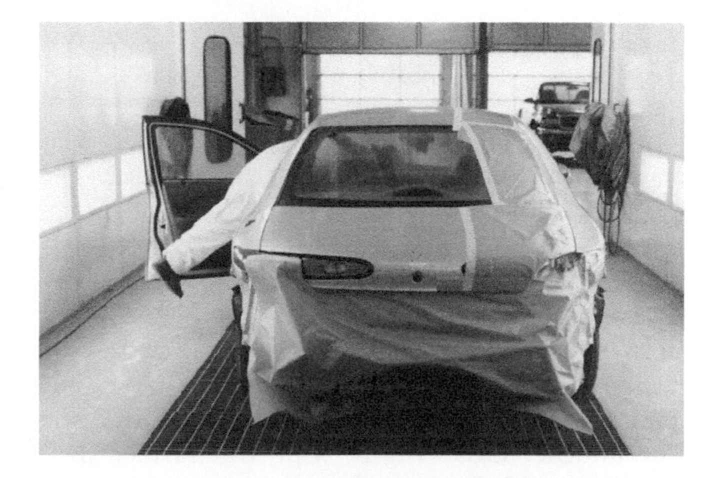

Figure 16–1. When it is ready for painting, pull the vehicle into a clean spray booth. Center it in the booth so you have adequate distance around the vehicle to work.

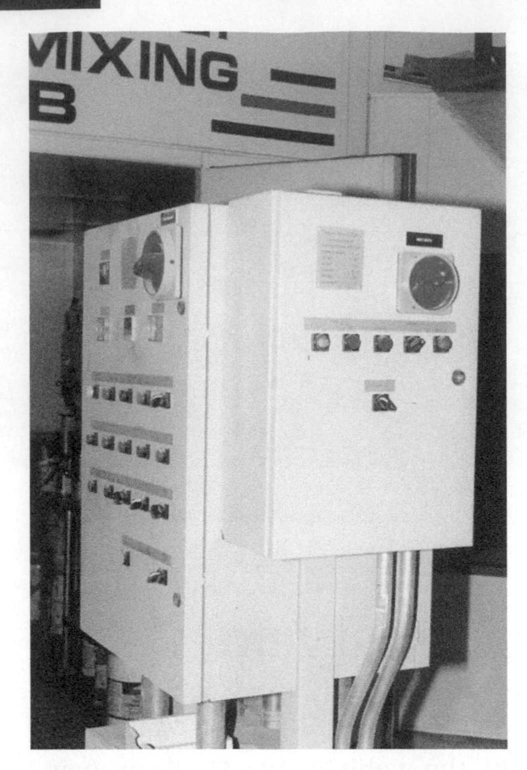

Figure 16–2. Make sure the air circulation system in the spray booth is turned on before refinishing/painting.

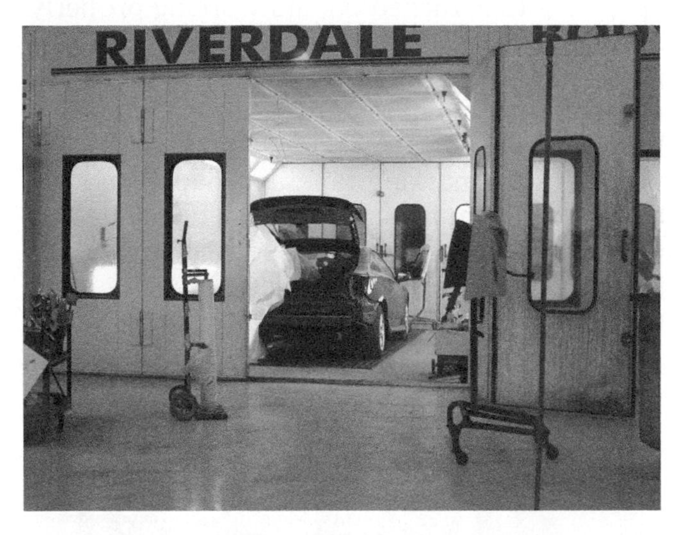

Figure 16–3. A paint booth, if maintained and used properly, will result in a quality paint job with minimum problems.

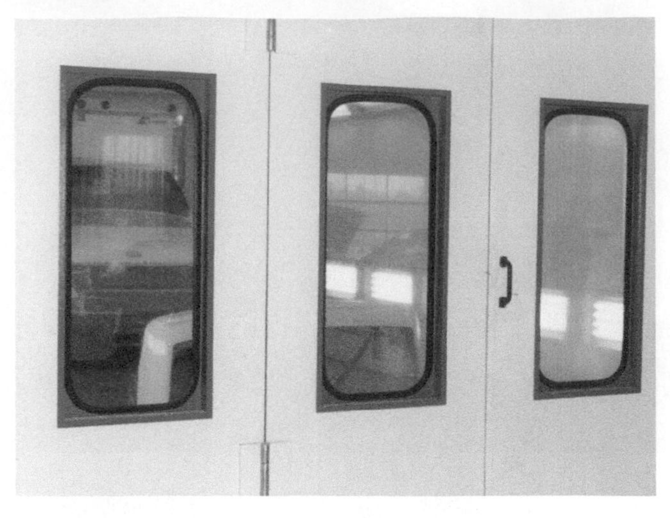

Figure 16–4. Keep the doors on the spray booth closed so that the air circulation system can pull any airborne dust through the filters. If the doors are left open, dust will be pulled into the booth from outside work areas.

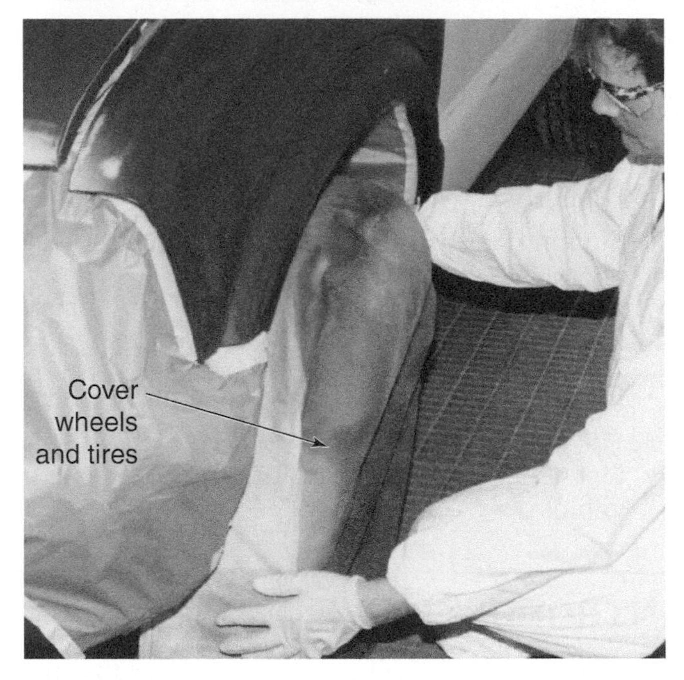

Figure 16–5. Double-check all masking closely. You do not want overspray to get on glass, lenses, and other surfaces not to be refinished. This technician is covering tires with wheel masks.

masks over the tires to protect them from overspray. Refer to **Figure 16–5.**

Wipe the surfaces to be painted with wax and grease remover (cleaning solvent). Use one clean rag to wipe on the wax and grease remover. Use another clean rag to wipe the surface dry. See **Figure 16–6.**

While wearing protective gear, blow off any remaining dust and lint with an air gun. Blow off all surfaces that might hold dust or debris that could get into the finish. As you blow off surfaces, wipe the vehicle down with a **tack cloth** (a rag with coating that holds dust and debris). Refer to **Figure 16–7.**

After wiping with a tack cloth, be careful NOT to touch the surface being refinished. Oil from your skin could contaminate the vehicle's surface.

Make sure the material has been reduced with the proper solvent to the desired viscosity. If needed, add the right amount of catalyst/hardener. Again, refer to the directions on the materials. See **Figure 16–8.** You may also want

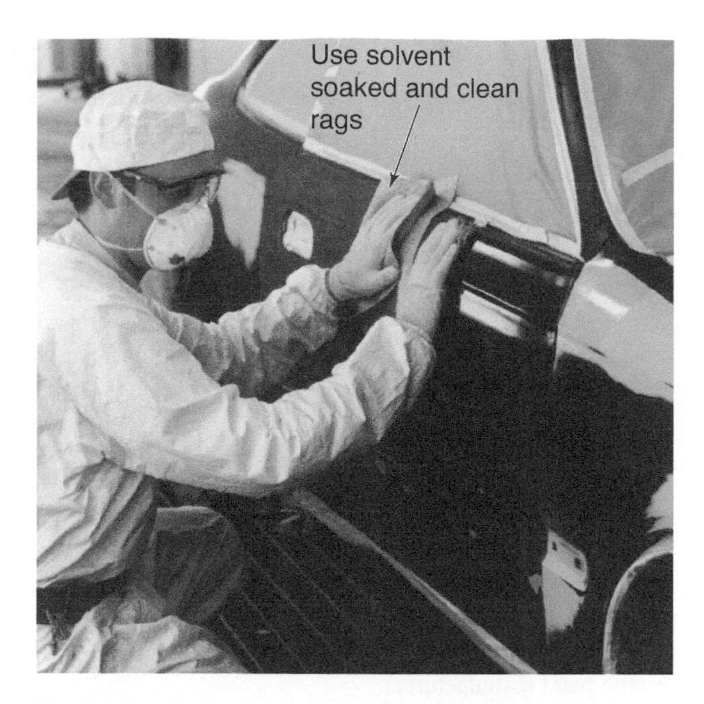

Figure 16–6. Wipe repair areas down with wax and grease remover (cleaning solvent). Use one clean rag to wipe solvent over the surface. Follow this with a clean, dry rag to wipe off cleaning solvent while it is still wet.

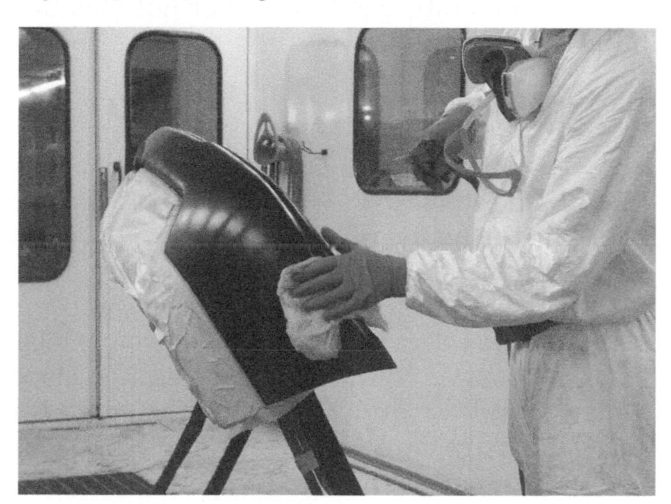

Figure 16–7. Wipe repair surfaces down with a tack rag while blowing with an air nozzle or the spray gun.

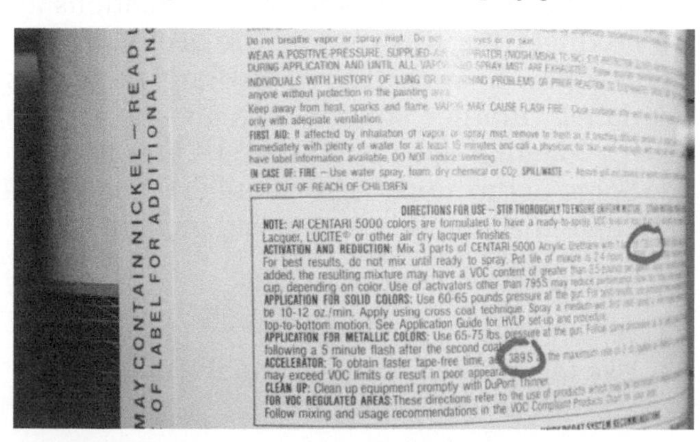

Figure 16–8. Always read finishing material direction. The label will give mixing and application information for the specific material to be sprayed.

to use a viscosity cup to check for proper material thickness or fluidity.

Make sure the material is mixed thoroughly. See **Figure 16–9.** A wide, flat bottom, stirring paddle or steel spatula of at least 1 inch (25 mm) works well. You can also use a mixing machine

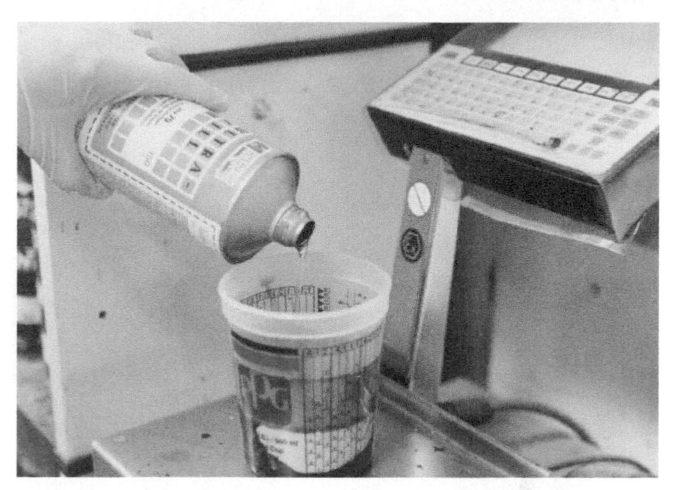

(A) Here a technician is using a computerized scale to add the recommended ingredients for the specific paint color.

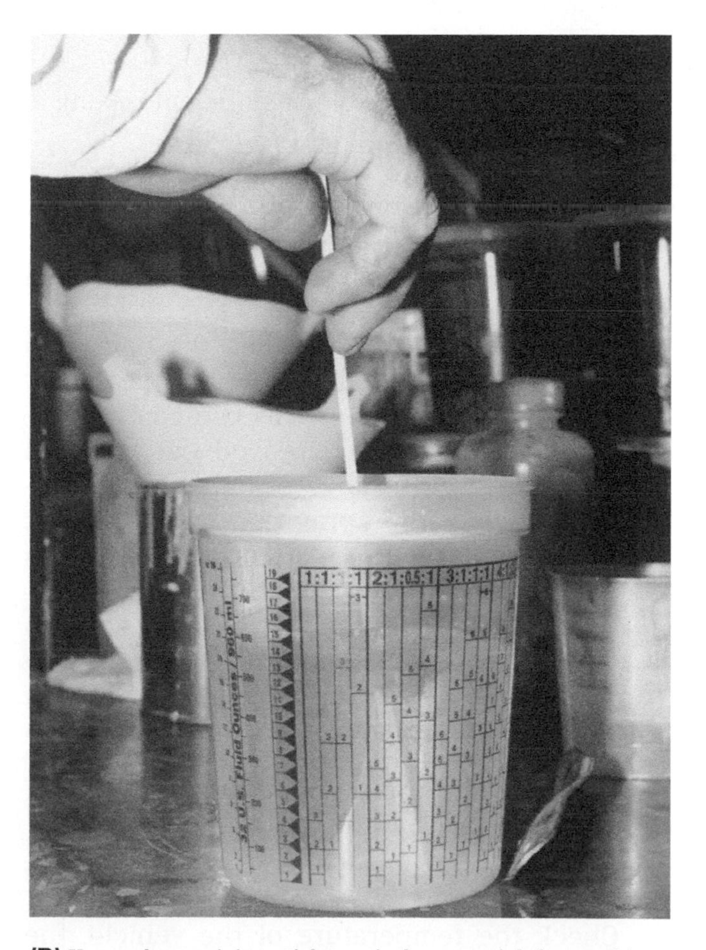

(B) Use a clean mixing stick to stir the material thoroughly.

Figure 16–9. Proper paint mixing is essential to a good paint job.

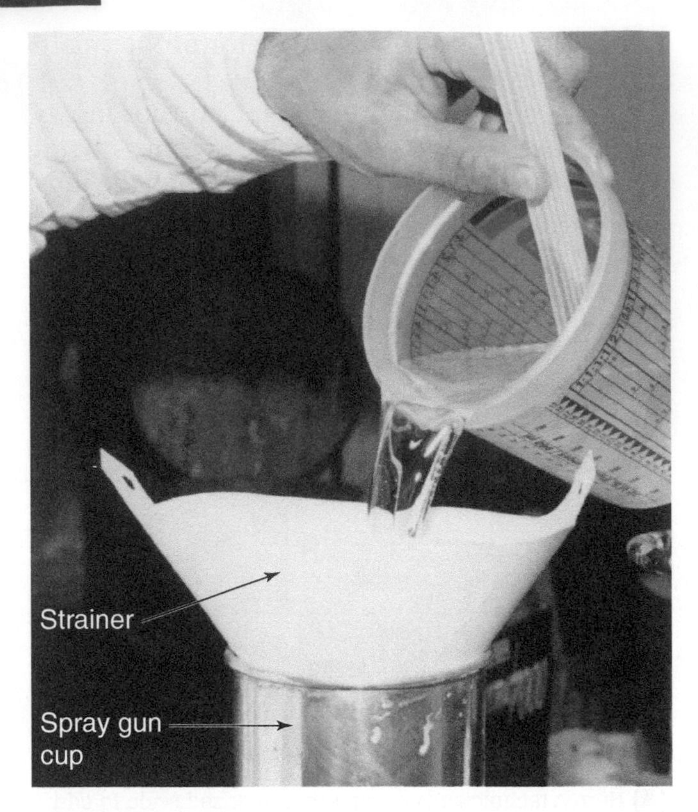

Figure 16–10. Filter all material being poured into your spray gun. This is "a must" to prevent paint problems.

(shaker) if one is available. Insufficient mixing is a common reason for paint problems.

Use a strainer to filter the material as it is poured into the spray gun. See **Figure 16–10.** This will remove any larger particles that might have entered the mixing container and would cause paint problems.

Paint settling occurs when the paint sits idle and pigments, metallic flakes, or mica particles settle to the bottom. This can cause problems because the color sprayed out first will contain a high percentage of these heavier ingredients. When the spray gun cup is almost empty, the paint will be lighter and have less metallic or mica in it.

Remember! If a color with heavy pigments is allowed to stand in your spray gun for 10 to 15 minutes without being stirred, the pigment will settle. This can cause color variations when sprayed.

Check that spray gun air pressure is correct. Perform a spray test pattern on a sheet of paper. Make sure the spray gun is working properly before applying paint to the vehicle.

Check the temperature of the vehicle, the spray booth, and spray materials. Refer to **Figure 16–11.** They should all be equalized and

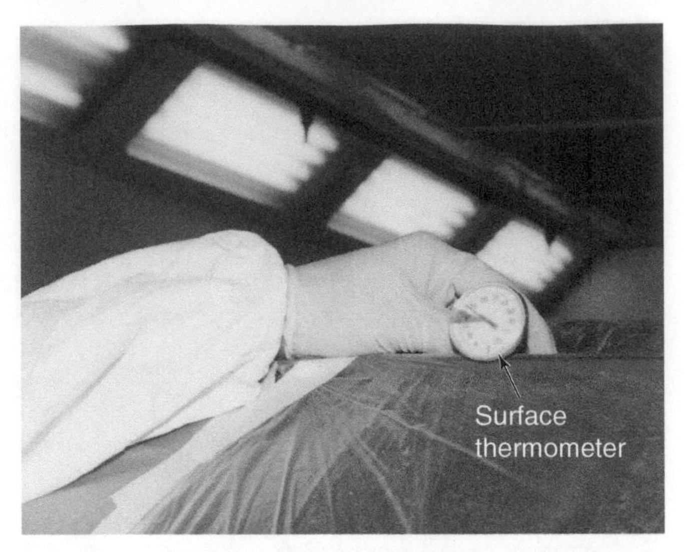

Figure 16–11. The technician is checking the surface temperature of a vehicle with a small thermometer. Vehicle surface temperatures should be within the range specified by the paint manufacturer.

within specs. Use a thermometer to check the surface temperature of the vehicle. If vehicle surface temperature is too cold or hot, painting problems will result.

REVIEW OF PAINT

The type of refinishing system or paint ultimately determines the attractiveness of the color, gloss, and overall finish. The type of paint also affects other variables.

Most vehicles are refinished with *acrylic urethane enamel* with a hardener or catalyst. A color basecoat is covered with a clearcoat to produce a high gloss, yet durable finish. The hardener helps the paint cure so that the vehicle can be released to the customer in less time.

Before applying the paint, carefully read the paint manufacturer's directions that appear on the paint can. Each has specific formulations for its products. For this reason, the best source of data on how to apply a specific brand of paint is the label. Another source of good information can be found in the manufacturer's literature.

Some of the more important label and literature data that should be checked include:

1. Viscosity recommendations
2. Air pressure recommendations
3. Use of additives, reducers, solvents, activators, and hardeners
4. Application techniques
5. Number of coats required

6. Blending and mist coat procedures
7. Polishing and compounding recommendations
8. Cleanup procedures

Make sure you are using the correct type of refinishing materials for the job. Refer to the paint code information on the body plate to find the correct paint color and type needed. The *body ID number* or *service part number* gives information about how the vehicle is equipped. It will give paint codes or numbers for ordering the right type and color paint. Lower and upper body colors will be given if it is a two-tone paint. The body ID number will also give trim information. This number will be on the body ID plate on the door, console lid, or elsewhere on the body.

Typical locations for paint codes are shown in **Figure 16–12.** An example of an actual body ID plate is given in **Figure 16–13.**

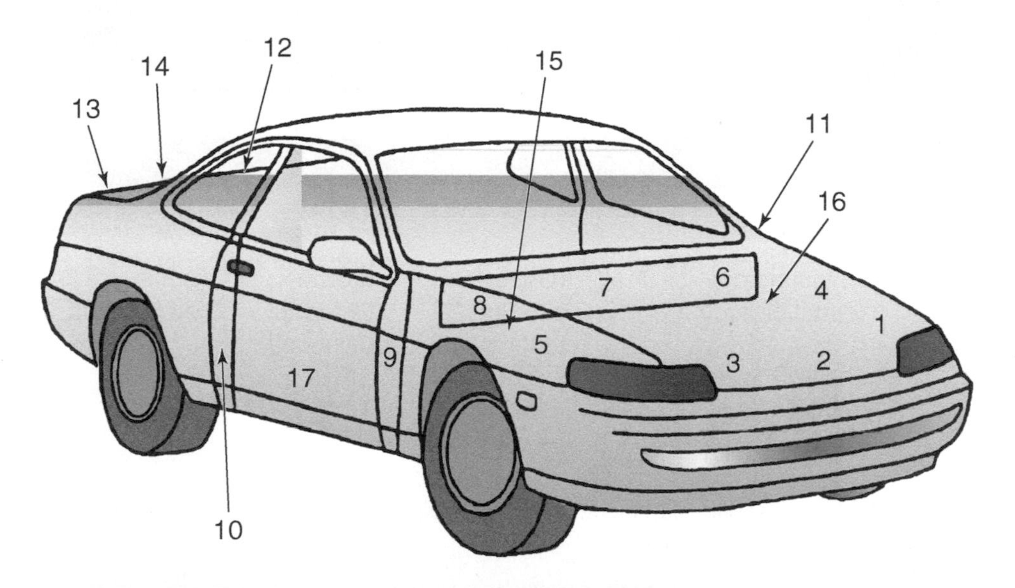

Model	Position	Model	Position
Acura	9	Honda	8,10
Alfa Romeo	4,13	Hyundai	6,7
AMC	9,10	Isuzu	2,10
Audi	12,13	Lexus	7,8
Austin Rover	17	Mazda	1,2,3,4,6,8
BMW	4,5	Mercedes	2,7,9
Chrysler	3,5,16	Mitsubishi	7
Chrysler Corp.	3,5	Montero/Pickup	3
Caravan/Voyager/Ram Van	6	Cordia/Tredia	4
Chrysler Imports	1,2,4	Others	1,2,3
Colt Vista	16	Nissan	1,3,4,6,8,15,*
Conquest	7	Peugeot	2,3,4,5,8
Daihatsu	1,6,7	Porsche	9
Datsun	2	Renault	1,3,4,5,8
Dodge D50	3	Rover	1,3,4,5
Ford	10	Saab	5,6,8
Ford Motor Co.	10	Subaru	2
General Motors		Suzuki	7,11
A, J and L Bodies	14	Toyota Passenger	7,8,14
E and K Bodies	12	Truck	4
B,C,H and N Bodies	13	Volkswagen	2,11
GM Imports	2,12,13,14	Volvo	6,7,8
		Yugo	12

* Under right front passenger seat

Figure 16–12. This chart shows typical locations for paint codes for major makes of vehicles. (Courtesy of Mitchell International, Inc.)

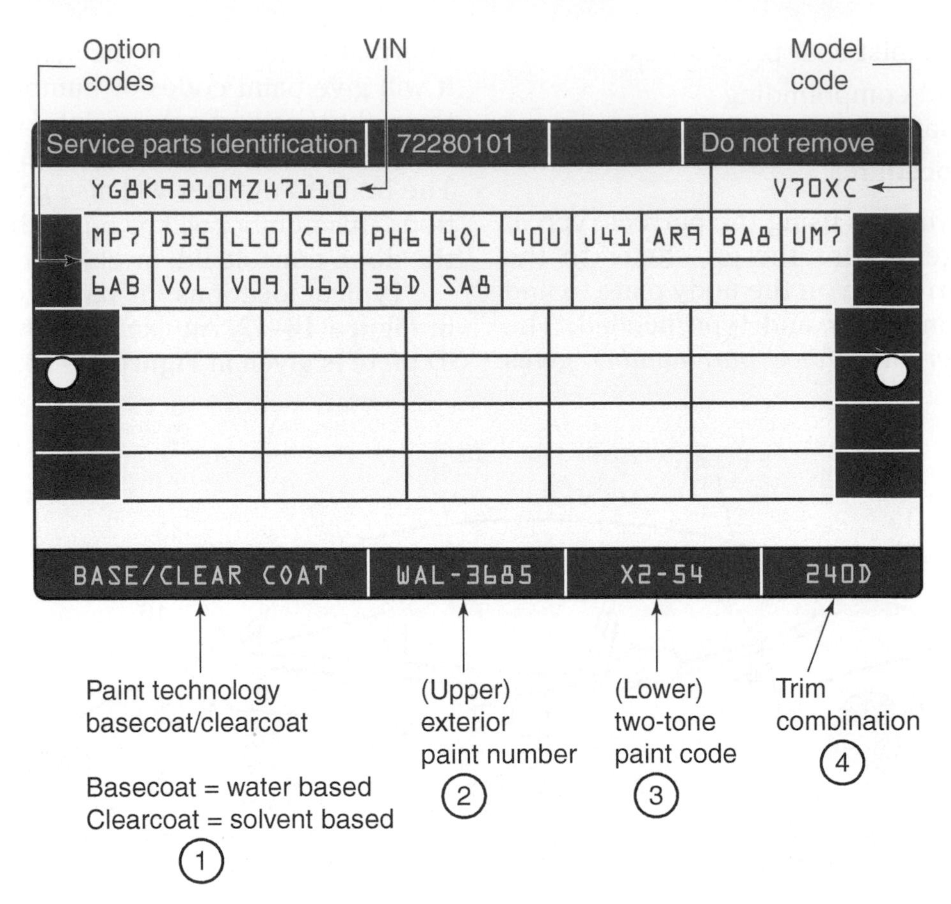

Figure 16–13. The body ID plate or service parts identification plate gives VIN and other data about the vehicle. Note the paint and trim code numbers.

DETERMINING TYPE OF FINISH

Before planning any refinishing job, you must find out what type of paint is on the vehicle. The vehicle might have its original finish, or it could have been repainted with a different type paint. Methods for finding out the type of paint on a vehicle include the following:

1. With the *solvent application method,* rub the paint with a white cloth soaked in lacquer thinner to see how easily the paint will dissolve. If the paint film dissolves and leaves a mark on the rag, it is a type of air-dried paint. If it does not dissolve, it is either an oven-dried or a two-part reaction type paint. Acrylic urethane paint film will not dissolve as easily as an air-dried paint, but sometimes the thinner will penetrate sufficiently to blur the paint gloss.
2. With a *heat application method,* wet sand an area with No. 2,000 grit sandpaper to dull the paint film. Then heat the area with an infrared lamp. If a gloss returns to the dulled appearance, the paint is acrylic lacquer.
3. With the *hardness method,* you must check the general hardness of the paint. Paints do not dry to the same hardness. Generally, two-part reaction and oven-dried paints dry to a harder film than air-dried paint.
4. With an *inspection method,* inspect closely for signs of repainting. Look for masking tape–created paint lines, overspray, and other signs of repairing. If the vehicle has not been repainted, you can use the body color code identification plate to determine the type of paint on the vehicle.

SPRAY GUN APPLICATION STROKE

The **application stroke** is a side-to-side movement of the spray gun to distribute the mist properly on the vehicle. The proper stroke is critical to the vehicle finish. Practice on masking paper. Any problems with the spray pattern must be corrected before painting the vehicle. Look at **Figure 16–14.**

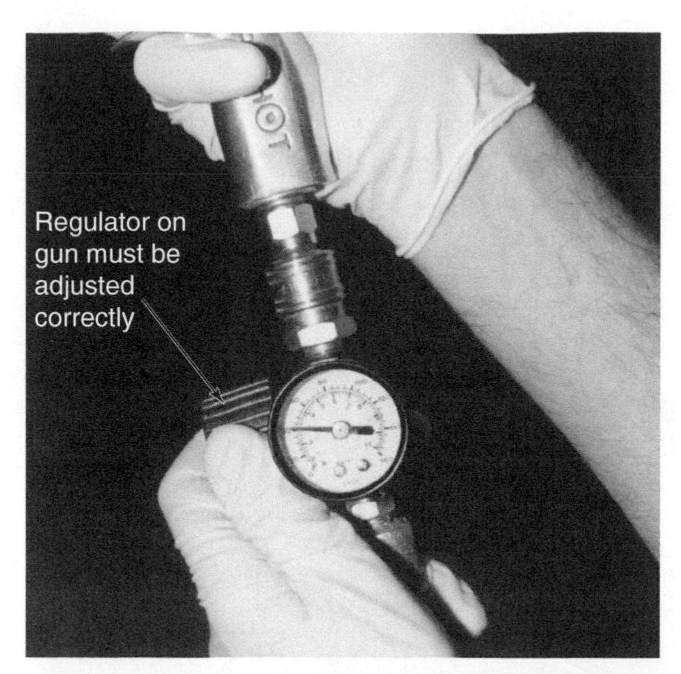
Regulator on
gun must be
adjusted
correctly

(A) Make sure air pressure to the spray gun is correct. Refer to recommendations from the spray gun and paint manufacturer.

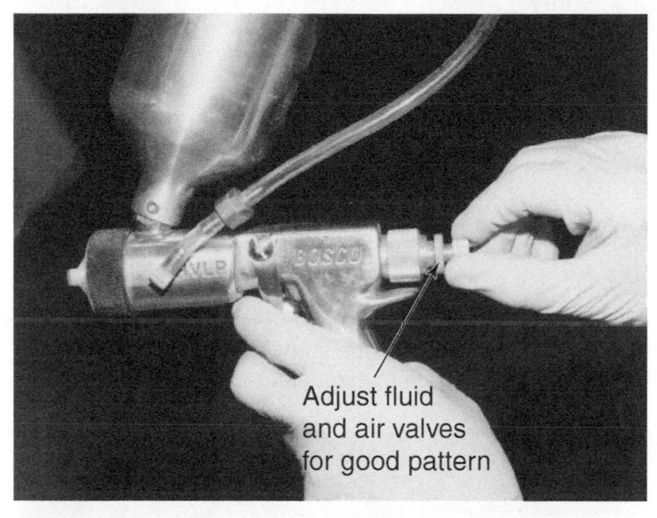
Adjust fluid
and air valves
for good pattern

(B) Adjust the spray gun fluid and air valves before spraying the vehicle.

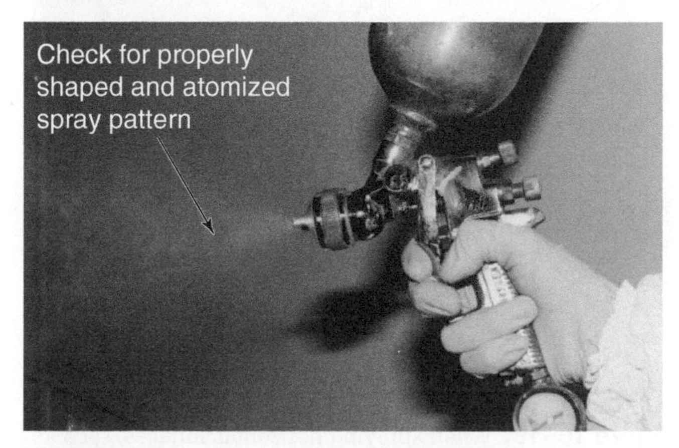
Check for properly
shaped and atomized
spray pattern

(C) Trigger the gun to check that the spray pattern is acceptable and that the gun is not spitting or leaking.

Figure 16–14. Check paint gun adjustments before trying to spray the vehicle body.

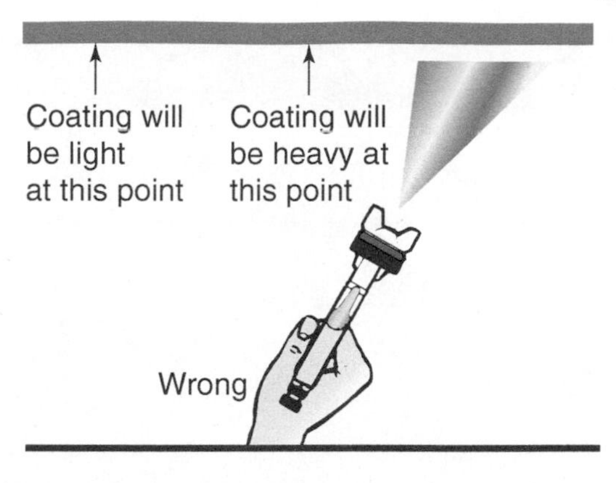
Coating will
be light
at this point
Coating will
be heavy at
this point
Wrong

(A) Wrong! If you fan the gun, the paint film will be thicker in the middle and thinner, drier on the sides. Only fan the spray gun when you want to blend and thin out the paint film.

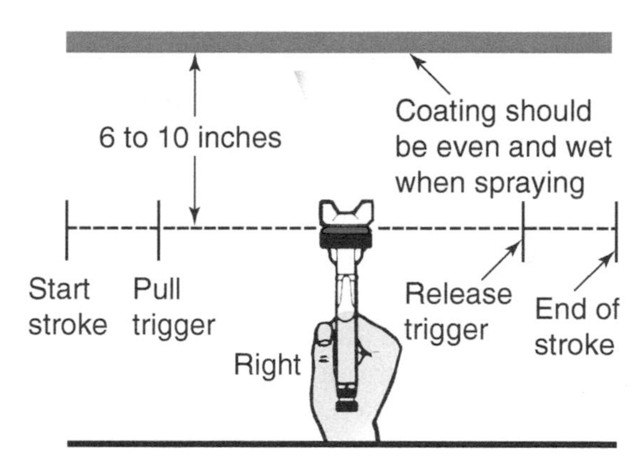
6 to 10 inches
Coating should
be even and wet
when spraying
Start
stroke
Pull
trigger
Right
Release
trigger
End of
stroke

(B) Right! Like a machine, hold the gun perfectly straight and at an equal distance from the surface as you move it sideways. Release the trigger before the end of each stroke.

Figure 16–15. Note the right and wrong ways of using a spray gun. (Illustration courtesy of ITW Automotive Refinishing, 1-800-445-3988)

To use a spray gun, hold the gun at the proper distance from the surface. Refer to **Figure 16–15.** **Spray gun distance** is measured from the gun tip to the surface being painted. Typically, hold the gun 6 to 8 inches (152 to 203 mm) away for lacquer and 8 to 10 inches (203 to 254 mm) away from the surface for enamel.

A **short spray distance** causes the high velocity mist to ripple the wet film. A **long spray distance** causes a greater percentage of the thinner to evaporate, resulting in orange peel or dry spray. See **Figure 16–16.**

A slower-drying thinner will permit more variation in the distance of the gun from the surface. However, it will produce runs if the gun gets too close. Excessive spraying distance also causes more overspray.

Spray gun angle refers to whether the gun is tilted up or down or sideways. Normally, hold

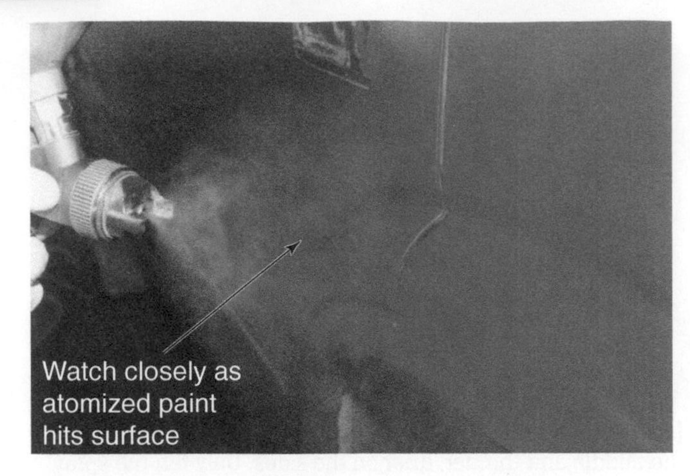

Figure 16–16. This photo shows how a spray gun atomizes paint into a fine mist that deposits smoothly on the vehicle surface.

the gun parallel and perpendicular to the surface. Keep the gun at a right angle to the vehicle. This should be done even when spraying curves in the body. Refer to **Figure 16–17.**

If you tilt the gun when spraying the sides of the vehicle, an uneven paint film will result. See **Figure 16–18.** On flat surfaces such as the hood or roof, the gun should be pointed almost straight down, as shown in **Figure 16–19.**

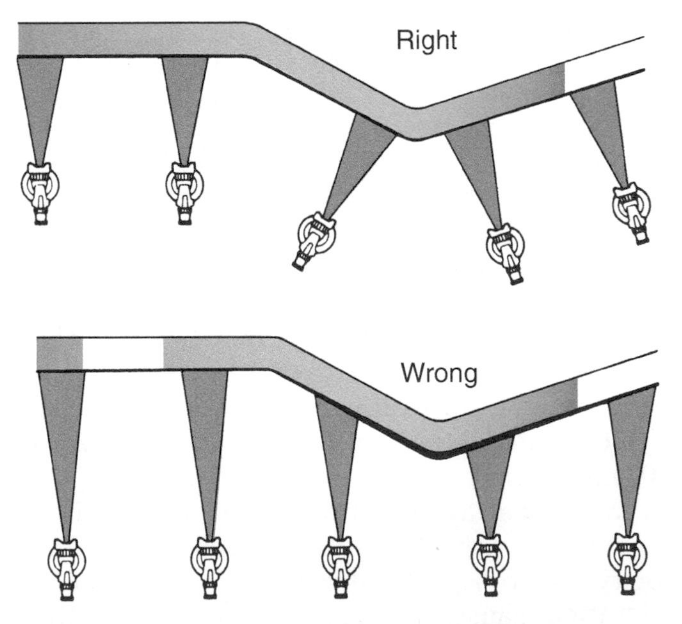

Figure 16–17. During normal painting, the spray gun should always be aimed directly at the surface and kept at an equal distance from the surface. If the surface curves, redirect the spray gun to spray right at the surface. **Right** The spray gun is rotated so that it stays aimed right at the surface. Note that the correct distance from the surface is also maintained. **Wrong** Since the spray gun is not kept aimed at the surface and distance decreases at the curved surface, the paint would be too thick at the curve. Run or sag might result.

WARNING

When painting a hood, roof, or deck lid, the spray gun cup must NOT leak. If the seal around the cup is faulty, paint will drip out of the gun and onto the vehicle. If the drip will NOT flow out, you might have to sand and repaint the panel.

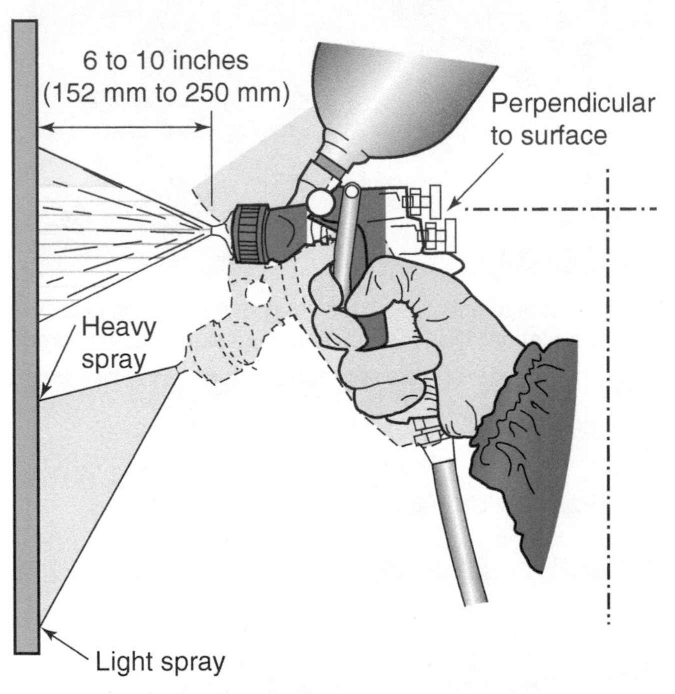

Figure 16–18. Do not let the spray gun tilt up or down. This would also result in uneven paint film.

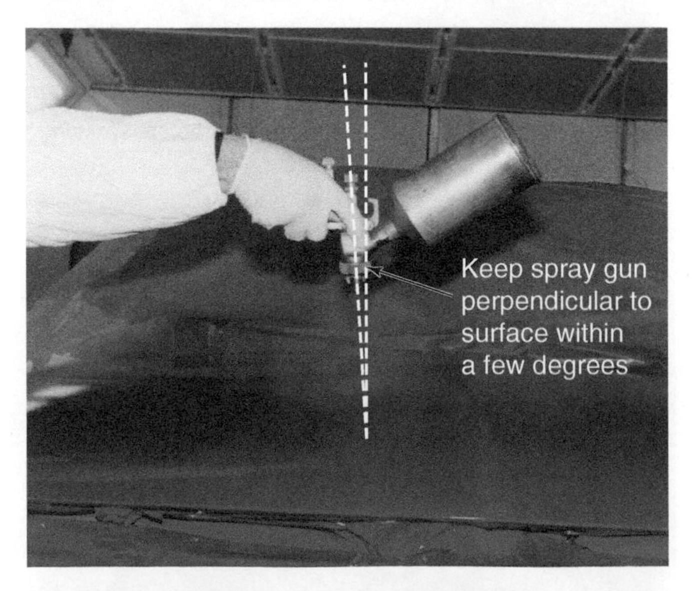

Figure 16–19. When spraying horizontal surfaces, such as the hood, roof, or trunk, hold the spray gun almost straight down. This will ensure that the pattern applies evenly to the surface. Make sure the cup is not leaking and cannot drip on the surface.

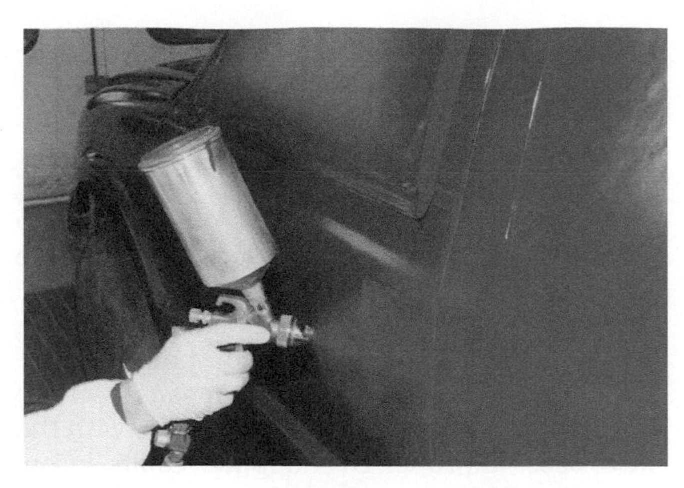

Figure 16–20. Normally, keep the spray gun aimed straight at the surface. Do not fan the gun unless you are blending the paint out over the next panel.

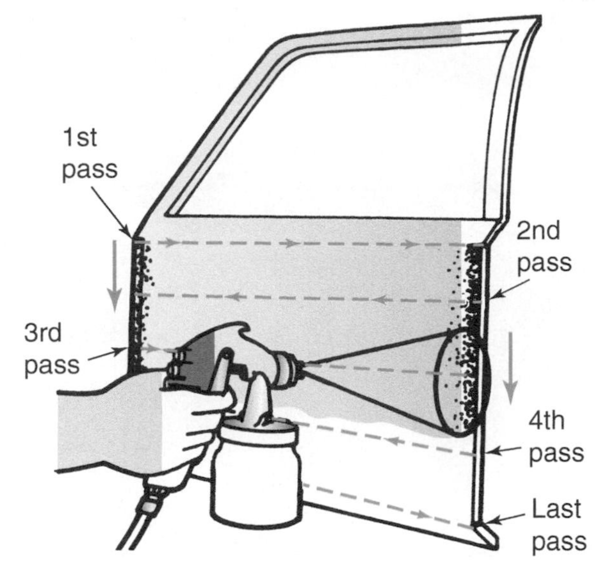

Figure 16–21. A banding or edge coat ensures that edges or ends of the panel receive enough coverage. After making banding coats on the edges, follow the arrows to spray the rest of the door or panel.

Avoid fanning the gun with your wrist. Fanning the gun will deposit an uneven paint film. The paint film will be thicker right in front of your gun and thinner on the sides. The only time it is permissible to fan the gun is when blending a small repair spot. With a spot repair, you want the paint film thinner at the edges to blend out the spray. See **Figure 16–20.**

Spray gun triggering involves stopping the paint spray before you stop moving the gun sideways. When you pull halfway back on the trigger, only air blows out of the nozzle. When you pull all the way back, material is atomized and sprayed out.

During the application stroke, release halfway on the trigger right before you stop moving the gun sideways. This will prevent too much material being deposited when the gun changes direction. It will also keep air moving through the nozzle to help prevent a sudden burst of paint. Release the trigger halfway at the end of each pass, then pull it back when beginning the pass in the opposite direction.

Spray gun speed refers to how fast the gun is moved sideways while spraying. Move the gun with a steady, deliberate pass, about 1 foot (0.3 m) per second. The speed must be consistent or it will result in an uneven paint film. If you move the gun too quickly, not enough paint will be deposited on the surface. If you move too slowly, too much paint will deposit on the surface. Never stop the gun while spraying, or a paint sag and run will result.

A **banding coat** is done to deposit enough paint on edges or corners of surfaces. Spray these difficult areas first. Refer to **Figure 16–21.** Aim directly at the corner or edge so that half of the spray covers each side of the corner or edge. Hold the gun an inch or 2 (25–50 mm) closer than usual while moving the gun up or down along the edge. After all of the edges and corners have been sprayed, spray the face or front of the panel.

Generally, start spraying at the top of any upright surface, such as a door panel. The gun nozzle should be level with the top of the panel. The upper half of the spray pattern should hit and cover the masking paper. Move the gun all the way across the top of the panel. Make sure you hold the gun square with the panel and keep it the same distance from the panel.

Overlap strokes involve making each spray gun coat cover about half of the previous coat of paint. Make each pass in the opposite direction. Keep the nozzle level with the lower edge of the previous pass. Thus, one half of the spray pattern overlaps the previous coat. The other half of the paint pattern is applied to the unpainted area.

Always blend your paint into the "wet edge" of the previously sprayed section. If you allow the wet edge to dry or cure too much before painting the panel next to it, an unwanted dry band of paint may occur where the two panels meet. By always spraying into the wet edge where you just painted, the paint will tend to melt together and not form a dry band.

Proper triggering where the sections meet will avoid a double coat and the possibility of paint sags or runs.

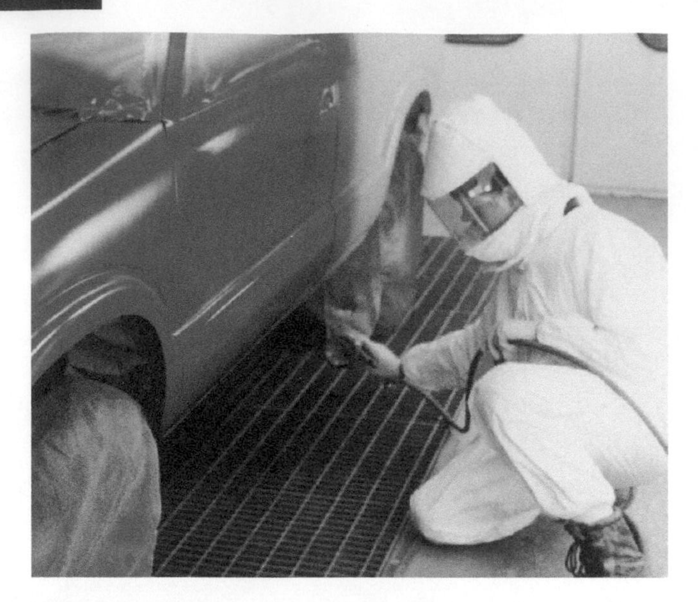

Figure 16–22. Make sure you apply enough color to the bottoms of panels. The spray gun may have to tilt upward to get under lower panels, like this rocker panel.

Continue the back-and-forth passes. Trigger the gun at the end of each pass and lower each successive pass one-half the top-to-bottom width of the spray pattern. Make your last pass with the lower half of the spray pattern hitting below the surface being painted. This will ensure enough paint film thickness at the bottom of the panel. Refer to **Figure 16–22.**

For a double coat, repeat the previous procedure. Allow flash time of several minutes between coats.

Two or three single coats may be required for clear paints. Allow the first coat to set up or become tacky before applying additional coats. Refer to the paint label for details.

For painting very narrow surfaces, switch to a gun with a smaller spray pattern. This can also be accomplished by reducing the air pressure and spray pattern on a full-size gun.

GUN HANDLING PROBLEMS

The inexperienced painting technician is prone to making spraying errors. These include the following:

Gun heeling occurs when the gun is allowed to tilt. Because the gun is no longer perpendicular to the surface, the spray produces uneven film thickness, excessive overspray, dry spray, and orange peel.

Gun arching occurs when the gun is NOT moved parallel to the surface. At the outer edges of the stroke, the gun is farther away from the surface than at the middle of the stroke. The result is uneven film thickness, paint runs, excessive overspray, dry spray, and orange peel.

Incorrect gun stroke speed means you are moving the gun too slowly or too quickly. If the stroke is made too quickly, the paint will NOT cover the surface evenly. If the stroke is made too slowly, sags and runs will develop. Proper stroke speed is something that comes with experience. Generally, you must watch the paint go onto the surface to carefully watch for a proper coat.

Improper spray overlap means you are NOT covering half of the previous pass with the next pass. Improper overlapping results in uneven film thickness, contrasting color hues, and sags and runs. If you overlap coats too much, the paint can run. If you do NOT overlap enough, poor coverage can result.

Improper coverage means the paint film thickness is NOT uniform or it is too thin. This is caused by NOT triggering exactly over the edge of the panel or from improper spray overlap.

TYPES OF SPRAY COATS

There are varying degrees of thickness for a spray coat: light, medium, or heavy. The easiest way to control thickness is by changing how fast you move the gun sideways. If you move the gun slower, a heavier, thicker coat will be applied. If you move more quickly, film thickness is decreased.

A *light coat* is usually produced by moving the spray gun a little more quickly across the surface of the vehicle. A thinner-than-normal coating of paint film will be deposited on the surface. A light coat is sometimes used when applying the colorcoat. The colorcoat can go on light, without a gloss. This will help you blend the new finish into the existing one with a less dramatic change of color. It will also distribute any metallic flakes more evenly. The wetter clearcoats will give the colorcoat its gloss.

A *medium wet coat* is produced by moving your spray gun at a normal speed over the surface being refinished. This is the most common coat used by the professional painter. It will produce a medium gloss with adequate coverage and will avoid runs and sags. A medium wet coat is the most common coat recommended by paint manufacturers on colorcoats and initial clearcoats.

A **full wet coat** is done by moving the spray gun slightly slower than normal. It will deposit more paint on the surface. A full wet coat is used when applying the final layer of clearcoat or single-stage colors. It is important that the last coat of clearcoat goes on wet to produce a high gloss or shine. Spraying a full wet coat requires skill and practice to prevent runs. The wet coat makes the paint lie down smooth and shiny. It prevents a dull, textured "orange peel" type paint film.

A *mist coat,* also called **dust coat,** *drop coat,* or **tack coat,** is a very light, thin coat. The spray gun pressure is reduced and it is held a little farther from the surface and moved more quickly from side to side. The mist coat cures or dries in a short period of time to bond and form a lightly textured paint film.

Mist coats can be used and are recommended to help avoid problems (mottling and blotching) with metallic paints. For example, some paint manufacturers recommend a mist coat as the last colorcoat with some metallics. Some painters also mist coat the first layer of clearcoat on troublesome metallics (troublesome silver and gold metallics) to prevent movement of the colorcoat flakes, which could affect paint matching.

Shading coats or *blend coats* are progressive applications of paint on the boundary of spot repair areas so that a color difference is not noticeable. They are applied in two or more coats. The second and third coats are lighter and sprayed over a wider area than the first.

PAINT BLENDING

Paint blending involves tapering or fanning the new paint gradually into the old paint to provide a smooth transition between the two finishes. This makes any difference in the new paint color or texture less noticeable. It helps hide any slight differences between the new and existing paints. Blending is the key to a successful spot repair. Look at **Figure 16–23.**

To blend paint, apply the colorcoat (basecoat-clearcoat) or topcoat (single-stage paint) with a fanning motion, working from the center outward. This allows each coat to be thinner at its outer perimeter and to blend out a bit farther than the previous one. Where the old and new paints meet, the existing paint will be visible through the thin layer of newly fanned paint. Any differences will be difficult to detect.

If you do NOT blend the paint, a marked contrast in paint color and texture will normally be obvious. Paint blending is commonly done when applying the colorcoat on a spot repair. The colorcoat is applied only where needed to the repair area. The undamaged colorcoat is not painted. Then, when the whole panel is sprayed with the clearcoat, the old and new colors will show through the clearcoat. Any minute difference in the colorcoats will not be noticeable and more of the vehicle will retain its original color.

An alternative method is to apply the finish in short strokes from the center outward. Again, extend each coat so that it blends out farther than the previous one.

With either method, the spray pattern should be narrowed and the fluid delivery reduced. To minimize overspray, the air pressure may also have to be reduced, depending on the material being sprayed.

REFINISHING METHODS

Refinishing methods are selected according to several variables:

1. Condition of the original finish
2. Size of the area to be finished
3. Location of the repair on the vehicle

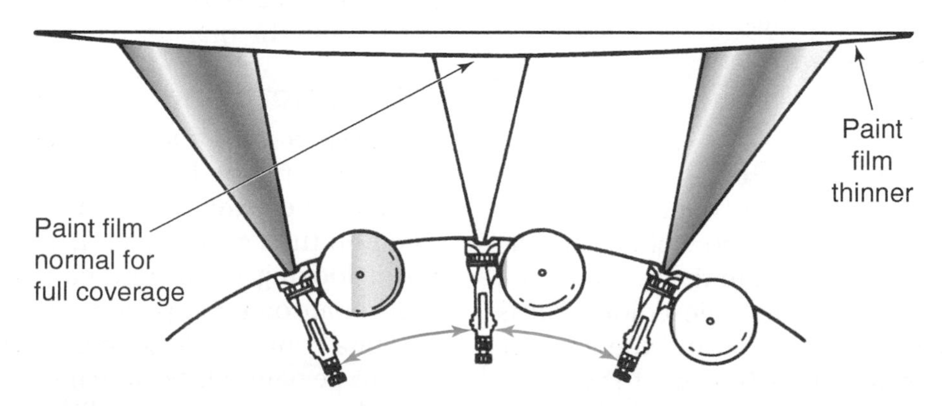

Figure 16–23. This view shows how fanning the spray gun at the wrist will blend the paint thinner near the outer edges of the repair area. Work the gun from the center outward. When the paint is thinner, it will gradually blend into the existing paint to hide the repairs.

From these variables, you must determine how much of the vehicle must be painted/refinished. The three categories of finish repair are spot repair (area of panel painted); panel repair (complete panel painted); and overall refinishing (whole vehicle painted).

SPOT REPAIRS

Spot repair involves painting an area smaller than the panel. The paint must be blended out to match the existing finish.

Spot repair generally involves:

1. Minor body repair
2. Application of primer or primer-surfacer.
3. Application of paint (colorcoat/clearcoat) to blend into the old finish surrounding the repair

Spot repairs are recommended where a complete panel repair is either uneconomical or impractical. This might be due to the tiny size of the damage, its hidden location, or another factor. It is also commonly used when two large panels have no break line. For example, when painting a quarter panel, the paint is blended into the sail panel where the roof joins the quarter panel. Look at **Figure 16–24.**

Solid Color Spot Repairs

You must use experience and common sense when deciding the range of blending needed for spot repairs with solid colors. Blending with a solid color of paint is used for situations such as light damage to the fender edge.

In this case, there are two methods of blending: at the hood-to-fender gap and at the body line. When blending at a body line, you do NOT have to paint the upper portion of the fender where paint shading shows more. This can help avoid problems with color and texture differences.

Metallic Color Spot Repairs

Matching metallic colors is complicated because you have to match the color and the density of the metallic flakes in the paint. If spot repairs are done with a metallic color, skill is required in matching the color and the metallic flakes through proper distribution of the paint. The blend area will be less noticeable if it is angled away from the body line.

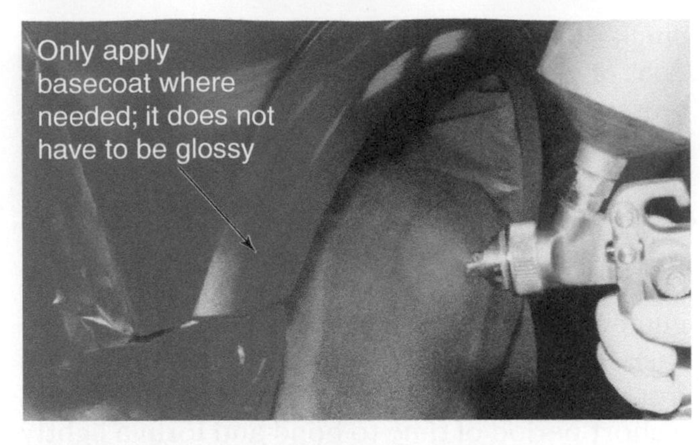

(A) Apply basecoat to the repaired area.

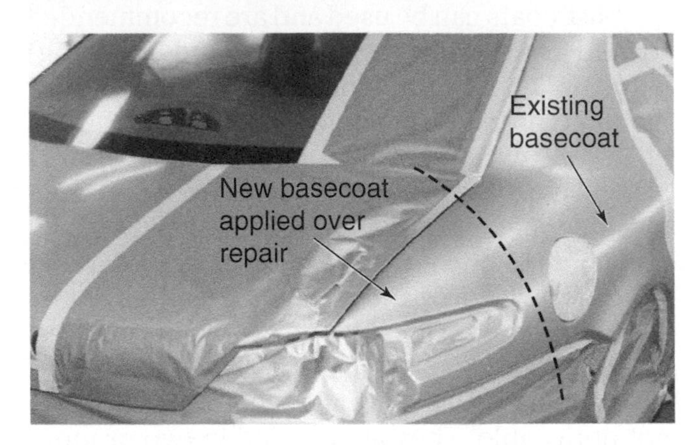

(B) Apply basecoat to the area just beyond the repaired area, and then apply clearcoat to the entire quarter panel.

Figure 16–24. Study how to spot repair a quarter panel.

PANEL REPAIRS

Panel repairs involve painting/refinishing a complete body part separated by a definite boundary, such as a door or fender. Usually, you do NOT have to blend the paint with panel repairs. Blending is only needed when it is difficult to match the paint, as with a metallic color. However, blending is routinely done for such areas as between the quarter panel and roof panel.

Solid Color Panel Repairs

Panel repair with a solid color covers an entire panel (door, hood, etc.). The color match is made at the panel joints. Panel repair is more common than spot repair. It usually results in a better looking repair and can be just as fast as spot repair on most panels.

For a complete panel repair, mask off the area NOT to be painted, as shown in **Figure 16–25.** If a panel has damage at two different locations, the whole panel should be repaired. Blending can

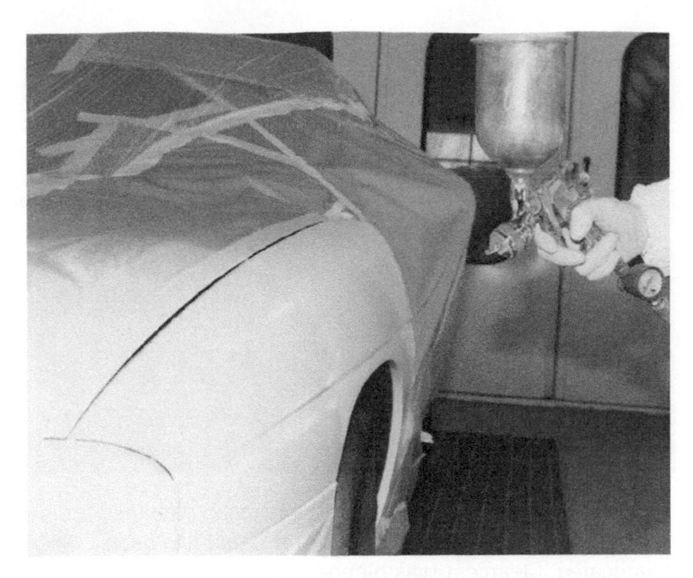

Figure 16–25. This technician is doing a complete panel repair on the front fender.

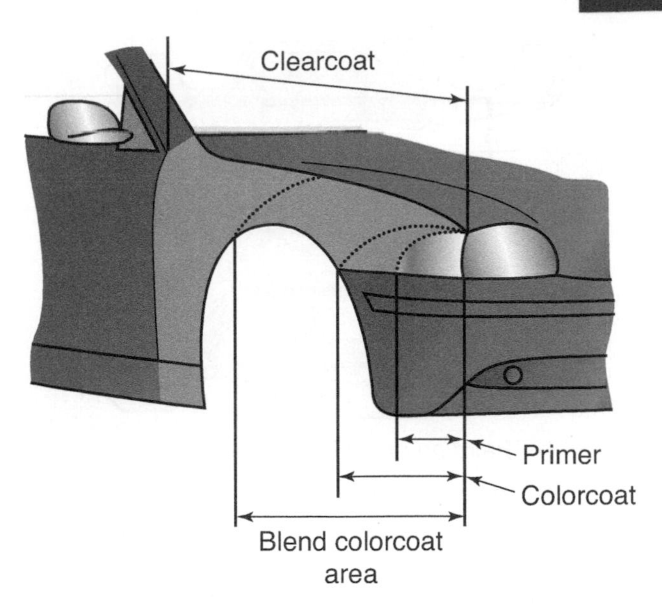

Figure 16–26. Note how to do a panel repair with a colorcoat-clearcoat paint. Colorcoat is applied and blended over the filler or repair area only. Then the whole fender must be sprayed with clearcoat to make the old and new colorcoats match.

be done to the molding or extended below the molding.

When blending new color into old, you must use common sense to determine where to blend the paint. Try to find a body section that gives a natural break line or small area for blending.

Metallic Color Panel Repairs

New and old paint differences tend to be very noticeable with bright metallic colors. It is almost impossible to match the new metallic finish exactly with the previous one. You must extend the blending over a wide area to help hide the differences. This will make the repair less visible. See **Figure 16–26.**

If a panel has damage at both ends, or if the whole panel is to be refinished, the blending may have to extend onto adjacent panels.

OVERALL REFINISHING

Overall refinishing involves painting/refinishing the whole vehicle. This is usually done when the surface has weathered and deteriorated. Surface prep is time consuming since the entire surface must be cleaned and sanded or scuffed. Any damage must be straightened. Also, all parts NOT to be painted (trim, glass, mirrors, etc.) must be masked or removed. There are several things you must remember when refinishing the whole vehicle.

For overall refinishing, keep a wet edge while maintaining minimal overspray on the horizontal surfaces. This prevents spray from settling onto dry surfaces, which would cause a gritty surface.

Avoid paint runs or sags by changing the point of overlap on each coat. **Paint overlap** refers to the area where one vertical painted area overlaps the new area being painted.

There is no universal sequence for overall refinishing of a vehicle. However, most experienced painting technicians agree that the following method is an excellent technique for nondowndraft spray booths.

Start by painting the roof, then the rear, then the driver's side, then the front, and finally the passenger side. It will produce minimum overspray on horizontal surfaces. This will also help keep a wet edge when starting a new section.

The term **wet edge** means that the area just sprayed will still be wet when starting on a new adjoining area.

When using a downdraft spray booth, overall paint sequence is different. See **Figure 16–27.** This is because of the direction of the airflow (top to bottom). Following this procedure allows the three main horizontal surfaces to remain wet while maintaining minimum overspray.

APPLYING BASECOAT-CLEARCOAT

Basecoat-clearcoat systems pose a major challenge to painting technicians. Since most vehicles now have basecoat-clearcoat finishes, it is very important to become familiar with them.

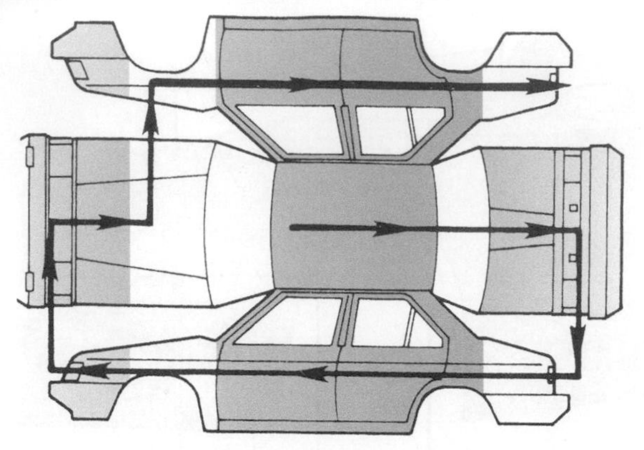

Figure 16–27. This is a typical sequence for doing an overall refinishing job when using a downdraft spray booth. Some painting technicians like to use a slightly different sequence.

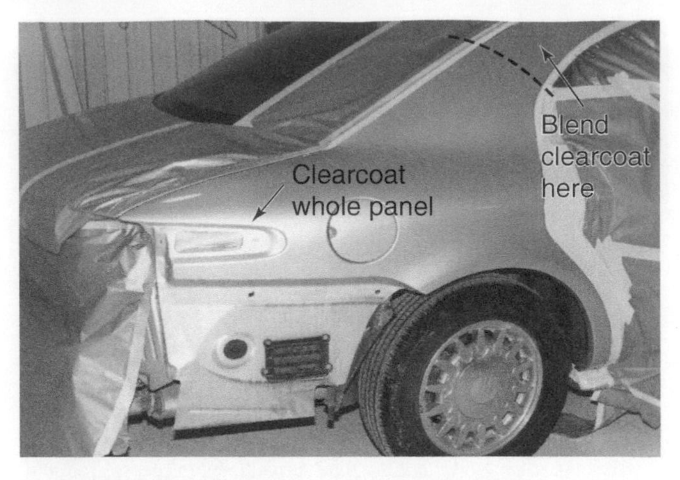

Figure 16–29. After colorcoating the small damaged area to cover the primer, the whole quarter panel has been clearcoated. Clearcoat was blended at the small sail panel area where the roof meets the quarter panel.

You must first spray the color basecoat over the repair or primed area. The basecoat does NOT have to be sprayed where the old color is acceptable. Blend the basecoat of color out around the repair. Then spray the whole panel with clear. This will normally make the old color and new basecoat blend and match.

When spraying, two medium coats of basecoat should be applied. The basecoat does NOT have to be glossy, and only enough should be used to achieve hiding. See **Figure 16–28.** Two or three medium wet coats of clear should be applied next. Allow at least 15 minutes flash time between coats.

Avoid sanding the basecoat. If sanding must be done because of dirt or imperfections, allow time for it to dry. Wet sanding with 800 to 1,200 grit sandpaper will minimize sand scratches. The sanded area must then be given another coat of basecoat to prevent streaking and mottling.

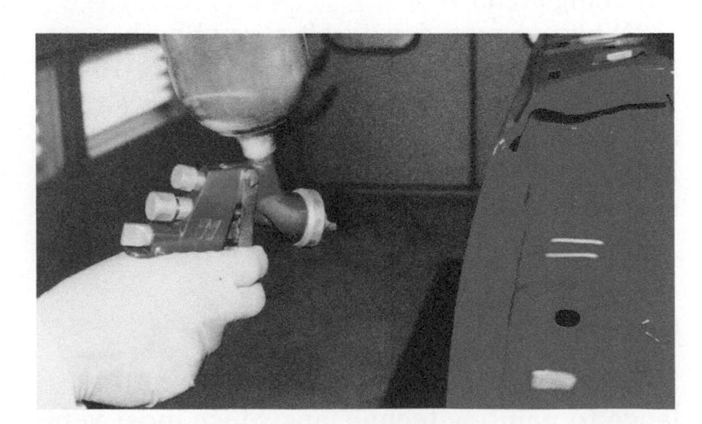

Figure 16–28. Colorcoats do not have to be glossy or shiny. Medium coats will help the new color match the existing color.

Several tips to remember when using basecoat-clearcoat finishes include:

1. On panel repairs, spray the basecoat only where needed. You do NOT have to basecoat the whole panel if the existing color is acceptable. Use as much of the existing color as possible to help avoid a color mismatch.
2. Do NOT load clearcoats on heavily. Because they are clear, it is easy to use too much trying to increase the desired glamour effect. As a result, the thick clear will "bury" the basecoat and hide the color.
3. Do NOT use over- or under-reduced clearcoats. Contrary to some opinions, clears do NOT perform better when they are under-reduced. Reduce clearcoats according to the label instructions. See **Figure 16–29.**

REFINISHING RULES

There are several rules you should remember when refinishing a vehicle. Ask yourself these questions and answer them before proceeding:

1. Are the vehicle surfaces straight and ready for refinishing? A common mistake is to overlook a surface problem. Since the surface is usually sanded dull, imperfections are easy to overlook. Double-check metal straightening work, body filler, and primer before proceeding. Even overlooking a small paint chip can ruin the job.

2. Are all surfaces perfectly clean and scuffed? Finish will NOT adhere to a dirty or glossy smooth surface. If the paint peels, you will have hours of rework. Blow off and tack-rag the vehicle before refinishing.
3. Are you working in an ideal environment? Are the spray booth and vehicle the right temperature? Are the booth filters and blower working properly? Do NOT try to paint a vehicle in an open shop. Dirt will almost always settle in the finish. Work only in a spray booth!
4. Is the mixing correct? Mix materials following label directions! Are all additives mixed into the paint? If you forget to add hardener, you will NOT be able to wet sand or buff the surface for weeks.
5. Is the spray gun working properly? Test and adjust the gun spray pattern on a sheet of paper or old part. If the gun is spitting or NOT working properly, you do NOT want to try to spray the vehicle. This would result in hours of rework.
6. Does the spray gun cup leak? A leaking cup can drip and ruin the job. You must tilt the gun down when spraying the roof, hood, and trunk lid. If the cup is leaking, material might drip out and onto these surfaces.
7. Are you allowing enough flash time between coats? Flash time is the time needed for a fresh coat of finish to partially dry. Flash time is needed to prevent the material from sagging or running.
8. Are you applying the material properly? Hold the gun the right distance from the surface, typically 8 to 10 inches (203 to 254 mm). Aim the gun directly at the surface while moving it at the correct speed. Do NOT fan the gun unless you are blending the paint.
9. Is the material going on the surface properly? Closely watch as it deposits on the surface. Check for application problems—dry coat, excessive wet coat, improper spray overlap, and so on. Constant inspection of the wet coat as it hits the surface is critical to doing high-quality work. Is the lighting good enough to see the material go onto all surfaces?
10. Are you applying the correct film thickness? A common mistake is to apply too much. Remember that "thin is in." You want to apply only enough material to provide good color coverage and gloss. Use the number of coats recommended by the manufacturer.
11. Could you accidentally touch the wet surface? Keep air hoses and yourself a safe distance away. It is easy to brush up against the wet finish and damage it.

REMOVAL OF MASKING MATERIALS

If the finish has been force dried, remove the masking tape while the finish is still warm. If the finish is allowed to cool, the tape will be difficult to remove. It can also leave adhesive behind.

Pull the tape slowly so that it comes off evenly. See **Figure 16–30.** Take care NOT to touch any painted areas, because the paint might not be completely dry. Fingerprints or tape marks could result.

If you used liquid masking material, wash it off with soap and water. Do NOT wash the freshly painted surfaces until they are fully dry.

WARNING

Never mask a vehicle and let it sit for a prolonged period. Also, do NOT let the masking paper and tape get wet. Either will cause problems. The tape edge can roll up and allow paint to spray onto parts NOT meant to be painted. Also, the tape can stick and be difficult to remove. You might have to carefully wash off the adhesive.

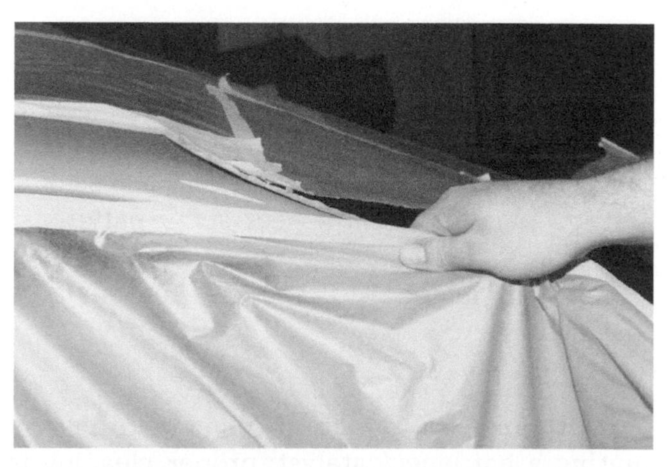

Figure 16–30. Remove masking tape slowly and pull it away form the new finish to keep it from peeling off new paint.

FINISHING URETHANE BUMPERS

Following is the procedure for finishing a colored urethane bumper:

1. Mask off the area to be finished. Clean it with a wax and grease remover. Insufficient cleaning will result in peeling or blistering.
2. Prepare the surface by wet sanding with 600 grit sandpaper.
3. Clean the surface again.
4. Apply the colorcoat over a section of or the entire bumper if needed. Use a two-part acrylic urethane with a flex agent added. For metallics, allow proper flash time after application. Then apply the clearcoat over the entire bumper.
5. Follow the drying time recommended by the manufacturer.

CLEANING THE SPRAY GUN

Like any precision piece of equipment, the refinisher's spray gun should be cleaned after use. Your livelihood depends on the proper care of your equipment, and your spray gun is a vital tool.

After you use a spray gun, always clean it and other equipment (mixing sticks, containers, viscosity cup, etc.) right away. Neglect and lack of care is responsible for most spray gun problems. Besides cleaning, you must also lubricate all bearing surfaces and packings at recommended intervals.

WARNING

If the gun is NOT cleaned right after use, passages will usually clog. When used the next time, the gun may spit (eject pieces of dried paint) or form a poor spray pattern. This is of particular importance when dealing with materials that have hardeners/activators.

With many of today's finishing materials requiring a hardener/catalyst, proper cleaning is essential. These painting/refinishing materials can set up (harden) in the spray gun. This could be a very expensive problem. Each spray gun MUST be properly and completely cleaned after each use.

DANGER

When cleaning spray guns, ALWAYS wear solvent-resistant gloves, proper eye protection, and an approved respirator. There are some painting/refinishing materials that pose a serious health risk!

SPRAY GUN CLEANING STEPS

1. Dispose of the remaining paint or refinishing materials in accordance with federal, state, and local laws and requirements.
2. Put a small amount of cleaning solvent into the paint cup.
3. Place the lid on the paint cup or place the paint cup on the bottom of the spray gun.
4. Shake the spray gun so that the cleaning solvent rinses the inside of the paint cup. On gravity-fed spray guns, pull the trigger all the way open and let some of the cleaning solvent come out of the spray gun and into a container for proper disposal later.
5. Remove the air cap. Take a cleaning brush and use some of the solvent in the paint cup to clean the air cap, fluid tip, and needle. See **Figure 16–31.**

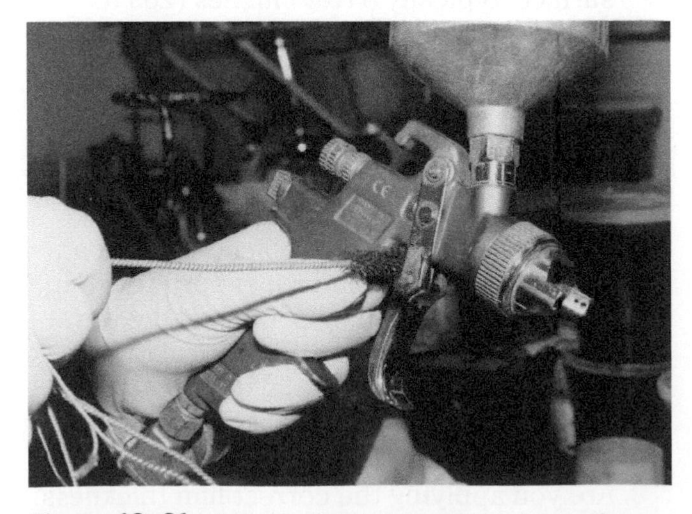

Figure 16–31. A small soft bristle brush can be used to keep the outside of the spray gun clean.

6. Reinstall the air cap.
7. Pour out the remaining (dirty) cleaning solvent into a container for proper disposal.
8. Place a small amount of fresh cleaning solvent in the paint cup.
9. While you are in the spray booth, spray this clean solvent through the spray gun.
10. Wipe the spray gun dry inside and out with a clean, dry, lint-free towel.

From time to time, every spray gun will need a more thorough cleaning. This will involve a full disassembly. For this type of cleaning, always refer to the spray gun manufacturer's instructions for the proper procedures.

Many shops have "automatic," or self-contained, spray gun cleaners. Since each one of these is different, always refer to the manufacturer's instructions. This will ensure proper cleaning of all spray equipment.

! WARNING !

Never use wire or nails to clean the precision opening in a spray gun. This could enlarge or damage the openings and affect spray gun operation.

To clean a pressure-feed spray gun, release the pressure in the cup first. Loosen the air cap. Then force the paint into the cup by triggering the spray gun. Empty the contents into a suitable container. Refill the cup with a clean, compatible solvent. The air cap can be left off. Spray the solvent out of the spray gun to wash out internal passages. If a tank is used, clean as directed by the manufacturer and reassemble.

Using a Spray Gun Washer

Areas in the United States with air pollution problems require the use of enclosed spray gun cleaning equipment. Spraying equipment (guns, cups, mixing sticks, and strainers) is placed in the tub of the **spray gun washer.** The spray gun washer will automatically clean them.

After the washer lid is closed, a pump circulates the solvent to clean the inside and outside of the equipment. In less than 60 seconds, the equipment is clean and ready for use. See **Figure 16–32.**

The spray gun washer saves time and increases safety. Compared with manual cleaning,

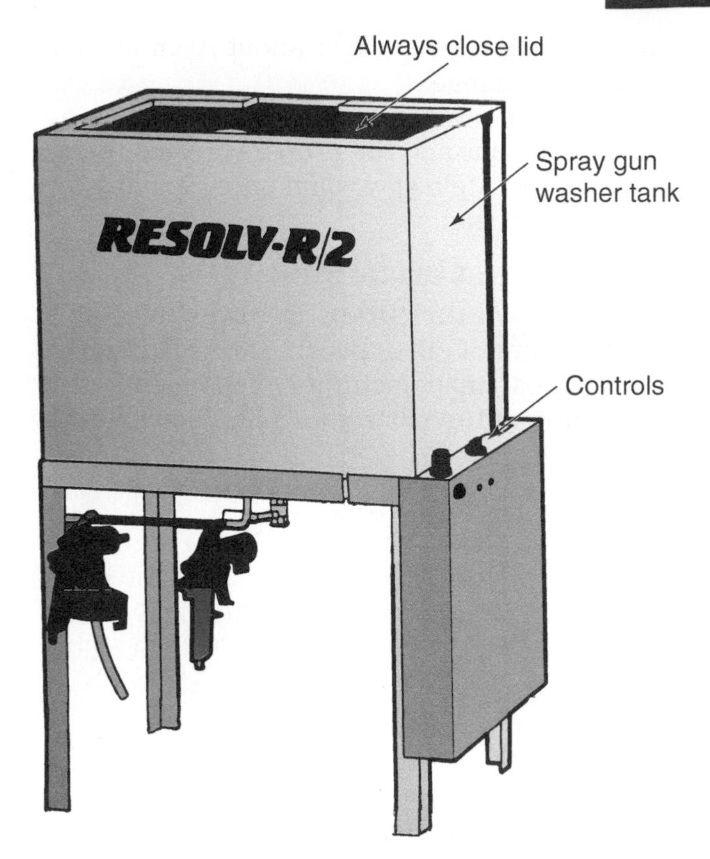

(A) A spray gun washer will quickly clean your spray equipment. Always keep the lid closed, even when it is not in use to keep solvent from evaporating.

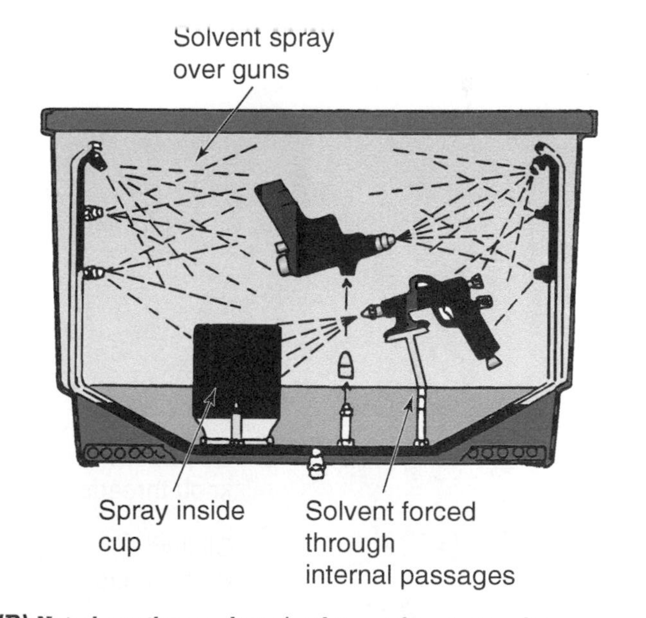

(B) Note how the washer circulates solvent over the outside of spray guns, inside the cup, and through internal passages. (Courtesy of PBR Industries)

Figure 16–32. To work properly, your spray gun must be maintained.

the spray gun washer saves about 10 minutes on each color change.

Check the owner's manual for complete operational details and the proper solvents to use. Always lubricate a spray gun after cleaning in a spray gun washer.

Spray Gun Lubrication

Spray gun lubrication involves placing a small amount of oil on packing and high friction points. Most manufacturers recommend daily lubrication of the parts shown in **Figure 16–33.**

> **WARNING**
>
> Do NOT overlubricate a spray gun. The excess oil could overflow into the fluid passages and mix with the paint. This could result in a defective paint job and "fisheyes" (small dimples in paint film).

Always examine the needle and nozzle periodically for excessive wear. Packings, springs, needles, and nozzles will have to be periodically replaced due to normal wear. This should be done only in accordance with the manufacturer's instructions.

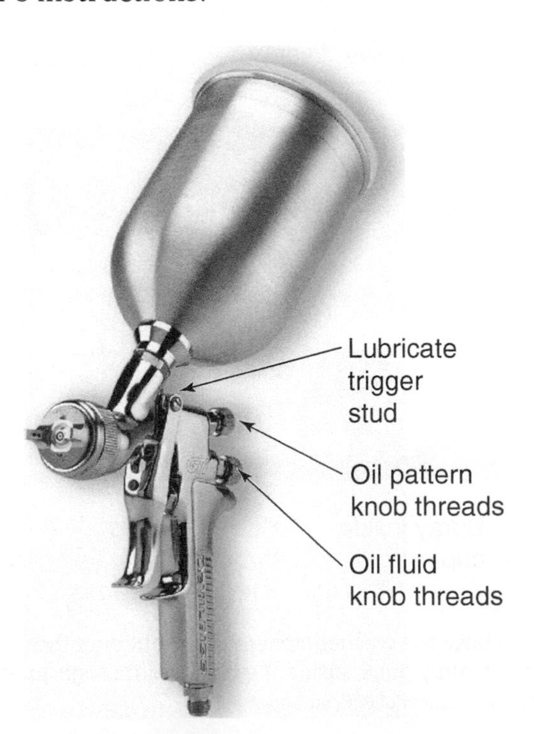

Figure 16–33. Note the points on the spray gun that should be lubricated. Use manufacturer-recommended spray gun lubricant, and do not use too much. Refer to your owner's manual for details. (Courtesy of ITW DeVilbiss)

Figure 16–34 shows how to use a spray gun equipped with a disposable plastic liner in its cup.

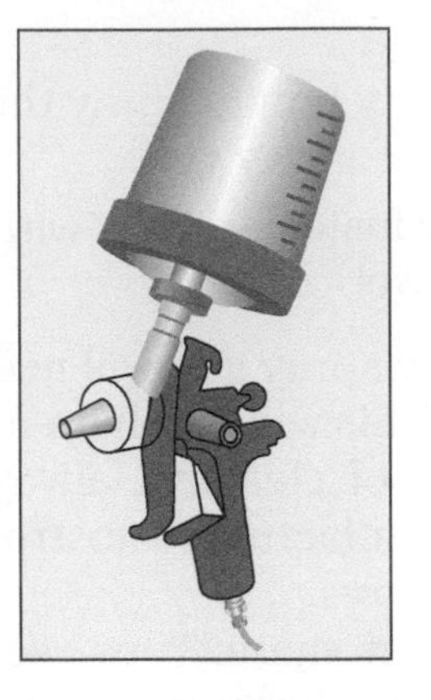

(A) The old metal cup has been removed and a new plastic cup and liner have been installed on the gun body.

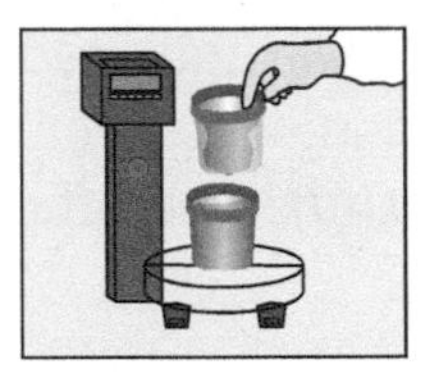

(B) Install the collapsible plastic liner into the plastic spray gun cup. Paint can then be filtered and mixed in the liner.

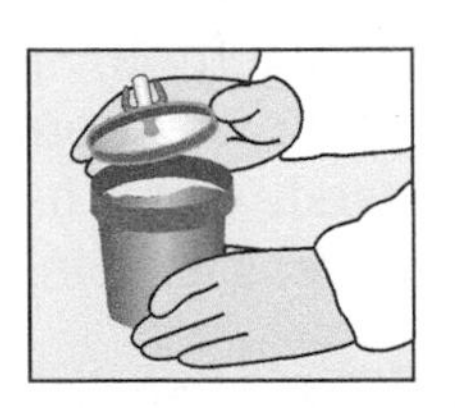

(C) Install and tighten the plastic lid onto the spray gun cup.

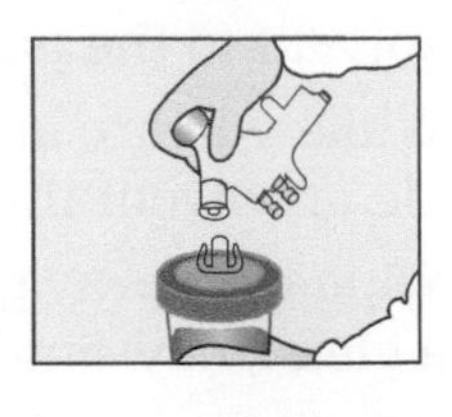

(D) Fit the gun body down over the plastic gun cup. Rotate to secure the gun body to the cup.

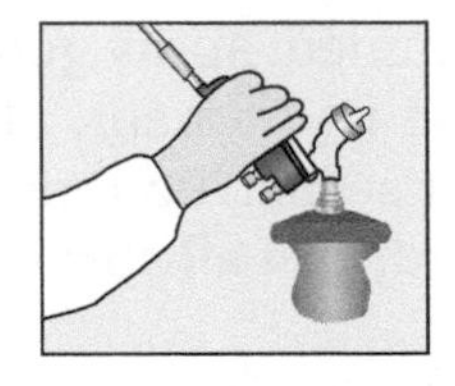

(E) Turn the gun upside down and trigger air out of the gun until the plastic liner collapses and all the air is out of the liner. The spray gun is now ready for use.

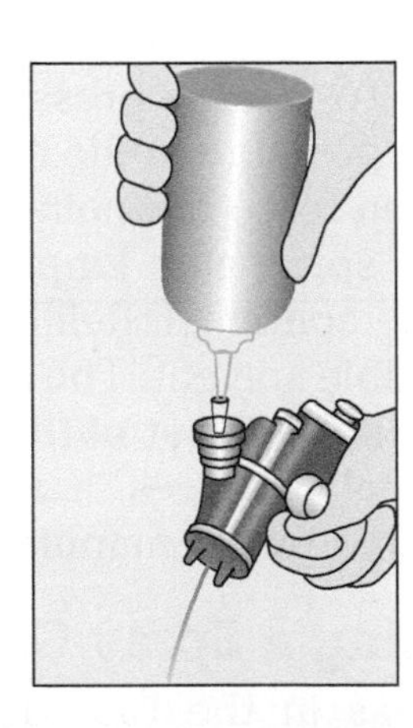

(F) When finished painting, remove and dispose of or store the plastic liner. Use solvent to clean the gun body. This saves from having to clean all of the unused paint from the gun cup, saving time and materials. (Courtesy of PPG Industries, Inc.)

Figure 16–34. This spray gun is equipped with a plastic cup with a collapsing plastic liner. This speeds cleanup and prevents spitting and dripping from the gun cup.

SUMMARY

- The most common types of paints are polyurethane enamels and acrylic urethane enamels.
- Spray gun distance is measured from the gun tip to the surface being painted. Typically, hold the gun 6 to 8 inches (152 to 203 mm) away for lacquer and 8 to 10 inches (203 to 254 mm) away from the surface for enamel.
- When applying basecoat, two medium coats are sufficient. Use enough to achieve hiding, no more.

TECHNICAL TERMS

tack cloth
paint settling
application stroke
spray gun distance
short spray distance
long spray distance
spray gun angle
spray gun triggering
spray gun speed
banding coat
overlap strokes
gun heeling
gun arching
incorrect gun stroke speed
improper spray overlap
improper coverage
full wet coat
dust coat
tack coat
shading coats
paint blending
spot repair
panel repairs
overall refinishing
paint overlap
wet edge
spray gun washer
spray gun lubrication

REVIEW QUESTIONS

1. From the customer's standpoint, the paint or colorcoat is the most important aspect of a painting/refinishing job. True or false?
2. How do you use a tack cloth?
3. What is some of the more important label information that should be checked before spraying?
4. A short spray distance causes the high-velocity mist to ______________ the wet paint ______________. A long spray distance causes a greater percentage of the thinner to ______________, resulting in ______________ ______________ or ______________ spray.
5. How do you properly trigger a spray gun?
6. Spray gun speed refers to how fast the spray gun is moved ______________ while spraying.
7. What are overlap strokes of a spray gun?
8. This refers to whether a paint film is uniform.
   a. Heeling
   b. Arching
   c. Spattering
   d. Coverage
9. *Technician A* says that the first coat of color on an overall finish should always be a very wet coat. *Technician B* says that the first coat of color depends on the paint manufacturer's directions and they usually recommend a medium wet coat. Who is correct?
   a. Technician A
   b. Technician B
   c. Both Technicians A and B
   d. Neither Technician
10. A spot repair is being made on the front of a fender using a silver metallic base-clear material. *Technician A* says to use a mist coat to help even out the metallic basecoat when blending over the existing finish. *Technician B* says to use a full wet coat of basecoat to ensure a good metallic match. Who is correct?
    a. Technician A
    b. Technician B
    c. Both Technicians A and B
    d. Neither Technician
11. ______________ ______________ or ______________ coats are progressive applications of paint on the boundary of spot repair areas so that a color difference is NOT noticeable.
12. Explain the difference between a spot repair and a panel repair.
13. How do you avoid runs and sags in paint during application?
14. When repairing a small area with basecoat-clearcoat, you need to spray the basecoat

only over the repair area, but the whole panel should be cleared. True or false?

15. List ten rules or questions you should remember when refinishing a vehicle.
16. When manually cleaning spray paint guns, it is wise to wear ______________, ______________, and a ______________.

ASE-STYLE REVIEW QUESTIONS

1. *Technician A* says that color variations can be caused if a color with heavy pigments is allowed to stand in a spray gun for 10 to 15 minutes without being stirred. *Technician B* says that all materials being poured into a spray gun should be strained. Who is correct?
   a. Technician A
   b. Technician B
   c. Both Technicians A and B
   d. Neither Technician

2. *Technician A* says to always read the labels on paint refinishing materials. *Technician B* says that procedures for mixing paint will vary with the manufacturer. Who is correct?
   a. Technician A
   b. Technician B
   c. Both Technicians A and B
   d. Neither Technician

3. A painter is having trouble with orange peel when spraying a vehicle. Which of these would be the most common cause of this problem?
   a. Spray gun held too close to the surface
   b. Spray gun held too far from the surface
   c. Spray gun moved too quickly
   d. Spray gun moved too slowly

4. A paint drip has been found on a freshly painted vehicle. Which of the following is a common source of this problem?
   a. Fluid nozzle
   b. Spray gun body
   c. Cup seal
   d. Packing

5. *Technician A* says to keep the spray gun trigger held down to prevent spitting. *Technician B* says to release halfway on the trigger right before you stop moving the gun sideways. Who is correct?
   a. Technician A
   b. Technician B
   c. Both Technicians A and B
   d. Neither Technician

6. Which of the following should be done to deposit enough paint on edges or corners of surfaces?
   a. Flood coat
   b. Double coat
   c. Band coat
   d. Cross coat

7. *Technician A* says to start at the bottom and work upward when painting a door. *Technician B* says that little or no paint should hit the masking paper. Who is correct?
   a. Technician A
   b. Technician B
   c. Both Technicians A and B
   d. Neither Technician

8. *Technician A* says that each spray gun coat should cover about half of the previous coat of paint when painting a panel. *Technician B* says to make each pass in the opposite direction when painting a panel. Who is correct?
   a. Technician A
   b. Technician B
   c. Both Technicians A and B
   d. Neither Technician

9. A hood is being painted. *Technician A* says to lean over so that the whole hood can be painted with continuous movements of the spray gun. *Technician B* says to blend the wet edge of the hood and to paint one side and then the other. Who is correct?
   a. Technician A
   b. Technician B
   c. Both Technicians A and B
   d. Neither Technician

10. Which of the following spray gun handling problems will deposit more paint at the top of the fan than at the bottom?

a. Fanning

b. Heeling

c. Arching

d. Stroking

ACTIVITIES

1. Practice spraying on a body part. Prepare its surface properly using information in previous chapters and this chapter. You might be able to obtain mismatched paint for free from a body shop or supplier. Write a report on what you learned and any problems that you encountered. List the materials used for the job.

2. Completely disassemble and reassemble a spray gun. Follow the manufacturer's instructions. Note if any parts are worn or dirty.

3. Practice spraying a metallic paint onto a part or a sheet of sandpaper. Intentionally apply too much paint so that it runs or sags in one location. In another location, spray a dry mist of metallic by holding the spray gun too far away from the surface. After drying, inspect the difference in the metallic. Make a report of your findings.

CHAPTER

17 Color Matching

OBJECTIVES

After studying this chapter, you should be able to:

- Describe color theory and how it relates to refinishing.
- Define the terms relating to color.
- Describe the use of a computerized color matching system.
- Make let-down and spray-out test panels.
- Explain how to tint solid and metallic colors.
- Summarize the repair procedures for multi-stage finishes.

INTRODUCTION

Color matching involves the steps needed to make the new paint look like the existing paint color. Even if you use the body color code numbers and correct paint formula to match the paint, the new paint may NOT be exactly the same color as the old. With today's multi-stage paints and factory robotic painting, it can be very difficult to match colors when making spot and panel repairs.

This chapter will help you develop the skills needed to match any type of paint. It summarizes color theory, evaluation, matching, computer analysis of paint, blending, tinting, and other factors. See **Figure 17–1.**

COLOR THEORY

Color is caused by how objects reflect light at different frequencies into our eyes. The color seen depends on the kind and amount of light waves the surface reflects.

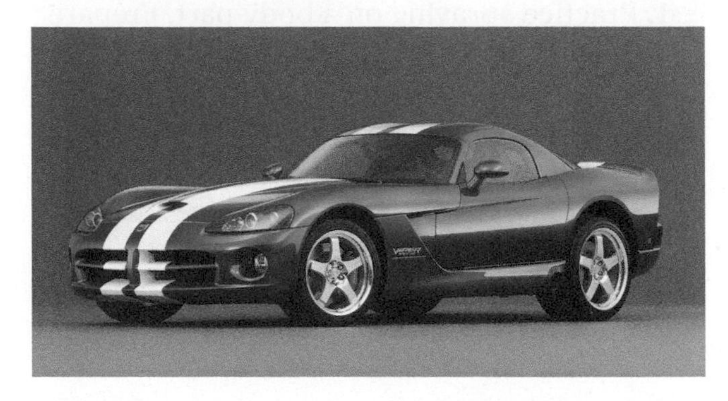

Figure 17–1. The paint color on today's vehicles is much more difficult to match than in the past. Paints with metal flakes and pearl colors can be a challenge to repair and match. (Courtesy of DaimlerChrysler Corporation)

When the eye sees a colored object, that object is absorbing all of the light except for the color that it appears to be. A red ball appears red because the ball absorbs all of the colors in the light shining on it except for the reds. In contrast, a black object absorbs almost all light, while polished chrome absorbs none.

White light is actually a mixture of various colors of light. By passing light through a prism, light is broken down into its separate colors, called the **color spectrum.**

LIGHTING

Sunlight contains the entire visible spectrum of light. It is the standard by which other light sources are measured. Since the vehicle will be seen in sunlight, you should always use sunlight, or daylight-corrected lighting, when making color evaluations.

Compared to daylight, **incandescent light** has more yellows, oranges, and reds. **Fluorescent light** can have more violets and reds. They should NOT be used when analyzing a color.

Lamps may also have a **lumen rating** for brightness. Lamps are normally between 1,000 and 2,000 lumens, with a higher lumen rating producing a brighter light.

Lamps may also be rated for **light temperature** in "Kelvin." Daylight is 6,200 Kelvin. For painting, a lamp rating of 6,000–7,000 Kelvin is recommended.

For this reason, choose lamps that are the closest to simulating actual sunlight. The spray booth manufacturer or representative may have recommendations. See **Figure 17–2.**

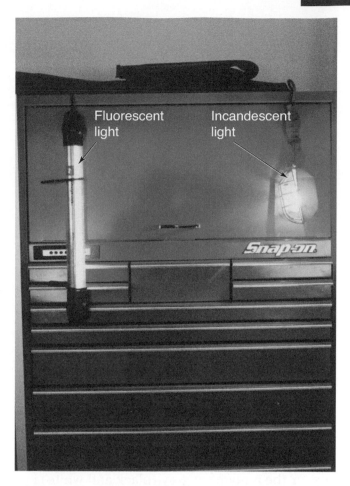

(A) Fluorescent and incandescent drop lights have been hung in front of a toolbox. Note how they make the red color of the toolbox look different.

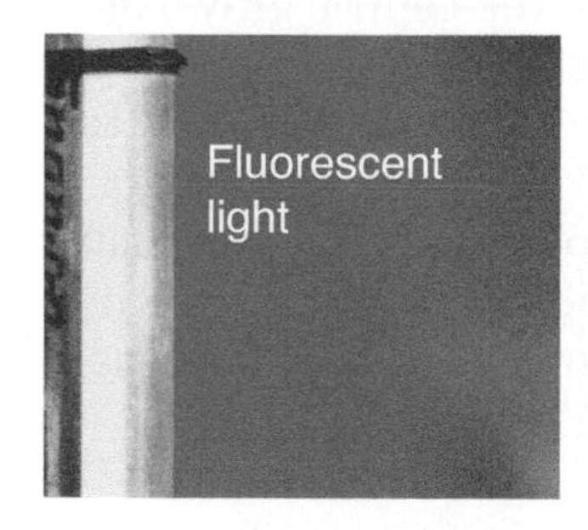

(B) This is a close-up of the color with fluorescent light.

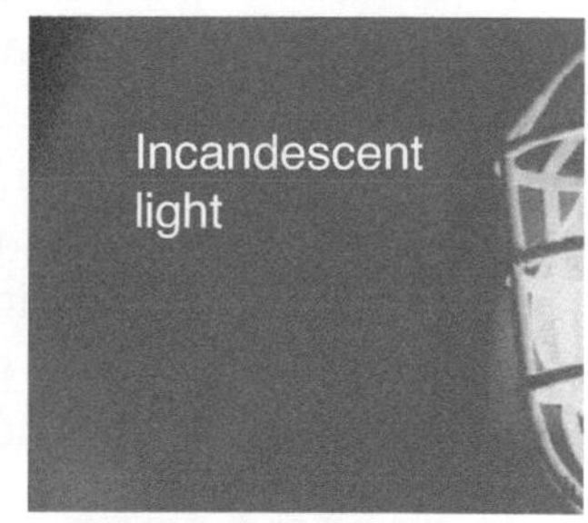

(C) This is a close-up of the color with incandescent light.

Figure 17–2. Sunlight is the best lighting to use when evaluating color. (Courtesy of Snap-on Tools Corporation)

COLOR BLINDNESS

Color blindness makes it difficult for a person's eye to see colors accurately. If problems arise when you are matching certain colors, it might be wise to have your eyes checked for color vision. Nearly 10 percent of all men have trouble seeing one or more colors.

To do finish matching, the technician must be able to recognize colors as they actually are. It is important not only to see the color that is to be worked on, but also the overtones within that color, including the shades of darkness or lightness and the richness or fullness of the color.

DIMENSIONS OF COLOR

Many people describe color in terms of what they see. For example, you might have heard these descriptions: sky blue, ruby red, grass green, or midnight blue. These terms cause confusion when describing colors.

To minimize the confusion when painting, color should be based on three *dimensions of color,* which are:

1. Value—lightness or darkness
2. Hue—color, cast, or tint
3. Chroma—saturation, richness, intensity, muddiness

These three dimensions are used to organize colors into a logical sequence on a color tree. The **color tree** is used to locate colors three-dimensionally when matching colors. Colors move around the color tree in a specific sequence—from blue to red to yellow to green. Refer to **Figure 17–3.** This sequence is easier to remember if you think of "BRYG." These are the first letters of blue, red, yellow, and green.

Value refers to the degree of lightness or darkness of the color. It is one dimension of color. When using the color tree, the value scale runs vertically through the tree. It is white at the top and black at the bottom. It is neutral gray at the center.

Hue, also called color, cast, or tint, describes what we normally think of as color. Hue is the color that is seen, moving around the outer edge of the color tree. It moves from blue to red to yellow to green.

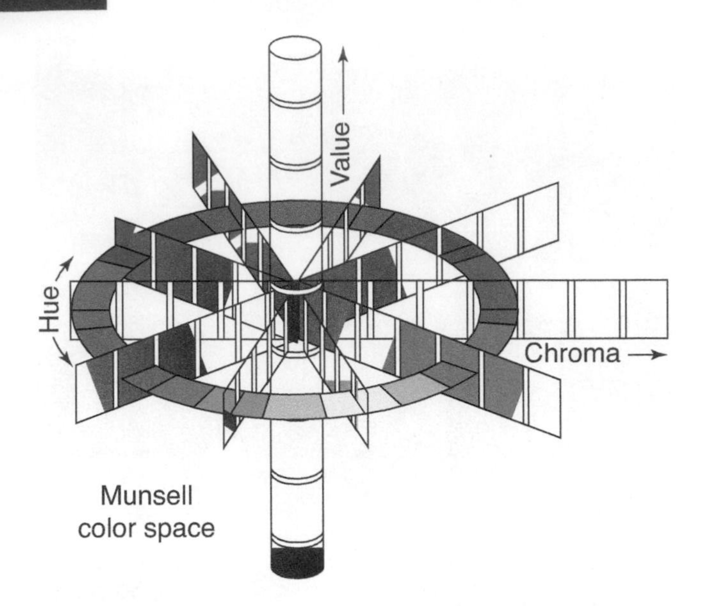

Figure 17–3. Note this graphic representation of the three dimensions of color. All three dimensions must match when repainting only a portion of a vehicle body. (Courtesy of Munsell Color Group)

When using the color tree, the hue scale shows color position around the color tree. It uses four main colors: blue, red, yellow, and green.

Chroma refers to the color's level of intensity, or the amount of gray (black and white) in a color. It is also called saturation, richness, intensity, or muddiness. It moves along the spokes that radiate outward from the central gray axis of the color tree. Weak, washed-out colors with the least chroma are at the core of the color tree. Highly chromatic colors that are rich, vibrant, and intense are at the outer edge. When using the color tree, chroma increases as it moves outward from the neutral gray center. It decreases as it moves closer to the neutral gray center.

METAMERISM

Metamerism is how different light sources affect the appearance of paint pigments and metallics. A paint may have some red in it NOT noticeable in daylight, but the red becomes very evident under street lights. The color change results from the new paint and OEM color formulas NOT being made of the same pigments. This causes the pigments to look different under different light sources.

COLOR MATCHING

Because many factors can cause a color mismatch problem, you must follow a step-by-step sequences on every job. OEM or factory original paint colors can vary slightly from area to area. For example, plastic bumpers often have a noticeable color variance. This is especially true with metallics, because metal body panels will attract the metal flakes more than a plastic part or panel.

There can be a difference in the two finishes even though they are officially the same color. This can pose problems when trying to satisfy customers.

Whatever the reason for color variance, you must match the only color standard that really matters—the vehicle color itself. For better or worse, the vehicle color is the standard!

Color Directory

A **color directory** contains color chips, paint mixing formulas, and other paint-related information for most makes and models of vehicles.

To use a color directory, locate the vehicle manufacturer's paint code. Then you can identify the color chip next to it. It is wise to compare the color chip with the vehicle color. There is always the chance that the vehicle has been repainted with a different color.

Figure 17–4 shows an actual page from a color matching manual (or color chip book). Note how it gives several chips for the same color.

PAINT FORMULAS

The **paint formula** gives the percentage or amount of each ingredient needed to match an OEM color. The formula will be available from

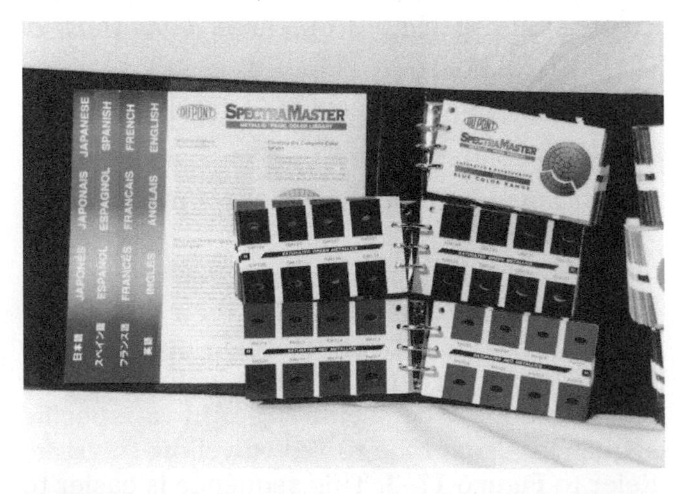

Figure 17–4. Color manuals from the paint manufacturer give color chip samples, instructions, and charts for mixing and matching colors. Study typical pages from a color manual. Chips are placed on the vehicle paint to find a color match. You can then use the formula for the matching chip to mix the paint.

the paint manufacturer, mixing system, or from the local paint jobber.

A **basecoat patch** is a small area on the vehicle's surface without clear to enable the technician to check for color match with tricoat colors. The manufacturer masks the patch before clearcoating to help you match the color more easily. The basecoat patch is sometimes located under the deck lid or hood. If the color match is correct, order the paint by color stock number.

Refinish suppliers supply paint (colors) in two ways—factory colors and custom colors. If it is a recent model or a popular color, chances are they will have the paint ready-mixed. These ready-mixed paints are called **factory packaged colors.**

If it is an older color, they might have to mix it. **Custom-mixed colors** are those colors that are mixed to order at the paint supply distributor. Custom-mixed colors can always be identified easily. The contents of the can must be written or typed on the label by the person who mixed the paint.

An **intermix system** is a full set of paint pigments and solvents that can be mixed at the collision repair shop. Most paint manufacturers have made a color mixing system available to painters. With an in-house paint mixing system, it is possible to mix thousands of colors. An in-shop mixing system also allows you to better match the color on the vehicle more easily.

COMPUTERIZED COLOR MATCHING SYSTEMS

Computerized color matching systems use data from the (electronic device for reading color) to help match the vehicle's color. Many spectrophotometer systems can input color data into a computer. The computer can then use its stored data to help determine how to mix or tint the color.

Depending on the sophistication of the system, a computerized color matching system may be able to:

1. Compare the actual color of the vehicle to a computer-stored set of color formulations.
2. Make a recommendation on which tint in the formula will move the sample panel closer to the vehicle.
3. Automatically keep a record of the mixing or tinting procedure. This will let you quickly match the paint if the vehicle returns for another repair.

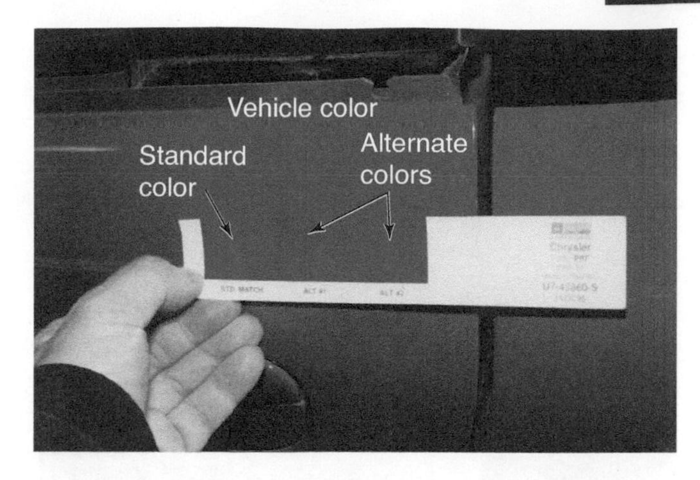

Figure 17–5. Alternate chips, or variance paint chips, are often provided so you can more closely match the formula to the actual color on the vehicle. Hold alternate or variance chips next to the vehicle paint and select the one closest to the vehicle's color.

COLOR VARIANCE PROGRAMS

Color variance programs compare the color of refinish paints to OEM color standards and actual painted parts and panels obtained from collision repair shops. If a particular OEM finish variation is noted often enough, a paint manufacturer may develop a *color variation formula* to match the OEM finish.

Variance chips are several samples of slightly different colors to help match paint colors. One paint code will have a series of variance chips on each side of a typical color. They can be used to adjust the color formulation more precisely than by just using one chip. See **Figure 17–5.**

To use variance chips, lay the chips on the vehicle under proper lighting. Find the chip that best matches the color on the vehicle. Using the number code for this chip, the computer will then give instructions for mixing the color to match that chip and the vehicle. Computerized formulas will give a percentage of each pigment color to change the paint color as needed. See **Figure 17–6.**

SPRAY METHODS AFFECT COLOR

Although a technician cannot control the variables that can affect colors at the manufacturing plant, there are variables in the shop that can be controlled. For example, a refinishing technician can control:

1. Paint agitation
2. Spray techniques

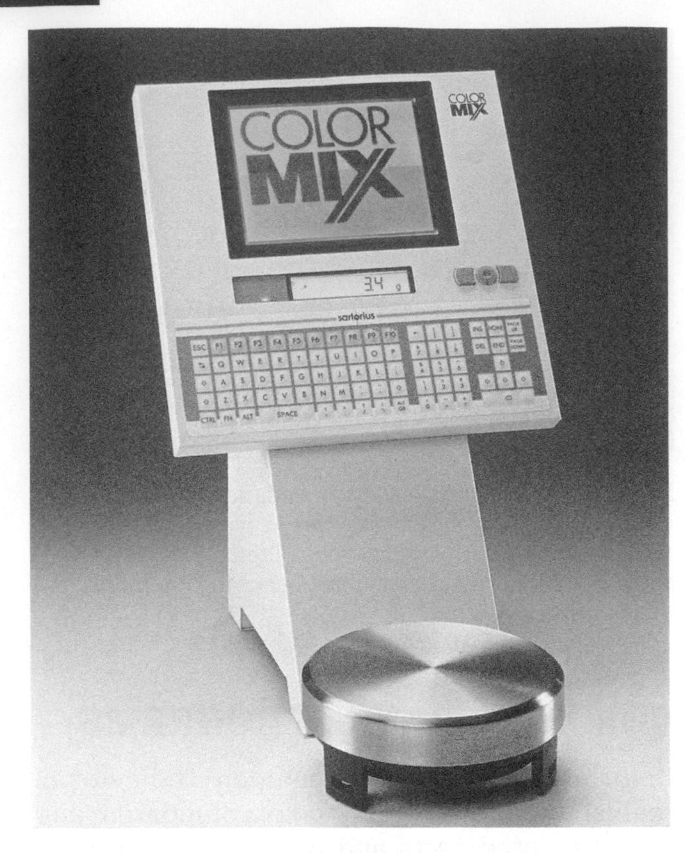

(A) Electronic scales will then give a readout of each ingredient needed to mix the color properly. After selecting the correct paint chip and its formula, the screen will prompt you to pour in each ingredient in the paint color.

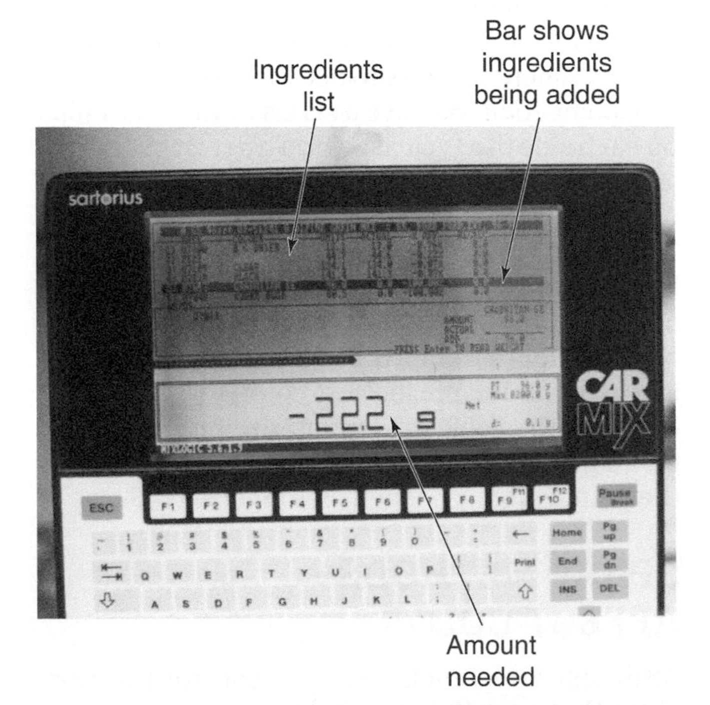

(B) By watching the readout on the computerized paint mixing scales, you know when you have poured in enough of each ingredient to produce the correct color of paint.

Figure 17–6. Computerized mixing systems will give amounts of each ingredient to use when matching color.

3. Amount of material applied
4. Spray gun design
5. Spray gun adjustments
6. Wetness of spray coats
7. Amount and type of solvent used for paint reduction
8. Paint mixing formula

All of these will help you make the new color match the existing finish.

Varying the spraying technique can affect color. That is, the application technique could cause the color to vary. Technicians who spray wet end up with a darker color than those who spray drier, especially with metallics.

MATCHING SOLID COLORS

For many years vehicles were solid colors, such as black, white, tan, blue, green, maroon, and so on. Solid colors reflect light in only one direction. Solid colors are still used on vehicles, but to a lesser degree when compared with a few years ago.

Matching solid colors is easier than matching metallic or mica paints. You only need to match the color pigment and NOT the metal or mica flakes suspended in the paint.

Oddly enough, a mismatch in a panel repair will usually show up more than a mismatch in a spot repair—even though the spot repair is smaller. That is because a panel, such as a vehicle door, has a distinct edge. And the repair, obviously, cuts off at that edge. Mismatched panels, as in the case of front and rear doors, will be right next to each other and will show a sharp contrast.

A spot repair, on the other hand, is performed by blending the repair into the surrounding area. In spot repairs, the first coat is applied to the immediate area being repaired. Subsequent coats extend beyond this area gradually. Finally, a blend coat extends beyond the colorcoats. Thus, if there is a slight mismatch, the blend coat and the last colorcoat will allow enough **show-through** of the old finish to make the color difference a gradual one.

MATCHING METALLIC FINISHES

Metallic colors contain small flakes of aluminum suspended in liquid, as illustrated in **Figure 17–7.** The position of the flakes and the

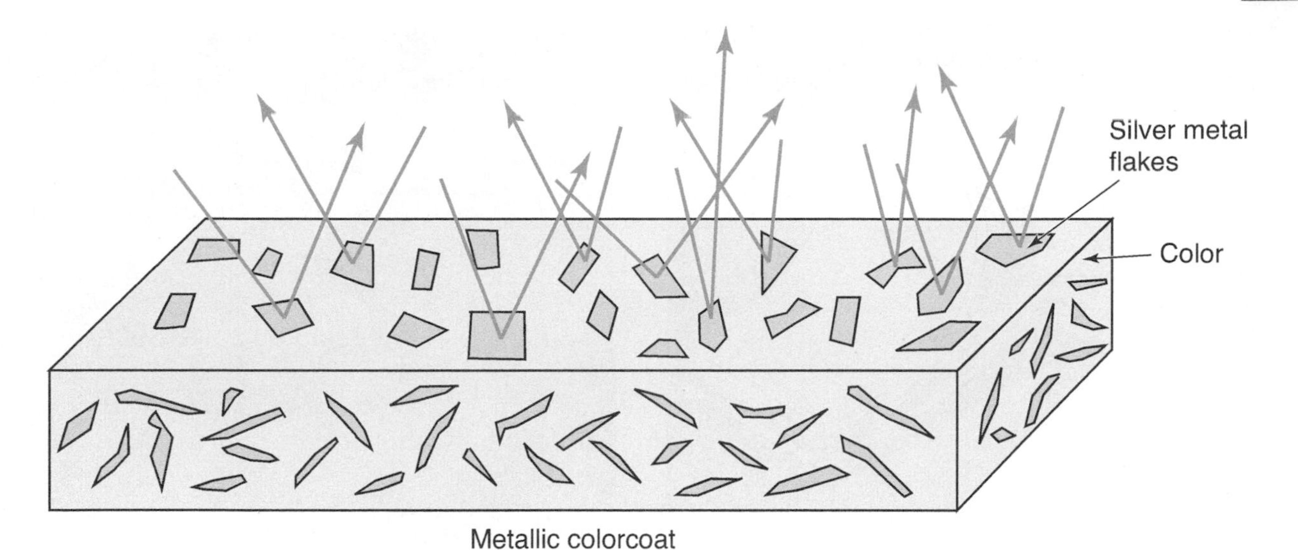

Figure 17–7. Metallic flakes in a color will reflect almost all light back out. The location and orientation of the flakes is critical to matching metallic finishes. If the metallic spray is too dry, the paint will look more silver because the flakes will not settle. If you spray too wet, the silver flakes will sink deeper into the color.

thickness of the paint affect the overall color. The flakes reflect light while the color absorbs a higher amount of the light. The thicker the layer of paint, the greater the light absorption.

A **dry application of paint** makes the color appear lighter and more silver. The aluminum flakes are trapped at various angles near the surface of the color film. Light reflection is NOT uniform. The light has less paint film to travel through; little of it is absorbed. The result is nonuniform light reflection and minimum light absorption.

A **wet application of paint** makes the color appear darker and less silver. The flakes have sufficient time to settle in the wet color. The flakes lie parallel to and deeper within the paint film. Light reflection is uniform and, because the light has to go farther into the paint film, light absorption is greater. The result is a painted surface that appears deeper and darker in color.

NOTE

Metallic colors must be stirred and mixed thoroughly before use. The pigment quickly settles below the binder. Also, the aluminum flakes settle below the pigment. If flakes stay at the bottom of the can, the paint will NOT match the same color on the vehicle being refinished.

A good technician must know how to handle metallic colors. They are very sensitive to the solvents with which they are reduced and the air pressure with which they are applied. Metallic colors are also affected by a number of variables. This would include spraying conditions such as temperature, humidity, and ventilation.

To darken a metallic color: (1) increase fluid flow; (2) decrease fan width; (3) decrease air pressure; (4) decrease travel speed; and (5) use a slower evaporating solvent. To lighten a metallic color, do just the opposite.

MATCHING MULTISTAGE FINISHES

Another type of glamour finish is the multistage finish. Shown in **Figure 17–8,** factory **multistage finishes** generally consist of:

1. E-coat (Electrostatic Metal primers)
2. Colored primer coats
3. Colored basecoats
4. Mica intermediate coats or pearlcoats
5. Clearcoats

Mica and carbon graphic pigments have special requirements when it comes to color evaluation. In vehicle finishes, mica may be coated with titanium dioxide. The thickness of the titanium dioxide coating determines the colors that are reflected and allowed to pass through.

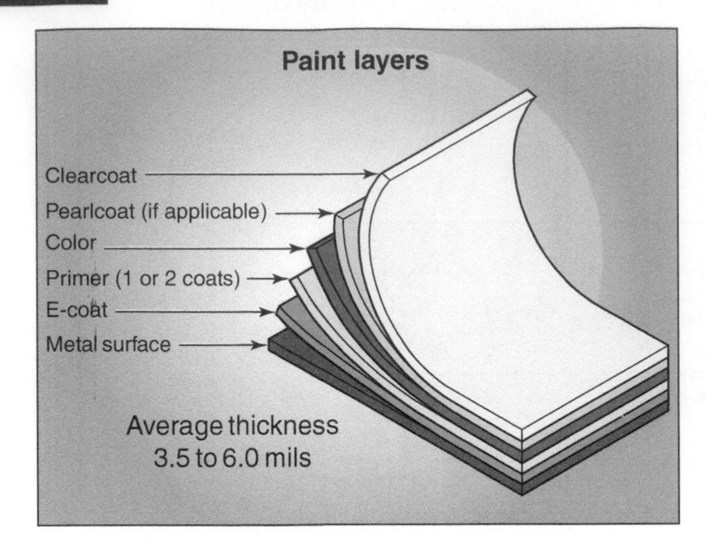

Figure 17–8. This cutaway shows the basic makeup of an OEM multistage finish. (Courtesy of Nissan North America, Inc.)

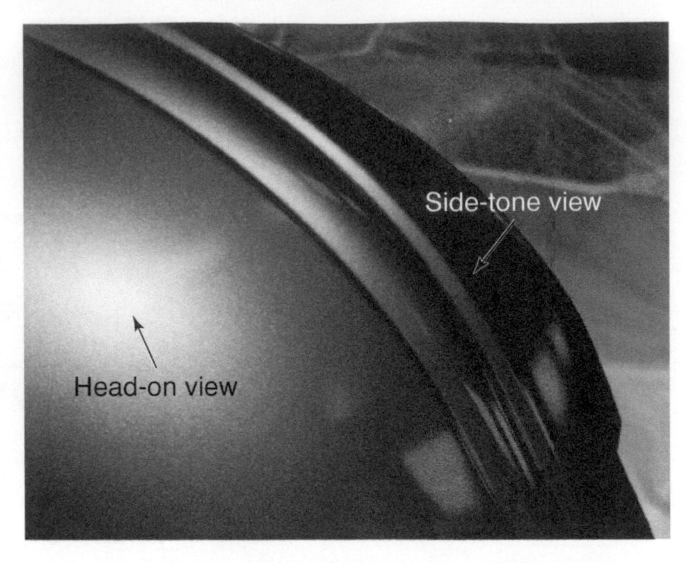

Figure 17–9. Flop occurs when a metallic or multistage color looks different when viewed at different angles. Note how this metallic color appears different on this curved bumper.

ZONE CONCEPT

The **zone concept** divides the horizontal surfaces of the vehicle into zones defined by character lines and moldings. It requires refinishing of an entire zone or zones with basecoat, mica intermediate coats, and clearcoats.

COLOR FLOP

Flop, also termed *flip-flop,* refers to a change in color hue when viewing from head-on and then from the side. The lightness or darkness of a color varies from head-on to side-tone views. Flop occurs most often in paints containing metallic pigments, but a type of flop can also occur in mica paints. Solid colors do NOT exhibit flop.

The direction and intensity of the light being reflected back by the flakes in the paint film is what causes the flop phenomenon. See **Figure 17–9.**

Head-on view compares the test panel to the vehicle straight on, or perpendicular. **Side-tone view** compares the test panel to the vehicle on a 45–60-degree angle. Compare the test panel to the vehicle on both angles with metallic finishes. The position of the metallics in the paint film can cause the color of the paint to change from head-on to side-tone.

The first approach to correcting the problem is to adjust the spraying technique to compensate for this effect. Spraying the fender a little wetter will slightly darken the appearance when looking directly into the panel. When viewed from an angle, the resulting appearance is lighter.

Spraying the panel slightly dryer reverses the effect, giving a lighter appearance when looking directly at the panel. This is because the aluminum flakes are close to the surface. The result is a darker appearance viewed at an angle, as light becomes trapped.

If spray techniques cannot correct the condition, the addition of a small amount of white will eliminate the sharp contrast from light to dark when the surface is viewed at various angles. The white acts to dull the transparency, giving a more uniform, subdued reflection through the paint film. Care should be taken when adding white since the change occurs quickly. Once too much white is added, recovering the color match becomes impossible.

CHECKING COLOR MATCH

Spraying test panels is the best way to check your color match before painting the vehicle. A test panel will check all variables.

Spray-out Panel

The **spray-out panel** checks the paint color and also shows the effects of the technician's technique on a test piece. See **Figure 17–10.** Spray-out panels are prepared by applying the paint as near to the actual spraying conditions as possible. When done properly, a spray-out panel shows the color exactly as it will look when sprayed on a vehicle.

Before making a spray-out panel, double-check the paint code. Reduce the paint correctly.

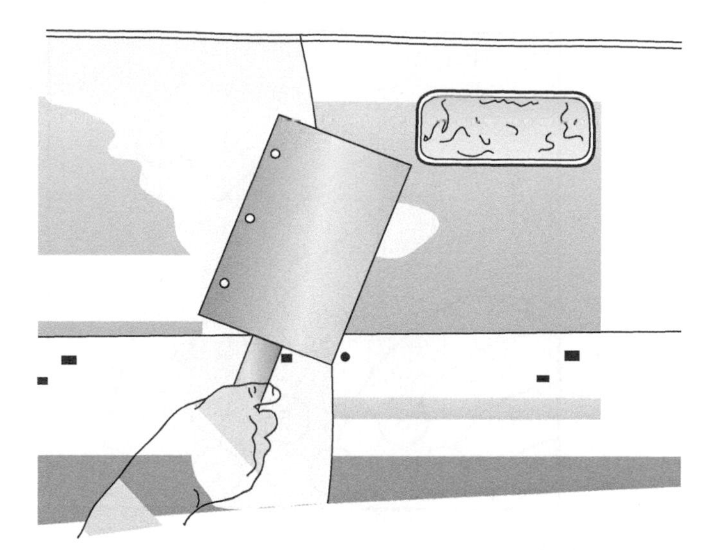

Figure 17–10. A spray-out panel tests the color match before applying the color to the vehicle. You must spray the test piece exactly as you are going to paint the vehicle body. By holding the test panel next to the vehicle color, you can see what the repair color will look like and whether the paint color must be changed.

Set up the spray gun with the material that will be sprayed. Adjust the air pressure at the spray gun for the material to be applied.

When making a spray-out panel, apply a primer that matches the primer on the vehicle. Apply basecoat to full hiding. Allow proper flash time between coats. Apply clearcoat to half the panel. The panel should be fully dry or cured prior to evaluating color match.

When evaluating color match on basecoat-clearcoat systems, apply clear to only half of the panel. The uncleared section can be used to check the color match of the basecoat prior to applying the clear. You can refer to any non-cleared patch on the vehicle.

Let-down Panel

A **let-down panel** is a spray test panel for evaluating the color match on tricoat and multistage paint systems. See **Figure 17–11.**

Here is how to make a let-down panel for a tricoat finish.

1. Spray the test panel (coated cardboard) with the same primers being used on the vehicle. After normal drying time, spray the primer-sealer over the let-down panel.
2. Spray the basecoat color to hide the test sheet, using the same air pressure and spray pattern that will be used on the vehicle. Duplicating your actual spray techniques when preparing the let-down panel is critical. Do NOT vary your procedures.
3. After the test panel has dried, mask it into four equal sections. See Figure 17–11. Then mask off the lower three quarters of the panel, exposing the top quarter.
4. Apply one coat of mica midcoat color over the top quarter of the test panel.
5. After the mica coat has flashed, remove the masking paper and move it down to the middle of the panel, exposing the top half.
6. Apply another coat of mica midcoat color over the exposed top half of the test panel.
7. After this second coat has flashed, remove the masking paper and move it down to expose three quarters of the panel.
8. Apply another coat of mica midcoat color over the exposed three quarters of the test panel.
9. After flashing, remove the masking paper entirely.

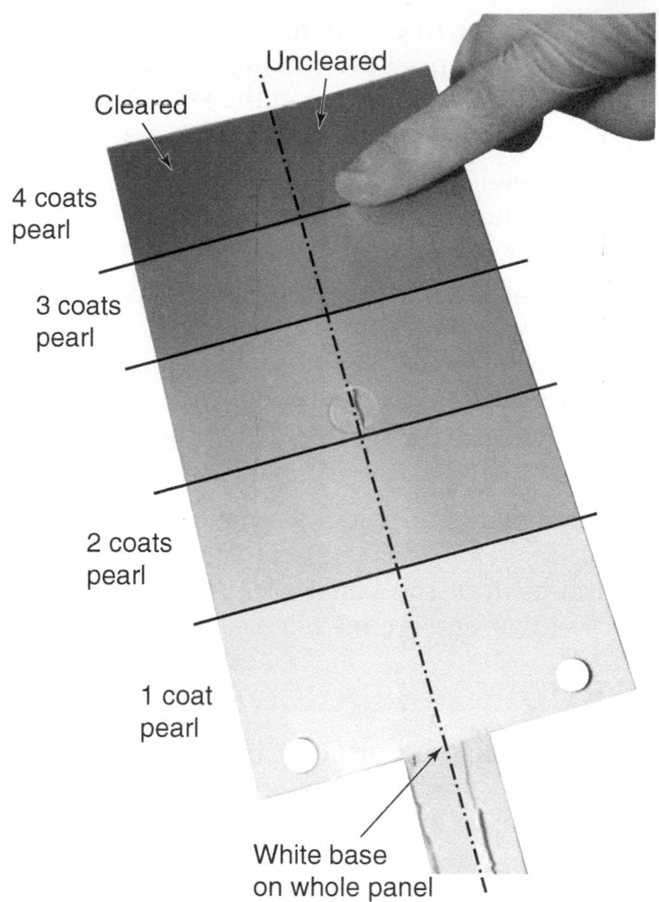

Figure 17–11. A let-down panel tests a multistage paint system for match before spraying the vehicle. You must mask each layer to apply different amounts of basecoat and clearcoat. You can then use the panel as a large paint chip for comparison to the vehicle's finish.

10. Apply a fourth coat of mica midcoat color. As always, spray the coating in the same way as would be done on the vehicle.
11. After the entire let-down panel has dried, mask off the panel lengthwise.
12. Apply the manufacturer's recommended number of clearcoats to the exposed half.
13. Compare the different shades on the let-down panel with the existing paint on the vehicle. Use the same number of coats used on the matching section of the let-down panel to achieve the correct paint match.

Once made, the let-down panel can be kept and used on vehicles with the same color code. On the back of the panel note the color code, gun settings, and technician's name.

BLENDING CLEARCOATS

Clearcoats may be blended by using additives provided by the manufacturer. When working with base-clear finishes, remember:

1. Clearcoats are NOT perfectly clear. They will change the appearance of a color.
2. Blend the basecoat and apply clear to the entire panel.
3. You may have to step-out the clear if it must be blended.
4. You should clear the entire surface of horizontal panels.
5. Blend into the smallest area possible to help hide the repair.

FLUORINE CLEARCOAT REPAIRS

The basic steps for spot repair with a fluorine clearcoat system are shown in **Figure 17–12.** They include:

1. Compound or sand with 1,200–1,500 grit sandpaper for better adhesion.
2. Apply first coat of basecoat.
3. Apply second coat of basecoat.
4. Apply third coat of basecoat or until hiding is obtained.
5. Apply color blender if necessary. Dry at 140°F (60°C) for 20 minutes.
6. Apply 3–4 coats of fluorine clearcoat. The area between numbers 5 and 6 in Figure 17–12 is faded out or blended if required. Dry at 60–70°F (16–21°C) for 10 minutes between coats. After applying final coat, force dry at 170°F (75°C) for 45 minutes.
7. Polish with fine compounds.

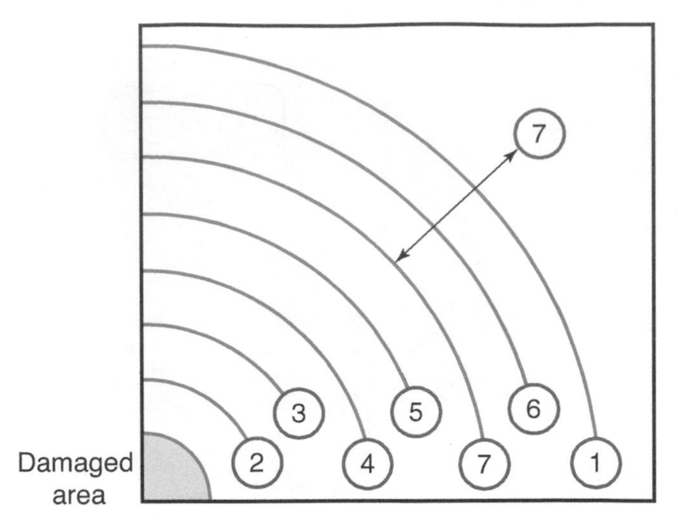

Figure 17–12. Compare the numbers on this illustration to the following: 1: Compound or sand with 1,200–1,500 grit sandpaper. 2: Apply the first coat of basecoat. 3: Apply the second coat of basecoat. 4: Apply the third coat of basecoat or until hiding is obtained. 5: Apply color blender if necessary. Dry at 140°F (60°C) for 20 minutes. 6: Apply 3–4 coats of clearcoat. Dry properly between coats. 7: Polish with fine compound. (Courtesy of Nissan North America, Inc.)

When working with tricoat and multistage finishes, a technician must match the basecoat prior to applying the intermediate and clearcoats. Some vehicle manufacturers leave an area of basecoat that is NOT coated with mica or clear for comparing the basecoat sprayout to the vehicle.

TRICOAT SPOT REPAIR

A **halo effect** is an unwanted shiny ring or halo that appears around a pearl or mica color repair. It is caused by the paint being wetter in the middle and drier near the outer edges of the repair.

Avoid a halo effect by applying the first coat of mica to the basecoat only. The more intermediate mica coats that are applied, the darker the finish will appear. Allow a larger area in which to blend the mica intermediate mica coats. They require more room to blend than a standard basecoat. Keep the tricoat repair area as small as possible.

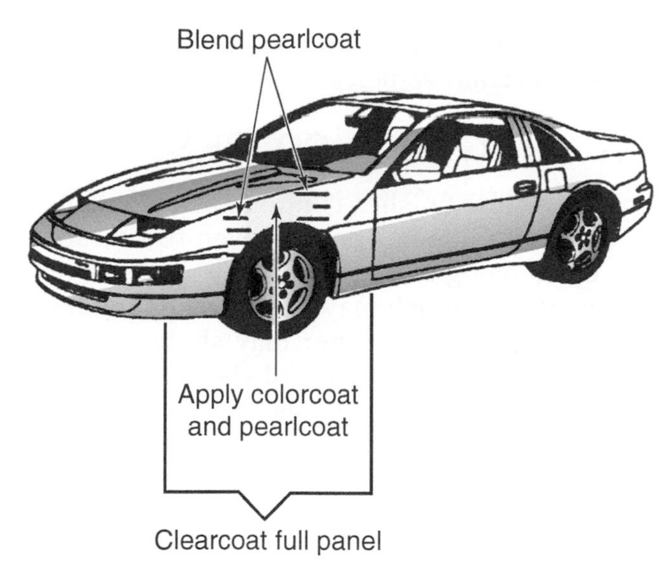

Figure 17–13. Note the coverage required for spot repairing a multistage finish. You must blend the pearlcoat over an area larger than the repair. Then clear the whole panel. (Courtesy of Nissan North America, Inc.)

This is one paint manufacturer's method for a spot or partial repair on a tricoat system:

1. Apply primer to area over the body filler.
2. Apply adhesion promoter to all unsealed panels. Adhesion promoter should extend beyond the repair area.
3. Apply two or more coats of basecoat to areas to full hiding. Extend each coat slightly beyond the previous one, allowing the surface to dry between coats. Look at **Figure 17–13.**
4. Check let-down panel for total number of coats of mica intermediate coats needed to match the OEM finish. Apply the intermediate coat to repair area, extending each coat beyond the last. Allow adequate flash time between coats.
5. Apply two coats of clear over entire panel. The clear may have to be blended into the sail panel. See **Figure 17–14.**

TRICOAT PANEL REPAIR

These are typical steps for a panel repair with a multistage finish:

1. Apply primer to area over the body filler.
2. Apply adhesion promoter to a large area to be repaired.
3. Apply two or more coats of basecoat to areas to full hiding. Extend each coat

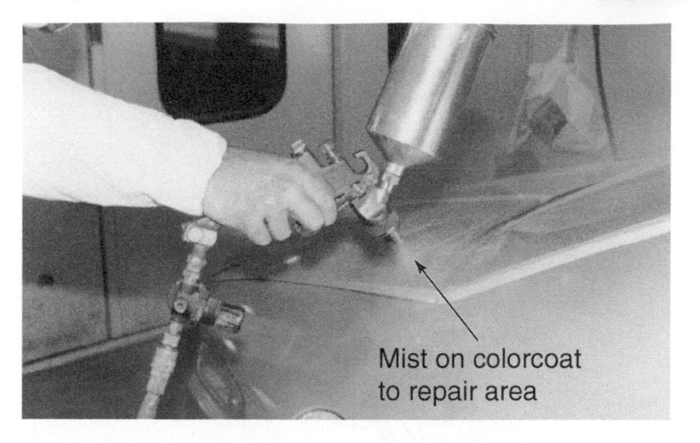

(A) Apply colorcoat only where it is needed, or over the repair area or primer. Mist metallic colors on lightly to help orient metallic flakes evenly.

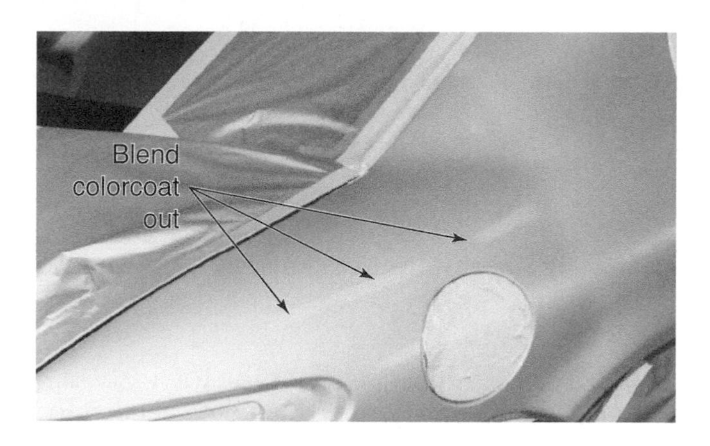

(B) Blend or fan the second colorcoat out away from the repair so the new paint and old paint gradually fade into each other.

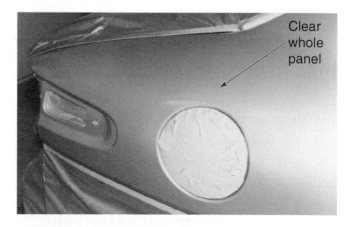

(C) Spray clear over the whole panel. If needed, blend the clear into a small, difficult to notice area, the sail panel between the roof panel and quarter panel in this example.

Figure 17–14. Study the basic steps for blending a metalic colorcoat/clearcoat spot repair.

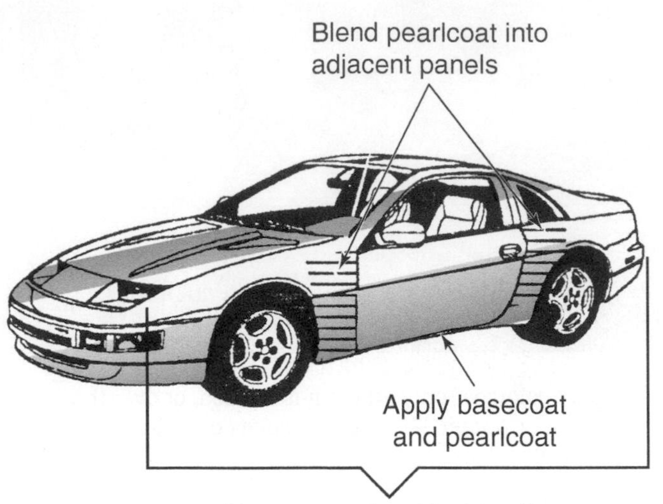

Figure 17–15. Note this panel repair of a multistage finish. You will usually have to blend the pearl into adjacent panels. Then clear the whole side of the vehicle to get a good match. (Courtesy of Nissan North America, Inc.)

slightly beyond the previous one, allowing the surface to dry between coats. See **Figure 17–15.**

4. Check the let-down panel for the total number of mica intermediate coats needed to match the OEM finish to areas. Extend each coat beyond the previous one, with only the last coat extending into adjacent panel. Allow adequate flash time between coats.
5. Apply two coats of clear to the entire repair area, ending at panel ends. (Edge to edge of doors, quarter panels, etc.)

BLENDING MICA COATS

This is a typical mica intermediate coat blending procedure:

1. Apply mica intermediate coat to the area covered by the basecoat.
2. Apply second mica intermediate coat well beyond the edge of the first coat.
3. Apply third mica intermediate coat so it extends just beyond the edge of the first coat but within the second coat.
4. Apply fourth mica intermediate coat to just beyond the edge of the second coat.

Spot repair recommendations for tricoats are now available. However, the zone repair is still a workable repair option and may be required on certain vehicles.

MATCHING MICA COLORS

Many base-clear finishes contain mica pigments. Some of these finishes have proven to be especially challenging to match.

Because the finish may NOT provide full hiding, the color of the primer may show through enough to change the look of the color. If the refinishing technician applies the color to full hiding, there may be a color mismatch because the primer color is no longer visible through the paint.

A color effect test panel is required for base-clear finishes that contain mica. To make this test panel:

1. Apply a primer that matches the primer color on the vehicle. Allow it to dry.
2. Mask the panel into thirds.
3. Apply one coat of basecoat to the exposed section. Allow it to dry.
4. Unmask the next section, and apply another coat of basecoat.
5. Unmask the last section of the panel, and apply an additional two coats of basecoat to the entire panel. Allow it to dry.
6. Apply two coats of clear to the panel. Allow it to dry.
7. Compare the test panel with the vehicle to determine the number of basecoat coats that provide the best match.

WHY A COLOR MISMATCH?

Tinting should be used only as a last resort. If the color of the refinishing varies from the original, check the following possible reasons for the mismatch:

1. Has the original finish faded? Check the color on unexposed areas such as door jambs or under the deck lid or hood to determine if the finish has faded. You can restore the luster by compounding the original finish beyond the repair area. This can remove chalking and oxidation before making a color comparison.
2. Was the wrong color used? Check the vehicle manufacturer's paint code and

the paint manufacturer's stock number of the color used to make sure that it is the right color.

3. Were the pigment and/or metallic flakes mixed thoroughly? Leaving pigment, metallic flake, or pearl in the bottom of the can could cause a mismatch. Be sure to agitate (mix) the paint thoroughly before and while spraying.
4. Has the amount of reducer been measured carefully? Over-reducing will lighten or desaturate a color. Remember that it is easy to add more reducer, but it cannot be taken out.
5. When using a test panel, was enough time allowed for the paint to dry? Be sure to allow proper flash and dry times for each coat. The paint usually gets darker as it dries. Dry time can be shortened by using heat lamps, heat guns, or other drying methods.
6. If using a clearcoat, remember that compounding the clear will make the paint appear darker. If testing a basecoat-clearcoat finish, color judgment cannot be made until the clear is applied to the basecoat.

TINTING

Tinting involves altering the color slightly to better match the new finish with the existing finish. Tinting may be one of the least understood tools of finish matching. There are three basic reasons for tinting:

1. To adjust color variations in shades to match the color from the manufacturer
2. To adjust color on an aged or weathered finish
3. To make a color for which there is no formula or for which there are no paint codes available

Some computerized paint systems provide color variance information. Before making the decision to tint, determine if a color variance chip or formula is available. These may provide a blendable match, and reduce or eliminate the need to tint. Computerized paint systems also provide tinting information. See **Figure 17–16.**

Some paint manufacturers produce metallic tinting bases designed to correct a specific problem, usually having to do with changes in side-tone. Use these products according to the manufacturer's recommendations. Using the color formula and tinting guide, select the tinting base that will move the color in the right direction. Refer to **Figure 17–17.**

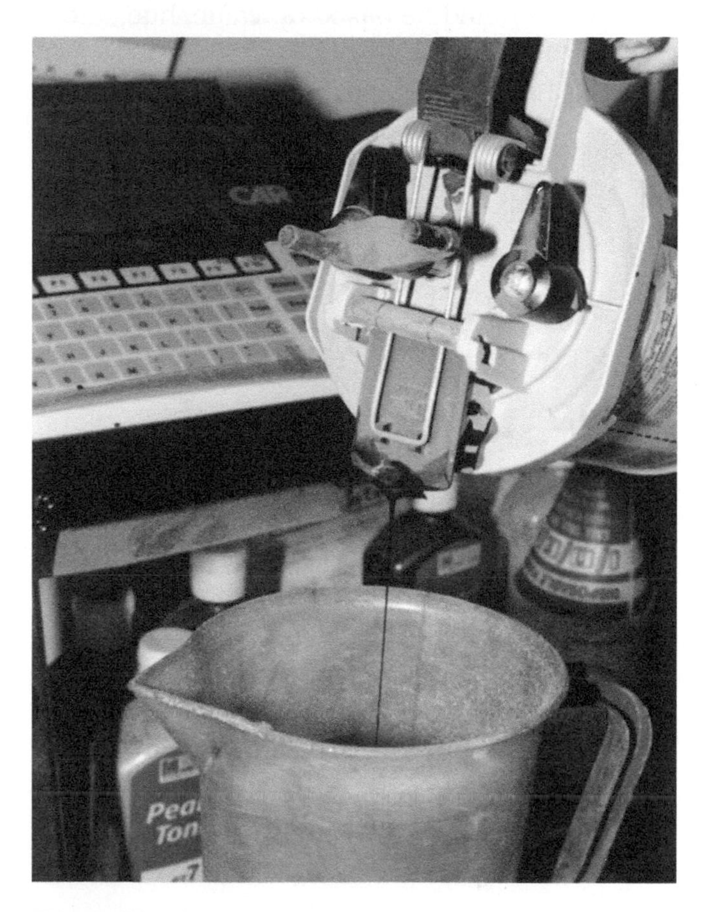

Figure 17–16. This technician is tinting a color by adding a tiny amount of the color pigment needed to make the test panel the same color as the color on the vehicle.

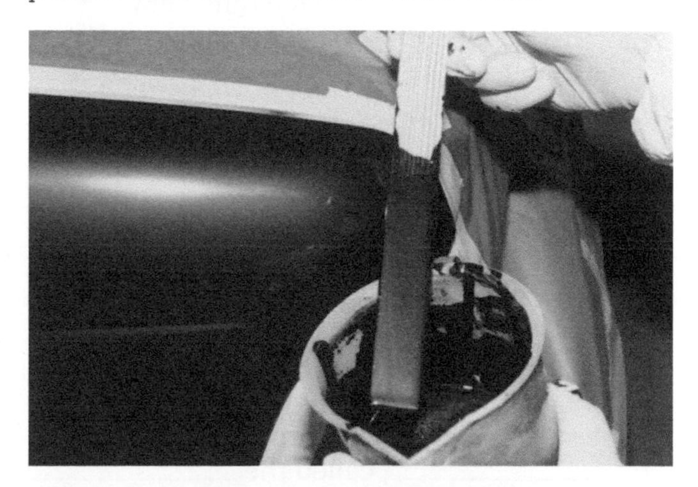

Figure 17–17. Tinting can be complex. Take your time and compare the tinted color to the color on the vehicle. One or more test panels may be needed on hard-to-match color, especially metallic and pearl colors.

SUMMARY

- The same shade of paint will look very different under incandescent and fluorescent lights. Therefore, it is very important to view a color in daylight or under a balanced artificial light.
- Color should be based on value, hue, and chroma.
- The two ways to check color match are:
  1. Spray-out panels—used with conventional paints
  2. Let-down panels—used with multistage paints

TECHNICAL TERMS

color matching
color
white light
color spectrum
sunlight
incandescent light
fluorescent light
lumen rating
light temperature
color blindness
color tree
value
hue
chroma
metamerism
color directory
paint formula
basecoat patch
factory packaged colors
custom-mixed colors
intermix system
computerized color matching systems
variance chips
show-through
dry application of paint
wet application of paint
multistage finishes
zone concept
flop
head-on view
side-tone view
spray-out panel
let-down panel
halo effect
tinting

REVIEW QUESTIONS

1. By passing light through a prism, light is broken down into its separate ______________, called the ______________.
2. When evaluating the color of a finish, it should be viewed under:
   a. Sunlight
   b. Incandescent light
   c. Fluorescent light
   d. Drop light
3. How do we see the color of a finish or any object?
4. ______________ refers to the degree of lightness or darkness of the color.
5. ______________, also called ______________, or______________, describes what we normally think of as color.
6. ______________ refers to the color's level of intensity, or the amount of gray (black and white) in a color.
7. What is a color directory?
8. A basecoat patch is a small area on the vehicle's surface without clear to enable the technician to check for color match. True or false?
9. This is a full set of paint pigments and solvents that can be mixed at the collision repair shop.
   a. Factory packaged colors
   b. Custom-mixed colors
   c. Intermix system
   d. Manufacturer system
10. List three tasks that a computerized color matching system may be able to do.
11. Explain variance chips in detail.
12. A dry metallic paint spray makes the color appear darker and less silver. True or false?
13. List six ways to darken a metallic color.
14. Define the term "flop."

ASE-STYLE REVIEW QUESTIONS

1. Which of these paints is the most difficult to match?
   a. Single-stage white
   b. Pearl paint
   c. Black/clearcoat
   d. White/clearcoat
2. *Technician A* says that sunlight should be used when evaluating color. *Technician B* says that when painting, a lamp rating of 6,000–7,000 Kelvin is recommended. Who is correct?
   a. Technician A
   b. Technician B

c. Both Technicians A and B
d. Neither Technician

3. Which of the following is NOT a dimension of color?
a. Value
b. Hue
c. Chroma
d. Gray scale

4. *Technician A* says that in order to use a color directory, locate the vehicle manufacturer's paint code. Then you can identify the color chip next to it. *Technician B* says that it is wise to compare the color chip with the vehicle color. There is always the chance that the vehicle has been repainted with a different color. Who is correct?
a. Technician A
b. Technician B
c. Both Technicians A and B
d. Neither Technician

5. *Technician A* says that paint can always be buffed so that the original paint code can be used. *Technician B* says that you may have to custom mix the paint to match the weathered paint. Who is correct?
a. Technician A
b. Technician B
c. Both Technicians A and B
d. Neither Technician

6. *Technician A* says that variance chips are no longer a viable way of selecting a paint color. *Technician B* says that spray methods affect color. Who is correct?
a. Technician A
b. Technician B
c. Both Technicians A and B
d. Neither Technician

7. *Technician A* says that matching solid colors is easier than matching metallic or mica paints. *Technician B* says that matching solid colors is more difficult than metallic, in which the flakes are all silver. Who is correct?
a. Technician A
b. Technician B
c. Both Technicians A and B
d. Neither Technician

8. *Technician A* says that spraying metallic colors dry makes the color appear darker and less silver. *Technician B* says that spraying metallic colors dry makes the color appear lighter and more silver. Who is correct?
a. Technician A
b. Technician B
c. Both Technicians A and B
d. Neither Technician

ACTIVITIES

1. Obtain a color matching manual. Read its directions and use it to find a color match for a vehicle. Write a report on your findings.
2. Locate a shop with a computerized color matching system. Write a summary on how to use the equipment.

CHAPTER

18 Paint Problems and Final Detailing

OBJECTIVES

After studying this chapter, you should be able to:

- List and explain the most common paint/refinish problems.
- Repair common finish problems.
- Use a sanding block.
- Wet sand to remove minor finish problems.
- Hand and machine compound a finish.
- Properly final detail a vehicle.

INTRODUCTION

After painting the vehicle and removal of masking materials, you must check your work quality. See **Figure 18–1.** Ideally, the vehicle can be released to the customer after a minor cleanup. Sometimes, however, you will find small imperfections in the paint film that must be corrected.

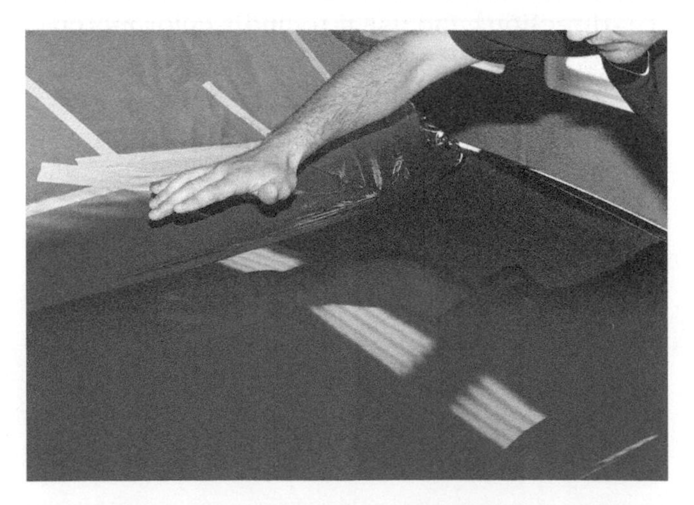

Figure 18–1. After painting the vehicle, inspect the paint film on all surfaces for problems. The slightest speck of dust or any other imperfection must be found and corrected before the customer inspects the repair. (Courtesy of DaimlerChrysler Corporation)

In rare occasions, you may have to solve major paint problems on existing or freshly painted surfaces.

This chapter provides you with the information needed to analyze, prevent, and correct paint problems. The last section of the chapter summarizes what must be done to final detail the vehicle. Since *first impressions* are important, you must know how to properly clean the vehicle before releasing it to the customer.

SURFACE IMPERFECTIONS

The steps for correcting surface imperfections include:

1. Examining the finish for imperfections
2. Correcting the imperfection
3. Finesse finishing
4. Final detailing

There are a number of defects in the repair area that must be corrected before the vehicle is delivered to the customer. A few of these paint problems include runs, sags, orange peel, dirt or dust, and overspray.

SURFACE FINISH MEASUREMENTS

A good panel repair will have several desirable characteristics. It should not be rough, wavy, nor have surface flaws.

Surface roughness is a measurement of paint film or other surface smoothness in a limited area. If you look at any paint surface with a magnifying glass, it will have some surface roughness. Ideally, you want the finish to be as smooth as possible. Paint film roughness is normally due to improper mixing or application (spraying).

Surface waviness is a measurement of an area's general levelness or trueness. If a panel is supposed to be perfectly flat, there should be no waviness when viewed from an angle. Improper sanding or blocking of plastic filler or primer is the main reason for waviness.

The first requisite for a high-quality refinishing job is a smooth body surface. The body technician will make extra work for the painting technician if the straightening/filling work is poor.

PAINT PROBLEMS

Paint problems include a wide range of troubles that can be found before or after painting. You must be able to inspect and analyze problems efficiently. If you fail to find a problem before spraying, you will have extra work fixing the mistake. You must also be able to solve finish problems that are found after you paint/refinish a vehicle.

Acid and Alkali Spotting

Acid and **alkali spotting** cause an obvious discoloration of the surface, as in **Figure 18–2.** Various paint pigments react differently when in contact with acids or alkalies. The cause of acid and alkali spotting is a chemical change of pigments. This chemical change results from atmospheric contamination in the presence of moisture. This problem is found on older finishes that have been exposed to industrial pollution.

To remedy acid spotting, wash the vehicle with detergent and water. Follow this with a vinegar bath. You might try wet sanding and compounding if there is only minor spotting. If the spots have absorbed deep into the finish, you will have to sand and refinish. If contamination has reached the metal or subcoating, the spot must be sanded down to the metal before refinishing.

To prevent acid spotting, steps should be taken to minimize contact between the vehicle finish and the contaminated atmosphere. Advise the customer to keep the vehicle in a protected area, such as a garage, as much as possible. In addition to this, the vehicle finish should be washed frequently and flushed vigorously with cool water to remove contaminants.

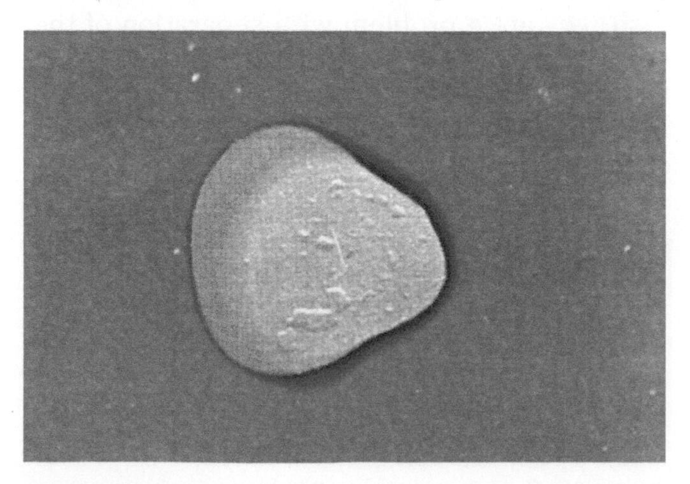

Figure 18–2. This is a close-up of acid or alkali spotting of paint. (Courtesy of PPG Industries, Inc.)

Bleeding

Bleeding is a discoloration of the new paint after refinishing. It results when solvent in the new finish penetrates the materials underneath the finish. This causes dyes or colors in the existing paint, filler, or putty to dissolve, and these are then absorbed up into the new finish. Usually, reds and maroons release a dye that comes to the surface of the fresh finish to cause a bleeding problem. An example of bleeding is shown in **Figure 18–3.**

To remedy bleeding, remove all colorcoats and refinish. You can also allow the surface to cure. Then apply bleeder sealer and recoat.

To prevent bleeding, apply bleeder sealer over suspected bleeder colors before spraying new color.

Blistering

Blistering shows up as small, swelled areas on the finish, like a "water blister" on human skin. There will be a lack of gloss if blisters are small.

Figure 18–3. This paint has suffered from bleeding or from the primer coming through the paint. (Courtesy of PPG Industries, Inc.)

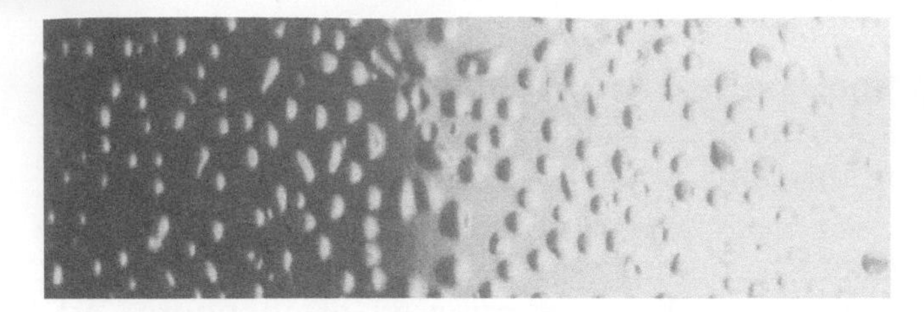

Figure 18–4. Here is a blistering paint problem. (Courtesy of PPG Industries, Inc.)

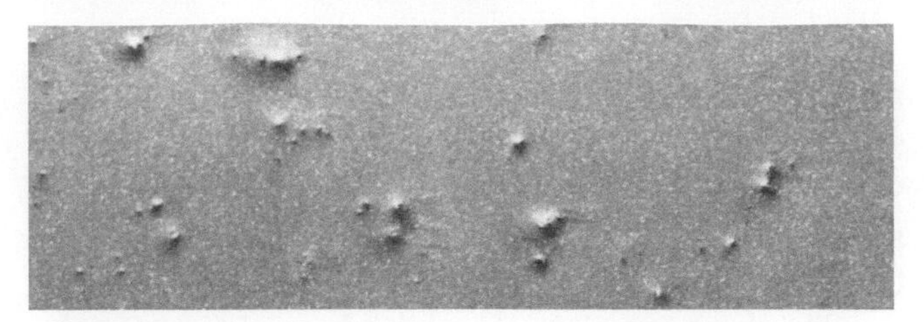

Figure 18–6. Dirt in the finish is a common problem that often results from not blowing off the vehicle while using a tack rag or from poor paint booth cleanliness. (Courtesy of PPG Industries, Inc.)

You will find broken-edged craters if the blisters have burst. See **Figure 18–4.**

Blistering is usually caused by rust under the surface. It is also caused by spraying over oil or grease, by moisture in spray lines, and trapped solvents. Blistering can also be due to prolonged or repeated exposure of the surface to high humidity.

To remedy blistering, sand and refinish the blistered areas. It can be prevented by thoroughly cleaning and treating metal.

Frequently drain your air lines of water. Avoid overly fast-drying solvents/reducers when temperature is high. Also allow proper drying time between coats.

Blushing

Blushing is a problem that makes the finish turn "milky." This is shown in **Figure 18–5.** It is caused by fast solvents/reducers in high humidity or condensation on the vehicle surface while painting.

To remedy blushing, use a slower-drying reducer or add retarder to the solvent/reducer and respray. You may also have to sand and refinish.

To prevent blushing, keep the material and the surface to be sprayed at room temperature. Select a good quality solvent/reducer. Use a retarder or reflow solvent when spraying in high humidity and warm temperatures.

Figure 18–5. Blushing makes the paint look "milky." (Courtesy of PPG Industries, Inc.)

Dirt in Finish

Dirt in finish is caused by foreign particles dried in the paint film. This is due to improper cleaning, not properly blowing off the vehicle, dirt on the technician, or failure to tack-rag the surface before spraying. This can also be due to a bad air regulator filter. A dirty work area or dirty spray gun can also deposit dirt in the finish. Refer to **Figure 18–6.**

To correct light dirt in the finish, rub out the finish with polishing compound. If the dirt is deep in the finish, sand and compound to restore gloss. Metallic finishes may show mottling with this treatment and will then require additional colorcoats.

To prevent dirt in the finish, blow out all cracks and body joints. Clean with solvent and tack-rag the surface thoroughly. Be sure all of your equipment and work area is clean. Replace inlet air filters if dirty or defective. Strain out foreign matter from the material. Keep all containers closed when they are not in use to prevent contamination.

Fisheyes

Fisheyes are a problem with separation of the wet film. Small indentations will form in the wet film. Sometimes, the previous finish under the new material can be seen in these spots. An example is in **Figure 18–7.**

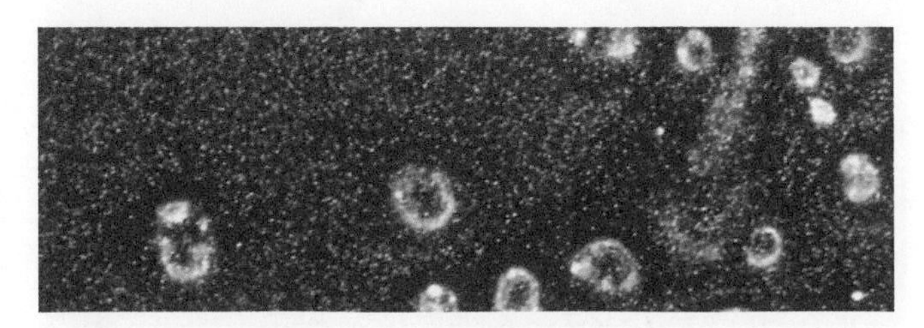

Figure 18–7. Fisheyes are small indentations in the surface film that look something like the eyes of a fish looking at you. (Courtesy of PPG Industries, Inc.)

Fisheyes are usually caused by improper cleaning of the old surface. They can also be due to spraying over finishes that contain silicone.

To correct a fisheye problem, wash off the new finish while it is still wet and respray. You can also add a fisheye preventer additive to the paint and respray over the problem. This will usually make the fisheyes flow out smooth. To prevent fisheyes, clean the surface with wax and grease remover.

Mottling

Mottling is a streaking of the color, usually with metallic finishes. It is caused by excessive wetting or a heavier film thickness in some areas. Look at **Figure 18–8.**

To remedy mottling of a freshly applied finish, back the spray gun away when spraying. Also increase air pressure for the final coat. Avoid overreduction. On a dried finish, scuff down the surface and apply additional color to correct mottling.

To prevent mottling, avoid excessive wetting or heavy film buildup in local areas. Be careful not to overreduce the color.

Orange Peel

Orange peel is a paint roughness problem that looks like tiny dents in the paint surface. It resembles the skin of an orange. An example is in **Figure 18–9.**

Figure 18–8. Mottling is a streaking problem common to metallic colors. (Courtesy of PPG Industries, Inc.)

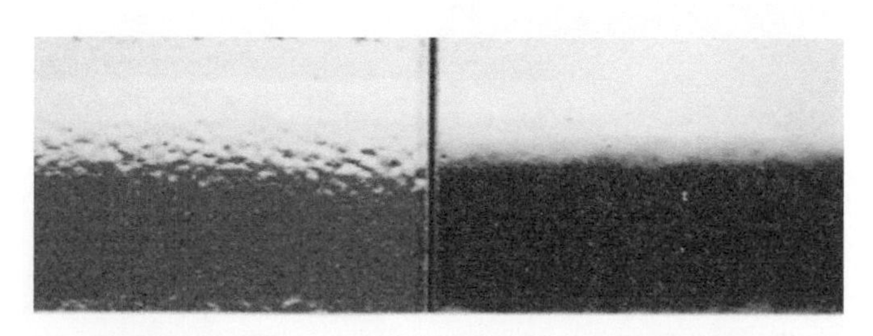

Figure 18–9. Orange peel is a rough, bumpy surface film. (Courtesy of PPG Industries, Inc.)

The droplets formed in the spray pattern hit the surface and dry before they have time to flow out. This causes a roughness in the surface.

When this occurs with primers, excessive sanding is required to make the surface smooth enough to apply the topcoats. While there is always a slight amount of orange peel in a film, too much will cause roughness, low gloss, or both.

Orange peel is commonly caused by underreduction or an improper solvent/reducer. The paint will lack proper flow. It can also be due to the surface drying too fast and improper air pressure at the spray gun.

To fix orange peel while you are still painting, you can often thin or reduce the final coat to its maximum limit and apply the last coat wet. This may make the orange peel flow out. If not, with enamel, rub the surface with a mild polishing compound. With severe cases, you may have to sand and refinish.

To prevent orange peel, properly adjust air pressure to the spray gun. Also make sure you have properly reduced the material.

Peeling

Peeling shows up as a separation of the surface film from the subsurface. It is caused by improper surface preparation or incompatibility of one coat to another. See **Figure 18–10.**

To repair a peeling problem, you must remove the peeling finish completely. Prepare the metal properly and refinish with compatible materials.

To prevent peeling, thoroughly clean and treat the surface. Use recommended primers for special metals. Follow acceptable refinish practices using compatible materials.

Pin Holes or Blistering over Plastic Filler

Pin holes or blistering over body filler are noticed as air bubbles raising the surface film.

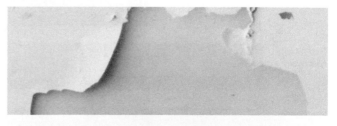

Figure 18–10. With peeling, a noticeable area of finish lifts. This problem is normally caused by improper surface sanding or a primer problem. (Courtesy of PPG Industries, Inc.)

These bubbles can then pop and cause craters when they erupt.

One cause for pin holes over body filler is excessive amounts of hardener. Vigorous stirring or beating of the hardener will also form bubbles in filler.

To fix this problem, sand thoroughly and recoat with a glaze coat of body filler or putty.

To prevent pin holes and blistering, mix in recommended quantities of hardener. Scrape the filler or putty back and forth, without stirring, to work out air bubbles.

Pitting or Cratering

Pitting or **cratering** is a problem where small holes form in the paint film. It can look like dry spray or overspray. It is caused by the same things as blistering (except, in this case, the blisters have broken). Corrections are also the same as for blistering. Refer to **Figure 18–11.**

Plastic Bleed-Through

Plastic bleed-through is a discoloration, often a yellowing, of the color due to chemicals from the body filler. Although it is very rare today, it may be caused by too much hardener or by applying the paint before the body filler is fully cured. See **Figure 18–12.**

Figure 18–11. Pitting, or cratering, looks similar to dry spray. If not a chemical problem with the paint, the surface may not have been sanded properly before painting. (Courtesy of PPG Industries, Inc.)

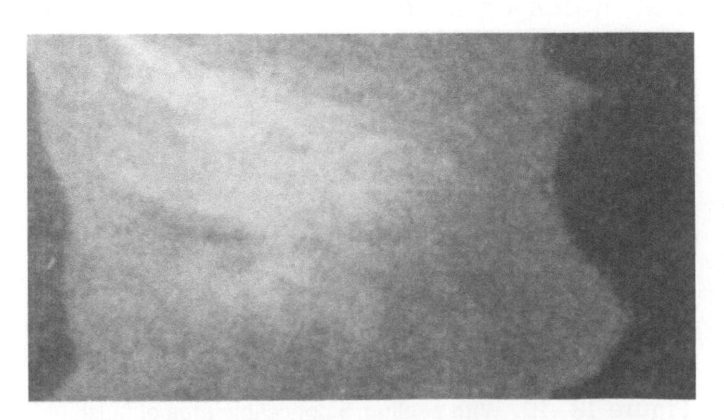

Figure 18–12. With a bleed-through problem, colors under the surface are visible. (Courtesy of PPG Industries, Inc.)

To remedy plastic bleed-through, allow the topcoat to cure and refinish. To prevent this problem, use the right amount of hardener in body fillers. Allow adequate cure time before refinishing.

Rust under Finish

Rust under finish will cause the finish to peel or blister. You can also have raised spots on the surface film. This problem is caused by improper metal preparation. Broken film has allowed moisture to creep under the surrounding finish. Rust can also be caused by water in air lines. Look at **Figure 18–13.**

To remedy rust under the finish, seal off the entrance of moisture from the inner part of panels. Sand down to the bare metal, prepare the metal and spray with a rust-preventative coating before refinishing. You can also prevent a rust problem by applying epoxy primer directly to the metal. Locate any source of moisture and stop it.

When replacing ornaments or molding, be careful not to break the film and allow dissimilar metals to come in contact with each other. This contact can produce electrolysis that may cause a tearing away or loss of good bond with the film.

Runs

Runs occur when gravity produces a mass slippage of an overwet, thick film. The weight of the film will cause it to slide or roll down the surface. A large area of finish will flow down and form large globules. See **Figure 18–14.**

Runs are caused by:

1. Overreduction with low air pressure
2. Extra slow-drying solvents/reducers

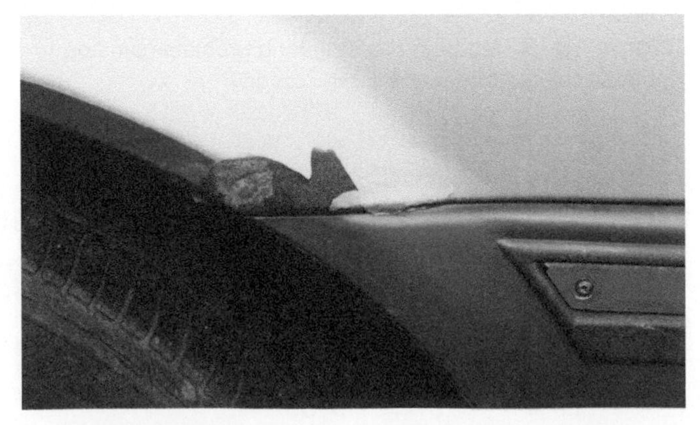

Figure 18–13. Rust under a finish is due to improper surface preparation.

Figure 18–14. Runs and sags are due to too much wet spray material in one place. (Courtesy of PPG Industries, Inc.)

3. Spraying on a cold surface
4. Improperly cleaned surface
5. Spray gun too close or moved too slowly
6. Too many coats

To fix a run in a metallic colorcoat, you must usually allow the finish to cure. Then sand and refinish the panel. If the run is only in the clearcoat and not in the metallic colorcoat, you can often wet sand to level the run without refinishing. On smaller parts or areas, you can also wash the wet paint off with solvent/reducer and start over.

With solid colors, you can also allow the finish to dry. Then wet sand the run or sag before buffing. This will not work with metallics.

To prevent runs, use the recommended reducer at specified reduction and air pressure. Do not spray over a cold surface. Clean the surface thoroughly. Allow sufficient flash time between coats. Use proper gun spray pattern, speed, and distance from the surface.

Sag

A **sag** is a partial slipping down of the surface film created by a film that is too heavy to support itself. It appears something like a "curtain." A large area of film is pulled down by gravity.

Sags are caused by:

1. Underreduction
2. Applying successive coats without allowing dry time
3. Low air pressure (lack of atomization)
4. Spray gun too close to surface
5. Spray gun out of adjustment
6. Moving spray gun too slowly

To fix a sag, sand or wash it off and refinish. To prevent sags, use the proper solvent/reducer at recommended reduction. Adjust the air pressure and the gun for correct atomization and move it at the right speed. Keep the gun at the the right distance from the work.

Primecoat Show-through

Primecoat show-through is a problem in which the color of the primecoat is seen through the paint. It is caused by insufficient colorcoats or repeated compounding. Primecoat show-through can also be caused by not having uniform color under the paint. To fix primecoat show-through, sand and refinish. Refer to **Figure 18–15.**

To prevent primecoat show-through, apply good coverage of color. Avoid excessive compounding.

Water Spotting

Water spotting is a dulling of gloss in spots. It can occur as a mass of spots that appear as a large distortion of the film. It is due to spots of water drying on a finish that is not thoroughly dry. It can be caused by washing the finish in bright sunlight. Refer to **Figure 18–16.**

To repair water spots, you can try wet sanding and polishing. However, you might have to sand and refinish.

To prevent water spotting, keep the fresh paint job out of the rain. Do not allow water to dry on the new finish.

Figure 18–15. This is a primecoat show-through problem. (Courtesy of PPG Industries, Inc.)

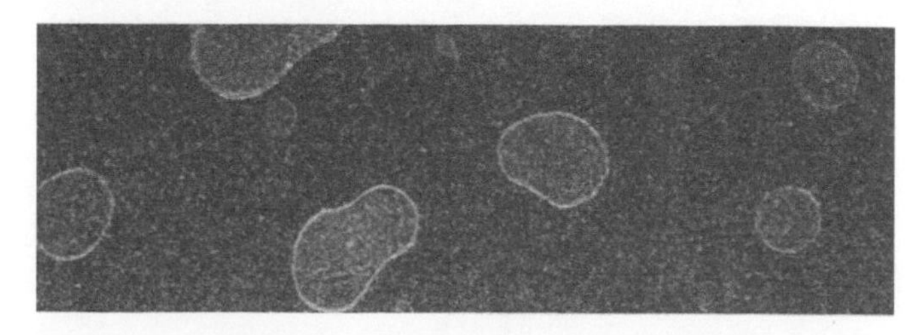

Figure 18–16. Water spotting dulls paint gloss. (Courtesy of PPG Industries, Inc.)

Wet Spots

Wet spots are a finish problem seen as off-colored and/or slow-drying spots of various sizes. It is usually due to improper cleaning. Heavy primecoats not properly dried is another reason. So is contamination with gasoline or other incompatible solvents.

To remedy wet spots, sand or wash the surface off thoroughly and refinish. To prevent this trouble, clean the surface with wax and grease remover. Allow primecoats to dry thoroughly. Use only water as a sanding lubricant.

Wrinkling

Wrinkling is a severe puckering of the film that appears like the skin of a prune (fruit). It is more common with enamel paints. There is a loss of gloss as the paint dries. Minute wrinkling may not be visible to the naked eye. See **Figure 18–17.**

Wrinkling is caused by:

1. Underreduction
2. Air pressure too low, causing excessive film thickness
3. Excessive coats
4. Fast reducers creating overloading
5. Surface drying trapping solvents
6. Fresh film subjected to heat too soon

To fix wrinkling, break open the top surface by sanding and allow it to dry thoroughly. Then remove the finish and refinish.

To prevent wrinkling, reduce and apply enamels according to directions. Do not force dry until solvents have flashed off.

Metal Dust Damage

Metal dust damage, also known as "rail dust," occurs when metallic particles from industrial fallout settle onto the paint. The particles soon begin to corrode, eating into the finish. Study **Figure 18–18.**

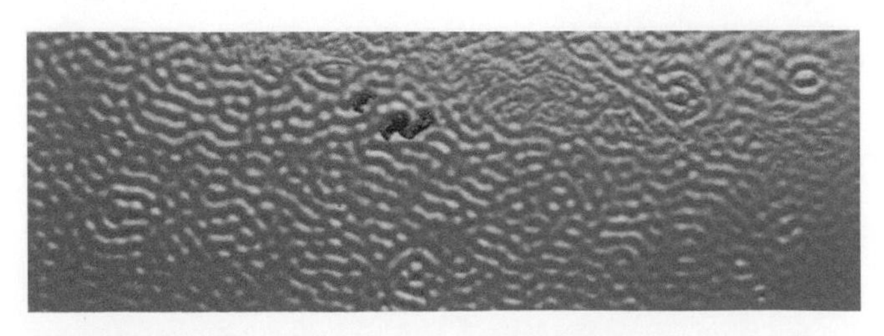

Figure 18–17. Wrinkling gives the paint a "prune" look. (Courtesy of PPG Industries, Inc.)

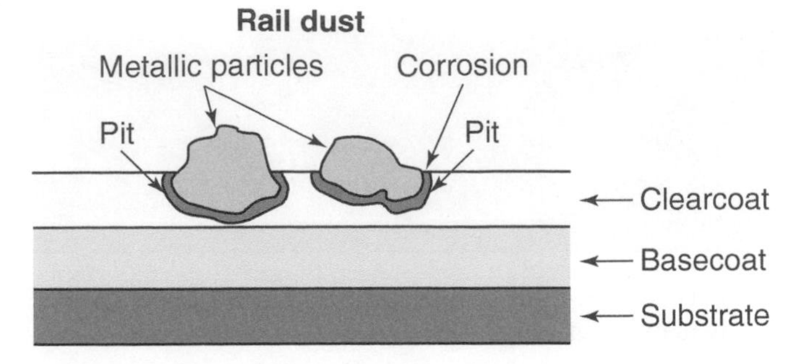

(A) Metal dust etched into the clearcoat can be felt with a hand or rag.

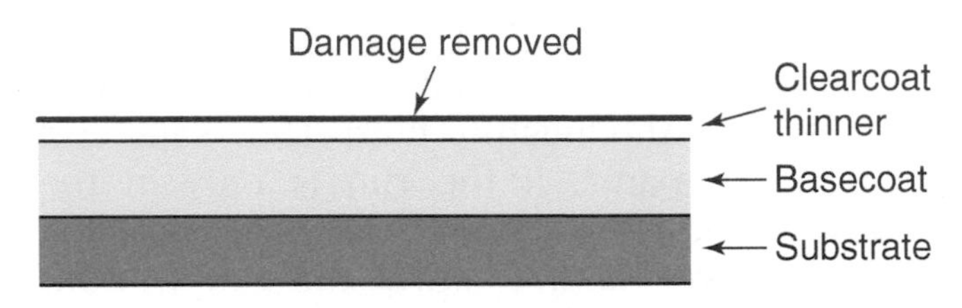

(B) After treatment, this damage can be repaired by wet sanding the clearcoat and compounding.

Figure 18–18. Metal dust fallout can etch into the finish.

Metal dust damage can be identified on light-colored finishes by the visible small brown or black specks. On darker-colored surfaces, you must feel for prickly protrusion in the paint film. You can also rub a cotton towel across the surface. The iron particles will snag bits of cotton in the rag.

Metal dust damage can sometimes be repaired by:

1. Blowing off the vehicle with compressed air
2. Washing and degreasing the vehicle
3. Treating with mild oxalic acid solution to dissolve the rust
4. Washing again to remove loose metallic particles
5. Color sanding, compounding, and glazing

Oxalic acid is also known as "industrial fallout remover." It works by dissolving the rust holding the particles to the paint. To use the oxalic solution:

1. Soak rags in the solution.
2. Lay the cloths over the affected area. Work in small areas.

3. Remove the cloths and rinse thoroughly with clean water. Remove excess water with clean towels.
4. Check the surface for remaining signs of iron particles.
5. If more particles are present, repeat the above steps.
6. If the solution does NOT dislodge all of the particles, wet sand the affected area. Then try machine compounding and polishing the area. If you do not cut through the finish or clear, this will repair the damage. The area must be refinished if it has gone through the topcoat.

DANGER

Wear, rubber gloves, a respirator, and a face shield when using oxalic acid. Protect yourself properly from the fumes and an accidental splash of acid.

Acid Rain Damage

Acid rain damage varies because it is chemical damage from industrial fallout. The contents of the fallout vary with geographic locations. Various types of minerals sit on top of the surface film and damage it. Refer to **Figure 18–19.**

Minor acid rain damage produces shallow craters, dulling, fading, and chalking that do not eat fully through the paint. Minor acid rain damage can be removed by:

1. Washing the vehicle.
2. Neutralizing the acid by using a baking soda solution. The solution is a mixture of 1 tablespoon of baking soda per quart of water. The solution is applied with a spray bottle or by laying a saturated cloth on the area.
3. Rinsing with clean water.
4. Wet sanding with 1,500 grit or finer sandpaper.
5. Compounding and glazing.

Test this in a small area on the worst acid rain damage first. If this does not restore the finish, there is major acid rain damage.

Major acid rain damage is severe chemical etching that has eaten completely through the paint. It may have eaten into the primer or all the way down to the body part. It requires that you strip all finish from the damaged areas. Otherwise, the acid residue will continue to eat through from beneath.

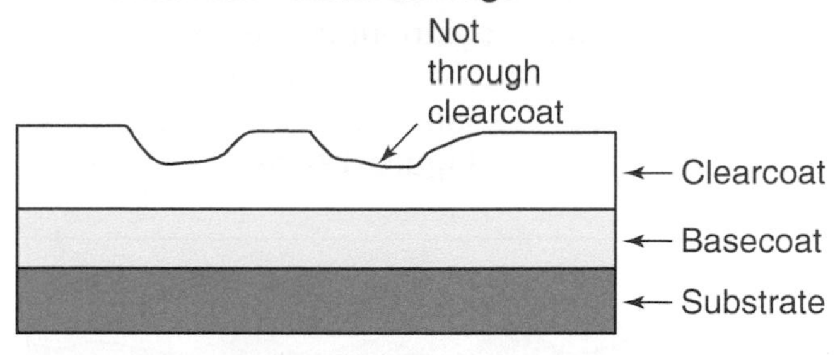

(A) With minor acid rain damage, the clearcoat is not penetrated. Wet sanding and buffing will usually fix the damage.

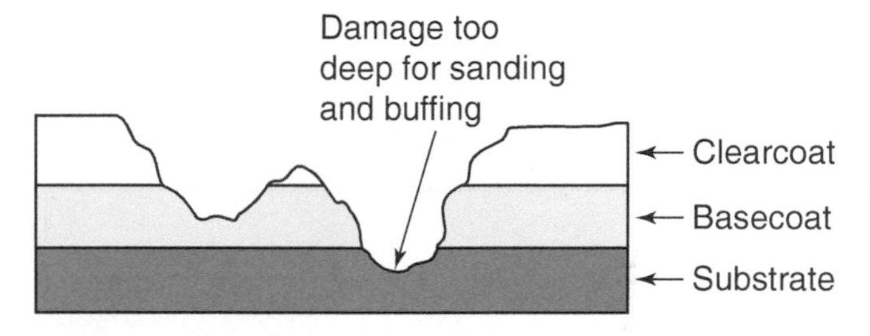

(B) Major acid rain damage is too deep and the area must be refinished.

Figure 18–19. Acid rain damage can also "eat" into the finish.

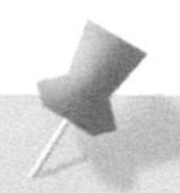

NOTE

Only horizontal surfaces (hoods, deck lids, roofs) usually suffer major acid rain damage and require stripping. The sides of the vehicle are usually unaffected and do NOT have to be stripped.

Sand Scratches

Sand scratches result from two sources:

1. Final sanding with incorrect (too coarse) sandpaper
2. Not allowing materials (usually primer or spot putty) to dry fully before painting/refinishing

If it is a solid color, you might be able to wet sand and machine compound the area. If the damage is in a colorcoat of a basecoat-clearcoat system, you will usually have to resand and refinish the area. See **Figure 18–20.**

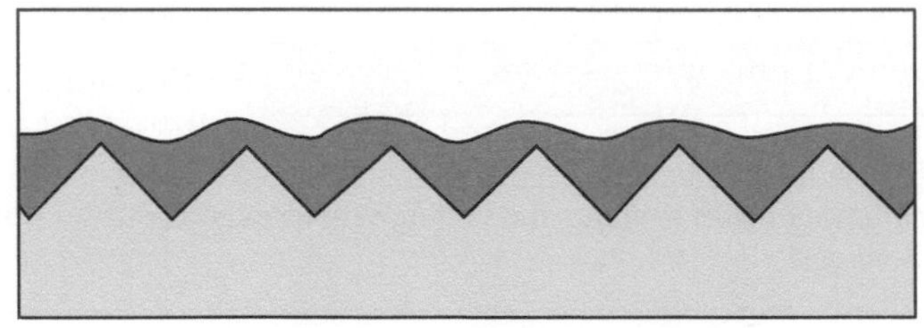

Primer-surfacer applied over sanded metal simulates the contours of the metal, with more shrinkage over deeper fills.

(A) Primer has been applied to a rough sanded surface.

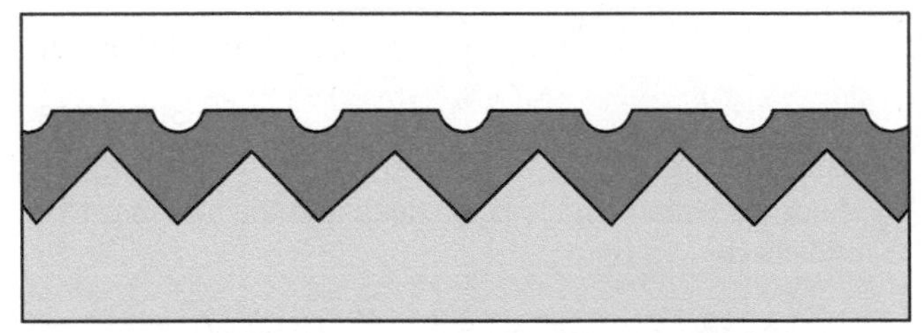

If sanded level before all solvents have evaporated, further evaporation of solvents will cause shrinkage, leaving furrows over the sanding marks in the metal.

(B) If sanded level before all solvents have evaporated, the primer will shrink more over sand scratches.

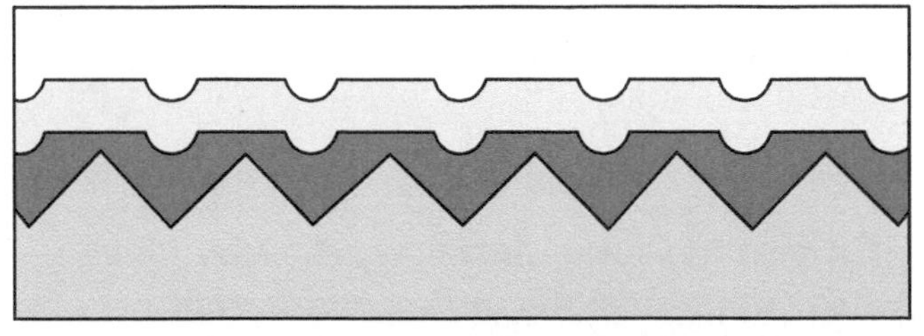

If the colorcoat is polished before all the thinner evaporates from the primer-surfacer and color, it will shrink back, showing sand scratches. This condition may also be caused by using coarse rubbing compounds, air pressure that is too high, or solvent that is too fast when applying printer-surfacer.

(C) If the paint (color and clear) is then applied, sand scratches will appear in the finish.

Figure 18–20. If damage is not due to too coarse a sandpaper, sand scratches can be due to not allowing materials under the surface to dry before refinishing. (Courtesy of PPG Industries, Inc.)

FINAL DETAILING

The objective in **final detailing** is to locate and correct any defect that may cause customer complaints. Corrective steps for final detailing are:

1. Wet sanding
2. Compounding
3. Machine glazing
4. Hand glazing

Each of these steps has its own requirements. As a general rule, finer and finer grades of products will be used for all of these steps. Progressively use finer wet sandpaper and compounds. Also, a single product line should be used throughout the repair. Manufacturer's recommendations should be followed.

Surface Paint Chips

Surface paint chips result from mechanical impact damage to the film: door dings, damage from road debris, etc. If the whole vehicle is not refinished, you should take the time to touch-up chips in the finish. Use the material mixed for the repair. It will usually have hardener in it.

Degrease the area with wax and grease remover. If you use a small paint brush, slowly move the touch-up paint straight into each chip. If you are using a solid color, use a thicker viscosity touch-up paint to fill the chip in one application. If you have metallic paint, use thinner touch-up paint and several coats to help match the color.

Allow the paint to cure sufficiently before wet sanding and polishing the chip repairs level.

Surface Protrusions

A **surface protrusion** (dirt) is a particle of paint or other debris sticking out of the film after refinishing. This problem results from a lack of cleanliness. Your spray gun, spray materials, or booth was contaminated.

Cut off the protrusion, being careful not to take off more finish than is necessary. The tip of the knife or razor blade should be pointed slightly upward. Smooth the area with a finesse sanding block or No. 3,500 grit sandpaper. Blow off any particles. Finish with an extra-fine rubbing compound.

Finesse Sanding

Finesse sanding can be used to level the protrusion with the surrounding film. Use a finesse sanding block as follows:

1. Dress the surface of the block with wet 220 grit sandpaper to make it smooth and flat. Thoroughly soak the block in clear water. Place the block over the protrusion and move it back and forth. If necessary, use a little water to help make the movement smoother. Refer to **Figure 18–21.** When the protrusion has all but disappeared, blow off the loose particles and finish the job with rubbing, then polishing compound.

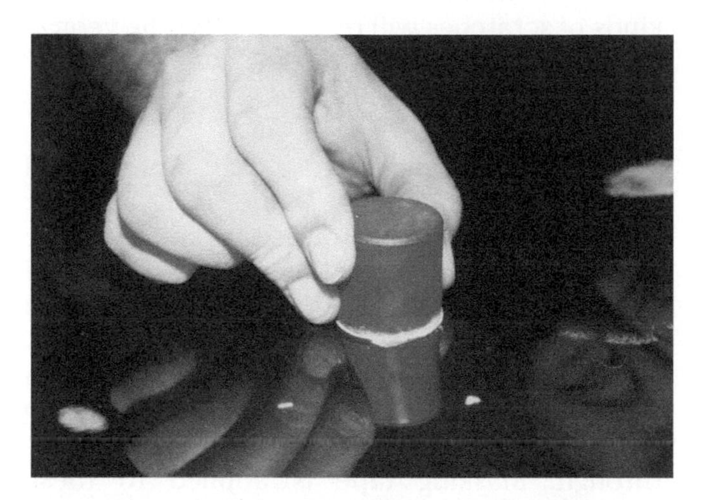

(A) Carefully rub a finesse sanding block over small imperfections in the film.

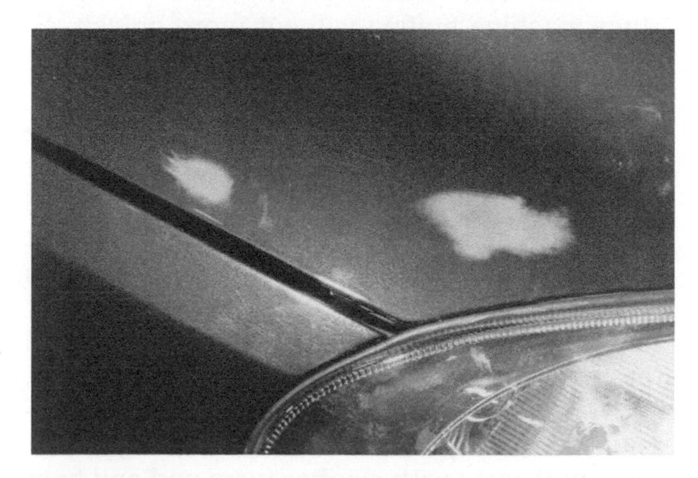

(B) Rub only until the raised imperfection is sanded level. Note the dull areas that have been finesse sanded.

Figure 18–21. Finesse sanding will quickly remove small paint film imperfections. Mark each paint flaw first with a water-based marker.

Wet Sanding

Wet sanding can be done to smooth the paint surface on larger areas, as when removing orange peel.

Wet sanding should normally be done with a *backing pad* or rubber *sanding block* to avoid crowning of the paint surface. A pad or block will help keep large, relatively flat surfaces level and uncrowned. On restricted and curved surfaces, you can use only your hand to wet sand.

Sanding blocks and sandpapers are available in a variety of grit sizes. For surface repairs, use coarser wet sandpapers, 500 to 600. For finesse finishing, 1,000, 1,200, and finer grits of wet sandpaper are typically used.

Wet sand in a small circular motion. Use plenty of water to flush away paint debris. Dip the block in a bucket of water or use a hose to flow water over the area. A sponge can also be used to help keep the sandpaper wet. Refer to **Figure 18–22.**

Check the defect often when using a sanding block. You do not want to cut too deep into the finish. If you cut through the clearcoat or color, repainting will be necessary. Wash surfaces thoroughly with clean water and a sponge after wet sanding.

Rubbing Compound

Rubbing compounds generally contain coarser grit abrasives than polishes. They are used to more rapidly cut the surface film by hand. Rubbing compounds produce a low surface gloss.

Rubbing compounds are available in various cutting strengths for both hand and machine compounding. *Hand compounds* are oil based to provide lubrication. Small areas or blended areas are best done by hand compounding. On large surfaces, machine compounding is recommended.

Rubbing compounds are used:

1. To eliminate fine sand scratches around a repair area
2. To correct a gritty surface
3. To smooth and bring out some of the gloss of paint
4. Sometimes as a final smoothing step to remove light scratches and small dirt particles before painting

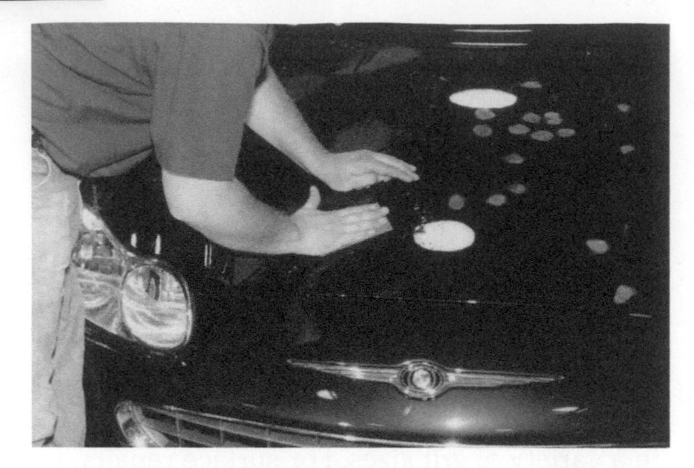

(A) Wet sand the problem area with water, a rubber sanding block, and extra fine wet sandpaper. Move the sanding block in a circular motion.

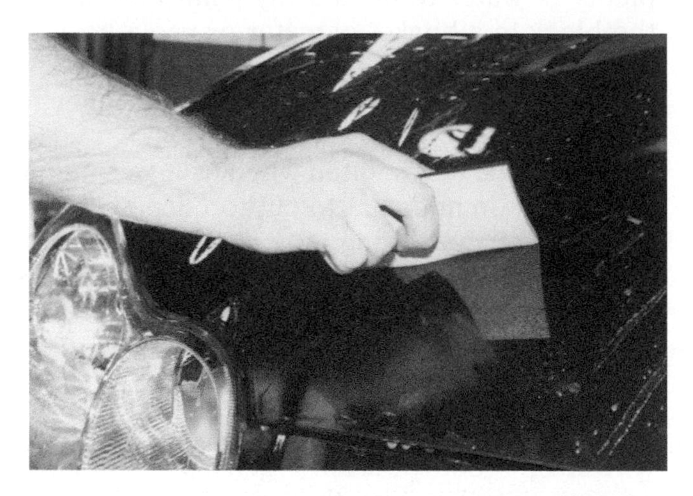

(B) Squeegee off the area to see if more sanding is needed.

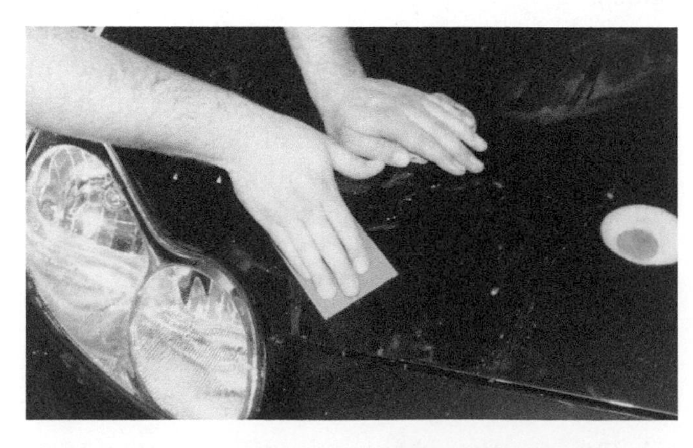

(C) A wet rag or sponge can be used to apply water to wash away sanding debris so the sandpaper will cut more quickly.

Figure 18–22. Study the basic steps for wet sanding a paint problem area.

Hand Compounding

Fold a soft, lint-free flannel cloth into a thick pad or roll it into a ball and apply a small amount of hand compound to it. Use straight, back-and-forth strokes and medium-to-hard pressure until the desired smoothness is achieved.

Hand compounding takes a lot of "elbow grease" and is time consuming. To keep the compounding of lacquer paints to a minimum, it is important to apply the finish as wet as possible (without sags or runs) by using the proper solvent/reducer for the shop temperature.

When using hand polishes or glazes, apply the glaze to the surface using a clean, dry cloth. Rub the glaze thoroughly into the surface. Then wipe it dry. Glazes can fill and cover up some scratches that should be buffed out. These kinds of scratches will reappear after the vehicle has been washed a few times.

Machine Compounding

Machine compounds are often water-based to disperse the abrasive while using a power buffer. A buffing pad is rotated by an electric or air (pneumatic) polisher to force the compound over the paint surface. If done properly, this will quickly bring it to a high gloss. See **Figure 18–23.**

Edge masking involves taping over panel edges and body lines prior to machine buffing or polishing to protect the paint from burn-through. Masking tape is applied to these surfaces to protect them.

Burn-through occurs when the pad removes too much paint on an edge, lip, or body surface. Since machine buffing will cut more quickly on these areas, always protect them with masking paper.

After the compounding is completed, remove the tape and compound the edge by hand—just enough to produce a smooth finish. Keep in mind that body lines usually retain less paint than flat surfaces and thus should get only minimum compounding.

Many finesse finishing systems recommend the use of specific buffing and polishing pads. Use a wool pad first with coarser machine compound to quickly remove the wet sanding marks. Then buff again with a softer foam pad and finer compound to bring out the paint gloss and to remove any swirl marks from the wool pad. Refer to **Figure 18–24.**

Apply machine compound over a small area. Then compound using a slow-speed power

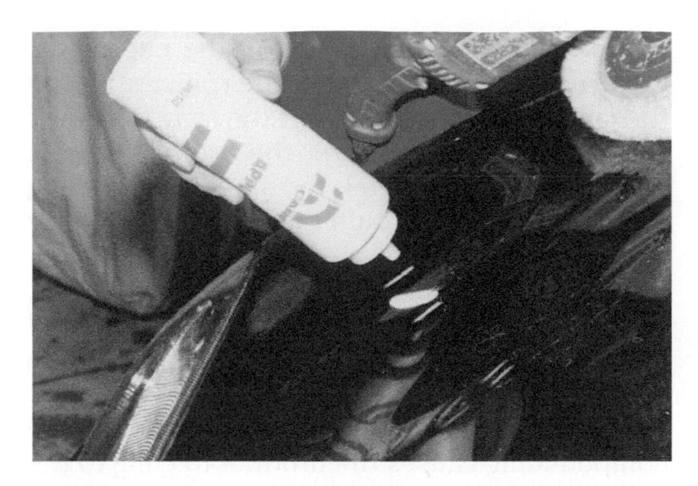

(A) Apply machine compound to a small area on the vehicle.

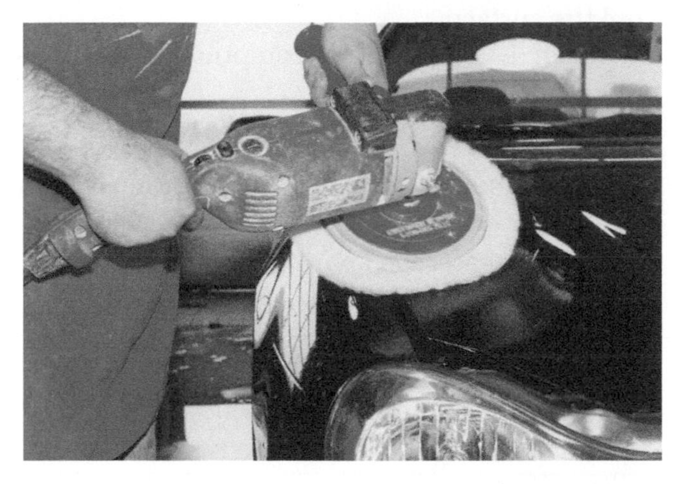

(B) To prevent the compound from flying all over, spread it out with the buffer pad before depressing the buffer trigger. Start the buffer. Do not press down on the buffer. Allow the weight of the tool to do the work.

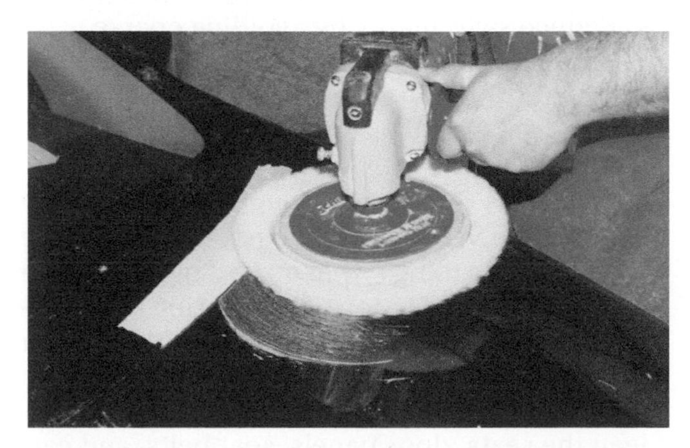

(C) Mask parts that could be damaged or sharp body lines. It is easy to cut through or burn through paint on sharp edges.

Figure 18–23. Note the major steps for buffing paint after wet sanding.

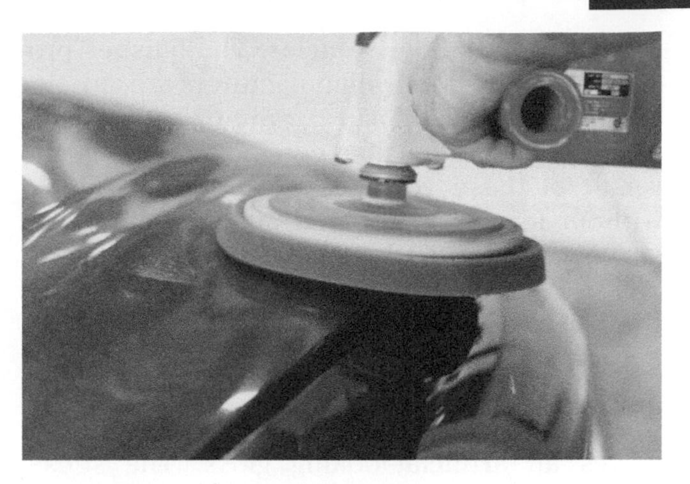

Figure 18–24. A foam pad is softer than a wool pad and will reduce swirl marks in the finish. It is often used after a wool pad. Use finer machine compound with a foam pad.

buffer. It is important to use a slow-speed machine to avoid static buildup and high surface temperatures. Do not push down on the buffer. Let the weight of the machine do the work.

Because the compound has a tendency to dry out, do not try to do too large an area at one time. Always keep the machine moving to prevent cutting through or burning the paint. As the compound starts to dry out, lift up a little on the machine so pad speed increases. This will make the surface start to shine.

Polishing

Polishing involves using very fine compound to bring the paint surface up to full gloss. It is usually done after compounding. You can hand polish small or hard-to-reach areas. Machine polish larger areas to save time.

Instead of a circular action buffer, you should use an orbital action machine for final polishing. An **orbital action polisher** will move the polishing compound in a random manner to prevent swirl marks left from machine compounding. Swirl marks are tiny lines in the surface film from the abrasive action of the coarser compound.

Slight defects in the paint can be repaired by polishing. The choice of rubbing compound depends on the extent of the damage. Final polishing should always be done with an extra-fine polishing compound.

Sponge Buffing Pads

A change in automobile finishes in recent years has led to the development of an entirely new technology in the buffing and final delivery prep of collision repaired vehicles. The finishes produced by automobile manufacturers are glossier and virtually free of any texture or orange peel. The high solids finishes commonly used in the repair of these vehicles are difficult to apply without leaving a textured appearance on the surface. In order to duplicate the manufacturer's finish, it is often necessary to buff or compound the finish to remove any surface blemishes and texture normally associated with spray painting operations.

Buffing with traditional wool pads often leaves an artificial-looking gloss. The subsequent development and the increased popularity of sponge pads for buffing operations has occurred for a variety of reasons. Sponge pads tend to be more user friendly and are less apt to damage the new finish than their wool counterparts. When buffing with a wool pad, both the compound and the fiber of the pad abrade and remove material from the surface. This can lead to excessive film removal, swirl marks, and even burning of the finish. When buffing with a sponge pad, the rubbing compound alone abrades the surface. Due to its softness and resilience, the sponge merely serves as the vehicle for the buffing action. This "softer" buffing action leaves the finish with a more natural-looking gloss, as it is less likely to leave swirl marks.

One of the major disadvantages of using sponge pads is the amount of heat they generate on the surface. Unlike the wool pad, which dissipates the heat through the fiber, the sponge pad transmits the heat back into the surface being compounded. Running the buffer at too high a speed may cause the surface to overheat, causing the rubbing compound to gum up and collect on the surface in a glue-like mass. This can readily be removed with water and a sponge, but if overdone, it can cause a blemish on the surface.

Using Buffers and Polishers. When using buffing and polishing pads:

1. Inspect, clean, or replace pads often to avoid residue buildup.
2. Use separate pads for different grades and types of products.
3. When applying the compound, apply an "X" of the product to the surface. Work it around the face of the pad before hitting the machine's trigger. This will help prevent compound from flying all over.

The buffer has an effect on the cutting action. For example, the higher the rpm, the higher the cutting rate and the lower the rpm, the lower the cutting rate. The faster the orbital buffer is moved across the panel, the slower the cutting rate. The slower the buffer is moved, the higher the cutting rate.

Excessive buffing heat can cause swirl marks, warping, discoloring, hazing, and the material can dry out too quickly. If the area is hot to the touch, there is too much heat. Cool it with water.

Static electricity created during machine compounding causes the product to cling to the surface being repaired. Avoid static by grounding the vehicle. You might also want to add 5 percent rubbing alcohol to the water used to cool the surface.

When using rubbing compounds and machine glazes:

1. Use a single manufacturer's product line.
2. Follow the manufacturer's recommendations for use.
3. Use the materials sparingly.
4. Use the buffing wheel to distribute the material evenly over the area to be repaired.
5. Keep the pad flat and directly over the surface being repaired.
6. Use a slow, circular motion.
7. Use the finest product possible. Using a finer product may take a little longer initially, but it will generally require less time to complete the repair.
8. Reduce swirl marks by avoiding coarse products and worn buffing pads.

GET READY

Get ready is the last, thorough cleanup before returning the vehicle to the customer. You must do all the "little things" that make a big difference to customer satisfaction. The interior and exterior of the vehicle should be cleaner than when the customer brought it in.

Vacuum the interior of the vehicle carefully. Clean the seats, door panels, seat belts, and carpets. If dusty, clean and treat the vinyl surface with a conditioner. Be sure to remove all excess reconditioner from the seat crevices and folds. Stubborn stains should be cleaned with a recommended cleaning solution.

WARNING

Avoid using strong cleaning agents on the plastic parts in the dashboard. Some will dissolve and damage plastic. Also avoid using anything containing silicone.

Carefully remove any overspray that may be on the vehicle. If it can be done without dripping on the new finish, use solvent (thinner or reducer). Clean body seams, moldings, and lights. Thoroughly clean all the glass, including windows, mirrors, and lights.

Use a brush with soap and water to clean the tires and wheels. Do not let dirty wheels spoil the appearance of an otherwise quality job. Coat them with a conditioner.

Chassis black can be used to blacken wheel openings and any other exposed undercarriage parts, since overspray often gets on these areas.

Replace wipers, moldings, and emblems that were removed before finishing. Take the time to clean off these items and be certain that everything is replaced.

As a finishing touch, clean the engine compartment. The easiest way to do this is to spray it with a heavy-duty engine cleaner. Then flush the engine compartment out with high-pressure water. A clean engine compartment usually makes a big impression on the customer.

Finally, inspect the vehicle with a careful eye for details. If a window is smeared, clean it again, (see **Figure 18–25**). If a piece of masking tape remains, remove it. If an emblem is missing, replace it before the customer asks where it is.

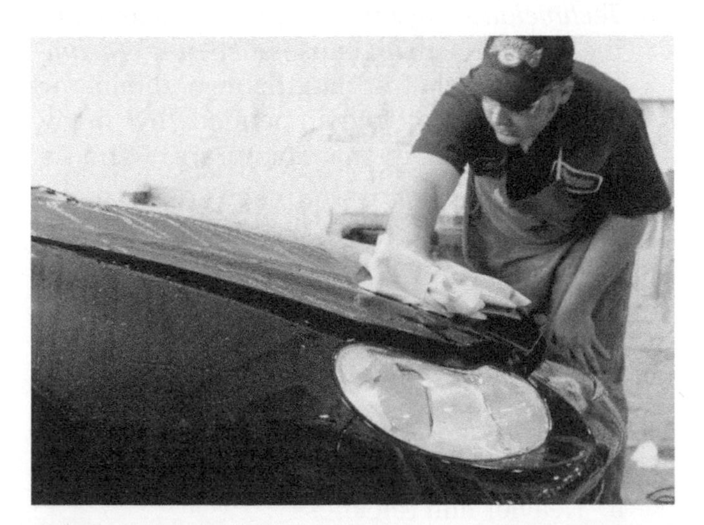

Figure 18–25. Make sure the vehicle is perfectly clean before releasing it to the customer. First impressions of the vehicle are very important.

If the vehicle gets dirty while waiting to be picked up, wipe it down. The number one objective should always be a satisfied customer.

CARING FOR NEW FINISH

A newly refinished vehicle must receive special care, as the finish can take several months to cure. Each paint manufacturer will have specific recommendations for caring for a new finish. Explain all precautions to the vehicle owner.

To care for a new finish, you and the customer should:

1. Avoid commercial car washes and harsh cleaners for 1–3 months.
2. Hand wash using only water and a soft sponge for the first month. Dry with cotton towels only. Do not use a chamois.
3. Avoid waxing and polishing for up to 3 months. After that time, use a wax designed for basecoat-clearcoat finishes, as they are the least aggressive.
4. Avoid scraping ice and snow near newly refinished surfaces.
5. Flush gas, oil, or fluid spills with water as soon as possible for the first month. Do not wipe them off.

SUMMARY

- Some of the most common paint problems include pinholes, mottling, runs, and sags.
- The steps for correcting surface imperfections include examining the finish for imperfections, finesse sanding, buffing, and final detailing.
- The objective in final detailing is to locate and correct any defect that may cause customer complaints. The four steps are sanding and filing, compounding, machine glazing, and hand glazing.

TECHNICAL TERMS

surface roughness
surface waviness
acid spotting
alkali spotting
blistering
blushing
fisheyes
mottling

orange peel
peeling
pin holes
pitting
cratering
plastic bleed-through
rust under finish
runs
sag
primecoat show-through
water spotting
wet spots
wrinkling
metal dust damage
acid rain damage
minor acid rain damage
major acid rain damage
sand scratches
final detailing
surface paint chips
surface protrusion
finesse sanding
rubbing compounds
edge masking
polishing
orbital action polisher
get ready

REVIEW QUESTIONS

1. List four steps for correcting surface imperfections.
2. ______________ shows up as small, swelled areas on the finish, like a ______________ ______________ on human skin.
3. What is paint blushing?
4. How can you correct a small amount of dirt on a painted surface?
5. What causes fisheyes and how can you prevent and fix them?
6. This is a paint roughness problem that looks like tiny dents in the paint surface.
   a. Paint protrusions
   b. Mottling
   c. Orange peel
   d. Peeling
7. List six reasons for paint runs.
8. Is fixing a run in a solid color and in a metallic the same? Explain your answer.
9. *Technician A* says to wet sand with a sanding block to keep from crowning the surface. *Technician B* says it is OK to use your hand to wet sand on curved surfaces. Who is correct?
   a. Technician A
   b. Technician B
   c. Both Technicians A and B
   d. Neither Technician
10. What is the difference between a rubbing compound and a polishing compound?
11. ______________ ______________ are water-based to disperse the abrasive while using a power buffer.
12. Why should you mask edges and body lines before buffing?
13. What is burn-through?

ASE-STYLE REVIEW QUESTIONS

1. *Technician A* says that dirt in the paint can be reduced with proper cleaning before refinishing. *Technician B* says that blistering is a problem that makes the finish turn "milky looking." Who is correct?
   a. Technician A
   b. Technician B
   c. Both Technicians A and B
   d. Neither Technician

2. A vehicle returns to the shop. The area painted seems to be suffering from a blistering problem. This could be caused by all of the following EXCEPT:
   a. Rust under the surface
   b. Painting over oil or grease
   c. Moisture in spray lines
   d. Improper reduction

3. *Technician A* says that improper cleaning of the surface usually causes fisheyes. *Technician B* says that adding fisheye eliminator additive is not recommended by many of today's paint manufacturers. Who is correct?
   a. Technician A
   b. Technician B
   c. Both Technicians A and B
   d. Neither Technician

4. Which of the following usually causes paint lifting?
   a. Heavier film thickness
   b. Improper drying of previous coatings
   c. Extreme temperature changes
   d. Slow-dry thinner

5. *Technician A* says that orange peel is commonly caused by underreduction. *Technician B* says that this problem can also be due to the surface drying too fast. Who is correct?
   a. Technician A
   b. Technician B
   c. Both Technicians A and B
   d. Neither Technician

6. Runs are caused by all of the following EXCEPT:
   a. Extra slow drying reducer/solvent
   b. Extra fast drying reducer/solvent
   c. Painting on cold surface
   d. Too many coats of paint

7. *Technician A* says that a small run in a solid color can often be repaired with wet sanding and buffing. *Technician B* says that a run in a metallic color cannot be repaired this way. Who is correct?
   a. Technician A
   b. Technician B
   c. Both Technicians A and B
   d. Neither Technician

8. *Technician A* says that sand scratches result from final sanding with too coarse a grit of sandpaper. *Technician B* says that it is from not allowing the primer to dry fully before painting. Who is correct?
   a. Technician A
   b. Technician B
   c. Both Technicians A and B
   d. Neither Technician

9. Which of the following would normally be used to correct a small protrusion in a paint film?
   a. Finesse sanding and buffing
   b. DA sanding and buffing
   c. Buffing only
   d. Repaint panel

10. *Technician A* says to use a cotton buffing pad before a foam pad. *Technician B* says a foam pad should be used first to eliminate swirl marks. Who is correct?
    a. Technician A
    b. Technician B
    c. Both Technicians A and B
    d. Neither Technician

ACTIVITIES

1. Inspect several vehicles. How many paint problems can you find? Make a report of your findings. Is there any industrial fallout problem in your area?
2. Obtain an old painted part. Intentionally paint the part to produce various paint problems. Allow the paint to dry and try to repair some of the problems without repainting. Write a report on this activity.
3. Final detail a vehicle. Clean all interior and exterior surfaces with recommended products.

CHAPTER

19 Decals, Custom Painting, and Trim

OBJECTIVES

After studying this chapter, you should be able to:

- Properly remove and install vinyl decals and striping.
- Prepare the surface before applying adhesive overlay material or before custom painting.
- Explain various techniques for doing custom paint work.
- Remove, align, and install molding and emblems.

INTRODUCTION

People of all ages often want their vehicles customized or personalized. Also, factory-installed pinstripes and decorative tape is now common. If you can do this kind of work, you will find it to be in high demand and very profitable.

OVERLAYS AND TAPE STRIPES

An **overlay** is a large, self-adhesive vinyl material applied to the finish. It provides an easy way to customize the looks of a vehicle. Overlays might be multicolor stripes, artwork, or artificial wood grain. Overlays can also be body color, mounting along the lower areas of the body to help protect the finish from stone chips.

Vinyl tape is a tough, durable decorative striping material adhered to the vehicle's finish. It has a pressure-sensitive backing that bonds securely to the finish.

Vinyl decals are generally more complex and decorative pressure-sensitive material than tape stripes. Both tape and decals can be original equipment or aftermarket installed.

When repairing collision damage, you may have to replace vinyl tape and decals. If you use established methods, this can be a rewarding task.

Overlay and Tape Stripe Removal

There are several ways to remove vinyl tape stripes and decals. These include:

1. Spray remover and plastic scraper
2. Heat gun and plastic scraper
3. Scuff pad (if repainting panel)
4. Rubber wheel (eraser wheel)

Vinyl overlay remover is a chemical that dissolves plastic vinyl to aid its removal. To use spray vinyl remover, mask the area around the stripe or decal with plastic, as shown in **Figure 19–1.** Scuff sand the decal with No. 220 grit sandpaper to help speed the action of the

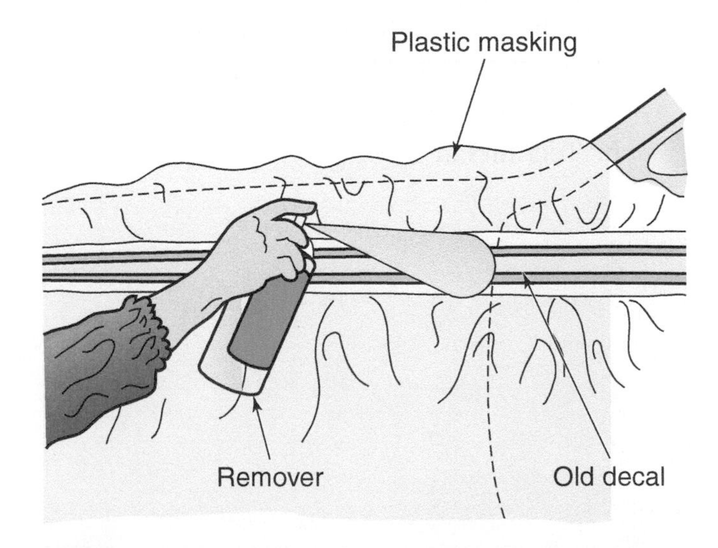

Figure 19–1. To remove vinyl stripes and decals, mask around the material. Then spray on two coats of remover. After soaking them, you can more easily peel off vinyl materials.

chemical. Do not cut through the vinyl or sand the paint, or you may have to repaint the panel.

If original equipment or if material on the other side of the vehicle is not going to be removed, measure the location of the existing stripe or decal before removal. Write down your measurements for later reference.

Spray the entire stripe or decal with remover spray. After a few minutes, spray the chemical on the vinyl again. Allow the remover to soak for about 15 minutes.

After allowing it to soak, peel the stripe or decal away from the panel. Start in one corner and try to peel it off in one piece. If needed, use a sharp plastic squeegee to help peel off the old material.

After removal of the stripe or decal, use the squeegee to remove any remaining adhesive from the panel. Then use a rag and **adhesive remover** to clean off the remaining vinyl glue.

On smaller pressure-sensitive overlays, a heat gun can sometimes be used to warm, soften, and remove the vinyl material. Without overheating, move the heat gun to gradually soften the stripe. As the vinyl and adhesive soften, slowly peel off the material. Then clean the area with adhesive remover.

An **eraser wheel** is a rubber wheel and arbor designed to remove tape stripes without damaging the paint. The wheel is mounted in an air drill or a small grinder. When spun against a stripe, the spinning wheel will abrade the tape and adhesive off the painted surface quickly and easily.

Overlay and Stripe Application

Use a water-soluble marker and tape measure to mark where you want to install the new striping or decal. Place tiny reference marks on the finish where needed.

Then place masking tape on the vehicle to serve as a guide. Align the tape with the marker reference marks.

Before tape or decal application, make sure the surface of the panel is ready. It should be wet sanded and buffed if needed. Also, clean the panel with wax and grease remover. This will remove any wax and other foreign matter.

Check to be sure that the temperature of the panel is about room temperature or warmer. It should be no cooler than 60°F (16°C) or no hotter than 90°F (32°C).

Installing Overlays

The **overlay wet method** of installation involves using soapy water to help simplify the application of larger decals and striping. Soapy water will allow you to shift and position the material without the adhesive instantly sticking to the panel. The water will also aid removal of the backing material from the overlay.

Fill a clean bucket with water. Then add some dishwashing liquid to the water and mix. Place the decal into the soapy water. Peel off the backing material carefully so that you do not tear the vinyl.

Position the overlay on the vehicle. Position it with masking tape. The soapy water will let you shift the overlay without it sticking tightly to the finish. Carefully straighten and align the material, removing any wrinkles. Working from the middle outward, use a rubber squeegee to flatten out the overlay. Make sure you have removed all air bubbles and wrinkles. Then use a rag or rubber roller to rub and adhere the overlay to the panel. As you rub toward the edges of the overlay, you will work any water out from under the vinyl. This will make the overlay stick to the finish.

Once the water is removed and almost dry, carefully peel off the carrier paper. Grasp at one edge of the carrier paper. Then slowly peel it off the vinyl. Go slowly so that you do not lift and tear the vinyl.

Next, if needed, cut off the ends of the overlay or stripe at the panel ends. Use a sharp razor blade knife to cut the material to the desired length. You may want the material to wrap around the panel edge, or you may prefer it to stop right at the edge.

Pierce any remaining air bubbles with a needle. Then rub the overlay with a rag to work the air out from under the vinyl.

Rubbing away from the overlay, double-check to be sure that all edges are adhered tightly to the finish. Rub over all edges a couple of times. The result will be a long-lasting, attractive addition to the vehicle's appearance. **Figure 19–2** shows how to install a small decal using the dry method.

Installing Vinyl Pinstripes

The **overlay dry method** of installation does not require soapy water to aid application. All surfaces must be clean and dry. Narrow pinstripe tape can be installed dry without wrinkling or bubble problems. Generally, if an overlay

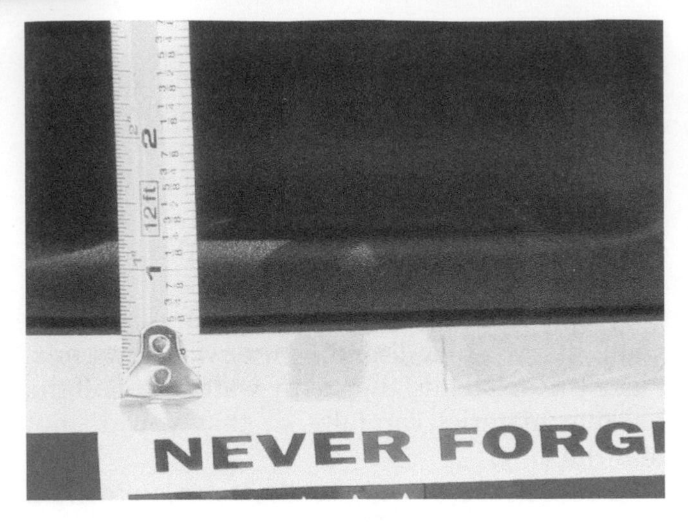

(A) Measure and mark the location of the decal so it is centered and straight or aligned as desired. Apply masking tape to the top of the decal to hold it in place.

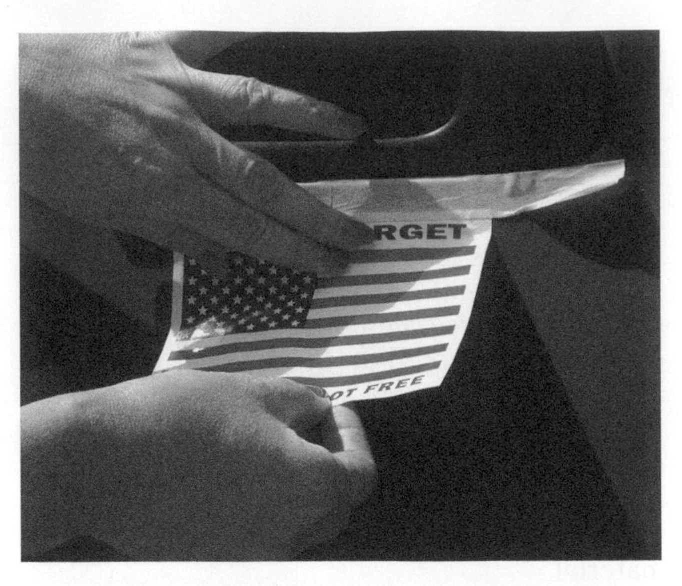

(C) Carefully lower the decal down onto the body surface. Rub outward to prevent air bubbles and wrinkles. Pull the decal back up and start over, if needed.

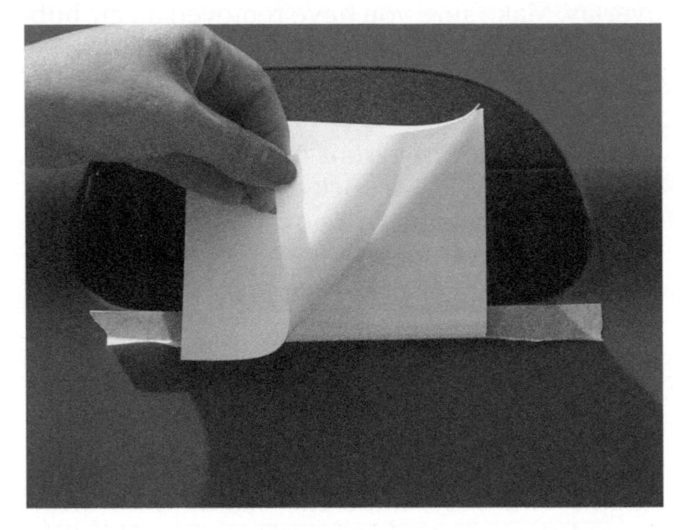

(B) Lift up the decal and peel off the backing material. Masking tape will hold the decal straight.

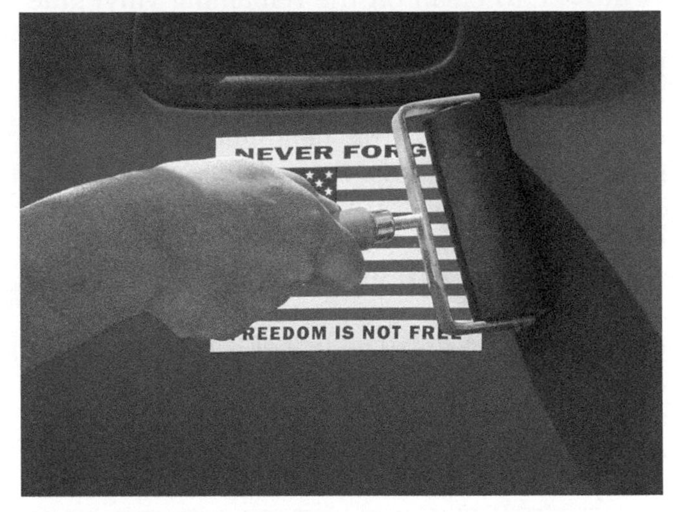

(D) Use a rubber roller, squeegee, or rag to rub the decal down onto the body surface.

Figure 19–2. Study the basic steps for installing a vinyl decal.

is narrower than about 2 inches (50 mm), you can use the dry method of installation.

Pinstripe tape may or may not have a carrier paper. Both types are installed in about the same way. With carrier paper, you will just have to peel off the paper after adhering the tape to the vehicle's surface.

A few rules for installing pinstripe tape include:

1. Make sure the surface is perfectly clean. Use soap and water. Then wash the area with wax and grease remover. If not, the tape will come off and your customer will return unhappy.
2. Use a grease pen or water-soluble marker to locate where you want the striping. If needed, you can also lay down masking tape as a guide. With the dry method, the tape will stick to the surface and can be difficult to reposition.
3. Position and adhere one end of the tape stripe. You might want to place masking tape over the end to keep it from pulling off.

4. Use one hand to lightly stretch the tape and the other to lightly push and tack the tape into position. You want to lightly stick the tape in position first. Then if it is not straight, you can pull the tape up and reposition it.
5. Never stretch the tape striping too tight. If you do, the tape will distort or come off after exposure to the heat of the sun.
6. Do not overstretch the tape when rounding corners. Again, this will thin the material and cause it to lift later.
7. After using your finger to lightly tack the tape into position, stand back and check its alignment and straightness. If it is not straight, pull the tape back off and realign it.
8. Once you are sure the tape is positioned properly, use a rubber squeegee or roller to bond the tape securely to the finish. Start at the center of the stripe and wipe toward the ends. Do not use too much pressure near the ends or you can tear the tape.
9. If the pinstripe tape has a carrier paper, slowly pull if off. Then check for kinks and air bubbles. Work them out. Again, rub a squeegee over the stripe to adhere it tightly to the finish.
10. Do not use your hand to try to bond pinstripe tape. It will tend to distort and wrinkle the tape. After using the squeegee, rub a soft rag over the tape to final bond it in place.

PAINTED PINSTRIPES

There are two common methods to paint on pinstripes. One uses vinyl masking tape to mask on each side of the paint stripe. The other uses a special striping tool to apply a thin line of paint over the finish. Painted-on pinstripes are sometimes requested for a custom paint job or during a restoration job. A painted stripe will generally last longer and look better than vinyl tape.

Using Pinstripe Tape

Pinstripe masking tape uses two pieces of vinyl tape held with a paper carrier. Position and apply the tape as you would pinstripe tape. Then remove the carrier paper.

Next, use a small pinstriping brush to apply the paint in the area between the tapes. Most painters use lacquer or catalyzed enamel so the strip will dry quickly. Use long smooth brush strokes parallel with the stripe. Using a brush saves time and material over a spray gun or airbrush because you do not have to mask large areas around the stripe.

When the paint stripe has flashed, carefully remove the masking tape. Slowly pull it straight back and off the vehicle. Do not pull sideways or you could peel off some of the freshly painted stripe. Wet sand and polish the painted stripes if needed.

Using Pinstriping Tool

A **pinstriping tool** uses a serrated roller to deposit a painted pinstripe. The tool holds the paint in a cylinder-shaped cup. The roller, when moved over the surface, deposits the paint onto the finish. Various widths of roller can be installed in the tool to change paint stripe widths.

A **magnetic guide strip** can be used to help guide the tool for making straight or slightly curved pinstripes. It is a flexible plastic material filled with magnets. When placed on a steel body part, the guide strip will stay in place without damage to the finish. A guide rod on the pinstriping tool contacts this guide when striping.

When the tool is held squarely and moved over the surface, it will make a uniform width pinstripe. If the tool is tilted, the width of the pinstripe will narrow. With practice, you will be able to make pointed or curly ends on the painted pinstripes.

Using Pinstriping Brushes

Pinstriping brushes have very long soft horse hairs on them. Special talent is needed to use them. Using a very steady hand, a freehand technique is sometimes used to pull the brush along the finish to apply painted pinstripes. Body lines or trim are often used as a guide when freehand striping.

Painting Wider Stripes

Wider painted stripes are done by spraying a different color or tint over the existing finish after masking. Before painting, wet sand the area to be painted with very fine (1,000 or finer grit) wet sandpaper. This will prepare the

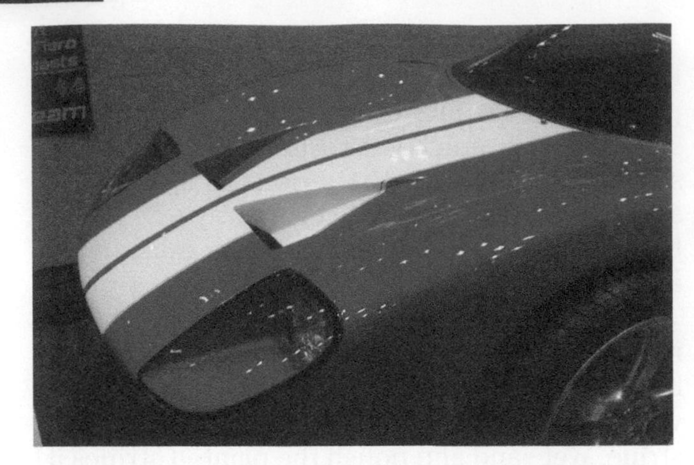

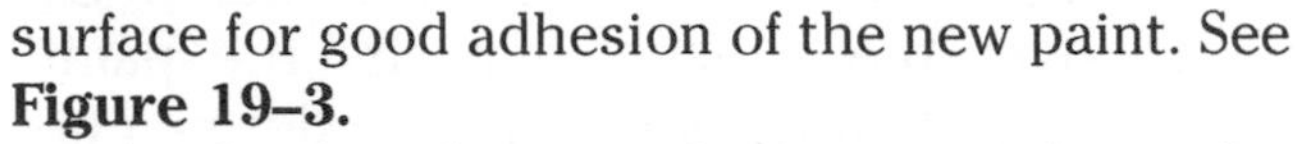

Figure 19–3. Larger decals, like these white stripes, should be applied using a mixture of dishwashing detergent and water. This will keep the large decal from sticking and aid in making it lay flat. As you work air and water from under the decal with a roller, it will stick to the body surface properly.

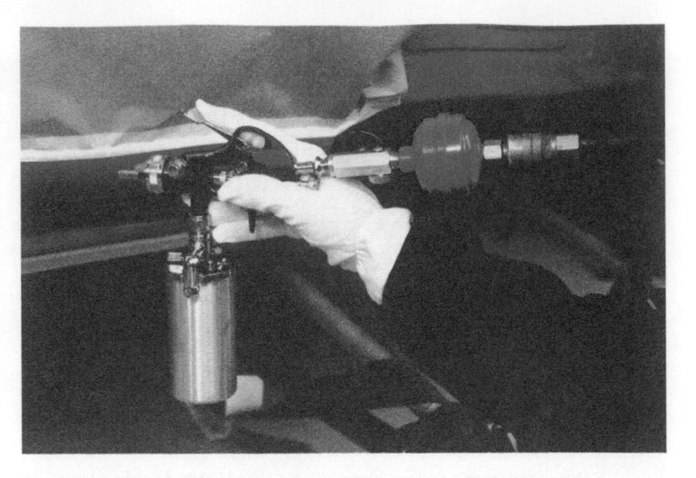

Figure 19–4. A small touch-up gun or an airbrush is commonly used when doing custom paint work. (Courtesy of Snap-on Tools Corporation)

surface for good adhesion of the new paint. See **Figure 19–3.**

Apply fine line masking tape where the stripes are wanted. Fine line tape is needed so the stripes have a smooth edge when the tape is removed. After carefully applying the fine line tape, mask the area on each side with paper or plastic and conventional masking tape.

Spray the color for the stripes onto the unmasked area. After drying, remove the masking material. Wet sand the area and buff it to a high gloss. If the stripe is wide, use a full-size spray gun. If the stripes are smaller, use an airbrush or touch-up gun to save materials and speed cleanup.

CUSTOM PAINTING

Custom painting can involve using multiple colors, metal flake paints, multilayer masking, and special spraying techniques to produce a personalized look. Multicolor stripes, flames, murals, landscapes, names, and other artwork can be added to the finish. Complex images require you to have special artistic talent. If you cannot paint an attractive image on paper, you will not be able to do it on a vehicle.

Custom painting requires considerable talent, skill, and knowledge. You need to plan the custom job carefully. This will let you determine how to mask and spray or apply each color. Custom painters are good at using airbrushes, striping tools, and masking materials. See **Figure 19–4.**

Before custom painting, make sure the base finish is in good condition. You do not want to waste your time trying to paint over a weathered or problem finish. Wet sand and clean the area to be custom painted. Use surface preparation methods detailed in other chapters.

To produce a feathered custom stripe on a van, the area to be striped is masked and painted with the main color for the stripe. Then an airbrush and a different color paint is misted around the outside edge of the stripe. This color is misted over the edge of the masking paper. Then, when the masking is removed, the two colors blend into each other for a custom stripe effect.

Custom masks can be made by drawing a design on thin posterboard and then cutting them out. The posterboard design is then taped onto the vehicle and spray painted. Using an airbrush and translucent paint, various attractive effects can be produced.

Card masking involves using a simple masking pattern to produce a custom paint effect. Usually, an airbrush is used to mist the paint over the edge of the masking card. The card can be moved to repeat the pattern to produce a wide range of paint effects.

Lace painting involves spraying through lace fabric to produce a custom pattern in the paint. Various lace designs can be purchased at fabric stores. The cloth pattern will allow the paint to pass through the holes in the lace but mask it in other areas.

A **marble effect** can be made by forcing crumpled plastic against a freshly painted stripe or area. When the plastic is lifted off, it will remove paint in random areas with a marble type effect.

Spider webbing is done by forcing paint through the airbrush in a very thin, fibrous type spray. Air pressure from the gun can also be used to spread and smear the wet paint to produce a varying effect.

Painted flames are a custom painting technique often used on "hot rods" or older street rods. First, fine line masking tape is used to form the outline of the flames. Then the area around this shape is covered with masking paper or plastic. See **Figure 19–5.**

First, the base color for the flames is applied. Then a second translucent color is blended. A third color may be used to darken the outer edges and center area of the flames. The flames are finally wet sanded and polished when dry.

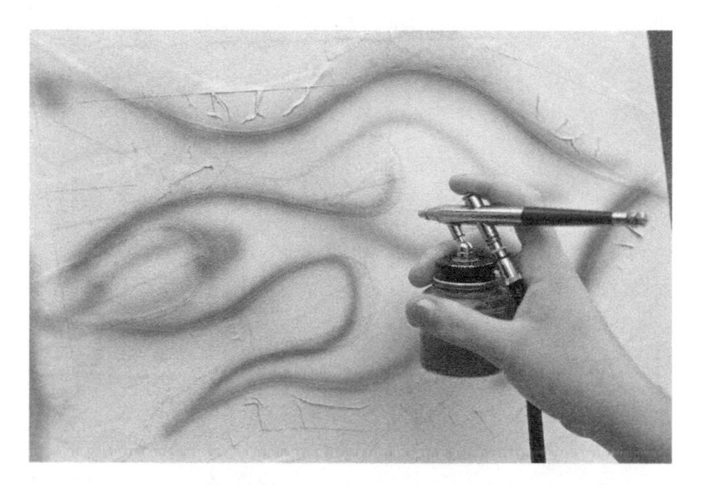

(A) The area to be painted must be masked to expose the desired shape to be painted. An airbrush is being used to apply custom paint to the flames.

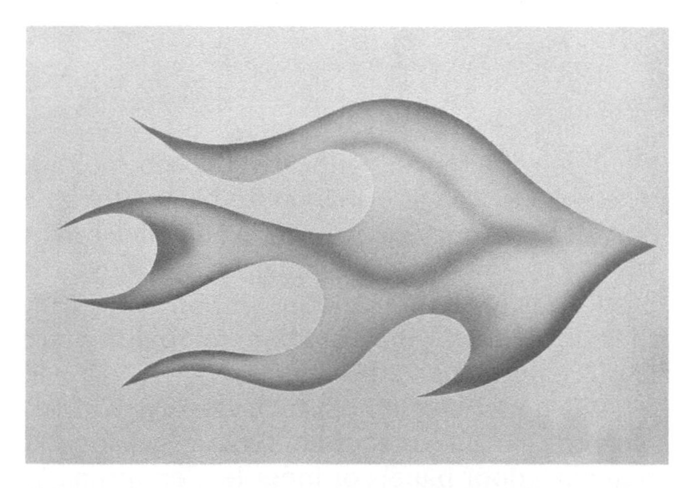

(B) Note how the whole flame was painted yellow. Then red was added to the edges of the flame to give it a custom effect.

Figure 19–5. Flames are a very common example of custom painting.

Painted lettering involves masking off letters over the finishing and spraying or brushing them on with a different color. This can be time consuming but is sometimes requested by customers.

When doing custom paint work, do not "bite off more than you can chew." Start out simple with minor complexity. As you learn to successfully do custom work, you can progress to more complex paint work. Experience is the best teacher with custom paint work.

A good idea is to practice techniques on old parts using leftover paint. Then you can learn from your mistakes and successes without working on a customer vehicle.

Figure 19–6 shows several custom motorcycle gastanks.

MOLDINGS AND TRIM

Moldings and trim can be held on with adhesive or mechanical fasteners, or both. If in doubt, your service manual or computer database will describe how each molding or trim is held in place.

To remove molding or trim that is held on by adhesive, place masking tape next to the molding or emblem to protect the surface from scratches. See **Figure 19–7.** Heat and warm the molding or emblem with a heat gun to soften the adhesive. Then force a **molding removal tool** or knife under the part to separate the adhesive from the body. Pull outward on the molding or emblem as you carefully work the tool behind the part. See **Figure 19–8.**

If a quantity of adhesive remains on the vehicle, you might want to cover the spot with a sheet of plastic and heat the adhesive again. This will soften the remaining adhesive and allow you to remove it easily with a putty knife or scraper. Be careful not to overheat the surface. Heating the old adhesive to about 104°F to 122°F (40°C to 50°C) should soften it enough for easy removal.

If you are reusing the old molding or trim, clean the remaining adhesive off its mounting surface. Scrape off the bulk of the old adhesive without cutting and damaging the molding or emblem. Then wrap the part in plastic film and

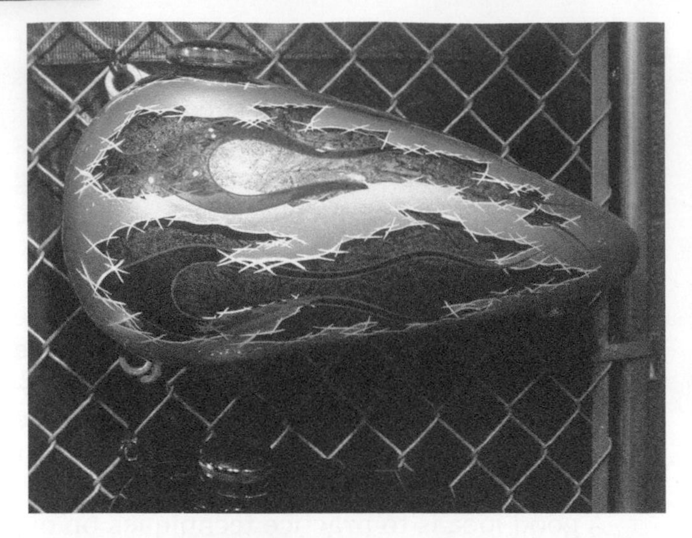

(A) Flames ripping through paint!

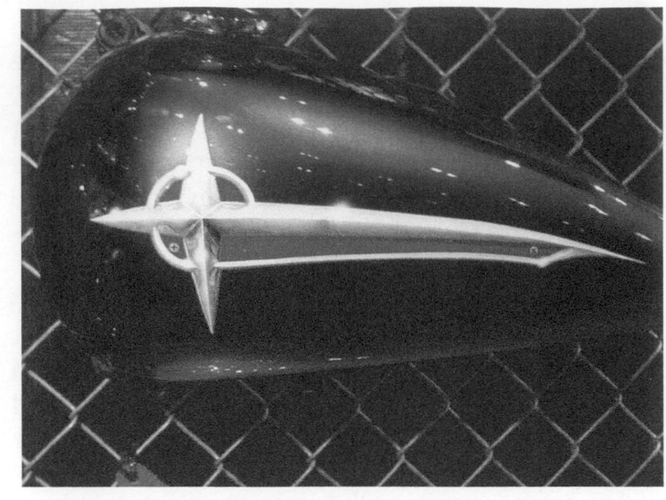

(C) Star of David with chrome trim.

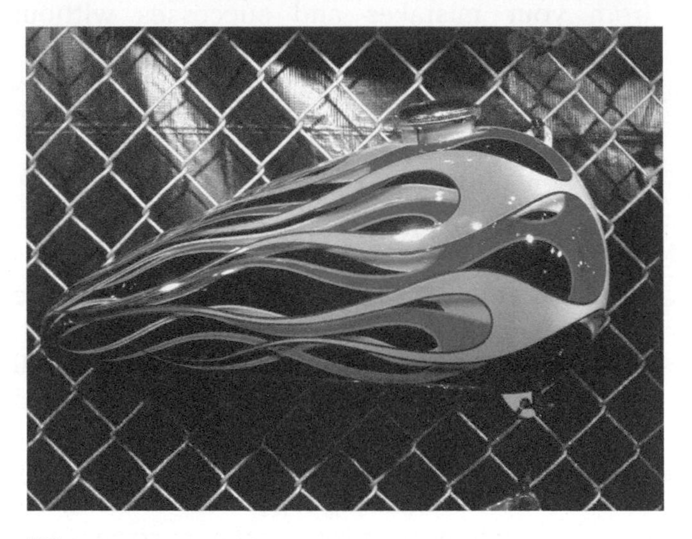

(B) Octopus or squid flames.

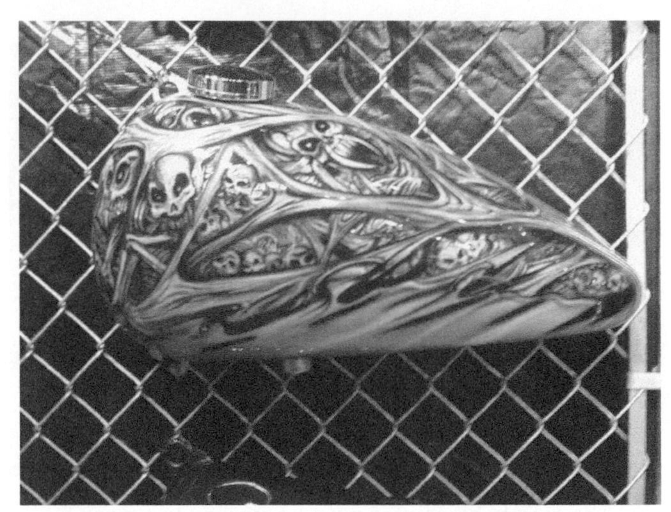

(D) Skulls in a hell cocoon.

Figure 19–6. Note the custom paint jobs on these gas tanks. How do you think each was done?

heat soften the adhesive. Scrape the remainder of the adhesive off the part. See **Figure 19–9.**

When installing an adhesive-backed molding or emblem, make sure the vehicle surface is perfectly clean. If not, the molding can come off.

If needed, use masking tape as a guide for molding installation. Carefully apply the masking tape to the vehicle in a perfectly straight line. Then position the molding next to the masking tape before pressing it into place.

Service publications will give measurements for locating the molding or trim properly. Use a pocket rule or measuring tape to mark where the molding or trim should be mounted. See **Figure 19–10.**

If you are reusing adhesive-backed molding or emblems, use aftermarket emblem adhesive. Spread a thin coating of emblem adhesive on the back of the molding or emblem. Then move the part straight into position without smearing the adhesive. Use masking tape to hold the part in place until the adhesive dries.

When molding is held by fasteners, you will have to gain access to them. This might involve removing door panels or inner fender aprons.

Attaching Moldings with Two-Sided Tape

The preferred method of securing moldings and trim has changed from using mechanical

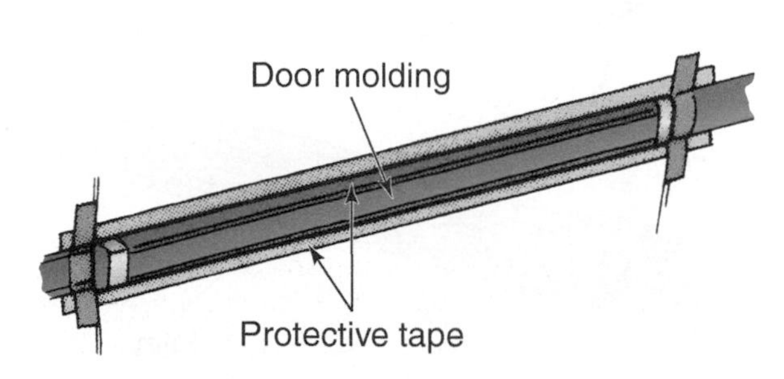

(A) Mask around the molding to protect the finish from damage.

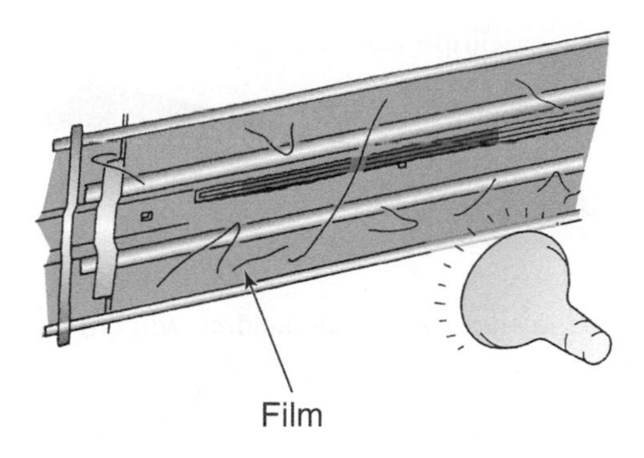

(C) Cover the remaining adhesive with film and heat soften it with a heat gun or lamp.

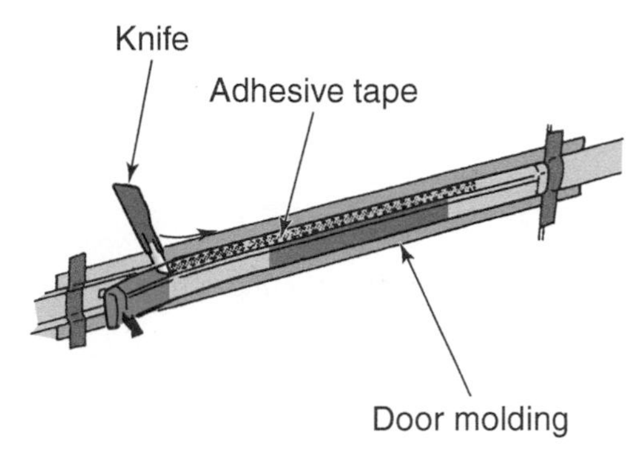

(B) Carefully push a knife between the molding and tape to free the molding from the body.

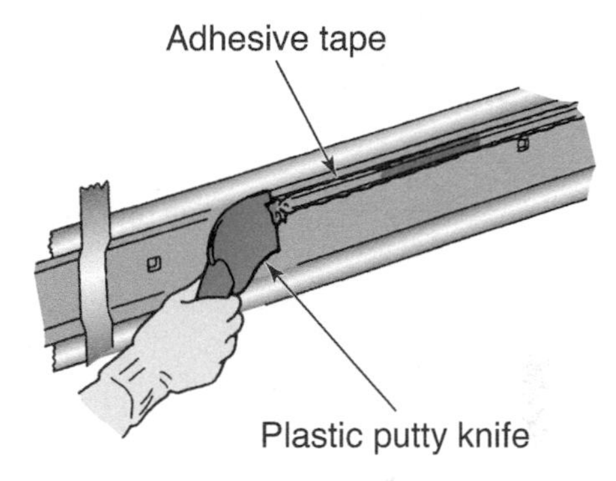

(D) Carefully remove the rest of the adhesive with a dull scraper to avoid paint damage.

Figure 19–7. Note the steps for removing molding held on with adhesive tape. (Reprinted with permission by American Isuzu Motors, Inc.)

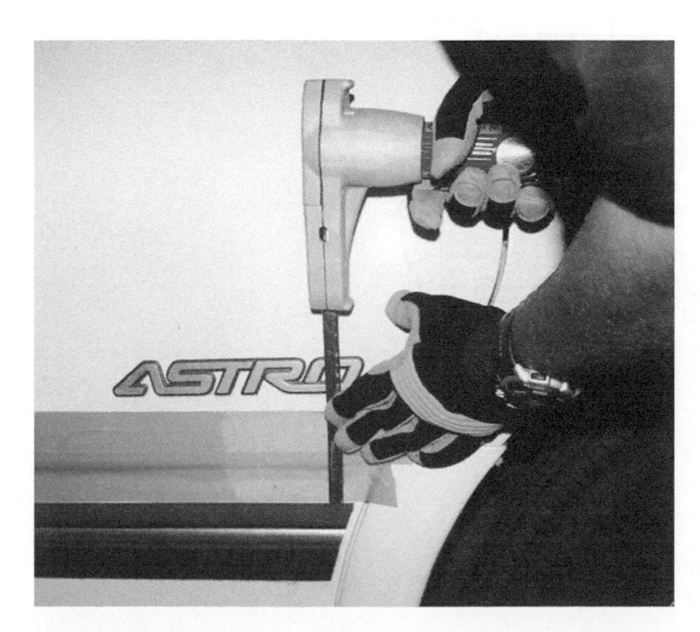

Figure 19–8. Here the technician is using an electric knife to remove an old emblem. Mask around the emblem to protect the paint from damage. (Courtesy of Equalizer Industries)

fasteners to the use of double-sided foam tape. The use and placement of the trim accessories has taken on a more diverse and integral function as they are often shaped to conform to the crowns, recesses, and irregular shapes of the surfaces to which they are applied. The double-sided tape holds the molding closer to the surface of the vehicle, reducing the possibility of its becoming snagged and pulled loose. The weight, mass, and often irregular shapes of these moldings do not lend themselves to being attached with traditional mechanical fasteners. Two-sided foam tape has become a very popular alternative because it is available in various sizes and can be used on virtually any size, shape, or trim configuration. In addition, it is no longer necessary to drill holes into the panels, which eliminates a source of rust.

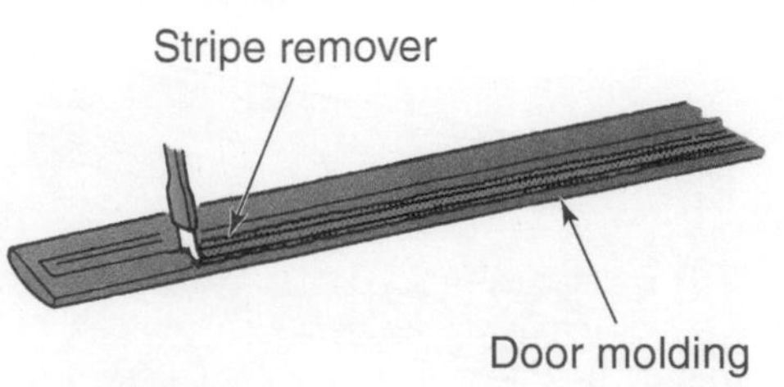

(A) Scrape the adhesive off the molding without marring the surface.

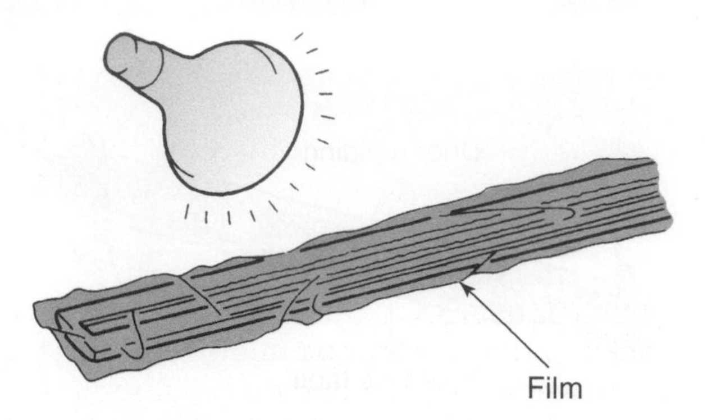

(B) Wrap it in plastic film and heat the molding to soften the remaining adhesive.

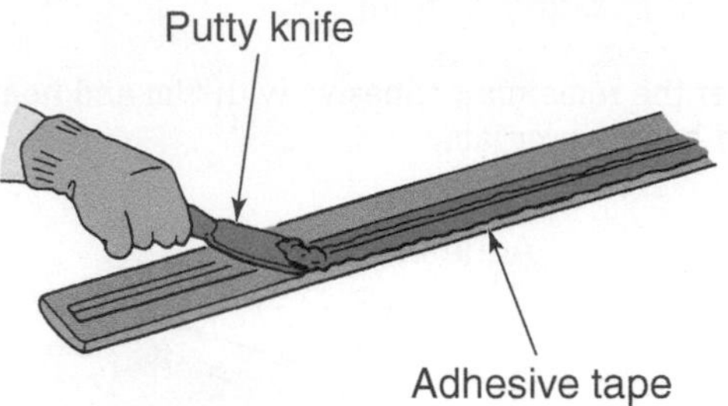

(C) Scrape the remainder of the adhesive off the part.

Figure 19–9. If the old molding is going to be reused, remove the excess adhesive from its mounting surface. (Reprinted with permission by American Isuzu Motors, Inc.)

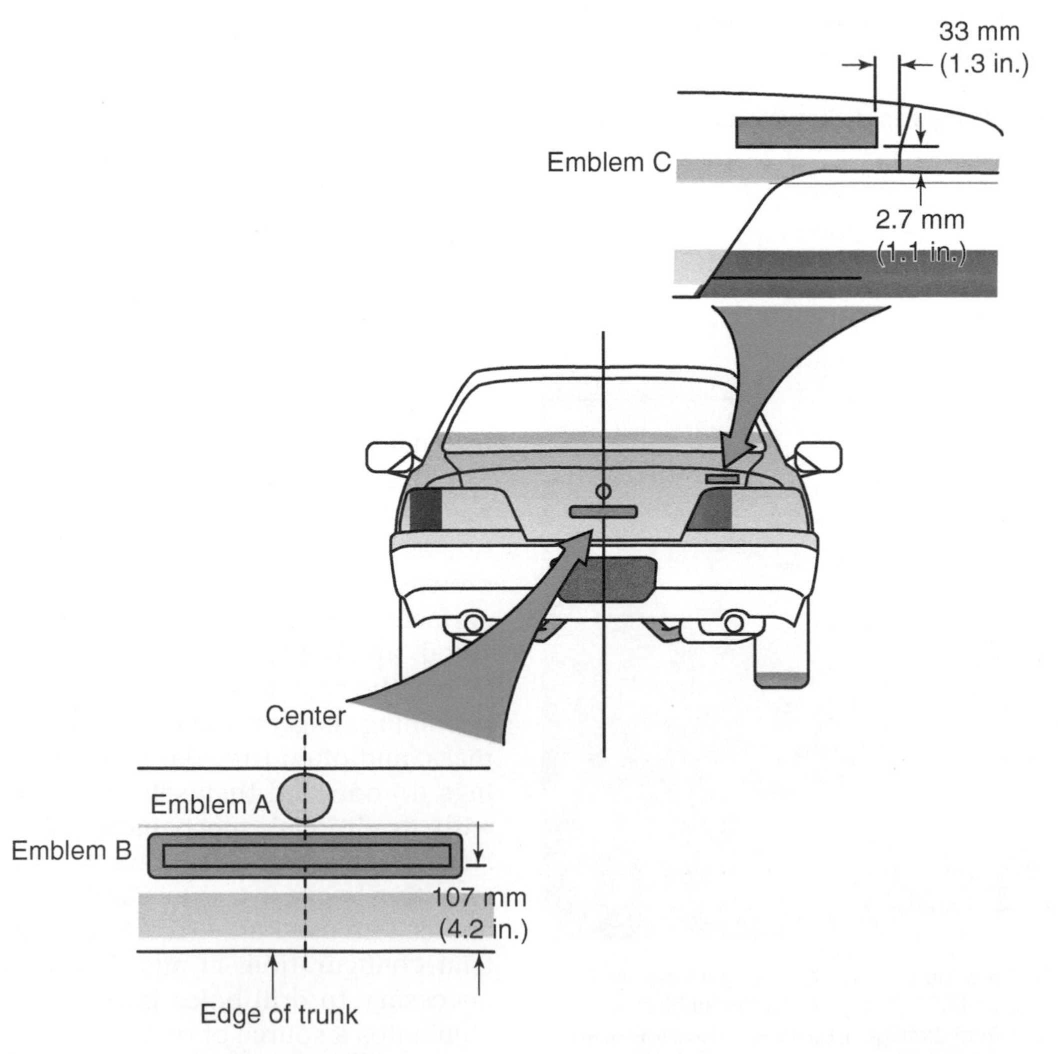

Figure 19–10. Note this service manual illustration showing how to locate emblems on this particular vehicle.

SUMMARY

- There are several ways to remove vinyl tape stripes and decals, including spray remover and scraper, heat gun and scraper, and scuff pad (if repainting the panel).
- The overlay wet method of installation involves using soapy water to help simplify the application of larger decals and striping. The overlay dry method does not require water. Generally, if an overlay is narrower than 2 inches (50 mm), you can use the dry method.
- Custom painting involves using multiple colors, metal flake paints, multilayer masking, and special spraying techniques to produce a personalized look. Stripes, flames, murals, or names may also be added.

TECHNICAL TERMS

overlay	magnetic guide strip
vinyl tape	pinstriping brushes
vinyl decals	custom masks
vinyl overlay remover	card masking
adhesive remover	lace painting
eraser wheel	marble effect
overlay wet method	spider webbing
overlay dry method	painted flames
pinstriping tool	molding removal tool

REVIEW QUESTIONS

1. What is a vinyl overlay?
2. Why do you sand vinyl overlays before using overlay remover?
3. List ten rules for installing pinstripe tape.
4. A ______________ ______________ uses a serrated roller to deposit painted pinstripes.
5. Explain card masking.
6. How do you do custom lace painting?
7. How do you produce a spider webbing effect when custom painting?
8. What is a molding removal tool?
9. Custom paint work is easy if basic methods are followed. True or false?

ASE-STYLE REVIEW QUESTIONS

1. Pinstripe tape must be removed from a fender before painting. *Technician A* says to use a sharp putty knife to remove the pinstripe. *Technician B* says to use a rubber wheel in an air drill. Who is correct?
   a. Technician A
   b. Technician B
   c. Both Technicians A and B
   d. Neither Technician

2. *Technician A* says to measure the location of the existing stripe or decal before removal. *Technician B* says that service information might publish stripe or decal locations. Who is correct?
   a. Technician A
   b. Technician B
   c. Both Technicians A and B
   d. Neither Technician

3. *Technician A* says that vinyl remover is not harmful. *Technician B* says that there is no need to wear eye protection when using vinyl remover. Who is correct?
   a. Technician A
   b. Technician B
   c. Both Technicians A and B
   d. Neither Technician

4. Which of the following will allow you to shift and relocate large overlays or decals?
   a. Adhesive remover
   b. Rubber wheel
   c. Solvent
   d. Soapy water

5. An air bubble is found near the middle of a large overlay or decal. *Technician A* says to poke a hole in the air bubble with a needle. *Technician B* says to use a razor blade to cut an opening in the air bubble. Who is correct?
   a. Technician A
   b. Technician B
   c. Both Technicians A and B
   d. Neither Technician

6. *Technician A* says that narrow pinstripe tape can be installed with the body surface dry. *Technician B* says that large decals or overlays can be installed with the body surface dry. Who is correct?
   a. Technician A
   b. Technician B
   c. Both Technicians A and B
   d. Neither Technician

7. Newly installed pinstripe tape is coming off when in the hot sun. Which of the following might be the problem?
   a. Tape not stretched enough
   b. Tape stretched too tight
   c. Heat gun not used
   d. Not installed straight enough

8. *Technician A* says that you can use special masking tape before painting on pinstripes. *Technician B* says that you can use a special pinstripe tool or roller. Who is correct?
   a. Technician A
   b. Technician B
   c. Both Technicians A and B
   d. Neither Technician

9. When painting very wide stripes, which of the following sandpaper grits should you use to sand the area?
   a. 80 grit
   b. 120 grit
   c. 500 grit
   d. 1,000 grit

10. When heating adhesive for molding removal, which of the following is the maximum temperature commonly recommended to prevent part warpage or damage?
    a. 74°F–80°F (23°C–27°C)
    b. 84°F–90°F (29°C–32°C)
    c. 94°F–104°F (34°C–40°C)
    d. 104°F–122°F (40°C–50°C)

ACTIVITIES

1. Obtain a body part with an overlay on it from a salvage yard. Use proper methods to remove the vinyl overlay without damaging the finish.
2. Using a scrap part, practice doing custom paint work. Try doing lacing, flames, and other effects.
3. Attend a custom car show. Using a camera, document the types of custom paint effects found. Ask the car owners about their custom paint effects. Write a report on how some of the custom paint jobs were done.

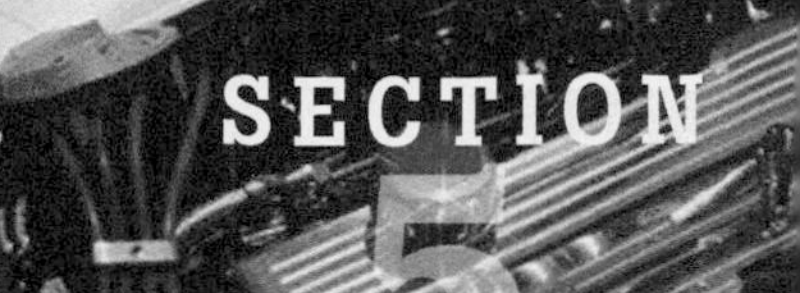

CHAPTER 20 Measuring Vehicle Damage

OBJECTIVES

After studying this chapter, you should be able to:

- Explain how impact forces are transmitted through both frame and unibody construction vehicles.
- Describe how to visually determine the extent of impact damage.
- List the various types and variations of body measuring tools.
- Analyze damage by measuring body dimensions.
- Explain the importance of the datum plane and centerline concepts as related to unibody repair.
- Interpret body dimension information and locate key reference points on a vehicle, using body dimension manuals.
- Discuss the use of tram bars, self-centering gauges, and strut tower gauges.
- Diagnose various types of damage, including twist, mash, sag, and side sway.
- Given a damaged vehicle and a body specification manual, locate and measure key points using a tape measure, tram bar, and self-centering gauges.
- Explain the operation of electronic laser, ultrasonic, and robotic arm measuring systems.

INTRODUCTION

When a vehicle is in a high-speed collision, powerful impact forces can bend the frame or unibody structure. The frame, body, or unibody is designed to absorb some of the energy of the collision and protect its occupants. When a heavily damaged vehicle enters the shop, the extent of the damage must be carefully evaluated. Sometimes, measurements are needed to help the estimator calculate the costs of the repairs.

Vehicle measurement involves using specialized tools and equipment to measure the location of reference points on the vehicle. These measurements are then compared to published dimensions from an undamaged vehicle. By comparing known good and actual measurements, you can determine the extent of damage. The difference in the two measurements indicates the direction and amount of frame or body misalignment.

WHY IS MEASUREMENT IMPORTANT?

There is good reason for close body structure tolerances. Steering and suspension systems, for instance, are mounted to the frame or unibody structure. Severe body or frame damage can change steering or suspension geometry or misalign mechanical parts. This can result in poor handling, vibration, and noise problems.

Thus, the tolerances of critical manufacturing dimensions must be held to within a maximum value of less than ⅛ inch (3 mm).

To correctly analyze damage on a unibody vehicle, the entire structure must be considered. To do this, it is necessary to be able to take proper measurements to locate damage. It will also help to plan where to pull.

Measurement gauges are special tools used to check specific frame and body points. They allow you to quickly measure the direction and extent of vehicle damage.

Control or **reference points** are specific locations on the frame or body for making measurements. They may be holes, specific bolts, nuts, panel edges, or other locations on the vehicle. To repair a badly damaged vehicle, you must restore the reference points to their factory dimensions. This must be done while reference points in the undamaged area remain in their correct locations.

DAMAGE DIAGNOSIS

To repair a vehicle properly, you or the estimator must first accurately diagnose the collision damage. Someone must assess the severity and extent of damage and find all parts that have been affected. Once this has been determined, a plan can be made for repair.

Damage found from an inaccurately diagnosed vehicle will be uncovered during repair. When this happens, the repair method or procedure must be changed.

Generally, physical damage is rarely missed during an inspection by a competent estimator or body technician. However, the effects of the damage on unrelated systems and damage next to the impacted part can be accidentally overlooked. A visual inspection alone is inadequate. Accident damage should be assessed by measurements with the proper tools and equipment.

The following is a basic diagnosis procedure:

1. Know the type of vehicle construction (full frame, partial frame, unibody).
2. Visually locate the point of impact.
3. Determine the direction and force of the impact. Once this is determined, check for possible damage.
4. Determine if the damage is confined to the body, or if it involves mechanical parts (wheels, suspension, engine).
5. Systematically inspect damage to the parts along the path of the impact and find the point where there is no longer any evidence of damage. For example, pillar damage can be determined by checking the door opening alignment.
6. Measure the major parts and check body height by comparing the actual measurements with the values in the body dimensions chart. Use a centering gauge to compare measurements of the height of the left and right sides of the body.
7. Check for suspension and overall body damage with the proper fixtures.

IMPACT EFFECTS

A modern vehicle is designed to withstand the shocks of normal driving and to provide protection for the occupants during a collision. Special consideration is given to designing the body so that it will collapse and absorb the maximum amount of energy in a severe collision.

In the body-over-frame construction, the passenger (pay-load) area is enclosed with panels of steel attached to a structural frame. The frame also supports most of the drivetrain and mechanical accessories. In the unibody construction, the metal body panels are welded together, making a structural unit.

Under the force of collision impacts, the frame-type vehicle and the unibody-type vehicle react quite differently. Also, damage assessment and repair techniques are different, even though the basic repair skills are similar.

When the collision damage has been identified using the proper identification and analysis procedures, anyone skilled in the mechanics of collision damage repair is capable of repairing the damage successfully.

ANALYZING COLLISION FORCES

The impact force of a collision and the extent of damage differ depending on how the collision occurred. The damage can be partly determined by understanding how the collision happened.

The body technician may need to know the following items:

1. The size, shape, position, and speed of the vehicles involved in the collision
2. Speed of the vehicle at the time of the collision

3. Angle and direction of the vehicle at the time of the impact
4. The number of passengers and their positions at the time of the impact

A good body/frame technician can usually determine what actually happened to cause the damage. Certain types of collision damage often occur in a predictable pattern and sequence.

If a driver's first reaction is to turn away from the danger, the vehicle will be forced to take the hit on the side, as in **Figure 20–1.** If the driver's reaction is to slam on the brakes, the direction of impact would be frontal. A frontal collision where the point of impact is high on the vehicle could cause the cowl and roof to move rearward and the rear of the vehicle to move downward. If the point of impact is low at the front, the inertia of the body mass could cause the rear of the vehicle to distort upward, forcing the roof forward. This could leave an excessively large opening between the front upper part of the door and the roof line. See **Figure 20–2.**

Given vehicles with similar weights traveling at the same speed, vehicle damage will vary depending on what is struck—another vehicle, a utility pole, or a wall.

If the impact is spread over a larger area (as in hitting a wall), damage will be minimal (**Figure 20–3A**). Conversely, the smaller the area of impact, the greater the severity of the damage, (**Figure 20–3B**). In this example, the bumper, hood, radiator, and so forth have been severely damaged. The engine has been pushed back and the effect of the collision has extended as far as the rear suspension.

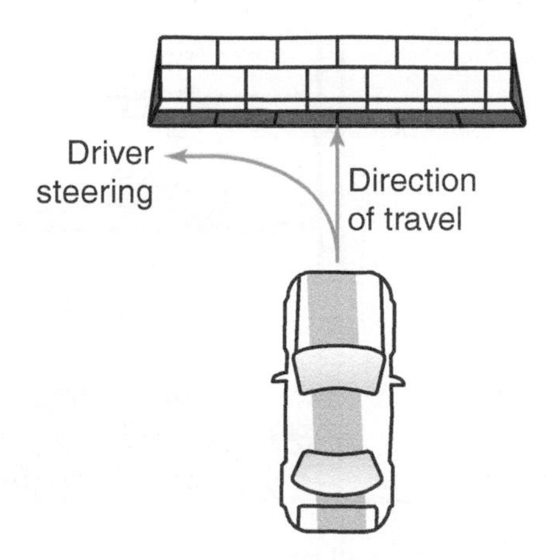

(A) The obstruction is directly in front of the car. The driver would then turn the steering wheel to swerve away from the obstruction to try to avoid impact.

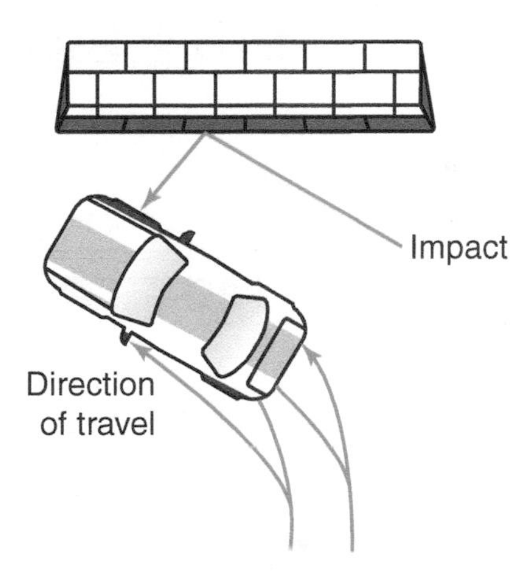

(B) Swerving changes the direction and angle of impact. Impact to the side of the body structure would normally cause side sway damage.

Figure 20–1. The example shows a typical collision because of the vehicle skidding sideways into an obstruction.

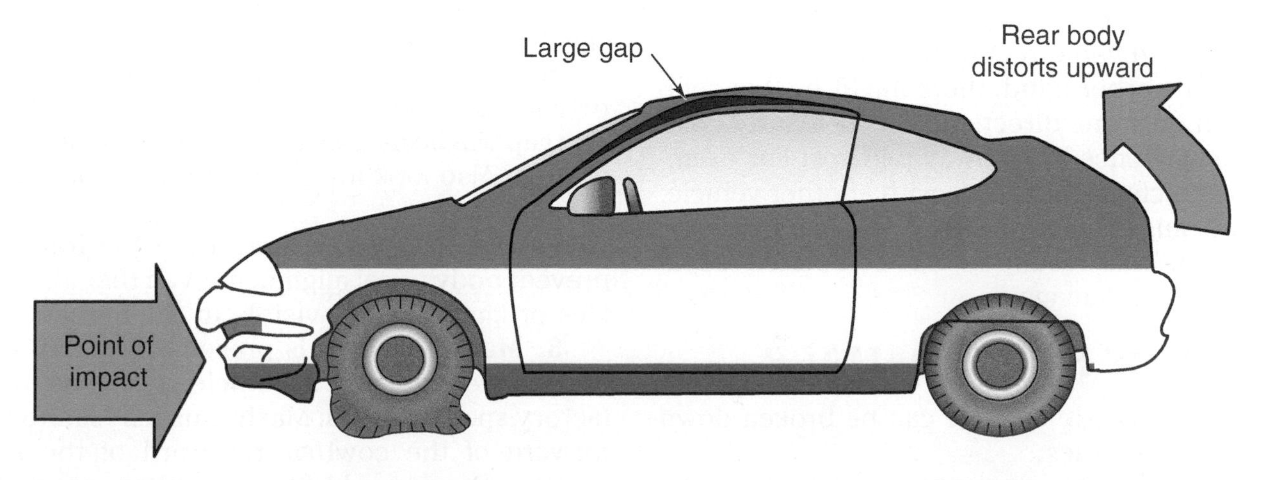

Figure 20–2. A hard frontal impact causes major or primary damage to the front end. Minor, secondary damage occurs elsewhere from the shock wave flowing through the body.

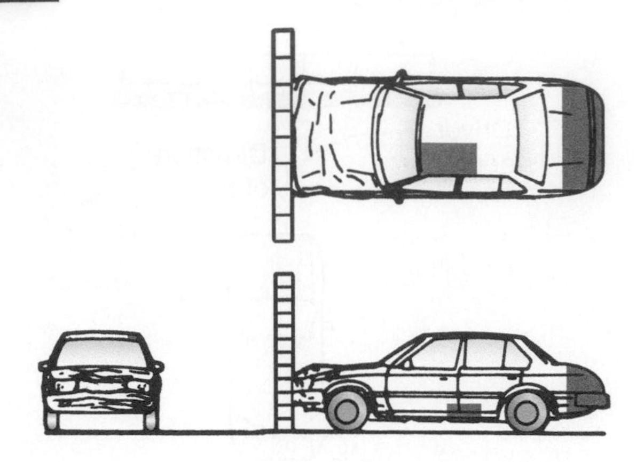

(A) The vehicle hits a wall straight on. The large area absorbs energy, and damage is limited to the front body parts.

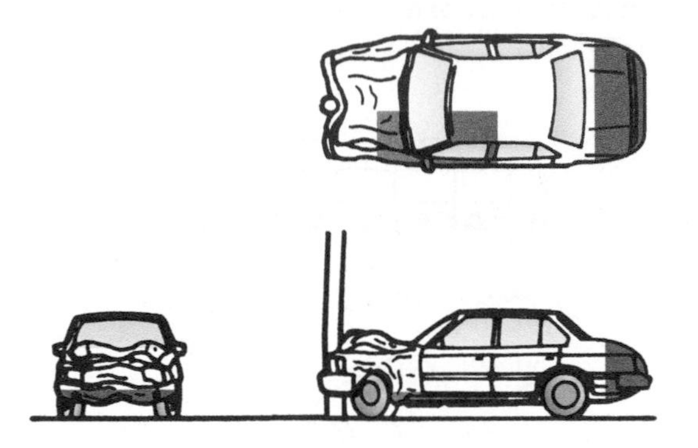

(B) Another vehicle hits a utility pole. The small area must absorb all the energy, so the damage travels much deeper into the engine compartment.

Figure 20–3. Note impact damage differences.

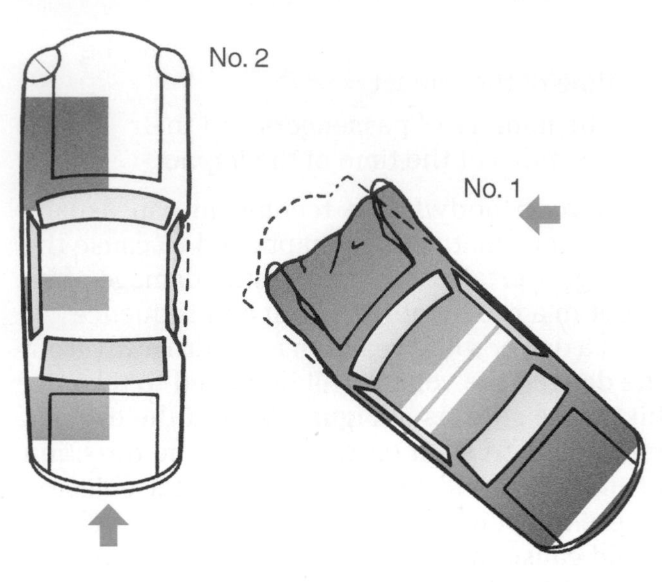

Figure 20–4. A broadside or "t-bone" collision often causes heavy frame or unibody damage. Vehicle Number 1 would suffer side sway and front end damage. Vehicle Number 2 would suffer major side sway damage in the central section.

Another consideration is when one vehicle hits another while moving. If vehicle Number 1 in **Figure 20–4** drives into the side of vehicle number 2 while Number 2 is moving, the motion of the first vehicle will drive the front end of the vehicle back. However, the motion of vehicle Number 2 will also "drag" that same front end to the side. There is only one collision, but the damage is in two directions.

On the other hand, there might be two collisions in only one direction. This is a fairly common occurrence in highway pile-ups. For example, a vehicle might collide with another vehicle. Then it might leave the road and hit a pole or guardrail. This results in two completely separate types of damage.

TYPES OF FRAME DAMAGE

Full frame vehicle damage can be broken down into five categories:

1. Side sway damage results from collision impacts that occur from the side. It often causes side bending of the frame. Side sway usually occurs in the front or rear of the vehicle. Generally, it is possible to spot side sway damage by noting if there are buckles on the inside of one rail and buckles on the outside of the opposite side rail.

Side sway can be recognized by abnormalities such as a gap at the door on the long side and wrinkles on the short side. Look for impact damage obviously from the side. For example, hood and deck lid will not fit into proper opening.

2. Sag damage is a condition where a section of the frame is lower than normal. See **Figure 20–5.** The structure has a swayback appearance. Sag damage generally is caused by a direct impact from the front or rear. It can occur on one side of the vehicle or on both sides.

Sag can usually be detected visually by an irregular gap between the fender and the door. The gap will be narrow at the top and wide at the bottom. Also look for a door hanging too low at the striker.

Enough sag can be present in the frame to prevent body panel alignment even though wrinkles or kinks are not visible in the frame itself.

3. Mash damage is present when any section or member of the vehicle is shorter than factory specifications. Mash is usually limited to forward of the cowl or rearward of the rear window. Doors could fit well and appear to be undisturbed. See **Figure 20–6.**

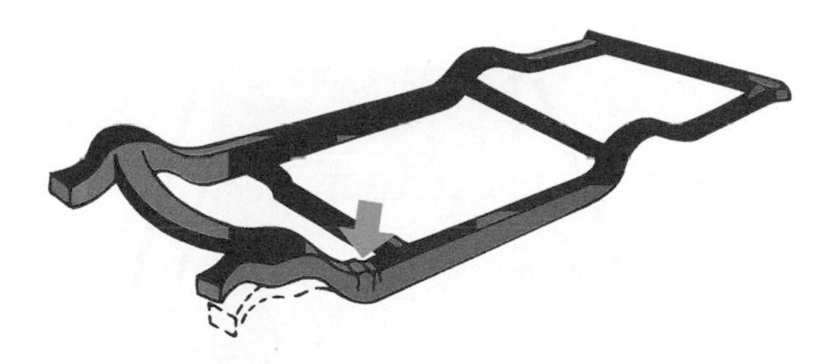

(A) Front sag is often in the cowl area from the buckling of frame rails.

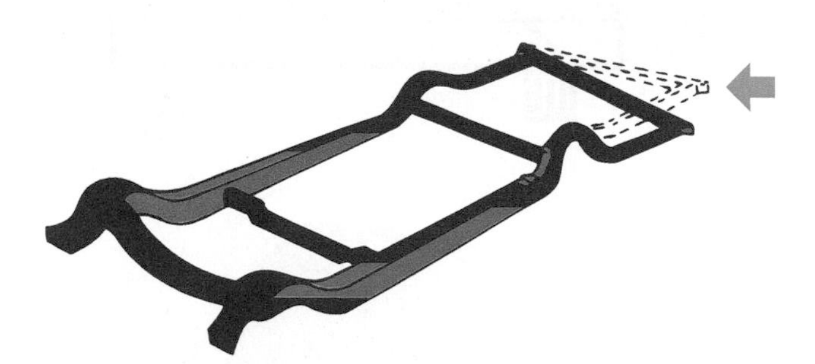

(B) Rear sag is similar, but at the rear rails.

Figure 20–5. Sag causes the frame members to drop lower from severe impact.

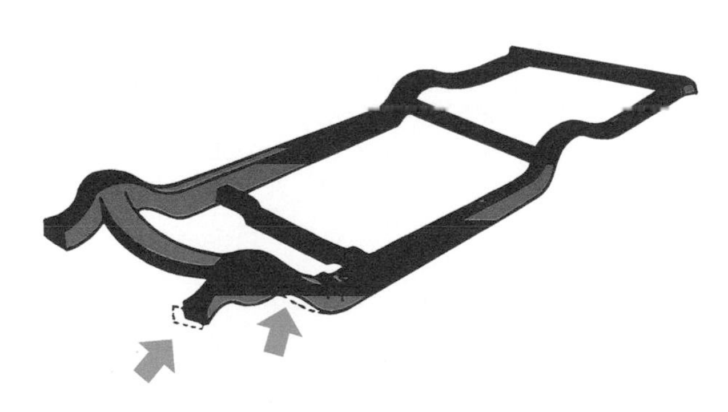

(A) Note the mash damage on the left front rail.

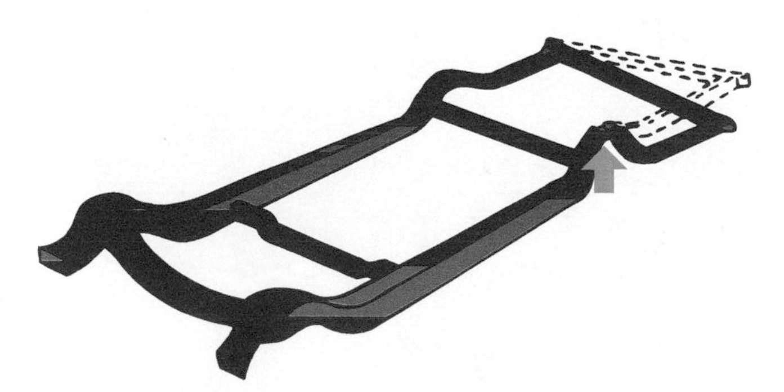

(B) Note the mash damage on the left rear rail.

Figure 20–6. Mash damage results from crushing-in of structural panels and members.

Mash is indicated by wrinkles and severe distortion in fenders, hood, and possibly frame horns or rails. The frame will rise upward at the top of the wheel arch, causing the spring housing to collapse.

With mash damage, there is very little vertical displacement of the bumper. The damage results from direct front or rear collisions.

4. Diamond damage is a condition where one side of the vehicle has been moved to the rear or front. This type of damage causes the frame to be out of square. It will form a parallelogram and is caused by a hard impact on a corner or off-center from the front or rear. Refer to **Figure 20–7.**

Diamond damage affects the entire frame or unibody, NOT just the side rails. Visual indications are hood and trunk lid misalignment. Buckles might appear in the quarter panel near the rear wheel housing or at the roof to quarter panel joint. Wrinkles and buckles probably will appear in the passenger compartment and/or trunk floor. There usually will be some mash and sag combined with the diamond.

5. Twist damage is a condition where one corner of the vehicle is higher than normal; the opposite corner might be lower than normal. It is another type of total frame damage. Twist can happen when a vehicle hits a curb or median strip at high speed. It is also common in rear corner impacts. Look at **Figure 20–8.**

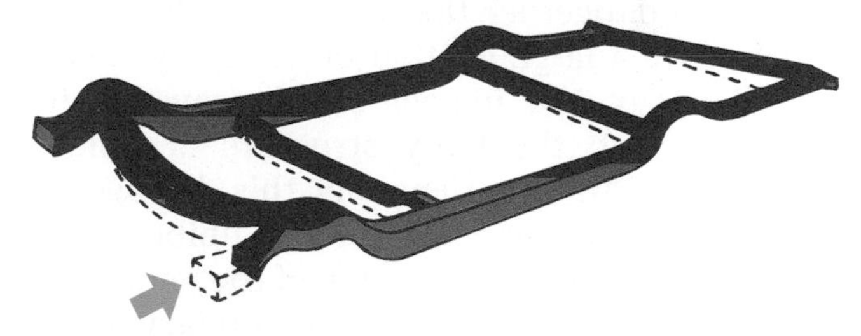

Figure 20–7. Diamond damage forces only one side of the frame rearward. The hard impact to the left frame rail may affect both sides.

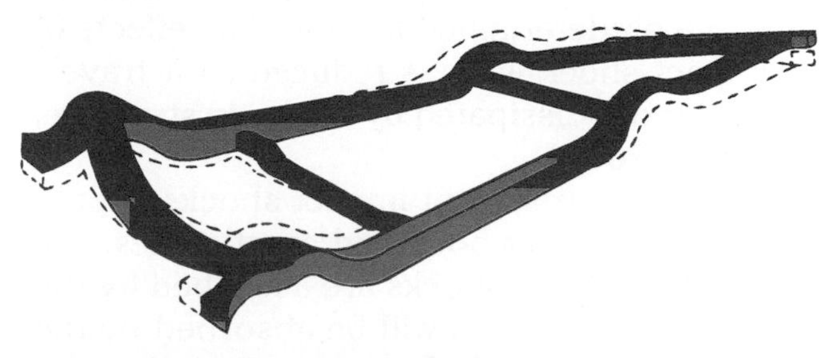

Figure 20–8. Twist damage forces one side of the frame up and the other side down. This is very difficult and expensive to repair.

Unfortunately, most accidents result in a mix of one or more of these damage problems. Side sway and sag frequently occur almost simultaneously. Also, some of these collision solutions affect crossmembers, especially the front member. In a rollover accident, for example, the front crossmember on which the motor mounts are attached will be pulled or pushed out of shape because of the engine's weight. This will result in a sag of this crossmember.

UNIBODY VEHICLE DAMAGE

The damage that occurs to a unibody vehicle as the result of an impact can best be described by using the **cone concept.** The unibody vehicle is designed to absorb a collision impact. When hit, the body folds and collapses as it absorbs the impact. As the force penetrates the structure, it is absorbed by an ever increasing area of the unibody. This characteristic spreads the force until it is completely dissipated. Visualize the point of impact as the tip of the cone.

The centerline of the cone will point in the direction of impact. The depth and spread of the cone indicate the direction and area that the collision force traveled through the unibody. The tip of the cone and point of impact is the **primary damage** area. See **Figure 20–9.**

Since unibodies are pieces of thin sheet metal welded together, the shock of a collision is absorbed by a large portion of the body shell. The effects of the impact shock wave as it travels through the body structure is called **secondary damage.** Generally, this damage is toward the inner structure of the unibody or toward the opposite end or side of the vehicle.

To provide some control on secondary damage and to provide a safer passenger compartment, a unibody vehicle is designed with **crush zones.** These crush zones are engineered to collapse in a predetermined fashion. The effects of the impact shock wave is reduced as it travels through and is dissipated by the body structure. See **Figure 20–10.**

In other words, front impact shocks are absorbed by the front body and crush zones. See **Figure 20–11.** Rear shocks are absorbed by the rear body. Side shocks will be absorbed by the rocker panel, roof side frame, center pillar, and door.

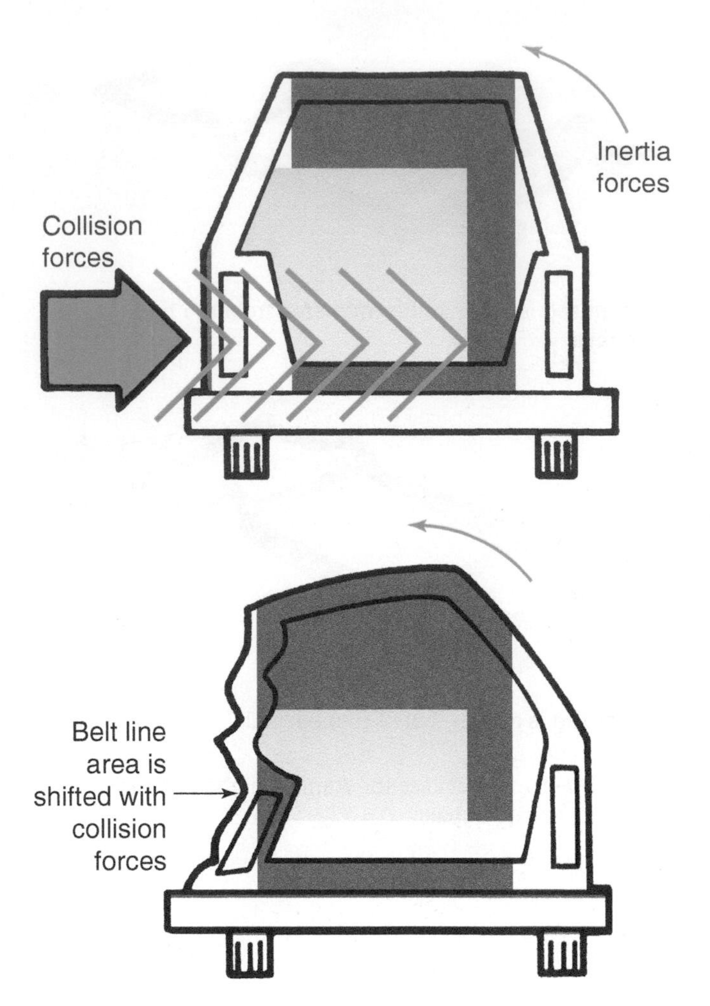

Figure 20–9. Unibody vehicles use the cone or egg shell principle to help absorb the energy of the impact. Note how the roof has shifted sideways because its inertia tried to keep it from rapidly moving with the impact. (Courtesy of Babcox Publications)

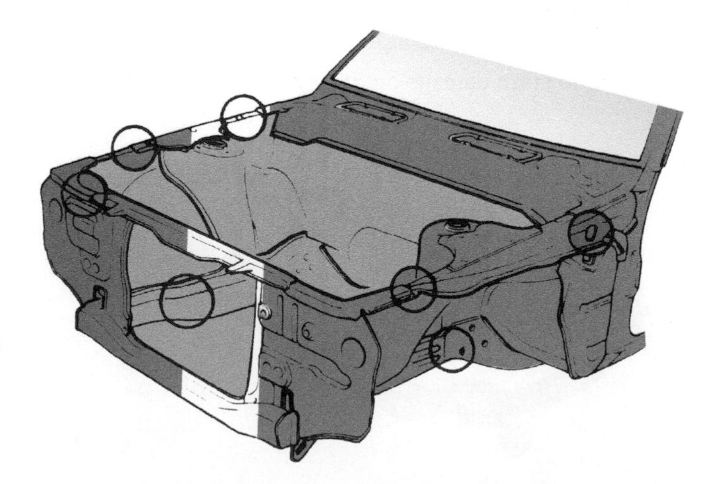

Figure 20–10. These are typical crush zones on a unibody vehicle. They should be checked closely for buckles, bends, paint or sealer cracks, and other signs indicating damage.

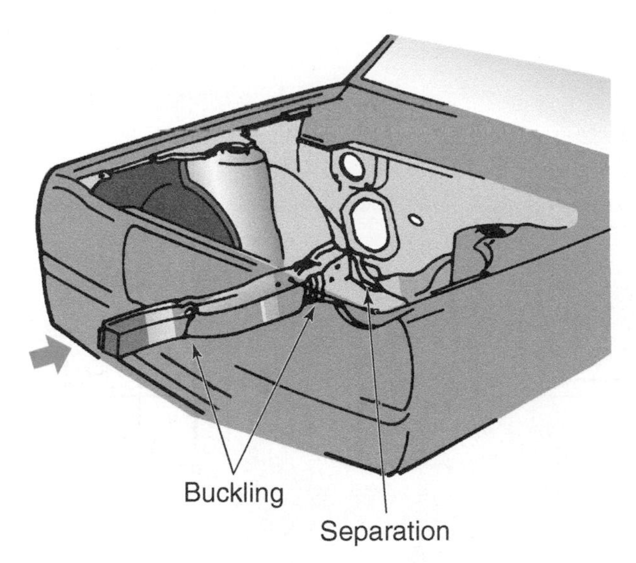

Figure 20–11. With a hard collision, unibody frame rails can buckle and even separate or tear away from other parts. They are designed to absorb energy and protect the passenger compartment.

Impact damages on unibody vehicles can be described as follows.

Frontal damage results from a head-on collision with another object or vehicle. The impact of a collision depends on the vehicle's weight, speed, area of impact, and the source of impact. In the case of a minor impact, the bumper is pushed back, bending the front side members, bumper stay, front fender, cone support, radiator upper support, and hood lock brace.

If the impact is further increased, the front fender will contact the front door. The hood hinge will bend up to the cowl top. The front side members may also buckle into the front suspension crossmember, causing it to bend. See Figure 20–11. If the shock is great enough, the front fender apron and front body pillar (particularly front door hinge upper area) will be bent, which will cause the front door to drop down. In addition, the front side members will buckle. The front suspension member will bend. The instrument panel and front floor pan may also bend to absorb the shock.

If a frontal impact is received at an angle, the attachment point of the front side member becomes a turning axis. Lateral as well as vertical bending occurs (sway). Since the left and right front side members are connected together through the front crossmember, the shock from the impact is sent from the point of impact to the front side member of the opposite side of the vehicle.

Rear damage occurs if the vehicle is moving backward and hits something or if it is hit by another vehicle from behind. When the impact is comparatively small, the rear bumper, the back panel, trunk lid, and floor pan will be deformed. Also, the quarter panels will bulge out.

If the impact is severe enough, the quarter panels will collapse to the base of the roof panel. On four-door vehicles, the center body pillar might bend. Impact energy is absorbed by the deformation of the above parts and by the deformation of the kick-up of the rear side member.

Side damage will cause the door, front section, center body pillar, and even the floor to deform. When the front fender or quarter panel receives a large perpendicular impact, the shock wave extends to the opposite side of the vehicle.

When the central area of the front fender receives an impact, the front wheel is pushed in. The shock wave extends from the front suspension crossmember to the front side member. If severe, the suspension parts are damaged and the front wheel alignment and wheelbase may be changed. The steering gear or rack can also be damaged by side impacts.

Top impacts can result from falling objects or from a rollover of the vehicle. This type of damage involves not only the roof panel, but also the roof side rail, quarter panels, and possibly the windows as well.

When a vehicle has rolled over and the body pillars and roof panels have been bent, the opposite ends of the pillars will be damaged as well. Depending on the manner in which the vehicle rolled over, the front or back sections of the body will be damaged, too. In such cases, the extent of the damage can be determined by the deformation around the windows and doors.

DIMENSIONAL REFERENCES

Two major dimensional references are indicated in all body dimension manuals: the datum plane and centerline.

A **datum line,** or **datum plane,** is an imaginary flat surface parallel to the underbody of the vehicle at some fixed distance from the underbody. It is the plane from which all vertical or height dimensions are taken. It is also the plane that is used to measure the vehicle during repair. The datum is normally shown on dimension charts from the vehicle's side view.

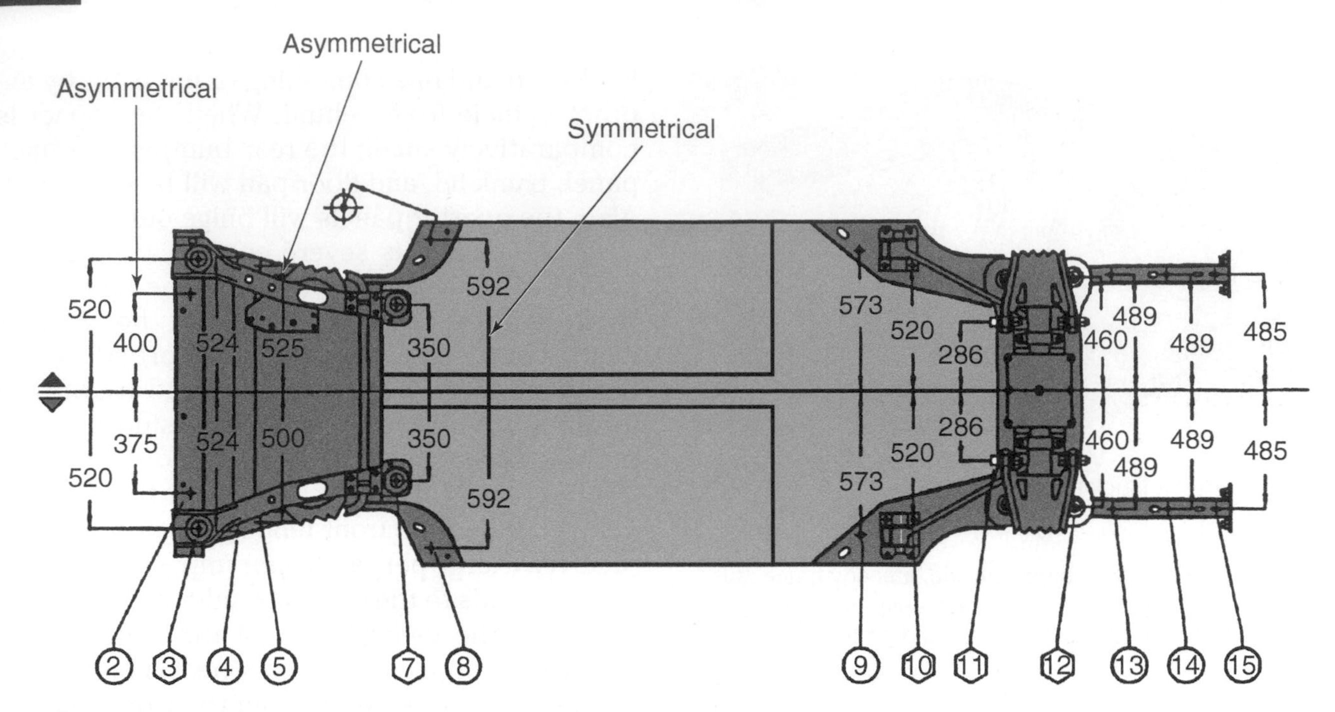

Figure 20–12. A body dimension manual will give measurements and reference points for a specific make and model vehicle. If symmetrical, measurements on both sides are the same. If asymmetrical, measurements will be different on each side. (Courtesy of Hein-Werner® Corporation)

The **center plane,** or **centerline,** divides the vehicle into two equal halves: the passenger side and the driver side. The centerline is shown on dimension charts in either the bottom or top views. It can sometimes be found on some vehicles in the form of body center marks. **Body center marks** are stamped into the sheet metal in both the upper and lower body areas of the vehicle. They can save time when taking measurements.

All width or **lateral dimensions** of symmetrical vehicles are measured from the center. That is, the measurement from the centerline to a specific point on the right side will be exactly the same as the measurement from the centerline to the same point on the left side. One side of the structure would be a perfect mirror image of the other. Most vehicles are built symmetrically. But if the vehicle is NOT symmetrical (asymmetrical), the self-centering gauges will NOT align and will NOT indicate a true center reference.

It is usually necessary to think of the vehicle as a rectangle divided into three zero plane sections. The *three zero plane sections* break the vehicle into three areas—front, center, and rear. The torque box location is used as the dividing lines. This three-section principle is a result of the vehicle's design and the way it reacts during a collision.

Symmetrical means that the dimensions on the right side of the vehicle are equal to the dimensions on the left side of the vehicle. If the vehicle is **asymmetrical,** these dimensions are NOT the same. In such a case, use gauges that can be adjusted to compensate for the asymmetry. See **Figure 20–12.**

VEHICLE MEASURING BASICS

In unibody construction, each section should be checked for diagonal squareness by comparing diagonal lengths. Length and width should also be compared. The center section should be used as a base when reading structural alignment. All measurements and alignment readings should be taken relative to the center section.

Start measuring in the center or middle section. If it is NOT square, then move to the undamaged end of the vehicle to find three correctly positioned reference points. See **Figure 20–13.**

Keep in mind that to accurately measure a vehicle, you must start with at least three dimensions you know are undamaged. The way to do this is to check the squareness of the vehicle. If the vehicle is NOT symmetrical, refer to the dimension chart for correct measurements.

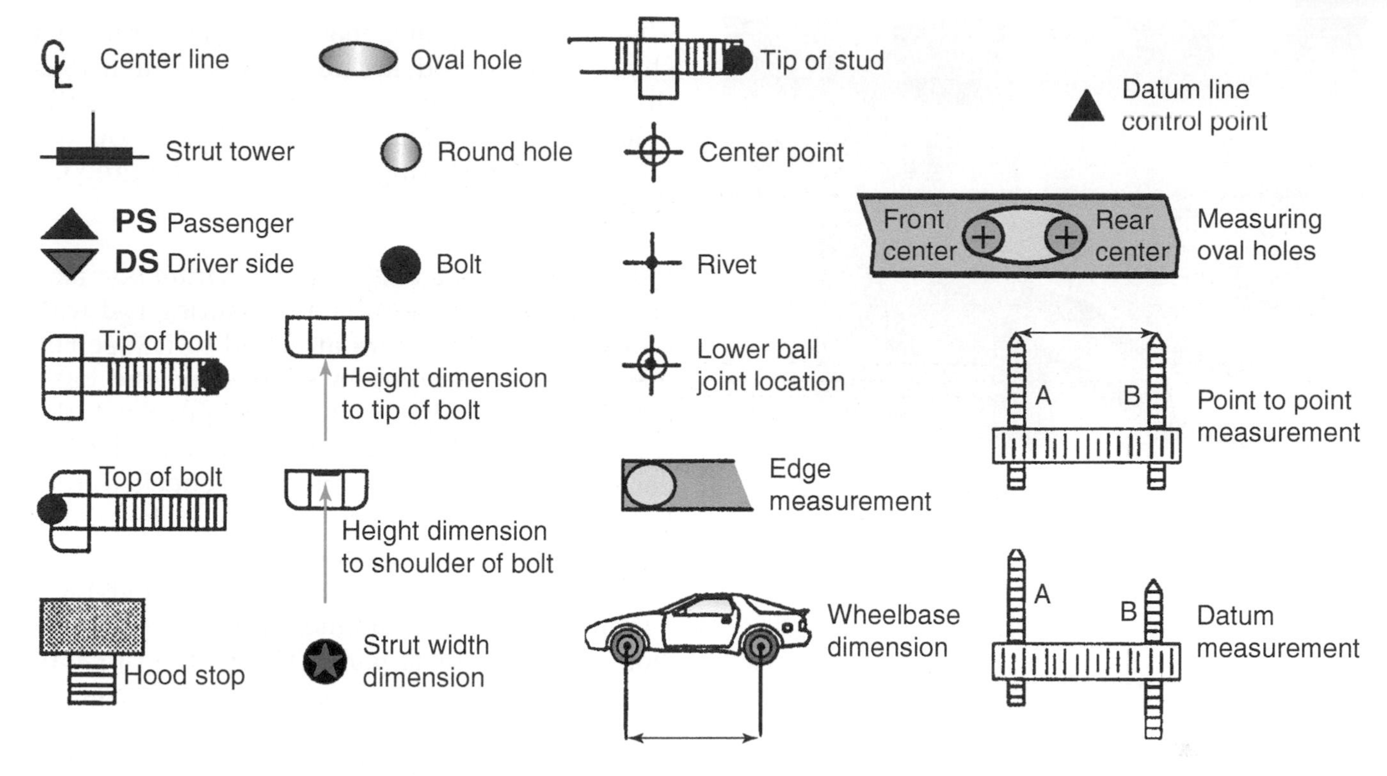

Figure 20–13. These are common symbols used when reading dimension manuals. They show you which points on a wrecked vehicle must be measured to determine structural damage. (Courtesy of Hein Werner® Corporation)

Remember! The terms "control point" and "reference point" have different meanings. The *control points* used in manufacturing are NOT necessarily the same as the reference points the collision repair technician uses to measure the vehicle. *Reference points* refer to the part of panel locations (bolts, holes, etc.) used to give unibody dimensions in body specification manuals. The distance between reference points can be measured with either a tram bar or a tape measure to analyze damage. See **Figure 20–14.**

TYPES OF MEASURING EQUIPMENT

Because of the importance of measuring during repairs, many kinds of special equipment have been developed by manufacturers. Each provides the capability to measure very quickly and accurately. Although a number of styles of measuring equipment can be found in collision repair shops, most of it can be divided into four basic systems:

1. Gauge measuring systems
2. Universal measuring systems
3. Dedicated fixture systems
4. Electronic measuring systems

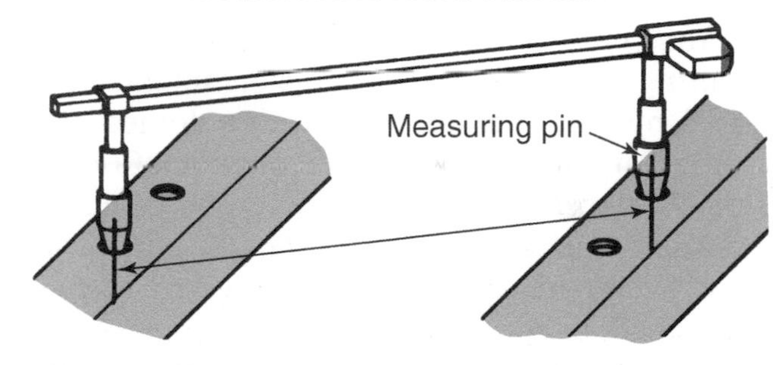

(A) Tram bar tips are touched on specified reference points. The length of the tram bar should equal the spec measurements given in the manual.

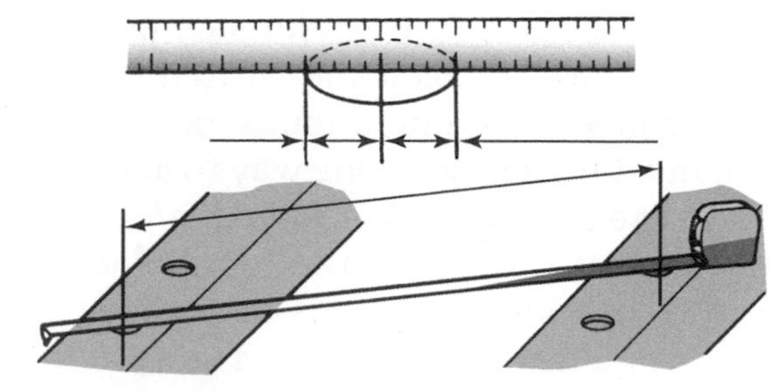

(B) A tape measure is also used to make measurements between reference points.

Figure 20–14. These are two basic methods of measuring on a vehicle.

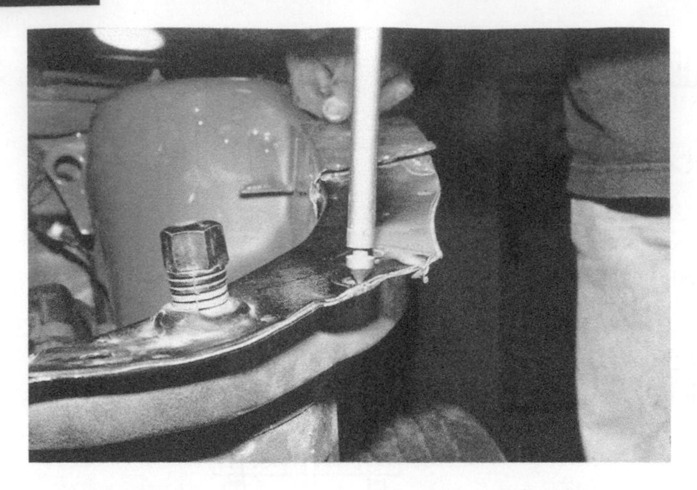

Figure 20–15. Here the tram bar tip is touching the reference point on the damaged vehicle's radiator support. It is not centered in the hole so the unibody must be straightened.

Gauge Measuring Systems

Gauge measuring systems use sliding metal rods or bars and adjustable pointers with ruled scales to measure body dimensions. The tape measure, tram bar, the self-centering gauge, and the strut tower gauge can be used separately or in conjunction with one another. See **Figure 20–15.**

Tram bars are used for measurement; self-centering gauges check for misalignment. Supported by MacPherson strut tower domes, the strut tower gauge allows visual alignment of the critical reference points of unibody vehicles. The tram bar, self-centering gauge, and strut tower gauge are available as a unit or as separate vehicle diagnostic tools.

The tracking gauge is used to check alignment of the front and rear wheels. It is another popular measuring gauge. If the front and rear wheels are NOT in alignment, the vehicle will NOT handle properly.

Keeping Records. Since reference point measurements must be taken and written down several times in a repair operation, a method of tabulation must be devised. One way to accomplish this is to use a *data chart* or *tabulation chart.*

In the first column of the tabulation chart, write the location of what is being measured. Numbers or letters can be used. The second and third columns contain the manufacturer's specifications taken from the body dimension manual and actual distance as it exists on the damaged vehicle. The 1-2-3 are the readings taken at measurement step 1, measurement step 2, and so on. That is, as each pull is made, the measurements should be recorded, including those dimensions that have been corrected. This chart tells the collision repair technician at a glance how the job stands in restoring the vehicle to its precollision state.

Using Tram Bars and Tapes. A *tram bar,* also known as a *tram gauge* is a measuring rod with two adjustable pointers attached to it (see Figure 20–14). The pointers slide along the bar's length and are adjustable for height. Since the tram bar measures one dimension at a time, each must be recorded and cross checked from two additional reference points. At least one must be a diagonal measurement.

The best areas to select for tram bar measurements are the attachment points for suspension and mechanical parts. These are critical to alignment. Throughout the pulling and straightening process, critical reference points must be measured (and recorded) repeatedly with the tram bar to monitor progress and to prevent overpulling.

The tram bar might have a scale superimposed on it. However, since almost all dimension charts list measurements in metric, use a tape measure with both English and metric scales to set up the tram bar. The tape measure can also be used to take quick measurements between reference points. Be sure the tape measure has been checked for accuracy before using it.

Reference point holes are frequently larger in diameter than the tram bar tip. To measure accurately with the tram bar when the holes are the same diameter, measure like edge to like edge. Study **Figure 20–16.**

When the holes are NOT the same size, they will usually be the same type of hole: round, square, or oblong. To find the center-to-center measurement, measure inside edge to inside edge, then outside edge to outside edge. Add the results of the two measurements and divide by 2.

The term **point-to-point measurement** refers to the shortest distance between two points, as shown in **Figure 20–17.** The term **datum measurement** refers to the distance between two points when measured from the datum plane/line.

A few body dimension manuals give the measurements based on the bar's length. Here, the bar of the tram becomes the datum plane beneath the vehicle. The pointers are set at the

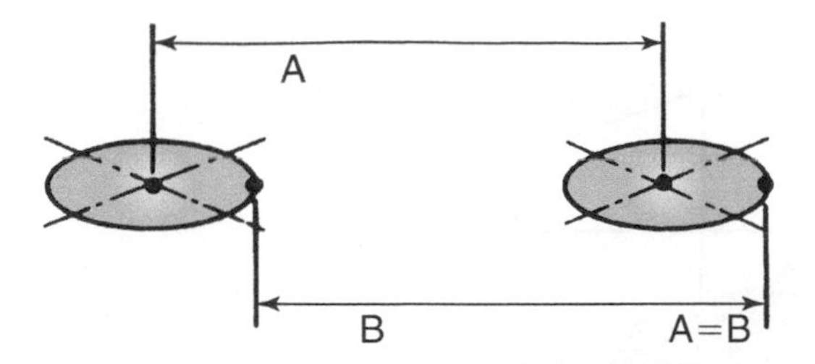

(A) You can measure from center to center or edge to edge if the holes are the same size. Both would read the same.

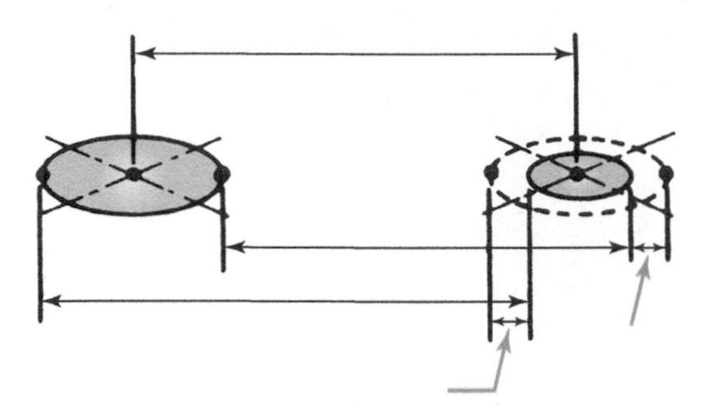

(B) If the reference holes are different sizes, it would be best to measure from center to center.

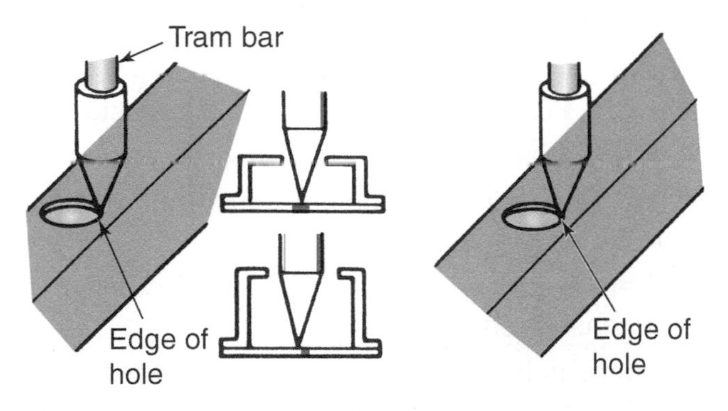

(C) If the tram bar does not fit into the holes tightly, use tips to measure edge to edge for accuracy.

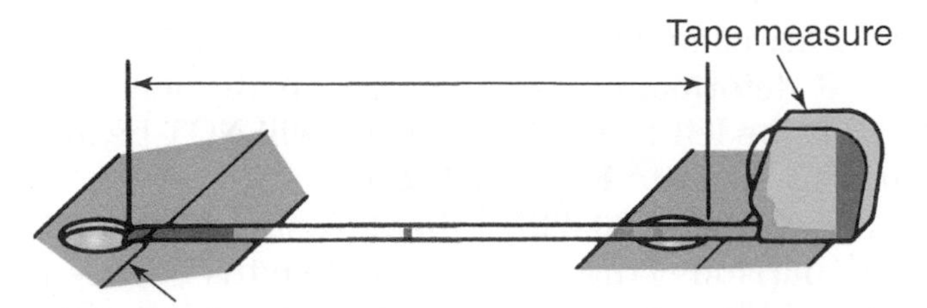

(D) A tape measure is handy when measuring equal sized holes edge to edge, especially when working under the vehicle.

Figure 20–16. Note various methods for measuring the distance between reference points.

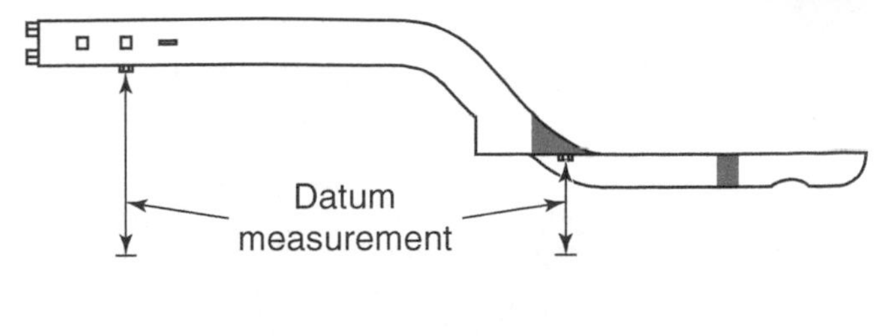

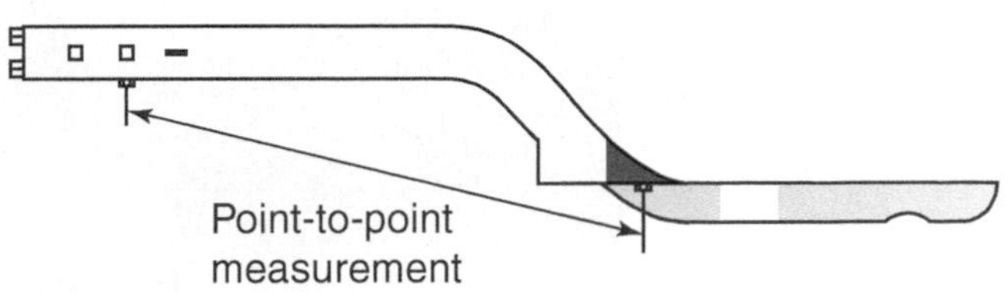

Figure 20–17. When specs are given, they can be point-to-point or datum measurements.

horizontal height dimensions specified on the dimension chart. It is important to always check the method used on the dimension chart because the two distances are NOT the same.

Upper Body Measurement. Upper body damage can also be determined by the use of a tram bar and a steel measuring tape. Their use is basically the same as when doing an underbody evaluation. Dimension charts have measurements for many upper body reference points.

Front Body Measurement. When a damaged vehicle needs the hood and front side member replaced, you should take measurements during the repair. Even if only the front, right side of the vehicle body received the impact, the left side will usually be damaged also. Therefore, the extent of deformation must be checked before pulling.

Figure 20–18 shows the typical front body reference points. They should be measured and checked against the dimension chart for the specific vehicle.

When checking front end dimensions, measure the attachment points for suspension and mechanical parts. These are critical to proper alignment. Each dimension should be checked from two additional reference points with at least one reference point being a diagonal measurement.

Note that the longer the dimension, the more accurate the measurement. A measurement from the lower cowl to the engine cradle is a better gauge than a measurement from a lower cowl to another lower cowl area. This is because the longer dimension takes in a larger area of the

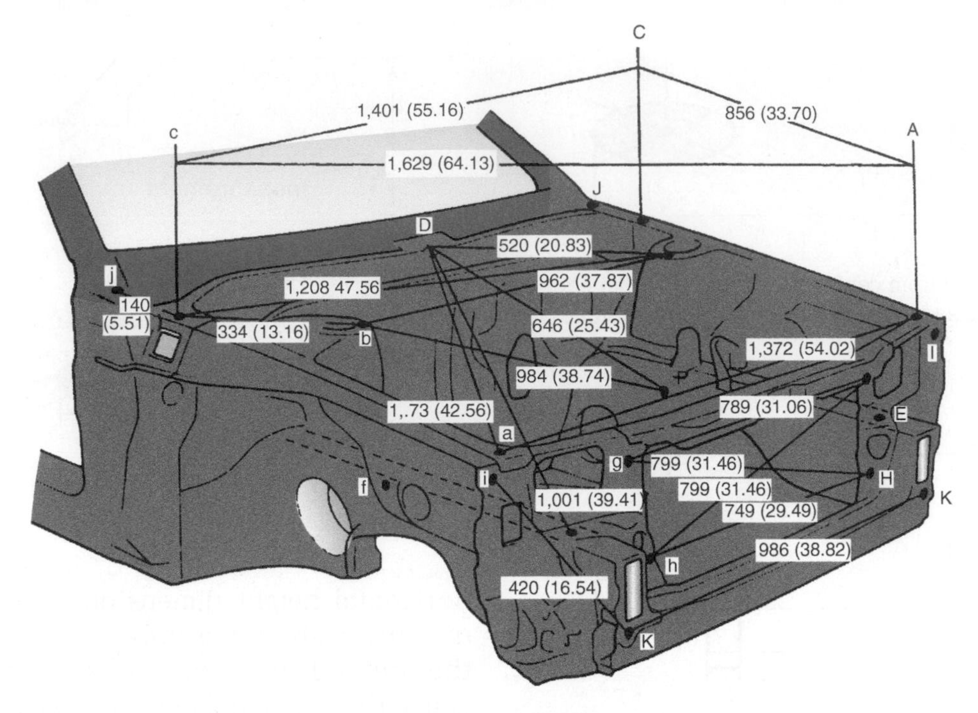

Figure 20–18. A dimensions manual will give front end body reference points like these. Most of these would have to be measured after a major front end collision.

vehicle. The use of two or more measurements from each reference point assures greater accuracy. It also helps identify the extent and direction of any panel damage.

Body Side Panel Measurement. Body side structure damage can be evaluated by the fit and operation of the doors when opened and closed. Deformation around the door openings can cause an uneven gap and air or water leaks. Thus, accurate measurements must be taken. The tram bar is used to measure the body side panel. See **Figure 20–19.**

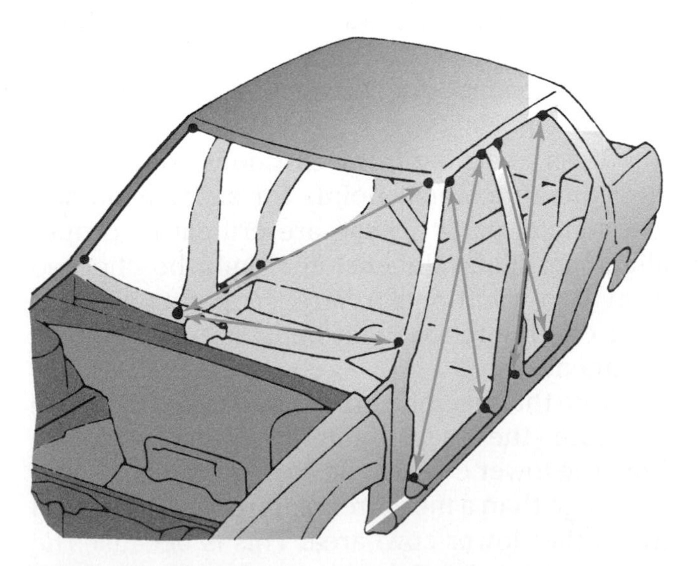

Figure 20–19. Note typical side reference points.

Diagonal line measurement compares reading across an opening or between four reference points to determine damage. Damage can be detected if the left-to-right symmetry of the body is used for measuring diagonal lines, as shown in **Figure 20–20A.** Use this measuring method if:

1. The data on the engine compartment and underbody are missing.
2. There are no data available in the body dimension chart.
3. The vehicle has been severely damaged in a rollover.

The diagonal line measurement method is NOT adequate when inspecting damage to both sides of the vehicle or in the case of twisting. This is because the left-to-right difference in the diagonal lines cannot be measured. See **Figure 20–20B.**

If deformation is the same on the left and right, the left to right difference will NOT be apparent. Refer to **Figure 20–20C.**

In **Figure 20–20D,** the measurement and comparison of the left and right lengths between yz and YZ will give an even better indication of damage conditions. This method should be used in conjunction with the diagonal line measurement method. This method can be applied where there are parts that are symmetrical on the left and right sides.

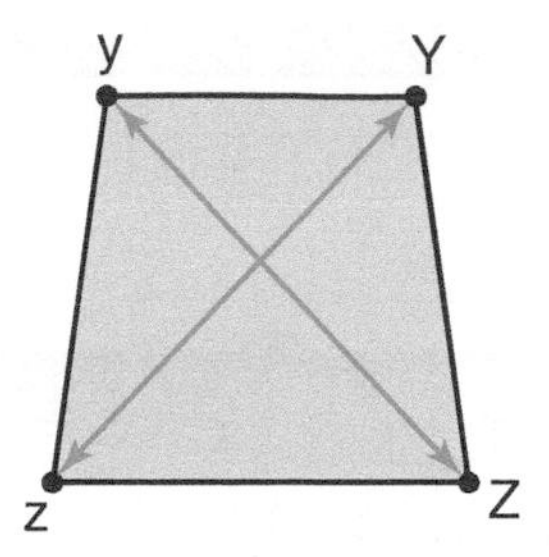

(A) Yz equals yZ; no warping or damage present in this example.

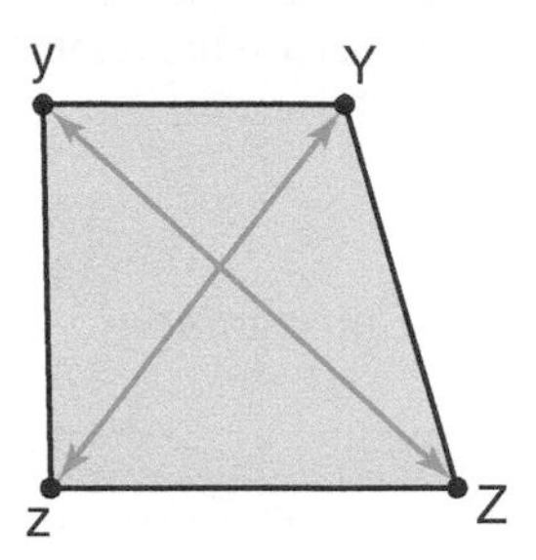

(B) Yz is less than yZ, which indicates deflection damage to the left.

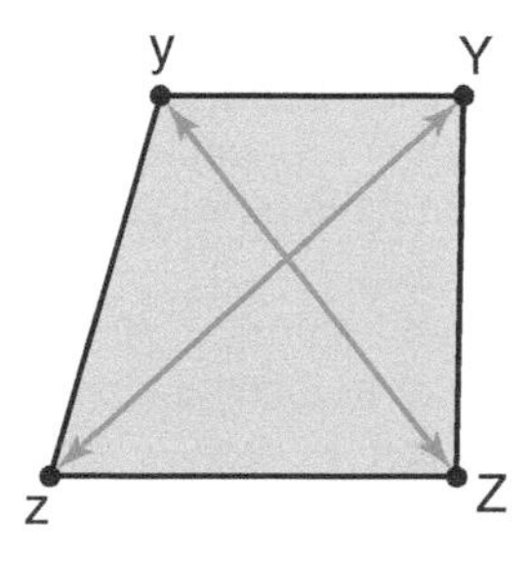

(C) Yz is greater than yZ; the measurement would show deflection damage to the right.

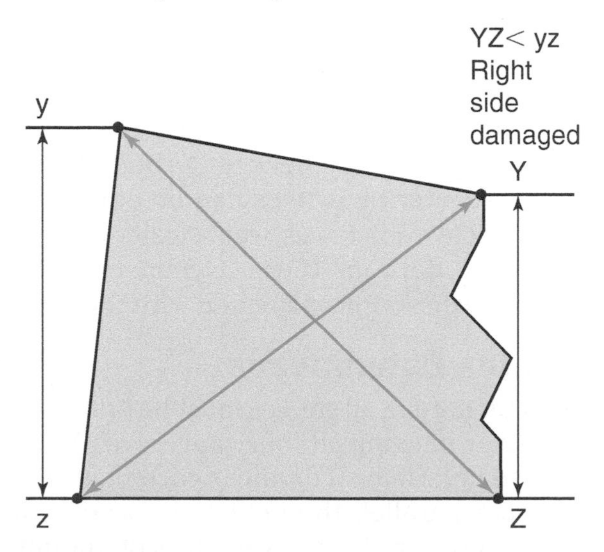

(D) YZ should equal yz. Damage on the right has pushed the YZ dimension smaller than yz. The damage would have to be pulled out until both dimensions are equal and within specs.

Figure 20–20. Study the use of the diagonal line measuring technique for finding collision damage.

Rear Body Measurement. Damage to the rear body can be analyzed by the fit and action when the deck lid is opened and closed. Damage to this area can cause water leakage around the deck lid seal. Any wrinkle in the rear floor is usually due to buckling of the rear frame rail, a major problem. Thus, measure the rear body together with the underbody. In this way, the straightening work can be performed effectively.

Keep in mind that all reference points need to be checked from two or more reference points. Diagonal measurements are a good way to cross-check dimensional reference points. Correct use of self-centering gauges will also reveal the kind of misalignment that would be shown by diagonal tram bar measurements.

Self-centering Gauges

Self-centering gauges show alignment or misalignment by projecting points on the vehicle's structure into the technician's line of sight. See **Figure 20–21.**

Self-centering gauges are installed at various control areas on the bottom of the vehicle. They have two sliding horizontal bars that remain parallel as they move inward and outward. This action permits adjustment to any width for installation on various areas of the vehicle.

Self-centering gauges are used to establish the vehicle centerline and datum plane. Use the gauges in sets of four or more. Adjust and hang them at the locations indicated in the dimensional data manual to establish the datum plane. The body manual will also give information for adjusting them to hang on the same plane under the vehicle. Scales are provided for adjusting

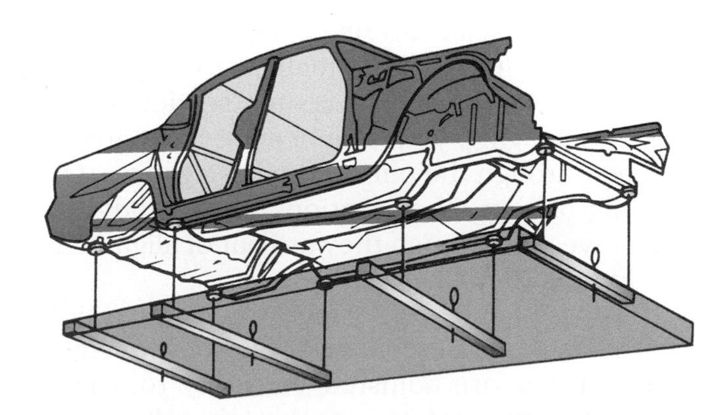

Figure 20–21. A self-centering gauge is used to check for major frame and unibody damage. Four self-centering gauges are often suspended under a vehicle to form a datum plane and center plane. (Courtesy of Blackhawk Collision Repair, Inc., Subsidiary of Hein-Werner® Corporation)

the gauges to hang the correct distance down under the vehicle.

Begin by setting up the **base gauges,** or the two gauges hung near the center off the vehicle. Usually, the torque box area is used. Generally, these will be gauges numbered 2 and 3. Add other gauges as needed and use the base gauges for reference.

When inspecting for damage, first hang self-centering gauges from two places where there is no visible damage, then hang two more gauges where there is obvious damage. Then sight the gauges hung at both the undamaged and damaged locations and check to see if the gauges are parallel to each other or if the centering pins are misaligned.

The gauges are also equipped with center pins or sights, which remain in the center of the gauge regardless of the width of the horizontal bars. This allows the technician to read centerline throughout the length of the vehicle.

When sighting gauges for parallel, always stand directly in the middle, scanning with both eyes. To ensure accuracy, readings should be made at the outer edge of the self-centering gauge, NOT in the middle.

The farther one stands from the gauges while reading, the more accurate the reading will be. Standing close changes the line of sight to the front gauges so drastically that an accurate reading is nearly impossible.

Self-centering gauges should always be set at the same height or plane. Different heights will change the angle of sight and give a false reading. Sighting from the end of the vehicle opposite the damage can make readings more accurate. With practice, you can improve the damage analysis with self-centering gauges.

The sighting of centerline pins must be done with one eye. Since the center section is the base for gauging, your line of sight must always project through the pins of the base gauges. Observing pins in other sections of the body will then reveal how much they are out of alignment. See **Figure 20–22.**

Each self-centering gauge has two vertical scales—one on the left side, one on the right. These scales are adjusted vertically to assure that the horizontal bars accurately reflect true positions.

Once hung in specific locations, the gauges generally remain on the vehicle throughout the entire repair operation. This is true unless they interfere with straightening, anchoring, or with the tram bar.

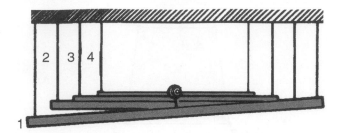

(A) The front view of the gauges shows that the front frame rails have been pushed out of alignment. Sight straight down gauges like looking through the sights or scope of a gun. The rear three gauges are in alignment, indicating no damage are in the rear of the car.

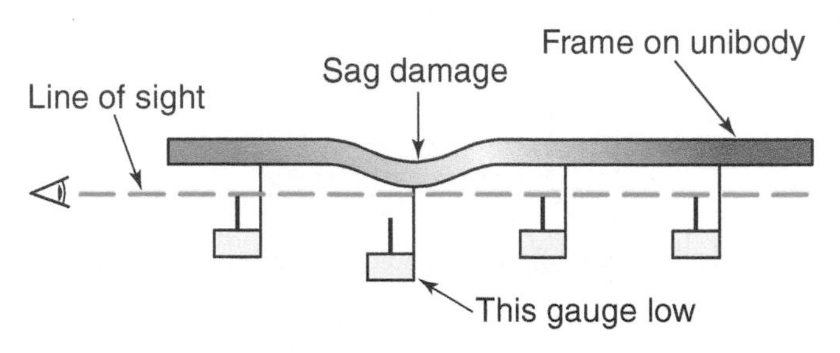

(B) The side view of self-centering gauges shows sag damage near the cowl or fire wall area of the vehicle. The front frame rails might have buckled from frontal impact.

Figure 20–22. If self-centering gauges are out of alignment, the frame or unibody is damaged and must be pulled on a frame rack.

Special centering gauges are available that can be used to check such items as body pillar damage.

The same system of alignment is employed when using gauges to check underbody damage. Some self-centering gauges can be adjusted for asymmetrical vehicles as well. Again, check the dimensional data for these asymmetrical vehicles. Follow directions provided with the gauges.

Using the Datum Plane

To read for datum, all gauges must be on the same plane. After hanging all four gauges, read across the top to determine if datum is correct. If all four gauges are parallel, the vehicle is on datum. If they are NOT parallel, the vehicle is off datum.

Since the datum line is an imaginary plane, datum heights can be raised or lowered to facilitate gauge readings. Just remember that if the datum height is changed at one gauge location, all the gauges MUST be adjusted an equal amount to maintain accuracy.

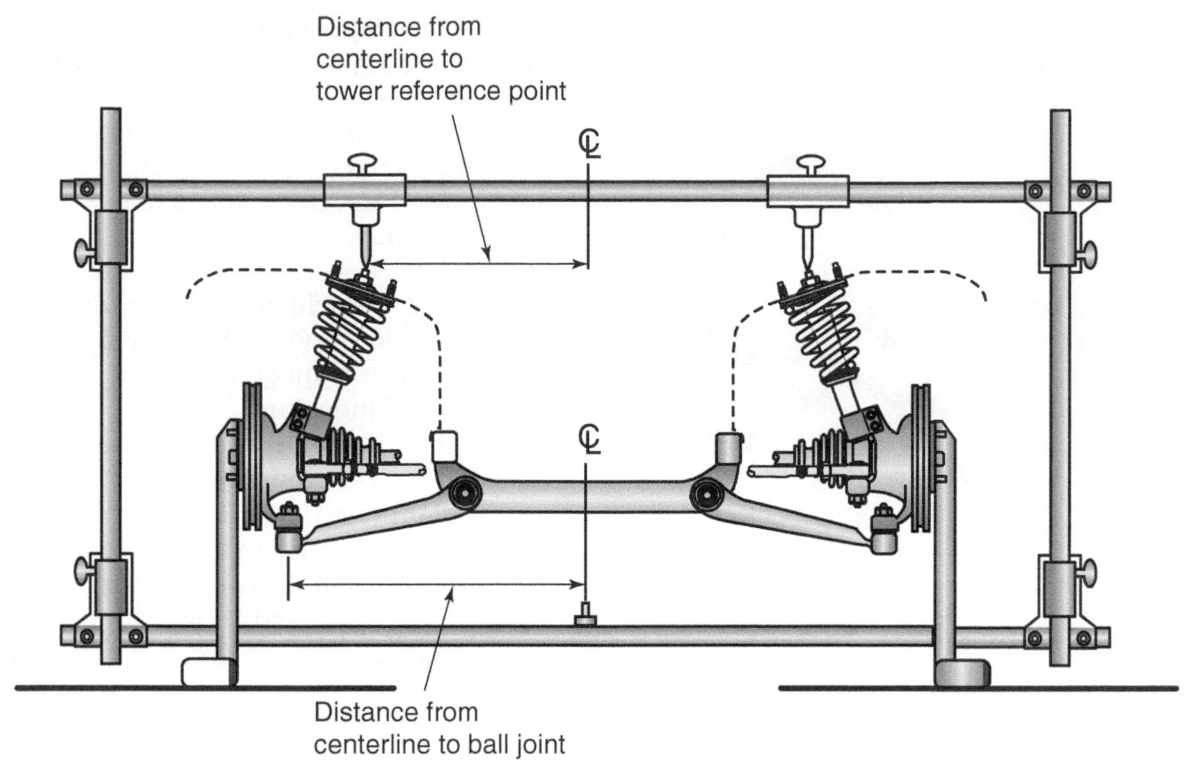

Figure 20–23. A strut tower gauge is designed to measure damage around the engine compartment quickly and accurately. Measurements should generally be at equal distances from the centerline.

While datum readings are usually obtained from self-centering gauges, there are individual gauges available for measuring datum heights. These datum gauges are usually held in position by magnetic holders. Remember that the dimensions that allow the vehicle to be level with the road are measured from the datum plane.

Using the Centerline

To check for centerline misalignment, use the four self-centering gauges hung on the datum. To establish the true centerline, the center pin on the No. 2 gauge must be lined up with the center pin on the No. 3 gauge. Then the center pins of No. 1 and No. 4 can be read relative to the centerline of the base.

Frame or unibody damage will affect the centerline reading. If a vehicle has a diamond condition, a shortened rail or subrail, or an out-of-level condition, the centerline reading may be affected. Further inspection by gauging or measuring will be necessary.

Using Strut Tower Gauges

Supported by the shock-spring towers, the **strut tower gauge** allows visual alignment of the upper body area. It shows misalignment of the strut tower/upper body parts in relation to the vehicle's centerline plane and datum plane. See **Figure 20–23.**

The strut tower gauge features an upper and lower horizontal bar, each with a center pin. The upper bar is usually calibrated from the center out. Pointers are used to mount the gauge to the strut tower/upper body locations.

Using dimension charts, the strut tower gauge is adjusted to the correct dimensions. You must use the vertical scales that link the upper and lower horizontal bars to set the lower bar at the datum plane. With the lower bar set to align properly, the upper pointers should be located at reference points on the strut towers. If they are NOT, the strut towers are damaged and pushed out of alignment. This would tell you that straightening would be needed so that the front suspension and wheels could be aligned properly.

Universal Measuring Systems

Universal measuring systems have the ability to measure several reference points at the same time, making the job much easier and more accurate. See **Figure 20–24.** However, universal systems still require a degree of skill and

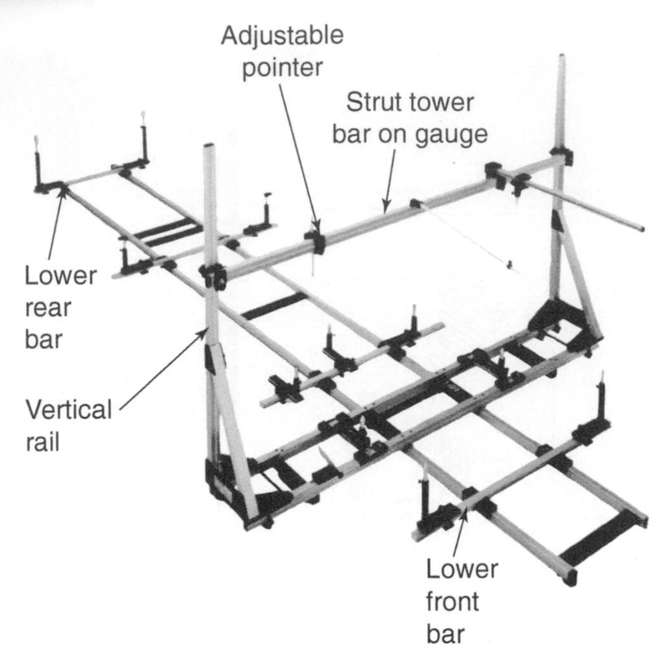

Figure 20–24. Study the major parts of this universal measuring system. By aligning the bars and pointers with reference points on the undamaged area of the vehicle, pointers will not line up with the damaged areas and their reference points. (Courtesy of Chief Automotive Systems, Inc.)

attention to detail to operate properly. And to get the proper readings, the equipment must be set using the manufacturer's specifications.

Universal measuring systems can be mechanical or laser, or a combination of the two.

With a universal measuring system, all the reference points can be checked by just moving around the vehicle. You can quickly determine where each reference point on the vehicle is in comparison to the measuring system.

If a reference point on the vehicle is NOT in the same position as the dimension chart says it should be, the reference point on the vehicle is wrong. When the system is set up properly, you can monitor the key points by simply looking at the pointers. If the pointers are out of position, then the vehicle is NOT dimensionally correct. Thus, that reference point is out of position and must be brought back to precollision specifications.

WARNING

The pointers can be damaged during pulling/straightening. Lower the pointers, if necessary, to clear the way for the pull. This will avoid damaging or misaligning the measuring system.

While the important vehicle dimensions can be found in body dimension manuals, most universal measuring equipment manufacturers have specific dimension charts for their equipment. These charts, one for each vehicle model manufactured, serve as guides to use before and during the repair.

The dimension chart usually illustrates two views of the vehicle underbody. Some charts also give underhood and upper body dimensions. The latter is most important with the mill and drill pad dimensions.

Remember! Many equipment manufacturer's dimension charts are intended for that specific piece of equipment only. Because of this variation between systems, it would be difficult to explain how each manufacturer's system measures a vehicle. You will need to read the equipment owner's manual for these details.

Mechanical Measuring Systems

A typical mechanical system consists of:

1. A bridge(s) that runs the length of the vehicle from front to back.
2. Sliding arms that mount to the bridge. They can be moved from front to back on the bridge for length measurements. They can also be moved outward or inward for width measurements.
3. Pointers that are mounted on the arms. They can be adjusted up or down for height measurements.
4. Specific fixtures for the make and model vehicle.

The pointer may accept special adapters to fit over a bolt head or into a reference point hole. The equipment manufacturer will provide instructions for this type of setup.

Mechanical measuring systems are designed and used according to guidelines found in the equipment manufacturer's publications. They are written for each family of body styles. Mechanical measuring systems look complicated, but they are easy to use after reading their directions carefully.

Dedicated Bench and Fixture Measuring Systems

The **dedicated bench and fixture system** acts as "go-no-go" gauge. It is a completely different type of measuring method. Instead of taking actual measurements, dedicated fixtures are used to check body or frame alignment.

The **dedicated bench** consists of a strong, flat work surface to which fixtures are attached.

Fixtures are thick metal parts that bolt between the vehicle and bench to check alignment. They are designed from the vehicle manufacturer's drawings and specifications. The fixtures physically check mountings or other key locations of the underbody.

If the fixtures fit the vehicle properly, the technician knows that the underbody, strut towers, and so forth are in perfect alignment. All that is necessary is to straighten the vehicle until the reference points match the fixtures. Other underbody measurements are usually not required.

The dedicated bench and fixture measuring system requires a specific set of fixtures for each family of body styles. If the collision repair shop does not own the required fixtures, they can be rented. The bench has built-in reference positions, and the fixtures are positioned to the specific references according to instructions supplied by the manufacturer. At least three fixtures must be positioned on the bench before the vehicle is mounted. Generally these are the torque-box fixtures. However, the damage to a specific vehicle will dictate which fixtures should be used.

Figure 20–25 shows four of the more common types of fixtures. They are:

1. *Bolt-on Fixtures*—used when attachment is required to steering or suspension mountings. The studs or bolts on the vehicle are used to attach the fixtures. Depending on the damage, the fixtures can either be bolted to the vehicle first and lined up with the bench during the repair, or they can be attached to the bench first and lined up with the vehicle during repair.
2. *Pin-type Fixtures*—used most often to mate with reference point holes in the underbody. They can also be used to mate with suspension mounting holes.
3. *Strut Fixtures*—used in the same manner as a pin-type fixture. A typical strut fixture consists of a bottom plate assembly as with the other fixtures, an adjustable shaft with a cross pin, and a bolt-on top plate.
4. *Bench Extensions*—included where the length of the vehicle requires that fixtures be positioned beyond the bench surface. The extensions are always used at the rear of the vehicle. Each extension is drilled with holes on top and on the bottom.

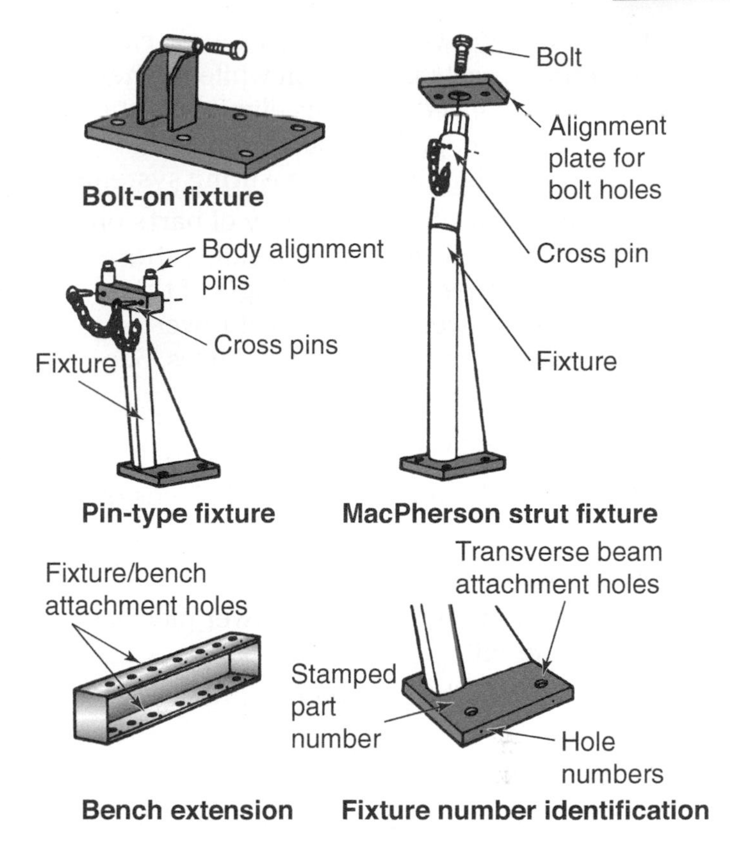

Figure 20–25. Note various fixture types. Fixtures mount on the frame rack and fasten to major structural panels on the vehicle. If the bolts or pins on the fixtures do not line up, the vehicle unibody is not aligned and is damaged.

Most fixtures share a common attachment method to the transverse beams. The base plate for each fixture is drilled with holes and is marked with a part number and the location on the transverse beam. Stamped at the rear of each fixture base are the numbers that correspond to the numbers on the transverse beam.

Once the vehicle is mounted on the bench, at least three fixtures should be set up on the undamaged area of the vehicle. Then place as many fixtures as possible in the damaged area of the vehicle. The fixtures perform a number of functions:

1. They show where a reference point should be located.
2. They provide gauging of all the reference points at the same time. No measuring is required. If all the points line up, the steering, suspension, engine mounts, and so on are in alignment.

3. Once lined up with the fixtures, they can hold these parts in position while further straightening is done. This eliminates the "pull-measure, pull-measure" sequence required with universal measuring systems.
4. They allow accurate assembly of parts on the vehicle before actually welding those pieces together. A good example of this would be a lower rail and strut tower assembly on some unibody vehicles. See **Figure 20–26.**

The sequence is as follows:

1. Position and hold the lower rail pieces on the fixtures.
2. Weld them together.
3. Position and hold the strut tower pieces on top of the rail.
4. Weld them in their correct position.

Electronic Measuring Systems

Electronic measuring systems use a computer, or PC, to control the operation of the measuring system. Computerized measuring systems can use:

1. Laser scanner and reflective targets
2. Ultrasound generating probes and receiver beam
3. Robotic measuring arm

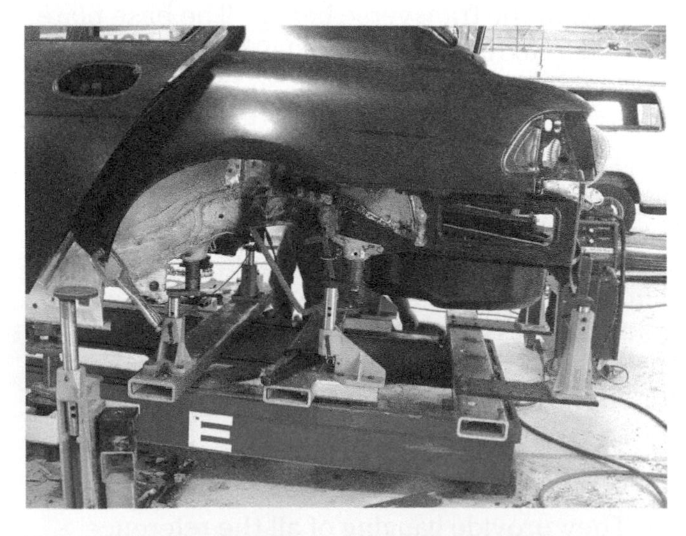

Figure 20–26. Some high-end auto manufacturers require a fixture system to correct major structural damage. Fixtures are often rented for the exact vehicle being repaired. Panels are properly measured and aligned when they will fit and align with fixtures.

Any of these system variations can input accurate measurements for computer analysis. A PC provides for fast entry and checking of vehicle dimensions against electronic specifications.

Laser Measuring Systems

The laser measuring system uses a strong beam of light, beam splitters, and targets to measure vehicle damage. It is extremely accurate when properly installed and used. See **Figure 20–27.**

The word **laser** is an acronym for "light amplification by stimulated emission of radiation." All laser measuring systems operate in basically the same way. The laser unit is aimed at a target or measuring scale. See **Figure 20–28.** The target or scale is either hung from or attached to the vehicle. Some systems even use parts of the vehicle as targets. Look at **Figure 20–29.**

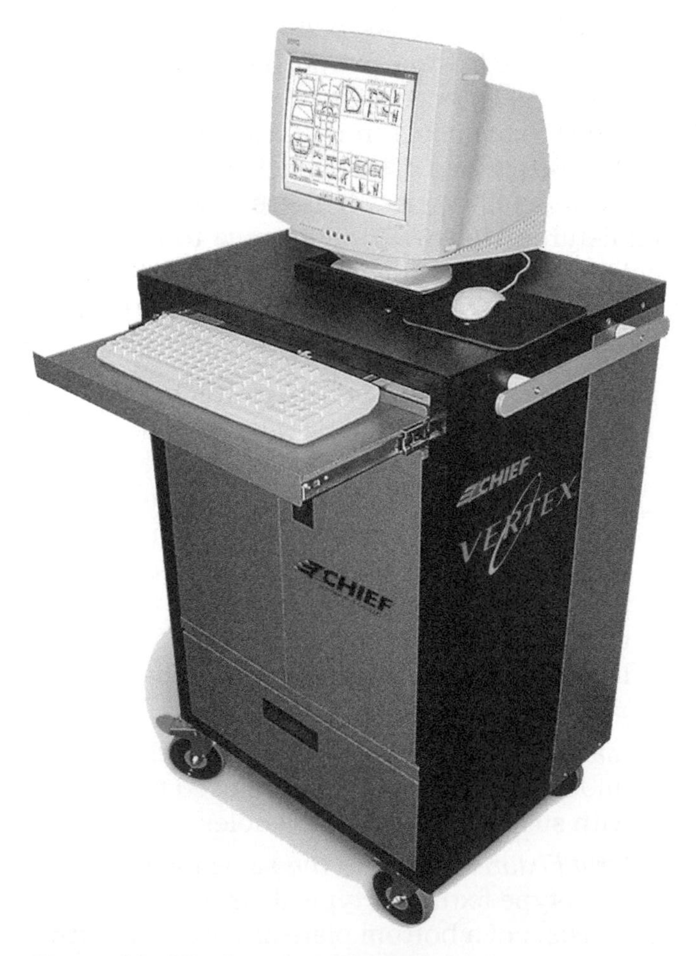

Figure 20–27. This three-dimensional computerized laser measuring system can take length, width, and height measurements at one time. A personal computer can display the dimensions manual, give instructions for use, show locations of reference points, and even tell you which points on a specific vehicle are not aligned properly. (Courtesy of Chief Automotive Systems)

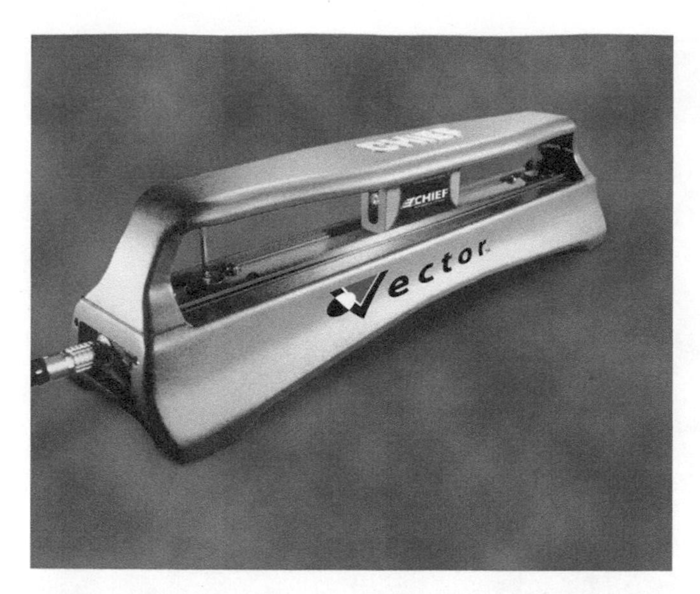

Figure 20–28. A laser unit throws out a rotating beam of light that can be used to measure accurately. (Courtesy of Chief Automotive Systems)

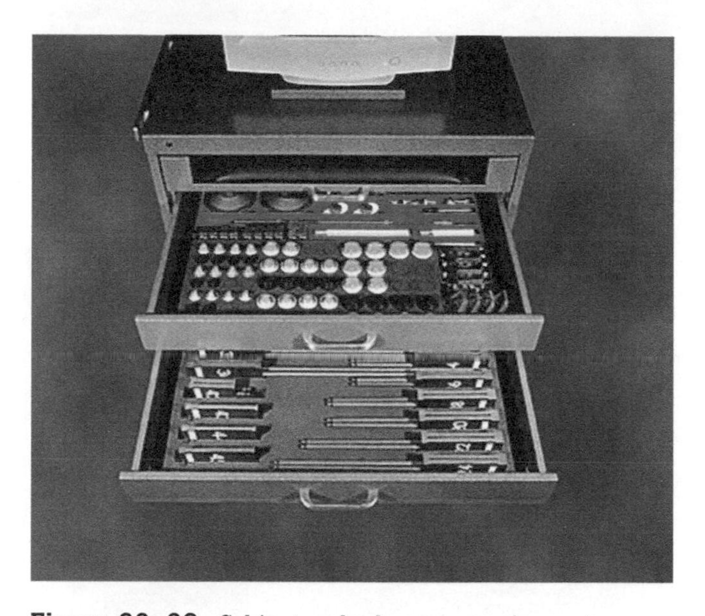

Figure 20–29. Cabinet under laser measuring system holds magnets, clips, rods, and reflectors that must be mounted on reference points of the damaged vehicle. (Courtesy of Chief Automotive Systems)

There are several types of systems available. However, all laser systems work either from the centerline or from the datum plane reference. See **Figure 20–30.**

Measurements are taken by observing the laser beam on the targets. Some targets are clear, allowing the laser beam to pass through them. Several *clear targets* can be used with one laser light source.

Beam splitters, or **laser guides,** are capable of reflecting the laser beam to additional targets. Using combinations of transparent targets and beam splitters, it is possible to measure several dimensions on a vehicle at the same time using a single laser source.

Three-dimensional laser systems use up to three laser units to give length, width, and height coordinates anywhere on the vehicle. They will check deck lid openings, cowls, door openings, hinges, pillars, and roof lines. With such a system, a single laser unit can be used to make measurements in conjunction with measuring devices such as a tape measure or calibrated bar.

Other items used with laser measuring devices include calibrated bars. They attach to the vehicle or act as support devices for the laser unit itself. Scales are hung from reference points on the underside of the vehicle. The laser beam passes through the center of the scale on the target when the measuring point is in its correct position.

Some laser measuring systems permit the technician to monitor upper body dimensions. For instance, pillar locations and window openings can be checked easily with a laser.

Some laser systems also offer an integral four-wheel alignment capability. Wheel alignment on the measuring system is beneficial. Suspension problems can be measured and corrected during frame or unibody repairs.

When properly set up, the laser system can generally stay with the vehicle during the pulling and straightening process, like the mechanical systems. However, if the laser or mounting bars are in danger of being damaged during the pull, they must be moved. See **Figure 20–31.**

Laser measuring systems provide direct, instantaneous dimensional readings so that the reference points in both the damaged and undamaged areas of the vehicle can be monitored continually during the pulling and straightening operation. Look at **Figure 20–32.**

Laser targets are special reflective mirrors that mount on reference points of the vehicle. Targets can be hung on reference points using snap-in clips, nylon bolt clips, plugs, and magnets. This allows you to mount targets quickly and easily.

The **body scanner,** or laser assembly, has two spinning lasers that strike and reflect off each target. The body scanner usually mounts on the rack under the vehicle center section. Rotating lasers send out perfectly straight light

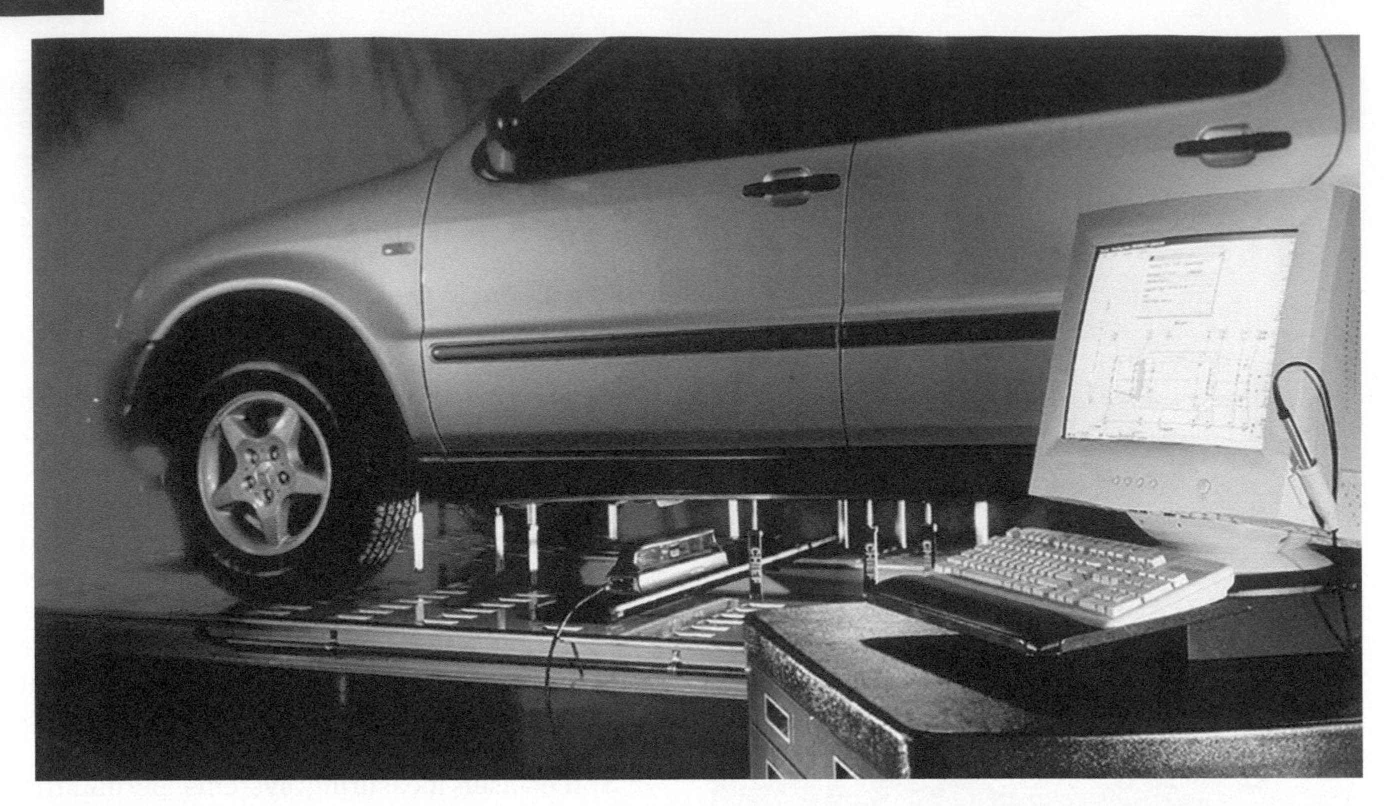

Figure 20–30. Note how reflectors have been hung under the vehicle on specified reference points. When laser bounces off reflectors, measurements are taken almost instantaneously. The computer monitor will then display which points are damaged and pushed out of alignment. (Courtesy of Chief Automotive Systems)

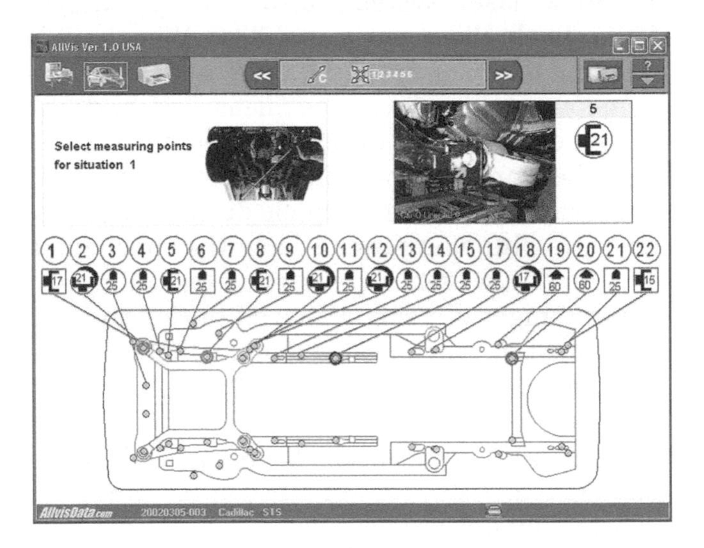

Figure 20–31. Here the computer measuring system is showing reference points and which adapters are needed to hang reflectors. (Courtesy of Laser Mate)

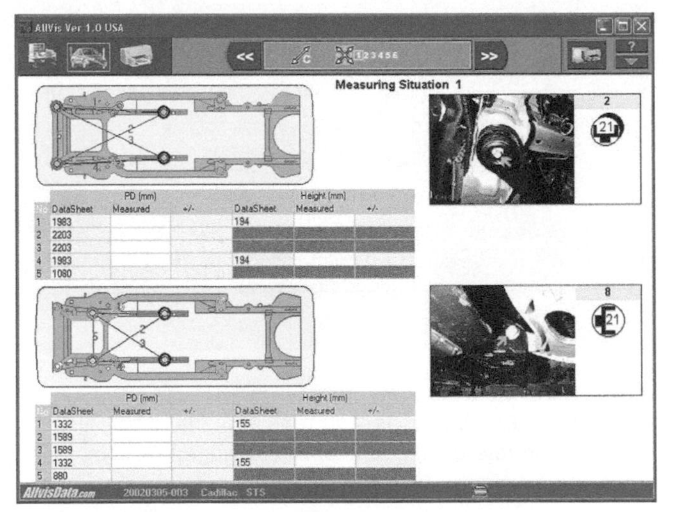

Figure 20–32. The computer measuring system is displaying data or specs for the undamaged vehicle. If the vehicle is undamaged, measurements should read within 2 mm of known good measurements. (Courtesy of Laser Mate)

beams that hit and reflect off the targets. This allows the scanner to accurately measure the location of the targets to determine if the vehicle has frame or unibody damage.

The lasers spin at approximately 850 rpm. Each revolution of a laser is divided into more than one million counts (divisions of a circle). The number of counts made while the laser beam travels out to a target and back to the laser hub is monitored by the computer. This allows the system to triangulate the distance of each target from the laser scanner or hub.

The distances to each target can be mathematically calculated by the computer into length and width measurements for damage analysis. This can be done simultaneously for all targets on the vehicle. The computer can compare these live measurements with electronically stored dimensions to quickly display the amount and direction of frame or unibody damage on the computer monitor.

A graphic display of the frame or unibody is shown on the monitor in **Figure 20–33.** Small boxes or circles next to the drawing will give numbers that represent the amount and direction of damage in millimeters. Small arrows will point in the direction of damage.

As you straighten the damage, the monitor will display numbers that change to show how much each target and reference point has moved. When the numbers next to each target read zero (or within specs), the vehicle has been straightened and all measurements are correct. This provides constant measurement feedback as you straighten the damage. Refer to **Figure 20–34.**

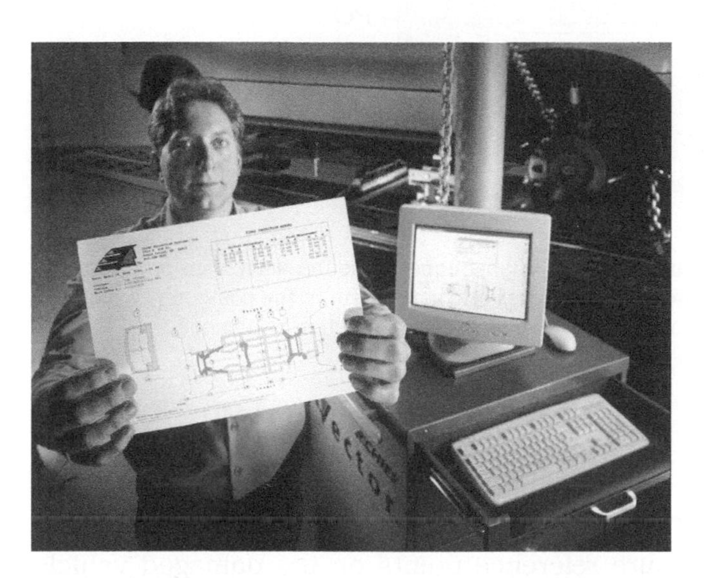

Figure 20–33. The printout of computer displays can be used when taking tram bar or tape measure readings of the damage without the laser system in place.

Ultrasound Measuring Systems

Ultrasound measuring systems use many of the same principles as electronic laser systems. However, sound waves, not light beams, are used to measure vehicle reference point locations. This is illustrated in **Figure 20–35.**

A lightweight aluminum receiving device known as an **ultrasonic receiver beam** mounts under the vehicle center section. Instead of targets, high-frequency emitters or **ultrasound probes** that generate high-frequency sound waves are mounted on vehicle reference points and then connected to the receiver beam and the computer with leads. Each probe produces high-frequency sound waves, which are heard as clicking sounds. The receiver has high-frequency microphones that detect when each probe's sound wave returns to the beam. This allows the computer to calculate the exact location of each probe and reference point being measured.

This system also uses a graphic display of the vehicle unibody or frame to show whether each probe and reference point is within specifications. The computer can compare actual readings to its electronic dimensions manual to

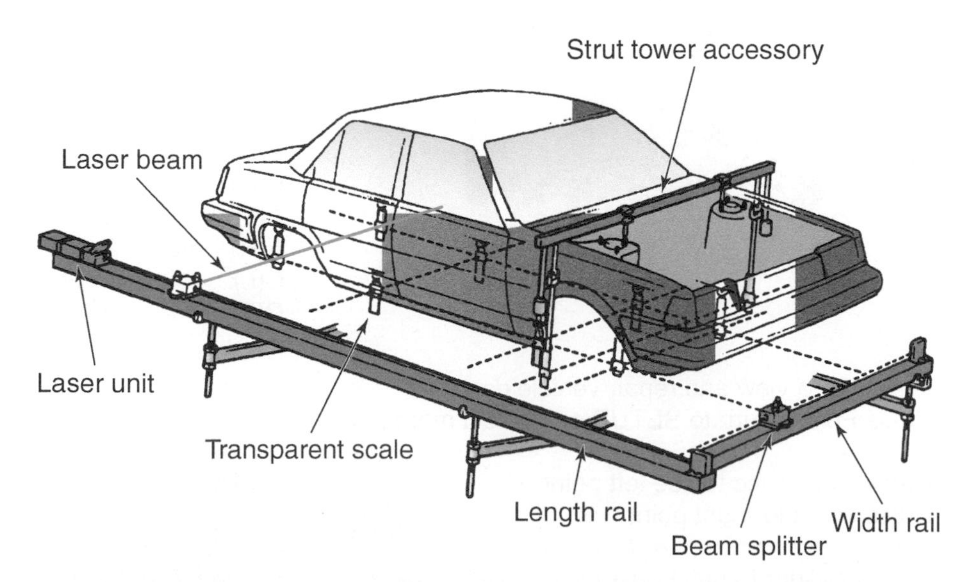

Figure 20–34. Study the basic parts of a laser measuring system. Laser directs beam or beams of light under and around the vehicle. Reflectors or beam splitters then show the locations of reference points on the vehicle.

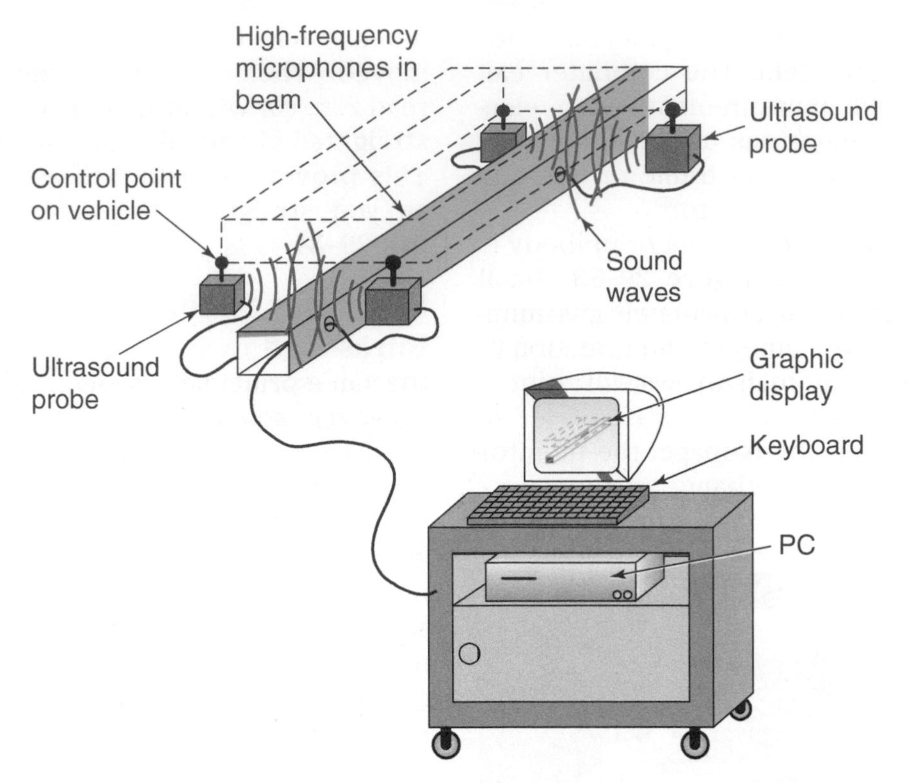

Figure 20–35. Note the basic operation of an ultrasonic measuring system. High-frequency sound waves are produced by probes at reference points. Microphones on a receiver pick up these sound waves and send them to the computer, which can then calculate the locations of the probes and reference points to determine the extent and direction of damage.

show the direction and extent of damage. As the vehicle is straightened, you can change to real-time display to watch as the points are pulled back to zero, which indicates perfect alignment. See **Figure 20–36.**

Computerized Robotic Arm Measuring Systems

A **computerized robotic arm measuring system** uses a track-mounted robot arm to measure reference points on the damaged vehicle.

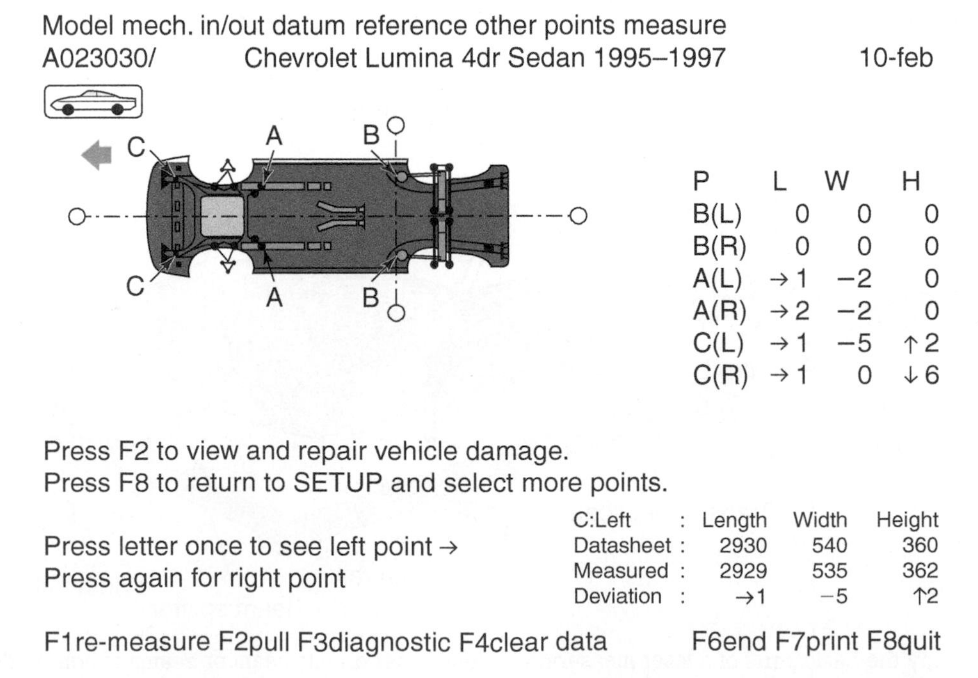
Model mech. in/out datum reference other points measure
A023030/ Chevrolet Lumina 4dr Sedan 1995–1997 10-feb

P	L	W	H
B(L)	0	0	0
B(R)	0	0	0
A(L)	→1	−2	0
A(R)	→2	−2	0
C(L)	→1	−5	↑2
C(R)	→1	0	↓6

Press F2 to view and repair vehicle damage.
Press F8 to return to SETUP and select more points.

Press letter once to see left point →
Press again for right point

C:Left	Length	Width	Height
Datasheet :	2930	540	360
Measured :	2929	535	362
Deviation :	→1	−5	↑2

F1re-measure F2pull F3diagnostic F4clear data F6end F7print F8quit

Figure 20–36. This printout shows reading from an ultrasonic measuring system. Note how points C left and C right are not within specifications.

The robot must be moved by hand into contact with each reference point. A button is then pushed on a remote control unit to store the reading in the computer.

With the control unit connected to the computer, measurements appear immediately on the computer screen. The control unit has storage capacity for data and specifications of up to four different vehicle models. The vehicle measurements can be quickly compared with specifications. Deviations are also displayed.

If the measurements and deviations need to be documented, the control unit can be connected to a printer to provide a printout. Measurements are available either on disk or via modem from the manufacturer's main computer. All data and specifications can be stored in the shop's personal computer.

SUMMARY

- There are two basic types of automotive construction: body-over-frame (BOF) vehicles and unibody (or monocoque) vehicles.
- Vehicle damage is broken down into five categories: side sway, sag, mash, diamond, and twist.
- The four basic measuring equipment systems are gauge, universal, dedicated, and electronic.
- Universal measuring systems have the ability to measure several reference points at the same time, making the job easier and more accurate. Universal measuring systems can be mechanical or electronic, or a combination of the two.
- The laser measuring system uses a strong beam of light, beam splitters, and targets to measure vehicle damage. It is extremely accurate when properly installed and used.

TECHNICAL TERMS

vehicle measurement
measurement gauges
control points
reference points
side sway damage
sag damage
mash damage
diamond damage
twist damage
cone concept
primary damage
secondary damage
crush zones
datum line
datum plane
center plane
centerline
body center marks
lateral dimensions
symmetrical
asymmetrical
gauge measuring systems
point-to-point measurement
datum measurement
diagonal line measurement
self-centering gauges
base gauges
strut tower gauge
universal measuring systems
dedicated bench and fixture system
dedicated bench
fixtures
electronic measuring systems
laser
beam splitters
laser guides
body scanner
ultrasound measuring systems
ultrasonic receiver beam
ultrasound probes
computerized robotic arm measuring system

REVIEW QUESTIONS

1. On some unibody designs, which has a fixed (nonadjustable) value?
   a. Camber
   b. Caster
   c. Toe
   d. Offset
2. The ______________ is a measuring rod with two adjustable pointers attached to it.
3. From what part of a unibody vehicle are all height dimensions taken?
   a. Datum plane
   b. Center plane
   c. Centerline
   d. Reference point
4. Explain the difference between control points and reference points.
5. All unibody measurements and alignment readings should be taken relative to what section?
   a. Front
   b. Rear
   c. Center
   d. Side

6. Where are body center marks located?
7. The ______________ ______________, or ______________, divides the vehicle into two equal halves: the passenger side and the driver side.
8. Define the term "datum plane" and explain how it is used.
9. When checking front end dimensions, *Technician A* measures from the lower cowl area to the front mount of the engine cradle. *Technician B* measures from one lower cowl area to another. Whose measurement will provide a better reading?
   a. Technician A
   b. Technician B
   c. Both Technicians A and B
   d. Neither Technician
10. What are self-centering gauges used to establish?
   a. Datum plane
   b. Vehicle centerline
   c. Mash
   d. Sag
11. List five safety rules to follow before starting a vehicle damage evaluation.
12. ______________ ______________ are special tools used to check specific frame and body points. They allow you to quickly measure the direction and extent of vehicle damage.
13. What is sag damage?

ASE-STYLE REVIEW QUESTIONS

1. *Technician A* says that most computerized measuring systems will show live readouts giving the direction and extent of damage. *Technician B* says that computerized measuring systems store dimensions for the undamaged vehicle. Who is correct?
   a. Technician A
   b. Technician B
   c. Both Technicians A and B
   d. Neither Technician
2. Which of the following types of damage is a condition in which a section of the frame or unibody is lower than normal?
   a. Sway
   b. Crush
   c. Mash
   d. Sag
3. *Technician A* says that diamond damage can occur in body-over-frame construction. *Technician B* says that diamond damage may be severe on a unibody vehicle. Who is correct?
   a. Technician A
   b. Technician B
   c. Both Technicians A and B
   d. Neither Technician
4. When inspecting for damage with self-centering gauges, *Technician A* says to first hang gauges from two places where there is no visible damage. *Technician B* says to hang two more gauges where there is obvious damage. Who is correct?
   a. Technician A
   b. Technician B
   c. Both Technicians A and B
   d. Neither Technician
5. An electronic laser measuring system is being used to determine the extent of vehicle damage. *Technician A* says that the lasers rotate at several million rpm. *Technician B* says that each rotation of the laser is divided into over a million counts. Who is correct?
   a. Technician A
   b. Technician B
   c. Both Technicians A and B
   d. Neither Technician
6. An ultrasonic measuring system is being used. *Technician A* says that the probes emit a clicking sound. *Technician B* says that the receiver beam contains high-frequency microphones that measure the probe locations. Who is correct?
   a. Technician A
   b. Technician B

c. Both Technicians A and B
d. Neither Technician

7. An electronic measuring system shows a sideways arrow and a small 7 in a box next to the arrow and target. What should you do?

a. Pull 7 mm in the same direction as the arrow.
b. Pull 7 mm in the opposite direction of the arrow.
c. Pull 7 inches in the same direction as the arrow.
d. Pull 7 inches in the opposite direction of the arrow.

8. An electronic measuring system shows zeros for all targets except one, which shows a reading of 1. What should be done?

a. Nothing; this is within specs.
b. Pull the target 1 mm in the direction of the arrow.
c. Pull the target 1 mm in the opposite direction of the arrow.
d. Pull all targets until readings are correct.

9. An electronic measuring system shows a minus 5 for a width reading. What does this mean?

a. Width is too small by 5 inches.
b. Width is too small by 0.5 inch.
c. Width is too small by 5 millimeters.
d. Width is too small by 5 meters.

10. *Technician A* says that spring clips can be used to mount targets on reference points. *Technician B* says that magnets can be used to mount targets when holes are not available on a reference point. Who is correct?

a. Technician A
b. Technician B
c. Both Technicians A and B
d. Neither Technician

ACTIVITIES

1. Obtain and study the operating manual for several types of measurement systems. Write a report or summary of unique methods for using each type of equipment.
2. Using a body dimensions manual, locate the data for one specific make and model vehicle. Note the locations of the reference points. Make a few practice measurements on this vehicle.
3. Visit collision repair shops. Ask the owners if you can watch a technician measuring damage on an actual vehicle. Write a report on your visit.

CHAPTER

21 Straightening Full-Frame and Unibody Vehicles

OBJECTIVES

After studying this chapter, you should be able to:

- List the types of straightening equipment and explain their operation.
- Describe basic straightening and aligning techniques.
- Identify safety considerations for using straightening equipment.
- Plan and execute repair procedures.
- Identify signs of stress/deformation and make the necessary repairs.
- Determine if a repair or replacement can be done before, during, or after straightening.

INTRODUCTION

The major steps for repairing a heavily damaged vehicle are given in **Figure 21–1.** Study them!

Vehicles with major damage must often have their frame, body, or unibody structures straightened. Vehicle straightening involves using high-powered hydraulic equipment, mechanical clamps, chains, and measuring systems to bring the frame, body, or unibody structure back to its original shape. At the same time, it might involve the replacement of welded panels that are damaged.

ALIGNMENT BASICS

The term **straightening** refers to using alignment equipment to pull the damaged metal back out to its original shape. The vehicle is secured and held stationary on the equipment. Then clamps and chains are attached to the damaged area. When the hydraulic system is activated, the chains slowly pull out the damage. Measurements are made at unibody/frame reference points while pulling to return the vehicle to its original dimensions. See **Figure 21–2.**

When realigning a vehicle, a pulling force or *traction* should be applied in the direction opposite the force of the impact. This is illustrated in **Figure 21–3.** When determining the direction of a pull, you must set the equipment to pull perpendicular to the damage.

The **single pull method** uses only one pulling chain, and it works well with damage on one part. A small bend in a part can often be straightened with a single pull.

With damage to several panels, a **multiple pull method** with several pulling directions and steps are needed. See **Figure 21–4.** With major damage, body panels are often deformed into complex shapes with altered strengths in the damaged areas. To pull in only the opposite direction would not work, because of the differences in the strength and recovery rates of each panel.

Use the method that works best for the given situation. Since applying force in only one place will not always work, you often have to exert pulling force on many places at the same time. For convenience, the term "direction opposite to input" will be used to describe the effective pulling direction.

To alter the direction while pulling, divide the pulling force into two or more directions. This will allow you to change the direction of the **composite force,** that is, the force of all pulls combined. Look at **Figure 21–5.**

STRAIGHTENING EQUIPMENT

Straightening equipment is used to apply tremendous force to move the frame or unibody structure back into alignment. Straightening equipment includes anchoring equipment, pulling equipment, and other accessories.

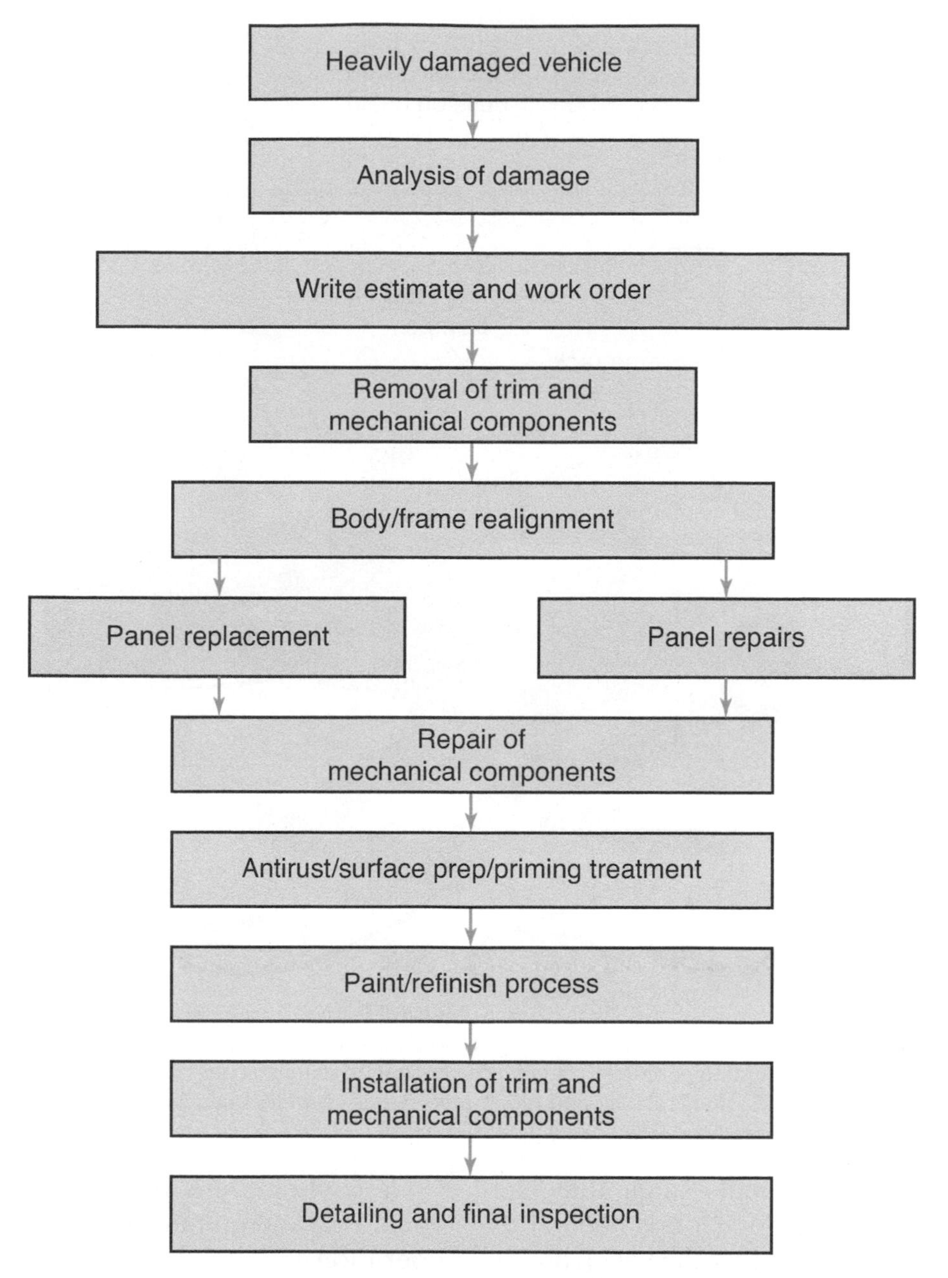

Figure 21–1. Study the major steps for major collision repair to the body/frame structure. Note that panel replacement is done after frame or unibody straightening.

The **anchoring equipment** holds the vehicle stationary while pulling and measuring. Anchoring can be done by fastening the frame or unibody of the vehicle to anchors in the shop floor or to the straightening equipment rack or bench. The objective of the anchoring system is to hold the vehicle solidly in place while pulling forces are applied. It must also distribute pulling forces throughout the vehicle.

The **pulling equipment** uses hydraulic power to force the body structure or frame back into position. There are many different types of pulling equipment available. Regardless of their design or operating features, each system uses the same basic pulling theory and is used in a similar manner. Refer back to Figure 21–2.

Hydraulic rams use oil under pressure from a pump to produce a powerful linear motion. When you electrically activate the system, oil is forced into the ram cylinder. The ram is then pushed outward with tremendous force. This pulls on the chain attached to the vehicle (often with a powerful clamp or strong hook) to remove the damage. The rams can be mounted in or on the pulling towers, posts, or between the vehicle and anchoring system.

Pulling posts or towers are strong steel members used to hold the pulling chains and hydraulic

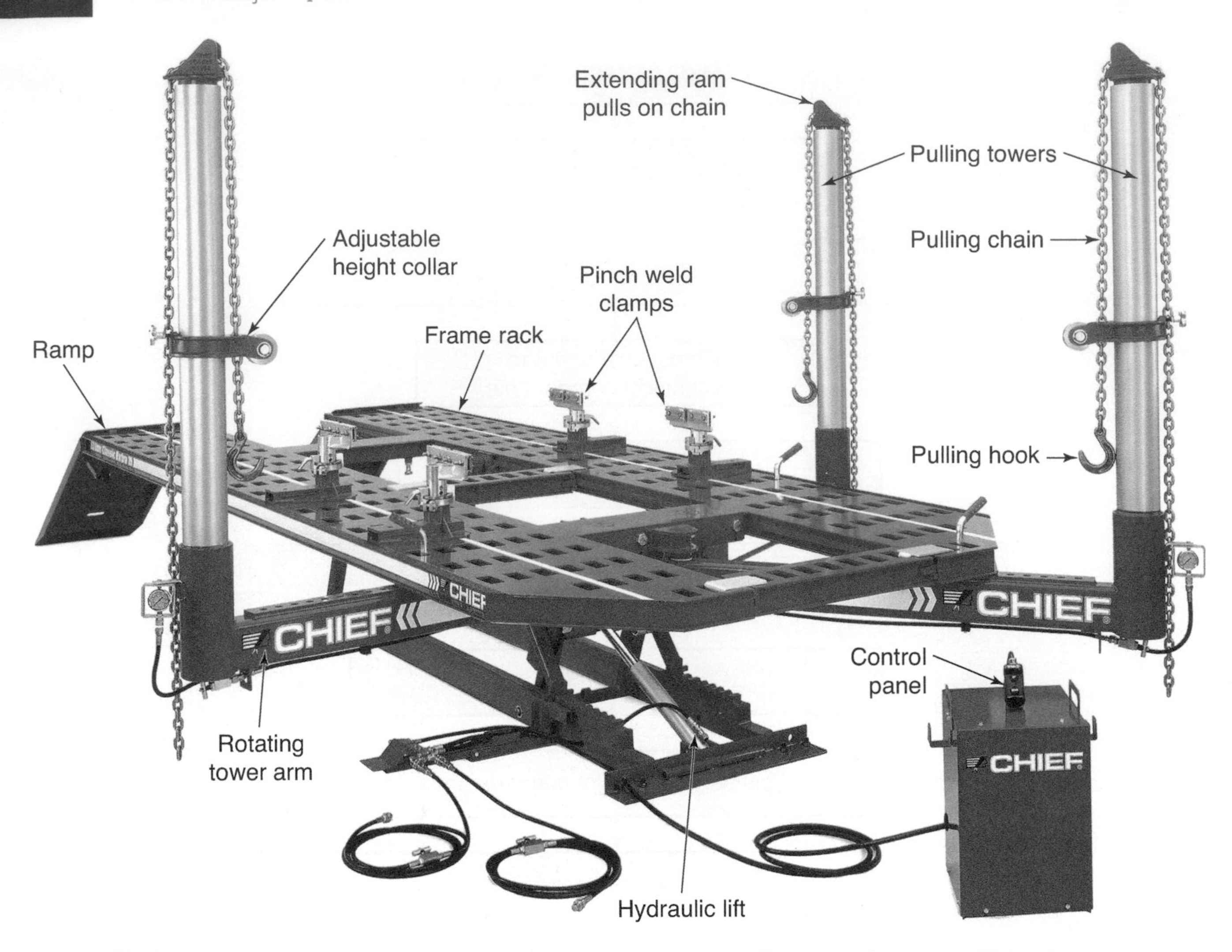

Figure 21–2. Straightening or aligning equipment is powerful enough to pull out even the worst collision damage. Knowledge of the equipment, vehicle construction, and repair procedures, as well as common sense, are needed to repair badly damaged vehicles. (Courtesy of Chief Automotive Systems, Inc.)

rams. Depending on equipment design, they can be positioned at whatever location is needed to make the pull. They push against the bench as the pull is made. This eliminates the need for separate anchoring to keep the pulling equipment from sliding under the bench as the pull is made.

DANGER

The amount of straightening pressure required to remove damage should not be too high. If the straightening equipment is straining during the pulling process, something is wrong. If this happens, stop pulling! Release tension, and reevaluate the setup to find the problem. If too much pressure is applied, parts or equipment can be damaged and serious injuries could result.

You should be familiar with a variety of anchoring and pulling systems and their general operation.

In-Floor Straightening Systems

In-floor straightening systems have anchor pots or rails cemented or mounted in the shop floor. Some use **anchor pots** or small steel cups in various locations in the shop floor. See **Figure 21–6.** Others use a system of steel **anchor rails** in the floor so that an infinite number of pulling-holding locations can be used. Both systems must be balanced both in direction and force of the pull.

To provide the pulling force for straightening, the anchor pot system can use hydraulic rams and pulling posts or towers. The floor grid system generally uses hydraulic rams to provide the pulling force.

An in-floor system is ideal for a small collision repair shop. After the rams and the other

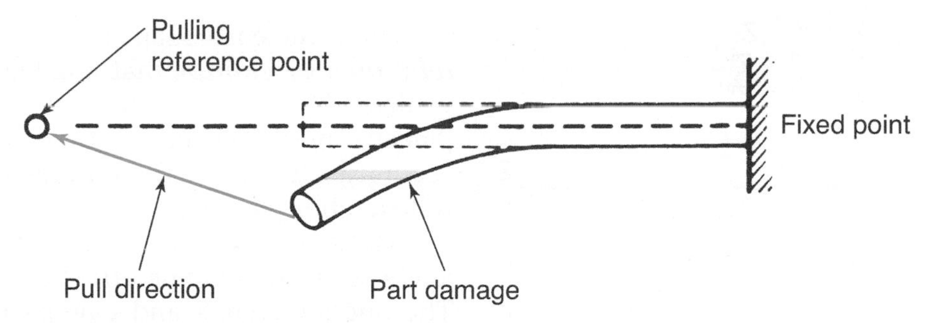

(A) Think of how you would need to pull on the component to return it to its original position.

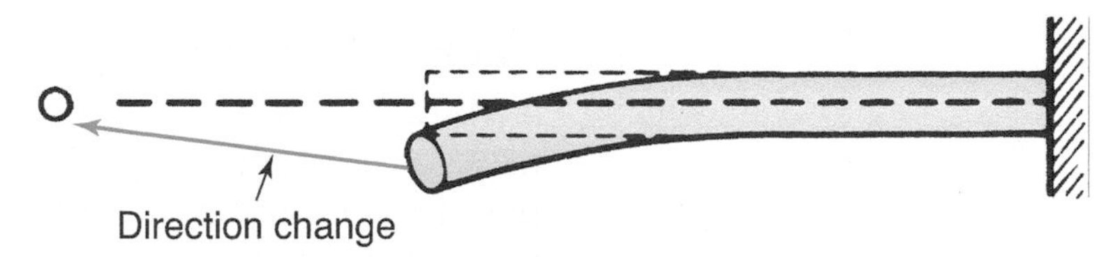

(B) As you pull on the component, the angle of pull might change slightly.

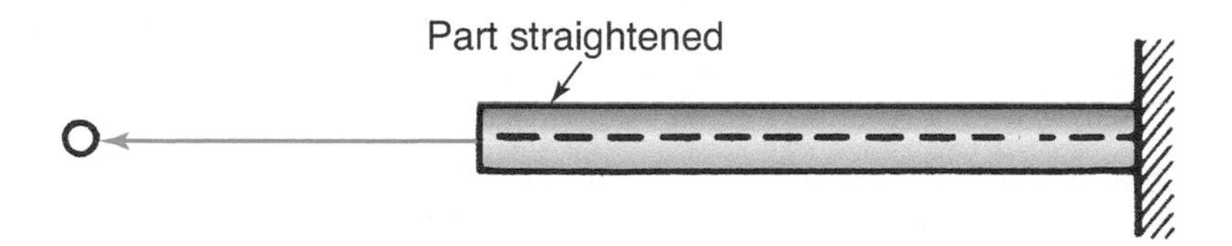

(C) The component has been pulled back to its original shape.

Figure 21–3. Study the basic pulling action.

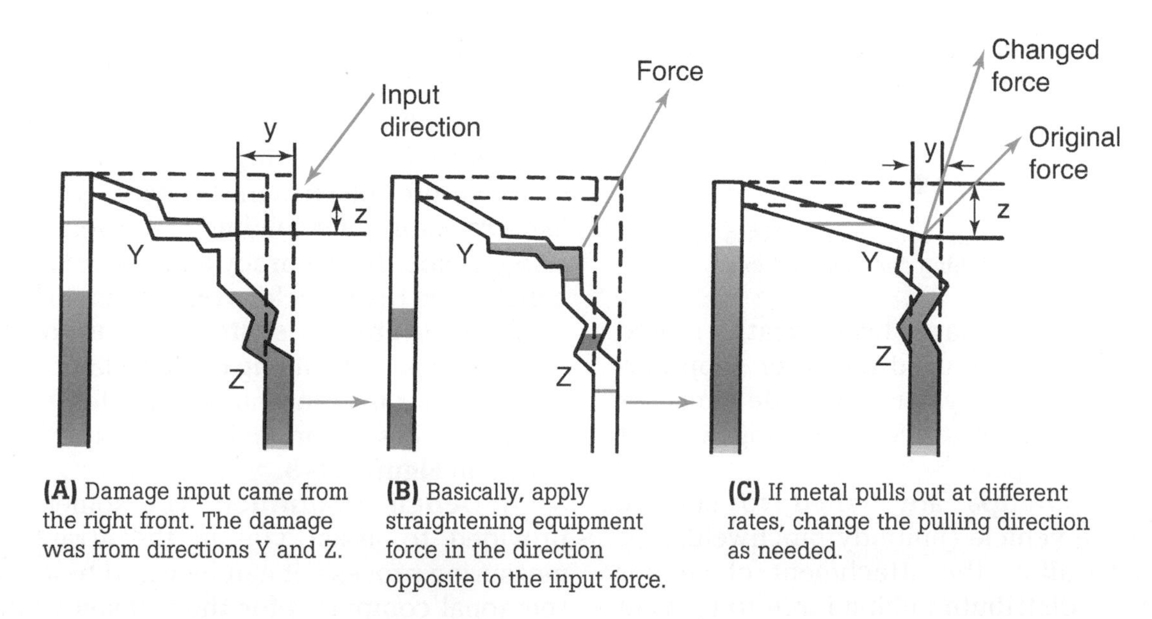

(A) Damage input came from the right front. The damage was from directions Y and Z.

(B) Basically, apply straightening equipment force in the direction opposite to the input force.

(C) If metal pulls out at different rates, change the pulling direction as needed.

Figure 21–4. Note how to find the general pulling direction.

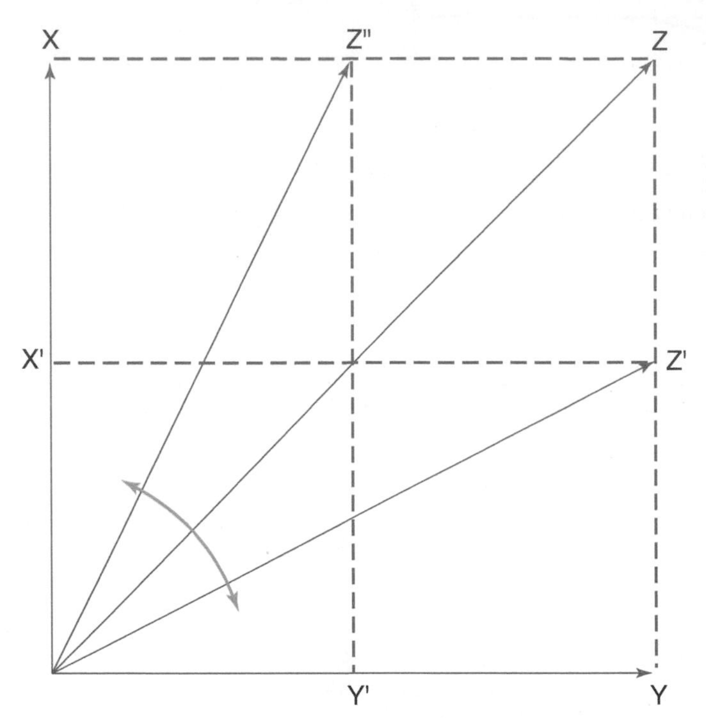

Figure 21–5. If pulling force is divided between two directions (X and Y), the composite, or total, force direction (Z) will change freely with adjustments to force in the two directions. This shows that using two chains to pull allows for better adjustment of pulling direction.

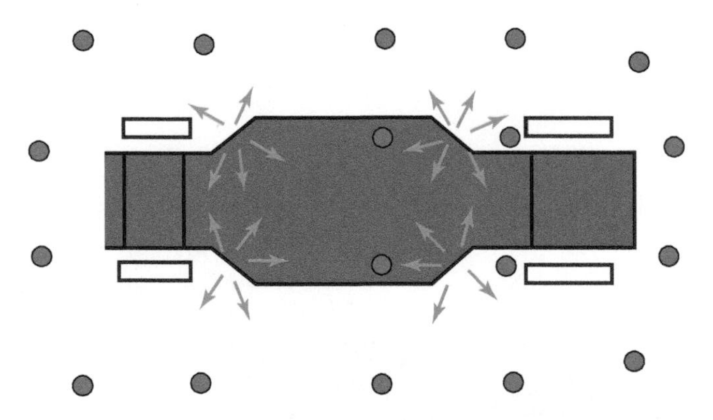

Figure 21–6. The anchoring setup must balance holding power as needed for the pulling direction and force.

power accessories have been neatly stored away, the area can be used for other shop purposes. Also, in-floor systems provide single or multiple pulls and positive anchoring without sacrificing shop space.

Anchor clamps are bolted to specific points on the vehicle (unibody pinchwelds, for example) to allow the attachment of anchor chains. They distribute pulling force to prevent metal tearing.

The vehicle is usually supported using *cross tube anchor clamps* that link both sides of the vehicle. The cross tube anchor clamps are placed over the cross tube and tightened securely. Chains are then attached to the cross tube anchor clamps.

Anchor chains are attached from the floor anchors to the clamps attached to the vehicle. The anchor chains and clamps must hold the vehicle securely while straightening. *Chain tighteners* or shorteners are used to take slack out of the anchor chains.

Rack Straightening Systems

A **rack straightening system** is generally a drive-on system with a built-in anchoring and pulling mechanism. Most racks tilt hydraulically so that vehicles can either be driven on or pulled into position with a power winch.

A **power winch** normally uses an electric motor and steel cable to provide a means of pulling the damaged vehicle onto the rack.

Rack straightening systems are generally stationary. They are capable of making multiple pulls. Pulling towers are generally attached to the rack. Depending on the system, there can be two or more towers. On some systems, the towers can be positioned 360 degrees around the rack. In other systems, the positioning is limited to the front and sides of the rack.

Bench Straightening Systems

A **bench system** is a portable or stationary steel table for straightening vehicle damage. Some benches tilt. Others have drive-on ramps and the bench can be raised straight up or down as needed. Refer to **Figure 21–7.**

A **bench-rack system** is a hybrid machine that allows quick loading like a rack but has the other features of a bench. The table will often tilt like a rack for quick loading of the vehicle. It will also provide the accuracy and convenience of a bench once the vehicle is on the machine.

Straightening system accessories include the various pulling chains, clamps, hooks, adapters, straps, and stands needed to mount various makes and models of vehicles. Some are shown in **Figure 21–8.**

A **bench computer** can sometimes be provided to assist you in the straightening-measuring process. It can be wired to a main PC (personal computer) for the transfer of data to and from the office. The computer might be

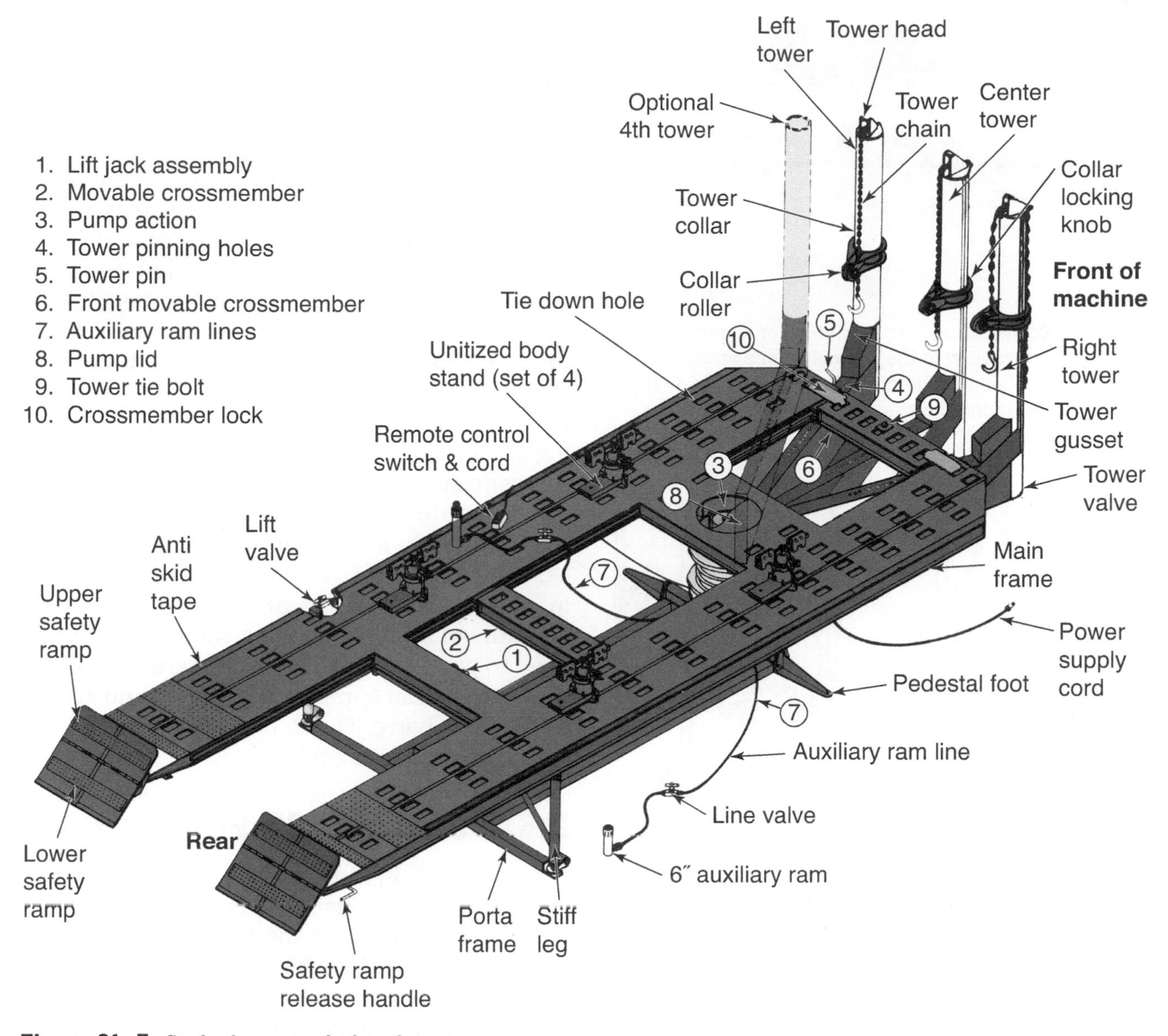

Figure 21–7. Study the parts of a bench system. (Courtesy of Chief Automotive Systems, Inc.)

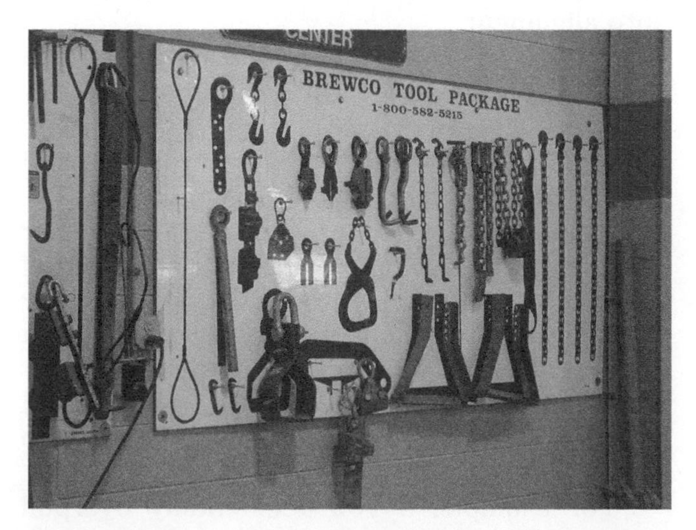

Figure 21–8. Note the various accessories used during straightening.

used to retrieve body dimension specifications and also do other functions.

An **operating manual** and other publications are provided to give detailed information on using the exact type of straightening equipment properly. You must always refer to these materials when working. They give anchoring and pulling instructions, the accessories needed for each vehicle, and other essential information. See **Figure 21–9.**

Portable Pullers

A **portable puller,** sometimes called a "damage dozer," is a hydraulic ram and post mounted on caster wheels. This type of pulling of equipment can be easily rolled around the vehicle to

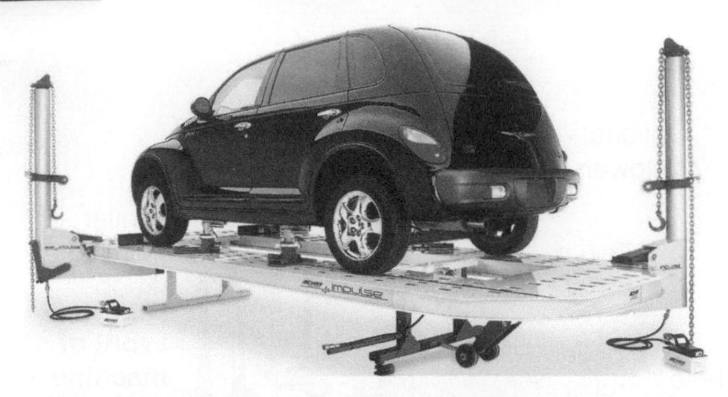

Figure 21–9. When using straightening or alignment equipment, always refer to the manufacturer's instructions. This vehicle has been anchored to the rack or frame so that it will not move during the straightening process. (Courtesy of Chief Automotive Systems)

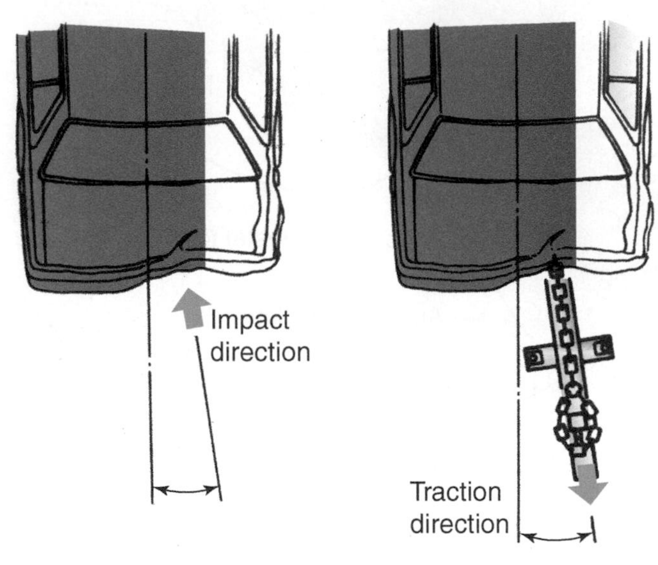

Figure 21–10. With a portable puller (dozer), you can easily set traction or pulling direction. (Courtesy of Nissan North America, Inc.)

extract damage by means of chains and clamps. It is often used to repair or pull minor damage. See **Figure 21–10.**

Being easily movable, this equipment can easily set the traction direction to the damage input. Many units of this type will pull in only one direction.

Other Straightening Equipment

An **engine crane** can be formed on most racks or benches to raise and remove an engine. A bar is added to the post or tower to provide a vertical pulling action for engine removal.

An **engine stand** is sometimes needed to hold a power plant after removal from the vehicle. It will hold the engine on a small rollaround framework for convenience.

An **engine holder** can be used to support the engine-transmission assembly when the cradle must be unbolted or removed. It rests on the inner fenders and is adjustable in width. A chain(s) is (are) used between the holder and engine to keep it from falling down while working.

A **portable pulling/pushing arm** can be anchored next to the vehicle to remove damage. With a pulling/pushing arm, the unit can pivot completely around the end of the bench from the center position on the special flange. In the other positions, it can reach the end and one side of the bench. The unit can also be used anywhere along the side of the bench by hooking the inner clamp on the outer flange on the opposite side.

Portable hydraulic rams or **portable power units** are small piston and cylinder assemblies for removing minor damage. Shown in **Figure 21–11,** they are possibly the most versatile of all body aligning tools. They can be used to push or pull in restricted areas. Portable power units can spread, clamp, pull, and stretch parts. See **Figure 21–12.** In **Figure 21–13,** some actual repairs are being done.

MEASURE AS YOU PULL!

As discussed in Chapter 20, *vehicle measurement* is done by using specialized tools and equipment to measure the location of reference points on the vehicle. These measurements are then compared to published dimensions from an undamaged vehicle. After studying damage measurements, straightening equipment can then be used to pull the frame or body back into alignment.

Always measure as you pull! This is critical for competent work. You must monitor how the vehicle is reacting to the pulling operation. This will let you modify pulling directions and locations as needed.

The challenge faced by the collision repair industry is to find out which panels are out of alignment, and in which direction and how far they have moved. Only then can a proper plan be devised to bring the vehicle back to proper dimensions. You must accurately measure and monitor the entire vehicle while pulling. Refer to **Figure 21–14.**

For example, if you accidentally overpull parts, you may have to replace them. Since replacement was not initially required on the

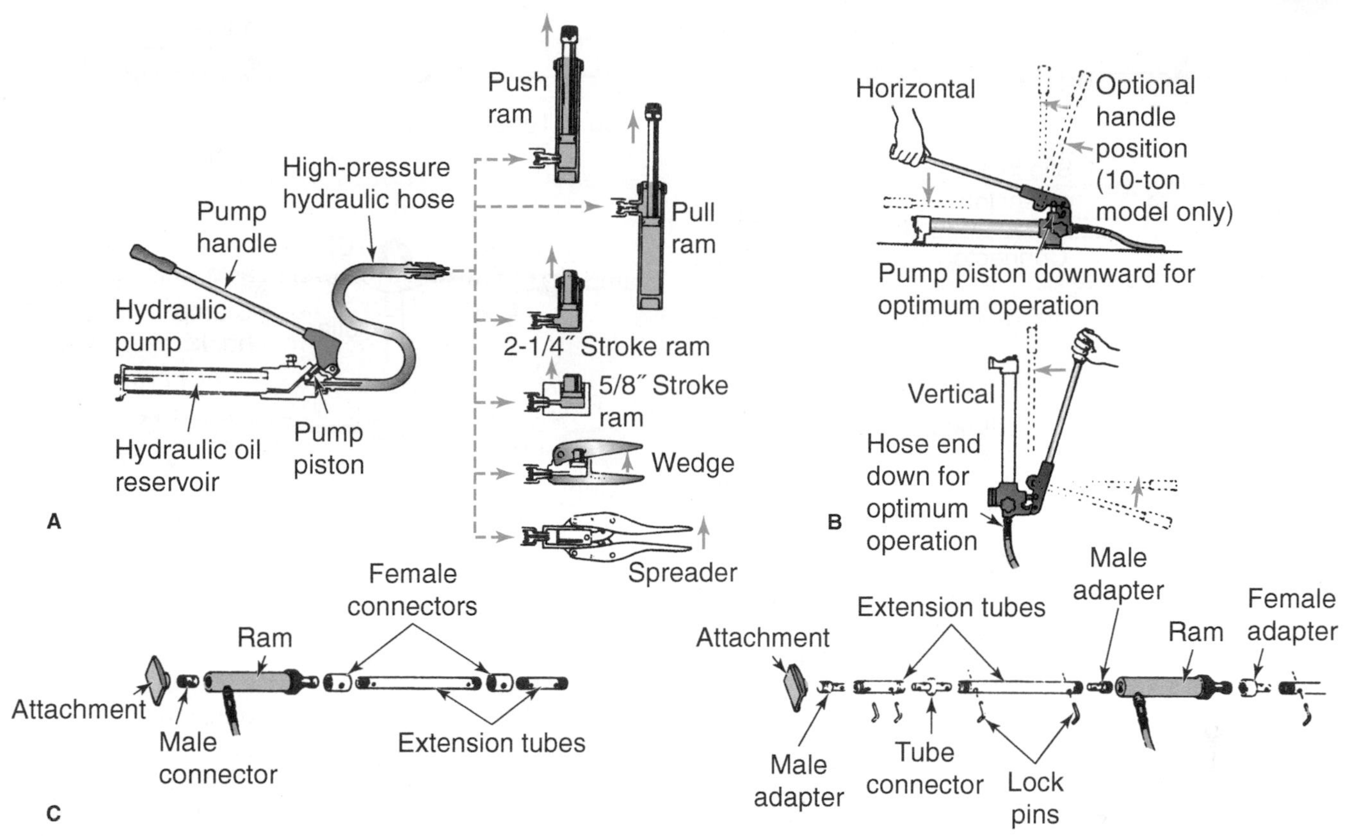

Figure 21–11. Study the parts of a portable hydraulic ram system. (Courtesy of Hein Werner Corporation) **(A)** The hydraulic pump is the heart of the system. When the handle is moved up and down, hydraulic pressure flows out of the hose to various attachments, like the ram. Note the various attachments for the ram. **(B)** When in use, the hose must not face upward or air can enter the system. **(C)** Threaded connections and pins hold the attachments on the ram.

estimate, you may have to do this extra work free of charge. Both you and the shop would lose money and time. Remember! Always measure as you pull! See **Figure 21–15.**

PART REMOVAL

A general rule: Remove only the parts that prevent you from getting to the area of the vehicle being repaired. Major straightening operations can be done with major mechanical parts intact.

Depending on the construction of the vehicle and the location and degree of damage, there will be cases where it will be more convenient to remove parts before proceeding with the repair. Carefully analyze the vehicle and the damage to determine what must be removed. It is sometimes best to remove parts before putting the vehicle on the bench. You might have better access to the fasteners.

Take the time to carefully study the locations of the engine and transmission mounts, suspension mounts, and whether or not these parts themselves are damaged. See **Figure 21–16.**

PLANNING THE STRAIGHTENING

When planning the straightening process, the technician should determine the following:

1. The direction of the "pulls"
2. How to repair the damage in the reverse (first-in, last-out) sequence to which it occurred during the collision
3. Plan the straightening sequence with the "pulls" in the opposite direction from those that caused the damage
4. The correct attachment points of the pulling clamps
5. The number of "pulls" required to correct the damage
6. Which parts must be removed to make the pulls

Many times it may be best to draw out the repair plan prior to actually straightening the vehicle. This drawing should show OEM and actual dimensions, anchoring, and pulling locations.

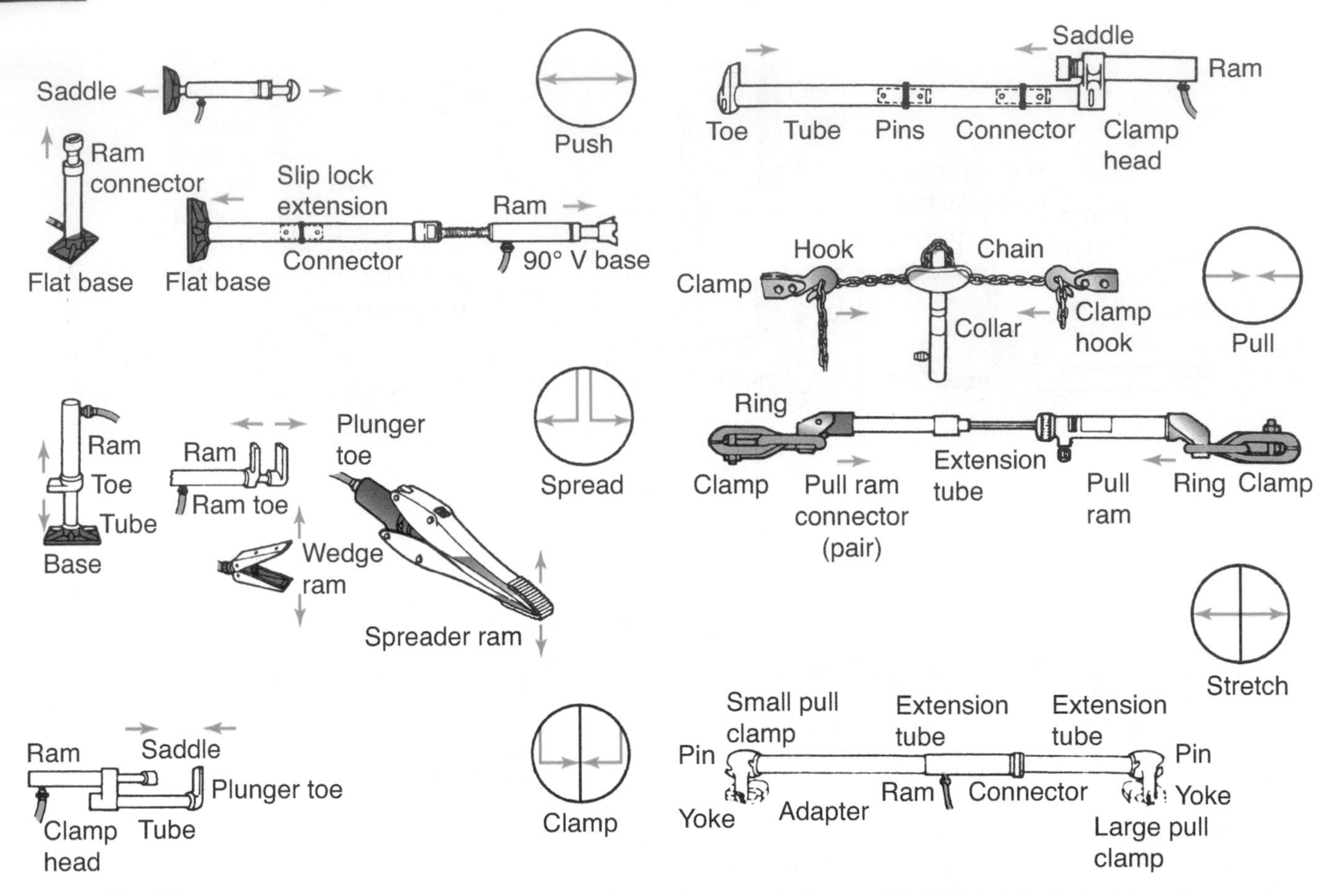

Figure 21–12. Study how the portable ram can be used to push, spread, clamp, pull, and stretch damaged parts. (Courtesy of Blackhawk Collision Repair, Inc., Subsidiary of Hein-Werner® Corporation)

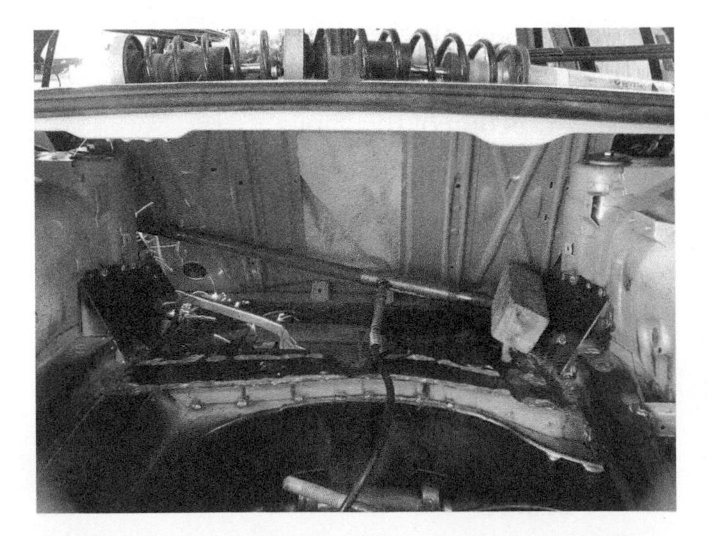

(A) The ram is positioned to push on the rear shock towers.

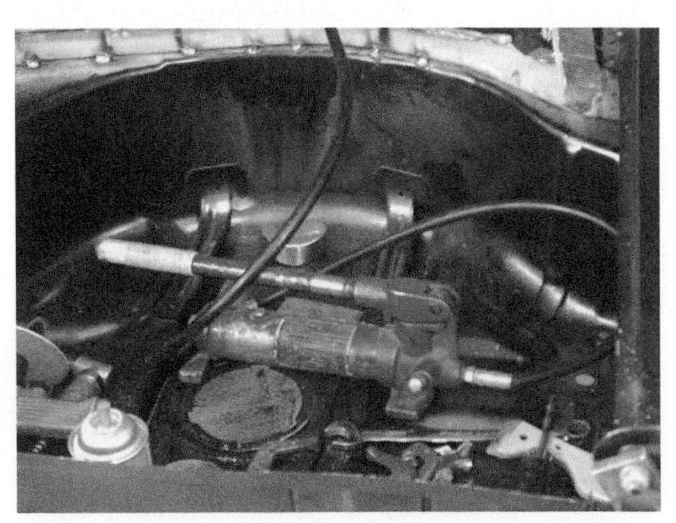

(B) By pumping the handle or portable power unit, the ram will extend with tremendous force, pushing the parts back into alignment.

Figure 21–13. Here a portable power unit is being used to force the trunk area outward before welding of new panels.

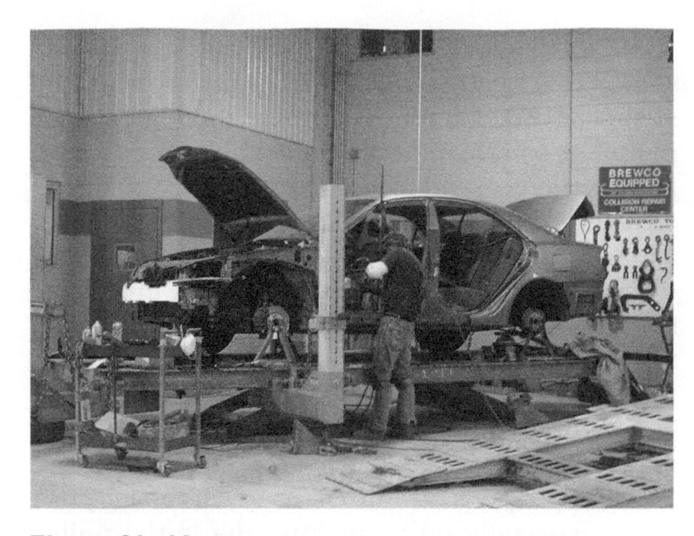

Figure 21–14. Measurement is a vital aspect of straightening. Measurements give you feedback about the progress of the pull.

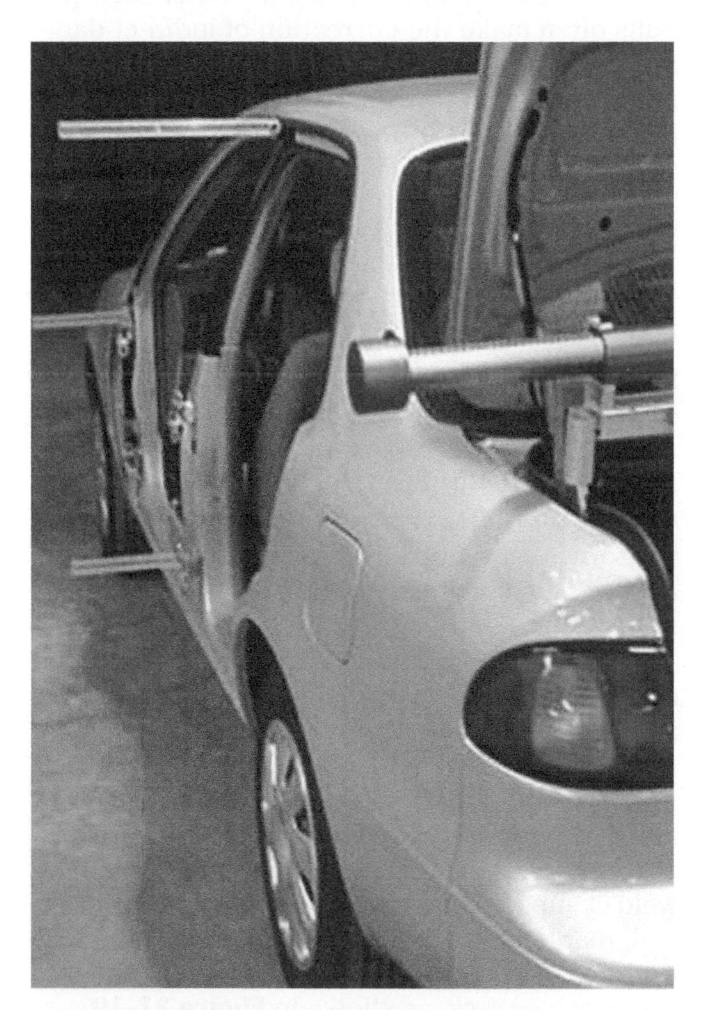

Figure 21–15. Measurement is done before pulling so the technician can develop a plan for removing the damage. Measurement is also done while pulling to check the progress of the straightening equipment. (Courtesy of Laser Mate)

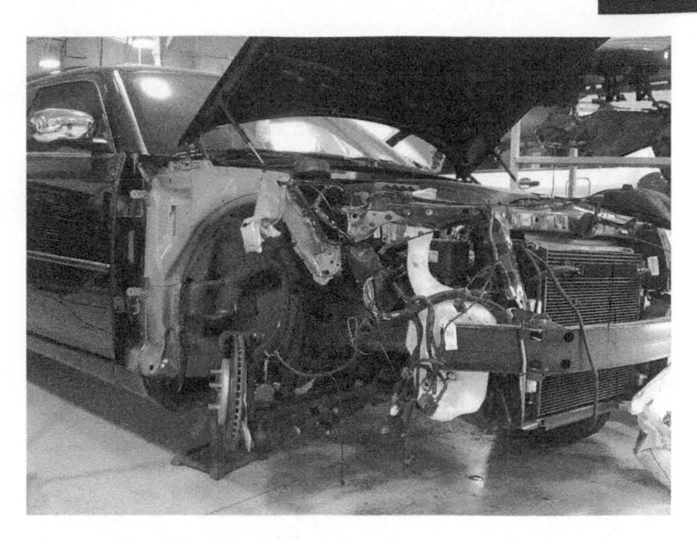

Figure 21–16. Before straightening, it may be necessary to remove some parts so you can properly repair the damage. Here the fender and front bumper have been removed.

The easiest way to determine where to straighten from is to picture the damage being removed by pulling with "your bare hands." The pulling process will work in the exact same manner.

Before attempting any repair work, determine exactly the collision procedures that should be taken. A little extra time spent on such an analysis and operational plan can save hours of work.

As a general rule, vehicle straightening is needed whenever the damage involves the suspension, steering, or powertrain mounting points. This, of course, would include situations such as a side collision where the suspension parts and their mountings are not damaged directly, but because of deformation in the center section of the vehicle's structure, the whole body is out of alignment.

STRAIGHTENING SAFETY

When using straightening equipment, inadequate attention to safety can result in part damage and serious injury.

1. Use the straightening equipment correctly according to the instruction manual.
2. Never allow unskilled or improperly trained personnel to operate straightening equipment.
3. Make sure the rocker panel pinchwelds and chassis clamp teeth are tight.

4. Always anchor the vehicle securely before making a pull. Check that the chassis clamps and anchor bolts are tightened.
5. Always use the size and grade (alloy) chain recommended for pulling and anchoring. Use only the chain supplied with the straightening equipment.
6. Drawing chains must be positively attached to the vehicle and/or anchoring locations so that they will not come off during the straightening operation. Avoid placing chains around sharp corners.
7. Before pulls are made, apply counter supports so you do not pull the vehicle off the bench or rack.
8. Never use a service jack (floor jack) for supporting the vehicle while working on or under it. Always use jack stands (safety stands) for supporting the vehicle.
9. A pull clamp can always slip and cause sheet metal tear. Prevent bodily harm and material damage by always using safety wires.
10. Never stand in line with a pulling chain or clamp. Chain breakage, clamp slippage, or sheet metal tearing could cause injury or damage. Remember, it can be dangerous to work inside the vehicle when pulls are being made.
11. Cover pulling chains with a heavy blanket. If a chain breaks, this will keep the chain from being thrown.

Before doing any straightening work, protect the vehicle and externally attached parts as follows:

1. Remove or cover interior parts (seats, instruments, carpet).
2. When welding, cover glass, seats, instrument panels, and carpet with a heat-resistant material.
3. Be careful not to scratch or damage parts that do not require painting. If the painted surface is scratched, be sure to repair that portion. Even a small flaw in the painted surface might cause corrosion and an unhappy customer.

STRAIGHTENING BASICS

Body-over-frame (BOF) vehicles can usually be straightened and realigned with a series of single-direction pulls.

Remember that a unibody vehicle is designed to spread collision forces throughout the structure. Most unibody repairs demand multiple pulls, which sometimes means four or more pulling points and directions during a single straightening and alignment setup.

Remember! A single, hard pull in one direction on a unibody vehicle can tear the metal before it is straight. There simply is not enough material available in any one place to transmit sufficient force to complete a repair. Again, as in the anchoring system, the pulling force must be distributed through several attaching points.

Multiple pulls should be used whenever possible, especially when making the initial pulls. This will spread the force of the pull over a larger area to minimize tearing. They will also allow the technician to "pull" on several areas, and at different angles, at one time. Multiple pulls often make the correction of indirect damage easier. They can be made using one or more pulling posts or towers, hydraulic rams, or adjustable pulling towers on racks or benches.

Making a light "pull" first, holding the pressure, then pulling on another area, allows damage to be removed in a more controlled manner.

ANCHORING PROCEDURES

If there are four anchoring points used during straightening operations, the anchoring points must be able to withstand the total pulling force applied without damaging them. See **Figure 21–17.** Depending on the angle of the pull, the forces may not be distributed equally. The anchoring points nearest the pull may be loaded more than the others.

Multiple anchoring systems are available in many different designs. The anchoring systems are designed for use on different designs of equipment and type of vehicle to be anchored.

On most unibody vehicles, multiple anchoring is accomplished using four **pinchweld clamps,** as shown in **Figure 21–18.** The pinchweld clamps are attached to the body at the front and rear of the rocker panel pinchwelds. The bottoms of the pinchweld clamps are fastened to the bench or rack, as shown in **Figure 21–19.**

Some floor grid or anchor pot systems use pinchweld clamps and cross tubes. The *cross tubes* pass through the pinchweld clamps and run from one side of the vehicle to the other. They are supported by four safety stands. One safety stand is positioned at each pinchweld

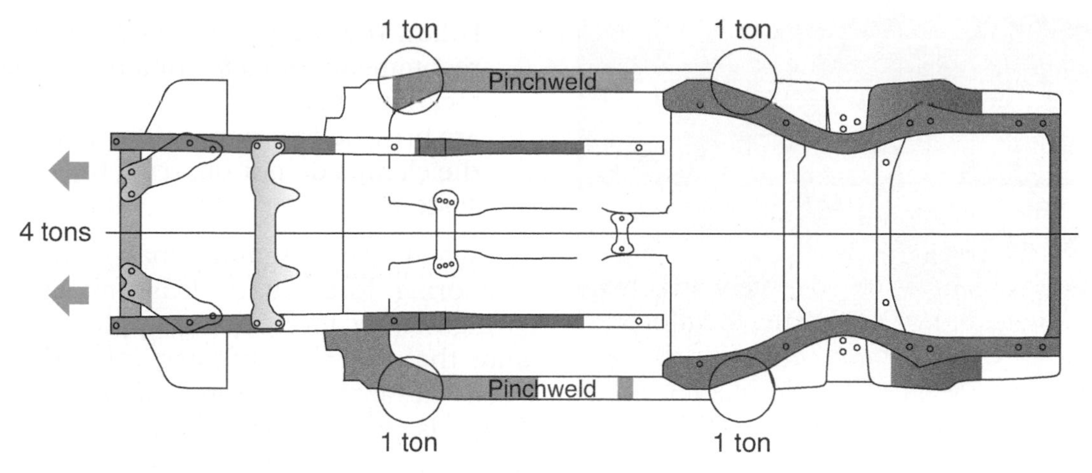

Figure 21–17. When anchoring a vehicle, remember that anchoring strength must be equal to or greater than the pulling force that will be applied.

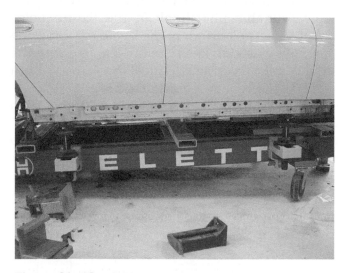

Figure 21–18. Unibody cars are anchored using pinchweld clamps. Four are normally used in the center section of the vehicle.

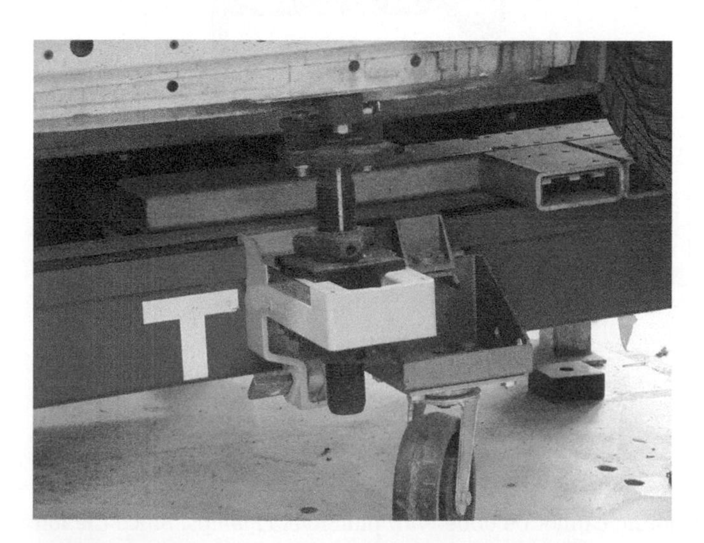

Figure 21–19. The pinchweld clamps must be securely tightened to the lower underbody of the vehicle. The bottom of the clamps are fastened to the bench.

clamp location. They are anchored to a floor grid or anchor pots using chains or a lock arm and wedges. This is also called *chainless anchoring.*

Some unibody vehicles do not have pinchwelds, or they are too weak to withstand pulling forces. These vehicles require the use of a different type of anchoring system that attaches to suspension or mechanical parts mounting locations. Many equipment manufacturers have special anchoring adapters available for these vehicles. If the equipment manufacturer does not have specific anchoring recommendations for the vehicle being repaired, a creative anchoring solution will be needed.

Sandwich clamps can be used to anchor the vehicle if they are installed in areas where there are double or triple layers of structural metal. If anchoring in this manner, always use caution and common sense when anchoring the vehicle. Monitor the anchoring locations closely.

On body-over-frame vehicles, multiple anchoring is accomplished by using chains. The anchoring chains are attached to the frame in the four torque box areas. These are often the strongest points on the frame. The other ends of the chain are attached to the bench, rack, floor grid, or anchor pots in the floor. See **Figure 21–20.**

Here are some common cautions and tips to be used when anchoring vehicles:

1. Do not wrap chains around suspension parts.
2. Always remove all slack from anchoring chains prior to pulling.
3. Always follow equipment manufacturer's pinchweld clamp tightening sequences.

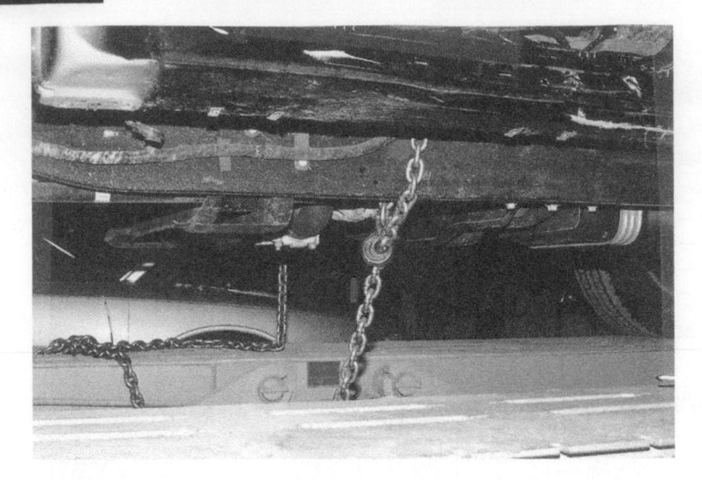

Figure 21–20. This truck frame is being anchored with large chains.

4. Always remove all grease, undercoating, and dirt from the pinchweld flanges and the clamp jaws before installing clamps.
5. Do not use chains that are not designed for pulling and anchoring equipment; for example, do not use tow chains.
6. Make sure that fuel and brake lines will not be crushed by the pinchweld clamps or straightening equipment.
7. Follow the equipment manufacturer's recommendations for pinchweld clamp locations. Many times the clamp locations are provided on dimension charts so that the clamps do not obstruct the measuring system.

When straightening, make sure that the anchoring force is at least as great as the straightening force being applied. Also, make sure that the straightening force does not exceed the anchoring force. If the straightening force is greater than the anchoring force, anchoring points on the vehicle will be damaged. Monitor the pinchwelds during the entire straightening process. Make sure pinchwelds are not straining, buckling, or distorting.

A full-frame vehicle can be anchored by placing a suitable plug hook in the fixture holes located on the bottom of the frame rail. Blocking should be used to keep the hook in line with the frame rail. Make an identical hookup on both sides of the vehicle. See **Figure 21–21.**

When anchoring the vehicle in preparation for straightening, lean toward "overanchoring" or "overclamping." An extra anchor point or two takes very little time and surely cannot hurt anything.

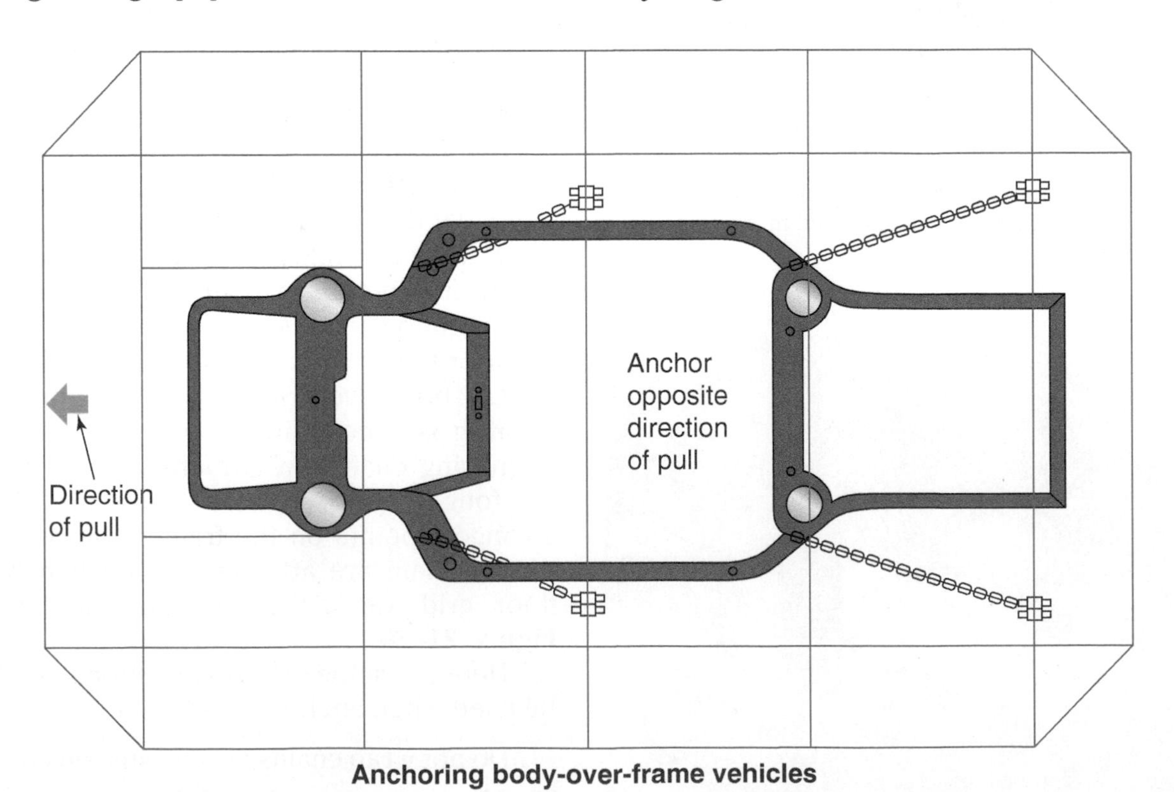

Figure 21–21. With body-over-frame/full-frame vehicles, anchoring cannot be done with pinchweld clamps. Since the full frame is thick and strong, chains are secured to the frame for straightening. (Courtesy of Blackhawk Collision Repair, Inc., Subsidiary of Hein-Werner® Corporation)

WHEEL CLAMPS

Wheel clamps are used to load the suspension with the wheel and tires removed with the vehicle on the rack or bench. They allow you to access parts behind the wheels and tires. They also provide more accurate measurement of body alignment because the suspension is not left hanging unsupported.

After raising the suspension with a jack and removing the wheel, bolt the wheel clamp over the lug studs. You can then lower the wheel stand onto the surface of the bench or rack.

When anchoring a vehicle, remember that the anchoring force must oppose the pulling force. See **Figure 21–22.** Remember! It is critical that the vehicle is anchored securely. Always check anchoring chains or clamps before pulling (see **Figure 21–23**).

ATTACHING PULLING CHAINS

Pulling chains transfer pulling force from the straightening equipment to the damaged area on the vehicle. One end of the pulling chain is fastened to the hydraulic ram, post, or tower, and the other end to the pulling clamps or adapters.

Pulling clamps bolt around or onto the vehicle so a pulling chain can be attached to the vehicle. See **Figure 21–24.** After determining where to pull from, the pulling clamps can be attached to any point that can withstand the force of the pull. Examples of where to attach the pulling clamps are:

1. Bumper energy absorber mounts and bolt holes
2. Steering, suspension, and mechanical mounting points
3. Damaged sheet metal
4. Weld-on tabs
5. Pinchweld flanges

Do not attach a "pull" to any suspension or mechanical parts; use only the mounting points.

Body-over-frame vehicles have frames that are ⅛–¼ inch (3–6 mm) thick.

On unibody vehicles the technician must use more care when pulling. Single hard "pulls" can tear the thin metal. To prevent tearing, multiple "pulls" should be used. If needed, use more than one clamp to ensure that the metal does not tear.

Set the pulling clamp so that the line extending along the path of the pulling force passes through the middle of the teeth of the clamp. If this is not done, rotational force will act on the clamp to pull it off, further damaging the section.

Nylon pull straps provide an additional means of making pulls in difficult areas. They are sometimes used on double pull hook-ups.

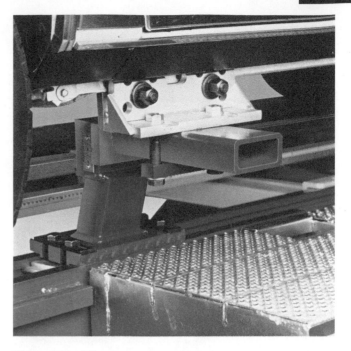

Figure 21–23. Always check that all anchoring clamps or chains are tight before starting the pull. (Courtesy of Car-O-Liner)

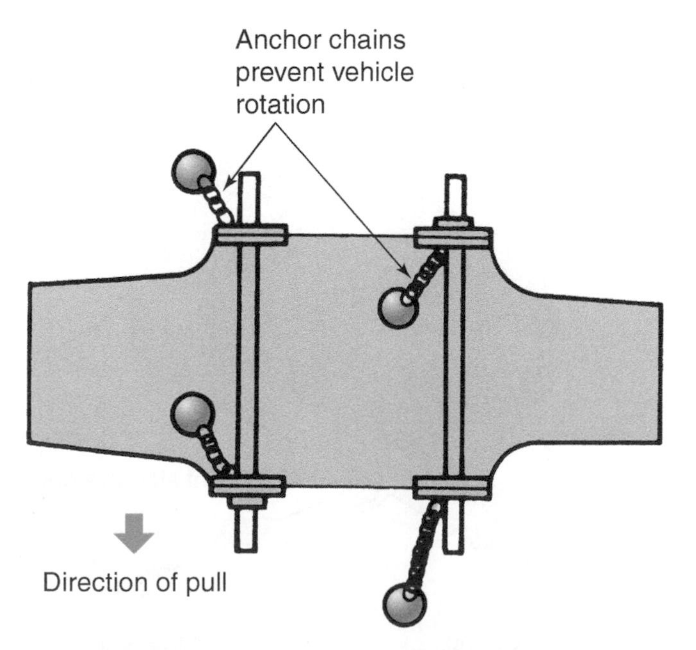

Figure 21–22. Note the position of the chains for anchoring a front, side pull. This will keep the vehicle from rotating. (Courtesy of Blackhawk Collision Repair, Inc., Subsidiary of Hein-Werner® Corporation)

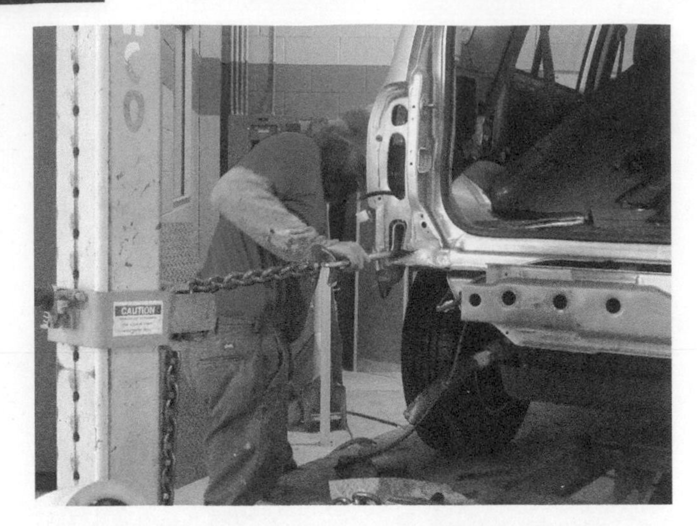

(A) Determine the direction of pull and find the best location on the vehicle for pulling out damage.

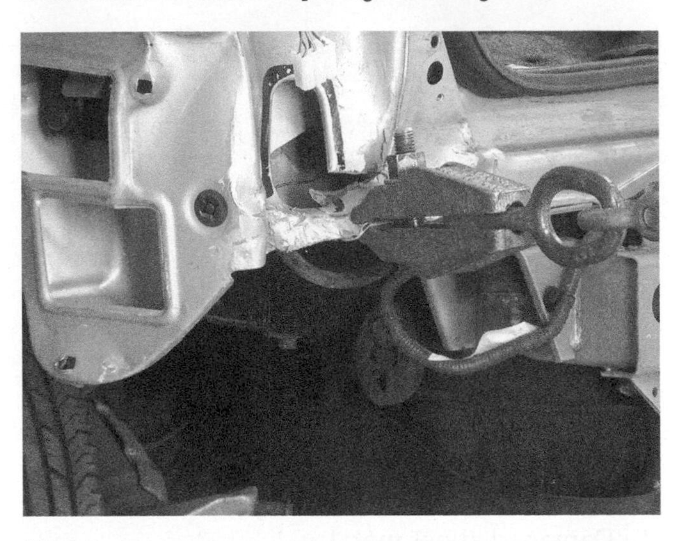

(B) The clamp has been tightened and secured to the rear frame rail to pull minor damage.

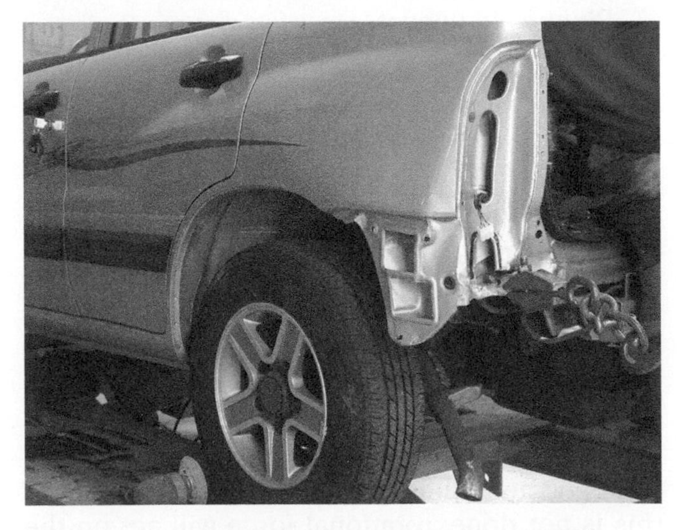

(C) Stand to one side and watch the metal as you pull. Avoid metal tearing and overpulling.

Figure 21–24. Pulling clamps bolt to the structure of the vehicle. Then pulling chains can be attached to these clamps.

When you are straightening a bend in a frame rail, make sure the clamp is attached to the correct portion of the rail, as shown in **Figure 21–25.** This will help stretch and pull out the damage. With this type of damage, you might use a second pulling chain from the side to help straighten the damage. See **Figure 21–26.**

A **welded pull-tab** can be used if you need to pull where there is no place to attach a clamp. Illustrated in **Figure 21–27,** weld a small piece of steel plate onto the vehicle unibody where

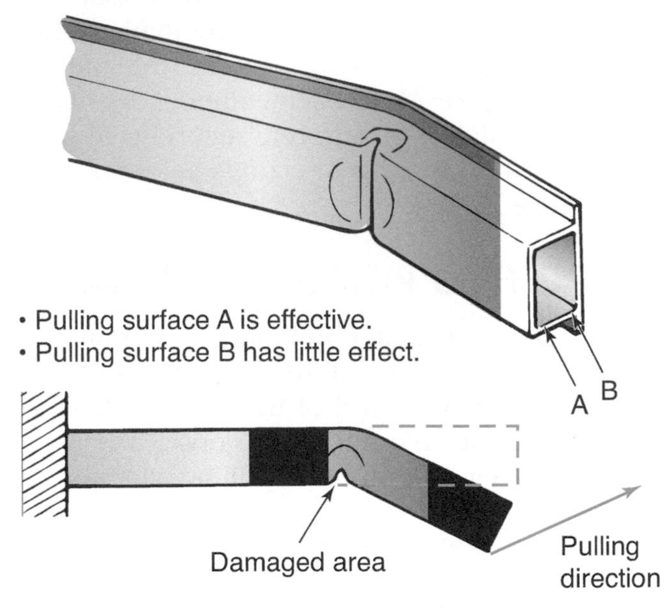

Figure 21–25. When straightening a bent box section, clamp on the side of the component that is bent. This will help stretch and straighten the component better than clamping on the other side of the box section.

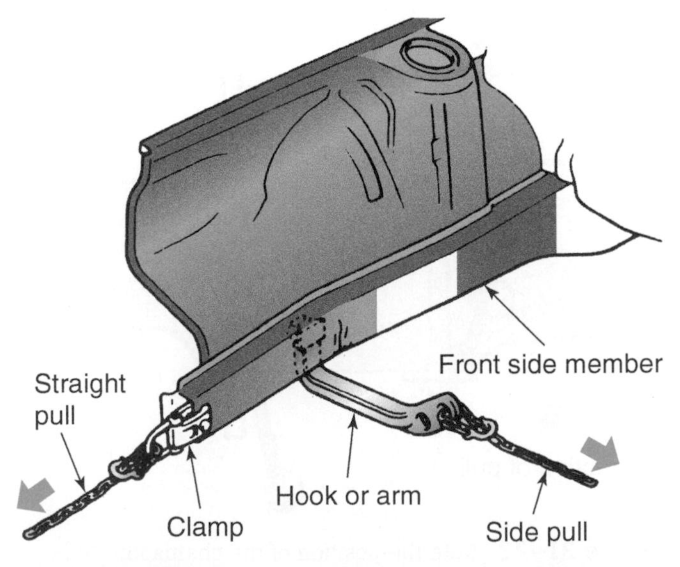

Figure 21–26. When straightening a part like this front rail, pulling from two directions is an efficient method of straightening. Note the pulling arm on one pulling chain.

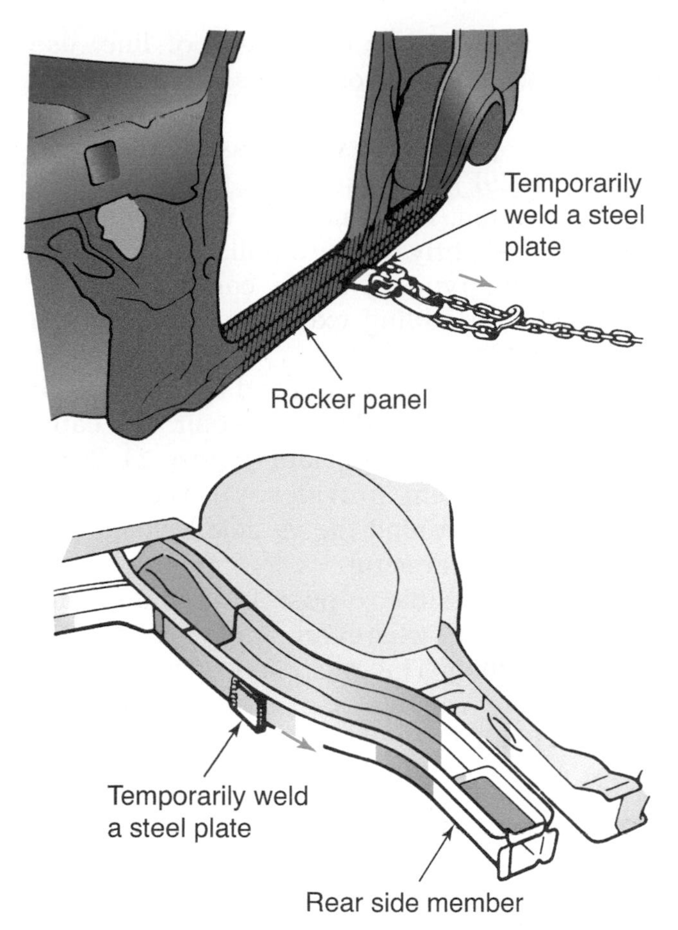

Figure 21–27. When you need to "pull" and there is no place to attach clamps, weld small metal tabs onto the body structure. Then you can attach a clamp and chain to the metal tab.

needed. Then you can bolt the pulling clamp onto the metal tab. After pulling, use an air cut-off tool to carefully remove the weld without damaging the body.

Pulling adapters are special straightening equipment accessories that allow you to pull in difficult situations. They come in various shapes and sizes for specific tasks.

Strut pulling plates are designed to bolt onto the top of strut towers for pulling. Spacers and hardened bolts are used to secure the strut pulling plate to the threaded holes in the strut tower. Then the pulling chain can be attached to the plate.

EXECUTING A PLANNED STRAIGHTENING SEQUENCE

The progress toward alignment should be monitored with the measuring system during the "pull." Since the body (sheet metal) has elasticity, the structure will partially return to its postdamaged condition even if the body is pulled back to the prescribed dimensions. Therefore, estimate the amount of return in advance and make allowance for it during the straightening operations.

Because of the power of the rams, the metal will begin moving as soon as the chain slack is taken up. There is no need to worry whether or not the ram has the capability to move the metal. This frees up the technician to concentrate on the straightening problem.

Simply make the "pulls" a little at a time, relieve the stress, take a measurement. When using a bench, check how close the fixtures are to their corresponding reference points on the unibody, and start the sequence again.

Normally, work from the center section outward. First, correct the length. Then correct side sway damage. Finally, correct height.

Remember! Approach the straightening operation as though it was going to be done with your bare hands. Determine how the metal should be moved to mold it back into shape if the only tools available were your hands. How many areas could be moved at one time and in which directions? This is the key to effective straightening.

Due to the high-strength and heat-sensitive characteristics of many unibody vehicles, do not attempt to make an alignment or straightening pull in one step. Instead, use a sequence that consists of a pull, hold the pull, more pull, hold, and so on. This will allow more time for working the metal, allow the metal more time to "relax," and allow more time for the process of alignment for clamping, repair or reattachment by welding, and so on.

That is, start the hydraulics moving, slowly and carefully. Watch the movement closely. Is it doing what it is supposed to do? If it is on the right track, keep on going. If not, determine why and make the angle or direction adjustment and try again.

STRAIGHTENING DIRECTIONS

There are a number of setups for "pulling" and "pushing" in different directions. We will review the most common ones.

The "pulling" (straightening) arrangement with the *vector system* is determined by a simple triangle. By changing the shape of the triangle formed by the pulling equipment and chains, you can alter straightening directions.

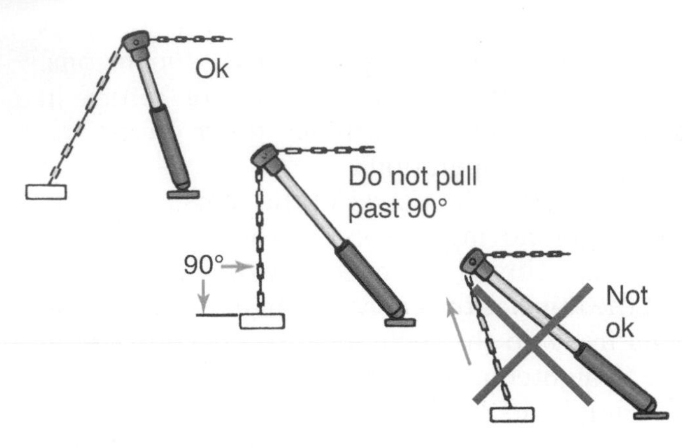

Figure 21–28. When setting up equipment, do not allow the angle of pull to go beyond 90 degrees or a strain can break the pulling chain or other parts. (Courtesy of Blackhawk Collision Repair, Inc., Subsidiary of Hein-Werner® Corporation)

Figure 21–28 shows a triangular arrangement that will provide more of a straight out pull. Note that the ram is placed at an angle to the right of true vertical. As force is applied, the ram will swing to the right pulling the damaged sections with it. When setting up a pull, make sure the ram is at the proper height. This can be controlled by adding the proper length of tubing onto the ram.

Remember! At no time should pulling continue if the chain between the ram and the anchor goes beyond perpendicular (see Figure 21–28). If this occurs, chain overloading could result because of the added stress placed on the anchored end of the chain. To avoid this condition, be sure that the chain lock head is not placed behind the chain anchor.

In a typical pull setup at frame rail height, the power ram is set so that the angle between the ram and the pulling chain is equal to the angle between the ram and the anchor. With several tons (kilograms) of force and a large amount of chain travel, you can easily make lower, tough, structure pulls.

For an out and down pull, less tubing is needed (**Figure 21–29A**). Another way to make a down pull is to attach a chain between the vehicle and floor anchors. By pulling on the chain bridge, the vehicle is forced down (**Figure 21–29B**).

A horizontal pull on a rail can be accomplished by placing the ram at about a 45-degree angle (**Figure 21–29C**).

By adding tubing to the ram, a straight outward pull on the cowl can be accomplished (**Figure 21–29D**).

To pull straight out at the roof line, use the ram with extension tubes as shown in **Figure 21–29E.**

Upward pulls are very easy to set up (**Figure 21–29F**). In most cases, the ram is in a vertical position. This pull setup will produce an upward and slightly outward pull.

The same type of setup can be used at roof height by adding extensions to the ram (**Figure 21–29G**).

Although pushing is not used to the extent it once was in collision damage repair, the capability to push is still important (**Figure 21–29H**). The vector system provides push capability from any angle around the vehicle by means of a simple triangular setup.

It is also possible to push from underneath the vehicle at whatever angle is needed (**Figure 21–30A**). This push setup can be used to effectively remove sag at the cowl area (**Figure 21–30B**).

OVERPULLING

Overpulling is done by pulling the damage slightly beyond its original dimension. If done in a controlled way, the metal will flex back slightly when tension is released. The unibody/frame reference points will then line up properly. If done too much, overpulling might not be a correctable error. See **Figure 21–31.**

Overpulling damage results from failing to measure accurately and often. To prevent overpull damage on unibody vehicles, measure the progress when pulling the damaged area.

Remember, you can stretch a piece of string into a straight line, but there is no way to push it straight back. Any damaged metal that is pulled or stretched beyond the critical control dimension is difficult to shrink or compress back. In most instances, the only way the overpulled panel can be repaired is by replacement of body parts. This is a very time-consuming and costly mistake.

When straightening damage, the metal will creep or spring back when the pulling tension is released. A slight overpull may be necessary to obtain the desired dimensions. Use the following straightening sequence when intentionally overpulling:

1. "Pull" the damage.
2. Stress relieve.

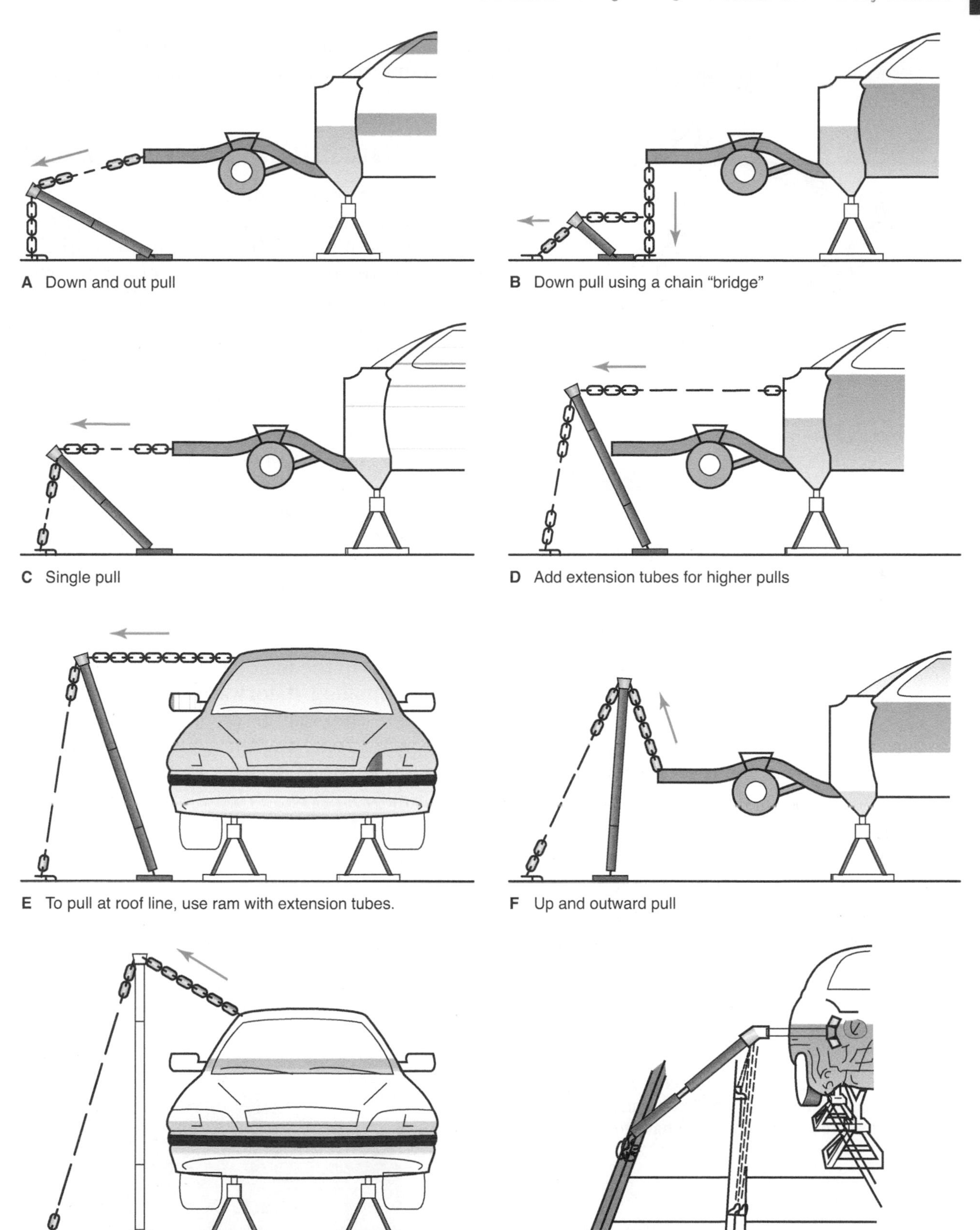

A Down and out pull
B Down pull using a chain "bridge"
C Single pull
D Add extension tubes for higher pulls
E To pull at roof line, use ram with extension tubes.
F Up and outward pull
G Upward roof line pull
H Typical push setup

Figure 21–29. Study these single-pull setups. (Courtesy of Blackhawk Collision Repair, Inc., Subsidiary of Hein-Werner® Corporation)

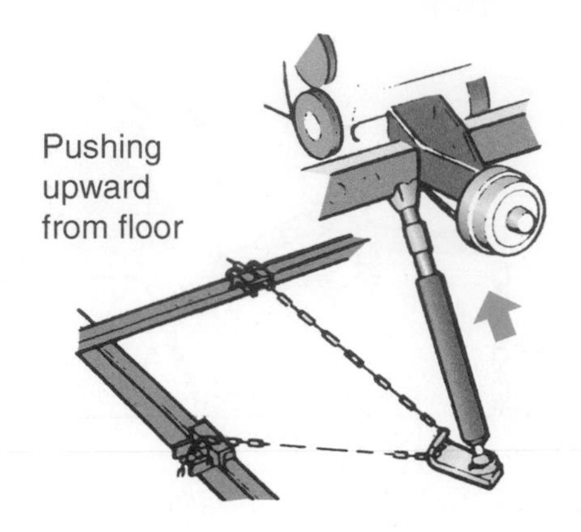

(A) The ram is being used to push up and sideways on the vehicle.

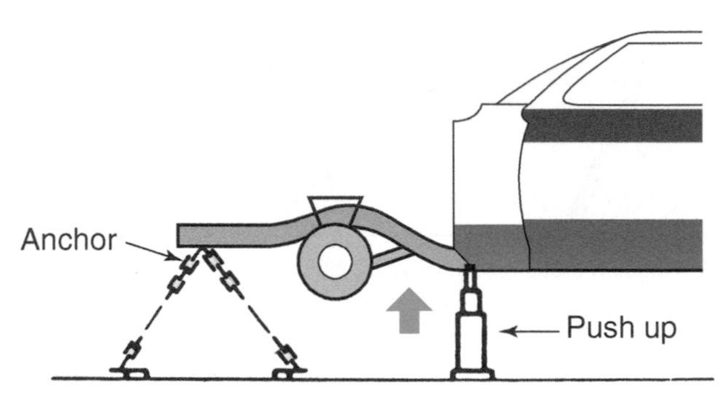

(B) With the front of the frame rails anchored, the ram is being used to remove sag at the cowl area.

Figure 21–30. Note these two setups for pushing. (Courtesy of Blackhawk Collision Repair, Inc., Subsidiary of Hein-Werner® Corporation)

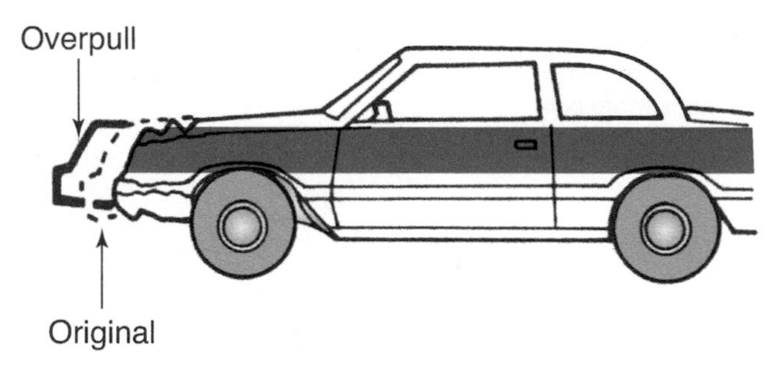

Figure 21–31. Overpulling stretches parts beyond their original dimensions. If done in a controlled manner, it can speed repairs. If done too much, parts will have to be replaced.

3. Release the pulling tension to allow the metal to return.
4. Measure.
5. Repeat as needed to obtain the desired dimensions.

The key is to "pull" and measure during the entire straightening process. Failure to do so can result in an area being overpulled. An overpull occurs to the point where the metal will not spring back.

ALIGNING FRONT END DAMAGE

First, "pull" the side member on the replacement side in the direction opposite to the impact direction. Then repair the fender apron and side member on the repair side. Also, repair the front fender apron and side member installation areas on the replacement side.

There are many cases where the entire inner fender apron or side member on the repair side is deflected left or right only. Measure the diagonal dimensions A and B, as shown in **Figure 21–32.** Then correct that distance while keeping an eye on the repair condition. The operation can be done efficiently if the fender apron upper reinforcement is pulled at the same time as the side member.

If there is severe damage to the side member on the repair side, separate the front crossmember and radiator upper support and repair them separately. Grip the inside face of the side member. While pulling it forward, pull the broken piece from the inside or push it from the outside. After repairing the bent portion, match up the dimensions to the standard diagonal dimensions.

To repair the other front fender apron and side member area, the main repairs are near the instrument panel and the cowl panel. If the impact was severe, the damage will extend into the front body pillar (the door would fit poorly in this case). Simply gripping the front edge of the side member of the fender apron and pulling will not repair this damage. See **Figure 21–33A.**

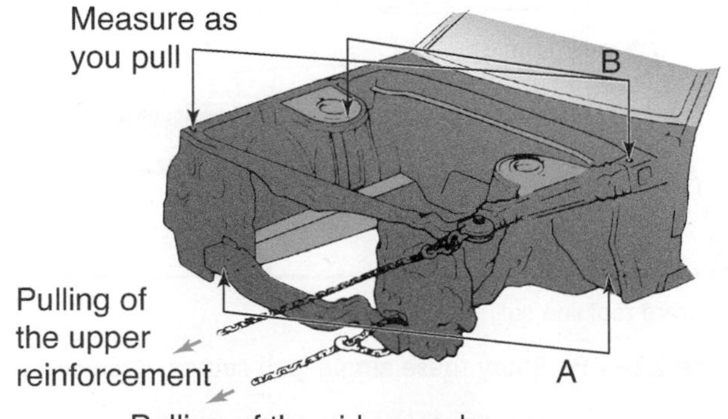

Figure 21–32. As you pull out front damage, measure your progress.

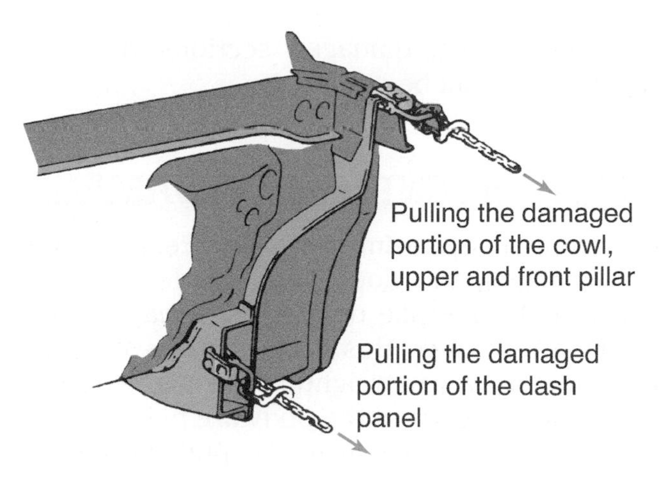

(A) With the fender apron cut off, attach clamps next to the cowl and pull.

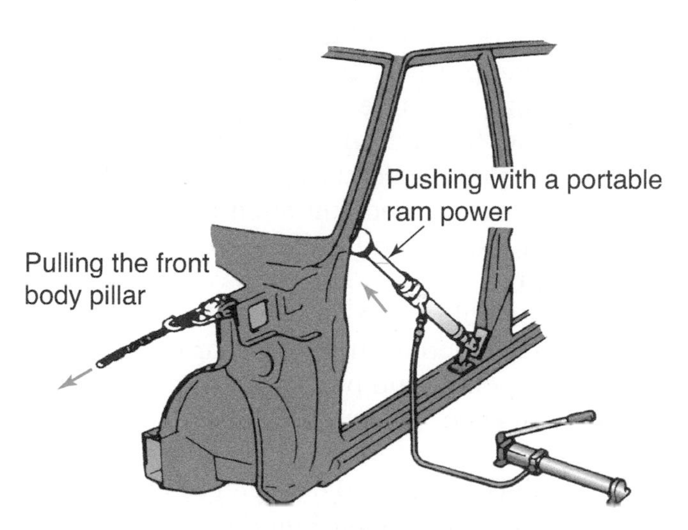

(B) Pulling at the cowl and pushing from behind with a portable power unit may be needed.

Figure 21–33. With major front damage, you may have to cut away damaged parts so you can pull near the cowl area.

In this case, cut the inner fender apron and side member near the installation area, clamp near the major panel damage, and pull (keep an eye on the door fit conditions).

At the same time that the pillar is being pulled forward, pushing can be done from the interior side with a power ram. See **Figure 21–33B.**

During front unibody aligning, confirm pulls by measuring the dimensions at reference holes. This is often done at the front floor reinforcement and rear of the front fender installation holes.

If the impact to the front side member structure is severe, there is a tendency for it to take the shape shown in **Figure 21–34.** The height of the standard measuring point might be distorted. Further, the front side member often has a reference point in the rear that has a

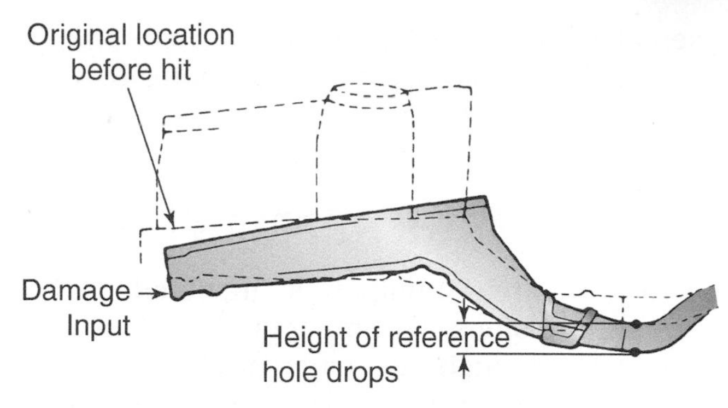

Figure 21–34. During a front collision, this frame rail was pushed back and down.

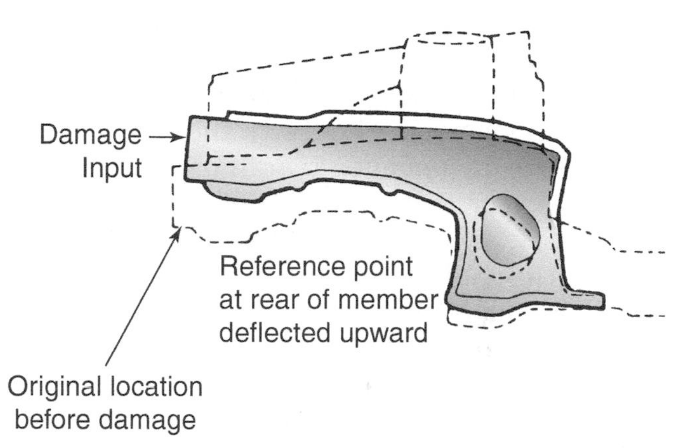

Figure 21–35. During a front collision, this frame rail was pushed back and up.

tendency to be deflected upward when damaged. See **Figure 21–35.**

To correct lateral bending damage of the front, the clamping point receiving the greatest force is point B in **Figure 21–36,** which must be clamped securely. If point C is not secured, point A cannot be pulled. A blocking device should be

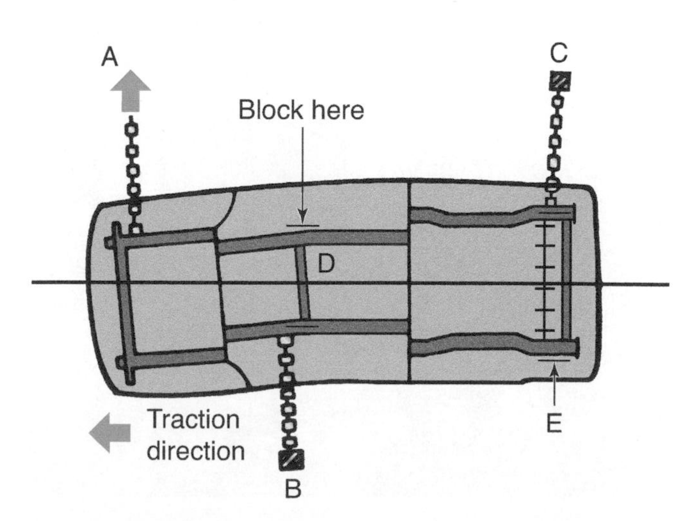

Figure 21–36. Note the setup and "pull" for correcting lateral damage. Blocking devices should be used to link the side rails together.

used at points D and E. Holding devices should also be placed across the underbody to help transmit pulling force to both sides of the vehicle.

REAR DAMAGE REPAIRS

Usually, the rear bumper is impacted during rear-end collisions. The impact force will usually propagate through the ends of the rear side members or nearby panels. The rear collision will also cause damage to the kick-up area. The wheel housings may deform causing the entire quarter panel to move forward. If the impact is severe enough, it will have an effect on the roof, door panels, and center body pillar.

Attach clamps or hooks to the rear portion of the rear side member, rear floor pan, or quarter panel rear end portion. See **Figure 21–37.** "Pull" while measuring the dimensions of each part of the underbody and door openings. As you "pull," inspect panel fit and part clearances.

Relieve the stress in the quarter panel by pulling on the side member only. If the wheel housing or the roof side inner panel is clamped and pulled along with the rear side member, the clearances with the door panel can be corrected.

With rear structure twist from a front impact, the rear lower preliminary pulling will restore some of the lower alignment points. Moving forward with subsequent "pulls," the alignment and number of anchoring points will, of course, move right along with them.

After pulling, damaged sections requiring replacement can be cut away.

STRAIGHTENING SIDE DAMAGE

If there is a severe impact to the center of the rocker panel, the floor pan will deform. The entire body will take on a curved shape, like a "banana." To align this type of damage, use a method similar to straightening a piece of bent wire. The two ends of the body are pulled apart, and the side that is caved in is pulled outward. This can often be repaired with three-way pulling, as shown in **Figure 21–38.**

Anchoring unitized body vehicles for side "pulls" can be very difficult due to the limited chain hook-up areas. See **Figure 21–39.** When straightening the side of a vehicle, the center section can be anchored by passing a chain around the pinchweld clamp and hooking to the edge of the bench. Tension/anchoring can be applied by attaching the pull chain to the pinchweld clamp.

The portable beam and knee can be used as a side anchor with either inside or outside contact. By attaching the pull chain to the portable beam and knee, it can be used as a pulling attachment.

It is advisable to make an end-to-end stretch pull when pulling outward on the center section of a vehicle. This is shown in Figure 21–39.

If pulling high on the body, tie the vehicle down on the opposite side. See **Figure 21–40.**

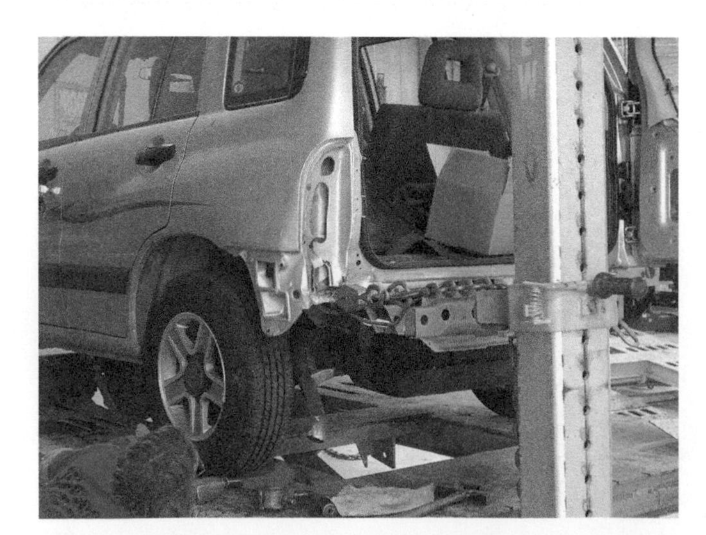

Figure 21–37. Straightening rear damage is not as complex in most instances because you do not have to deal with the steering and the engine.

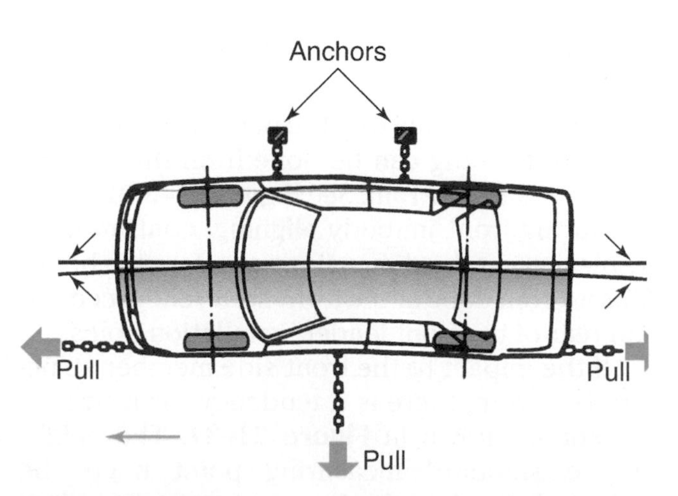

Figure 21–38. For inside damage, you may have to pull in three directions as shown. (Courtesy of Nissan North America, Inc.)

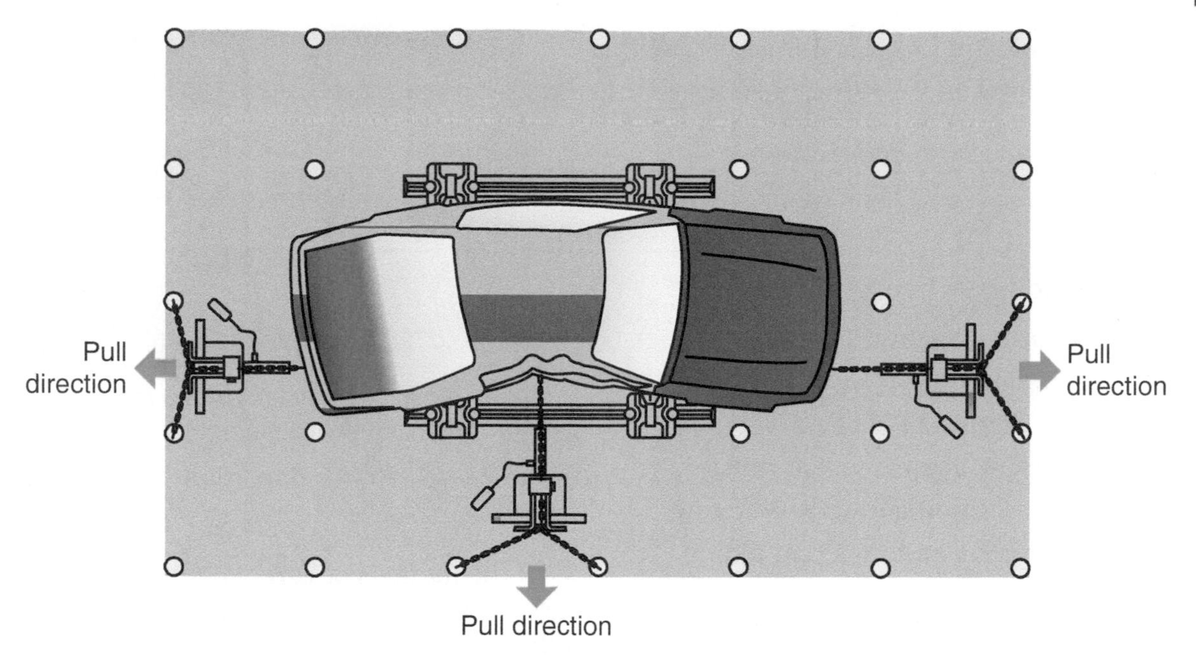

Figure 21–39. Study how this car is being pulled to remove major damage from a side impact. It is being pulled from the front and rear, as well as from the side. (Courtesy of Wedge Clamp International, Inc.)

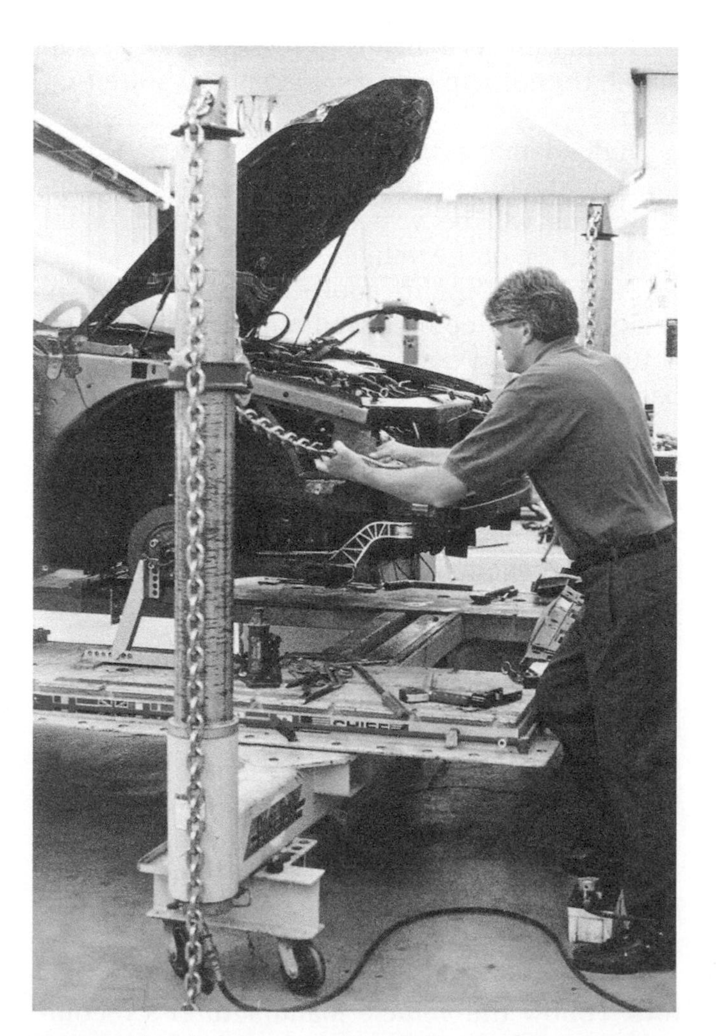

Figure 21–40. When pulling high on a vehicle, make sure the vehicle is anchored securely.

STRAIGHTENING SAG

Blocking under the low area and pulling down on the high end will correct sag. The vehicle must also be tied down to the straightening system at the opposite end.

Anchoring the high portion of the vehicle to the straightening system with chains and pushing up at the low spot will also remove the sag. When using the pulley and base for the downward pull, the tower pull chain must be in the lowest position.

Sag can also occur at the front frame crossmember. The ends of the crossmember will be closer than normal and the center will be too low. This condition can be corrected by using three hydraulic rams and two chains.

STRAIGHTENING DIAMOND DAMAGE

To straighten a diamond condition, place a pulling tower or ram on each end of the bench base on opposite sides. Adjust chain height and attach chains to the vehicle as described for end pull corrections. Block or anchor one side of the vehicle to prevent side movement. Activate the pull ram while measuring the results.

STRESS RELIEVING

Stress is defined in metallurgical books as the internal resistance a material offers to being deformed when subjected to a specific load (force). In the collision repair industry, **part stress** can be defined as the internal resistance a material offers to corrective techniques. This resistance or stress can be caused by:

1. Deformation
2. Overheating
3. Improper welding techniques

Indicators of stress include:

1. Misaligned door, hood, trunk, and roof openings (see **Figure 21–41**)
2. Dents and buckles in aprons and rails
3. Misaligned suspension and motor mounts
4. Damaged floor pans and rack and pinion mounts
5. Cracked paint and undercoating
6. Pulled or broken spot welds
7. Split seams and seam sealer

Stress relieve locked-up metal by hammering and/or heating while pulling. See **Figure 21–42.** First, mark the creases or folds to make them more visible. Pull the damaged metal to tension, then loosen it up with hammering and heat if needed. Increase the tension and loosen it again.

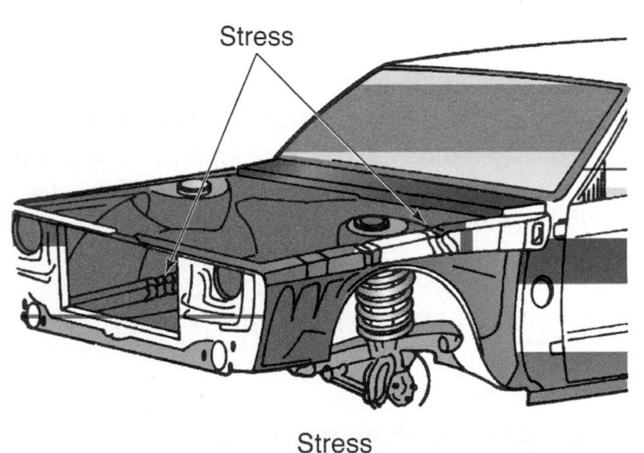

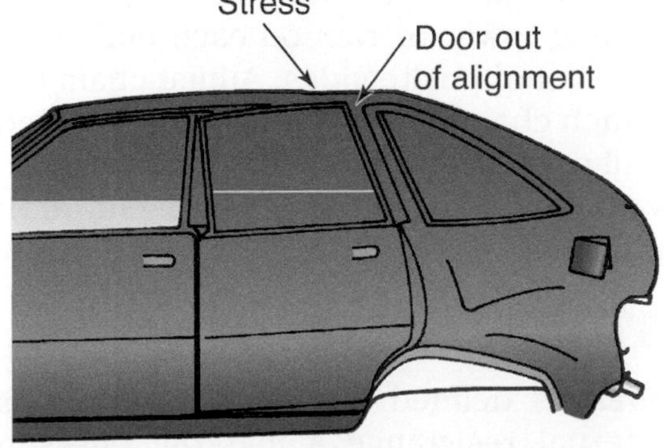

Figure 21–41. These are signs of stress and deformation.

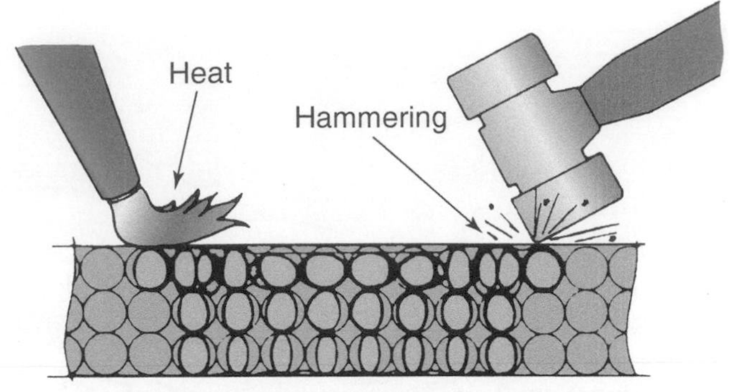

Figure 21–42. Stress can be relieved with hammering and/or heat.

If the metal is severely bent, it may be necessary to use a little heat. However, use heat carefully. Some components should NOT be heated. Check with the vehicle manufacturer for heating procedures.

Heat only on the corners and double panels where there is sufficient strength. Use heat carefully and only as a means of releasing locked-up metal. Do not use heat as a means to soften up an area.

If the damage requires the use of heat, follow the manufacturer's recommendations. These instructions will be written for the exact metal composition of the vehicle.

Never attempt to cool the heated area by using water or compressed air. Allow it to cool naturally. Rapid cooling can cause the metal to become hard and, in some cases, brittle.

The best way to monitor heat applications is with a *heat crayon,* **thermal melt stick,** or *thermal paint.* Stroke or mark the cold piece with the crayon. When the stated temperature has been reached, the mark will liquefy. Heat crayons are quite precise and far more accurate than watching for specific color change.

STRESS CONCENTRATORS

Stress concentrators are designed into unibody vehicles to control and absorb collision forces, minimize structural damage, and increase occupant protection. They result in a localized concentration of stress as a load is applied.

Do not remove designed stress concentrators. Follow the vehicle manufacturer's recommendations for straightening or replacing of parts that have designated stress concentrators.

FINAL STRAIGHTENING/ ALIGNMENT CHECKS

Once the repair is completed, including all straightening and welding operations, the alignment procedures are ready for a final check. Final measurements should be made and compared to the unibody/frame dimensions book.

Begin the final checks by slowly walking around the vehicle looking for obvious signs of misalignment.

Review the repair order or estimate to be sure everything was repaired. It is easier to straighten now than to wait until more steps have been completed and then find additional damage.

Among other items that should be carefully inspected are:

1. Check down low at the alignment between the door and rocker sill. This should be a straight gap.
2. Check the general alignment of all the upper body areas. Make sure everything looks as though nothing was ever out of alignment.
3. Open and close the doors and deck lid. Do they feel tight and secure when latched? Make sure they close smoothly and open easily.
4. If applicable, trial install large bolt-on parts, like the fenders and the hood. This will determine if all the bolt holes are aligned or if further pulling is needed. If needed, make final adjustments. Make sure everything aligns properly before removing the vehicle from the straightening equipment.

SUMMARY

- Vehicle straightening involves the use of high-powered hydraulic equipment, mechanical clamps, chains, and a measuring system to bring the frame back to its original shape.
- Straightening equipment includes anchoring equipment, pulling equipment, hydraulic rams, and pulling posts.
- Stress is the internal resistance a material offers to being deformed when subjected to a specific force. It can be caused by deformation, overheating, or improper welding techniques.
- Indicators of stress include misaligned doors, dents in aprons and rails, cracked paint and undercoating, and split seams and seam sealer.
- Once repairs are complete, it is time for a final alignment check. All measurements must be checked against factory specifications to ensure quality work.

TECHNICAL TERMS

straightening
single pull method
multiple pull method
composite force
anchoring equipment
pulling equipment
hydraulic rams
pulling posts
anchor pots
anchor rails
anchor clamps
anchor chains
rack straightening system
power winch
bench system
bench-rack system
straightening system accessories
bench computer
operating manual
portable puller
engine crane
engine stand
engine holder
portable pulling/pushing arm
portable hydraulic rams
portable power units
pinchweld clamps
wheel clamps
pulling clamps
welded pull-tab
pulling adapters
strut pulling plates
overpulling
overpulling damage
part stress
stress relieve
thermal melt stick
stress concentrators

REVIEW QUESTIONS

1. Which of the following is not an in-floor system?
   a. Anchor-pot system
   b. Modular rail systems
   c. Chainless anchoring system
   d. None of the above
2. Generally, how should you apply straightening force to a damaged vehicle?

3. Portable hydraulic rams have the capability to:
   a. Pull
   b. Push
   c. Spread
   d. All of the above
4. Define the term "anchoring equipment."
5. Define the term "straightening equipment."
6. Why are anchor clamps used instead of hooks when pulling?
7. When should the repair or replacement of severely damaged sections that cannot be restored by the straightening operation take place?
8. How is a power winch used in a collision repair shop?
9. When planning the straightening process, list six rules to remember.
10. List eleven basic safety rules for pulling out damage.
11. What are the four most important points to remember when pulling/straightening?
12. On most unibody vehicles, multiple anchoring is accomplished using four ______________ ______________.
13. ______________ ______________ ______________ are designed to bolt onto the top of shock towers for pulling.
14. What are stress concentrators?

ASE-STYLE REVIEW QUESTIONS

1. *Technician A* says that you never overpull. *Technician B* says that overpulling is needed since the frame tends to snap back when pulling tension is released. Who is correct?
   a. Technician A
   b. Technician B
   c. Both Technicians A and B
   d. Neither Technician

2. *Technician A* says that it is ideal to have at least four undamaged reference points on the vehicle that can be used to set the vehicle up properly on the straightening equipment. *Technician B* says a straightening system should be used whenever the damage involves the suspension, steering, or powertrain mounting points. Who is correct?
   a. Technician A
   b. Technician B
   c. Both Technicians A and B
   d. Neither Technician

3. *Technician A* always removes the suspension and driveline completely from a unibody vehicle before putting it on a straightening bench. *Technician B* says that single-pull systems cannot be used on unibody vehicles. Who is correct?
   a. Technician A
   b. Technician B
   c. Both Technicians A and B
   d. Neither Technician

4. When anchoring a unibody vehicle in preparation for pulling, *Technician A* leans toward "overanchoring." *Technician B* sometimes temporarily welds a piece of steel to a section to be pulled. Who is correct?
   a. Technician A
   b. Technician B
   c. Both Technicians A and B
   d. Neither Technician

5. *Technician A* says that the only way that overpull damage can be repaired is by part replacement. *Technician B* says heat can be used to correct an overpull. Who is correct?
   a. Technician A
   b. Technician B
   c. Both Technicians A and B
   d. Neither Technician

6. Which of the following is true?
   a. Cracked paint and undercoating is a sign of stress.
   b. Most of the stress relieving will be "cold work."
   c. The best way to monitor heat applications is with a heat crayon.
   d. High-strength steel (HSS) can be heated.

7. Technicians are planning to straighten a badly damaged vehicle. *Technician A* says to

pull the damage in the same sequence as it occurred during the collision. *Technician B* says to straighten a damaged vehicle it should be pulled in the reverse sequence that the damage occurred. Who is correct?

a. Technician A

b. Technician B

c. Both Technicians A and B

d. Neither Technician

8. *Technician A* says never to stand in line with a pull chain. *Technician B* says to cover pull chains with heavy blankets. Who is correct?

a. Technician A

b. Technician B

c. Both Technicians A and B

d. Neither Technician

9. *Technician A* anchors a unibody vehicle with chains. *Technician B* uses pinchweld clamps. Who is correct?

a. Technician A

b. Technician B

c. Both Technicians A and B

d. Neither Technician

10. An inner fender apron is resisting straightening force. A minor buckle is found in the apron. *Technician A* says to use controlled heat and hammer blows to remove the stress from the panel. *Technician B* says to replace the panel. Who is correct?

a. Technician A

b. Technician B

c. Both Technicians A and B

d. Neither Technician

ACTIVITIES

1. Visit a collision repair shop. Observe an experienced technician using straightening equipment. Write a report on your visit.
2. Read the operating manuals for different types of straightening equipment. Compare their differences and similarities.
3. Inspect several badly damaged vehicles. Write a report on what repairs would have to be made.

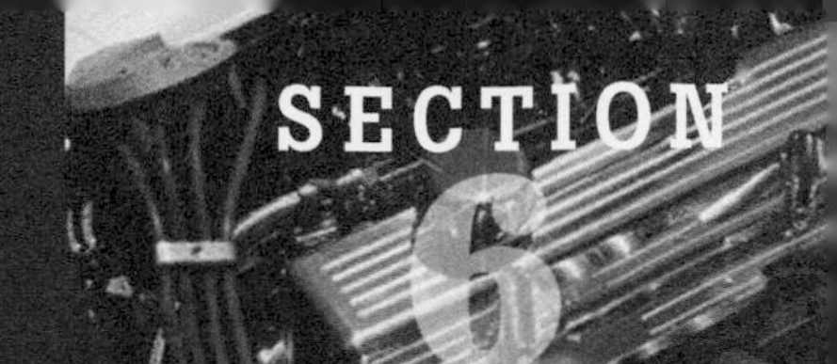

CHAPTER 22

Replacing Structural Parts and Rust Protection

OBJECTIVES

After studying this chapter, you should be able to:

- List the parts of the vehicle that are considered structural.
- List the steps necessary for replacing a part along factory seams.
- Describe how spot welds are separated.
- Explain how new body panels can be positioned on a vehicle.
- List the steps for welding new body panels in place.
- Describe how to install foam panel fillers.
- Section rails, rocker panels, A- and B-pillars, floor pans, and trunk floors.
- Define rust and describe the common factors in its formation.
- Identify the principal methods of rust protection.
- Choose the correct antirust materials and equipment.
- List common types of seam sealers and explain where each should be used.

INTRODUCTION

Most collisions will involve at least some parts replacement (see **Figure 22–1**). While many parts on a vehicle add to its structural integrity, some parts play a greater role. These parts are known as structural parts.

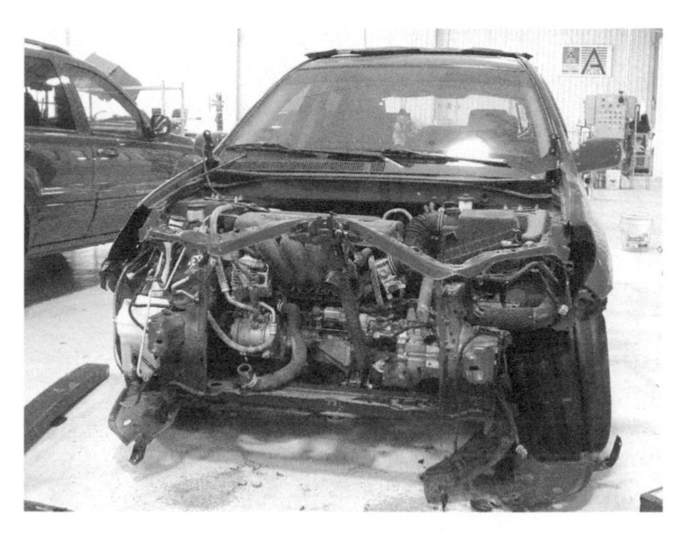

Figure 22–1. Badly damaged parts, especially when kinked and crushed, must be cut off so a new panel can be welded on. This frontal collision required that a new radiator support be welded in to repair damage.

Structural parts can be defined as those parts of the vehicle that:

1. Support the weight of the vehicle
2. Absorb collision energy
3. Absorb road shock

Parts that are generally considered to be structural include:

1. Core support/tie bar
2. Front rails
3. Strut towers
4. Rocker panels
5. A-pillar (hinge pillar)
6. B-pillar (center pillar)

7. Rear rails
8. Rear strut towers
9. Suspension crossmembers

Restoring rust protection is also a vital aspect of collision repair. Failing to do so can result in major structural failure. Corrosion of structural parts can severely impair the handling and crash worthiness of the vehicle. This damage may not be evident until a collision, but then it will be too late.

REPAIR OR REPLACE GUIDELINES

The decision to repair or replace a structural part will be based on the judgment and skill of the technician/appraiser. A simple rule is:

If the part is bent, repair it.
If the part is kinked, replace it.

Whenever possible and practical, the part should be repaired rather than replaced.

TYPES OF STRUCTURAL REPLACEMENTS

Structural replacement can take one of two forms: replacement at factory seams and sectioning.

Replacement of panels along **factory seams** (the end or edge of a panel) should be done when practical and economical. The result is almost identical to factory production in both strength and appearance. Replacement of damaged parts along factory seams is a common practice in collision repair. Parts should be replaced along factory seams whenever it is practical and possible.

Sectioning involves cutting the part in a location other than a factory seam. This might or might not be a factory-recommended practice. Special care must be taken. Sectioning a part should be analyzed to make sure it will NOT jeopardize structural integrity.

There are three general types of structural parts:

1. Closed sections, such as rocker panels, front rails, A-pillars, and B-pillars
2. Hat channels, such as rear rails
3. Single-layer, flat parts, such as floor pans and trunk floors

Most manufacturers have specific recommendations for parts replacement. Always follow the procedures described in the body repair manual.

When planning to section a structural part:

1. Check the body repair manual for model-specific sectioning procedures.
2. If specific sectioning recommendations do NOT exist, follow the general guidelines presented here. Body repair manuals are available through various publishers and vehicle manufacturers.

Keep in mind that the vehicle must be returned to precollision condition. Failure to restore precollision crushability may affect future air bag deployment, leading to liability exposure.

When choosing a sectioning location, look for a uniform area with enough clearance to perform welding operations.

You should NOT section in or near:

1. Suspension mounting locations
2. Structural part mounting locations
3. Dimensional reference holes
4. Compound shapes
5. Reinforcements (except as noted)
6. Compound structures
7. Collapse/crush zones
8. Engine or drivetrain mounting locations

DETERMINING SPOT WELD LOCATIONS

To start removal of a structural component, you usually must first locate all factory spot welds. Remove the paint, sealer, or other coatings covering the joint area to find the spot welds. A course scuff wheel mounted in a air tool is often used to remove the paint so you can locate the spot welds on the damaged component.

Another way to do this is to heat the paint film. It is the best choice for loosening the paint film. A coarse wire wheel or brush attached to an air drill or grinder can be used to remove the paint, sealers, and other coatings.

Scrape off thick portions of primecoating or seam sealer before scorching the paint. Do NOT overheat the paint film so that the sheet metal panel begins to turn color. Heat the area only enough to soften the paint and then brush or scrape it off. It is NOT necessary to remove paint from areas where the spot welds are visible through the paint film.

In areas where the spot weld locations are NOT visible after the paint is removed, carefully drive a chisel between the panels. Doing so will cause an outline of the spot welds to appear.

SEPARATING SPOT WELDS

After the spot welds have been located, there are several methods of separating them. You can use a hole saw, compound drill bit, conventional drill bit, cutoff tool, or spot weld cutting tool. Regardless of which is used, be careful NOT to cut into the lower panel if it is to be used. Also be sure to cut out the spot welds without creating an excessively large hole.

If needed, center punch each spot weld before drilling. This will keep the bit from wandering. See **Figure 22–2.**

Make sure the bits are sharp, and use the same pressure on the drill as if you were drilling mild steel. The speed at which the bit turns should be slower than for mild steel. This will keep the heat from affecting the metal.

Figure 22–3 shows how a cutoff tool can be used to remove spot welds.

After the spot welds have been removed, drive a chisel between the panels to separate them. Be careful NOT to cut or bend the undamaged panel. Look at **Figure 22–4.**

Remember! A chisel should never be used by itself to remove spot welds. This will create excessive damage to adjacent panels.

SEPARATING CONTINUOUS WELDS

In some vehicles, panels are joined by continuous MIG welding. Since the welding bead is long, use a grinding wheel or cutoff tool to cut through the weld. Be careful NOT to cut into or through the undamaged panels. Hold the cutoff tool at a 45-degree angle to the joint. After grinding through the weld, use an air chisel to separate the panels.

PREPARING VEHICLE FOR NEW PANEL

Always refer to the appropriate body repair manual for the type and placement of welds. The manual will also give other details for the specific vehicle.

After removing the damaged panels, prepare the vehicle for installation of the new panels:

1. Grind off the welding marks. See **Figure 22–5.** Use a wire brush or scuff wheel to remove dirt, rust, paint, sealers, and so on from the joint surfaces. Zinc coatings should NOT be removed.

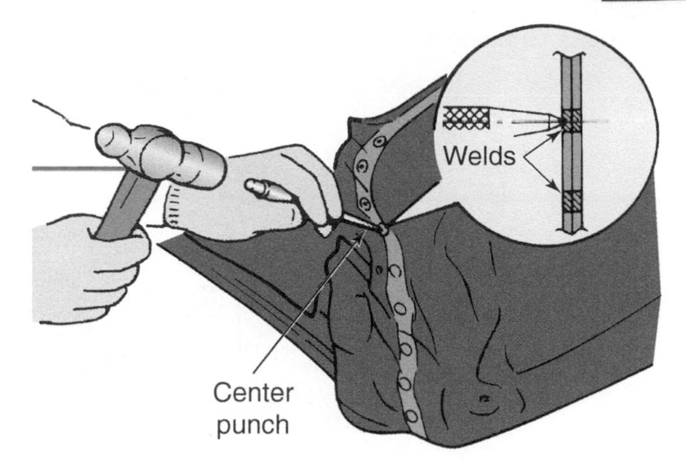

(A) Center punching will help the drill stay in the center of spot welds.

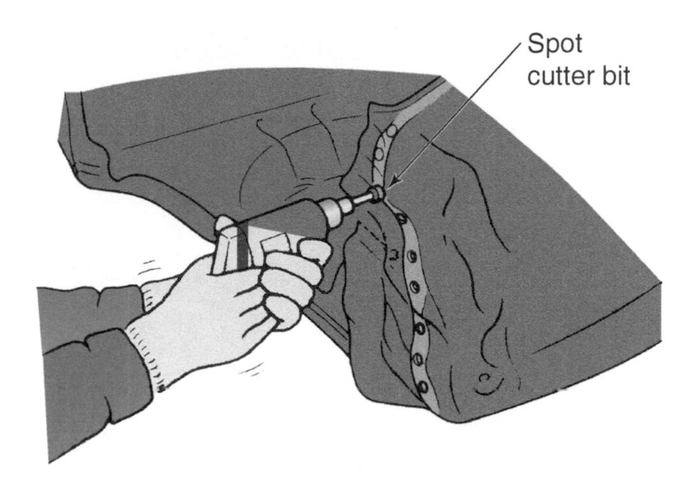

(B) Use a drill to cut out the spot weld. Do not drill through the lower panel if it is to be reused.

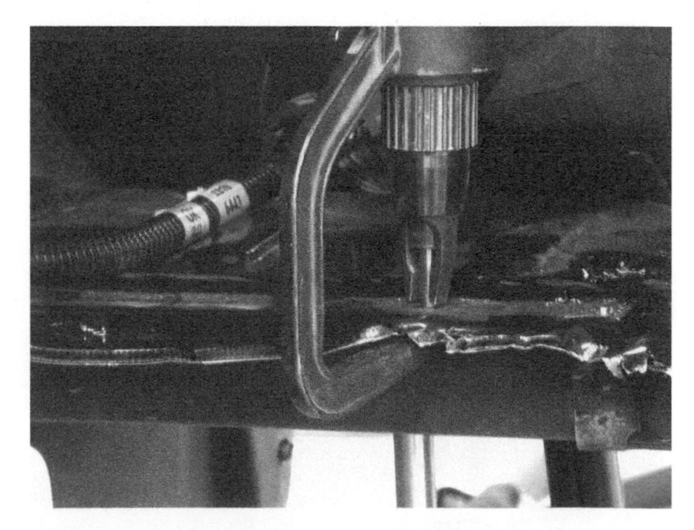

(C) Here a technician uses a spot weld drill to remove welds for trunk floor pan removal.

Figure 22–2. Spot welds can easily be seen and removed after any paint or caulking hiding them is removed. (Courtesy of Nissan North America, Inc.)

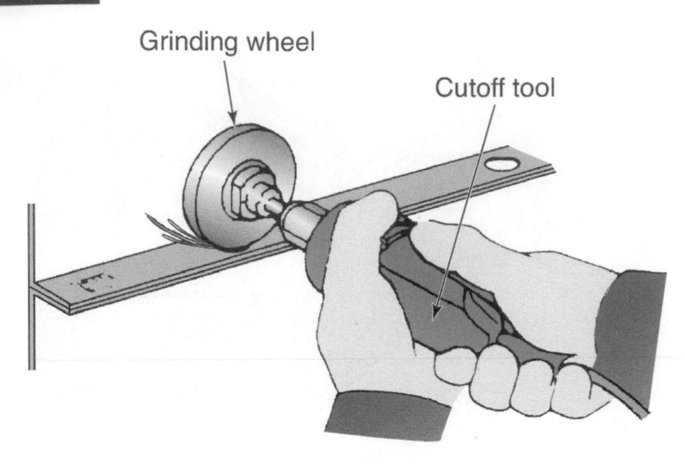

(A) Carefully hold the cutoff tool over the spot weld to grind it away.

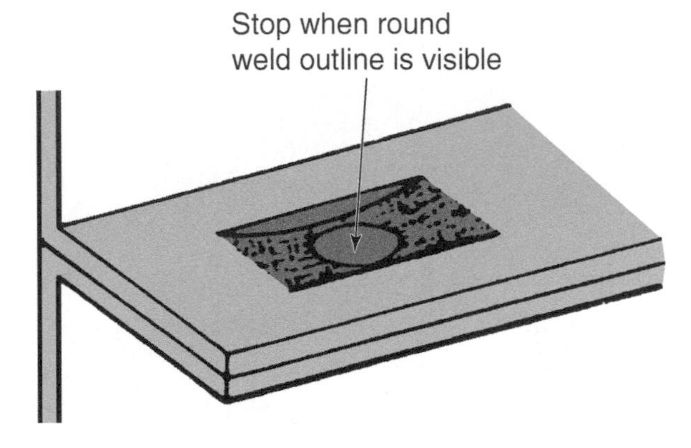

(B) To prevent panel damage, stop grinding when you reach the lower panel.

Figure 22–3. A cutoff tool provides another way of removing spot welds.

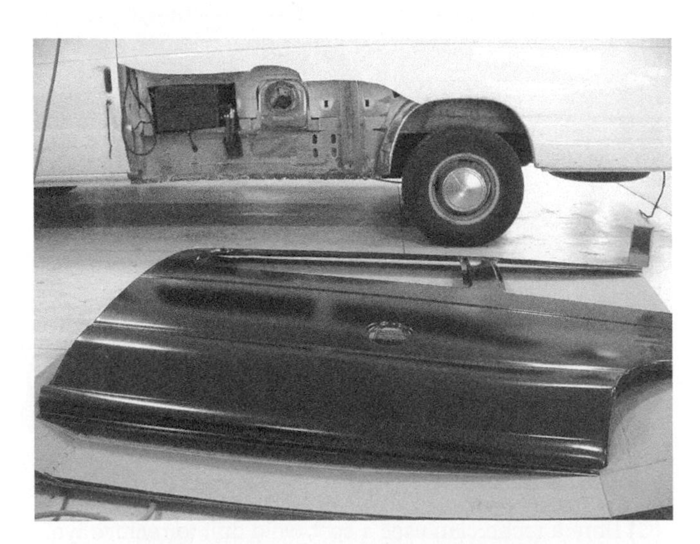

Figure 22–4. Here the technician has started cutting off an old panel on the side of a van. The new replacement panel is lying on a protective piece of cardboard to avoid damaging it.

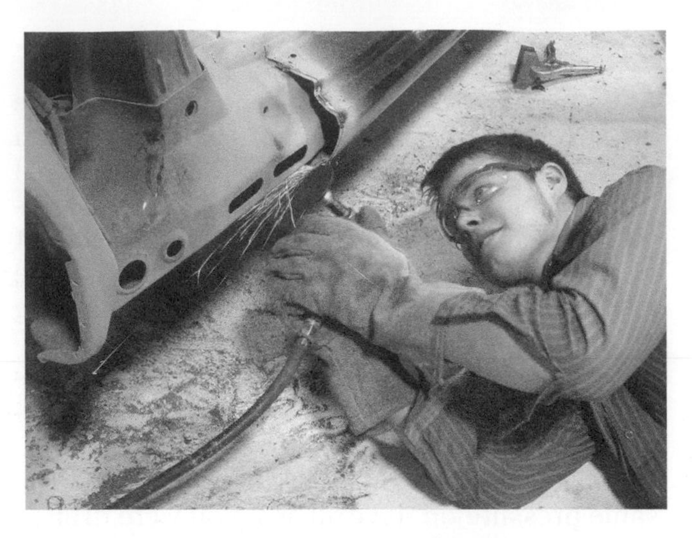

Figure 22–5. Grind off small nuggets from existing spot welds so flanges on the existing panels are smooth and clean.

2. Remove paint and primecoating from the backsides of the panel joining surfaces on parts that will be spot welded during installation.
3. Smooth the mating flanges with a hammer and dolly. See **Figure 22–6.**
4. Apply weld-through primer to areas where bare metal is exposed. Refer to **Figure 22–7.**

PREPARING REPLACEMENT PANEL/PART

Since all new parts are coated with primer, it is important that this coating be removed from the flanges to allow the welding current to flow properly. Also, holes for plug welds must be drilled precisely.

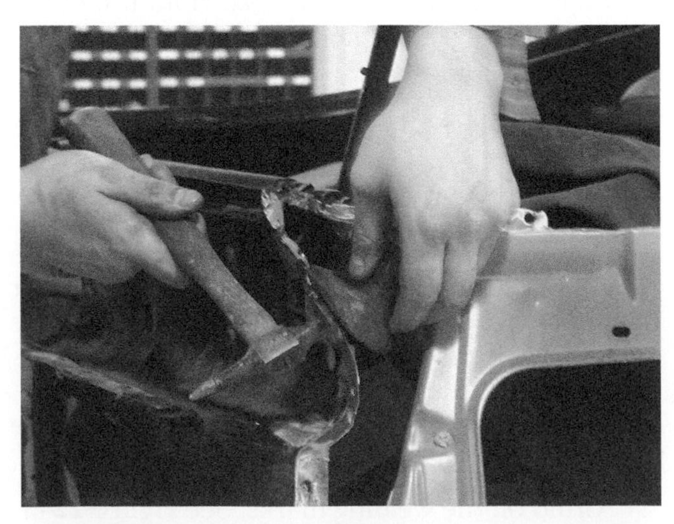

Figure 22–6. After removing the damaged panel, straighten the flange on the other panels so they will fit against the new panel properly.

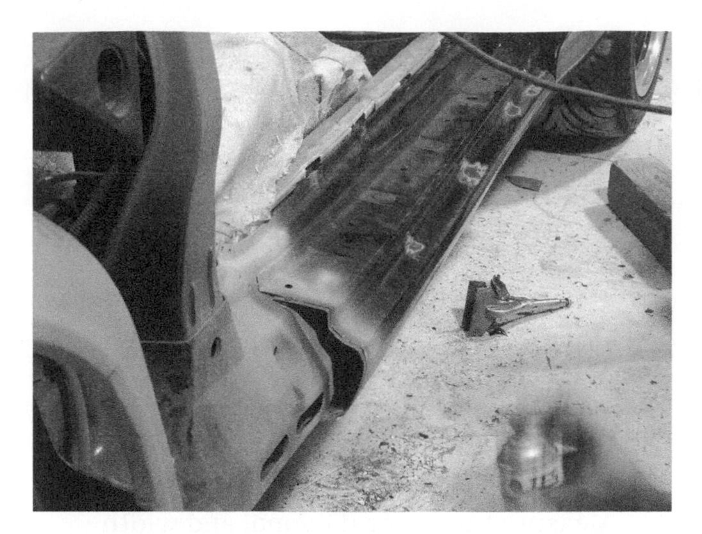

Figure 22–7. Spray weld-through primer on the flanges of all panels to be welded. This will protect them from rust and corrosion.

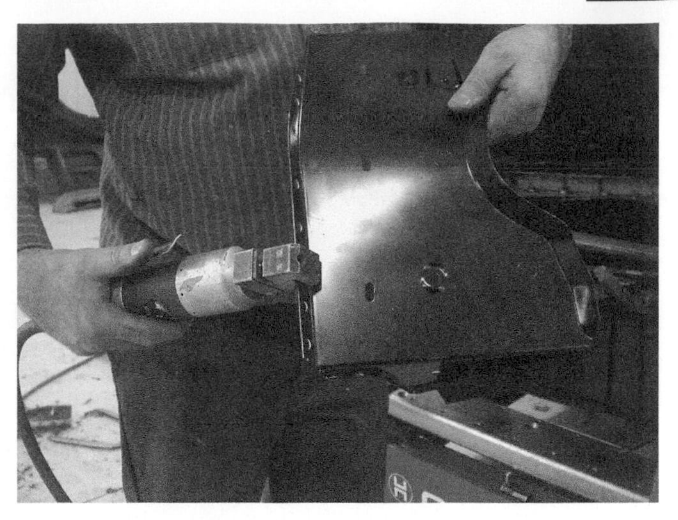

Figure 22–8. The correct number and size of holes should be drilled or punched in the replacement parts. Holes should be positioned on the old panel as explained in factory service literature.

To prepare a replacement panel for welding, follow these steps:

1. Use a disc sander to remove the paint from both sides of the spot weld area. Do NOT grind into the panel. Do NOT heat it too much. You do NOT want the panel to turn blue or warp.

DANGER

Whenever possible, grind so that sparks fly down and away. Always wear proper eye and hand protection when grinding.

2. Drill or punch holes for plug welding. Always refer to the body repair manual for the size of plug weld holes. Always be sure to duplicate the location and number of spot welds used at the factory. See **Figure 22–8.**
3. Apply weld-through primer to the welding surfaces where the zinc coating was removed.
4. Be sure all plug weld holes are of the proper diameter. If a recommended hole size is NOT given in the repair manual, drill $\frac{5}{16}$-inch (8 mm) holes.
5. If the new panel is sectioned to overlap any of the existing panels, rough cut the new panel to size using an air saw or a cutoff wheel. The edges should overlap the portion of the remaining panel by $\frac{3}{4}$ to 1 inch (19 to 25 mm). See **Figure 22–9.**

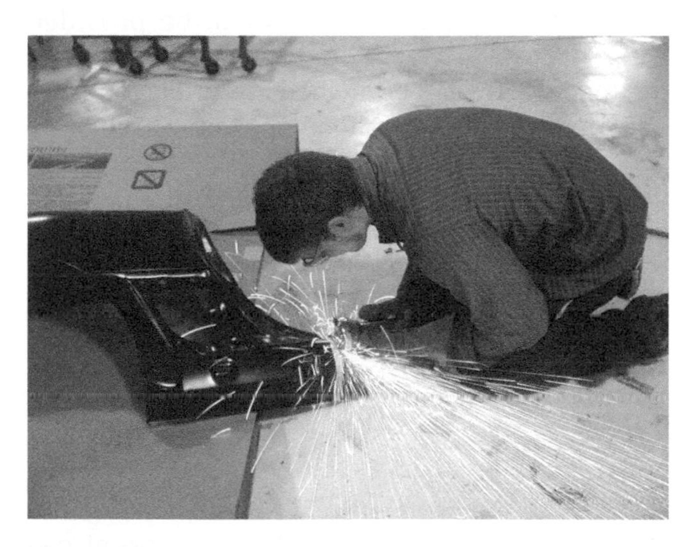

Figure 22–9. Cut the new panels to size with a cutoff wheel or other power tool. Mark the panel with tape or a marker so it is cut correctly.

Remember! If the overlap portion is too large, it will make positioning of the panel difficult. If the overlap is too small, structural integrity will suffer.

POSITIONING NEW PANELS

Aligning new panels is a very important step in repairing unibody vehicles. Improperly aligned panels will affect both the appearance and quality of the repaired vehicle.

Use a measuring system to determine the installation position. Remember that the fit of the new and old parts must be within specifications. Whether structural or cosmetic panels are being replaced, proper measurement and fit are critical.

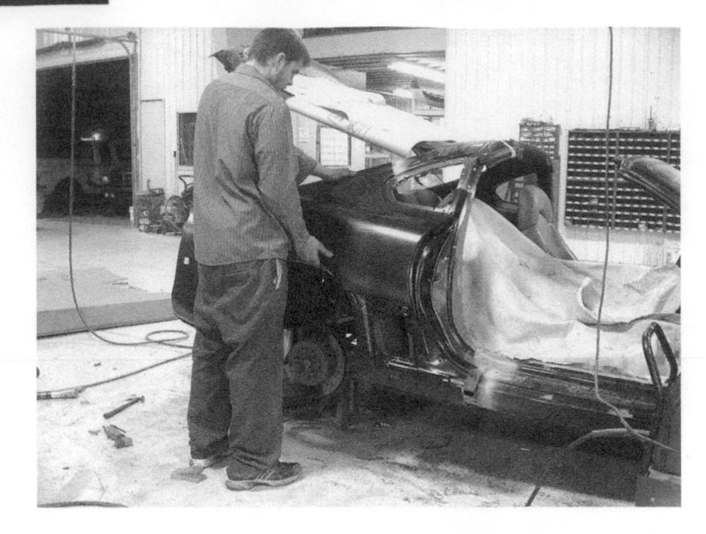

Figure 22–10. Fit the new panel into position on the vehicle. Locking pliers are initially used to hold it in place.

Panel alignment marks can be provided to help position parts before welding. Refer to the manufacturer's published materials for more information on panel alignment marks.

Once you have the part in relative position, use locking pliers or self-tapping screws to hold it in place. Use self-tapping screws only in places where there is not sufficient room for locking pliers. You will have to remove and weld each hole made by a self-tapping screw. Measure the position of the panel and adjust its location if needed. See **Figure 22–10.**

Panel Positioning and Measurement

The vehicle must be properly positioned on the straightening bench before the new panel can be correctly aligned. All straightening must be done before replacing panels. Otherwise, proper alignment of the new panels will be impossible.

As an example of a typical procedure for structural part replacement, we will describe the replacement of a front fender apron, front crossmember, and core support/tie bar.

1. Match the assembly reference marks on the installation areas of the front fender apron and the rail. Secure them with locking pliers. Parts that have no assembly reference marks should be positioned in the same location as the old parts.
2. Align the parts by measuring the distance between reference points. Temporarily install the front crossmember by tack welding one spot. Make any length adjustments by light tapping. Use a hammer against a wood block to adjust the panel without damage (**Figure 22–11A**).
3. Mark a positioning line at the end of the part that is NOT welded. Use locking pliers to hold the parts together. You can also drill small holes and fasten them together with sheet metal screws. Mark a line on the apron area but do NOT weld the panels together.
4. Use a measuring system to match the height of the new parts to the parts on the opposite side of the vehicle (**Figure 22–11B**). Support the new parts with a jackstand to make sure that the height does NOT change at all.
5. Measure the lower diagonal and width dimensions (**Figure 22–11C**). Support the parts with jack stands so that the height does NOT change. Then adjust the rail as needed to obtain the correct dimensions. Confirm the height dimensions again.
6. Take care to position the front crossmember so that both the left and right ends are uniform.
7. Once the dimensions of the rail match the dimensions found on the dimension chart, secure the part in place. The suspension crossmember can also be installed with fixtures. Use a sufficient number of plug welds to fasten the joining area of the rail to the front crossmember.
8. Make sure that the apron's upper length has NOT changed. Confirm by checking for shifting of the marked line.
9. Measure the diagonal dimensions between the fender rear installation hole and the strut tower hole or fender front installation hole (**Figure 22–11D**).
10. Measure the width dimension of the strut tower and the front fender bolt hole and fasten them together. If the width dimension does NOT match the body dimension manual, make a small adjustment. Be careful of changes in diagonal dimensions. Temporarily install and fasten the upper core support and the core support (**Figure 22–11E**).
11. Measure the rail width dimensions. Set the measuring system to the proper measurement and adjust the apron as needed. Lightly fasten the support with locking pliers and tap it softly by hand to move it into place.

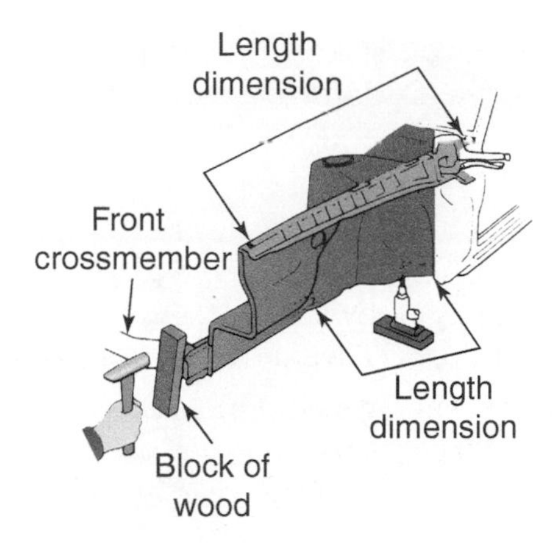

(A) Us a wood block and light blows to adjust the panel as needed.

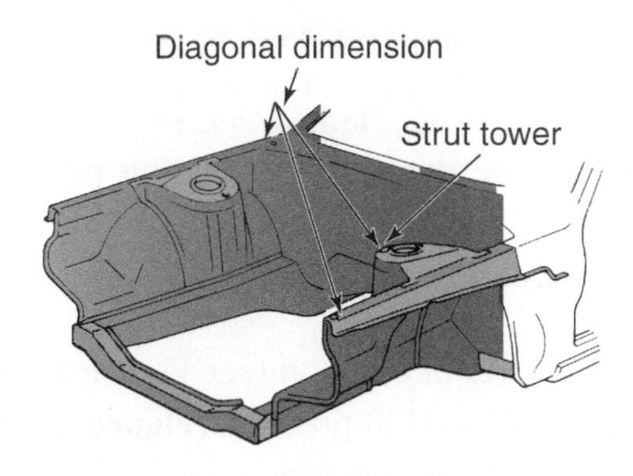

(D) Note the basic method for measuring fender apron dimensions.

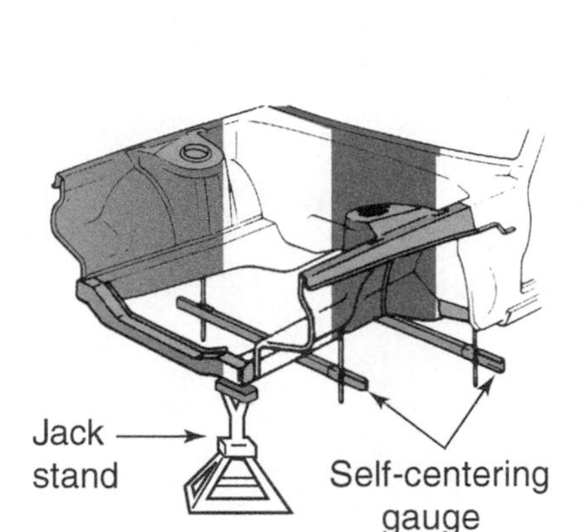

(B) Jack stands should be used to support the panel. Use a measuring system to check panel positioning.

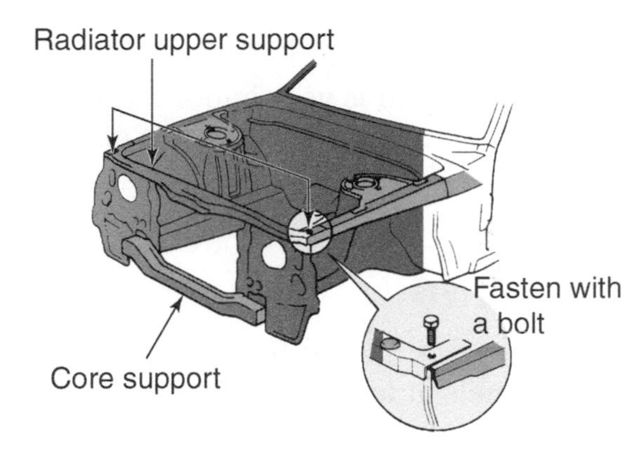

(E) After the inner component, the apron in this example, is secured, install the next component, core support.

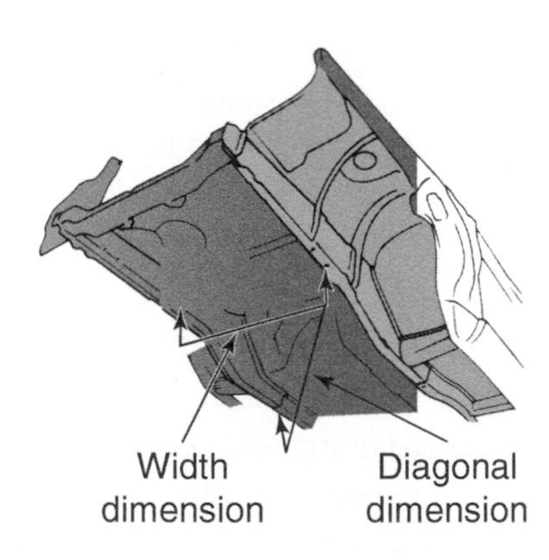

(C) Measure the lower diagonal and width dimensions.

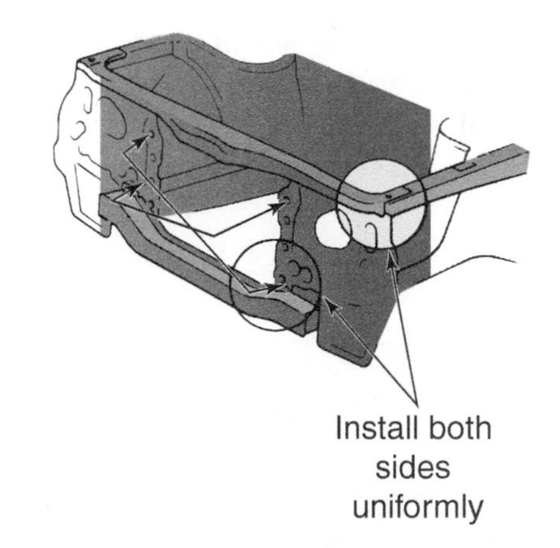

(F) Measure each component's location before final welding.

Figure 22–11. Carefully measure and position the panel before welding.

12. Measure the diagonal dimensions for the side supports (**Figure 22–11F**). Be sure these dimensions match.
13. Temporarily install the front fender and inspect it for proper fit with the door and hood. If the clearance is NOT correct, it might be because the fender apron or the rail height is NOT correct.
14. Measure as previously described, and verify the overall dimensions once more before welding.

WELDING NEW PANELS/PARTS

When the position and dimensions of the new panel are satisfactory, it can be permanently welded in place. See **Figure 22–12.** Under ideal circumstances, the general welding procedure for panels should be:

1. Apply weld-through primer to bare metal surfaces.
2. Clamp parts in position (see **Figure 22–13**).
3. Tack weld parts in position (**Figure 22–14**).
4. Remeasure part positions.
5. Weld parts in final position. See **Figure 22–15** through **Figure 22–18.**
6. Grind cosmetic weld surfaces.

Remember that it is very important to duplicate exactly the location and number of original factory spot welds.

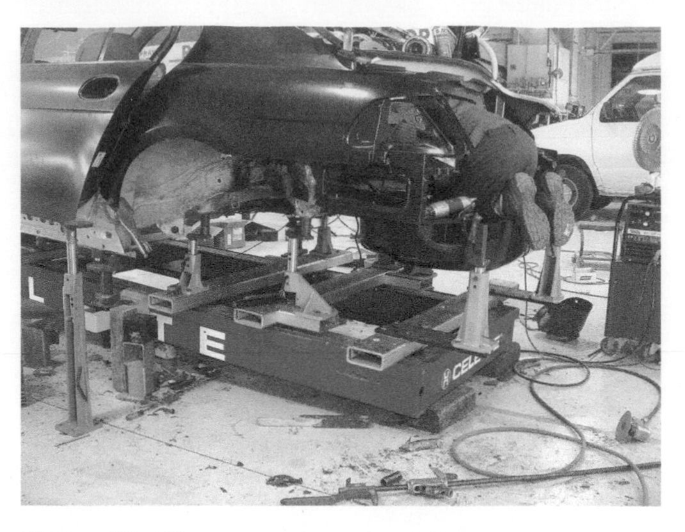

Figure 22–13. A frame rack and fixtures are being used to hold the panels in alignment before and during welding.

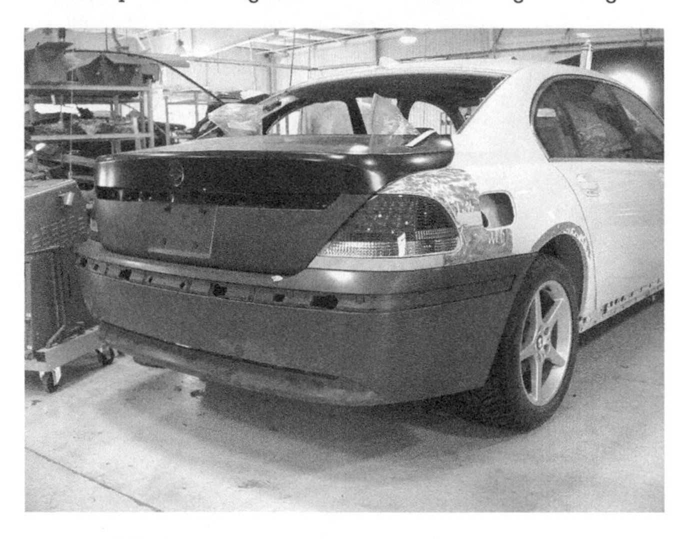

Figure 22–14. After tacking, screwing, or clamping the panels in place, many technicians like to fit on the doors, lids, bumpers, and other parts to make sure everything aligns before final welding.

SECTIONING

As mentioned, sectioning involves cutting and replacing panels at locations other than factory seams. When body parts need to be replaced, replacing them at factory seams is the logical first choice. However, this is impractical when many seams have to be separated in undamaged areas. In some repairs, sectioning of parts such as rails, pillars, and rocker panels may be required to make their repair economically feasible. See **Figure 22–19.**

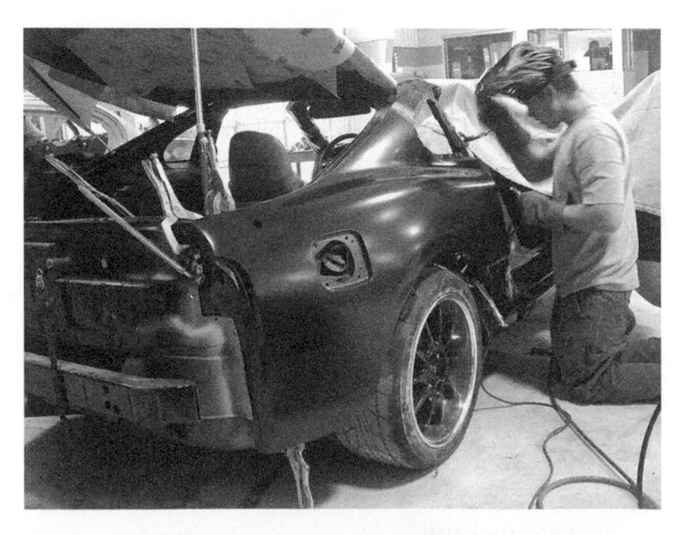

Figure 22–12. Once aligned with adjoining panels, plug, resistance spot, and continuous welds are then used to install the new panel

Using New Versus Recycled Assemblies

Recycled assemblies are undamaged parts from another damaged vehicle that are used for repairs. The use of recycled assemblies in collision repair makes sense for a number of reasons:

1. Fewer welds need to be made when using recycled assemblies compared to new, separate parts.
2. Less factory corrosion protection is disturbed.
3. Less measuring is required than when welding separate new parts and attaching them to the vehicle.
4. There is an abundance of recycled assemblies available in most areas.

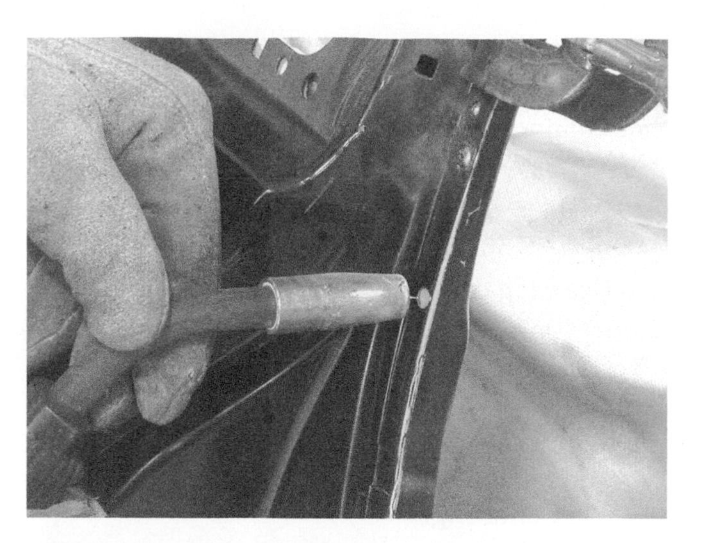

(A) With the new panel clamped and aligned, hold the welder gun straight over the hole to be filled with weld bead.

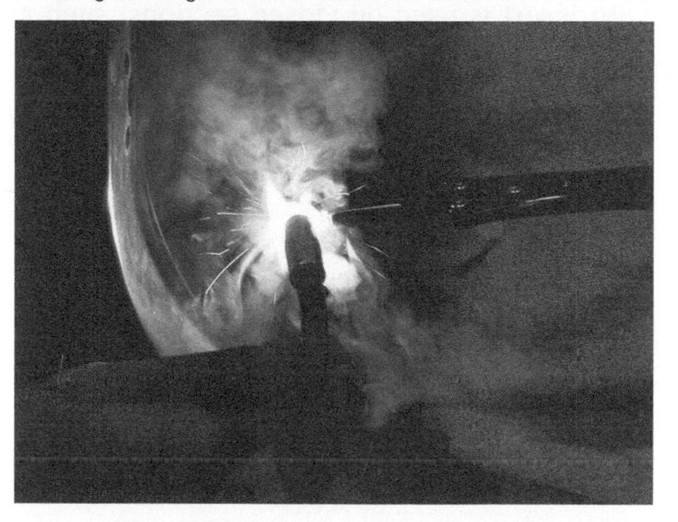

(B) Make your plug weld by moving the welder gun in a small circular motion while triggering the machine.

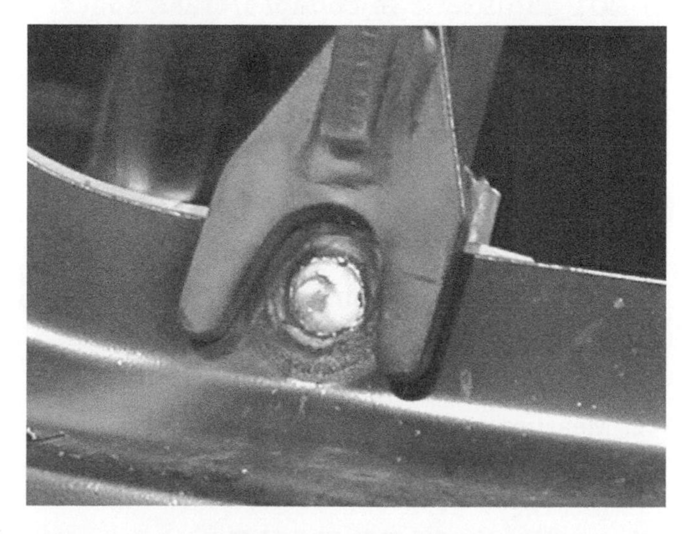

(C) Special plug weld pliers hold the panels tightly together while making the plug weld. Note the good penetration and how the weld nugget is almost flush with the flange.

Figure 22–15. Plug welds are the most common type used to install structural parts. Study the basic steps.

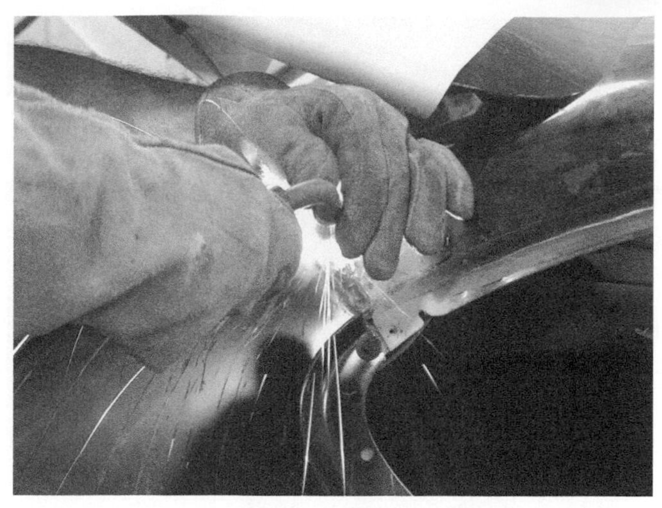

Figure 22–16. Continuous welds are needed on the exposed surfaces of the replacement panels. Avoid excessive heat buildup that will warp sheet metal.

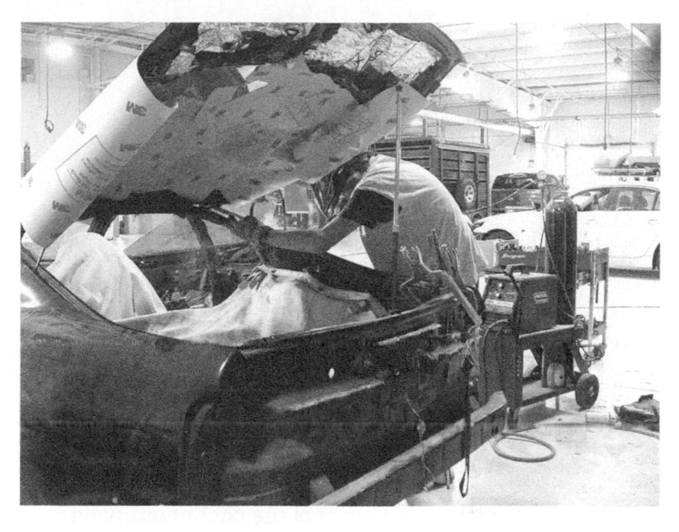

Figure 22–17. Weld blankets and welding paper have been used to cover the interior and glass on this vehicle. Welding and cutting sparks will pit glass or burn holes in upholstery.

Section Joints

A butt joint with insert is used mainly on closed sections, such as rocker panels, A- and B-pillars, and rails. *Inserts* make it easy to fit and align the joints correctly. They also help make the welding process easier. Refer to **Figure 22–20.**

Another basic joint is an **offset butt joint** without an insert. This type is also known as a *staggered butt joint.* The staggered butt joint is used on A- and B-pillars and front rails.

The third type is a lap joint, which is used on rear rails, floor pans, trunk floors, and B-pillars.

The configuration and makeup of the part being sectioned might call for a combination of joint types. Sectioning a B-pillar, for instance, might require the use of an offset cut with a butt joint in the outside piece and a lap joint in the inside piece.

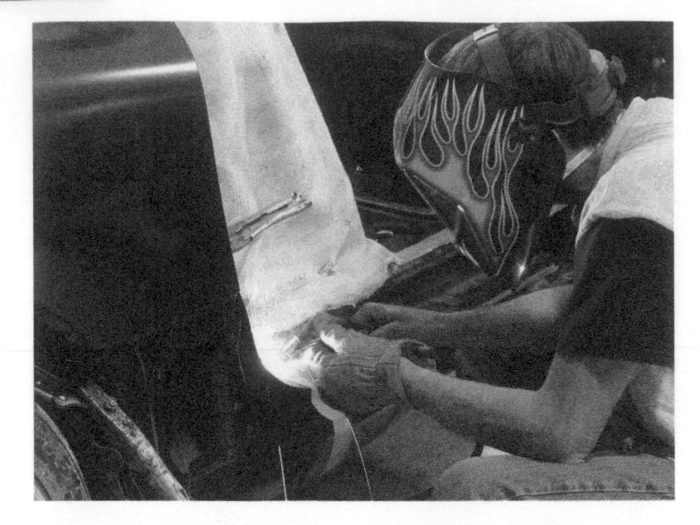

(A) When making a continuous weld bead, only weld an inch or so at a time to avoid too much heat transfer into the panels.

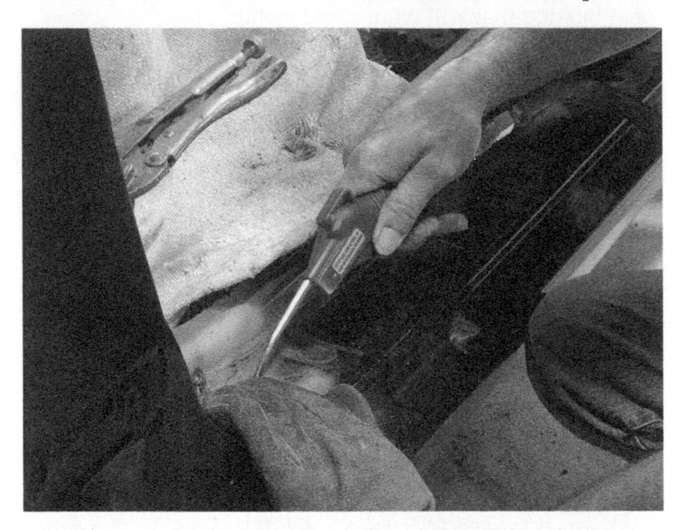

(B) An air blow gun will help cool the continuous weld bead quickly.

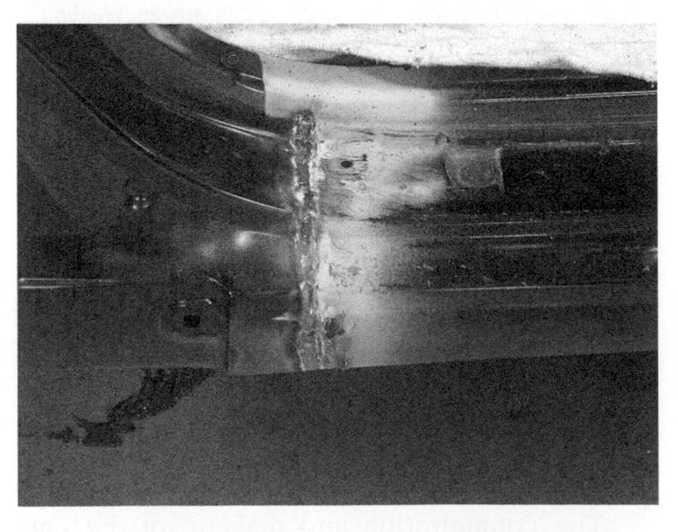

(C) Complete the continuous weld in sections, allowing it to cool before continuing.

Figure 22–18. Here the technician is welding a new quarter panel to the rocker panel.

Using Lap Joints. Lap joints are used on floor pans, trunk floors, rear rails, and other flat or hat channel shaped parts.

When welding lap joints:

1. Parts should be overlapped ¼ inch to 1 inch (6 to 25 mm) or as specified.
2. Use plug or resistance spot welds in the overlap area. Weld from the top piece down.
3. Close the bottom edge of the panels with a continuous weld bead.
4. Apply seam sealer to lap joints in floor pans and trunk floors to prevent water and fumes from entering.

Using Butt Joint with Insert. The butt joint with insert is used on closed sections, such as rocker panels, sail panels, A-pillars, B-pillars, and front rails.

The insert is made from a section of either the replacement or damaged part. Refer to **Figure 22–21.** The insert is used for the following reasons:

1. It provides a backing for the MIG butt weld.
2. It keeps burn-through to a minimum.
3. It ensures a completely closed joint.
4. It aligns the parts for the best possible fit.

NOTE

When sectioning front and rear rails, DO NOT put inserts in collapse/crush zones. Strengthening these parts will change the way collision damage is absorbed, possibly endangering the passengers.

Sectioning Front Rails—Insert Method

The procedures for front rail sectioning using a butt joint with insert are as follows:

1. Decide where to section the damaged part.
2. Measure and mark cuts on both panels. Make cuts along the marked lines. See **Figure 22–22.**

! WARNING !

Do NOT throw any parts away until the repair is finished.

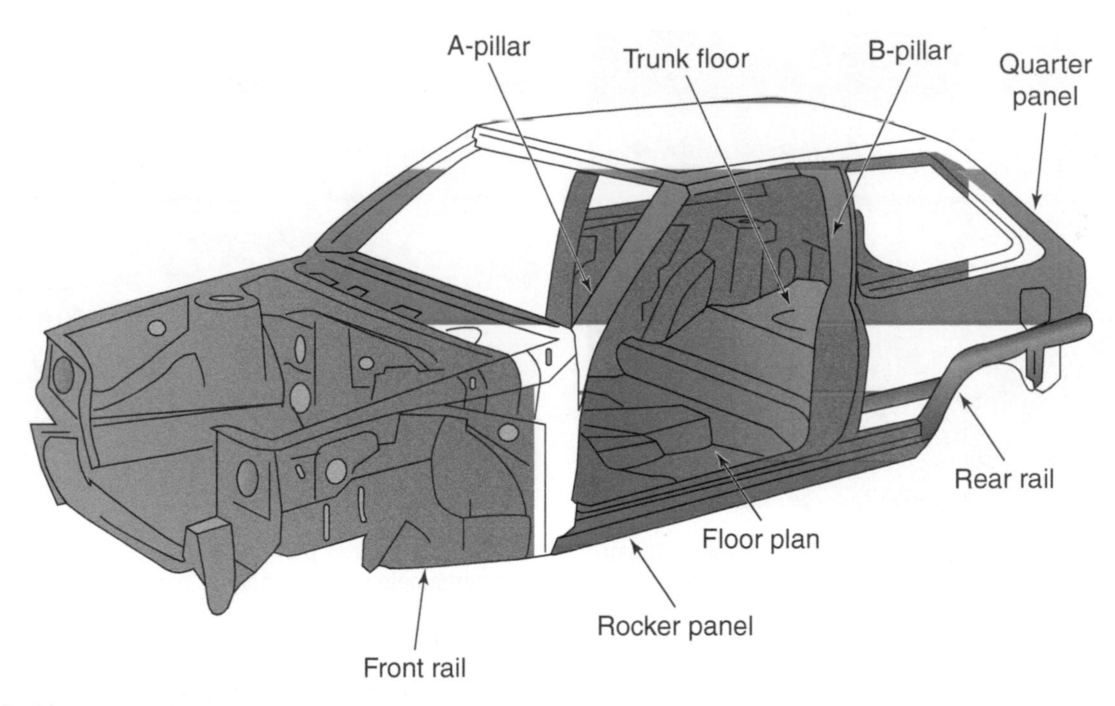

Figure 22–19. Note these common sectioning areas on a vehicle.

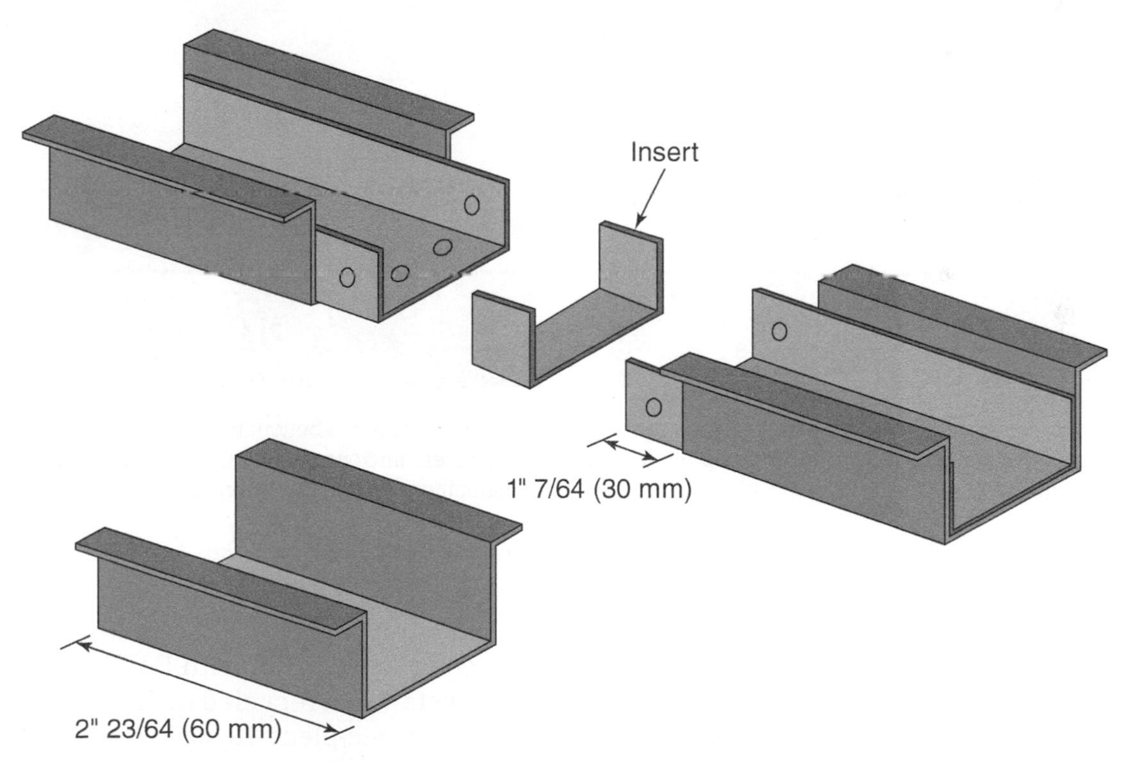

Figure 22–20. An insert can be made by cutting off excess material from the new or old part. It makes the weld much stronger and lowers the weld bead more flush with the top of the panels. (Courtesy of Nissan North America, Inc.)

3. Make and fit an insert into the rail sections.
4. Drill plug weld holes as needed.
5. Grind down burrs from all panel flanges.
6. Remove all paint, undercoating, and seam sealers but do NOT remove galvanizing.
7. Apply weld-through primer to bare metal flanges.
8. Fit the insert into place and tack weld it.
9. Butt the pieces, leaving a gap the thickness of the panels being welded.

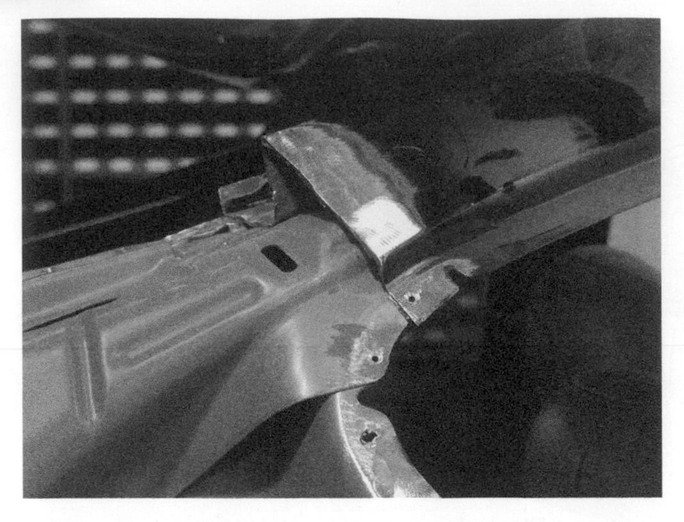

(A) The sail panel has been cut so that about a 1/8-inch gap exists between it and the new quarter panel. The weld surface has been ground clean.

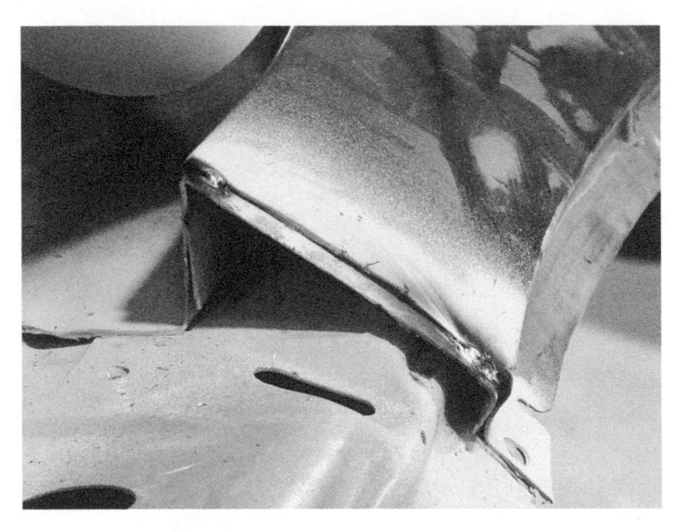

(B) An insert has been tack welded into place under the sail panel. The existing panel and insert have been sprayed with weld-through primer.

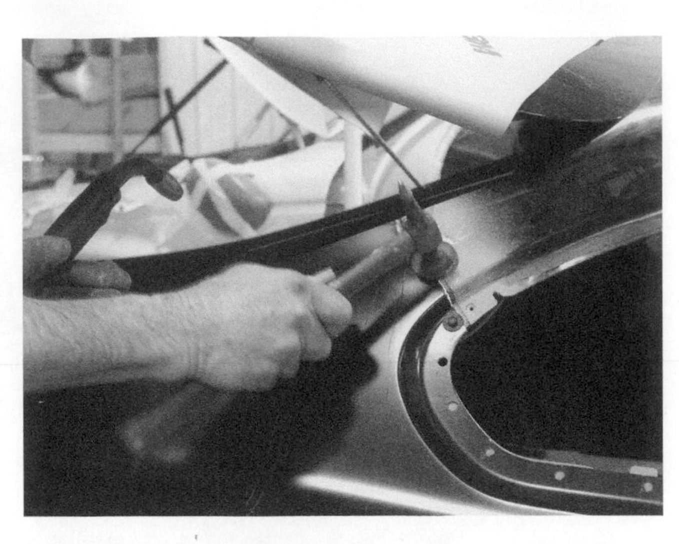

(C) The new quarter panel has been positioned. A body hammer is being used to final fit parts before welding.

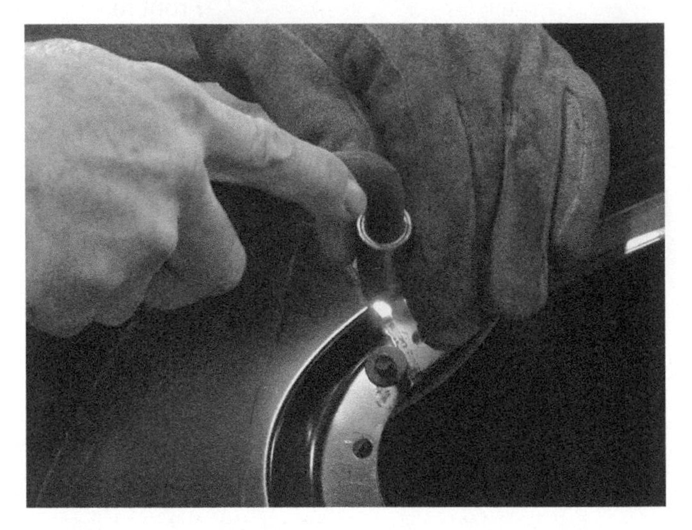

(D) Weld a small gap between the panels to join the roof panel, insert, and quarter panel. Cool the panels several times while doing your continuous weld to avoid panel warpage.

Figure 22–21. Note the major steps for using an insert when making a continuous weld at the top of a quarter panel.

10. Tack weld and measure alignment of parts.
11. Final weld parts.
12. Prep for rust protection, primer, and paint.

Sectioning Rocker Panels

When sectioning rocker panels, the two joints most commonly used are a butt joint with insert or a lap joint. In some cases, only the outer panel is replaced or the rocker may be replaced with or without the B-pillar attached. If the B-pillar is attached, then a B-pillar section will have to be made at the same time.

Use a butt weld with insert when installing a recycled rocker panel with B-pillar attached, or when installing a recycled quarter panel. If working on a three-piece design, remove the outer panel first.

Sectioning Multi-Part Rocker Panels

The **multiple part rocker** assembly is made up of several pieces of sheet metal with internal reinforcements. Reinforcements make it more difficult to use inserts. It is also more important to plan the exact order the work will be done. This will ensure that all the welding will be done in the right sequence. Also, the various rocker

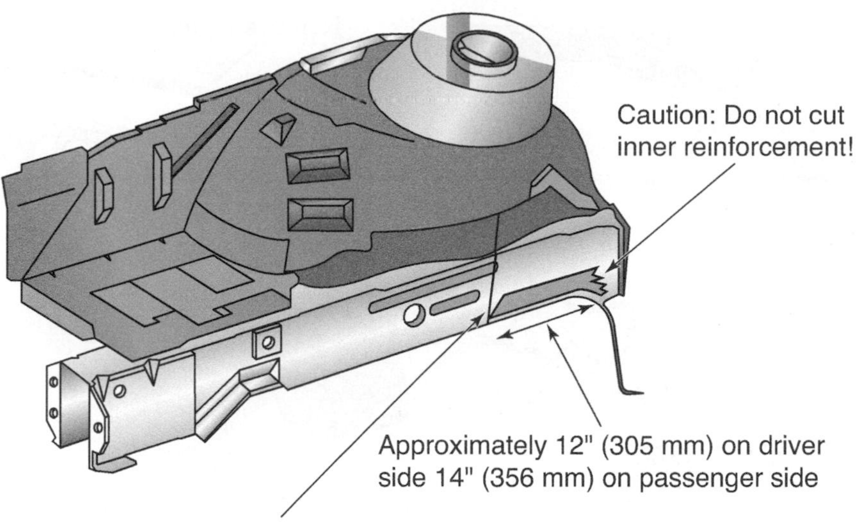

Figure 22–22. Since the sectioning of the front frame rails is critical to the integrity of the vehicle, use great care. This is a typical example on a unibody vehicle. Always refer to the manufacturer's procedures and do not cut inner reinforcements. (Courtesy of Tech-Cor, Inc.)

parts will be cut so as to provide maximum reinforcement to one another.

Sectioning A-Pillars

A-pillars use either two- or multiple-piece construction. They can be sectioned using a butt joint with insert or an offset butt joint.

A butt joint with insert or an offset butt joint can be used on two-piece A-pillars. On multiple-piece A-pillars, the design of the part will guide repair planning. There is often an inner reinforcement at the upper and lower ends, so an offset butt joint may be the only choice. Reinforcement locations vary, so refer to a body repair manual to properly plan the repair. Use an insert if the design of a multiple-piece pillar allows.

Sectioning A-Pillars—Insert Method

Sectioning an A-pillar is similar to sectioning other closed sections. To section an A-pillar using a butt joint with insert:

1. Plan the cut near the middle of the pillar. See **Figure 22–23.**
2. Remove the damaged part section.
3. Measure and cut the replacement part.
4. Make and fit the insert.
5. Drill plug weld holes as needed.
6. Fit the insert into place and secure it.
7. Butt the pieces together, leaving a gap about the thickness of the panels being welded.
8. Tack weld and measure alignment of panels.
9. Final weld panels.
10. Prep for rust protection, prime, and paint.

Replacing Foam Fillers

Some manufacturers place foam inside panels/components. **Foam fillers** are used to add rigidity and strength to structural parts. They also reduce noise and vibrations. Cutting and welding will damage the foam filler. Replacing the foam fillers must be part of the repair procedure.

Some vehicle manufacturers are using urethane foam in A- and B-pillars, and other locations. The manufacturer may or may not consider the foam filler to be structural. The use and location of foam fillers are different from vehicle to vehicle. Follow manufacturer's recommendations for replacing or sectioning foam-filled panels.

Some OEM replacement parts come with the foam already in the part. When the parts come without foam filler, or foam filler needs to be replaced, a product designed specifically for this application must be used to fill the panel.

! WARNING !

Single-part urethane foams made for home use CANNOT be used for replacing automotive foam fillers.

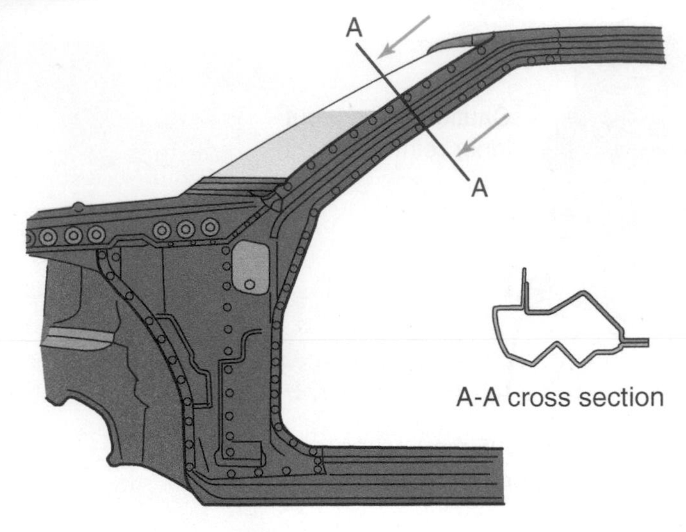

(A) Note a typical location of the area to be cut and of the spot welds that must be removed to replace an A-pillar.

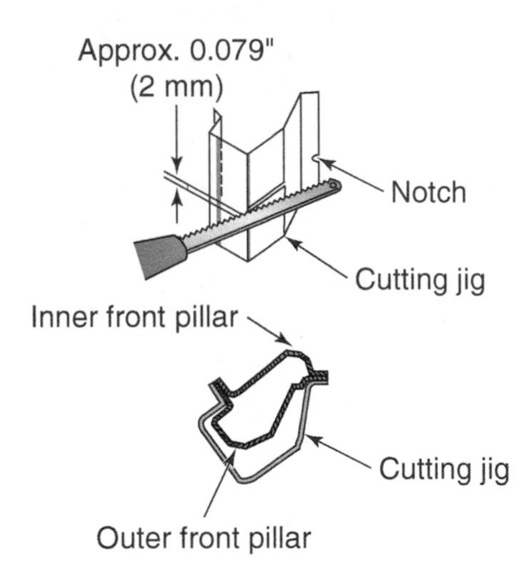

(B) A cutting jig can be made and placed over the component to help you make a straight cut through the pillar.

Figure 22–23. Sectioning A-pillars is similar to sectioning other parts. Check the manufacturer's recommendations for the exact procedure. (Courtesy of Nissan North America, Inc.)

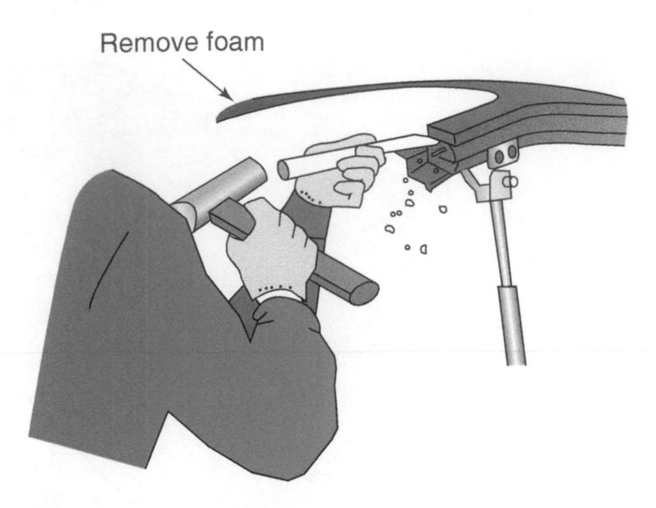

(A) After cutting off the damaged component, remove the foam from the area to be welded.

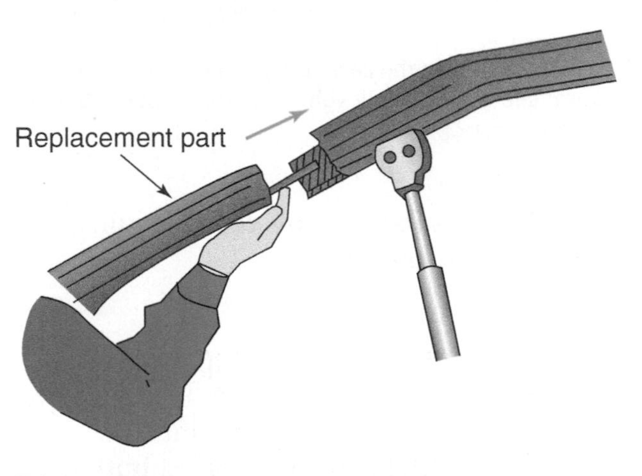

(B) Fit the replacement component with cut on the vehicle.

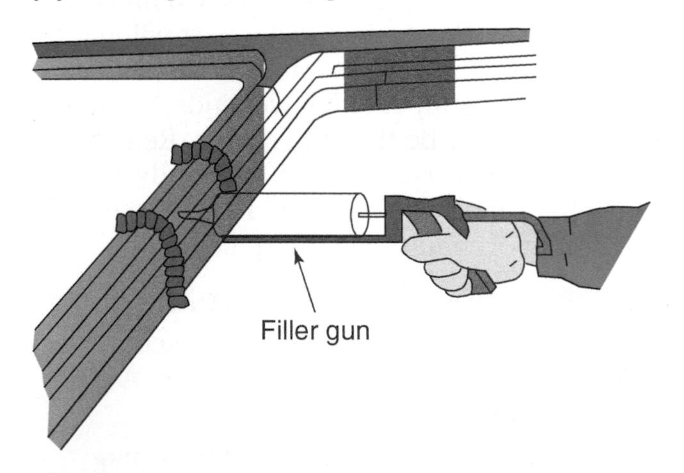

(C) After welding, inject the recommended type of foam into the panel.

Figure 22–24. Study the basic steps for replacing a part filled with foam. (Used with permission from Nissan North America, Inc.)

Remember! Cutting and welding will damage the foam. Replacing the foam fillers must be part of the repair procedure. When sectioning foam-filled A-pillars, the foam filler is removed in the repair area. It is then replaced after all welding is completed. See **Figure 22–24.**

Sectioning Floors

Floor pans and trunk floors are sectioned using lap joints. It is critical to completely seal the joints following the sectioning procedure to keep moisture and exhaust gases out of the passenger compartment. Do NOT cut through any reinforcements or critical areas, such as seat belt anchoring points.

When sectioning floor pans and trunk floors, the rear section always overlaps the front section. This allows road splash to stream past the bottom edge of the joint and NOT strike the joint head on.

Full Body Sectioning

One of the most drastic repairs that can be performed is full body sectioning. **Full body sectioning** is replacing the entire rear section of a collision damaged vehicle with the rear section of a salvage vehicle. It may be more economical than trying to rebuild the damaged vehicle using new parts. Full body sectioning requires the highest-quality workmanship possible.

Jigs are often used to help locate and guide the cut when sectioning. They are used on any sectioning procedure where an offset butt joint is used. Precise cuts are essential when sectioning.

Full body sectioning procedures require sectioning the two A-pillars, two rocker panels, and the floor pan. When this procedure is properly performed, sectioned vehicles have been shown to be as strong and serviceable as an undamaged vehicle.

Full body sectioning is complicated by antilock brake systems (ABS). The replacement vehicle must be so equipped, or the ABS parts must be retrofitted.

Location and function of body computers may change, even within the same production year of a given vehicle. Check the locations of these computers on both the damaged vehicle and the salvage section.

When performing a full body sectioning, complete disclosure must be made to the vehicle owner. A conference between the owner, insurance appraiser, and repairer is suggested. Then all parties will be aware of exactly what will be done to repair the vehicle.

Replacing Adhesives

Some vehicle manufacturers use structural adhesives along certain weld seams. These two-part epoxy adhesives are sometimes called **weld-bond adhesives** because spot welds are placed through the adhesive.

Weld-bond adhesives are used to add strength and rigidity to the vehicle body. They also improve rust protection in weld seams. Adhesives also help control noise and vibrations.

Parts most commonly weld-bonded are:

1. A- and B-pillars
2. Rocker panels
3. Roof panels
4. Rear quarter panels

If adhesives are disturbed by repairs, they must be replaced. Follow recommendations in the body repair manual.

Some manufacturers use *structural adhesives* in place of welds. One example is around the wheel openings and sail panel reinforcement. This is a different type of adhesive than the weld-bond adhesive. Check the body repair manual for information on the use of structural adhesives.

RUST (CORROSION)

Rust, or *corrosion,* is a chemical reaction, called **oxidation,** formed when three ingredients are present:

1. Oxygen
2. Exposed metal
3. Moisture

Oxidation occurs in two steps:

1. Stable metal and oxygen atoms break down into positively and negatively charged particles called ions.
2. These ions are unstable, and they combine with each other to form metal oxides, which are more stable.

A necessary ingredient for oxidation to occur is an electrolyte.

1. An electrolyte usually is moisture.
2. Moisture is the only part of the oxidation process that repair shops can do anything about.
3. Moisture is controlled by applying coatings to the metal surface to act as a moisture barrier.
4. Coatings do break down with weather exposure.
5. The best coating systems are those that last the longest.
6. Coatings only slow down the process of corrosion. Stopping it permanently is a difficult challenge.

Rust Protection

Even with all of the care taken to protect vehicles, corrosion protection breakdown still occurs. The breakdown falls into three general categories:

1. Paint film failure
2. Collision damage
3. Repair process

During a collision, the protective coatings on a vehicle are damaged. This occurs not just in the areas of direct impact, but also in the indirect damage zones. Seams pull apart, caulking breaks loose, and paint chips and flakes. Locating the damage and restoring the protection to all affected areas remains a key challenge for the collision repair technician.

Even touching a bare metal surface with bare hands adds corrosion-causing agents. Make sure bare hands do NOT contact bare metal that has been cleaned for refinishing.

When dealing with the zinc coating on a galvanized body structure, there are two important things to remember:

1. If at all possible, do NOT remove it.
2. If it must be removed, replace it. See **Figure 22–25.**

To be effective, the coating must be applied to a clean surface. The coating must also be tight and unbroken.

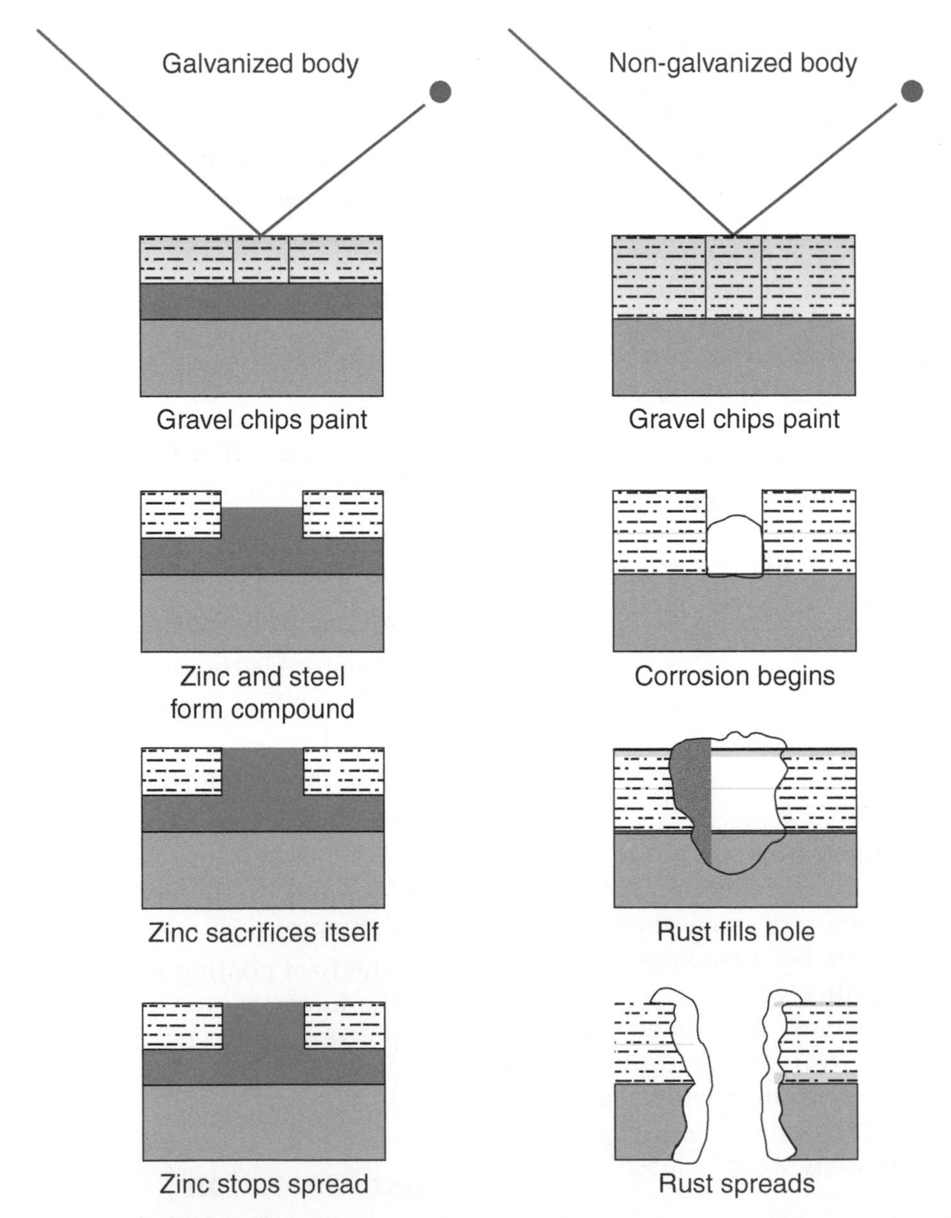

Figure 22–25. Note how corrosion attacks galvanized and nongalvanized parts. (Courtesy of Volkswagen of America)

When performing collision repairs:

1. Preserve the original coating as much as possible.
2. Use conversion coatings to create a zinc phosphate coating on the steel surface.
3. Use weld-through primers on bare steel in weld areas.

The collision repair shop's interest in corrosion is twofold. First, the technician must be able to repair corrosion damage. Second, the technician must be able to provide treatment that will prevent corrosion from recurring.

When restoring corrosion protection:

1. Use a complete system.
2. Do NOT mix different manufacturers' products.
3. Follow manufacturer's instructions.
4. Do NOT skip steps.

Corrosion Protection Safety

As with other materials used in collision repair, the use of corrosion protection materials requires that you follow safety rules. The most basic rules are:

1. Epoxy systems can create skin irritation, so wear gloves and avoid skin contact.
2. If skin contact has occurred, wash the affected area with soap and hot water. Then apply a skin cream.
3. If adhesive accidentally contacts the eyes, wash immediately with clean water for 15 minutes. Then consult a physician.
4. Spot welding in weld-bond joints can generate gases that can be harmful if inhaled. Be sure to work in a well-ventilated area and wear a respirator.

Anticorrosion Materials

Anticorrosion or rust-proofing materials can be divided into four broad categories:

1. **Anticorrosion compounds** are either wax- or petroleum-based anticorrosion compounds resistant to chipping and abrasion. They can undercoat, deaden sound, and completely seal the surface. They should be applied to the underbody and inside body panels so that they can penetrate into joints and body crevices to form a pliable, protective film.
2. *Seam sealers* prevent the penetration of water, mud, and fumes into panel joints. They serve the important role of preventing corrosion from forming between adjoining surfaces.
3. *Weld-through primers* are used between the two pieces of base metal at a weld joint.
4. *Corrosion converters* change ferrous (red) iron oxide to ferric (black/blue) iron oxide. Rust converters may also contain some type of latex emulsion that seals the surface after the conversion is complete. These products offer an interesting alternative for areas that cannot be completely cleaned.

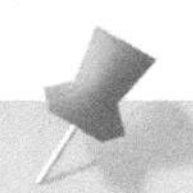

NOTE

Some manufacturers do not recommend the use of corrosion converters.

Applying Corrosion Protection Materials

Care is needed when applying anticorrosion compounds. Keep the material away from parts that conduct heat, electrical parts, labels and identification numbers, and moving parts. Avoid applying corrosion protection materials to:

1. Seat belt retractors and passive restraint guide rails
2. Hidden headlamp assemblies
3. Power window motors and cables
4. Exhaust system
5. Engine and accessories
6. Air filter
7. Air lift shock absorbers
8. Transmission parts
9. Shift linkages
10. Speedometer cables
11. Brake parts
12. Locks, key cylinders, and door latches

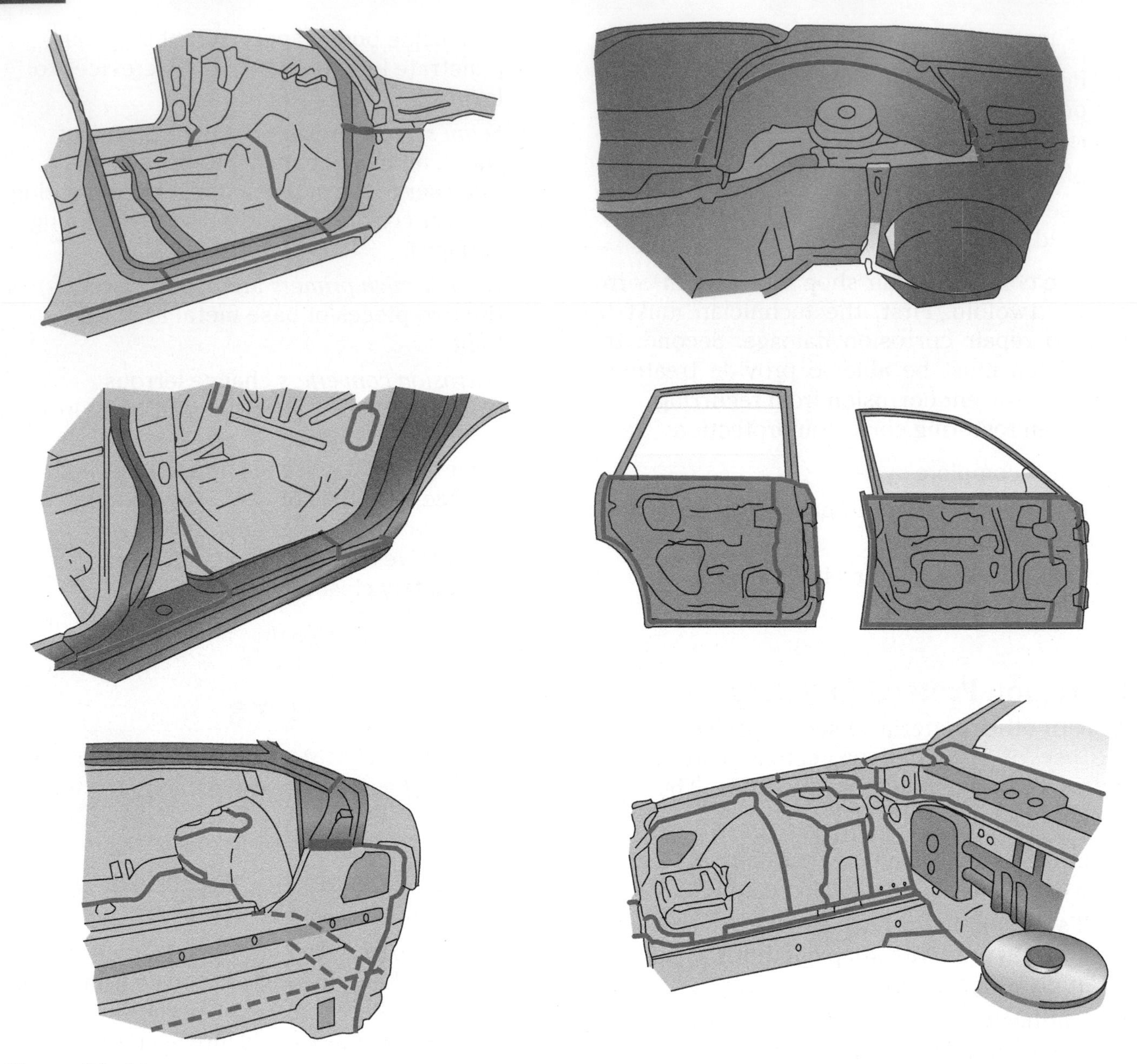

Figure 22–26. Seam sealers must be applied in a continuous bead along the edges of panels. (Courtesy of Nissan North America, Inc.)

13. Power antennas
14. Theft prevention labels
15. Drive shaft

The corrosion protection process for exposed joints and seams can be summed up as follows:

1. Thoroughly clean the joint or seam.
2. Apply primers and seam sealers (see **Figure 22–26**).
3. Apply final primer coat(s).
4. Apply paint.

In general, anticorrosion procedures for exposed exterior underbody surfaces are as follows:

1. Clean with a wax and grease remover. If needed, remove any loose sound-deadening materials. They can create moisture pockets for corrosion.
2. Prime with self-etch or epoxy primer.
3. Apply sealer and paint to primed areas.

Figure 22–27 shows how to install seam sealer to adjoining panels.

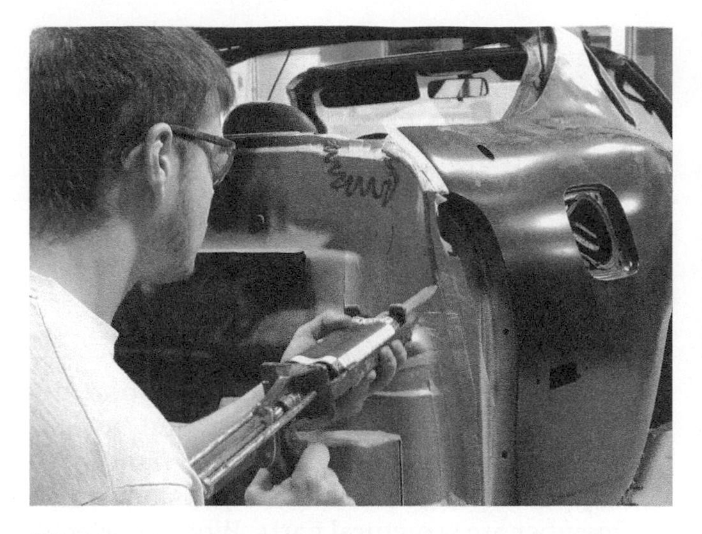

(A) After the self-etch primer has dried overnight, mask the area to be sealed. Leave an opening next to the panel flanges. Use your sealer gun to apply a generous bead of sealer.

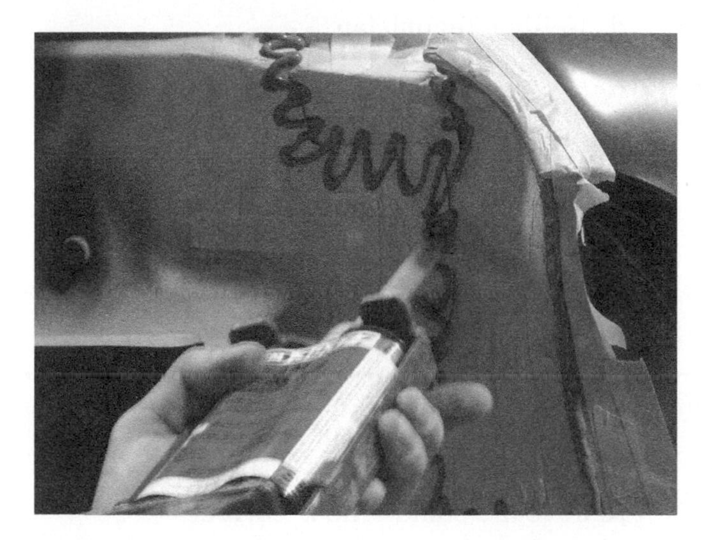

(B) Use a zigzag motion to apply the sealer to the panel flanges.

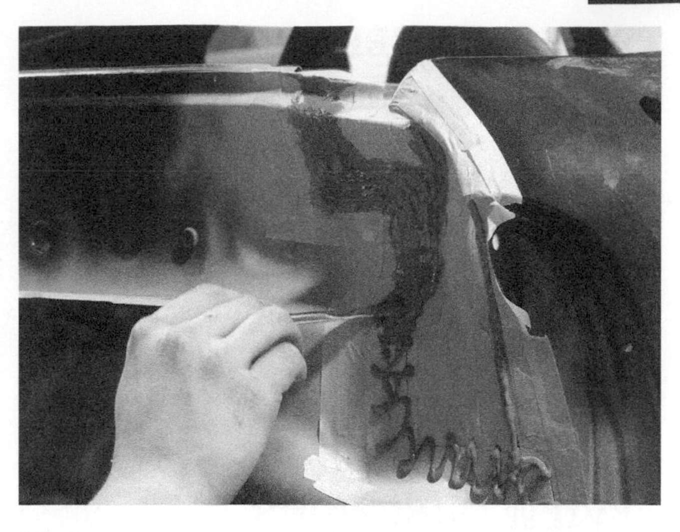

(C) Brush the sealer out smooth to match the appearance of the original sealer.

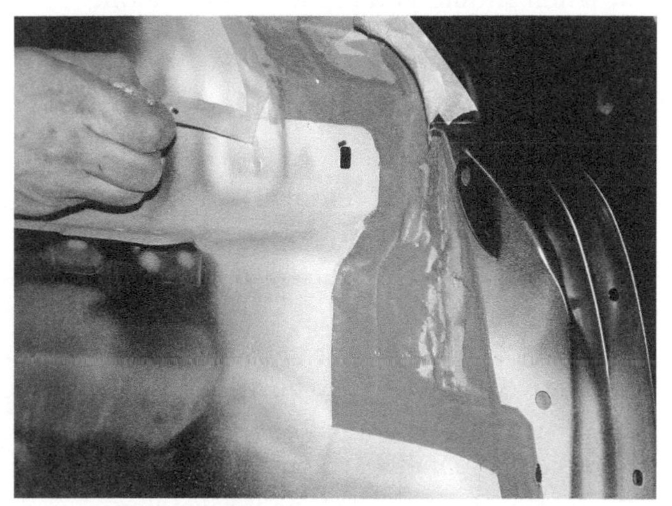

(D) Remove the masking and the area is ready for paint.

Figure 22–27. Study the major steps for installing seam sealer to protect welded panels from corrosion and to prevent water and air leaks.

SUMMARY

- Structural parts are those parts of a vehicle that support the weight of the vehicle, absorb collision energy, and absorb road shock.
- A simple rule regarding repairing versus replacement is:
  If the part is bent, repair it.
  If the part is kinked, replace it.
- Sectioning involves cutting and replacing panels at locations other than at factory seams. Sectioning of parts such as rails, pillars, and rocker panels may be required to make their repair economically feasible.
- Full body sectioning is replacing the entire rear section of a collision damaged vehicle with the rear section of a salvage vehicle. It may be more economical than trying to rebuild a damaged vehicle with new parts.
- Corrosion breakdown falls into three general categories: paint film failure; collision damage; and the repair process.

TECHNICAL TERMS

structural parts
factory seams
sectioning
panel alignment marks
recycled assemblies
offset butt joint
multiple part rocker
foam fillers
full body sectioning
jigs
weld-bond adhesives
oxidation
anticorrosion compounds

REVIEW QUESTIONS

1. List three functions of structural parts.
2. If the part is bent, ______________ it. If the part is kinked, ______________ it.
3. When should you replace panels along factory seams?
4. What is sectioning?
5. You should not section in or near these eight areas.
6. How do you start removal of a structural panel?
7. List five tools that can be used to remove spot welds.
8. A chisel should never be used by itself to remove spot welds. True or false?
9. All straightening must be done before replacing panels. True or false?
10. List the six general steps for welding panels.
11. These are three basic types of sectioning joints.
    a. Lap joint
    b. Offset butt joint
    c. Butt joint with insert
    d. All of the above
    e. None of the above
12. When cutting panels, *Technician A* uses a template. *Technician B* uses a jig. Who is correct?
    a. Technician A
    b. Technician B
    c. Both Technicians A and B
    d. Neither Technician
13. ______________ ______________ are used to add rigidity and strength to structural parts.
14. Avoid applying corrosion protection materials to these 15 areas or parts.

ASE-STYLE REVIEW QUESTIONS

1. *Technician A* says that the core support tie bar, front rails, strut towers, and rocker panels are structural parts. *Technician B* says that pillars and the suspension cross-member are structural parts. Who is correct?
    a. Technician A
    b. Technician B
    c. Both Technicians A and B
    d. Neither Technician

2. Which of the following locations can be sectioned?
    a. Suspension mounting locations
    b. Structural part mounting locations
    c. Dimensional reference holes
    d. Uniform area with clearance

3. To find spot welds on a damaged panel, *Technician A* uses a coarse scuff wheel mounted in an air tool. *Technician B* heats the panel until the metal glows red hot to remove the paint. Who is correct?
    a. Technician A
    b. Technician B
    c. Both Technicians A and B
    d. Neither Technician

4. When removing spot welds, *Technician A* drills through the top and bottom panel. *Technician B* drills through the top panel only. Who is correct?
    a. Technician A
    b. Technician B
    c. Both Technicians A and B
    d. Neither Technician

5. When preparing a new structural panel for installation, *Technician A* applies weld-through primer to areas where bare metal is

exposed. *Technician B* duplicates the location and number of spot welds used at the factory. Who is correct?

a. Technician A
b. Technician B
c. Both Technicians A and B
d. Neither Technician

6. *Technician A* says to remove the vehicle from the straightening bench before starting installation of new parts. *Technician B* says that further straightening may be needed after installation of new structural parts. Who is correct?

a. Technician A
b. Technician B
c. Both Technicians A and B
d. Neither Technician

7. When determining where to use new or recycled assemblies for structural repairs, *Technician A* says that less factory corrosion protection is disturbed when using recycled parts. *Technician B* says that more measuring is required when welding separate new parts and attaching them to the vehicle. Who is correct?

a. Technician A
b. Technician B
c. Both Technicians A and B
d. Neither Technician

8. *Technician A* uses a butt joint with insert rocker panels, A-pillars, B-pillars, and front rails. *Technician B* uses a butt joint with insert on floor pans and hoods. Who is correct?

a. Technician A
b. Technician B
c. Both Technicians A and B
d. Neither Technician

9. A-pillars with multiple piece construction must be sectioned. *Technician A* is going to use a butt joint with insert. *Technician B* is going to use an offset butt joint. Who is correct?

a. Technician A
b. Technician B
c. Both Technicians A and B
d. Neither Technician

10. A floor is going to be sectioned. *Technician A* says to cut the replacement panel to overlap the existing panel by at least 1 inch (25 mm). *Technician B* says to tack weld the panel in place and remeasure before final welding. Who is correct?

a. Technician A
b. Technician B
c. Both Technicians A and B
d. Neither Technician

ACTIVITIES

1. Inspect a damaged vehicle. List the structural parts that would require replacement.
2. On the same vehicle, summarize the procedures for structural part replacement.
3. Visit a collision repair shop. Ask the owner to allow you to watch a technician replacing a structural part.

CHAPTER

23 Interior Repairs

OBJECTIVES

After studying this chapter, you should be able to:

- Identify the major parts of a vehicle's interior.
- Remove and replace seats, seat covers, and carpeting.
- Service an instrument cluster and other dashboard parts.
- Explain how to replace headliners.

INTRODUCTION

During a collision, interior parts can be damaged. The dashboard, steering wheel, and other parts can all be damaged. This would include headliners, seats, and other related parts. Interior parts may need to be removed and reinstalled when replacing quarter panels, door panels, roof panels, and other structural parts. For this reason, you should be familiar with procedures for replacing interior parts.

SEAT SERVICE

Seats are often damaged during a collision. They can be damaged by the inertia of the occupant, by side impact intrusion into the passenger compartment, or by stains. You might also have to remove seats for carpet replacement or floor panel repairs.

A **bucket seat** is a single seat for one person. A **bench seat** is a longer seat for several people. Both require similar methods during service.

Seat Removal

Four bolts normally secure the seat to the floor. To remove the front seat hold-down bolts, slide the seat fully backward. This will allow easier access to the front bolts. Then slide the seat forward to remove the two rear hold-down bolts.

After disconnecting any wiring and other parts attached to the seat, carefully lift it out of the vehicle.

A rear bench seat is often held in position by screws or spring-loaded clips. The screws are normally at the front bottom of the seat. When removed, the seat can be pushed back and lifted up and out.

With spring clips, use your hands to force the seat down and back. This will free the hidden clips and allow you to lift the bench seat out.

Seat Parts

Figure 23–1 shows the parts of a typical front seat:

1. **Seat cushion**—bottom section of the seat, which includes cover, padding, and frame

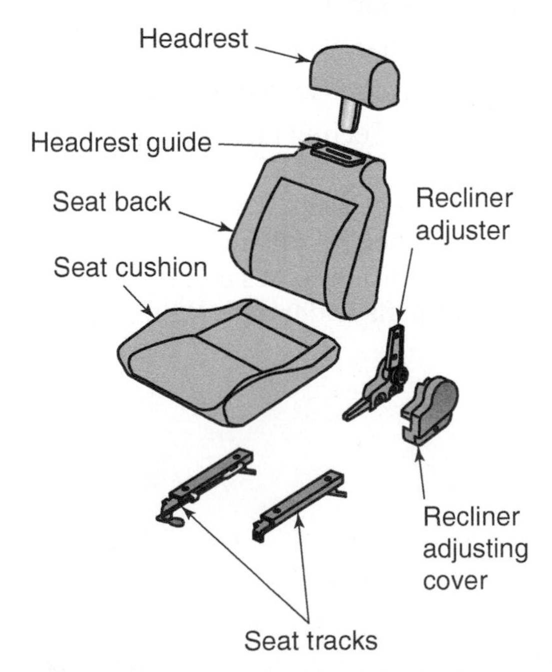

Figure 23–1. Note the major parts of a typical bucket seat. Seat tracks wear out and can be damaged in collision. Four bolts normally secure the seat tracks and seat to the vehicle floor.

2. **Seat back**—rear assembly that includes cover, padding, and metal frame
3. **Headrest**—padded frame that fits into the top of the seat back
4. **Headrest guide**—sleeve that accepts headrest post and mounts in the seat back
5. **Recliner adjuster**—hinge mechanism that allows adjustment of the seat back to different angles
6. **Seat track**—mechanical slide mechanism that allows seat to be adjusted forward or rearward

Seat Cover Service

The seat cover is a cloth, vinyl, or leather cover over the seat assembly. The cover may require replacement when damaged. You must disassemble the seat to replace the covers. See **Figure 23–2.**

Hog rings and clips normally stretch and hold the seat cover over the seat frame and padding. They are located on the bottom of the seat cushion or rear of the seat back. Remove them and you can lift off the seat cover. The new cover can then be installed in reverse order of removal. Refer to Figure 23–2.

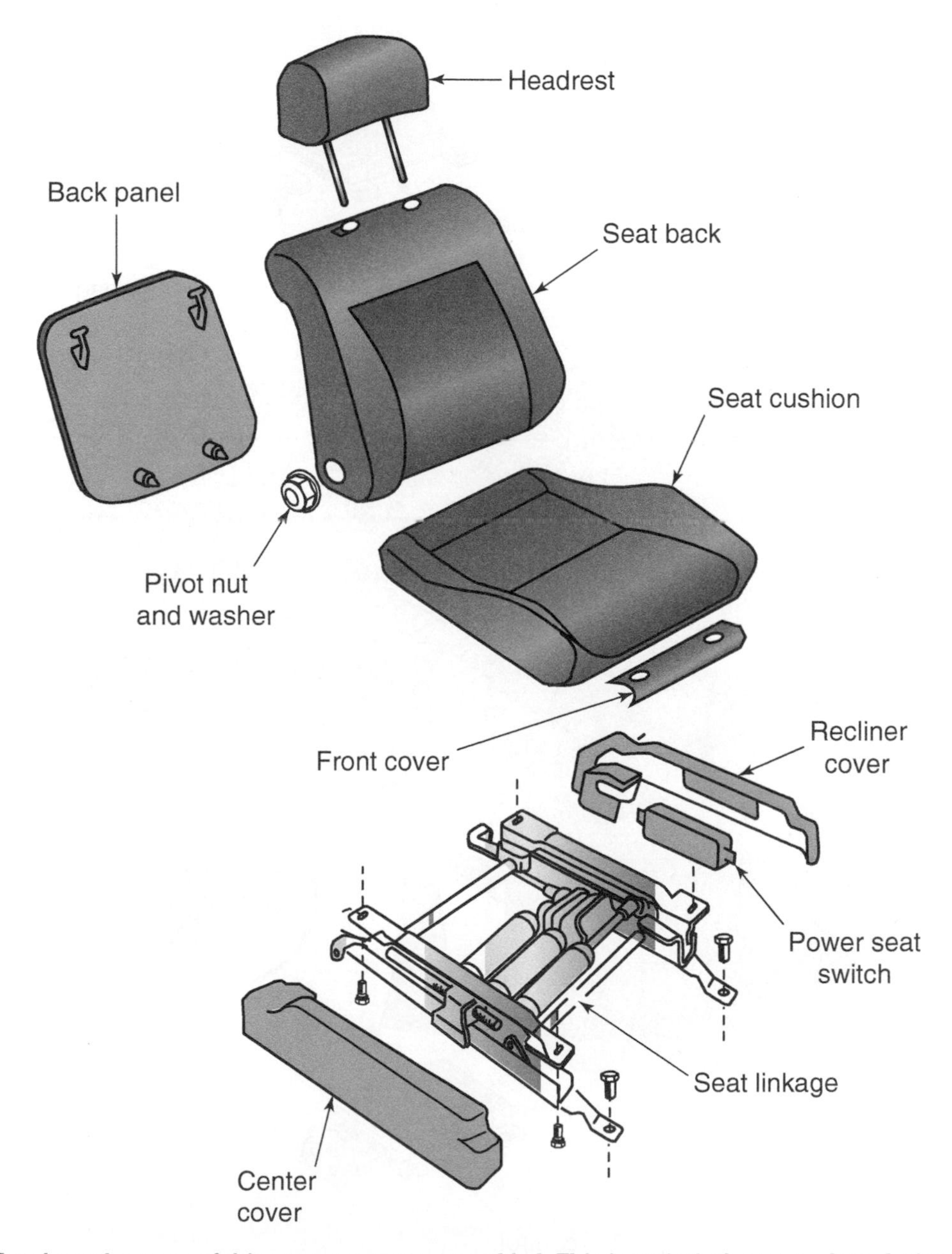

Figure 23–2. Note how the parts of this power seat are assembled. This is typical of most modern designs. The seat track or linkage assembly contains electric motors and a small transmission for seat movement.

CARPETING SERVICE

Carpeting can be stained or torn during a collision. If it cannot be cleaned with a strong carpet cleaner or if torn, the carpeting must be replaced. The major parts of *interior carpeting* are shown in **Figure 23–3.**

To replace carpeting, you must remove the seats, seat belt anchors, trim pieces, and any other parts mounted over the carpeting. This might include the console, any electronic control units, and wiring harness bolted down to the carpet. Screws and clips hold these parts and the carpet down into place. See Figure 23–3.

After removal, the new carpet is installed in the reverse order of removal. Make sure the new carpet is stretched out smooth and properly centered before installing any fasteners. An adhesive may be required between the carpet and floor in some locations. Refer to the service manual if in doubt.

HEADLINER SERVICE

A **headliner** is a cloth or vinyl cover over the inside of the roof in the passenger compartment. It can be torn or damaged during a collision. Some thick cloth or vinyl-covered foam

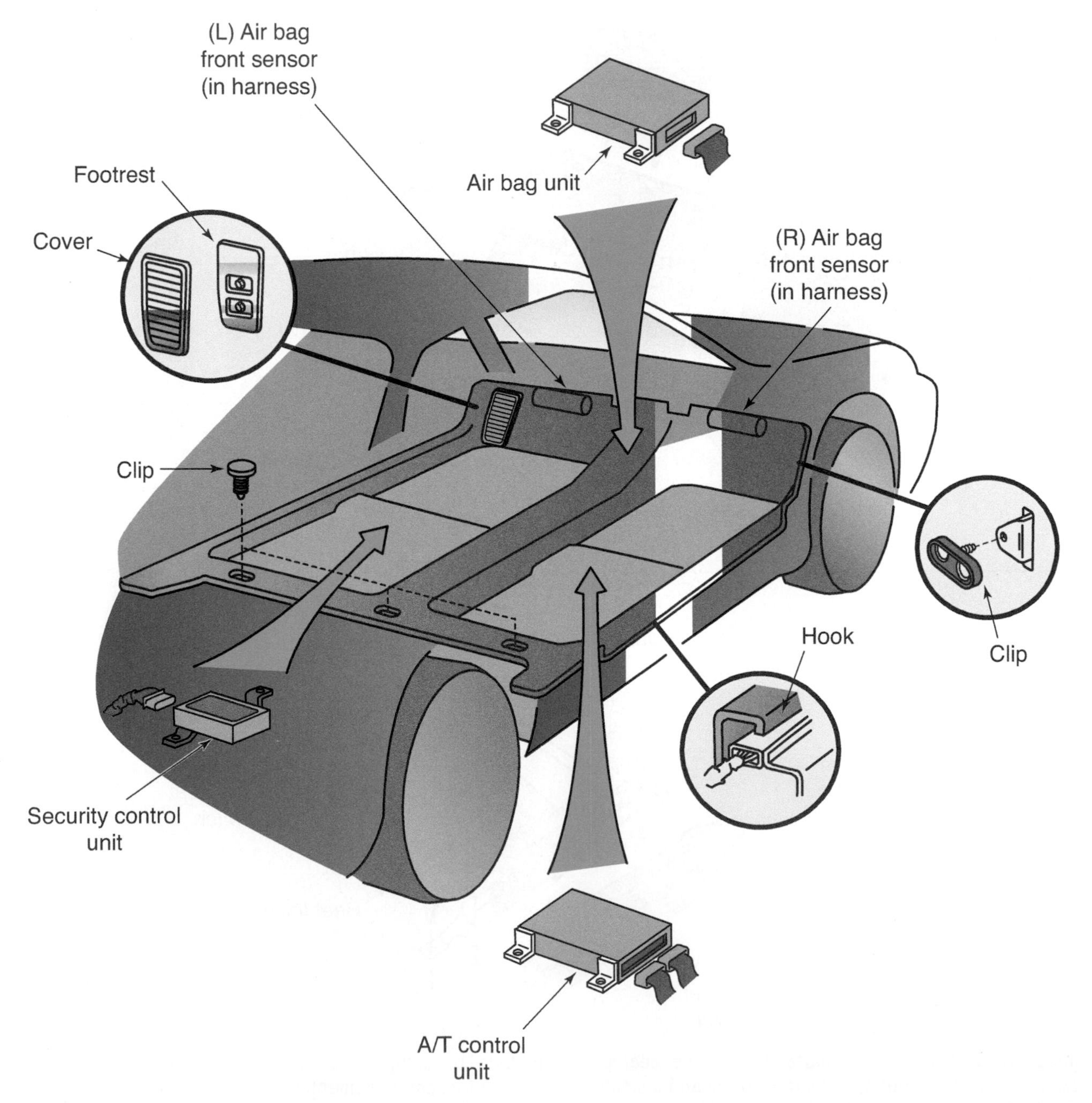

Figure 23–3. Note the various pads, clips, screws, tape, and control units that must be removed to replace carpeting in this vehicle.

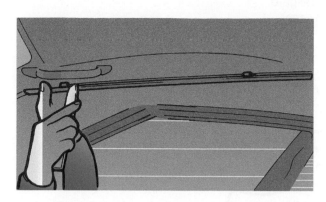

(A) Remove the roof side trip. A clip release tool is needed.

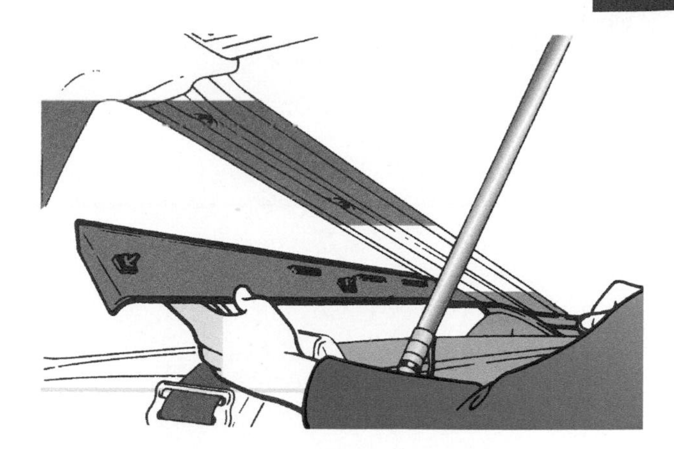

(C) Remove the rear pillar trip. Note the clips in the center of the trim piece.

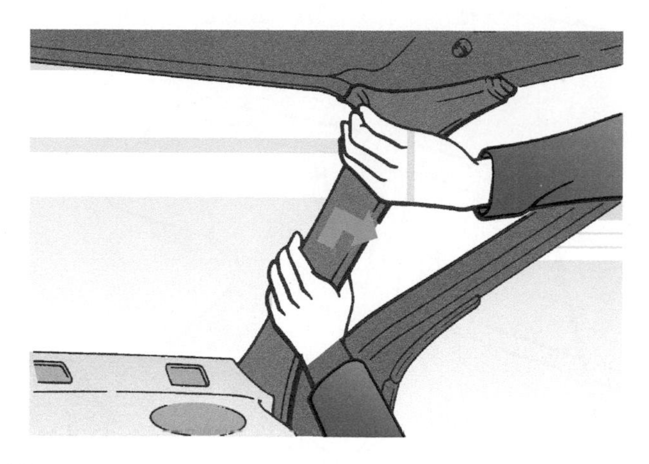

(B) Remove the front pillar trim. It is often held on with screws and/or plastic clips.

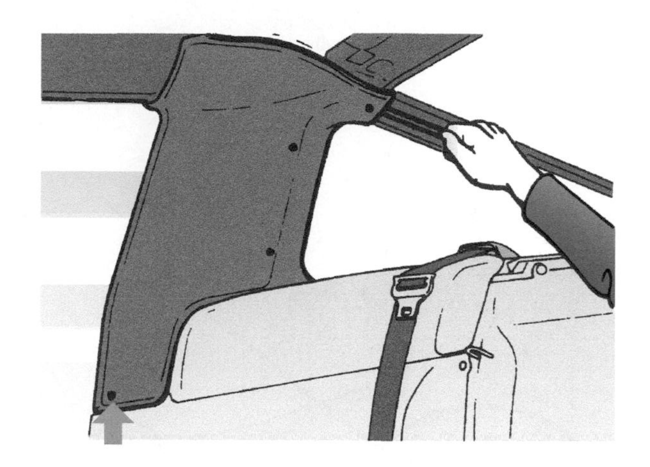

(D) Remove the upper quarter trim. Screws and clips may secure this piece.

Figure 23–4. These are parts that typically must be removed to replace a headliner. (Courtesy of DaimlerChrysler Corporation)

headliners are bonded directly to the roof panel. Others are thin vinyl suspended by metal rods and bonded around the edges of the roof.

To service a headliner, first remove all of the trim pieces around the edges of the roof. Various screws and clips secure the trim pieces. Refer to **Figure 23–4.** You may also have to remove the sun visors, grab handles, and other parts for headliner service. See **Figure 23–5.**

When installing a foam-backed headliner, be careful not to overbend and kink it. Center it in position. Then install it in reverse order of removal. Again, refer to the service manual if in doubt.

INSTRUMENT PANEL SERVICE

The *instrument panel* bolts in the front of the passenger compartment on the fire wall or cowl. It contains the instrument clusters, radio, glove box, vents, vinyl or leather-covered pad, and other parts.

When the instrument panel is damaged in a collision, it must be removed and replaced. An exploded view of a typical instrument panel is shown in **Figure 23–6.** Study the relationship of the parts.

Many instrument panel parts can be replaced without unbolting the dash pad. The instrument cluster, vents, and many trim pieces can be removed and replaced with the main part of the dash intact. Vents often snap into place. A thin screwdriver can often be used to release and remove most vents.

Some of the screws and bolts that secure the instrument panel parts can be difficult to find and remove. Some are along the bottom of the dash. Others are on the sides. A few fasteners can be inside openings in the instrument panel. You will have to remove parts to access these fasteners.

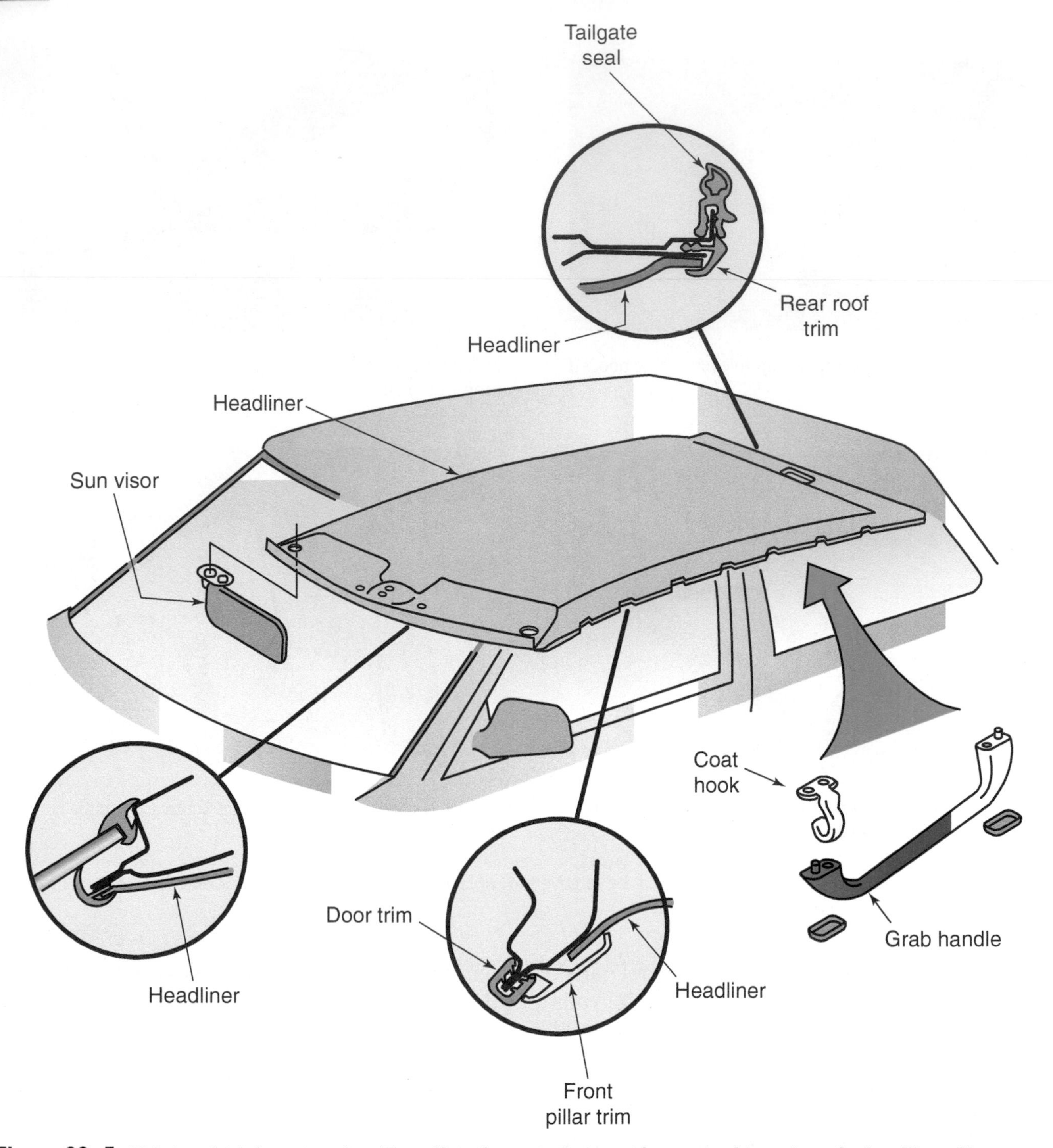

Figure 23–5. This is a thick foam-type headliner. Note the parts that must be serviced to replace the headliner. Also note how the headliner is held secure by trim pieces.

INSTRUMENT CLUSTER SERVICE

An **instrument cluster** contains the speedometer, gauges, indicator lights, and similar parts. It may require service when damaged in a collision or when parts are not working.

To service an instrument cluster, first disconnect the battery. This will prevent the chance of an electrical fire if wires short to ground.

Remove the instrument panel cover. Several screws secure it. Next, remove the screws that hold the cluster to the dash. Pull the cluster out far enough to disconnect the wires and speedometer cable. Then lift the cluster out. Bulbs can be replaced from the rear of the cluster.

To replace gauges or the speedometer, you must disassemble the cluster. To disassemble the instrument cluster, remove the small screws that hold the plastic lens plate over the housing.

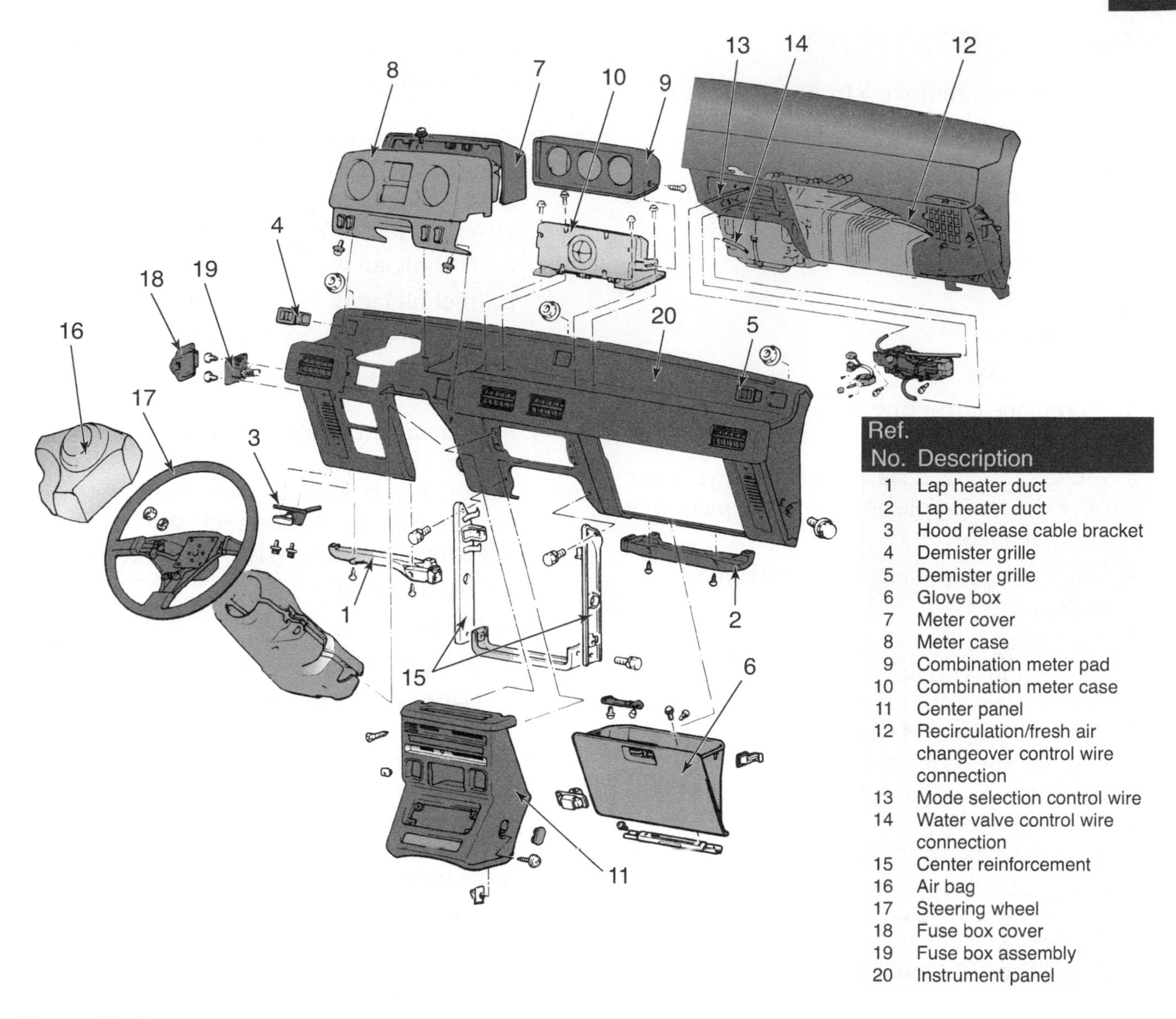

Ref. No.	Description
1	Lap heater duct
2	Lap heater duct
3	Hood release cable bracket
4	Demister grille
5	Demister grille
6	Glove box
7	Meter cover
8	Meter case
9	Combination meter pad
10	Combination meter case
11	Center panel
12	Recirculation/fresh air changeover control wire connection
13	Mode selection control wire
14	Water valve control wire connection
15	Center reinforcement
16	Air bag
17	Steering wheel
18	Fuse box cover
19	Fuse box assembly
20	Instrument panel

Figure 23–6. Study the major parts of an instrument panel. Bolts and screws that hold the instrument panel can be hard to find. The service manual will give details about fastener locations. (Courtesy of DaimlerChrysler Corporation)

With the lens removed, you can then replace gauges and speedometer head. Screws on the rear of the cluster normally hold each unit in place. Again, keep fingerprints off the faces of the gauges and speedometer. They will show up easily after installation.

Install the instrument cluster parts in reverse order of removal. Remember to connect all wires and the speedometer cable, if used, to the cluster. Check the operation of all dash lights and gauges after installation.

SUMMARY

- The typical parts of a front seat include the seat cushion, seat back, headrest, headrest guide, recliner adjuster, and seat track.
- To replace carpeting, you must remove the seats, seat belt anchors, trim pieces, and any other parts mounted over the carpeting. This might include the console, any electronic control units, and wiring harness bolted down under the carpet.

TECHNICAL TERMS

bucket seat
bench seat
seat cushion
seat back
headrest
headrest guide
recliner adjuster
seat track
hog rings
headliner
instrument cluster

REVIEW QUESTIONS

1. How do you remove a front bucket seat?
2. List and explain the six basic parts of a front bucket seat.
3. These are used to stretch and hold the seat covers on the seat.
   a. Hog rings
   b. Screws
   c. Bolts
   d. Adhesive
4. To replace carpeting, you must typically remove which parts?
5. A ______________ is a cloth or vinyl cover over the inside of the roof in the passenger compartment.
6. List the typical parts of an instrument panel.
7. A vehicle needs to have its instrument cluster lens replaced. *Technician A* says to keep fingers off the inside of the instrument lens. *Technician B* says to disconnect wires and the speedometer cable before pulling the cluster too far out of the dash. Who is correct?
   a. Technician A
   b. Technician B
   c. Both Technicians A and B
   d. Neither Technician

ASE-STYLE REVIEW QUESTIONS

1. *Technician A* says that four bolts normally secure the seat to the floor. *Technician B* says that the seats are welded to the floor. Who is correct?
   a. Technician A
   b. Technician B
   c. Both Technicians A and B
   d. Neither Technician

2. *Technician A* says that rear bench seats can be held in position by screws. *Technician B* says that spring-loaded clips can hold them. Who is correct?
   a. Technician A
   b. Technician B
   c. Both Technicians A and B
   d. Neither Technician

3. *Technician A* says that seat covers are usually bonded to the cushions. *Technician B* says that hog rings and clips hold the seat covers in place. Who is correct?
   a. Technician A
   b. Technician B
   c. Both Technicians A and B
   d. Neither Technician

4. An instrument cluster is being repaired. *Technician A* says to first disconnect the battery. *Technician B* says to pull the cluster out far enough to disconnect the wires and speedometer cable. Who is correct?
   a. Technician A
   b. Technician B
   c. Both Technicians A and B
   d. Neither Technician

5. *Technician A* says to keep your hands clean when touching the back of an instrument cluster lens. *Technician B* says to keep your fingers off the inside of the instrument lens at all times. Who is correct?
   a. Technician A
   b. Technician B
   c. Both Technicians A and B
   d. Neither Technician

6. *Technician A* says that to replace carpeting the technician must remove the seats, seat belt anchors, trim pieces, and any other parts mounted over the carpeting. *Technician B* says that the carpeting is put in the vehicle last and can be removed with just removing the door trim plates. Who is correct?
   a. Technician A
   b. Technician B
   c. Both Technicians A and B
   d. Neither Technician

7. *Technician A* says that seats are seldom damaged in a collision and they never need to be checked. *Technician B* says that the seats should be checked not only for visible damage but they should also be operated

through their complete range of movement to ensure full operation. Who is correct?
a. Technician A
b. Technician B
c. Both Technicians A and B
d. Neither Technician

8. *Technician A* says that all headliners are bonded directly to the roof. *Technician B* says that some are mounted on metal rods and bonded around the edge of the roof. Who is correct?
a. Technician A
b. Technician B
c. Both Technicians A and B
d. Neither Technician

9. When removing an instrument cluster, *Technician A* says that some of the fasteners may be hard to locate and remove. *Technician B* says that the service manual will give locations of the fasteners. Who is correct?
a. Technician A
b. Technician B
c. Both Technicians A and B
d. Neither Technician

ACTIVITIES

1. Inspect several vehicles. List any damage or deterioration to the interior. Make a damage report.

2. Remove and replace vehicle seats. Refer to a service manual for specific directions.

CHAPTER 24 Mechanical Repairs

OBJECTIVES

After studying this chapter, you should be able to:

- Explain the basics of front, rear, and computer-controlled suspension systems.
- Describe the design and operation of steering systems.
- Understand how various brake systems work, and describe the procedures for manual and pressure bleeding.
- Perform key cooling and air-conditioning system repairs and maintenance.
- Inspect an exhaust system, and describe the guidelines for working on an emission control system.

INTRODUCTION

After a collision, it is often necessary to remove mechanical parts. This would include suspension, steering, drivetrain, and engine parts.

With a front hit, parts right behind the grille are often damaged. The air-conditioning (A/C) condenser, radiator, engine mounts, water pump, engine accessory units, antilock brake system (ABS) controller, and other mechanical parts can be damaged. With body panels removed, it is much easier to service these parts. See **Figure 24–1.**

If a vehicle hits a curb or other stationary object with its tires during a collision, tremendous force is transmitted through the wheels and into the steering and suspension systems. Control arms, steering rods, and related parts are often damaged. Other parts on the bottom of the vehicle (engine oil pan, transmission pan, exhaust system, etc.) can also be damaged from the impact.

! WARNING !

When diagnosing and repairing mechanical parts, always refer to the service manual for the specific vehicle. Never attempt to work with mechanical components without the aid of a service manual. It will give the detailed procedures and specifications.

POWERTRAIN

The **powertrain/drivetrain** is all of the parts that produce and transfer power to the drive wheels. This includes the engine, transmission or transaxle, drive axle, and other related parts. See **Figure 24–2.**

Engine

The **engine** provides energy to move the vehicle and power all accessories. See **Figure 24–3.** Most vehicles use gasoline engines, while some use diesel engines. The basic parts of a typical internal combustion, piston engine include:

Block—the foundation of the engine; all the other engine parts are either housed in or attached to the block. A **cylinder** is a round hole bored (machined) in the block that guides piston movement.

Piston—transfers the energy of combustion (burning of an air-fuel mixture) to the connecting rod. *Rings* are circular seals installed around the top sides of the piston. They keep combustion pressure and oil from leaking between the piston and cylinder wall (cylinder surface). A **connecting rod** is a link that attaches the piston to the crankshaft.

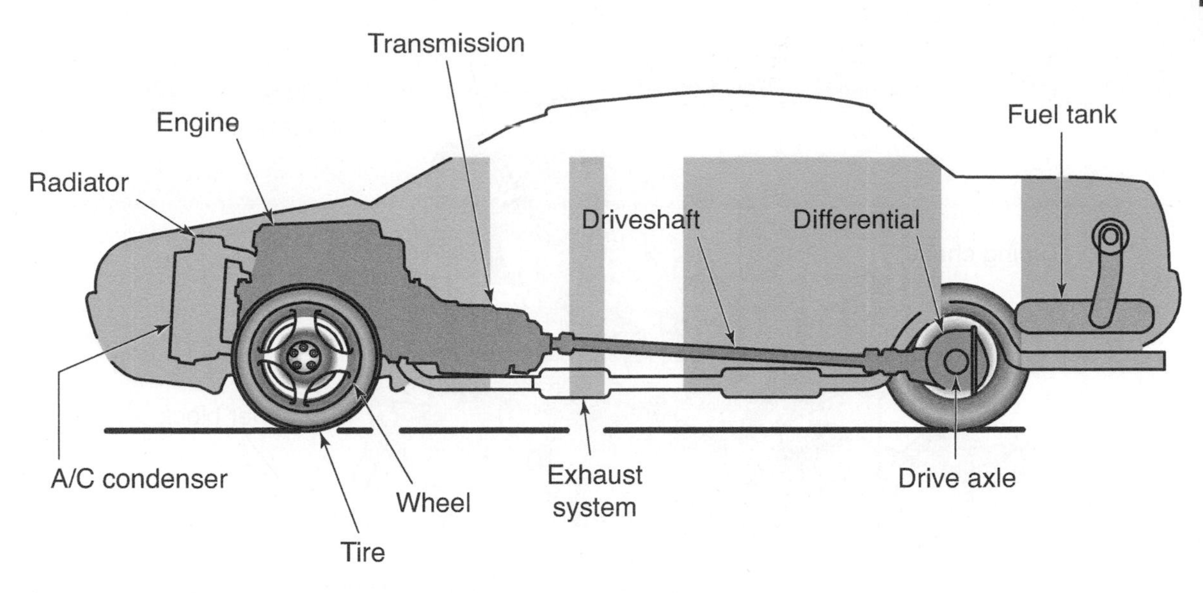

Figure 24–1. Mechanical parts (radiators, engine pulleys, wheels and tires, etc.) are often damaged in a collision. Collision repair technicians should be able to remove and replace most mechanical parts on a vehicle.

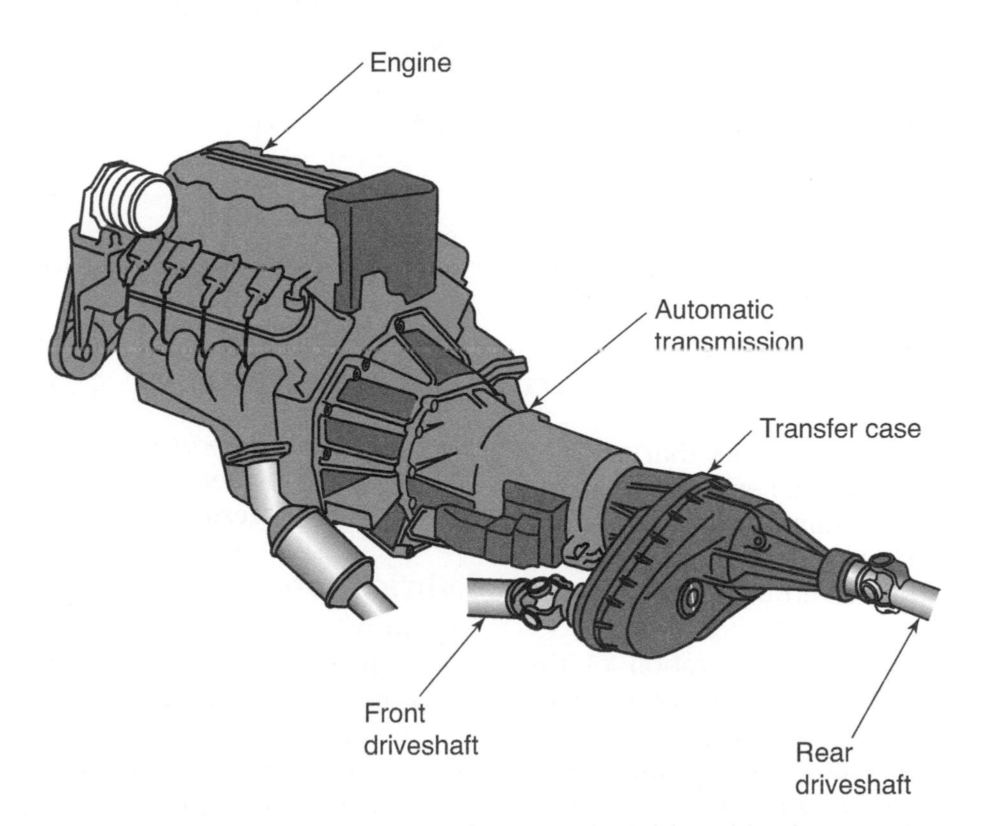

Figure 24–2. The rear view shows how the transmission for an all-wheel-drive vehicle fastens to the rear of the engine.

Crankshaft—changes the reciprocating (up and down) motion of the piston and rod into more useful rotary (spinning) motion. Power to turn the driving wheel comes from the rear of the crank, and accessories are driven off the front.

Cylinder head—covers and seals the top of the cylinder. It contains valves, rocker arms, and sometimes the camshaft. The **combustion chamber** is a small enclosed area between the top of the piston and bottom of the cylinder

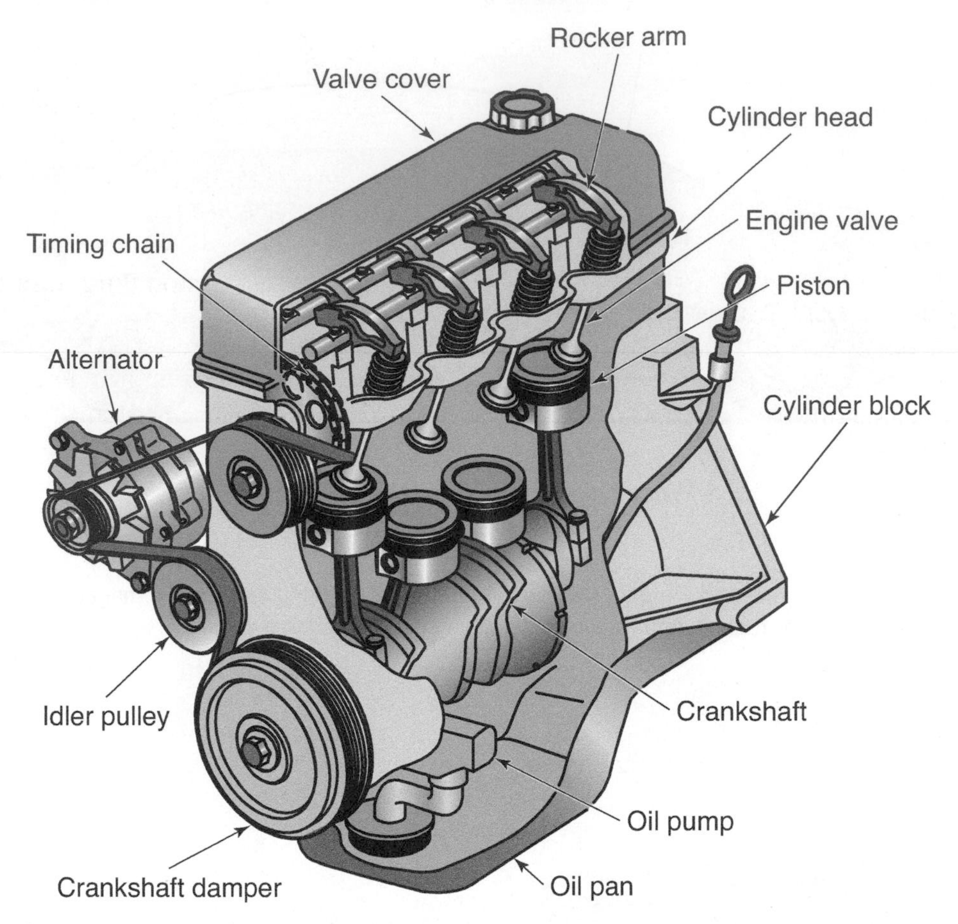

Figure 24–3. Study the basic parts of an engine. The intake valve allows air and fuel to enter the combustion chamber. When the spark plug fires, the mixture burns and forces the piston and rod down. This spins the crankshaft to produce usable power for the drivetrain. (Courtesy of General Motors Corporation, Service Operations)

head. The burning of the air-fuel mixture occurs in the combustion chamber.

Valves—flow control devices that open to allow air-fuel mixture into and exhaust out of the combustion chamber. Valve springs hold the valves closed when they do not need to be open. They also return the valvetrain parts to the at-rest position.

Camshaft—controls the operation of the valves. It can be located in the block or the cylinder head. A **lifter** is a cylindrical part that rides on the camshaft lobes and transfers motion to the pushrods. The **pushrods** are hollow tubes that transfer motion from the lifters to rocker arms. The **rocker arms** are levers that transfer camshaft action from the pushrods to the valves.

Flywheel—a heavy metal disc used to help keep the crankshaft turning smoothly. It also connects engine power to the transmission. A larger gear on the outside of the flywheel engages the starting motor when cranking the engine for starting.

ENGINE SUPPORT SYSTEMS

Various *engine support systems* are powered by the engine to protect the engine from damage and to power accessory systems.

Lubrication System

The **lubrication system** forces oil to friction points in the engine. This keeps the moving parts from quickly wearing and failing.

The *oil pump* forces motor oil through passages inside the engine. It can be driven by the crankshaft or by a gear on the camshaft. Oil *galleries* are the passages through the block, heads, and other parts for oil flow through the engine. An *oil pickup* is a tube with a filter screen for drawing oil out of the pan and into the pump. A *pressure relief valve* limits the maximum amount of oil pressure. See Figure 24–3.

The **oil pan** holds a supply of motor oil. Also called the *sump,* it often bolts to the bottom of the engine block. An oil drain plug is provided in the oil pan for draining and changing the engine oil. The **oil filter** traps debris and prevents it from circulating through the engine oil galleries.

Lubrication System Service. In a collision, the oil filter, oil pan, and related parts are sometimes damaged. They can be made of thin metal and can be crushed and ruptured easily.

When starting an engine before or after repairs, check the oil level with the **oil dipstick.** Also, always look under the vehicle for oil leakage. If you find an oil leak, shut the engine off immediately. Find and fix the source of the oil leak.

Cooling System

A **cooling system** maintains the correct engine operating temperature. It is often damaged in a collision and must be restored to its precollision condition. The basic parts of a cooling system are shown in **Figure 24–4.**

Antifreeze is used to prevent freeze-up in cold weather and to lubricate moving parts. Antifreeze also prevents engine overheating. A *coolant recovery system* stores an extra supply of coolant for the system.

The **radiator** transfers coolant heat to the outside air. The **radiator pressure cap** prevents the coolant from boiling. A **radiator fan** draws outside air through the radiator to remove heat.

The **water pump** circulates coolant through the inside of the engine, hoses, and radiator. The *water jackets* are passages in the engine for coolant. The **thermostat** regulates coolant flow and system operating temperature.

A **heater system** uses coolant heat and a heater core (small radiator under the dash) to warm the passenger compartment. The *automatic transmission cooler* uses the radiator to reduce automatic transmission fluid temperature.

Cooling System Service. Cooling system problems normally result in engine overheating. In collision repair, problems may be due to a crushed water pump, bent drive pulleys, damaged thermostat housing, or large leak. Always inspect closely for these problems and proper coolant level before starting the engine.

Antifreeze should NOT be reused. Antifreeze contains additives, lubricants, and corrosion inhibitors that break down over time. Antifreeze should be replaced with a 50/50 mixture of antifreeze and water. Always follow antifreeze manufacturer's recommendations. Some warranties will NOT be honored if the antifreeze recommended by the manufacturer is NOT installed. See **Figure 24–5.**

An *antifreeze tester,* commonly called a *hydrometer,* is used to determine the freeze-up protection of the coolant mixture. Pull a sample of the vehicle's coolant solution into the tester. Then read the lowest temperature the coolant will withstand without freezing.

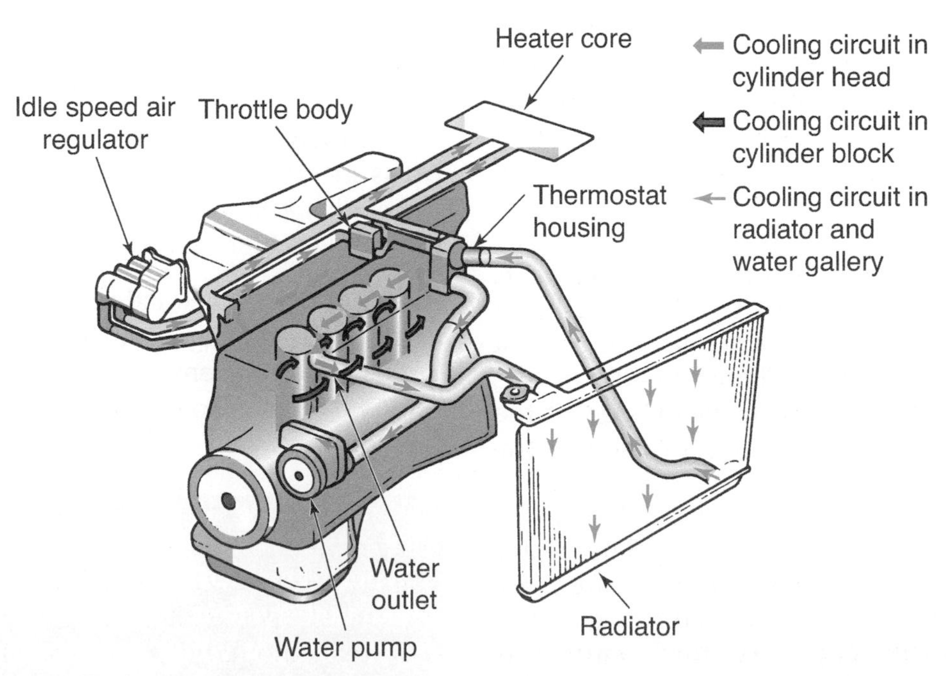

Figure 24–4. Study the basic parts of a cooling system and trace flow. With a front hit, the water pump can often be cracked, requiring replacement. (Courtesy of Nissan North America, Inc.)

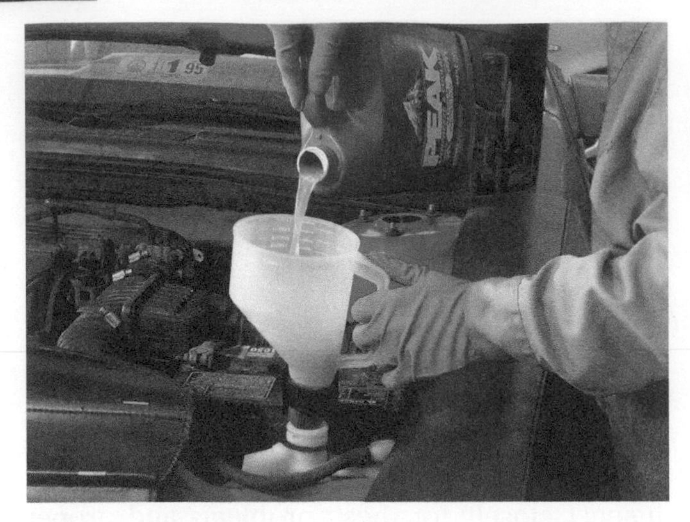

Figure 24–5. If the cooling system has been drained for major repairs, refill it with a 50/50 mix of water and antifreeze. Run and warm the engine before checking the reservoir level. Do not remove the radiator cap with a warm system or steam can cause severe burns.

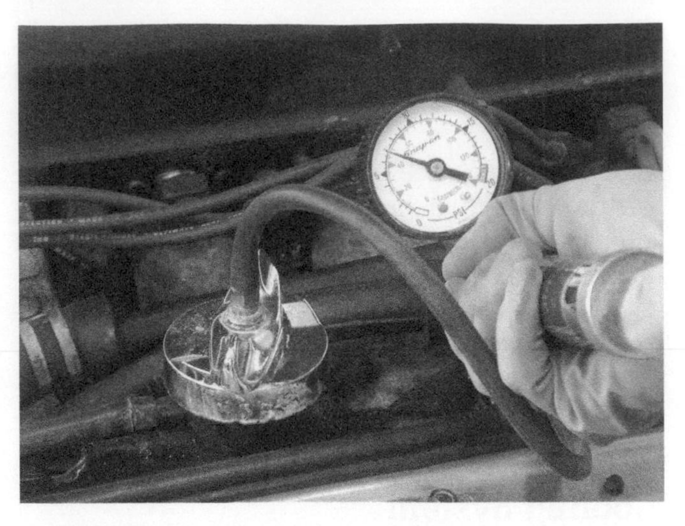

Figure 24–6. A cooling system pressure tester is commonly used to check the condition of the system. With the tester mounted on the radiator, pump in the cap-rated pressure. Then check for leakage under the engine compartment. The system should hold the pressure without leakage.

Cooling fans are either belt driven or electric. Their operation is critical for proper cooling of both the cooling and A/C systems.

When inspecting belt-driven fans, inspect the belts for cracks, tears, glazing, and proper tension. Check the fan blades for cracks and the fan clutch for leaks.

When inspecting electric fans, check electrical connections for corrosion and reconnection following repairs. Look for cut, pinched, or burned wires. Make sure the fan comes on when the engine reaches normal operating temperature and when the A/C is turned on.

Radiator caps should be inspected for calcium deposits, which could prevent the cap from operating. They are rated to maintain different pressures and should be replaced according to the pressure recommended by the manufacturer.

A **cooling system leak test** is performed by installing a pressure tester on the radiator neck. Pump the tester handle until its gauge equals the cap pressure rating. A loss of pressure or coolant means there is a leak (see **Figure 24–6**).

When mounted on the front or side of the engine, the thermostat housing can also be damaged during a collision.

A **radiator cap pressure test** is done using a cooling system pressure tester. The tester gauge should stop increasing its pressure reading when the cap rating is reached.

The **radiator cap pressure rating** is stamped on the cap. If the cooling system is disassembled during repair or parts are replaced, a pressure test should be performed.

Exhaust System

The **exhaust system** collects and discharges exhaust gases caused by the combustion of the air-fuel mixture within the engine. It also quiets the noise of the running engine. Refer back to Figure 24–1.

The **header pipe** is a steel tubing that carries exhaust gases from the engine's exhaust manifold to the catalytic converter. The **catalytic converter** is a thermal reactor for burning and chemically changing exhaust byproducts into harmless gases. The *intermediate pipe* is tubing that is sometimes used between the header pipe and catalytic converter or muffler.

A **muffler** is a metal chamber for dampening pressure pulsations to reduce exhaust noise. The *tailpipe* is a tube that carries exhaust gas from the muffler to rear of the vehicle.

Exhaust System Service. The exhaust system can also be damaged during a collision, requiring partial replacement. Its parts may also need removal during major collision repairs.

DANGER

When inspecting or working on the exhaust system, remember that its parts get very hot when the engine is running. Contact with them could cause a severe burn.

Because of constant changes in recommended catalytic converter servicing and installation requirements, check with the vehicle manufacturer for the latest data regarding replacement.

To check the exhaust system's condition, grab the tailpipe (when cool). Try to move it up and down and side to side. There should be only slight movement in any direction.

Remember! There is only one way to repair faulty exhaust system parts: replace them. It might not be necessary to take off all exhaust system parts. You can usually separate parts and replace them individually.

Fuel System

The vehicle's **fuel system** must carefully feed the correct amount of fuel into the engine. If too much or too little fuel is admitted, the engine will NOT run efficiently.

A **gasoline injection system** has sensors and a computer to control electrically operated fuel valves, called **fuel injectors.** The injectors are located in the intake manifold. When the intake valve opens, the fuel is sprayed into the intake port and pulled into the combustion chamber by airflow.

A **diesel injection system** uses a high-pressure, mechanical pump to force fuel directly into the engine's combustion chambers. No spark plugs are needed. The pistons squeeze the intake air, which gets heated enough to start the fuel burning.

A *fuel tank* is a container that stores fuel. The **fuel pump** is a mechanical or electric part for forcing fuel to the engine. *Fuel lines* are tubing and hoses that route fuel from tank to engine. A **fuel filter** is used for straining out debris in the fuel. The **fuel pressure regulator** is a part that controls the amount of fuel pressure at the fuel injectors.

DANGER

Before disconnecting any part of a fuel system, you may have to relieve fuel pressure. Many fuel injection systems retain pressure even when the engine is not running. If this pressure is not relieved, it will cause fuel to spray in the work area and create a fire hazard.

DRIVETRAIN

The *drivetrain* uses engine power to turn the drive wheels. It includes everything after the engine—the clutch, transmission, drive shaft, drive axles. Drivetrain designs vary. Some cars use a **manual transmission** (hand shifted). Others use an **automatic transmission** (shifts gear automatically using internal oil pressure).

The **transmission** is an assembly with a series of gears for increasing torque to the drive wheels so the car can accelerate properly. It provides high power for acceleration in lower gears and good gas mileage in higher gears. With an automatic transmission, a **torque converter** (fluid coupling) is used in place of a clutch. Refer back to Figure 24–2.

A **transaxle** is a transmission and differential combined into a single housing or case. Both automatic and manual transaxles are available.

A **clutch** is a device used to couple and uncouple engine power to a manual transmission or transaxle. It uses a friction disc, pressure plate, flywheel face, and release bearing for activation.

Front-wheel drive vehicles use a transaxle to transfer engine torque to the front drive wheels. *Constant velocity axles,* or **CV-axles,** transfer torque from the transaxle to the wheel hubs. They can be found on rear-wheel drive (RWD), four-wheel drive (4WD), all-wheel drive (AWD), and front-wheel drive (FWD) vehicles.

Front-engine, **rear-wheel drive** vehicles use a conventional transmission, drive shaft, and rear axle assembly to transfer power to the rear drive wheels.

A **drive shaft** is a long tube that transfers power from the transmission to the rear axle assembly. It has *universal joints* at both ends that allow flexibility of the suspension while maintaining driving force.

The **rear axle assembly** is the housing that contains the ring gear, pinion gear, differential assembly, and axles. Rear suspension springs attach to the housing.

A **differential assembly** is a unit within the drive axle assembly. It uses gears to allow different amounts of torque (turning force) to be applied to each drive wheel while the vehicle is making a turn.

Drivetrain/Powertrain Service

Begin drivetrain/powertrain inspection by checking the condition of the CV-joint boots.

Splits, cracks, tears, punctures, or thin spots require replacement. If the boot appears corroded, this indicates improper greasing or excessive heat. Squeeze-test all boots. If any air escapes, replace the boot. Also replace any boots that are missing.

On FWD transaxles with equal-length half shafts, inspect the intermediate shaft U-joint, bearing, and support bracket for looseness by rocking the wheel back and forth and watching for any movement.

Various drivetrain and suspension problems can be confused with symptoms produced by a bad CV-joint. The following list of symptoms should help guide the technician to a proper diagnosis.

A vibration that increases with speed is rarely due to CV-joint problems or FWD half shaft imbalance. An out-of-balance tire or wheel, an out-of-round tire, or a bent rim are the more likely causes. It is possible that a bent half shaft as a result of collision or towing damage could cause a vibration, as could a missing damper weight.

A drive shaft should be checked for signs of contact against the chassis or rubbing. Rubbing can be a symptom of a weak or broken spring or engine mount, or chassis misalignment.

It may be required to remove the drivetrain to make structural repairs. Because modern unibody vehicles tend to have very crowded engine compartments, removal of the drivetrain allows ready access to structural panels.

When servicing parts of a drivetrain in collision repair, always refer to the service manual. It will give the instructions and specs needed to do proper repairs. See **Figure 24–7.**

Label all wires, hoses, and other parts to help with reassembly. This will save time and prevent confusion later.

Sometimes, only engine and transmission removal are needed during collision repair. This might be needed for major frame or unibody straightening or structural part replacement.

When removing a drive shaft, mark its alignment in the rear axle assembly. Some shafts are factory balanced on the vehicle. If you change its orientation, vibration can result.

Brake System

The **brake system** uses hydraulic pressure to slow or stop wheel rotation with brake pedal application.

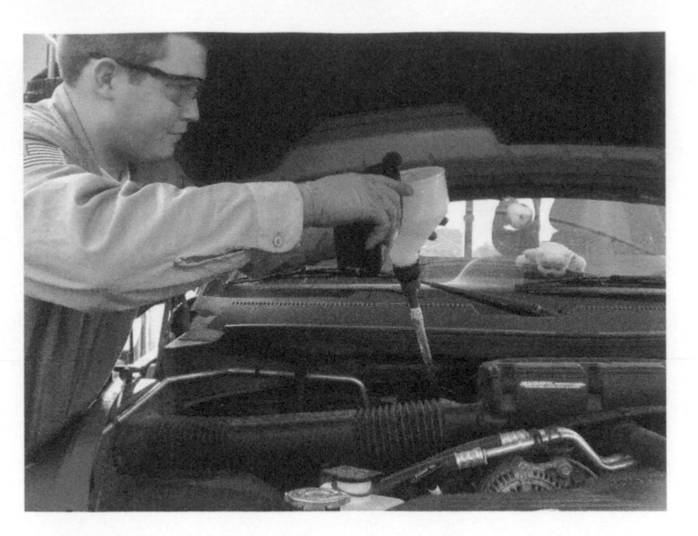

Figure 24–7. The automatic transmission level should normally be checked with the engine idling. If needed, use a long funnel to add the correct amount and type of transmission fluid.

The *brake pedal* transfers the driver's foot pressure into the master cylinder. The **master cylinder** develops hydraulic pressure (oil pressure) for the system.

Brake lines and *hoses* carry fluid out to the wheel cylinders. The **wheel cylinders** use hydraulic pressure to push the brake pads or shoes outward.

The **brake pads** or **shoes** have a friction lining for rubbing on the brake rotor or drum. The **brake rotors** or **drums** provide heavy metal friction surfaces bolted between the hub and wheel. A **caliper** holds the piston(s) and brake pads on disc brakes. Refer to **Figure 24–8** and **Figure 24–9.**

The *parking* or *emergency brake* uses a steel cable to physically apply the brake shoes or pads.

Power brakes are a standard hydraulic brake system with a vacuum, hydraulic, or electric assist. A booster unit is added to help apply the master cylinder and brakes.

Brake System Service

When applicable, inspect the brake system for:

1. Kinked or bent brake lines
2. Cut hoses
3. Damaged rotors or drums
4. Backing plate interfering with drum
5. Damage to caliper or mounting area
6. Damage to master cylinder or booster
7. Dash lamp operation if equipped with ABS

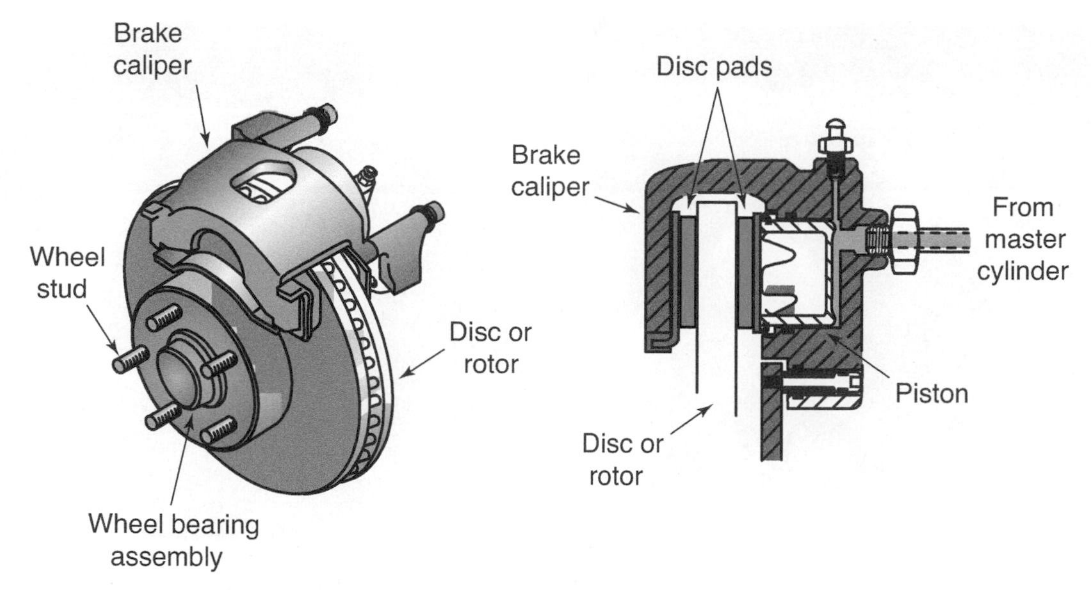

Figure 24–8. With disc brakes, the caliper mounts over the disc. When fluid pressure enters the caliper, the piston is pushed outward. This applies the brake pads to the spinning rotor or disc to slow or stop the vehicle.

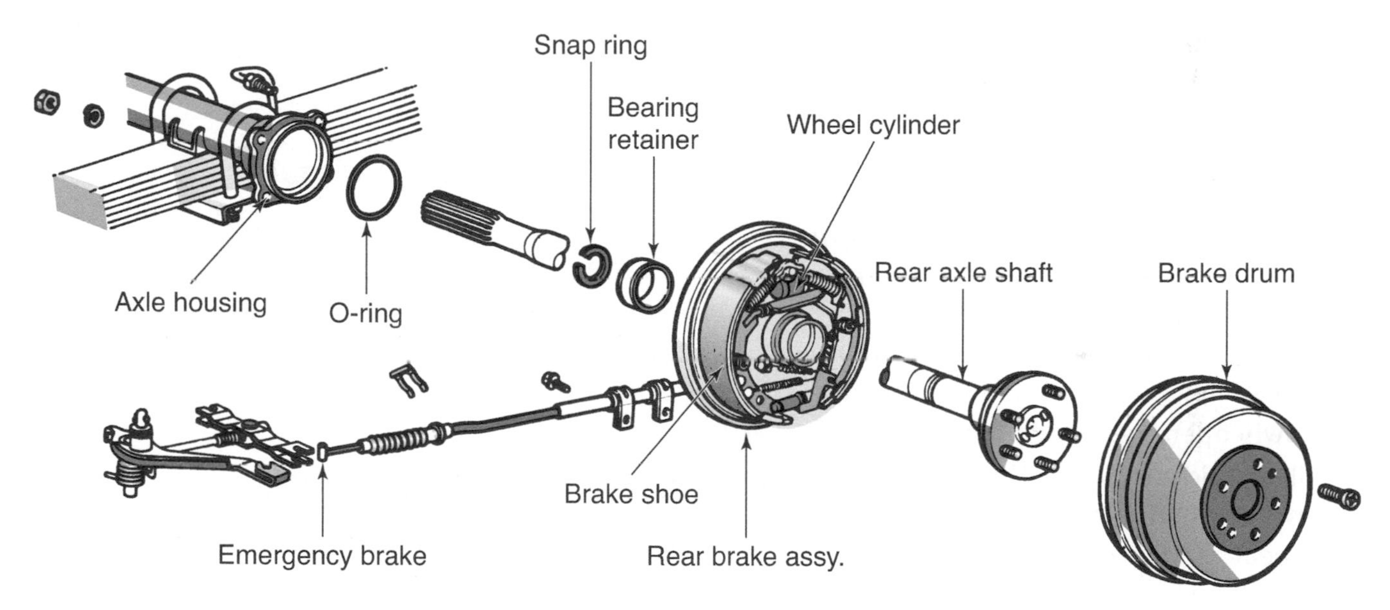

Figure 24–9. With drum brakes, the drum mounts over the brake shoes and wheel cylinders. The wheel cylinders push out on the shoes to apply the brakes. (Courtesy of Toyota Motor Co.)

Brake lines are seamless steel, reinforced flexible rubber, or nylon. They use two types of flared ends, metric bubble flare or double flare. Brake lines must be replaced with the same material as used by the factory. Brake lines should be replaced if kinked or severely bent.

When servicing brake lines:

1. Do NOT use copper, aluminum, or rubber hoses.
2. Do NOT repair nylon brake lines.
3. Do NOT use compression fittings.
4. Route in the same locations as the factory.
5. Reinstall all supporting clamps and springs that were removed during repair.

Brake fluid absorbs moisture. Its container should NOT be left open to the atmosphere. Make sure to use the proper type of brake fluid. Vehicles can require DOT 3, 4, or 5. Check the master cylinder label or markings for the type used. See **Figure 24–10.**

Do NOT reuse fluid drained from system. It may contain contaminants that will damage the system.

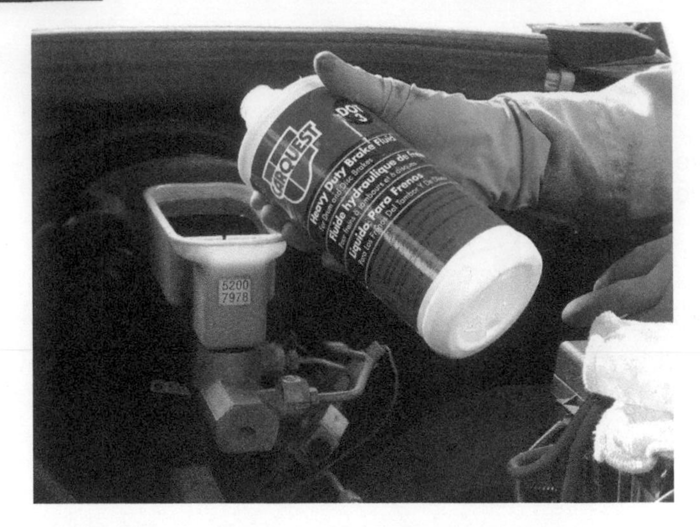

Figure 24–10. Always make sure that the brake master cylinder is full before releasing the vehicle to the customer.

Brake system bleeding is done to remove air from the brake fluid. To do this:

1. Clean the bleeder screw.
2. Attach a drain hose to the bleeder screw and submerge the other end in a clear jar partially filled with brake fluid.
3. Bleed one wheel at a time.
4. Start with the wheel closest to, or farthest from, the master cylinder (follow the manufacturer's recommendations).
5. Have a helper pump the brake pedal several times, then hold it with moderate pressure.
6. Slowly open the bleeder screw.
7. Allow fluid/air to flow through it, then close the bleeder screw.
8. Repeat as needed until fluid runs clear without air.
9. Repeat at all wheels, following manufacturer's recommended order, making sure that the master cylinder does not run dry.
10. Refill the master cylinder.

Antilock Brake System Service

Antilock brakes service is similar to conventional brakes. However, electronic parts are added to operate the system. Most ABS brakes have self-diagnosis. The computer will output a trouble code if an electrical-electronic malfunction develops. You can refer to charts in the service manual to see what each number code means. This will tell which part might be at fault.

For example, if a trouble code indicates a problem with one of the wheel speed sensors, make sure it is adjusted properly and undamaged. You may also need to test the sensor and its wiring.

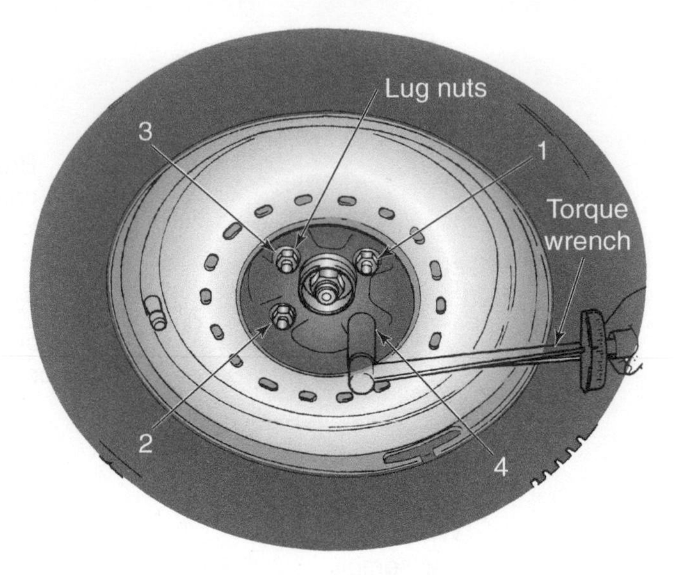

Figure 24–11. To avoid warpage of the brake drum, rotor, hub, and wheel, torque the lug nuts to specifications in a crisscross pattern. (Courtesy of DaimlerChrysler Corporation)

WARNING

When installing the wheels back onto a vehicle, torque the lug nuts to specs. Use a crisscross pattern as shown in **Figure 24–11.** The service manual will give lug nut torque values.

STEERING SYSTEMS

The **steering system** transfers steering wheel motion through gears and linkage rods to swivel the front wheels. When you turn the *steering wheel,* a *steering shaft* that extends down through the **steering column** rotates the steering gearbox. The **steering gearbox,** either a worm or rack-and-pinion type, changes the wheel rotation into side movement for turning the wheels. A series of *linkage rods* connect the steering gearbox with the steering knuckles.

Parallelogram Steering

Parallelogram steering uses two tie-rod assemblies connected to the steering arms to support a long center link. The **center link** holds the tie-rods in position. An **idler arm** supports the center link on one end. The other end of the center link is attached to the **pitman arm** on the gearbox.

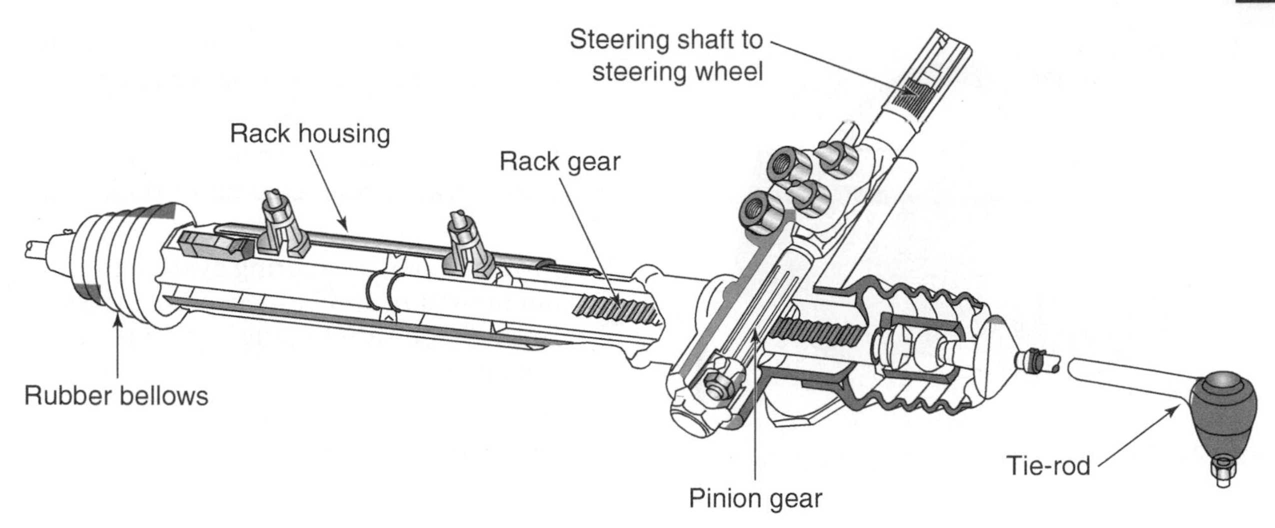

Figure 24–12. Note the parts of common rack-and-pinion steering. If damaged, the whole rack assembly is normally replaced.

The arrangement forms a parallelogram shape (each end moves equal and parallel to the other end).

Rack-and-Pinion Steering

Rack-and-pinion steering uses a simplified steering system that weighs less and takes up less space than parallelogram steering. For these reasons, it is used on most unibody vehicles. Refer to **Figure 24–12.**

The rack-and-pinion steering unit takes the place of the idler arm, pitman arm, center link, and gearbox used in parallelogram systems. It consists of a *pinion gear* at the end of the steering shaft, which meshes with a toothed shaft (a bar with a row of teeth cut into one edge) known as the **rack.** When the steering wheel is turned, the pinion rotates in a circle and moves the rack sideways—left or right—to turn the wheels.

Two inner **tie-rod ends** are threaded onto the end of the rack and are covered by rubber bellows boots. These **boots** protect the rack from contamination by dirt, salt, and other road particles. The inner tie-rods are threaded onto the outer tie-rod ends, which connect to the steering arms.

Power Steering

The power steering unit is designed to reduce the amount of effort required to turn the steering wheel. It also reduces driver fatigue on long drives and makes it easier to steer the vehicle at slow speeds, particularly during parking.

Power steering can be broken down into two design arrangements: conventional and electronically controlled. In the conventional arrangement, hydraulic power is used to assist the driver. An engine drive **power steering pump** forces pressurized oil through the system.

Power steering hoses carry the oil to and from the pump. A *hydraulic piston* on the steering linkage or in the gearbox helps turn the wheels. *Hydraulic valves* control power assist.

With a *computer-assisted steering* system, **sensors** provide feedback for the computer. The **computer** or electronic control unit can then precisely control power assist as variables change. Mechanical steering is still provided with an electrical failure.

With *electronically controlled power steering,* the conventional power steering parts are replaced with electronic controls and an electric motor. The electric motor is mounted in the rack assembly. A DC motor armature with a hollow shaft is used to allow passage of the rack through it. The outboard housing and rack are designed so that the rotary motion of the armature can be transferred to linear movement of the rack.

Collapsible Steering Columns

Collapsible steering columns crush under force to absorb impact. This reduces injuries to the driver. Steering column collapse is managed in two parts, upper and lower. The lower section of the column is linked to two or more universal joints. It uses universal joints that allow the section to fold.

A slight impact on the column end can collapse the steering shaft or loosen the plastic

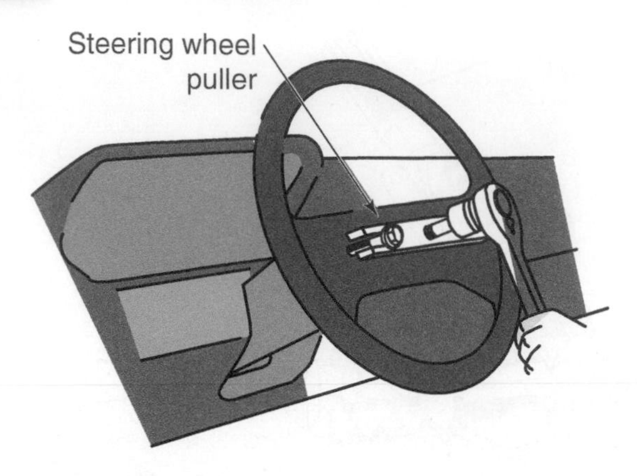

Figure 24–13. A wheel puller is needed to remove the steering wheel. Never hammer on a steering column or damage could result.

inserts that maintain column rigidity. When removing the steering wheel, use a puller. Do not hammer or pound on any components during removal. See **Figure 24–13.**

Steering System Service

To check a rack-and-pinion system, begin by raising the vehicle and taking the weight off the front suspension. Visually inspect the steering system for physical damage. Check the boots for leaks, and inspect the tie-rods. Examine the mounting points for any distortion. Inspect the tie-rod ends. Grab the tie-rod near the tire and try pushing it up and down. Any looseness indicates damage or wear.

Check the inner tie-rod socket by squeezing the bellows until the socket can be felt. With your other hand, push and pull on the tire. Looseness in the socket indicates damage or wear. With both hands, try to swivel a tire right and left while watching for play. If excessive movement is noted, wear or damage is likely. Observe the rack-and-pinion at the same time. Any movement might indicate a problem.

Remember that rack-and-pinion units must be mounted on a level plane. Misalignment of the rack-and-pinion will cause changes in the steering geometry during jounce/rebound. This condition cannot be corrected by changing the length of the tie-rods.

Here are some steering service tips that should be kept in mind:

1. Torque all steering system fasteners to specs with a torque wrench. Refer to the manual for an exact value.
2. Always install new cotter pins. Never reuse old cotter pins. If one were to fall out, a fatal accident could result.
3. Never try to straighten any steering system parts. Always replace bent or damaged parts.
4. Protect a power steering system from dirt and moisture at all times. If the system must be open, be sure to plug or tie off all openings with plastic.
5. Always replace the fluid lost with the recommended type.
6. Check the power steering hose routing when reassembling the system. Always route and hang hoses identical to the factory installation. Avoid contact with other parts. Watch for rubbing against moving parts.
7. Use proper tools when servicing a steering system. If you do not use the right tool, parts can be damaged.

SUSPENSION SYSTEMS

The **suspension system** allows the tires and wheels to move up and down with road surface irregularities. Its major parts are shown in **Figure 24–14.**

Control arms mount on the frame to swivel up and down. **Ball joints** on the out end of the control arms allow the steering knuckles to swivel and turn. The **steering knuckles** hold

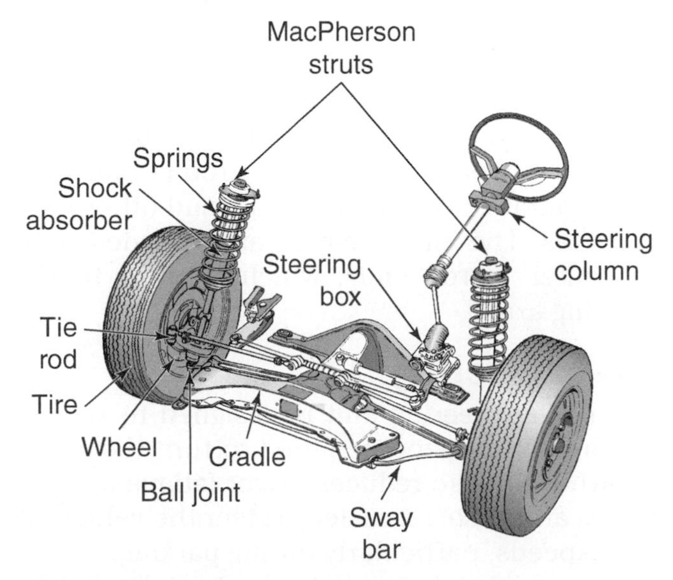

Figure 24–14. Study the major parts of a strut suspension. (Courtesy of McQuay-Norris)

the wheel bearings and wheels. The hubs mount on the wheel bearings to hold the wheels or rims. The *wheels* hold the tires. *Springs* support the weight of the car and allow suspension flexing. **Shock absorbers** are dampening devices that absorb spring oscillations (bouncing) to smooth the vehicle's ride quality. They may be gas, oil, or air filled.

Trailing arm rear suspension systems provide little, if any, independent movement of the rear wheels. They are commonly used on front drive vehicles. Also called a **dead axle,** a solid rear axle holds the two wheel assemblies.

Air spring suspension uses air springs to support the vehicle load. The air springs replace or supplement the conventional spring suspension. Air spring suspension provides for automatic front and rear load leveling. It will increase and decrease air pressure in the springs to raise, lower, or level the vehicle as needed.

Air spring suspension parts include a computer, air springs, air compressor, height sensors, and air lines. The sensors send signals to the computer about the ride height and attitude of the vehicle. The computer can then react to road and driving conditions. It sends out control signals to the compressor and valves to increase or decrease pressure in each air spring as needed.

Suspension System Service

Always inspect the suspension system for signs of damage from the collision. Damaged or worn suspension parts should be replaced. When worn or damaged, these parts can upset the settings of the entire suspension, steering, and drive line systems.

Loose, worn, or broken suspension parts will allow the wheels to shift out of alignment. This will cause premature tire wear and poor handling. A metallic thumping or knocking sound when driving over bumps or potholes, or unusual tracking indicates the need for service.

! WARNING !

The manufacturer has designed certain suspension, steering, and alignment features into the unibody vehicle. Do not try to straighten or bend any of the pieces that make up the suspension system.

AIR-CONDITIONING SYSTEMS

An **air-conditioning system** is designed to cool the passenger compartment. System designs vary. For example, some A/C systems use an accumulator, while others use a receiver-drier. Look at **Figure 24–15.**

Receiver-driers and **accumulators** serve the same basic purposes. They use a desiccant bag to remove moisture from the system. Their difference is their location. The accumulator is between the evaporator and compressor. The receiver-drier is between the condenser and expansion device. They act as storage tanks.

A/C systems are divided into two sides, high and low (see Figure 24–15). The dividing points are the compressor and the expansion device.

The **A/C high-side** contains high-pressure/high-temperature refrigerant. Its hoses feel hot to the touch. High-side hoses are generally smaller in diameter than the low-side.

The **A/C low-side** contains low-pressure/low-temperature refrigerant. Its hoses feel cold to the touch. Low-side hoses are generally larger in diameter than the high-side.

Air-Conditioning System Service

Discharging an A/C system removes refrigerant from the system and must always be done before parts are removed. Some compressors use a special back seating service valve that allows the compressor to be removed without completely discharging the system.

When removing refrigerant from the system, remember to use a recovery system. See **Figure 24–16.**

A **recovery system** will capture the used refrigerant and keep it from contaminating the atmosphere. Most will also filter the refrigerant for reuse. Since equipment varies, refer to the user's manual for detailed procedures.

Evacuating an A/C system is done to remove air and moisture from the system. It must be done any time air has entered the system. Evacuating is done by vacuum lowering the boiling point of the moisture, converting it to vapor (steam), and removing it.

Before **charging** (filling) the system with refrigerant, determine the amount and type of refrigerant used. This information is found in the service manual, on the label on the radiator support, or on the compressor. Do NOT

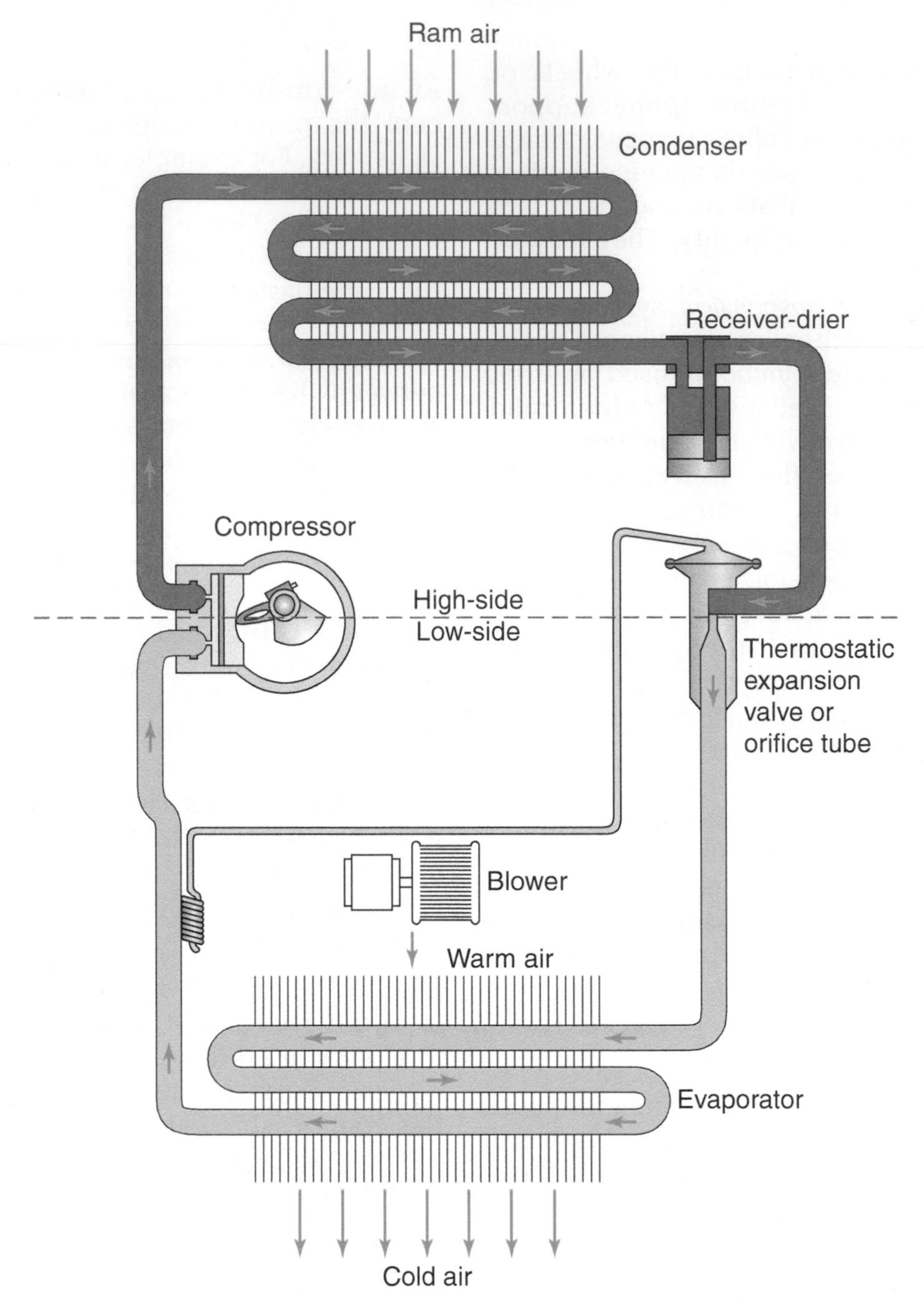

Figure 24–15. The high-side includes the condenser, receiver-drier, output side of the compressor, and connecting lines. The low-side includes the evaporator, expansion valve outlet, and inlet side of the compressor. The evaporator mounts under the dash of the vehicle. (Courtesy of Mitchell International, Inc.)

mix different types of refrigerants. Charging can be done with a gauge set or with a charging station.

Purging uses refrigerant to push air and dirt out of the hoses. It prevents air and other contaminants from being pushed into the A/C system. Always purge the gauge hoses before charging.

Refrigerant oil lubricates moving parts in the A/C system. Use only refrigerant oil. Make sure to use the type recommended for the system being serviced. Using a different type can result in damage to the compressor and seals and other parts.

There are several ways to find refrigerant leaks:

1. Electronic leak detector
2. Refrigerant cans with dye
3. Soap and water solution in a spray bottle

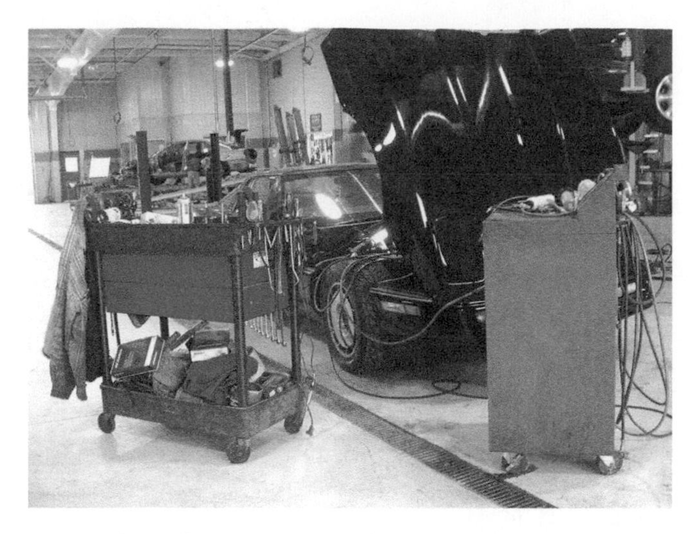

Figure 24–16. A recovery machine is needed to capture used refrigerant, which can then be recycled. This protects our atmosphere from damage.

A sight glass can often be used to check the amount of refrigerant in the system. It is located on the receiver-drier or in-line. When viewing the sight glass:

- Clear = completely full or completely empty
- Oil streaks = no refrigerant
- Foam or constant bubbles = low refrigerant charge
- Clouded = desiccant being circulated through system

Electronic leak detectors are battery-operated instruments that use an audio sound to alert you to the presence of a gas leak. They are designed to detect different types of gases.

When checking for refrigerant leaks, always check along the bottom of the hoses, fittings, seals, and other possible leakage points. This is because the refrigerant is heavier than air and is easier to detect below these parts.

Due to their possible depleting effect on the ozone layer, chlorofluorocarbon (CFC) and hydrochlorofluorocarbon (HCFC) are being phased out. This includes R-12 and other refrigerants used in A/C and refrigeration systems. **R-12,** also called CFC-12 or dichlorofluoromethane, is an older refrigerant used in vehicles manufactured before 1992.

R-134a, also called HFC-134A, is the refrigerant used in vehicles produced after 1992; it is the present replacement for R-12. It is less harmful to the ozone layer. New vehicles are being designed to run on this new refrigerant. The compressor and other parts are designed to be used with R-134a.

WARNING

R-134a is NOT compatible with R-12. Also, R-134a oils are NOT compatible with R-12 oils. They require separate service equipment. To avoid a mistake, R-134a uses metric quick-connect service ports. The high-side port is larger, so the same charging hoses cannot be used.

Mixing R-12 and R-134a, even in trace amounts, can be fatal to a system. This mistake can cause damage to seals, bearings, compressor reed valves, and pistons. Mixing refrigerants can also cause desiccants used in R-12 systems to break down and form harmful acids when used with R-134a.

DANGER

Wear hand and face protection when working on an A/C system. When refrigerant escapes from the system or the supply tank, it can cause severe frostbite burns.

The release of R-12 into the atmosphere is prohibited by current environmental regulations. Never vent the refrigerant into open air. Use a recovery/recycling machine.

When removing or opening up the A/C unit, seal all openings. This can be done with synthetic rubber, tight fitting caps, plugs, or plastic wraps. Use sturdy rubber bands or wire ties to hold plastic wraps in place securely.

EMISSION CONTROL SYSTEMS

Emission control systems are used to prevent potentially toxic chemicals from entering the atmosphere. The most common of these are the exhaust gas recirculation (EGR) valve, catalytic converter, air injection, and positive crankcase ventilation (PCV) systems. See **Figure 24–17.**

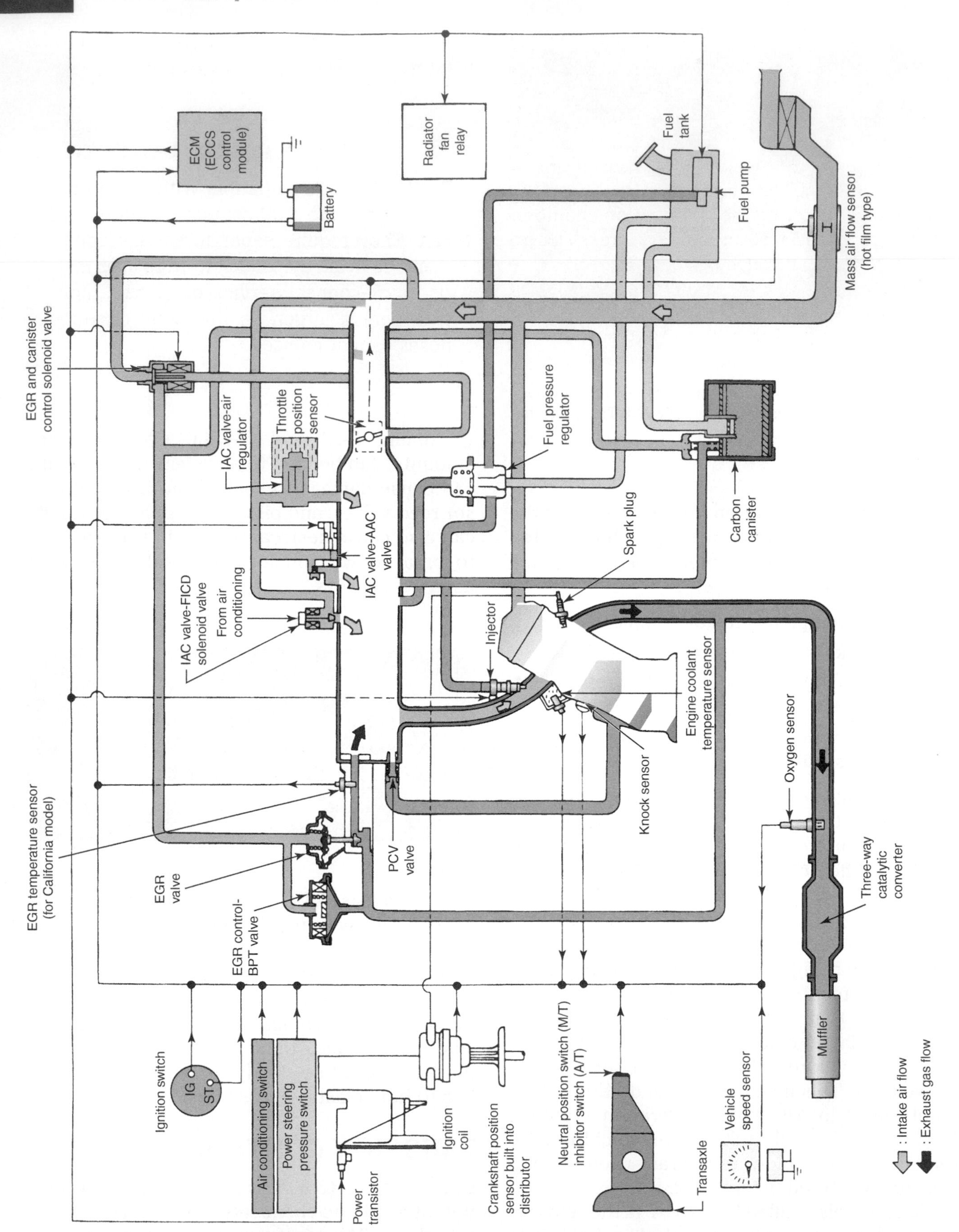

Figure 24–17. The emission control system helps prevent toxic emissions from entering Earth's atmosphere. Study this diagram, which shows several emission control systems. (Courtesy of Nissan North America, Inc.)

The **exhaust gas recirculation (EGR)** valve opens to allow engine vacuum to siphon exhaust into the intake manifold. The EGR valve consists of a poppet and a vacuum-actuated diaphragm. When ported vacuum is applied to the diaphragm, it lifts the poppet off its seat. Intake vacuum then siphons exhaust into the engine. The exhaust entering the combustion chambers lowers peak combustion temperatures. This reduces oxides of nitrogen pollution.

The **catalytic converter,** mounted in the exhaust system, plays a major role in emission control. The catalytic converter works as a gas reactor. Its catalytic function is to speed up the heat-producing chemical reaction between the exhaust gas and oxygen to reduce air pollutants in the exhaust.

The **fuel evaporative system** pulls fumes from the gas tank and other fuel system parts into a charcoal canister. The *charcoal canister* absorbs and stores vaporized fuel. When the engine is started, these vapors are drawn into the engine and burned. This prevents this source of pollution from entering our atmosphere.

The **positive crankcase ventilation system,** abbreviated **PCV,** channels engine crankcase blowby gases into the engine intake manifold. They are then drawn into the engine and burned. This prevents crankcase fumes from entering the atmosphere.

Emission Control System Service

Many times emission control systems are damaged in a collision. They must be serviced as part of the repair. The Clean Air Act, which is a federal law, makes the collision repair technician responsible for the emission control system. The law requires technicians to restore emission control systems to their original design. It also prescribes penalties for shops and technicians who alter emission control systems or fail to restore them to proper working condition.

The following guidelines must be strictly adhered to when working on emission control systems:

1. Damaged parts must be replaced with good parts. Eliminating damaged parts to avoid replacing them is against the law.
2. Using parts that prevent proper operation of the emission control system is also against the law.
3. Proper repairs to the emission control system must be made to manufacturer's specifications.
4. All replacement parts for emission control systems must satisfy the original design requirements of the manufacturer.

SUMMARY

- The powertrain/drivetrain is all of the parts that produce and transfer power to the drive wheels. This includes the engine, transmission or transaxle, drive axle, and other related parts.
- The suspension system allows the tires and wheels to move up and down with road surface irregularities. The types of suspension systems are front, rear, and computer controlled.
- Refrigerant leaks in an air-conditioning system may be found by using an electronic leak detector, refrigerant cans with dye, or soap and water solution in a spray bottle.

TECHNICAL TERMS

powertrain/drivetrain
engine
block
cylinder
piston
connection rod
crankshaft
cylinder head
combustion chamber
valves
camshaft
lifter
pushrods
rocker arms
flywheel
lubrication system
oil pan
oil filter
oil dipstick
cooling system
antifreeze
radiator
radiator pressure cap
radiator fan
water pump
thermostat
heater system
cooling system leak test
radiator cap pressure test
radiator cap pressure rating
exhaust system
header pipe
catalytic converter
muffler
fuel system

gasoline injection system
fuel injectors
diesel injection system
fuel pump
fuel filter
fuel pressure regulator
manual transmission
automatic transmission
transmission
torque converter
transaxle
clutch
front-wheel drive
CV-axles
rear-wheel drive
drive shaft
rear axle assembly
differential assembly
brake system
master cylinder
brake lines
wheel cylinders
brake pads
brake shoes
brake rotors
brake drums
caliper
power brakes
brake system bleeding
steering system
steering column
steering gearbox
parallelogram steering
center link
idler arm
pitman arm
rack-and-pinion steering
rack
tie-rod ends
boots
power steering pump
power steering hoses
sensors
computer
collapsible steering column
suspension system
control arms
ball joints
steering knuckles
shock absorbers
dead axle
air spring suspension
air-conditioning system
receiver-driers
accumulators
A/C high-side
A/C low-side
discharging
recovery system
evacuating
charging
purging
R-12
R-134a
emission control systems
exhaust gas recirculation (EGR)
catalytic converter
fuel evaporative system
positive crankcase ventilation system
PCV

REVIEW QUESTIONS

1. This would NOT be part of an engine.
   a. Block
   b. Control arm
   c. Connecting rod
   d. Cylinder head

2. An ____________________, commonly called a ____________, is needed to determine the freeze-up protection of the coolant mixture.

3. How do you test a cooling system for leakage?

4. Parallelogram steering is an older system being phased out by rack-and-pinion steering. True or false?

5. List seven steering service tips.

6. These mount on the out end of the control arms to allow the steering knuckles to swivel and turn.
   a. Bushings
   b. Coil springs
   c. Shocks
   d. Ball joints

7. Do not try to straighten or bend any of the pieces that make up the suspension system. True or false?

8. Explain the difference between the A/C high- and low-sides.

9. Why must you use a refrigerant recovery system?

10. Why should you evacuate an air-conditioning system?

11. What are three ways of finding refrigerant leaks?

12. Which emission control subsystem is responsible for channeling blowby gases into the fuel intake area?
   a. Engine control
   b. Positive crankcase ventilation
   c. Evaporative
   d. Exhaust gas recirculation

13. What is the engine's temperature control?
   a. Thermostat
   b. Radiator cap
   c. Cooling fan
   d. Coolant

14. When checking for refrigerant leaks, always check along the ____________ of the hoses, fitting, seals, and other possible leakage points.
15. Why must you wear hand and face protection when working on an air-conditioning system?
16. List four guidelines for working on emission control systems.

ASE-STYLE REVIEW QUESTIONS

1. *Technician A* says that antifreeze contains additives, lubricants, and corrosion inhibitors that break down over time. *Technician B* says that antifreeze should be replaced with a 50/50 mixture of antifreeze and water. Who is correct?
   a. Technician A
   b. Technician B
   c. Both Technicians A and B
   d. Neither Technician

2. Upon examining a collapsed steering column, *Technician A* decides to attempt a repair of the collapsed portion. *Technician B* says the collapsed portion must be replaced. Who is correct?
   a. Technician A
   b. Technician B
   c. Both Technicians A and B
   d. Neither Technician

3. Which of the following is a replacement for R-12?
   a. R-13a
   b. X-29a
   c. R-22
   d. R-134a

4. When evacuating an A/C system that has been open to the atmosphere for an extended period, *Technician A* holds the system at high vacuum for 30 minutes. *Technician B* replaced the receiver-drier. Who is correct?
   a. Technician A
   b. Technician B
   c. Both Technicians A and B
   d. Neither Technician

5. Which of the following parts would not normally be damaged during a frontal collision?
   a. Radiator
   b. Condenser
   c. Fuel tank
   d. Water pump

6. A brake line is found to be damaged following a collision. *Technician A* says that the line should be repaired with a spliced-in section. *Technician B* says that a new copper line must be formed. Who is correct?
   a. Technician A
   b. Technician B
   c. Both Technicians A and B
   d. Neither Technician

7. *Technician A* says that many fuel injection systems retain pressure when the engine is not running. *Technician B* says that there is never fuel pressure when the engine is not running. Who is correct?
   a. Technician A
   b. Technician B
   c. Both Technicians A and B
   d. Neither Technician

8. *Technician A* says to begin drivetrain inspection by checking the condition of the CV-joint boots. *Technician B* says that splits, cracks, tears, punctures, or thin spots in CV-joint boots require replacement. Who is correct?
   a. Technician A
   b. Technician B
   c. Both Technicians A and B
   d. Neither Technician

9. A vehicle suffers from a vibration that increases with speed. *Technician A* says that this symptom is normally due to CV-joint problems. *Technician B* says that an out-of-balance tire or wheel, an out-of-round tire, or a bent rim is the more likely cause. Who is correct?
   a. Technician A
   b. Technician B

c. Both Technicians A and B
d. Neither Technician

10. Which of the following parts should be marked for alignment before removal from the rear axle assembly?
a. Drive shaft
b. CV-joint
c. Axle shaft
d. Brake housing

ACTIVITIES

1. Inspect a vehicle with collision damage. Use the methods in this chapter to find mechanical damage. Make a report of your findings.
2. Refer to manufacturer's service manuals. Read about the troubleshooting and repair of mechanical systems.

CHAPTER

25 Wheel Alignment

OBJECTIVES

After studying this chapter, you should be able to:

- Define the term "wheel alignment."
- Inspect tires, steering, and suspension systems before alignment.
- Check and adjust caster, camber, and toe.
- Summarize alignment equipment variations.

INTRODUCTION

In collision repair, **wheel alignment** involves positioning the vehicle's tires so that they roll properly over the road surface. Wheel alignment is essential to safety, handling, fuel economy, and tire life. See **Figure 25–1.**

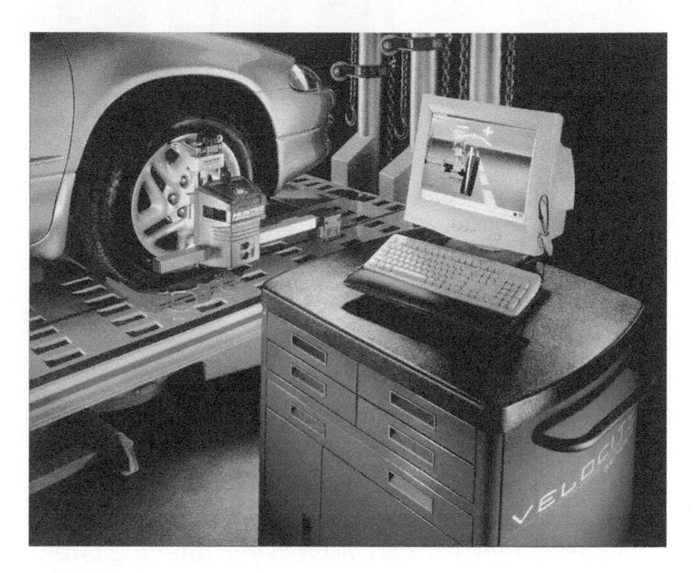

Figure 25–1. Wheel alignment involves final adjustment of the steering and suspension systems to make the tires roll properly over the road surface. If structural repairs were made properly, this is a relatively simple task using modern equipment. (Courtesy of Hunter Engineering Company)

Following collision repair, a vehicle may require an alignment if:

1. There is damage to any steering and suspension parts.
2. There is damage to any steering or suspension mounting locations.
3. There was engine cradle damage or a position change.
4. Suspension or steering parts were removed for access to body parts.
5. There was damage to major structural components.

WHEEL ALIGNMENT BASICS

Improper wheel alignment will cause rapid tire wear and poor handling.

Caster

Caster is the angle of the steering axis of a wheel from true vertical, as viewed from the side of the vehicle. It is a directional stability adjustment. Caster is measured in degrees.

Caster has little effect on tire wear. Caster affects where the tires touch the road compared to an imaginary centerline drawn through the spindle support. Caster is the first angle adjusted during an alignment.

Positive caster tilts the tops of the steering knuckles toward the rear of the vehicle. See **Figure 25–2.** It aids in keeping the vehicle's wheels traveling in a straight line. The wheels resist turning and tend to return to the straight-ahead position.

Negative caster is just the opposite (see Figure 25–2). It tilts the tops of the steering knuckles toward the front of the vehicle. Negative caster makes the wheels easier to turn. However, it produces less directional stability. The wheels tend to follow imperfections in the road surface.

Caster is designed to provide steering stability. The caster angle for all wheels should be

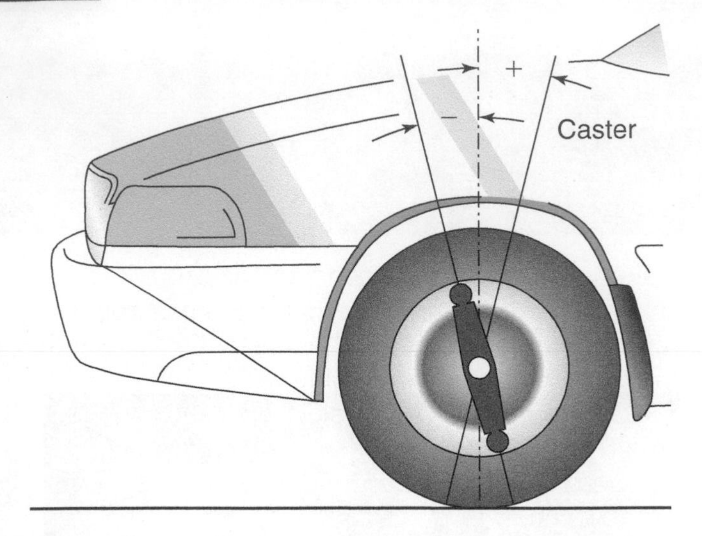

Figure 25–2. Note the difference between positive and negative caster. Caster affects whether the car's steering wheel pulls to the left or right while driving.

almost equal. Unequal caster angles will cause the vehicle to steer toward the side with less caster. Too much negative caster can cause the vehicle to have "sensitive" steering at high speeds. The vehicle might wander as a result of too much negative caster.

Several factors can adversely affect caster. The most common problem is worn or loose strut rod bushings and control arm bushings. Caster adjustments are not provided on some strut suspension systems. Where they are provided, they can be made at the top or bottom mount of a strut suspension.

Caster is measured in degrees from true vertical. Specifications for caster are given in degrees positive or negative. Typically, more positive caster is used with power steering. More negative caster is used with manual steering to reduce steering effort. Also, a vehicle pulls to the side with the least amount of caster.

Camber

Camber is the angle represented by the tilt of the wheels inward or outward from vehicle centerline when viewed from the front of the vehicle. It ensures that all of the tire tread contacts the road surface. Camber is measured in degrees. It is usually the second angle adjusted during a wheel alignment. See **Figure 25–3.**

Camber is usually set equally for all wheels. Equal camber means each wheel is tilted outward or inward the same amount.

Positive camber has the top of the wheel tilted out, when viewed from the front. The outer edge of the tire tread contacts the road.

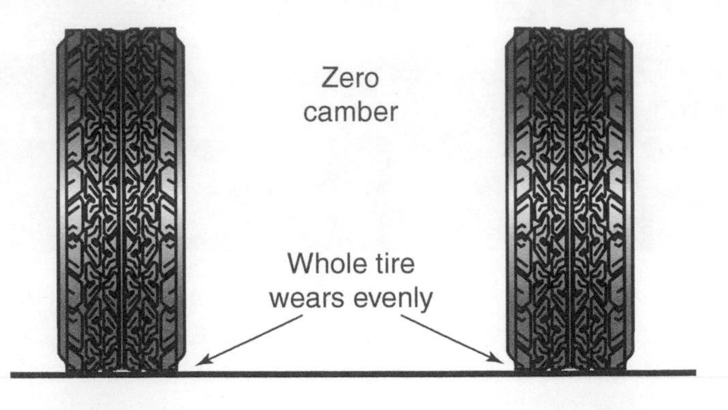

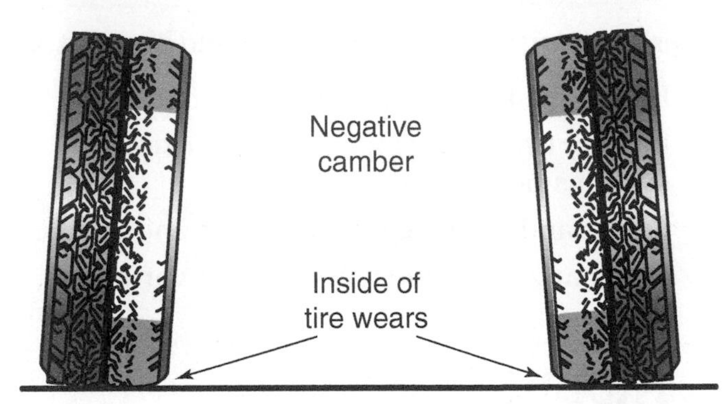

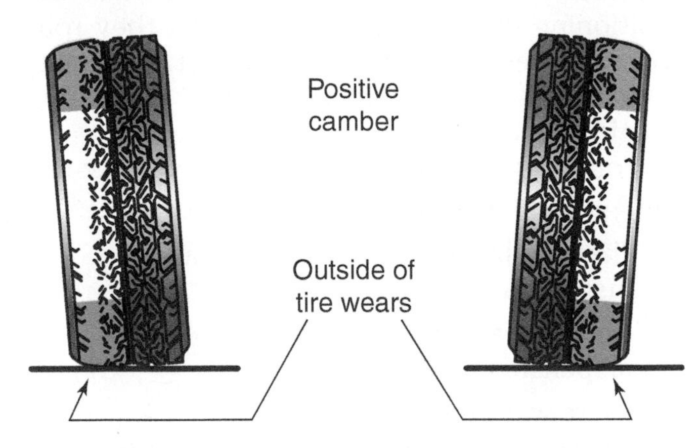

Figure 25–3. Camber is the tilt of the wheel in or out from the centerline when viewed from the front of the vehicle. Check with vehicle manufacture specs for camber settings. Camber affects whether the whole tire tread or just the edges of the tread wears.

Negative camber has the top of the wheel tilted inward when viewed from the front. The inner tire tread contacts the road surface more.

Camber is controlled by the control arms and their pivots. It is affected by worn or loose ball joints, control arm bushings, and wheel bearings. Anything that changes chassis height will also affect camber.

Camber is adjustable on most vehicles. Some manufacturers prefer to include a camber adjustment at the spindle assembly. Camber adjustments are also provided on some strut suspension systems at the top mounting position of the strut. Remember that camber adjustment also changes steering axis inclination (SAI) or the included angle.

Very little adjustment will be required if the strut tower and lower control arm positions are in their proper place. If you find serious camber error and suspension mounts have not been damaged, it is an indication of bent suspension parts. In this case, diagnostic angle and dimensional checks should be made to the suspension parts. Damaged parts must be replaced.

Toe

Toe is the difference in the distance between the front and rear of the left- and right-hand wheels. Toe can be measured in inches or millimeters or degrees, depending upon the equipment used. See **Figure 25–4.**

Toe adjustment is critical to tire wear. If properly adjusted, toe makes the wheels roll in the same direction. If toe is NOT correct, the misaligned wheels will scuff or drag the tires sideways, causing rapid tire wear.

Remember! *Excessive toe* (in or out) will cause a sawtooth edge on the tire tread from dragging the tire sideways.

Toe-in results when the front of the wheels are set closer than the rear. The wheels point in at the front. **Toe-out** is the just the opposite. It has the front of the wheels farther apart than at the rear. The wheels point out at the front.

Toe is a very critical tire-wearing angle. Wheels that do not track straight ahead have to drag as they travel forward.

Rear-wheel-drive vehicles are often adjusted to have toe-in at the front wheels. Toe-in is needed to compensate for tire rolling resistance, play in the steering system, and suspension system action. The tires tend to toe-out while driving. By setting the wheels for a small toe-in of about 1⁄16 inch (1.5 mm), the tires will roll straight ahead over the road surface.

Front-wheel-drive vehicles need to have their front wheels set for a slight toe-out. The front wheels pull and propel the vehicle. As a result, they are forced forward by drivetrain torque. This tries to make the wheels point inward while driving. Front-wheel-drive toe-out of 1⁄16 inch (1.5 mm) is typical.

Steering Axis Inclination

Steering axis inclination (SAI) is the angle between true vertical and a line through the upper and lower pivot points, as viewed from the front.

On collision damaged vehicles, SAI can help in diagnosing misalignment of a vehicle structure. For example, SAI can be used with structural measurements to diagnose:

1. Strut tower misalignment
2. Shifted engine cradle or crossmember
3. Control arm mounting location damage
4. Misaligned frame or body structure

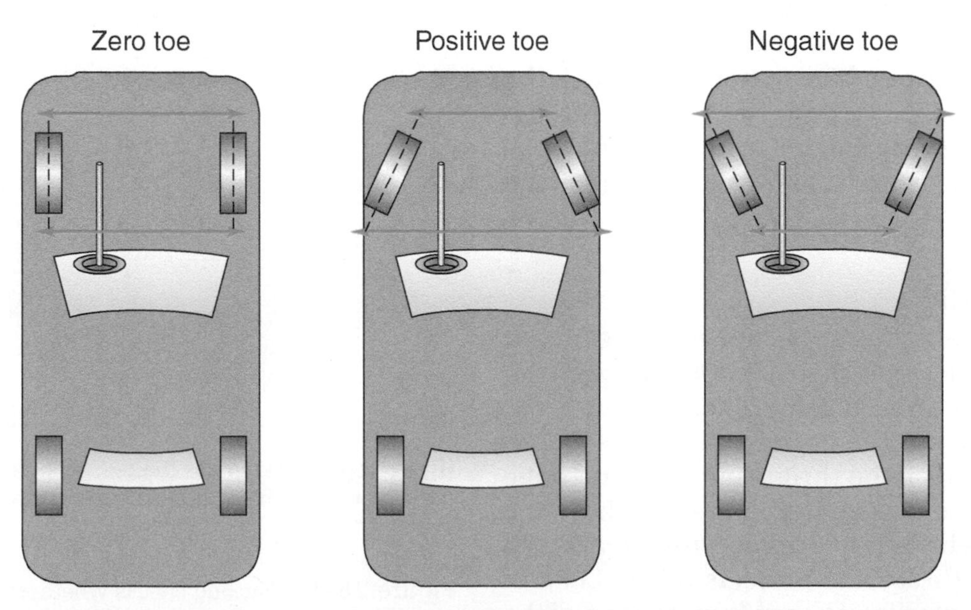

Figure 25–4. Toe is the most important wheel alignment adjustment to prevent rapid tire wear. Rear-wheel-drive cars require positive toe. Front-wheel-drive cars often need negative toe. You want zero toe when the vehicle is moving down the road under its own power. (Courtesy of Hunter Engineering)

Turning Radius

Turning radius, called *toe-out on turns,* is the different amount each wheel moves during a turn. It is built into the steering geometry. Turning radius is designed to allow the inside wheel to turn a few degrees more than the outside wheel during a turn. This makes the inside wheel turn in a smaller circle.

As an example, during a left turn, the left wheel will turn approximately 20 degrees while the right wheel will turn approximately 18 degrees. A bent steering arm will affect turning radius.

Thrust Line/Centerline (Tracking)

Tracking is the parallel alignment of the rear wheels, the vehicle centerline, and the front wheels. If a vehicle is tracking properly, its rear wheels will follow the centerline of the vehicle when moving straight ahead. Tracking problems require the driver to turn the steering wheel to have the vehicle travel in a straight line. See **Figure 25–5.**

To check tracking, wet an area of roadway, and drive the vehicle through it. Then continue driving out of the water, far enough to make measurable tracks. The rear-wheel tracks should be an equal distance from the front-wheel tracks on both sides. Incorrect tracking is often caused by worn springs, offset rear axle, or rear toe problems.

You must make sure the vehicle runs straight down the road. The rear tires must track (follow) directly behind the front tires when the steering wheel is straight. The geometric centerline of the vehicle should parallel the road direction. This will be the case when rear toe or the rear axle is parallel to the vehicle's geometric centerline in the straight-ahead position.

Thrust Angle

Thrust angle is the angle between the thrust line and vehicle centerline. It should be zero if it aligns with the vehicle centerline.

With most manufacturers, a *positive thrust angle* (+) results if the thrust line projects to the RIGHT of the vehicle centerline as seen from the top of the vehicle. A *negative thrust angle* (−) results if the thrust line projects to the LEFT of the vehicle centerline as seen from the top of the vehicle.

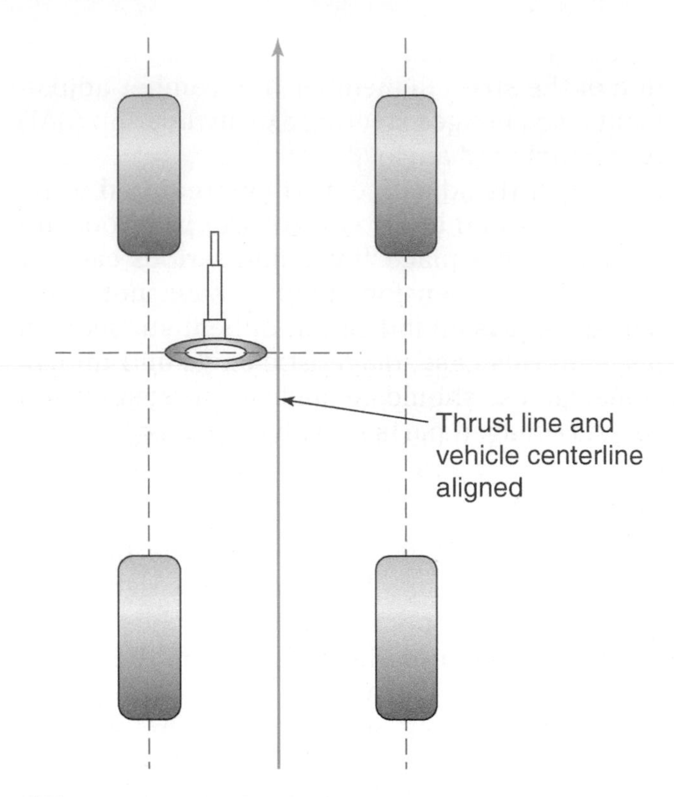

(A) Proper tracking has the rear wheels following in the tracks of the front wheels.

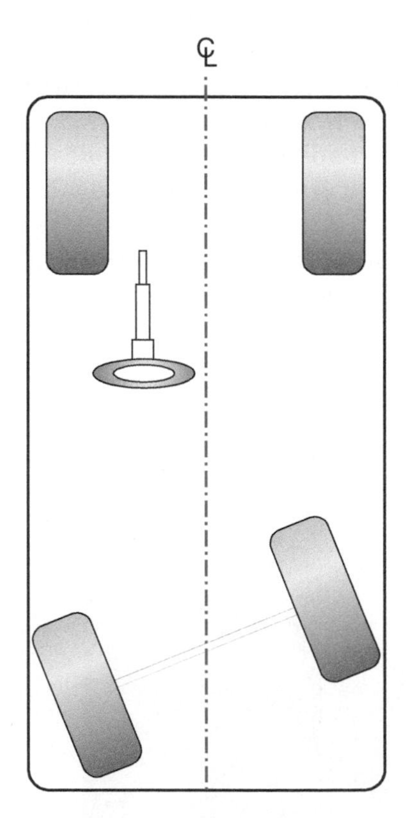

(B) Improper tracking has the rear wheels turned so they do not follow the front wheels. This is nicknamed "dog tracking."

Figure 25–5. Tracking checks whether the rear and front wheels are following each other. (Courtesy of Hunter Engineering Company)

Included Angle

Included angle is the sum of both camber and SAI angles. It is calculated by adding positive camber to the SAI angle. Included angle is calculated by subtracting negative camber from the SAI angle. It should generally be within ½ degree from side to side.

Wheelbase

Wheelbase is the measurement between the center of the front and rear wheel hubs. During collision repairs, individual wheelbase can be used as a diagnostic measurement. See **Figure 25–6.**

Wheelbase is measured to determine the forward and rearward position of each wheel. It is measured from identical known good points on the body structure or frame. Wheelbase measurements can be used to identify caster or axle positioning problems at each wheel.

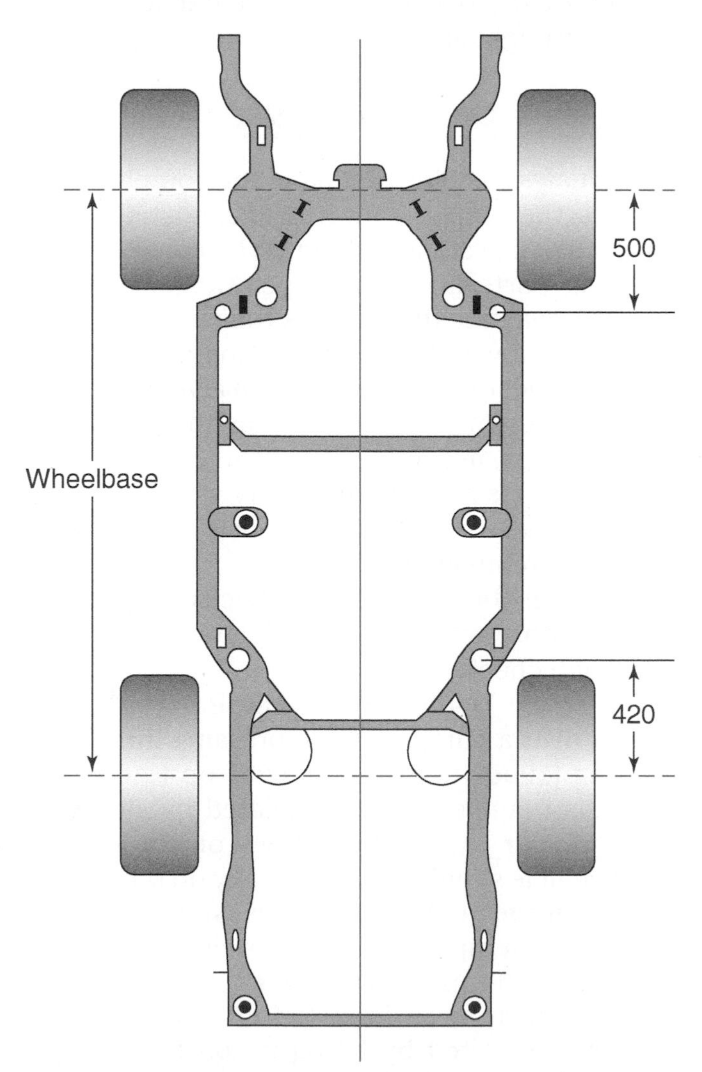

Figure 25–6. During wheel alignment, you may have to check the wheelbase to find the reason for improper wheel alignment. Set-back of one or more wheels may have resulted from collision. (Courtesy of Mitchell International, Inc.)

Wheelbase is generally acceptable if the difference is within ⅛ inch (3 mm) from side to side.

Different individual wheelbases from side to side:

1. Are generally created by frame or chassis misalignment following a collision
2. May be caused by the movement of an engine cradle
3. Will change caster by moving the lower ball joint or pivot point forward or rearward in relation to the upper pivot point
4. May be designed in by the vehicle maker on some vehicles

Set-Back

Set-back is when one wheel is moved back. It creates an unequal wheelbase between the left and right sides of a vehicle. Set-back may be caused by an impact to a front wheel assembly that moves a lower control arm, engine cradle, or radius rod backwards. It may be designed into some suspension systems.

PREALIGNMENT CHECKS

Before making adjustments, conduct the following prealignment checks:

1. VISUALLY INSPECT everything visible while the vehicle sitting on the shop floor: steering wheel effort, play in steering, and power steering fluid. This also includes checking for uneven tire wear and mismatched tire sizes or types. Look for normal wear as well as the results of collision damage. Look for towing damage as well.

Reading tires involves inspecting tire tread wear and diagnosing the cause. Improper camber and toe show up as specific tread patterns.

2. MEASURE RIDE HEIGHT. The vehicle is designed to ride at a specific height, sometimes referred to as **ride** or **curb height.** See **Figure 25–7.** Ride height specs are published in the service manuals and some alignment spec books.

Ride height is measured from the shop floor to specific points on the vehicle. Ride height should be correct before performing a wheel alignment. Various conditions that affect ride height and alignment include the following.

Vehicle load affects the weight on the front suspension and affects alignment angles. A heavy

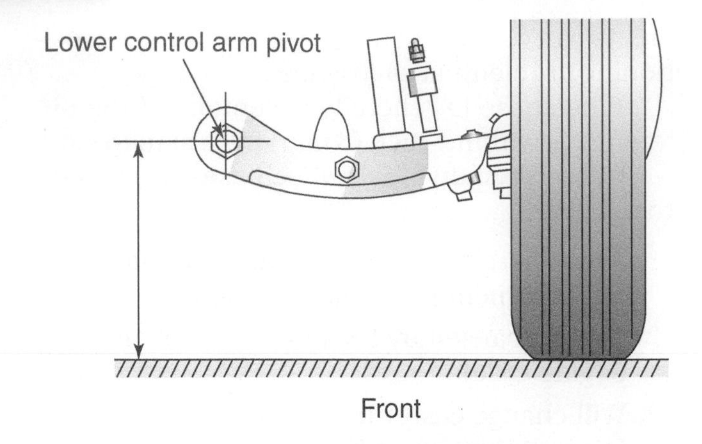

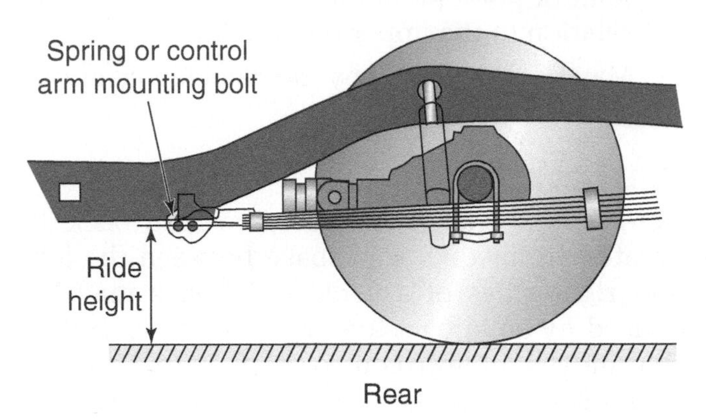

Figure 25–7. Curb height, or ride height, can affect wheel alignment. The vehicle should be at curb (empty) weight when measuring. Measure from specified points on the vehicle to a level shop floor. If curb height is not correct, springs may have weakened or suspension parts may have been damaged. (Courtesy of FMC Automotive Equipment Division)

load in the trunk takes weight off the front suspension and changes caster and camber angles. Coil and leaf springs should be checked and replaced if broken or sagged beyond tolerance. Torsion bars should be checked and adjusted if ride height is incorrect. Spring mounting locations, air spring suspensions, system faults, and shock absorbers can also affect ride height.

If the vehicle leans to one side or seems to be lower on one side than on the other, something is wrong. To isolate the problem, place the center of the main crossmember in the front of the vehicle on jack (safety) stands. Raise the front of the vehicle, and look at the rear of the vehicle. If the rear looks level, then the problem is in the front suspension, on the side of the vehicle that shows the lean. If the rear is not level, then the problem is with the low side of the rear suspension.

3. INSPECT THE UNDERSIDE of the vehicle for problems. With the vehicle raised, inspect all steering components such as the control arm bushings, upper strut mounts, pitman arm, idler arm, center link, tie-rod ends, ball joints (if equipped) for looseness, popping sounds, binding, and broken boots. Damaged parts must be repaired before adjusting alignment angles.

4. ROAD TEST the vehicle. Begin the alignment with a road test. While driving the vehicle, check to see that the steering wheel is straight. Feel for vibration in the steering wheel as well as in the floor or seats. Notice any pulling or abnormal handling problems, such as hard steering, tire squeal while cornering, or mechanical pops or clunks. This helps find problems that must be corrected before proceeding with the alignment.

Make sure the steering wheel is properly centered during your road test. If not, you will have to adjust the tie-rod ends to center it with the wheel straight ahead.

DIAGNOSTIC CHECKS

The analysis of ride and handling complaints involves the consideration of diagnostic angles. Suspension system parts must be considered as moving parts in vehicle operation; diagnostic checks evaluate the parts as they move.

When a vehicle has a steering problem, the first diagnostic check should be a visual inspection of the entire vehicle for anything obvious: bent wheels, misalignment of the cradle, and so on. If there is nothing obviously wrong with the vehicle, make a series of diagnostic checks without disassembling the vehicle.

One of the most useful checks that can be made with a minimum of equipment is a jounce-rebound check.

Jounce is the motion caused by a wheel going over a bump and compressing the spring. During jounce the wheel moves up toward the chassis. Jounce can be simulated by sitting on the bumper and pushing down on the vehicle. The vehicle should jounce equally on both sides.

Rebound is the motion caused by a wheel going into a dip or returning from a jounce and extending the spring. During rebound, the wheel moves down away from the chassis. Rebound can be simulated by lifting up on the bumper. The vehicle should lift equally on both sides.

A **jounce-rebound check** will determine if there is misalignment in the rack-and-pinion gear. For a quick check, unlock the steering wheel and see if it moves during jounce and/or rebound. For a more careful check, use a pointer and a piece of chalk. Use the chalk to make a reference mark on the tire tread and place the pointer on the same line as the chalk mark.

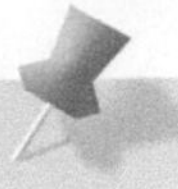

NOTE

Radial tires cause problems when they have defective belts, unusual wear patterns, uneven air pressure, or are mismatched. These tire problems can cause the technician to misdiagnose steering and alignment problems.

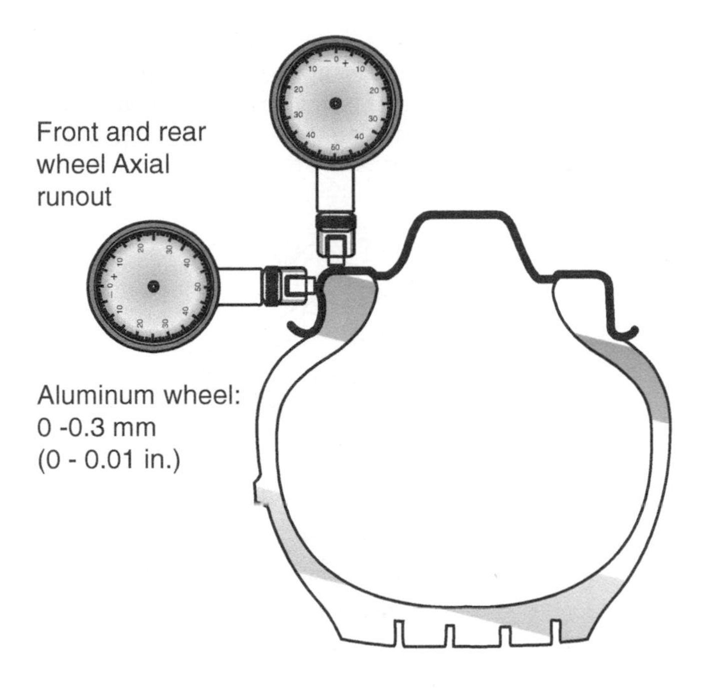

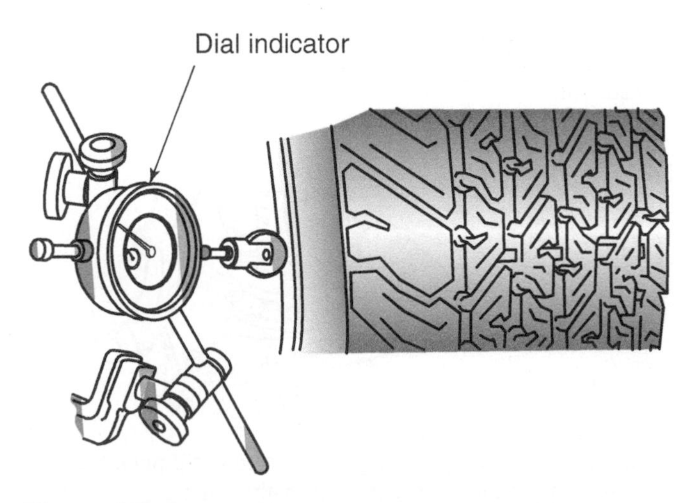

Figure 25–8. Bent wheels are a common problem in collision repair. A dial indicator will let you accurately check axial and radial runout of the wheels.

Bent wheels are common after a collision. Sometimes, wheel damage can be so small it is difficult to detect visually. A dial indicator can be used to measure actual wheel runout, as shown in **Figure 25–8.**

Loose tie-rod ends are another common problem. They can wear quickly and cause play in the steering. Never try to align wheels if there are loose, worn tie-rod ends. See **Figure 25–9.**

WHEEL ALIGNMENT PROCEDURES

After a thorough inspection and replacement of any damaged parts, wheel alignment adjustment is next. The main purpose of wheel alignment is to allow the wheels to roll without scuffing, dragging, or slipping on the road.

The order of adjustment—caster, camber and then toe—is recommended regardless of the make of vehicle or its type of suspension. Methods of adjustment vary. Refer to the manufacturer's service manual for details.

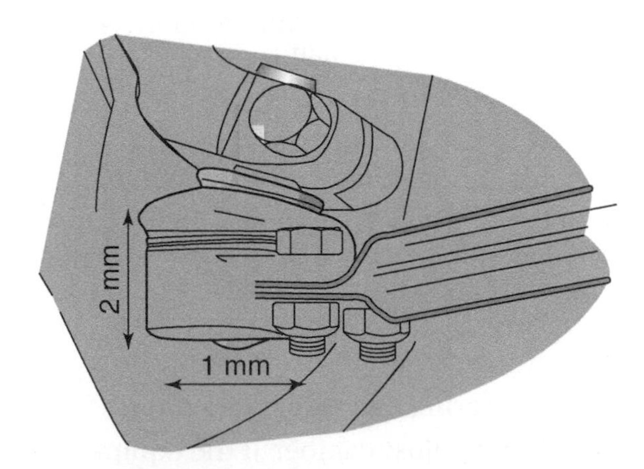

Figure 25–9. Always check the tie-rod ends for wear before adjusting wheel alignment. Play in the joint must be minimal. (Courtesy of Saab Cars USA, Inc.)

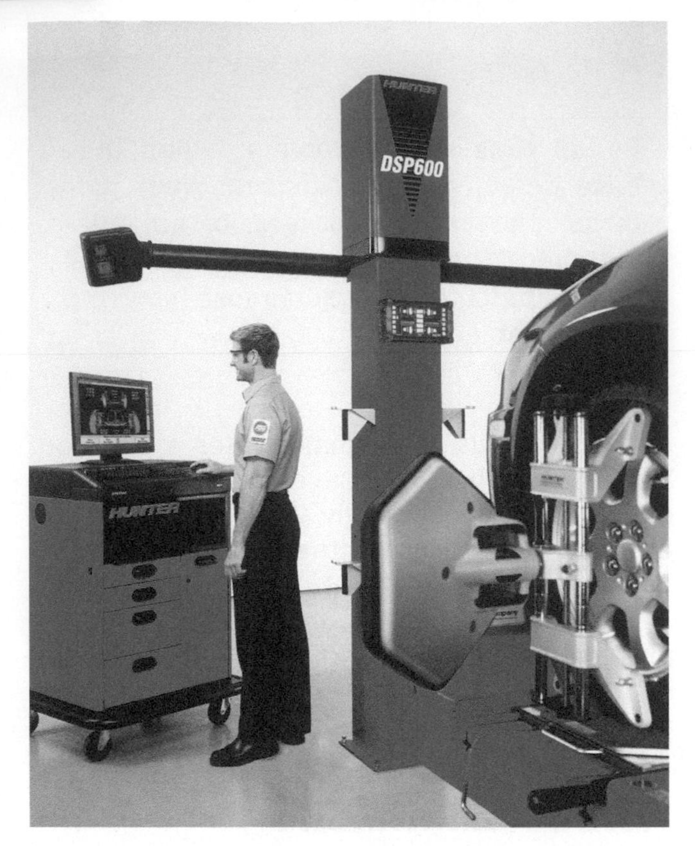

Figure 25–10. Alignment equipment basically uses a turning radius gauge (degree wheel) and a caster-camber gauge (level) to measure alignment angles. Tires are centered on top of the turning radius gauges. A wheel adapter holds the caster-camber gauge. (Courtesy of Hunter Engineering Company)

A typical procedure for a wheel alignment is as follows:

1. Obtain the manufacturer's specifications for the vehicle's wheel alignment checks and adjustments. Specs will vary depending on the design of the vehicle.
2. Mount the alignment equipment on the vehicle, following the equipment manufacturer's instructions. Equipment designs and operating procedures vary. Therefore, you must refer to the materials published by the equipment maker for proper use. See **Figure 25–10.**
3. Check steering and axis inclination.
4. Check and adjust camber. If the equipment shows camber to be within specs, no adjustment is necessary. If it is not within specs, you must change camber the right amount and direction. See **Figure 25–11.**

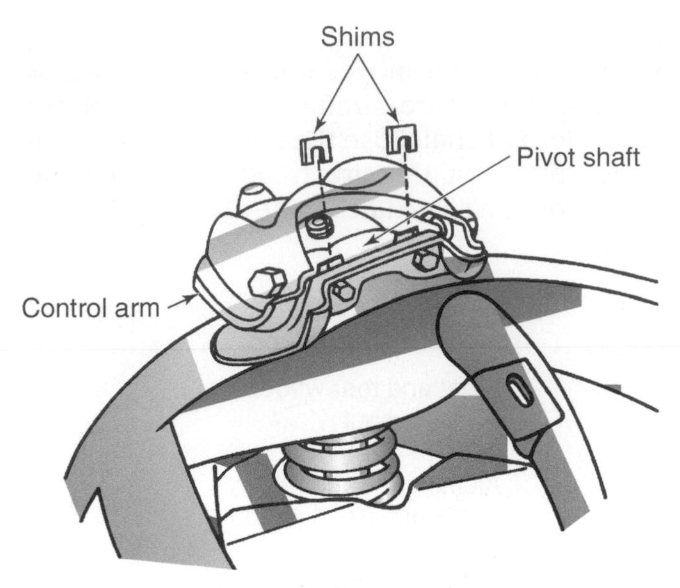

(A) Shims are often provided for upper/lower control arm suspension systems. Different thickness shims in front and rear will change caster. Inserting the same size shims only changes camber, SAI, and included angle.

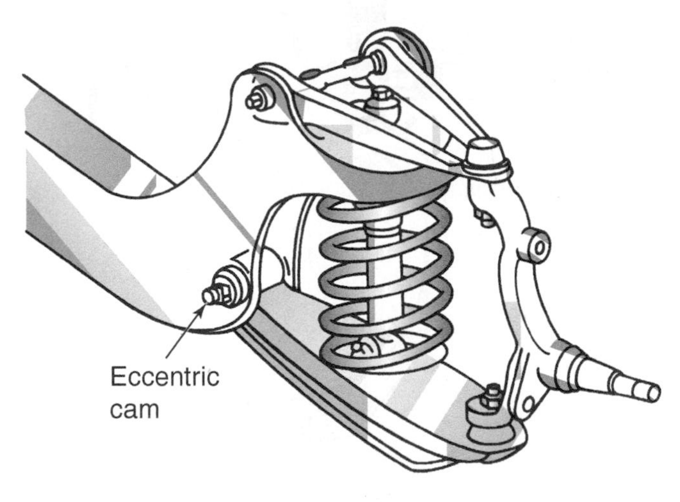

(B) Turning the eccentric cam bolt will pivot the control arm in and out for SAI, included angle, and camber-caster adjustment.

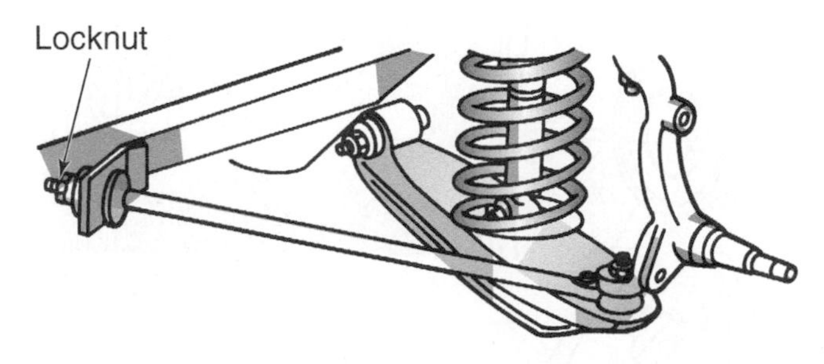

(C) Shortening or lengthening the strut rod will pivot the outer end of the lower control arm to alter caster.

Figure 25–11. Study various ways of adjusting caster, camber, SAI, and included angle. (Illustrations courtesy of Perfect Circle/Dana Corp.)

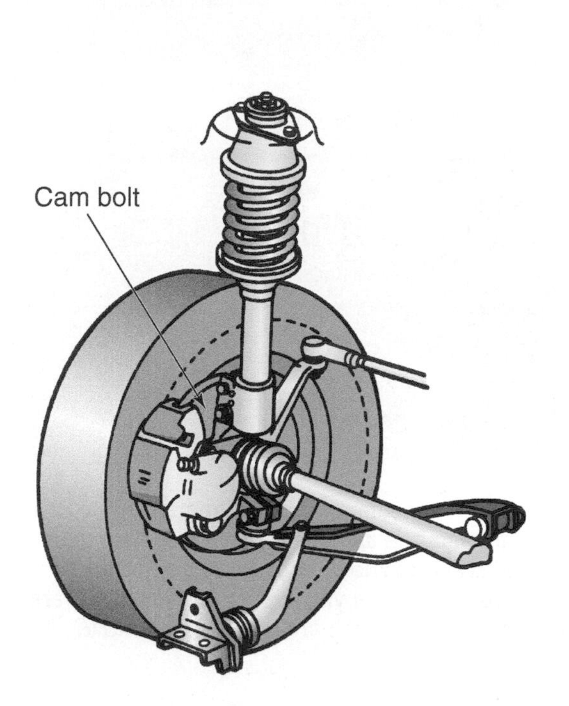

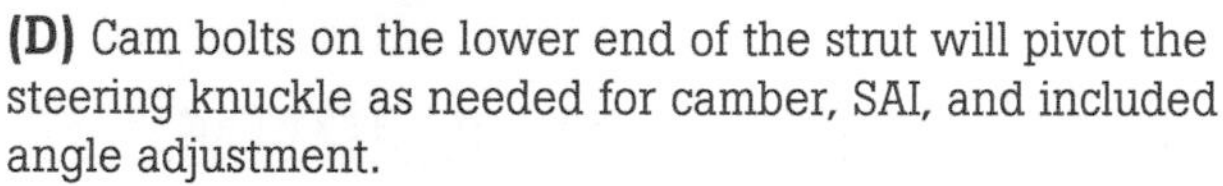
(D) Cam bolts on the lower end of the strut will pivot the steering knuckle as needed for camber, SAI, and included angle adjustment.

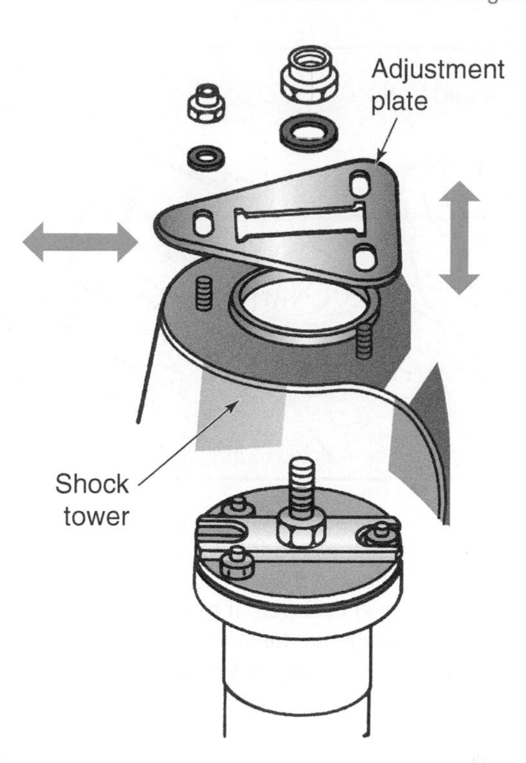

(E) Many strut suspensions have slotted holes for adjustment of caster, camber, SAI, and included angle. If they are not slotted, aftermarket kits are available to allow for adjustment.

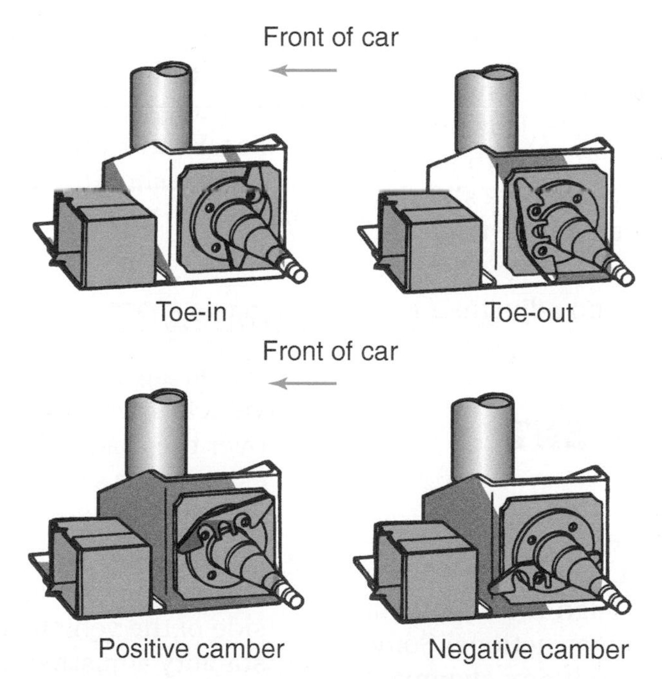

(F) Different thickness shims can be placed between the rear knuckle and the strut to adjust alignment.

Figure 25–11. ***(Continued)***

5. Check and adjust caster. If the car tends to pull to one side or if equipment readings are off, change caster. Again, see Figure 25–11 for adjustment methods.
6. Check turning radius. Replace parts if needed.
7. Check and adjust toe LAST. See **Figure 25–12.** Toe is the last adjustment made in an alignment. It is made at the tie-rods. Toe

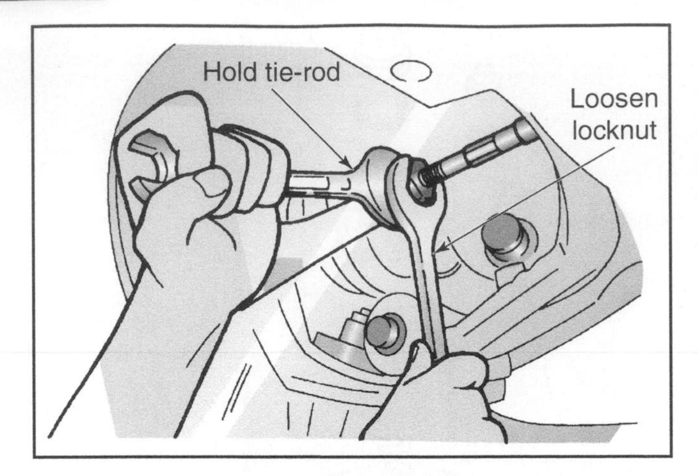

Figure 25–12. Toe is adjusted by shortening or lengthening tie-rod ends. If the steering wheel is centered, change the length of the right and left sides equally. This will keep the steering wheel centered. If the steering wheel is not centered, change the tie-rods differently to center the wheel. (Copyright Mazda Motor of America, Inc. Used by permission)

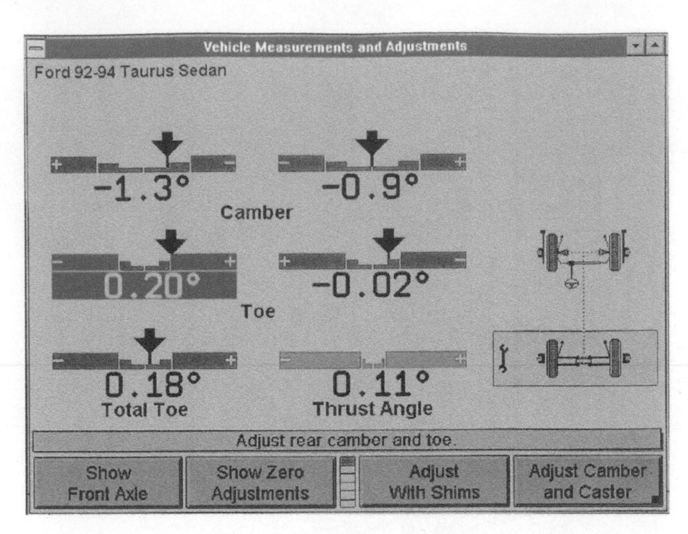

Figure 25–13. Today's computerized alignment equipment will guide you through the alignment procedure. This unit uses arrows and scales to show readings of alignment angles all at once. It also lets you know which readings are within specifications and which are not. (Courtesy of Hunter Engineering Company)

adjustments on a rack-and-pinion unit must be made evenly on both sides of the rack-and-pinion gear. If they are not made evenly, the rack assembly will be off-center in the gear. This can cause a pull due to the steering wheel being off-center. This pull condition is especially common with power-assisted rack-and-pinion gears. The steering assembly must be centered before these adjustments are made.

8. Document your readings and adjustment values.

ALIGNMENT EQUIPMENT VARIATIONS

Note that most modern wheel alignment equipment is computer controlled. See **Figure 25–13.** It will actually guide you through the alignment process, giving step-by-step instructions. Some equipment will even warn you if any alignment angle is not acceptable. This greatly simplifies the wheel alignment process.

Today most vehicles use a four-wheel alignment. Approximately 80 percent of today's vehicles require front- and rear-wheel alignment. This is due to the growing number of vehicles with independent rear suspensions. Collision repair of any magnitude usually requires at least a four-wheel alignment check.

ROAD TEST AFTER ALIGNMENT

After making your wheel alignment adjustments, road test the vehicle. Make sure the vehicle does not pull to one side of the road, vibrate, or exhibit other troubles.

See **Figure 25–14** and **Figure 25–15**. They are troubleshooting charts for the steering and suspension systems.

SUMMARY

- Wheel alignment involves positioning the vehicle's tires so that they roll properly over the road surface. Wheel alignment is essential to safety, handling, fuel economy, and tire life.
- Caster is the angle of the steering axis of a wheel from true vertical, as viewed from the side of the vehicle. It is a directional stability adjustment.
- Camber is the angle represented by the tilt of the wheels inward or outward when viewed from the front of the vehicle. It assures that all of the tire tread contacts the road surface. It is usually the second angle adjusted during a wheel alignment.
- Toe is the difference in the distance between the front and rear of the left- and right-hand wheels. It is critical to tire wear.

Suspension Problem Diagnosis						
	Problem					
Check	**Noise**	**Instability**	**Pulls to one side**	**Excessive steering play**	**Hard steering**	**Shimmy**
Tires/wheels	Road or tire noise	Low or uneven air pressure; radials mixed with belted bias ply tires	Low or uneven air pressure; mismatched tire sizes	Low or uneven air pressure	Low or uneven air pressure	Wheel out of balance or uneven tire wear or overworn tires; radials mixed with belted bias ply tires
Shock dampers (struts/ absorbers)	Loose or worn mounts or bushings	Loose or worn mounts or bushings; worn or damaged struts or shock absorbers	Loose or worn mounts or bushings	—	Loose or worn mounts or bushings on strut assemblies	Worn or damaged struts or shock absorbers
Strut rods	Loose or worn mounts or bushings	Loose or worn mounts or bushings	Loose or worn mounts or bushings	—	—	Loose or worn mounts or bushings
Springs	Worn or damaged	Worn or damaged	Worn or damaged, especially rear	—	Worn or damaged	—
Control arms	Steering knuckle control arm stop; worn or damaged mounts or bushings	Worn or damaged mounts or bushings	Worn or damaged mounts or bushings	—	Worn or damaged mounts or bushings	Worn or damaged mounts or bushings
Steering system	Component wear or damage	Component wear or damage	Component wear or damage	Component wear or damage	Component wear or damage	Component wear or damage
Alignment	—	Front and rear, especially caster	Front, camber and caster	Front	Front, especially caster	Front, especially caster
Wheel bearings	On turns or speed changes: front-wheel bearings	Loose or worn (front and rear)	Loose or worn (front and rear)	Loose or worn (front)	—	Loose or worn (front and rear)
Brake system	—	—	On braking	—	On braking	—
Other	Clunk on speed changes: trans-axle; click on turns; CV joints; ball joint lubrication	—	—	—	Ball joint lubrication	Loose or worn friction ball joints

Figure 25–14. Study this chart that shows suspensions system problems that can affect alignment.

TECHNICAL TERMS

wheel alignment
caster
positive caster
negative caster
camber
positive camber
negative camber
toe
toe-in
toe-out
steering axis inclination (SAI)
turning radius
tracking
thrust angle
wheelbase
set-back
reading tires
ride height
curb height
jounce
rebound
jounce-rebound check

REVIEW QUESTIONS

1. List four reasons a vehicle would require an alignment after collision repair.
2. Give six basic wheel alignment angles.

Steering Problem Diagnosis						
	Problem					
Check	Noise	Instability	Pull to one side	Excessive steering play	Hard steering	Shimmy
Tires/wheels	Road or tire noise	Low or uneven tire pressure; radial tire lead	Low or uneven tire pressure; radial tire lead	Low or uneven tire pressure	Low or uneven tire pressure	Unbalanced wheel; uneven tire wear; overworn tires
Tie-rods	Squeal in turns: worn ends	—	Incorrect toe: tie-rod length	Worn ends	Worn ends	Worn ends
Mounts or bushings	Parallelogram steering: steering gear mounting bolts, linkage connections; rack-and-pinion steering: rack mounts	Idler arm bushing	—	Parallelogram steering: steering gear mounting bolts, linkage connections; rack-and-pinion steering: rack mounts	Parallelogram steering: steering gear mounting bolts, linkage connections; rack-and-pinion steering: rack mounts	Parallelogram steering: steering gear mounting bolts, linkage connections; rack-and-pinion steering: rack mounts
Steering linkage components	Bent or damaged steering rack	Incorrect center link or rack height	Incorrect center link or rack height	Worn idler arm, center link, or pitman arm studs; worn or damaged rack	Idler arm binding	Worn idler arm, center link, or pitman arm studs
Steering gear	Improper yoke adjustment on rack-and-pinion steering	—	—	Improper yoke adjustment on rack-and-pinion steering; worn steering gear or incorrect gear adjustment on parallelogram steering; loose or worn steering shaft coupling	Parallelogram steering: low steering gear lubricant, incorrect adjustment; rack-and-pinion: bent rack, improper yoke adjustment	—
Power steering	—	—	—	—	Fluid leaks; loose, worn, or glazed steering belt; weak pump; low fluid level	—
Alignment	—	—	Unequal caster or camber	—	Excessive positive caster, excessive scrub radius (incorrect camber and/or SAI)	Incorrect caster

Figure 25–15. Study this chart for diagnosing steering system problems.

3. ______________ ______________ tilts the tops of the steering knuckles toward the rear of the vehicle, when viewed from the side of the vehicle.
4. ______________ ______________ has the top of the wheel tilted out, when viewed from the front. The outer edge of the ______________ ______________ contacts the road.
5. Camber is adjustable on most vehicles. True or false?
6. Explain the importance of proper toe adjustment.
7. *Technician A* says that rear-wheel-drive vehicles are often adjusted to have toe-in at the front wheels. *Technician B* says that front-wheel-drive vehicles need to have their front wheels set for a slight toe-out. Who is correct?
   a. Technician A
   b. Technician B

c. Both Technicians A and B
d. Neither Technician

8. SAI can be used with structural measurements to diagnose:
   a. Strut tower misalignment
   b. Control arm mounting location damage
   c. Misaligned frame or unibody structure
   d. Camber change
   e. Toe-out condition
9. Define the term "tracking."
10. This is the measurement between the center of the front and rear wheel hubs.
    a. Scrub
    b. Tracking
    c. Toe
    d. Wheelbase
11. How and why do you read tires?
12. How do you measure vehicle ride height?
13. In your own words, how do you inspect the underside of a vehicle before a wheel alignment?
14. Summarize the eight major steps for a wheel alignment.

ASE-STYLE REVIEW QUESTIONS

1. Following a collision, a vehicle would NOT require an alignment if:
   a. There is damage to any steering and suspension parts.
   b. There is damage to any steering or suspension mounting locations.
   c. There is engine cradle damage or a position change.
   d. There is damage to the deck lid.

2. Which of the following represents a directional stability adjustment?
   a. Toe
   b. Caster
   c. Camber
   d. Steering axis inclination

3. A customer complains of rapid tire wear. Which of the following is the most common cause of this problem?
   a. Toe
   b. Caster
   c. Camber
   d. Steering axis inclination

4. Which of the following should the front wheels of front-wheel-drive vehicles be set for?
   a. A slight negative camber
   b. A slight positive camber
   c. A slight toe-in
   d. A slight toe-out

5. *Technician A* says to check ride height before a wheel alignment. *Technician B* says to perform a road test before a wheel alignment. Who is correct?
   a. Technician A
   b. Technician B
   c. Both Technicians A and B
   d. Neither Technician

6. Which of the following is the normal sequence for a wheel alignment?
   a. Toe, caster, camber
   b. Camber, caster, toe
   c. Caster, inclination, toe
   d. Caster, camber, toe

7. At which of the following locations is toe adjusted?
   a. Tie-rod ends
   b. Top of strut towers
   c. Ball joints
   d. Steering knuckle

8. At which of the following locations is camber normally adjusted on most vehicles?
   a. Tie-rod ends
   b. Top of strut towers
   c. Ball joints
   d. Steering knuckle

9. A vehicle suffers from tire wear on the inner edge of the tire. *Technician A* says that the problem is caster. *Technician B* says that the problem is due to camber maladjustment. Who is correct?

a. Technician A
b. Technician B
c. Both Technicians A and B
d. Neither Technician

10. A vehicle steering wheel has a slight pull to the left. *Technician A* says to adjust caster. *Technician B* says to adjust toe. Who is correct?

a. Technician A
b. Technician B
c. Both Technicians A and B
d. Neither Technician

ACTIVITIES

1. Visibly inspect the alignment and tire wear on several cars. Try to find one with obvious misalignment. Write a report of your findings.

2. Refer to the operating manual for alignment equipment. Read through the specific procedures for the alignment equipment. Summarize any unique procedure and prepare to discuss it with the class.

CHAPTER

26 Electrical Repairs

OBJECTIVES

After studying this chapter, you should be able to:

- Use various kinds of electrical test instruments.
- Find electrical problems.
- Explain the operation of automotive electrical-electronic systems.
- Describe the operation of computer systems.
- Use scanners to find electrical-electronic problems.

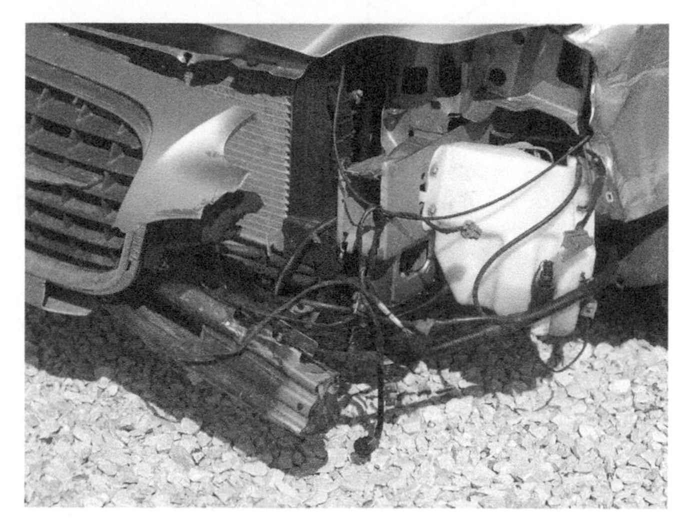

Figure 26–1. During a collision, the wires near the point of impact can be cut or crushed and damaged. As a technician, you should be able to locate and correct electrical problems.

INTRODUCTION

Electrical systems, such as the ignition, charging, starting, lighting, and computer systems, perform needed functions for a vehicle. It is almost impossible to work on any section of a vehicle without handling some type of electrical part. See **Figure 26–1.**

Electrical system repair is an essential aspect of repairing a collision-damaged vehicle. Electrical repairs are becoming more common due to the increased use of computer-controlled systems. These repairs can be made complicated by the many computer circuits running throughout the body structure.

ELECTRICAL TERMINOLOGY

Various vehicle systems are controlled by a series of electrical controls and devices. To understand electricity, you must become familiar with three electrical terms: current, voltage, and resistance.

Current is the movement of electricity (electrons) through a wire or circuit. It is measured in amperes, or amps, using an ammeter. The common electrical symbol for current is "A" or "I."

Voltage is the pressure that pushes the electricity through the wire or circuit. The *power source* generates the voltage that causes current flow. Voltage is measured in volts using a voltmeter. The symbol for voltage is "E" or "V." See **Figure 26–2.**

Resistance is a restriction or obstacle to current flow. It tries to stop the current caused by the applied voltage. Circuit or part resistance is measured in ohms using an ohmmeter. The symbol for resistance is "R" or "Ω."

A **conductor** carries current to the parts of a circuit. **"Hot wires"** connect the battery positive to the components of each circuit. **Insulation** stops current flow and keeps the current in the metal wire conductor. The body

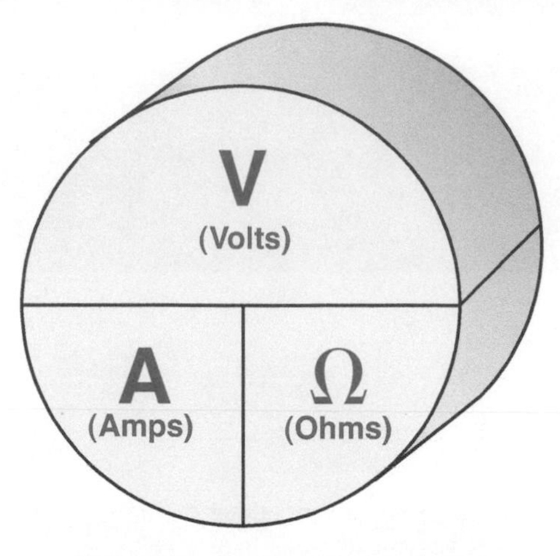

Voltage = Current × Resistance
Current = Voltage ÷ Resistance
Resistance = Voltage ÷ Current

Figure 26–2. Ohm's Law is a simple formula for calculating electrical values in a circuit.

structure provides the **ground** conductor back to the battery negative cable.

Electric Circuits

An **electric circuit** contains a power source, conductors, and a load. Some resistance is designed into a circuit in the form of a load. The **load** is the part of a circuit that converts electrical energy into another form of energy (light, movement, heat, etc.). Other parts are added to this simple circuit to protect it from damage and to do more tasks.

A **series circuit** has only one conductor path or leg for current through the circuit. Current must flow through the wires and components one after the other. If any part of the circuit is **opened** (disconnected), all of the series circuit stops working.

A **parallel circuit** has two or more legs or paths for current. Current can flow through either leg independently. One path can be **closed** (electrically connected) and the other opened, and the closed path will still operate.

A **series-parallel circuit** has both series and parallel branches in it. It has characteristics of both circuit types. All the circuits in a vehicle can be classified and tested using the rules of these three circuits.

Ohm's Law

Ohm's Law is a math formula for calculating an unknown electrical value (amps, volts, or ohms) when two values are known. If you know two values, you can mathematically calculate the third unknown value.

For instance, if you know that a circuit has 12.6 volts and 2 amps, what is the circuit resistance? Plug your two known values into Ohm's Law and you can find out (12.6 divided by 2 equals 6.3 amps). See Figure 26–2.

Magnetism

Magnetism involves the study of how electric fields act upon ferrous (iron-containing) objects. Many electrical-electronic parts use magnetism.

A **flux** or **magnetic field** is present around permanent magnets and current-carrying wires. This invisible energy is commonly used to move metal parts. An **electromagnet** is a set of **windings** or wires wrapped around an iron core. When current flows through the windings, a powerful magnetic field is produced. Electric motors, solenoids, relays, and other parts use this principle.

DIAGNOSTIC EQUIPMENT

Locating an electrical fault is not possible without using **diagnostic tools** (meters, test lights, jumper wires, etc.). Keep in mind that today's delicate electronic systems can be damaged if the wrong methods and equipment are used.

Multimeters

A **multimeter** is a voltmeter, ohmmeter, and ammeter combined into one case. Also called a **VOM** (volt-ohm-ammeter), it can be used to measure actual electrical values for comparison to known good values.

The **digital multimeter (DVOM)** has a number readout for the test value. This type is recommended by auto manufacturers because it will NOT damage delicate electronic components. A high-impedance (10 mega-ohm input) DVOM is recommended to avoid damaging sensitive components. Digital readouts give the precise measurement needed for proper diagnosis. DVOMs are used in conjunction with the vehicle's service manual.

An **analog multimeter (AVOM)** has a pointer needle that moves across the face of a scale when making electrical measurements. Use of an AVOM can damage sensitive electronic components. It should be used only when testing all-electrical, NOT electronic, circuits. AVOMs help show a fluctuating or changing reading, such as from an intermittent (changing) problem.

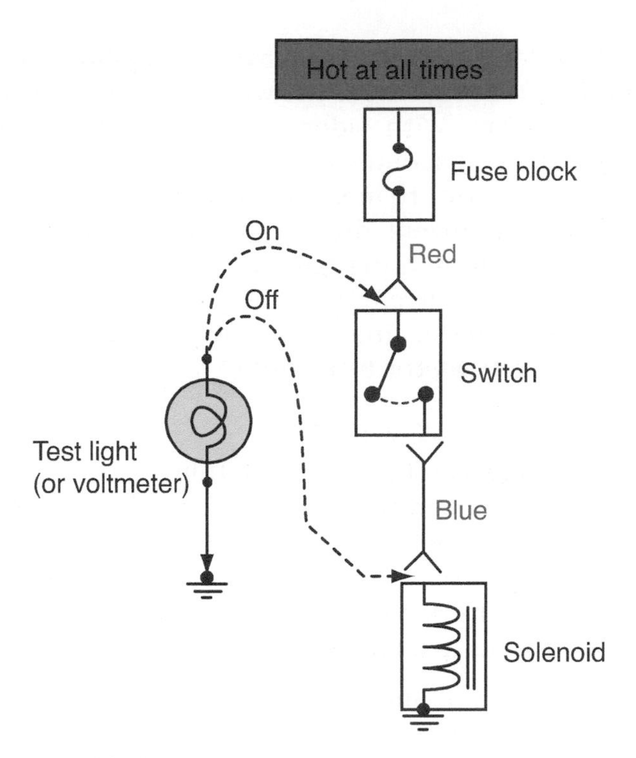

Figure 26–3. A test light provides a fast way of probing for voltage. Make sure you are using a high-impedance instrument when testing computer circuits. (Courtesy of General Motors Corporation, Service Operations)

Test Light, Jumper Wires

An externally powered **test light** is often used to determine if there is current flowing through the circuit. One lead of the test lamp is connected to a good ground. The other lead connects to a point in the circuit. If the lamp lights, current is present at that point. See **Figure 26–3.**

Whenever a technician has an electrical system problem that does not directly concern the computer, a test light is handy.

Connect the light to the voltage source and to ground. If the test light does not glow, there is an open circuit somewhere. If the light is on but the part does not work, the part is probably bad.

Jumper wires are used to temporarily bypass circuits or components for testing. They consist of a length of wire with an alligator clip at each end. They can be used to test circuit breakers, relays, lights, and other components. Refer to **Figure 26–4.**

Using Multimeters

When measuring resistance, always disconnect the circuit from the power source. The multimeter must never be connected to a circuit in which current is flowing. Doing so can damage the meter. See **Figure 26–5.**

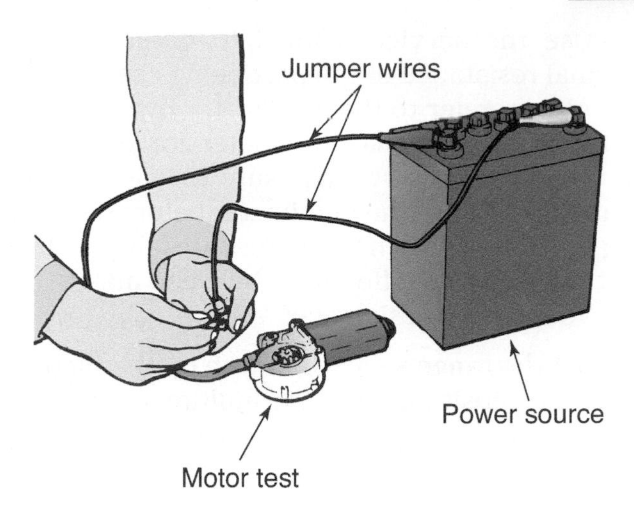

Figure 26–4. Jumper wires can be used to bypass resistive parts or to connect power directly to parts to check their operation. For example, if a motor runs when connected directly to voltage, you would know the circuit might not be providing power or a ground to the motor.

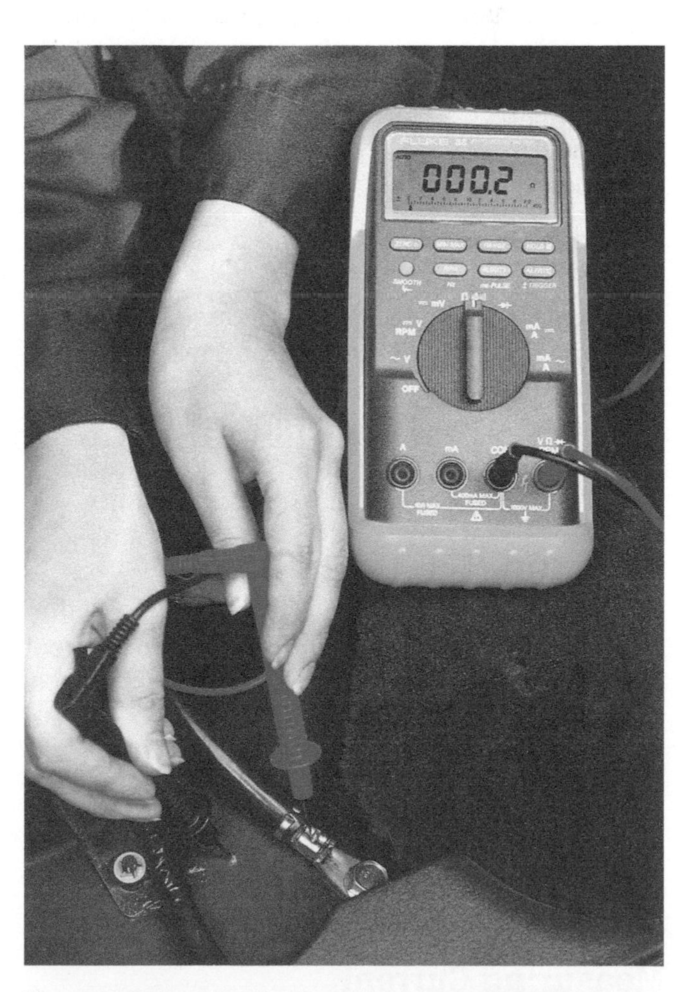

Figure 26–5. A VOM, also called a multimeter, is a voltmeter, ammeter, and ohmmeter in one case. It can be used to compare service manual electrical values with those on the vehicle being repaired. (Courtesy of Fluke)

Use the service manual to determine the normal resistance of the part being checked.

Always refer to the multimeter owner's manual before using the multimeter for diagnostic purposes. You must make sure that you understand how to use the multimeter before performing diagnostics. All multimeters are fairly similar, but there can be differences between makes.

To measure resistance:

1. Set the range selector switch on the highest range position. Turn the multimeter on.
2. Connect the multimeter test leads to opposite ends of the circuit or wire being tested.
3. Reduce the range setting until the meter shows a reading near the middle of its scale. Some DVOMs have an *auto ranging* function that adjusts the settings automatically.

Checking Continuity

A circuit remains closed and operational when it has **continuity,** or a continuous conductor path. Typically, the service manual will ask for a continuity check of a wire or part. The continuity check is done to see if the electrical circuit has a complete path without any opens.

1. Set the range selector switch on the highest resistance range position.
2. Connect the multimeter test leads to the opposite ends of the wire or part being tested.
3. Read the meter. An **infinite reading** (maximum resistance) shows an open circuit. A zero reading shows continuity.

Measuring Voltage

The multimeter allows you to select either alternating current voltage (ACV) or direct current voltage (DCV). The ACV is selected when measuring alternating current voltage. **AC current** is the type of current that is found in your home wiring.

DCV is selected when measuring direct current voltage. **DC current** is what is normally measured in the automobile. Some signals from sensors, however, can be AC.

Measuring Current

Current or amperage is sometimes measured to check the consumption of power by a load. For example, current draw is often measured when checking the condition of a starting motor.

Modern ammeters have an **inductive pickup** that slips over the wire or cable to measure current. With older ammeters, the circuit had to be disconnected and the meter connected in series to measure current.

A high current draw indicates a low resistance, like from a dragging or partially shorted motor. A low current draw means there is a high resistance in the circuit, like from a bad connection or dirty motor brushes.

Checking for Shorts

Many times adjoining wires within a wiring harness get pinched together or severed in a collision. A multimeter check will detect a severed wire.

When checking for a short between two adjoining wires in a harness:

1. Set the multimeter range selector switch the same as for a continuity check.
2. Connect the multimeter test leads to the opposite ends of the adjoining wires.
3. Because the wires are insulated, there should be a reading of almost infinity on the multimeter. If the multimeter reads zero, the wires are shorted to ground or another ground wire.

WIRING DIAGRAMS

To determine and isolate electrical problems, it is often necessary to trace through the electrical circuit using a **wiring diagram.** See **Figure 26–6.**

Abbreviations are used on wiring diagrams so that more information can be given. The service manual will have a chart explaining each abbreviation, number, and symbol on the diagram.

Electrical symbols are graphic representations of electrical-electronic components. Symbol charts can be found at the front of the wiring diagram section of the service manual. One is given in **Figure 26–7.**

Most wires on wiring diagrams will be identified by their insulation color. **Wire color coding** allows you to find a specific wire in a harness or in a connector. See **Figure 26–8.** The color code abbreviation chart can also be found at the front of the wiring diagram section of the service manual. Remember, different auto makers use different color coding abbreviations on their wiring diagrams.

Many wiring diagrams found in the service manuals also have circuits numbered. *Circuit*

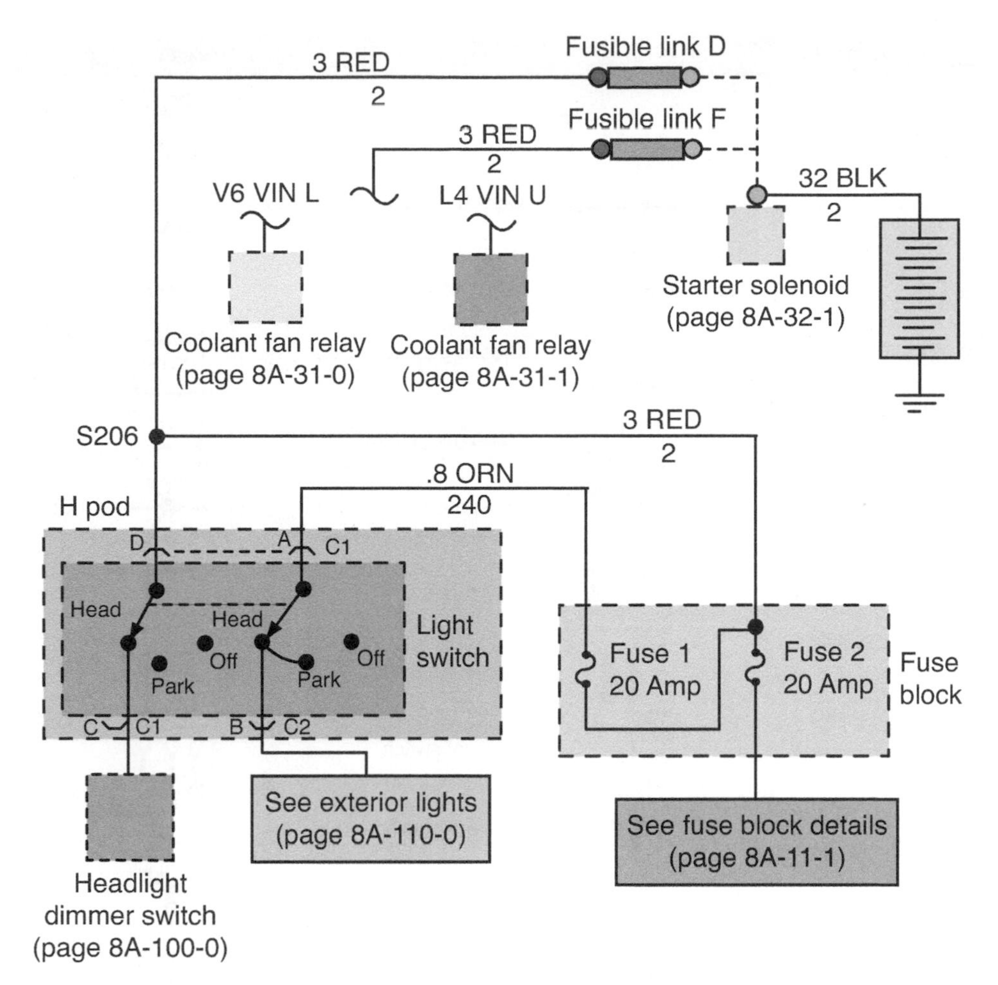

Figure 26–6. A wiring diagram is like a "road map" of the circuit being tested. It shows how wires lead to different locations or parts in the circuit. It also gives color codes, abbreviations, and other information for troubleshooting. (Courtesy of General Motors Corporation, Service Operations)

numbering is used to specify exactly which part of the circuit the service manual is referring to.

Remember! A wiring diagram is more like a "book" than a "picture." You can not understand a wiring diagram just by glancing at it. Like a book, you must read the diagram carefully all the way through for a complete understanding.

A **wiring harness** has several wires enclosed in a protective covering. A vehicle has several wiring harnesses, usually named after their location in the vehicle. The service manual will give illustrations with code numbers for locating parts and connections.

The service manual may also give a **part location diagram** for finding electrical parts (harnesses, sensors, switches, computers, etc.). Refer to **Figure 26–9** on page 446.

ELECTRIC COMPONENTS

A **switch** is used to turn a circuit on or off manually (by hand). When the switch is CLOSED (on), the circuit is complete (fully connected) and will operate. Various types can be found in today's vehicles.

A **solenoid** is an electromagnet with a movable core or plunger. When energized, the plunger is pulled into the magnetic field to produce motion. Solenoids are used in many applications: door locks, engine idle speed, emission control systems, etc. A bad solenoid can develop coil winding opens, shorts, or high resistance problems.

A **relay** is a remote control switch. A small switch can be used to energize the relay. The relay coil then acts upon a movable arm to close the relay contacts. This allows a small switch to control high current going to a load. A relay is commonly used with electric motors since they draw heavy current. See **Figure 26–10** on page 447. The service manual will often give relay locations for the specific make and model vehicle.

A bad relay will often have burned points that prevent current flow to the load. It can also develop coil opens and shorts that keep the points from closing.

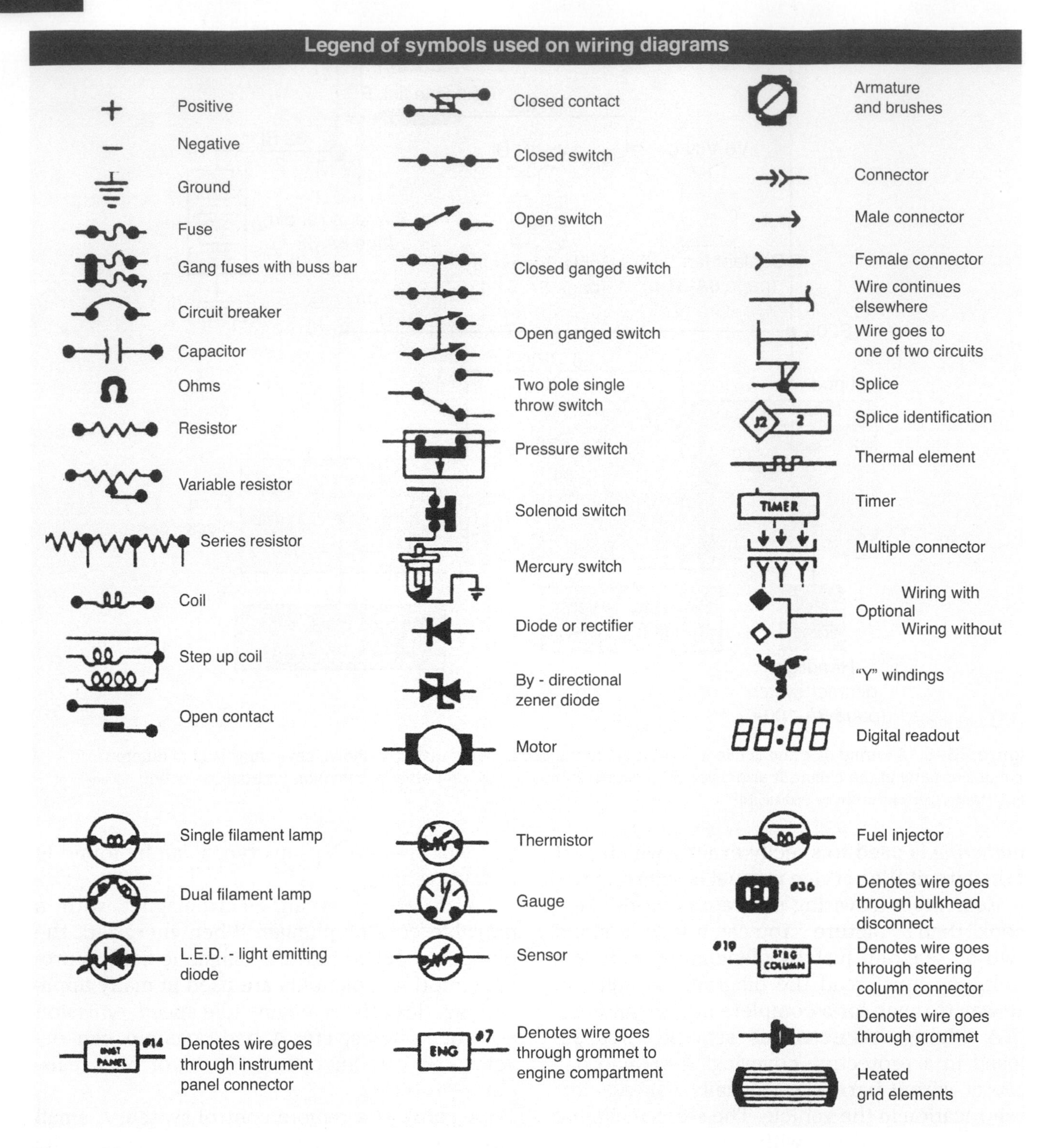

Figure 26–7. Study the symbols typically used on wiring diagrams. (Courtesy of DaimlerChrysler Corporation)

Motors use permanent and electromagnets to convert electrical energy into a rotation motion for doing work. Some examples are the electric starting motor for the engine, and stepper motors for computer control of parts.

Faulty motors can have worn bushings, brushes that decrease efficiency. They can also have winding shorts and opens that prevent motor operation.

CIRCUIT PROTECTION DEVICES

Circuit protection devices prevent excess current from burning wires and components. With an overload or short, too much current tries to flow.

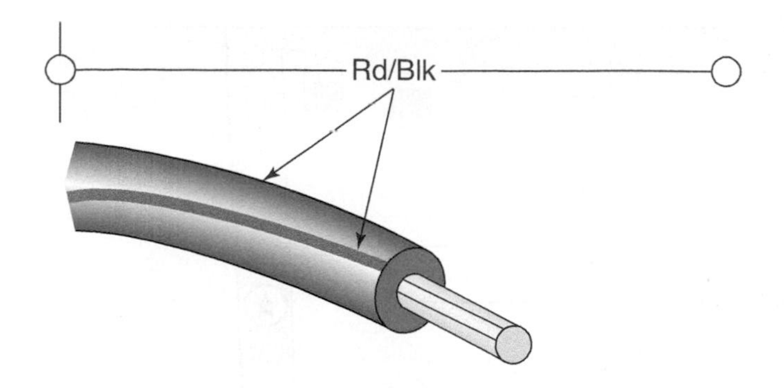

WHT.....White	ORN.....Orange
YEL......Yellow	PNK.....Pink
BLK......Black	BRN.....Brown
BLU......Blue	GRY.....Gray
GRN.....Green	PUR.....Purple
RED.....Red	LT BLU.....Light blue
	LT GRN.....Light green

Figure 26–8. Wire color codes are abbreviated on wiring diagrams. Study these common abbreviations. (Courtesy of American Honda Motor Co., Inc.)

Without a fuse or breaker, the wiring in the circuit would heat up. The insulation would melt and a fire could result.

FUSES

Fuses burn in half with excess current to protect a circuit from further damage. They are normally wired between the power source and the rest of the circuit. There are three types of fuses in automotive use: cartridge, blade, and ceramic. Refer to Figure 26–7.

The **cartridge fuse** is found on most older domestic vehicles and a few imports. It is composed of a strip of metal enclosed in a glass or transparent plastic tube. To check the fuse, look for a break in the internal wire or metal strip. Discoloration of the glass cover or glue bubbling around the metal end caps is an indication of overheating.

Late-model domestic vehicles and many imports use *blade* or *spade fuses.* To check the fuse, pull it from the fuse panel and look at the element through the transparent plastic housing. Look for internal breaks and discoloration.

The *ceramic fuse* is used on many European imports. The core is a ceramic insulator with a conductive metal strip along one side. To check this fuse, look for a break in the contact strip on the outside of the fuse.

All fuse types can be checked with a circuit tester or multimeter. A **blown fuse** will have infinite resistance.

Fuse ratings are the current at which the fuse will blow. Fuse ratings are often printed on the fuse. Always replace a fuse with one of the same amp rating. If you do NOT, part damage can result from excess current flow.

A **fuse box** holds the various circuit fuses, breakers, and flasher units for the turn and emergency lights. It is often under the instrument panel, behind a panel in the foot well, or in the engine compartment.

! WARNING !

Never permanently bypass a fuse or circuit breaker with a jumper wire. Do it only for test purposes.

FUSE LINKS

Fuse links or **fusible links** are smaller-diameter wire spliced into the larger circuit wiring for over-current protection. Fuse links are normally found in the engine compartment near the battery. They are often installed in the positive battery lead that powers the ignition switch and other circuits that are live with the key off.

Fuse link wire is covered with a special insulation that bubbles when it overheats. This indicates that the fuse link has melted.

CIRCUIT BREAKERS

Circuit breakers heat up and open with excess current to protect the circuit. They do NOT suffer internal damage like a fuse. Many circuits are protected by circuit breakers. They can be mounted on the fuse panel or in-line. Like fuses, they are rated in amperes.

Each circuit breaker conducts current through an arm made of two types of metal bonded together (known as a *bimetal arm*). If the arm starts to carry too much current, it heats up. As one metal expands farther than the other, the arm bends, opening the contacts and breaking the current flow.

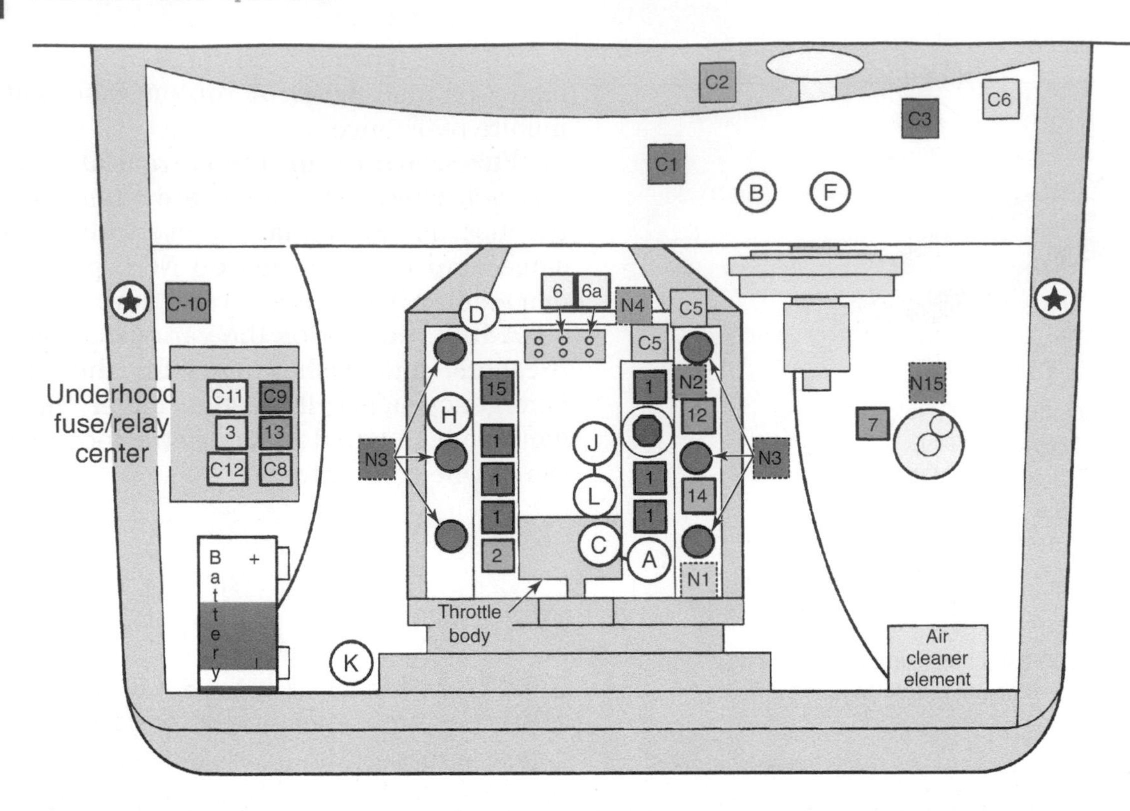

Computer harness

- C1 Engine control module (ECM)*
- C2 DLC diagnostic connector
- C3 "Check engine" malfunction indicator lamp
- C5 ECM harness ground
- C6 Fuse panel
- C8 ECM main relay
- C9 Fuel pump fuse 15A
- C10 Injector resistor
- C11 Oxygen 10A heater fuse
- C12 30A ECM main fusible link

ECM information sensors

- A Manifold absolute pressure
- B Heated oxygen sensor
- C Throttle position sensor
- D Engine coolant temperature
- F Vehicle speed sensor
- H Crank angle sensor
- J Knock sensor (under intake assembly)
- K Power steering pressure switch (in-line)
- L Intake air temperature

ECM controlled Components

- 1 Fuel injector
- 2 Idle air control
- 3 Fuel pump relay
- 6 Ignition control module ignition control
- 6a Ignition coils
- 7 Knock sensor module under charcoal canister
- 12 Exhaust gas recirculation (EGR) VSV
- 13 Air conditioning relay
- 14 Evaporate emission canister purge VSV
- 15 Induction air control plate system VSV

Emission components (not ECM controlled)

- N1 Crankcase vent valve (PCV)
- N2 Exhaust gas recirculation valve back pressure transducer
- N3 Spark plugs
- N4 Fuel rail test fitting (for fuel pressure test)
- N15 Fuel vapor canister

*The ECM is located behind the console in the lower dash.

EGR valve ★ Chassis grounds

Figure 26–9. Component location diagrams show where sensors and other parts are located on the vehicle. (Courtesy of American Isuzu Motors Inc.)

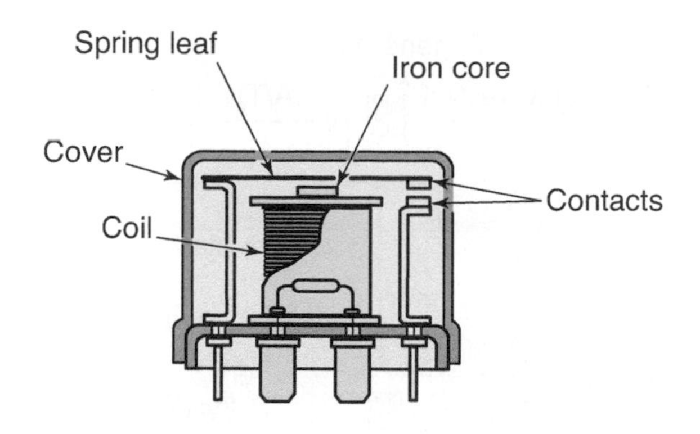

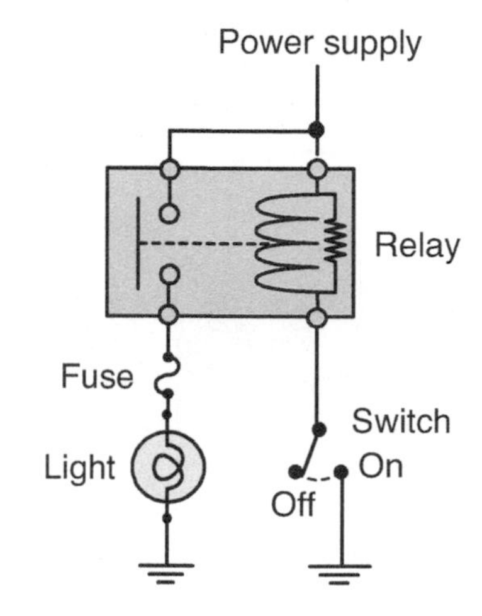

Figure 26–10. A relay is a coil mounted next to contact points. A small amount of current through the coil attracts and closes the points. Then a large load current flows through the contacts.

WARNING

When replacing fuses and circuit breakers, install one with the same amp rating. A higher rated unit could cause an electrical fire.

ELECTRICAL-ELECTRONIC SYSTEMS

The modern vehicle has numerous electrical-electronic systems, each designed to do a specific task. Some of these are discussed below.

Ignition System

The **ignition system** produces an electric arc (spark) in a gasoline engine to cause the fuel to burn. It must fire the spark plugs at the right time. The resulting combustion pressure forces the pistons down to spin the crankshaft.

The **ignition coil** is a step-up transformer that produces high voltage (30,000 volts or more) needed to make current jump the spark plug gap. A switching device is either contact points or an electronic circuit that causes the ignition coil to discharge its electrical energy. Either a distributor or the computer controls the operations of the ignition coil.

Spark plug wires are high-tension wires that carry coil voltage to each spark plug. The **spark plugs** use ignition coil high voltage to ignite the fuel mixture in the engine's combustion chambers.

Electronic Fuel Injection

Electronic fuel injection uses solenoid-type injectors (fuel valves) and computer control to meter gasoline into the engine. An in-tank electric pump pulls fuel out of the gas tank. A second, in-line fuel pump then pushes fuel up to the engine.

A *pressure regulator* on the **fuel rail** (large fuel log or line at engine) limits maximum system pressure.

Starting and Charging Systems

The **starting system** has a large electric motor that turns the engine flywheel. This spins or "cranks" the crankshaft until the engine starts and runs on its own power. See **Figure 26–11.**

The **ignition switch** in the steering column is used to connect battery voltage to a starter solenoid or relay. Other ignition switch terminals are connected to other electrical circuits. A **starter solenoid,** when energized, connects the battery and starting motor.

The **starting motor** is a large DC motor for rotating the engine flywheel. It normally bolts to the rear, lower, side of an engine. A few are mounted inside the engine, under the intake manifold. The **flywheel ring gear** meshes with the starter-mounted gear while cranking.

The **charging system** recharges the battery and supplies electrical energy when the engine is running. See **Figure 26–12.** An alternator or belt-driven DC generator produces this electricity.

A **voltage regulator,** usually mounted in the alternator, controls alternator output. **Charging system voltage** is typically 13 to 15 volts.

To quickly check the condition of a charging system, connect a voltmeter across the battery. With the engine off, you will read battery voltage. It should be above 12.5 volts. If it is not, the battery needs charging or is defective. When

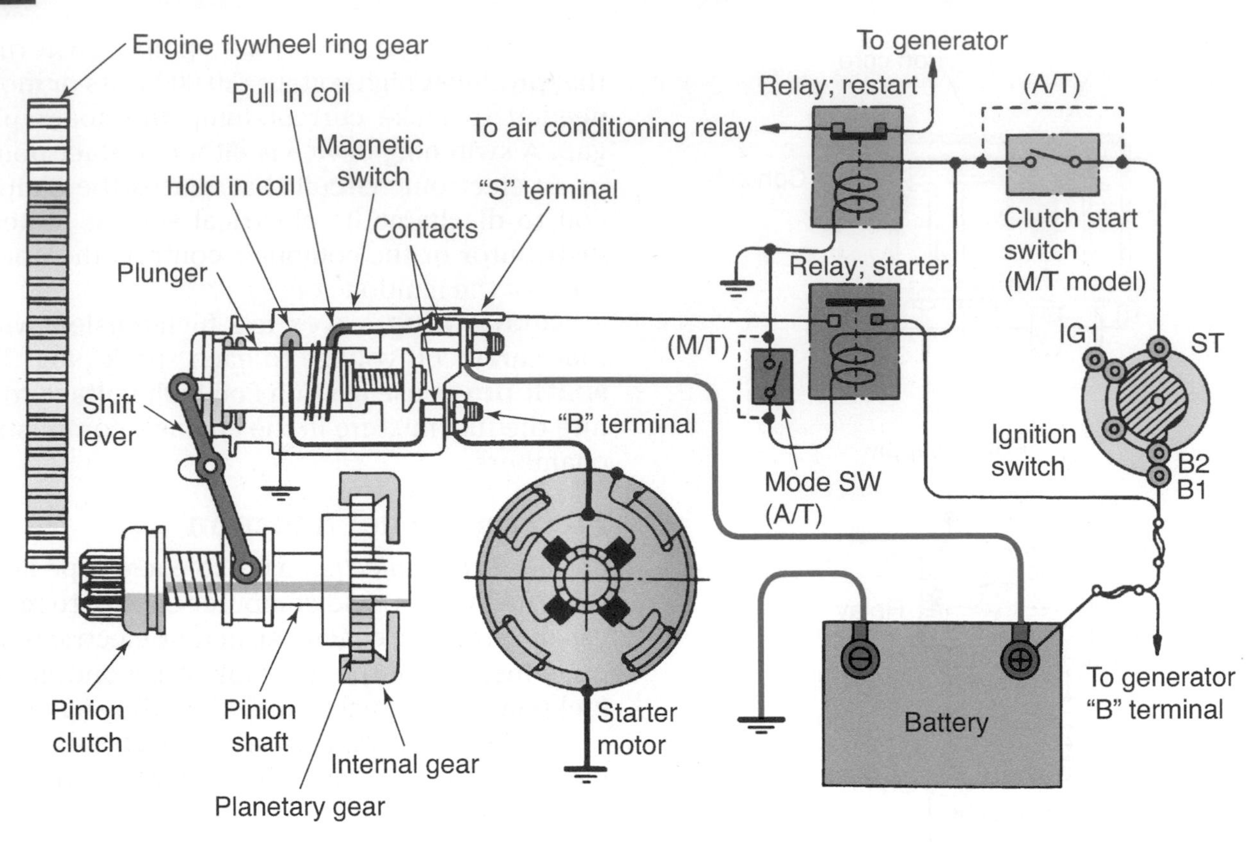

Figure 26–11. Study this typical starting system. Trace the wires from the battery, through the ignition switch, relay, solenoid, and motor. (Courtesy of American Isuzu Motors Inc.)

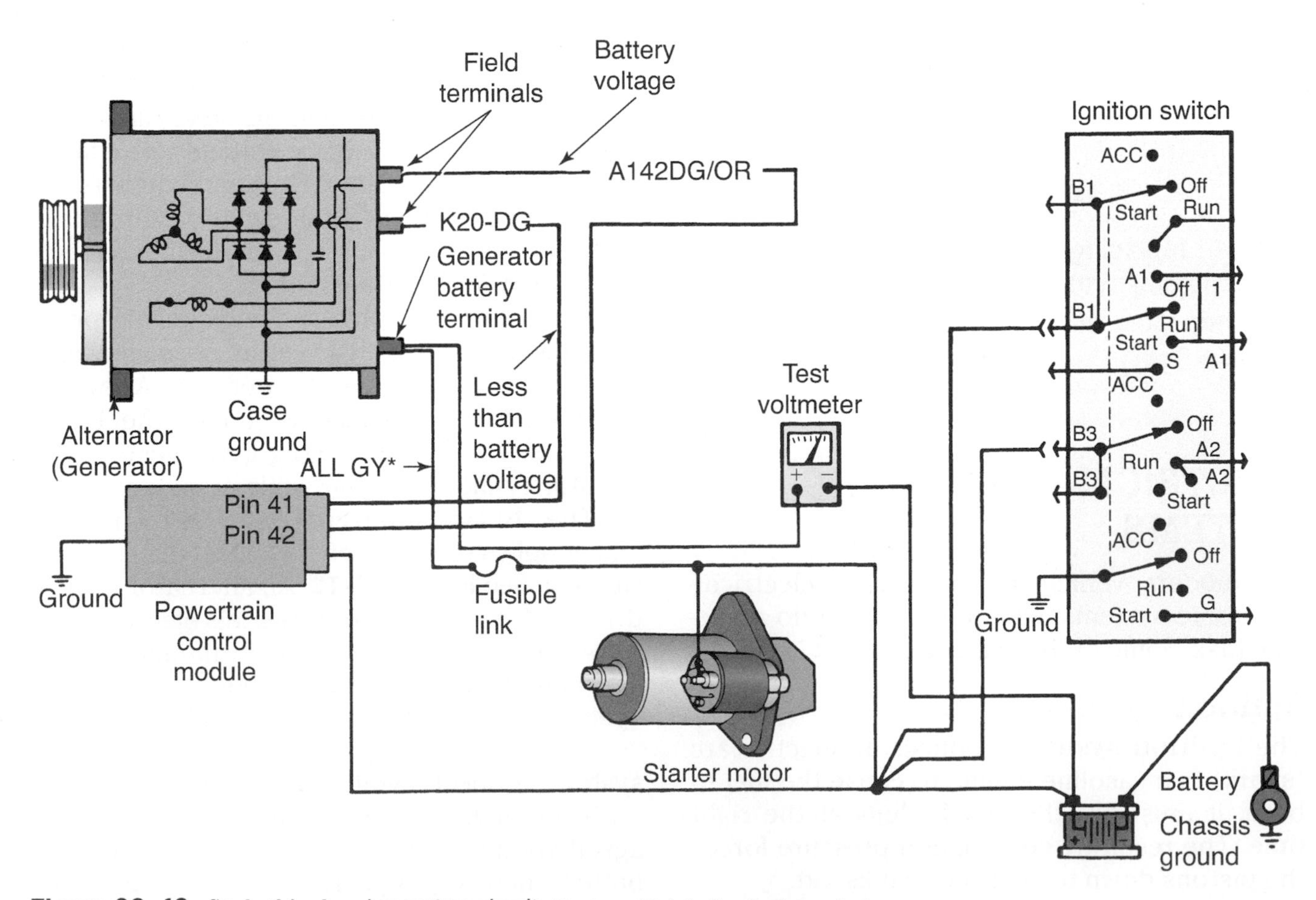

Figure 26–12. Study this charging system circuit. (Courtesy of DaimlerChrysler Corporation)

you start the engine with all electrical accessories ON (lights, radio, etc.), the voltage must stay above battery voltage. If it does NOT, there is something wrong with the charging system.

Engine No-Start Problem. Remember! If an engine cranks but fails to start, check for "spark" and "fuel." Both are needed for an engine to operate.

To CHECK FOR SPARK, pull off one of the spark plug wires. Install an old spark plug into the wire and lay the spark plug on the engine ground. When you crank the engine, a bright spark should jump across the spark plug gap. If it does not, something is wrong with the ignition system (blown fuse, damaged wires, crushed components, etc.).

If you have spark, CHECK FOR FUEL. This can often be done by installing a pressure gauge on the engine's fuel rail. A special test fitting is usually provided for a pressure gauge. With the engine cranking or the key on, the gauge should read within specs. If it does not, something is keeping the electric fuel pump(s) from working normally. Check for a clogged fuel filter, blown pump fuse, or wiring problem.

ELECTRICAL PROBLEMS

Common electrical problems in a collision damaged vehicle generally result from impact and crush damage to wires and electrical-electronic components. These problems can be classified as opens, shorts, grounds, and abnormal resistance values.

An **open circuit** is an unwanted break in an electrical circuit. With an open circuit, current flow ceases and the circuit is dead. This effect can occur in a wire or in an electrical part, such as a light bulb filament.

A **short circuit** is an unwanted wire-to-wire connection in an electrical circuit. A short occurs when the insulation is worn between two adjacent wires and the wires contact each other. Shorts often occur when wires are damaged or pinched due to collision damage.

A short can also result to ground, termed a **grounded circuit.** A grounded circuit condition occurs when the insulation on a wire is worn and the metal in the wire touches the metal of the vehicle body or frame.

When this occurs, the current is allowed to flow directly to ground without flowing to the electrical parts in the circuit. In other words, the current takes the *path of least resistance.* A low resistance or short to ground will blow the fuse or trip the circuit breaker for that circuit.

Bad grounds prevent current from returning to the battery. They are the most common cause of electrical system problems. If just the ground for one part is faulty, it will affect only the one circuit. If a major ground is faulty, many circuits will fail all at once. A major ground is one that connects the battery to the engine block or body. Sometimes a short is intermittent—it shorts momentarily when the vehicle bounces heavily or jars. A flickering dash light is an example of this.

An *abnormal resistance* is due to a bad connection or partial short. When tested, the circuit or component will show a value that is not within specs. For example, a high resistance in a light circuit will make the bulbs burn dimly. This is because the abnormally high circuit resistance is not allowing enough current to flow through the bulbs.

Diagnostic Charts

Diagnostic charts give possible causes for electrical problems and symptoms. They are important tools for collision repair technicians and insurance appraisers.

Most auto manufacturers use some type of diagnostic flow chart to aid technicians in the repair of electrical/electronically controlled systems. Diagnostic flow charts provide a systematic approach to troubleshooting and repair. They are found in service manuals and are given by vehicle make and model.

During the diagnosis, start at the top of the chart and follow the sequence down. The chart will point to the next area to move to after each check is performed. Work through the entire chart, step by step. Perform the repairs or parts replacements as indicated.

BATTERIES

A **battery** stores electrical energy chemically. It provides current for the starting system. It also provides current to all other electrical systems when the engine is not running.

Because of the potential electrical problems caused by a collision, always disconnect both battery cables right away. This will prevent the chance of an electrical fire while working.

When removing or disconnecting the battery, the ignition must be off to prevent voltage spikes. **Voltage spikes** are voltage surges that can destroy many microcircuits in today's electronic systems.

It is a good idea to remove the battery completely from the vehicle before doing any collision repair work. Once the battery has been placed on a bench, it should be checked for a cracked case and similar damage. In many cases with frontal collisions, the battery may need to be replaced.

A charge indicator that shows battery state of charge is often built into the top of the battery. It shows different colors to indicate battery condition.

A voltmeter or a specialized *battery tester* will also check battery condition (specific gravity or voltage). A good, fully charged battery will show 12.5 to 12.6 *open circuit volts* (nothing turned on).

Charging a Battery

The procedure for charging a battery with a battery charger is as follows:

1. Disconnect the negative battery cable.
2. Check the battery casing for damage.
3. Check the water level and add water if necessary.
4. Loosen the vent caps, if the battery is so equipped.
5. Attach the charger clamps to the battery. Connect the red cable to the battery positive. Connect the black cable to negative. See **Figure 26–13.**
6. Set the charger to the recommended settings.
7. Turn on the charger.
8. When charging is completed, turn off the charger.
9. Remove the charger clamps, negative first.
10. Replace the vent caps (if applicable).
11. Attach the negative battery cable.

Jump Starting

Although it is a common practice in some collision repair shops, avoid jump starting whenever possible. The discharged battery can explode. This is true of both the vehicle being started and the vehicle providing the jump.

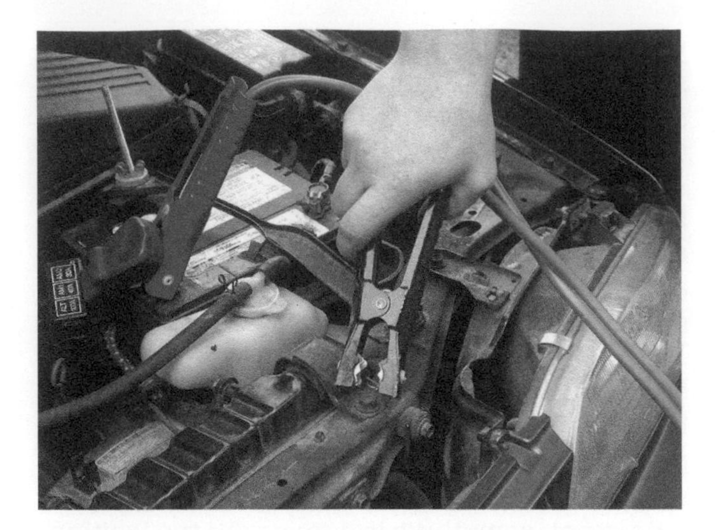

Figure 26–13. Jumper cables or a battery charger must be connected carefully to prevent sparks or electronic component damage. Connect positive to positive and negative to negative in the proper sequence: red to red, then black to any metal ground away from the battery.

Jumper cables are used to connect two batteries together when one is "dead" (discharged). Connect the jumpers positive to positive and negative to negative. Connect the last jumper to a negative ground away from the battery. This will prevent any spark near the battery (see Figure 26–13).

Special care is also necessary when charging or jump starting to avoid damaging computer circuits. Make sure everything is turned off and do not connect the jumper cables backwards.

Before reinstalling the battery after body work, clean its terminals. Use a battery post tool to remove a thin layer of oxidized metal from the terminals and battery cable ends. This will reduce resistance at the battery connections. See **Figure 26–14.**

When installing a battery, make sure the ignition is off. Reconnect the positive battery cable and then the negative battery cable.

Battery Safety

1. Keep batteries away from welding operations, open flames, sparks, or other heat sources.
2. Do NOT charge batteries with cracked cases.
3. Do NOT smoke near batteries.
4. Ventilate the area around dead or damaged batteries to avoid an explosion.
5. Do NOT charge a frozen battery.

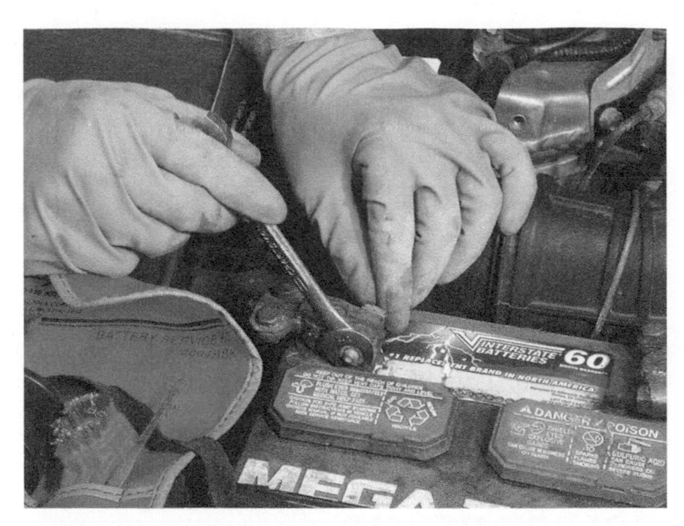

(A) Use a wrench and pliers to free the battery cable ends from the battery terminals.

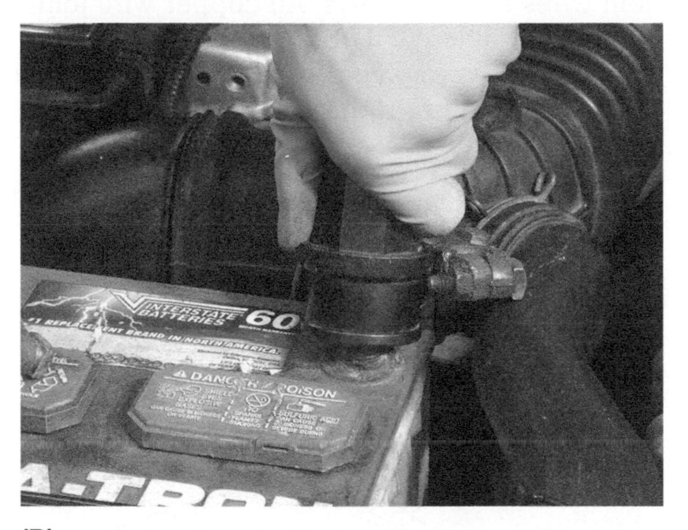

(B) Use the female end of the terminal cleaner on the battery post. Rotate the tool until the metal is shiny and clean.

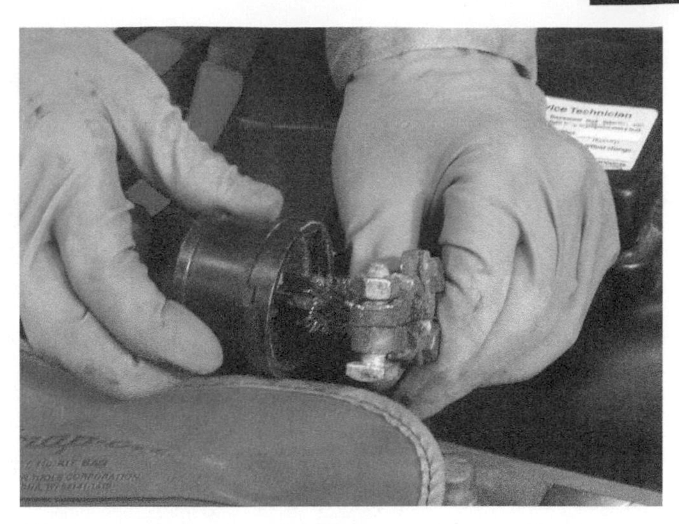

(C) Use the male end of the terminal cleaner on the inside of the cable ends. Rotate the tool until the corrosion or oxidation is removed from metal connections.

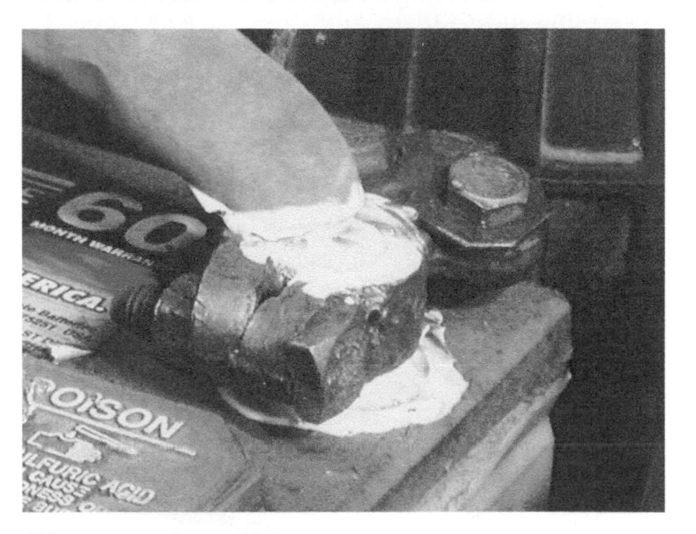

(D) Apply white grease to the battery terminals. Snug down the battery cable ends lightly or until the cable will not move or turn. Overtightening and cable end breakage is a common mistake.

Figure 26–14. Note the basic steps for servicing a battery with corroded terminals.

DANGER

Batteries produce hydrogen gas when discharging or being charged. This gas, if ignited, can make a battery explode! Acid and battery parts can fly into the shop. Charge only in a well-ventilated area.

Electrolyte in the battery is a mixture of water and sulfuric acid. When handling batteries, keep in mind that the electrolyte contains powerful sulfuric acid.

Wear eye protection whenever handling or charging the battery. Do NOT tilt the battery when carrying it. Be careful NOT to let electrolyte get on clothing, skin, or painted surfaces.

If the battery acid does spill, neutralize with baking soda. Immediately wash skin or eyes with water and seek medical attention.

LIGHTING AND OTHER ELECTRIC CIRCUITS

The *lighting system* feeds electricity to light bulbs throughout the vehicle. A few are the headlight, turn light, stop light, backup light, emergency flasher, and interior light circuits.

When lights fail to function, check the bulb first. If the bulb is good, trace for an open feeding current to the dead bulb.

Other electrical circuits (horn, power windows, etc.) use the same principles just discussed. If needed, refer to the service manual for diagrams of each circuit. Circuit designs vary from vehicle to vehicle.

REPAIRING WIRING AND CONNECTIONS

Some damaged wiring can be repaired if correct procedures are followed. See **Figure 26–15.** Be sure to follow the manufacturer's recommendations for wire repair.

When servicing electrical wiring, remember the following rules:

1. Never tug on the connectors. Use the special tools designed to separate the connectors. This will minimize the possibility of having electrical problems caused by intermittent contact.
2. Route wiring in the same location as the OEM.
3. Protect the electrical connectors from moisture and corrosion by using dielectric grease.
4. Use the same size and type of wiring for repairs. This is especially critical with sensor circuits that are affected by the slightest resistance change.

SOLDER REPAIR

Soldering uses moderate heat and solder to join wires or other parts. All copper wire joints should be soldered, if possible.

A pencil-type soldering iron is recommended for this procedure rather than a soldering gun.

Heat shrink tube
Terminal
Harness

(A) Slide a heat shrink tube over the wire.

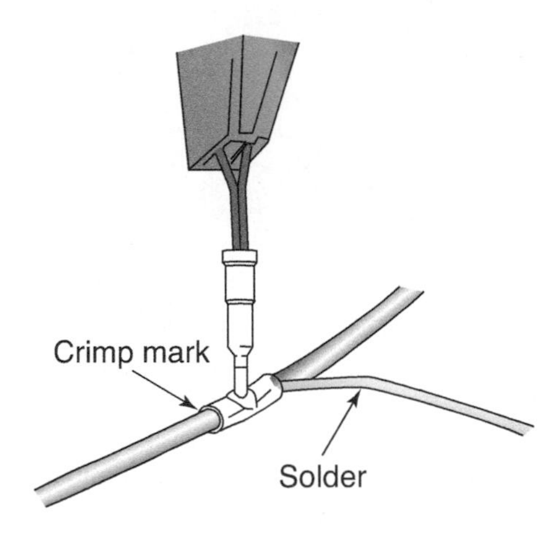

(C) Solder the connector to the wires to ensure good electrical connection.

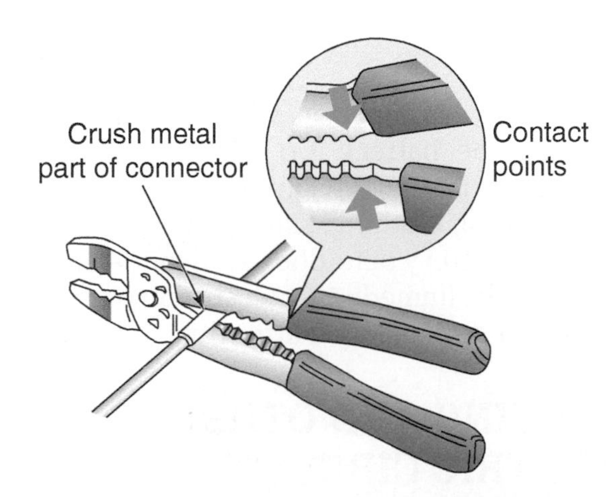

(B) Crimp the connector down over the wire ends.

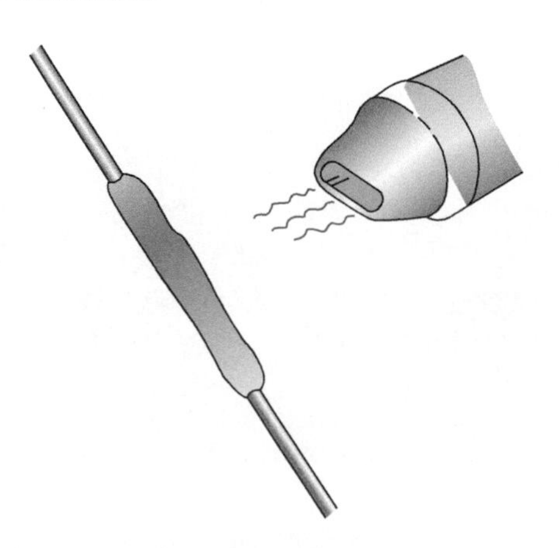

(D) Use a heat gun to shrink the plastic tube around the repair.

Figure 26–15. Note use of a connector to splice wire.

This is because guns have heavy coils that can create induced current in nearby components and damage them.

Be sure to use **rosin-core solder,** NOT acid-core, when soldering electrical connections. Acid fluxes create corrosion and can damage electronic components. In addition, dielectric grease is frequently used to protect connections from corrosion. When using this product, which has no acid content, follow the manufacturer's instructions and be sure NOT to cut into the moisture-sealed connector joints with test equipment probes.

Use the following procedure to make a solder connection:

1. Remove all traces of dirt and corrosion.
2. Strip the insulation back about ½ inch (13 mm) on each wire.
3. Wind the wires tightly together.
4. Heat the wire joint, NOT the solder. Touch the solder to the joint. Allow it to flow into the joint. Do NOT use too much solder.
5. Allow the joint to cool.
6. Gently pull on both ends of the wire to make sure the repair is secure.

A *shrink tube* can also be used over the joint to further protect the connection from corrosion. When heated, the tube shrinks in size and provides a coating over the repair much like the original insulation.

Liquid electrical tape can also be applied over the joint with a brush. This will help make the electrical connection waterproof.

Electrical tape is made of flexible, thin plastic. It can be used around wire splices when the connection will NOT be exposed to moisture.

ELECTRICAL CONNECTOR SERVICE

An automotive electrical connector includes two plastic, snap-together fittings. They allow several wires to connect together securely. Various connector designs are used on vehicles and each requires a different method for disconnection.

If needed, inspect electrical connectors when trying to find opens. They can be torn apart or damaged in the collision. **Figure 26–16** shows several ways to disconnect connectors.

COMPUTER SYSTEMS

Almost all vehicle systems are now controlled/monitored by computer. This would include the fuel, ignition, charging, suspension and brake, climate control, and other systems.

A basic **computer system** consists of:

1. Sensors (input devices)
2. Actuators (output devices)
3. Computer (electronic control unit)

The *sensors* are devices that convert a condition (temperature, pressure, part movement, etc.) into an electrical signal. They send electrical input signals back to the computer. See **Figure 26–17.** Once the computer analyzes the sensor data, it produces a preprogrammed output that is sent to system actuators.

Actuators are devices (solenoids or servo motors, for example) that move when responding to electrical signals from the computer. In this way, a computer system can REACT to sensor inputs and then ACT on these conditions by operating the motors or solenoids.

The *computer* is a complex electronic circuit that produces a known electrical output after analyzing electrical inputs. Today's vehicles can have one or more computers that monitor and control the operation of electrical systems.

SCANNING COMPUTER PROBLEMS

A **scan tool** is now the "most important tool" of the automobile technician. It provides the fastest way to use on-board diagnostics to find electrical-electronic problems in computer control systems. A scan tool "talks" to the vehicle's computers and can tell you if it detects any problems in the vehicle.

A scanner will convert computer or electronic control module (EMC) data into an alphanumeric display explaining the problem and service procedures in plain English.

Scan Tool Cartridges

Modern scan tools are removable cartridges that are small computer circuits that hold information about the specific vehicle. When the cartridge is installed into the scanner, the scanner has all the information needed to help analyze problems stored in the on-board computer system.

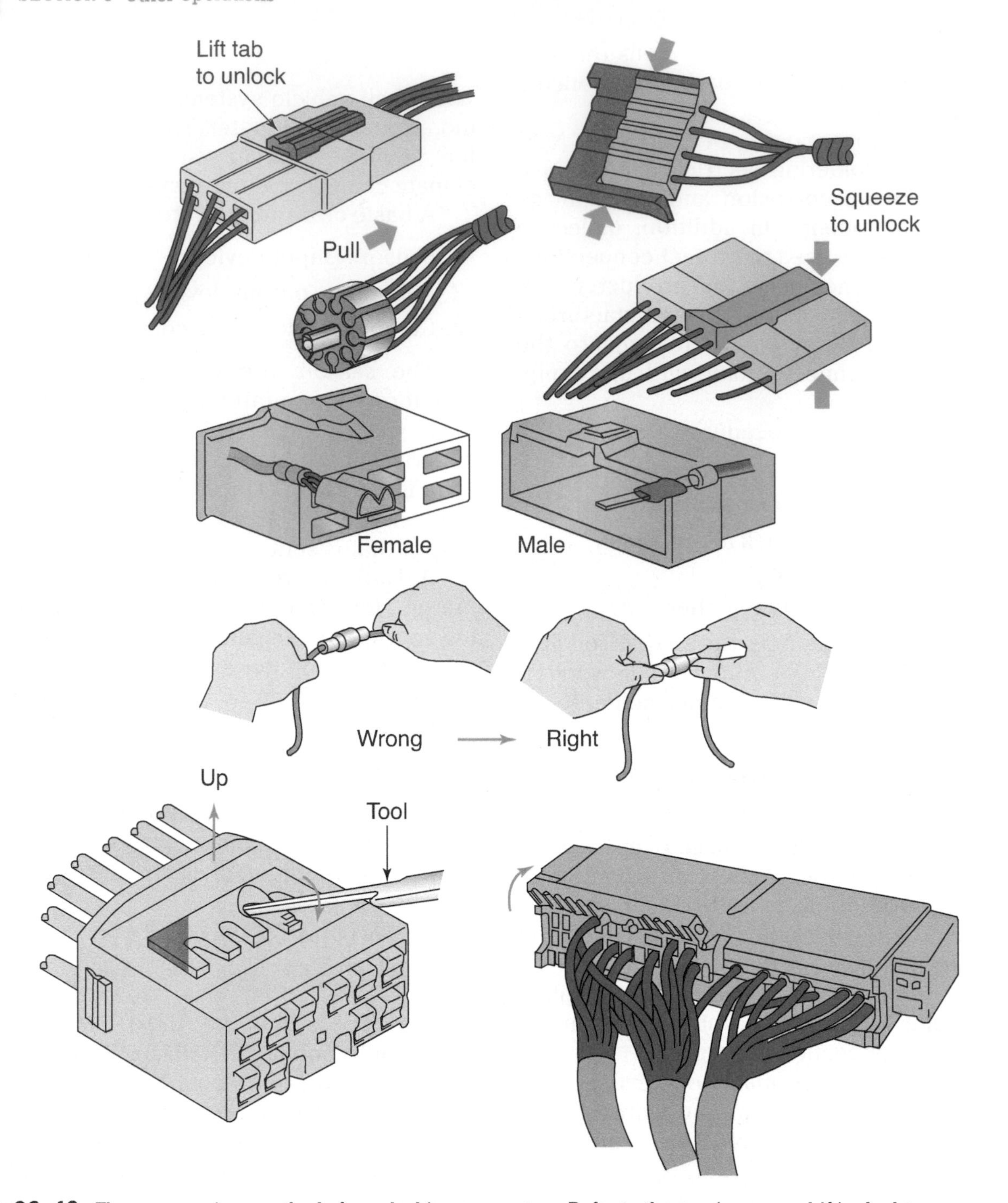

Figure 26–16. There are various methods for unlocking connectors. Refer to the service manual if in doubt.

A vehicle "make" cartridge provides data for each vehicle manufacturer (GM, Ford, Chrysler, foreign). New cartridges must be purchased as on-board diagnostic systems are improved.

Some scanners also come with a diagnostic or troubleshooting cartridge that gives extra information on how to verify the source of different problems. This is a handy resource when diagnosing hard-to-find problems.

Advanced scanners will hold two cartridges, one for the vehicle make and the troubleshooting cartridge. This scanner allows you to select different installed cartridges and even prompts you on the correct cable adapter and other essential information.

Scan Tool Control

The scan tool's menu allows you to scan different test functions: trouble codes and data, functional tests, custom setup, road test, and troubleshooter.

Codes and data allows you to retrieve stored trouble codes and electrical operating values

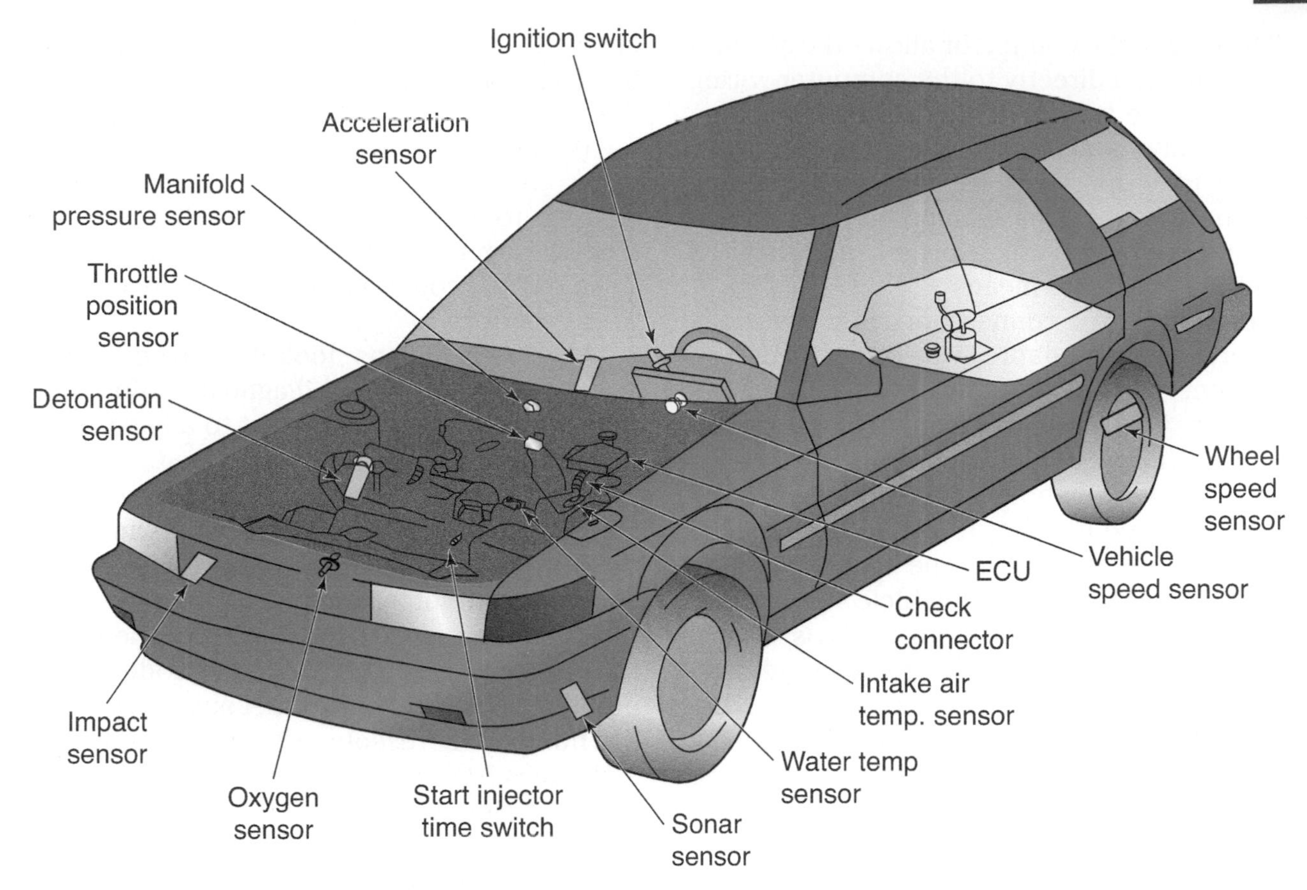

Figure 26–17. Numerous sensors provide inputs for the computer. The service information for the specific make and model vehicle would be required.

from the on-board computer. This is the most commonly used function.

Functional tests allows you to perform specialized tests of the computer, emission systems, ignition system, sensor circuits, fuel injectors, and other components.

Road test allows you to take an instantaneous "snapshot" of the data while driving the vehicle. When an intermittent problem occurs, activate the scanner and it will store operating values for later evaluation.

Troubleshooter will guide you through diagnosis of various problems. It will give hints about common problems, list tests that should be performed, and give other useful information.

Connecting the Scan Tool

If a malfunction indicator light (MIL) in the dash glows or if you cannot find the source of a performance problem, connect the scan tool to the diagnostic connector on the vehicle. See **Figure 26–18.**

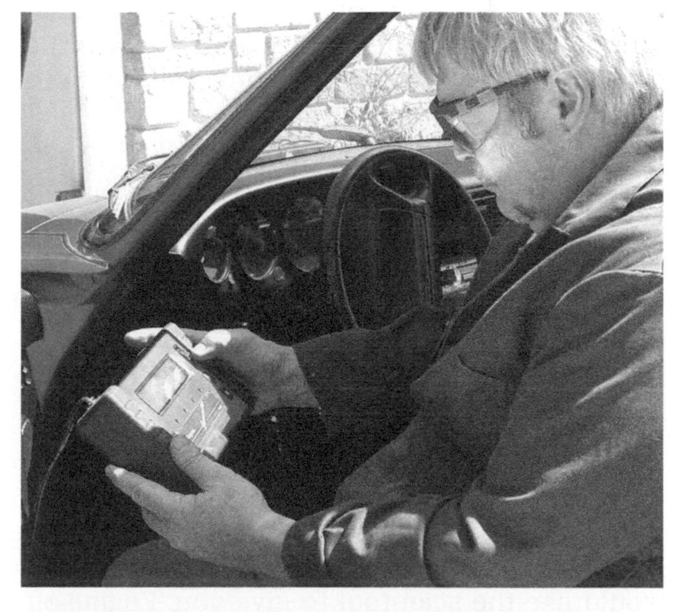

Figure 26–18. A scan tool, when connected to the vehicle's diagnostic connector, will allow you to retrieve trouble codes, perform sensor and actuator tests, erase trouble codes, and quickly analyze the conditions of most computer system circuits. (Courtesy of Snap-on Tools Corporation)

The diagnostic connector allows the scanner to be connected directly to the computer wiring harness on the vehicle. The scan tool can then automatically convert trouble code numbers into a display that gives information for finding problems quickly. This eliminates the need to refer to a service manual to find out what the trouble code number means.

Early diagnostic connectors came in various configurations. An adapter was often needed so the scanner connector would fit the vehicle's connector. Adapters are labeled for easy location for each make of vehicle.

With modern on-board diagnostics (OBD II), the standardized connector is a 16-pin personal computer–type connector. The scan tool cable should slide easily into the vehicle's diagnostic connector. If it does not, something is wrong. Never force the two together or you could damage the pins or terminals in the connectors. The most common location for the diagnostic connector is under the right side of the dash and visible (OBD II standard location).

Using the Scanner

Most manufacturers recommend that you start and fully warm the engine before scanning. However, if the problem symptoms occur only when the engine is cold, you may not want to warm the engine.

Turn off all accessories that could trip false trouble codes. Even opening the door while scanning could confuse the scanner. Lower the window so that you can start the engine without opening the car door.

Next, prepare the tool for the make of vehicle to be analyzed. The scanner will usually need you to input specific characters from the vehicle identification number (VIN). This will let the scanner know which engine, transmission, and other equipment are installed on the vehicle. The VIN plate is on the dash. You must input specific numbers and letters from the VIN. Scroll through the letters and press Y, or yes, when the character is correct or press the correct keypad character. Some vehicles will automatically download the VIN information into the scan tool for you. Next, select what information you would like the scan tool to give you. Engine-off diagnosis is done by triggering on-board diagnosis with the ignition key in the ON position but without the engine running. This pulls stored trouble codes out of the computer memory chips. This check is usually performed before the engine-running diagnostic, especially when the MIL in the dash is glowing.

When in the Engine-off/Key-on mode for more than 30 minutes, connect a battery charger to the vehicle. This will prevent extended current draw from draining the battery. False trouble codes could result from a partially "dead" battery.

Most technicians look for stored trouble codes first using stored diagnostic information. This is a quick way to go right to any hard (continuous) failure so it can be repaired.

A general rule is to correct the cause of the LOWER NUMBER CODE FIRST. Sometimes fixing the lowest code will clear other codes because of component interaction.

If a problem exists in any circuit, the scanner will not only give you a trouble code number, but it will also give you a brief summary of what the number represents. Always remember that code does NOT mean that a certain component is bad. It simply indicates the possible problem location or circuit. Multimeter testing of the component and circuit is still needed to verify the exact source of trouble. To prevent electronic control unit damage, always use a high-impedance, digital multimeter when testing.

Engine-running diagnosis has the engine warmed to full operating temperature and idling to check electrical values. It checks the condition of the sensors, actuators, computer, and wiring while they are operating under normal conditions of engine heat, vibration, and pressure.

Follow the scanner instructions to start this test. For example, the scanner instructions will typically say to run the engine for 2 minutes at 2,000 rpm. This will ensure that the engine and its components are fully warm and in closed loop mode. The scan tool will usually tell you whether the system is closed or open loop, whether the system is lean or rich, and other information related to system operation.

The troubleshooter cartridge might also give tips for finding a difficult-to-locate problem. If you have a code for a rich mixture, it might tell you to check the coolant temperature sensor, to check for high fuel pressure, or to check for leaking injectors. All could cause and trip a rich mixture trouble code. You might want to measure fuel pressure or do an injector leak down test.

The troubleshooter cartridge might even tell you to disconnect a questionable sensor and compare the readings with the circuit open. With the sensor disconnected, the scanner should read within the prescribed values for infinite resistance in the circuit. This will isolate the problem to either the wiring and ECM or the sensor quickly. If the reading does not change with the wiring disconnected, you know you have an open in the wiring. The troubleshooter cartridge might also inform you of an improved replacement sensor. A wiggle test is done by moving wires and harness connectors while scanning to find soft (intermittent) failures. If wiggling a wire produces a new trouble code, check that electrical connection more closely.

Erasing Trouble Codes

Erasing trouble codes, also termed clearing diagnostic codes, removes the stored codes from computer memory. There are various methods used to erase trouble codes from the computer:

- Use the scanner tool to remove stored diagnostic codes from the on-board computer. This is the best way to remove old codes after repairs.
- Disconnect the battery ground strap or cable. This will also erase digital clock memory and other memories, however.
- Unplug the fuse to computer or ECU.
- Codes will erase automatically after 30–50 engine starts.

After erasing trouble codes, you might want to again energize on-board diagnosis. If no trouble codes are then displayed, you have corrected the problem.

SUMMARY

- Current is the movement of electricity (electrons) through a wire or circuit. It is measured in amps.
- Voltage is the pressure that pushes the electricity through the wire or circuit. It is measured in volts.
- Resistance is a restriction or obstacle to current flow. It is measured in ohms.
- Some diagnostic equipment used in finding electrical faults includes the multimeter, test light, and jumper wires.
- Wires are often severed and electrical and electronic components damaged during a collision. A scan tool will help you quickly find the location of circuit faults. It will display which circuits or components are not operating within specifications.

TECHNICAL TERMS

electrical systems
current
resistance
conductor
hot wires
insulation
ground
electric circuit
load
series circuit
opened
parallel circuit
closed
series-parallel circuit
Ohm's Law
magnetism
flux
magnetic field
electromagnet
windings
diagnostic tools
multimeter
VOM
digital multimeter (DVOM)
analog multimeter (AVOM)
test light
jumper wires
continuity
infinite reading
AC current
DC current
inductive pickup
wiring diagram
electrical symbols
wire color coding
wiring harness
part location diagram
switch
solenoid
relay
motors
fuses
cartridge fuse
blown fuse
fuse ratings
fuse box
fusible links
circuit breakers
ignition system
ignition coil
spark plug wires
spark plugs
fuel rail
starting system
ignition switch
starting solenoid
starting motor
flywheel ring gear
charging system
voltage regulator
charging system voltage
open circuit
short circuit
grounded circuit
battery
voltage spikes
jumper cables
electrolyte
soldering
rosin-core solder

liquid electrical tape
electrical tape
computer system
actuators
scan tool

REVIEW QUESTIONS

1. Define the terms "current," "voltage," and "resistance."
2. A ______________ ______________ has only one conductor path or leg for current through the circuit.
3. A ______________ ______________ has two or more legs or paths for current.
4. If a circuit has 12.6 volts applied and 4.2 ohms, how much current would flow through the circuit?
5. What is a multimeter?
6. A lighting circuit has an intermittent problem. The bulbs go on and off. *Technician A* says to use a DVOM to find the trouble. *Technician B* says to use an AVOM. Who is correct?
   a. Technician A
   b. Technician B
   c. Both Technicians A and B
   d. Neither Technician
7. Why should you NOT use test lights on electronic circuits?
8. Explain the difference between AC and DC electricity.
9. The service manual may also give a ______________ ______________ ______________ for finding electrical components (harnesses, sensors, switches, computers, etc.).
10. How does a fuse operate?
11. With the engine running, how much voltage should be across the battery terminals?
   a. 12 to 15 volts
   b. 18 volts
   c. 12.6 volts
   d. 13 to 15 volts
12. If an engine cranks but fails to start, what should you do?
13. How do you use jumper wires?
14. Be sure to use ______________ ______________, NOT ______________, when soldering electrical connections. Acid fluxes create corrosion and can damage electronic components.
15. In your own words, explain the basic parts and operation of a computer system.
16. How do you use a scan tool?
17. Computers can be located:
   a. Under the dash
   b. Under the seats
   c. Under the hood
   d. Behind kick panels
   e. All of the above
   f. None of the above

ASE-STYLE REVIEW QUESTIONS

1. *Technician A* says that voltage is like electrical pressure that pushes current through a circuit. *Technician B* says that voltage is the flow of electrons through a circuit. Who is correct?
   a. Technician A
   b. Technician B
   c. Both Technicians A and B
   d. Neither Technician
2. Which of the following circuits will go completely "dead" if a load device burns open?
   a. Parallel circuit
   b. Series circuit
   c. Series-parallel circuit
   d. Hydraulic circuit
3. If a circuit is shorted to 0.1 ohm, how much current will try to flow through the circuit of 12.6 volts is applied?
   a. 0.126 amp
   b. 1.26 amps
   c. 12.6 amps
   d. 126 amps
4. A properly charged automotive battery should show how much open circuit voltage?
   a. 12 volts
   b. 12.1 volts
   c. 12.6 volts
   d. 12.8 volts

5. *Technician A* says to connect jumper cables positive to positive and negative to negative. *Technician B* says to connect the last jumper cable to a ground away from the battery. Who is correct?
   a. Technician A
   b. Technician B
   c. Both Technicians A and B
   d. Neither Technician

6. *Technician A* says that batteries can explode. *Technician B* says that battery acid can cause injury. Who is correct?
   a. Technician A
   b. Technician B
   c. Both Technicians A and B
   d. Neither Technician

7. A malfunction indicator light in the dash stays on after collision repair work is complete. *Technician A* says to connect a scan tool to the vehicle's diagnostic connector. *Technician B* says that it is better to connect a multimeter to the correct pins on the diagnostic connector for troubleshooting. Who is correct?
   a. Technician A
   b. Technician B
   c. Both Technicians A and B
   d. Neither Technician

8. A trouble code for an oxygen sensor circuit has been retrieved. *Technician A* says to replace the oxygen sensor. *Technician B* says to test the oxygen sensor and its circuit. Who is correct?
   a. Technician A
   b. Technician B
   c. Both Technicians A and B
   d. Neither Technician

9. After repairs, a vehicle's engine fails to idle normally and the scan tool finds a trouble code for the idle air motor. *Technician A* says to test the idle air motor with a multimeter. *Technician B* says to check for an opening in the wiring harness going to the idle air motor. Who is correct?
   a. Technician A
   b. Technician B
   c. Both Technicians A and B
   d. Neither Technician

10. On a late model vehicle, *Technician A* says that the diagnostic connector on OBD II vehicles should be visible on the fire wall of the vehicle. *Technician B* says that various scan tool connector configurations may be required. Who is correct?
    a. Technician A
    b. Technician B
    c. Both Technicians A and B
    d. Neither Technician

ACTIVITIES

1. Read the operating manual for a multimeter. Write a report on its use and safety rules.
2. Use a voltmeter to check the action of a charging system. How much voltage is the system producing across the battery? Discuss your findings with the class.

CHAPTER

27 Restraint System Repairs

OBJECTIVES

After studying this chapter, you should be able to:

- Explain the difference between an active and a passive restraint system.
- Learn how to service seat belts.
- Describe the operation of air bag systems.
- Repair air bag systems safely.

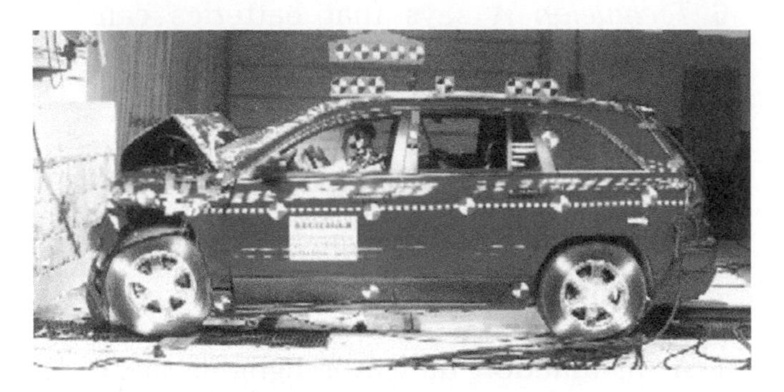

Figure 27–1. Modern restraint systems have saved thousands of lives in serious auto accidents. As a technician, you must learn how to service them properly after deployment. (Courtesy of DaimlerChrysler Corporation)

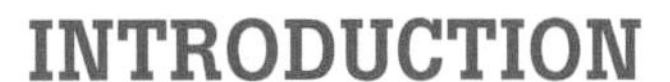

INTRODUCTION

A **restraint system** is designed to help hold passengers in their seats and prevent them from being injured during a collision. All new vehicles come equipped with some form of restraint system. See **Figure 27–1.**

ACTIVE AND PASSIVE RESTRAINTS

An **active restraint system** is one that the occupants must make an effort to use. For example, in most vehicles the seat belts must be fastened for crash protection. Conventional, manually operated seat belts would be classified as an active restraint system.

A **passive restraint system** is one that operates automatically. No action is required to make it functional. Two types are automatic seat belts and air bags.

SEAT BELT SYSTEMS

Seat belts are strong nylon straps with special ends attached for securing people in their seats. **Lap belts** are the seat belts that extend across a person's lap. **Shoulder belts** extend over a person's chest and shoulder. See **Figure 27–2.** A **seat belt buckle mechanism** allows you to put the seat belt on and take it off.

Seat belt anchors allow one end of the belts to be bolted to the body structure. A **belt retractor** is used to remove slack from the belts so they fit snugly. Various mechanisms are used in belt retractors. One is shown in **Figure 27–3.**

A *seat belt reminder system* uses sensors and a warning system to remind the driver to fasten his or her seat belt. On active systems, the driver's side front seat belt uses a 4- to 8-second fasten seat belt reminder light and sound signal. This is designed to remind you if the lap and shoulder belts are NOT fastened when the ignition is turned on. If the driver's seat belt is not buckled, the reminder light and sound signal will automatically shut off after a few seconds. See **Figure 27–4.**

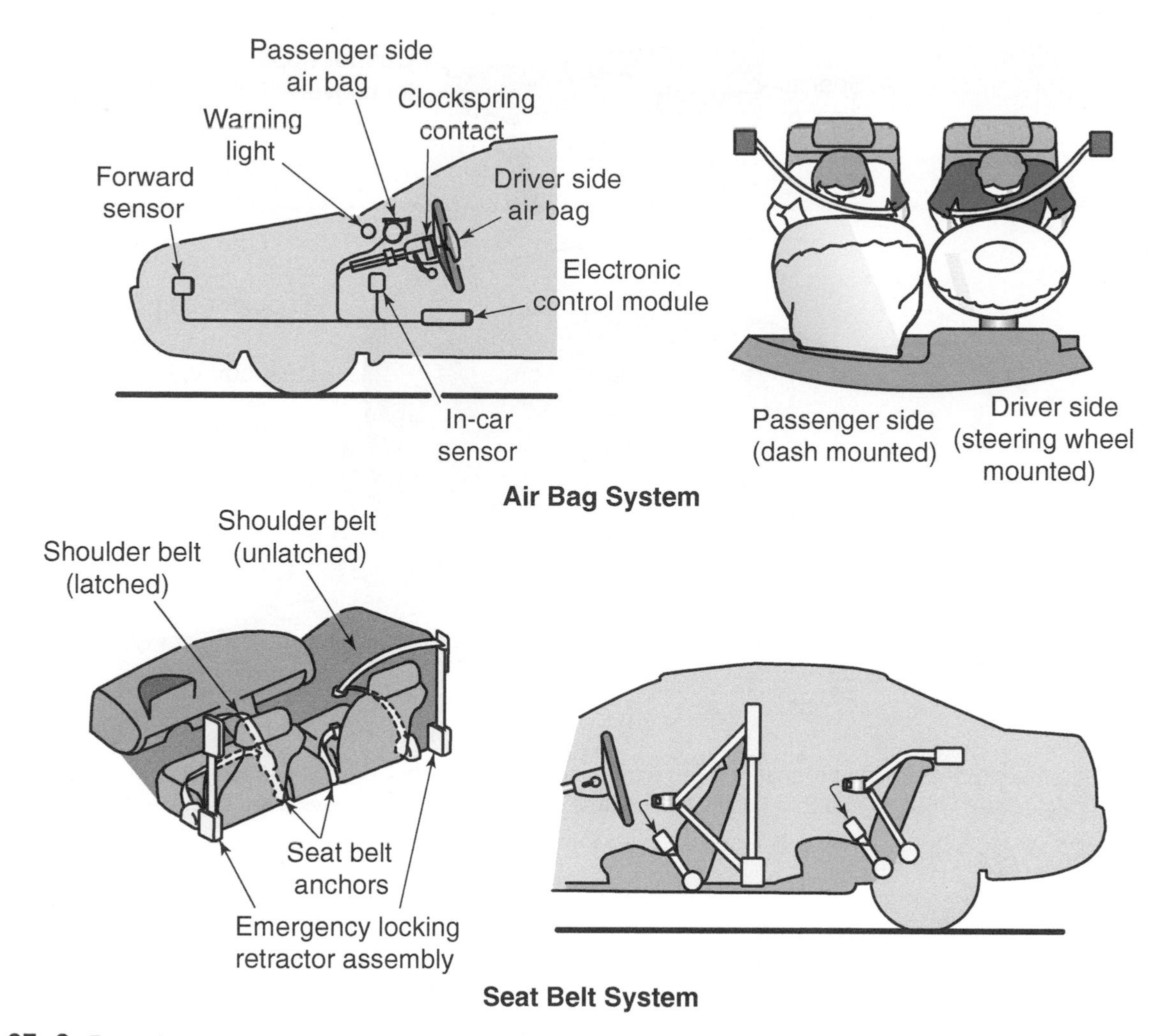

Figure 27–2. Restraint systems include seat belts and air bags, normally under computer control. Note the location of major parts.

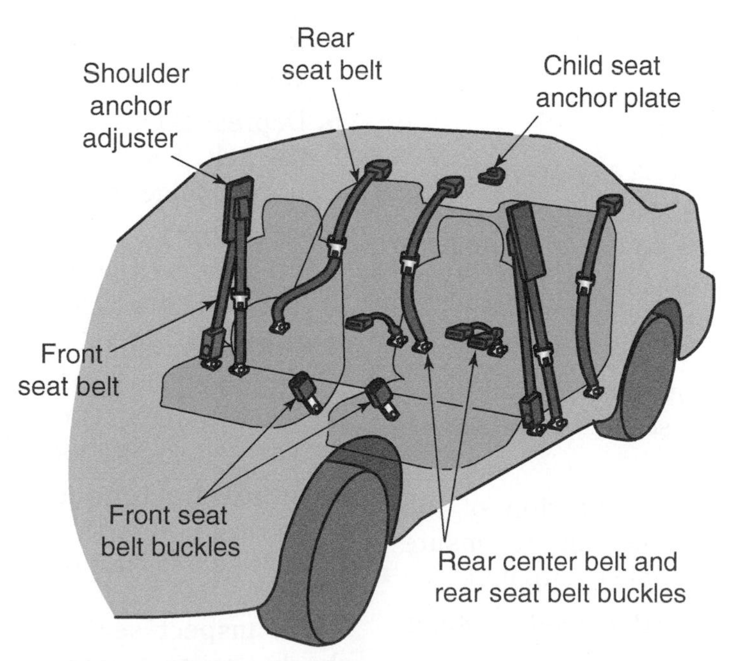

Figure 27–3. Study the major parts of the seat belt system. Buckles, latches, and belts themselves must be in good condition before release to the customer.

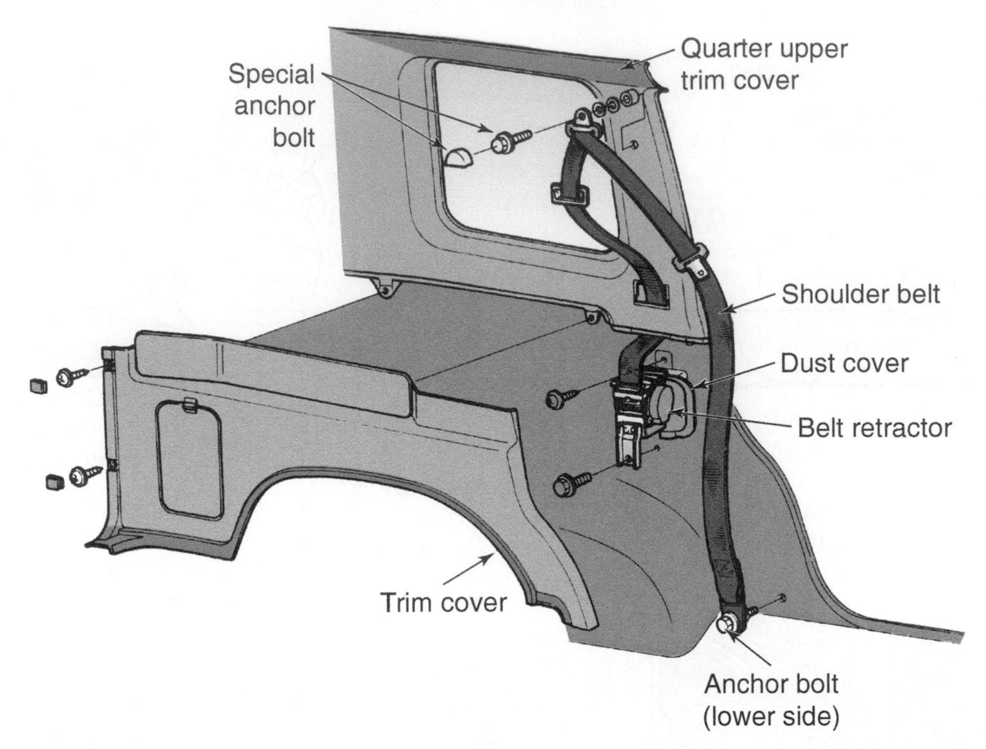

Figure 27–4. Always check the action of seat belt retractors after a collision. Inspect the webbing for cuts, tears, or frays. Make sure the retractors are working and that buckles install and release normally. (Courtesy of American Isuzu Motors Inc.)

Seat Belt Service

When servicing or replacing lap and shoulder belts, remember:

1. Do NOT intermix types of seat belts on front or rear seats.
2. Keep sharp edges and damaging objects away from belts.
3. Avoid bending or damaging any portion of the belt buckle or latch plate.
4. Do NOT attempt repairs on lap or shoulder belt retractor mechanisms or lap belt retractor covers. Replace with new replacement parts.
5. Tighten all seat and shoulder belt anchor bolts as specified in the service manual. Use a torque wrench.

A visual and functional inspection of the belts themselves is very important to ensure maximum protection for vehicle occupants.

1. Check for twisted, cut, or damaged webbing in all seat belts.
2. Fully extend the webbing from the retractor. Inspect the webbing and replace with a new assembly if needed.
3. Insert the tongue of the seat belt into the buckle until a click is heard. Pull back on the webbing quickly to ensure that the buckle is latched properly.
4. Replace the seat belt assembly if the buckle will NOT latch.
5. Depress the button on the buckle to release the belt. The belt should release with normal finger pressure.
6. Grasp the seat belt webbing. While pulling from the retractor, give the belt a fast jerk. The belt should lock up.
7. Drive the vehicle in an open area away from other vehicles. Drive at about 5 to 15 mph (8 to 24 km/h). Quickly apply the foot brake. The belt should lock up.
8. If the retractor does NOT lock up under these conditions, remove and replace the seat belt assembly.

To inspect seat belt anchors, you should check the seat belt anchorage for signs of movement or deformation. Replace if necessary. Position the replacement anchor exactly the same as in the original installation.

CHILD RESTRAINT SYSTEMS AND AIR BAG SAFETY

A **child restraint seat** is a small removable appliance available from most automobile dealers or through various retail outlets. These restraint seats are available in either rearward-facing or forward-facing models, and in some cases may be used in either way. The seat is intended to be tightly secured with the vehicle's shoulder or lap belt and held secure with a special locking clip supplied by the seat manufacturer. The seat should never be used without the special security clip or placed in the vehicle in a direction other than for which it is designed. Many late-model vehicles are equipped with integral seats built into the rear seat by the manufacturer.

DANGER

Children should NEVER be seated in the front.

AIR BAG SYSTEMS

An **air bag system** automatically deploys a large nylon bag during severe collisions. See **Figure 27–5.** One or more air bags can be used to help protect the driver and passengers from injury.

The **driver's-side air bag** is mounted inside the steering wheel center pad. It is activated during a frontal collision but may not deploy from side collisions.

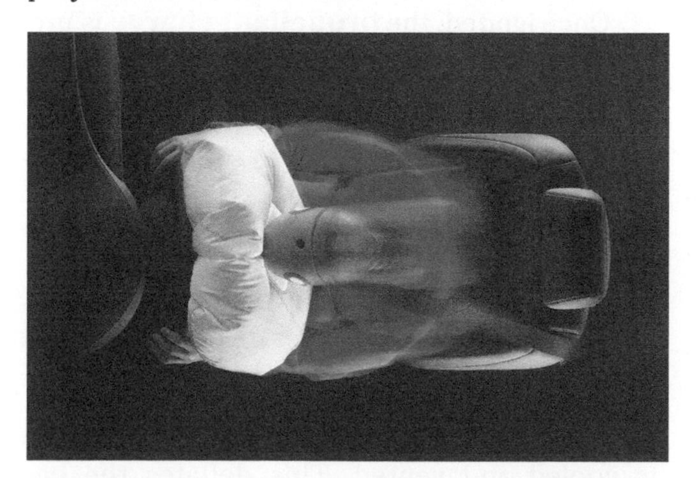

Figure 27–5. Driver and passenger air bags deploy during frontal collisions to keep occupants from hitting the steering wheel, instrument panel, and windshield. An air bag can deploy in a fraction of a second, before your body flies forward and hits the steering wheel or other parts in the passenger compartment. (Courtesy of DaimlerChrysler Corporation)

The **passenger-side air bag** is mounted behind a small door in the side of the instrument panel. This air bag also deploys during frontal impacts. The angle of impact and design of the system determines when the driver's and passenger's air bags deploy. Many systems operate with a frontal impact of within about 30 degrees of the vehicle's centerline.

Side impact air bags deploy from the door panels or from the side of the front seats. They may not deploy during a frontal impact. They are becoming more common and are used by several auto manufacturers. During a side impact from another vehicle, injury usually results when a passenger impacts the side window glass. Side impact air bags help protect people from this type of injury. See **Figure 27–6.**

Rear seat air bags fit into the rear cushion of the front seats. They inflate to protect the passengers in the rear seat from injury in a frontal collision. They are not very common but can be found in a few expensive luxury vehicles.

While the location and design of the air bag system varies from manufacturer to manufacturer, all air bag systems have similar parts, as shown in **Figure 27–7.** These include:

1. Air bag module—inflator mechanism and nylon bag that expand to protect the driver or passenger during a collision
2. Air bag system sensors—inertia sensors that signal the computer of a collision

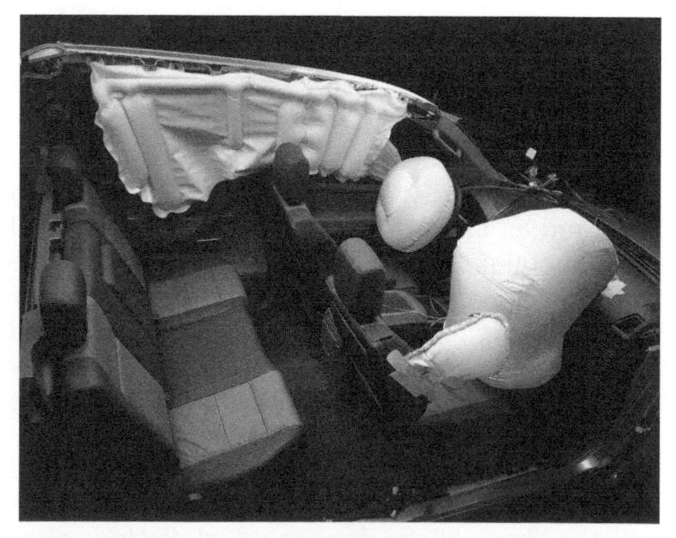

Figure 27–6. Many vehicles now have side air bags or air curtains that drop down to protect the driver and passengers during a side hit or "t-bone." Side air bags help keep the head and upper torso inside the passenger compartment. (Courtesy of Nissan Motor Co.)

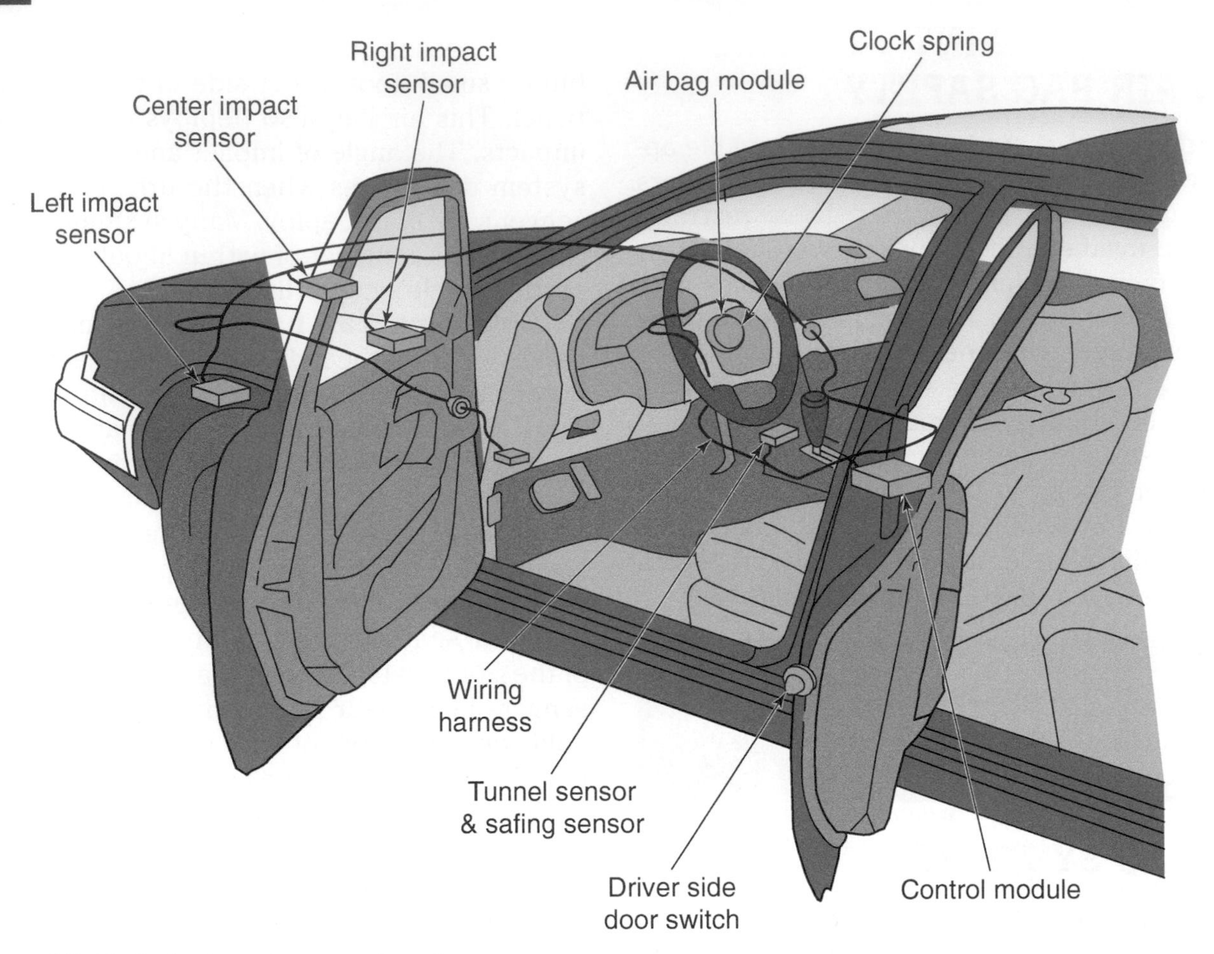

Figure 27–7. Study the major parts of an air bag system.

3. Control unit—computer that operates the system and detects faults
4. Wiring harness—wiring and connectors that link system parts
5. Dash indicator lamp—dash bulb that warns of system problem

Air Bag Module

The **air bag module** is composed of the nylon bag and an igniter-inflator mechanism enclosed in a metal-plastic housing. All air bag module components are packaged in a single container mounted in the center of the steering wheel pad or dash. See **Figure 27–8.** This entire assembly must be serviced as one unit when repair of the air bag system is required.

The **air bag** is a strong nylon bag attached to the metal frame of the module. Vent holes in the bag allow for rapid deflation after deployment.

The **air bag igniter** produces a small spark when an electrical signal is sent from the control unit. When the electrical current is applied, the igniter produces an electric arc across two small pins. This spark ignites an igniter charge. This charge rapidly burns and causes the gas-generating pellets to burn and produce rapid gas expansion.

Once ignited, the **propellant charge** is progressive, burning sodium azide, which converts to nitrogen gas as it burns. Heat causes the chemicals in the unit to produce a large amount of nitrogen gas. The nitrogen gas then fills the air bag in a fraction of a second. As the air bag inflates, the steering wheel cover is forced to split open allowing full inflation.

The occupant is then protected by the gas-filled bag instead of being restrained by the seat belts alone. In addition, there is some facial protection against flying objects.

Almost as soon as the bag is filled, the gas is cooled and vented. This deflates the bag right after the collision energy is absorbed. Vents allow rapid deflation. This prevents the driver or passenger from being pinned in the vehicle and also allows normal vision right after deployment.

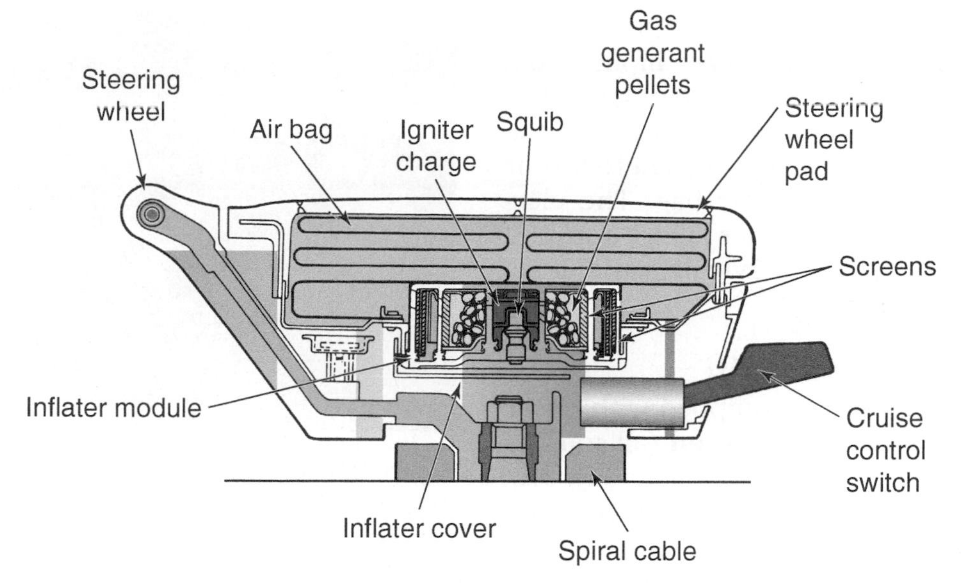

Figure 27–8. The driver air bag module mounts in the steering wheel. Note part names and locations.

Passenger side air bags are very similar in design to the driver's unit. The actual capacity of gas required to inflate the bag is much greater. The bag must span the extra distance between the occupant and the dashboard at the passenger seating location.

Another part relating to an air bag is the knee bolster. A **knee bolster** cushions the driver's knees from impact and helps prevent the driver from sliding under the air bag during a collision. It is located underneath the steering column and behind the steering column trim.

Air Bag Sensors

Two or more sensors are used in air bag systems, impact sensors and arming sensors.

Impact sensors are the first sensors to detect a collision because they are mounted at the front of the vehicle. Impact sensors are usually located in the engine compartment, while the safing sensor is usually located in the passenger compartment.

The *safing* or **arming sensor** ensures that the particular collision is severe enough to require that the air bag be deployed.

Both impact and arming sensors are inertia sensors. **Inertia sensors** detect a rapid deceleration to produce an electrical signal. Some air bag sensors use a small metal ball held in place by a permanent magnet. See **Figure 27–9.** The sensor ball is thrown forward by the inertia of the collision. It then touches two electrical terminals, which closes the sensor circuit to the computer.

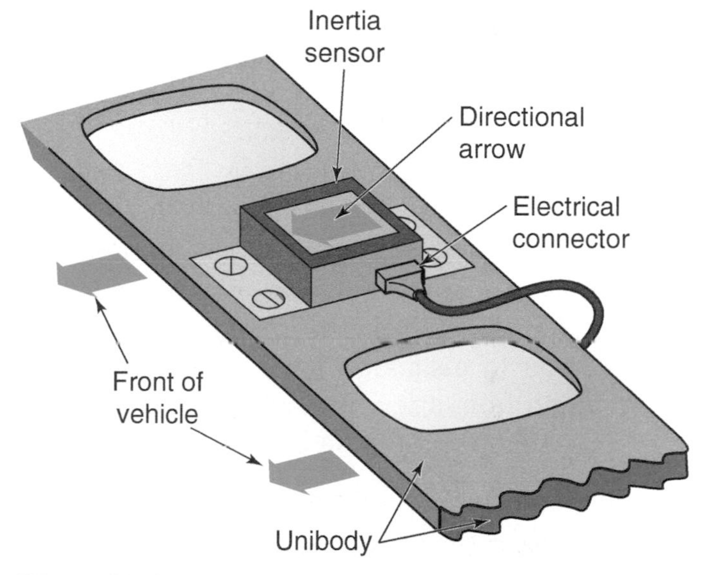

Figure 27–9. The inertia sensor detects rapid deceleration from hard impact on the front or side of the vehicle. It sends a signal to the computer to deploy the air bag. Inertia sensors must be installed with the arrow in the right direction. Also, make sure the system is disarmed so that the new air bag does not deploy while working.

Another air bag sensor design uses a weight attached to a coil spring. During impact, the weight is thrown forward. This overcomes spring tension, closing the sensor contact.

Seat cushion sensors detect the weight of a person sitting in the passenger seat. If no one is sitting in the passenger seat, the air bag system may not deploy the passenger air bag. This saves the considerable cost of having to replace the bag without its having protected someone.

Air Bag Controller

The **air bag controller** analyzes inputs from the sensor to determine if bag deployment is needed. If at least one impact sensor and the arm sensor are closed, it sends current to the air bag module. This fires the air bag. The electronic control unit also provides failure data and trouble codes for use in servicing various aspects of most systems.

Air Bag System Servicing

Before servicing a vehicle equipped with an air bag, the system must be **disarmed** (all sources of electricity for the igniter disconnected). Procedures for disarming the air bag system vary.

Manufacturers may specify removal of the system fuse or disconnection of the module. Always refer to the service manual for exact procedures for disarming the system. This will help prevent electrical system damage and accidental deployment of the new air bag. Always disconnect the negative battery cable.

WARNING

Air bag systems may be equipped with an energy reserve module that allows the air bag to deploy in the event of a power failure. It must be removed from the system or allowed to discharge for a period of time ranging from a few seconds to 30 minutes after disconnecting the battery.

DANGER

Even with the battery disconnected, an energy reserve module can deploy the air bag. If you are working near the bag, serious injury could result.

After air bag deployment, use a shop vacuum to clean the passenger compartment. Residual powder, which is an eye and skin irritant, can be present. Vacuum the instrument panel, vents, seats, carpet, and other surfaces contaminated with this powder. See **Figure 27–10.**

Air bag system parts replacement after a deployment will vary. Check for specific manufacturer recommendations on parts replacement. See **Figure 27–11.**

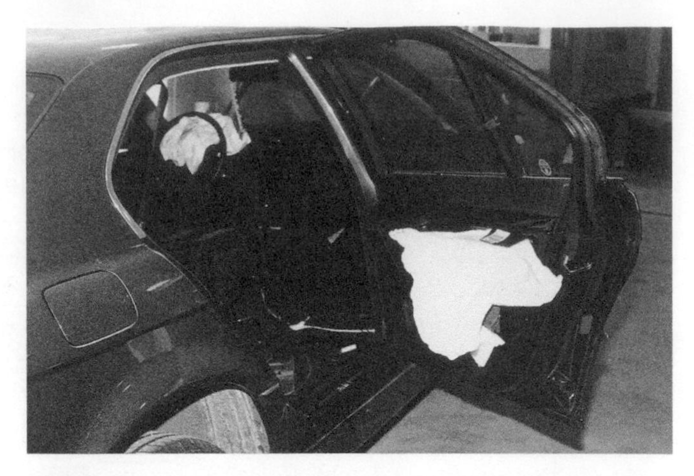

Figure 27–10. After air bag deployment, the passenger compartment should be vacuumed clean. Wear eye protection and a respirator before removing deployed air bags. Passenger air bag deployment often breaks the windshield. Side air bag deployment can damage the inner trim panel.

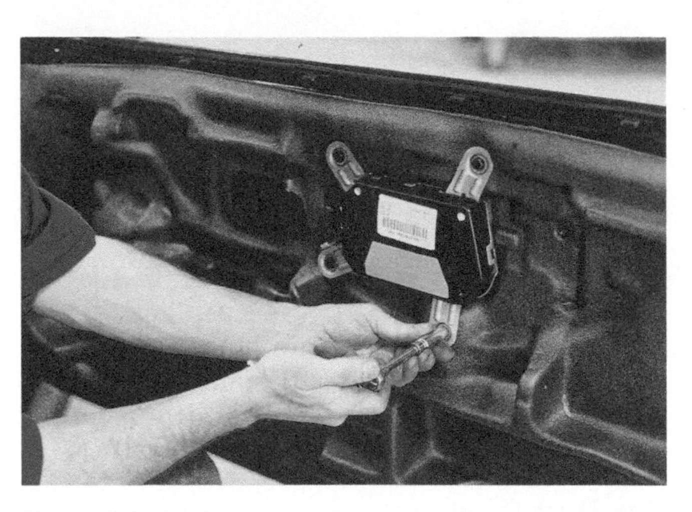

Figure 27–11. When installing new air bag parts, always follow the service manual instructions. Here a technician is installing a new side air bag on the door. Stay to one side and keep your head away from the bag during installation to avoid injury.

When replacing air bag system sensors, double-check that the system is disarmed before removing any sensor. The service manual will give sensor locations. Make sure you have the correct replacement sensor. During installation, check that the *sensor arrow* (directional arrow stamped on the sensor) is facing forward. If a sensor is installed backwards, the air bag will NOT deploy during the next collision.

To remove the deployed air bag, remove the small screws from the rear of the steering wheel. You can then lift out the module and disconnect its wires. Wear safety glasses and a respirator while removing the deployed bag. This will protect you from the residual powder.

Inspect all parts for damage. Parts that have visible damage should be replaced. This would include the steering wheel, steering column, and related parts. Damage to the electrical wiring may also require wiring harness replacement.

Obtain the correct replacement parts from the manufacturer. Also refer to the service manual for exact procedures. System designs vary.

DANGER

When carrying a live (undeployed) air bag module, be sure the bag and trim cover are pointed away from your body. This will help reduce the chances of serious injury if the bag accidentally inflates. When laying a module down on a work surface, make sure the bag and trim cover are face up to minimize a "launch effect" of the module if the bag suddenly inflates.

The air bag system performs a self-check every time the ignition is turned to the ON position. During the self-check the air bag dash lamp indicator will light steadily or blink. When the self-check is completed, the lamp should go OFF. If the lamp stays lit, there is a system fault present.

Make sure a final sweep is made for codes or collision information using the approved scan tool. Carefully recheck the wire and harness routing before releasing the car.

A final inspection of the repair should include checking to make sure the sensors are firmly fastened to their mounting fixtures, with the arrows on them facing forward. Be certain all the fuses are correctly rated and replaced.

SUMMARY

- An active restraint system is one that the occupants must make an effort to use, such as manually operated seat belts. A passive restraint system operates automatically, such as automatic seat belts and air bags.
- A child seat may be rear facing, front facing, or a combination. It is often secured with a lap and shoulder seat belt.
- Most air bag systems have these components: air bag module, air bag system sensors, control unit, wiring harness, and dash indicator lamp.

TECHNICAL TERMS

restraint system
active restraint system
passive restraint system
seat belts
lap belts
shoulder belts
seat belt buckle mechanism
seat belt anchors
belt retractor
child restraint seat
air bag system
driver's-side air bag
passenger-side air bag
side impact air bags
rear seat air bags
air bag module
air bag
air bag igniter
propellant charge
knee bolster
impact sensors
arming sensor
inertia sensors
seat cushion sensors
air bag controller
disarmed

REVIEW QUESTIONS

1. An active restraint system is one that the occupants must make an effort to use. True or false?
2. Seat belt ________ allow one end of the belts to be bolted to the body structure.
3. How does a seat belt reminder system operate?
4. What must you check when inspecting seat belts?
5. You should avoid placing children in the front seat. True or false?
6. List and explain the five major parts of an air bag system.
7. The ________ ________ ________ is composed of the nylon bag and an igniter-inflator mechanism enclosed in a metal-plastic housing.

8. How does gas cause an air bag to inflate?

9. Explain the operation of air bag system sensors.

10. Before servicing a vehicle equipped with an air bag, the system must be ____________. Even with the battery disconnected, the ____________ ____________ can fire the air bag.

11. How do you handle a live air bag module?

ASE-STYLE REVIEW QUESTIONS

1. *Technician A* says you can intermix types of seat belts on front or rear seats. *Technician B* says to tighten all seats and shoulder belt anchor bolts as specified in the service manual. Who is correct?

a. Technician A
b. Technician B
c. Both Technicians A and B
d. Neither Technician

2. *Technician A* says that you should NOT bleach or dye seat belt webbing. *Technician B* says to clean seat belts with a mild soap and water solution. Who is correct?

a. Technician A
b. Technician B
c. Both Technicians A and B
d. Neither Technician

3. *Technician A* says that child seats should only be used in the rear seat of a vehicle. *Technician B* says that child seats should be in the front seat. Who is correct?

a. Technician A
b. Technician B
c. Both Technicians A and B
d. Neither Technician

4. *Technician A* says that to disarm an air bag system you must usually remove the system fuse or disconnect the air bag module. *Technician B* says to always refer to the service manual for exact procedures for disarming the system. Who is correct?

a. Technician A
b. Technician B
c. Both Technicians A and B
d. Neither Technician

5. *Technician A* says that disconnecting the battery will disarm an air bag system. *Technician B* says to wait at least 1 minute after battery disconnection before working on the undeployed air bag system. Who is correct?

a. Technician A
b. Technician B
c. Both Technicians A and B
d. Neither Technician

6. After air bag deployment, *Technician A* says to use a shop vacuum to clean the passenger compartment. *Technician B* says to blow the compartment out with a blow gun. Who is correct?

a. Technician A
b. Technician B
c. Both Technicians A and B
d. Neither Technician

7. When installing impact sensors, *Technician A* says that you can install the sensors in any direction. *Technician B* says to check that the sensor arrow is facing forward. Who is correct?

a. Technician A
b. Technician B
c. Both Technicians A and B
d. Neither Technician

8. *Technician A* says that when carrying a live (undeployed) air bag module, be sure the bag and trim cover are pointed away from your body. *Technician B* says that when laying an air bag down on a work surface, make sure the bag and trim cover face up to minimize a "launch effect" of the module if the bag suddenly inflates. Who is correct?

a. Technician A
b. Technician B

c. Both Technicians A and B
d. Neither Technician

9. Which of the following should NOT be done following servicing of an air bag system?
a. Make a final sweep for trouble.
b. Watch for indicator light in dash.
c. Tap on impact sensor with a hammer.
d. Check wire and harness routing.

ACTIVITIES

1. Inspect a vehicle's restraint systems. List the types of restraints installed in the vehicle. Does it have shoulder harnesses and air bag(s)? List your findings.

2. Refer to a repair manual for a specific make and model vehicle. Summarize the procedures for service after air bag deployment.

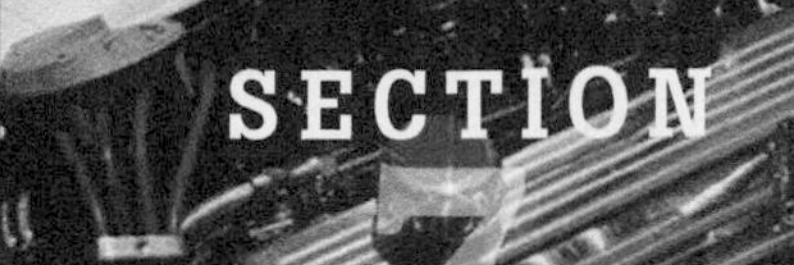

CHAPTER 28

Estimating Repair Costs

OBJECTIVES

After studying this chapter, you should be able to:

- Explain how damage repair estimates are determined.
- Identify and explain the most common abbreviations used in collision estimating guides.
- Make a rough estimate of the time required to refinish a given collision repair job.
- Explain the difference between direct and indirect damage and locate both types.
- Identify the key operating features of manual and computerized estimating systems.
- Compare manual and computerized estimating.

INTRODUCTION

An *estimate,* also called a *damage report* or *appraisal,* calculates the cost of parts, materials, and labor for repairing a collision damaged vehicle. Developed by the estimator, it is a written or printed summary of the repairs needed. The estimate is used by the customer, insurance company, shop management, and technician.

As you will learn, computerization has streamlined all aspects of collision repair shop operations. The computer-written estimate drives and integrates other aspects of the collision repair facility. Once initial vehicle and customer data are entered into the computer, everything from consulting estimating guides and vehicle dimension manuals to billing can be done electronically.

DAMAGE ANALYSIS

For an estimate to clearly establish a true cost of repairs, a thorough damage analysis must be performed on the vehicle. **Damage analysis** involves locating all damage using a systematic series of inspections, measurements, and tests. This allows repairs to be done right the first time and also prevents cost overruns. See **Figure 28–1.**

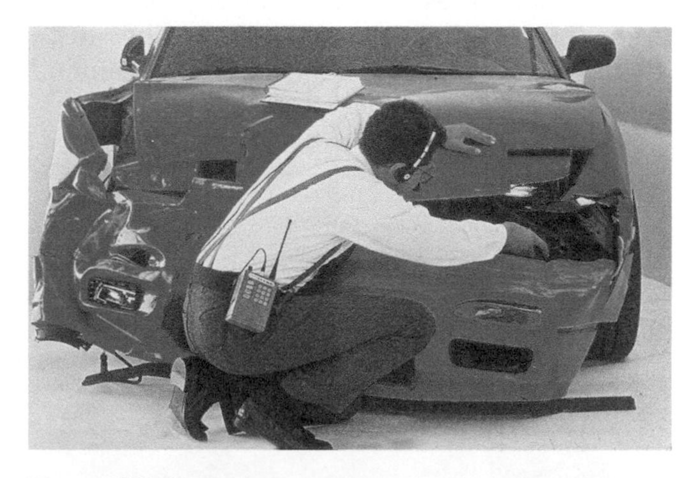

Figure 28–1. Estimating collision repair costs can be a challenge. You must evaluate many variables to determine what must be done to repair the vehicle. (Courtesy of Mitchell International)

Before starting damage analysis, you should:

1. If possible, discuss the collision with the owner or driver of the vehicle to obtain information that may help during damage analysis.
2. Identify the vehicle completely. Include vehicle identification number (VIN), year, make, model, engine, and optional equipment.
3. List mileage.
4. Identify and note all precollision damage.
5. Check wheels and tires, including the spare. Damaged wheels may provide clues about the collision.
6. Confirm the point of impact and analyze how the damage has traveled.

DIRECT AND INDIRECT DAMAGE

One of the reasons unibody vehicles are a challenge to repair is because of the way the body reacts to collision forces. There are two types of damage that must be identified. They are direct (primary) damage and indirect (secondary) damage.

Direct damage occurs in the area of immediate impact as a direct result of the vehicle striking an object. Direct damage is usually easy to locate and analyze. See **Figure 28–2.**

Indirect damage is caused by the shock of collision forces traveling through the body and inertial forces acting on the rest of the unibody. Indirect damage can be more difficult to completely identify and analyze. It may be found anywhere on the vehicle.

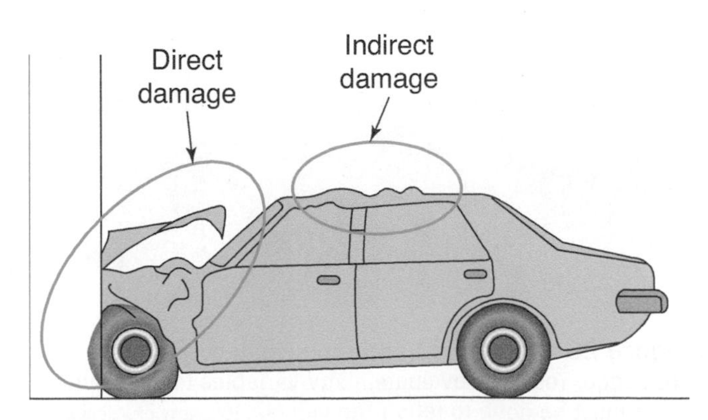

Figure 28–2. Direct or primary damage occurs at the point of impact. Indirect or secondary damage occurs elsewhere as forces travel through the vehicle structure. (Courtesy of Nissan North America, Inc.)

Before doing anything else, take time to carefully perform an overall visual inspection and try to determine the direction of impact and the areas of indirect damage.

VEHICLE INSPECTION

The direction of impact will affect the parts damaged. If the vehicle was hit in the front, side, or rear, you will know to check specific areas and parts for damage. See **Figure 28–3.**

You should use a damage analysis checklist to make sure nothing is overlooked.

Inspect the entire vehicle for damage, looking for:

1. Alignment of doors.
2. Alignment of the hood and deck lid.
3. Gaps between panels.
4. How the doors, hood, and deck lid open and close. See **Figure 28–4.**
5. Ripples in the roof, fenders, or quarter panels away from the direct impact.
6. Cracked or stressed paint.
7. Cracked seam sealers.
8. Cracked or broken glass.
9. Smooth operation of windows.
10. Damage to interior (instrument panel, seats, seat belts, etc.), deployed air bag, stained carpet, and other problems.
11. Indications of previous damage.
12. Remove parts if needed to analyze hidden damage. See **Figure 28–5.**

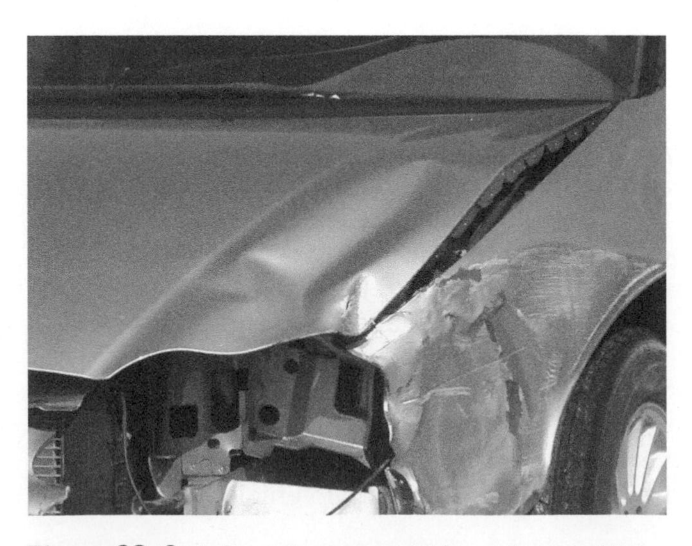

Figure 28–3. Indirect damage might be under or behind these damaged panels.

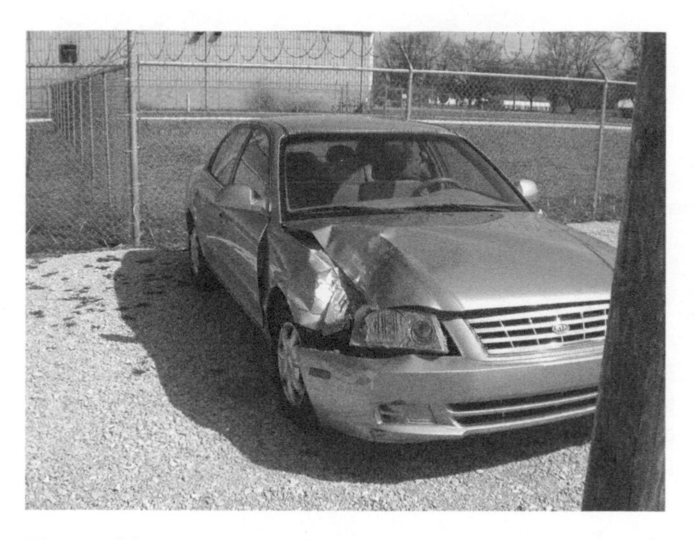

Figure 28–4. A hard hit to the right front of this vehicle could have resulted in secondary damage to many parts behind the point of impact.

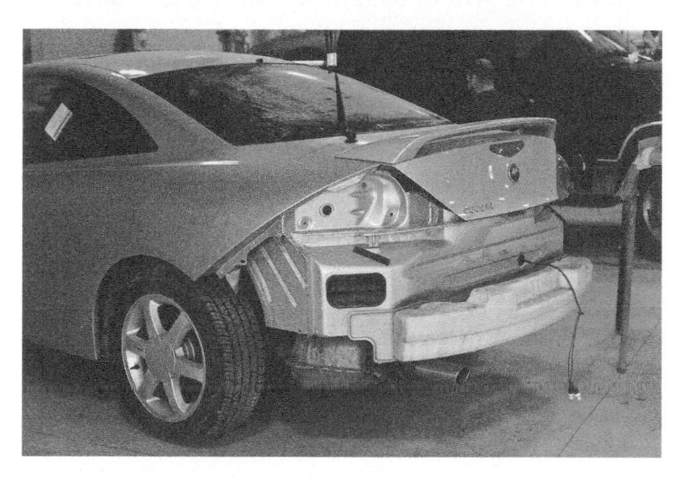

Figure 28–5. Sometimes parts must be removed to find hidden damage when writing an estimate.

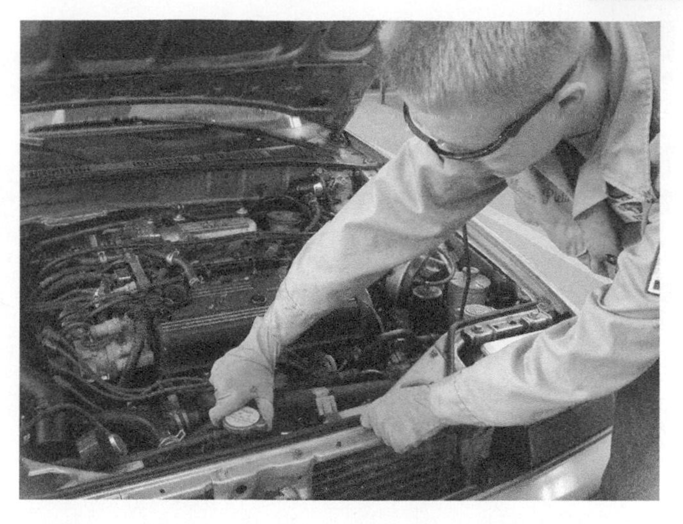

(A) The technician is removing the radiator cap (system cool to touch) to see if there has been a loss of coolant from damage to the radiator, engine water pump, or other parts.

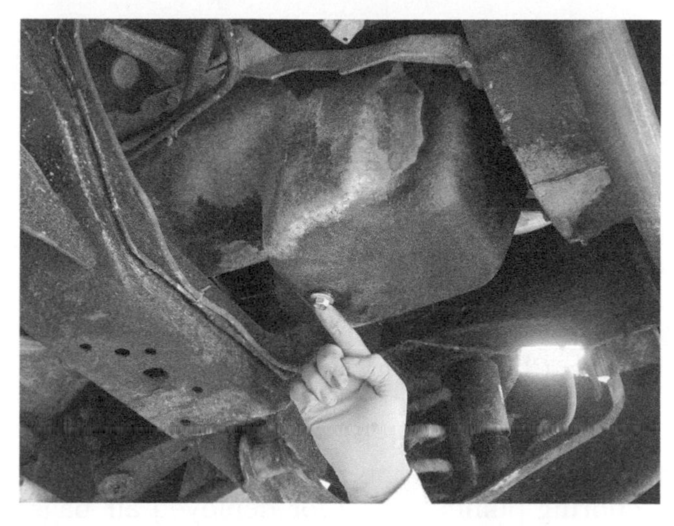

(B) Raising the vehicle on a lift is needed to check for damage to parts and panels on the bottom of the vehicle. The oil pan can be hit and damaged as the vehicle leaves the road during an accident.

Figure 28–6. Always inspect for damage to mechanical parts that must be included in the estimate.

13. If it was a frontal collision, inspect parts in the engine compartment for damage.
14. Check under the vehicle for fluid leaks, which are signs of mechanical damage. See **Figure 28–6.**

Always raise a badly damaged vehicle off the floor so that a good visual inspection can be made of all underbody and drivetrain parts. In some unibody vehicles, it might even be necessary to remove the drivetrain and suspension parts to make a thorough damage inspection.

In other words, the estimator must give the entire vehicle a thorough inspection—top to bottom and front to rear—and take nothing for granted. See **Figure 28–7.** If something is missed on the original estimate, it often becomes difficult to reopen it for further negotiations later. On the other hand, some estimates do include a hidden damage clause that permits added charges to the original estimate if hidden damages are discovered later.

Taking digital photographs of the vehicle to keep with the documentation is also a good idea. Photos can be useful if there are any questions about a repair. Videotaping the vehicle before and after repairs can also be helpful.

Modern computerized estimating systems can utilize electronic photos and digitize video footage for finalizing the estimate when at the office computer.

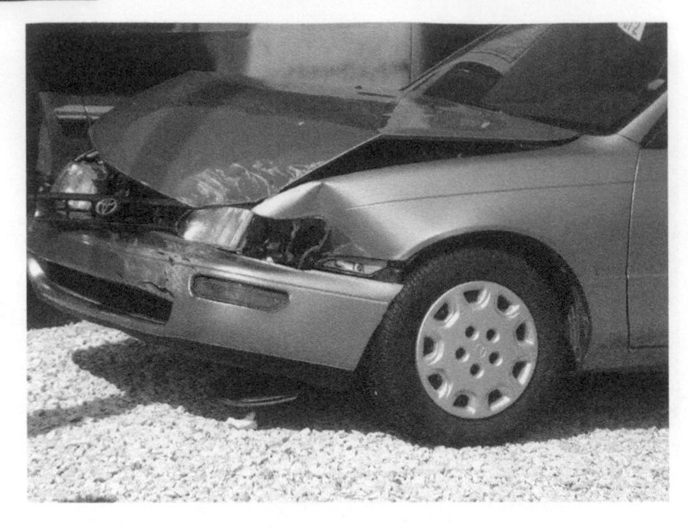

Figure 28–7. The estimator must have a thorough knowledge of vehicle construction and repair methods to develop an accurate estimate of repair costs.

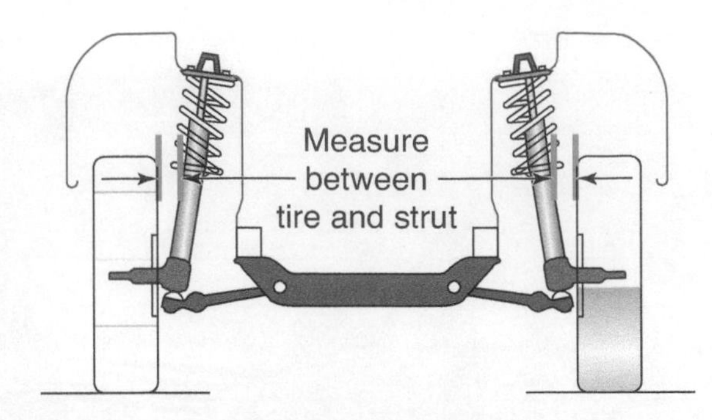

Figure 28–8. Measure between each tire and strut with a tape measure. Different measurements indicate damage. You can also measure curb height if major structural damage is possible. (Courtesy of Chief Automotive Systems, Inc.)

INTERIOR INSPECTION

The interior of the vehicle must also be inspected. Check for damage caused by collision forces, unrestrained passengers, or cargo. Inspect glass and mirrors. Check door handles and door locks for proper operation.

Inspect alignment of the glove box door. Misalignment may indicate instrument panel damage. Check interior controls for proper operation. Also inspect the console and shift lever.

Check seats and the restraint system for damage. Check seat belt buckles, webbing, and anchoring points. Check for deployed air bags and operation of motorized seat belts.

DAMAGE QUICK CHECKS

Damage quick checks can be done to analyze problems with the body structure, steering, and suspension systems. They can assist in determining if further steering system or suspension measurements are necessary.

A **steering wheel center check** involves making sure the steering wheel has not been moved off center due to part damage.

If the steering wheel looks centered and the front tires point straight ahead, steering gear, steering column, and steering arms are probably NOT damaged.

If damage is suspected, inspect the strut carefully for signs of impact, bent housing, or other obvious damage. This check will NOT work with struts that do not have an accessible strut shaft. See **Figure 28–8.**

A **wheel run-out check** will show if there is damage to a rotating part of a wheel assembly. To do this:

1. Raise the wheel assembly off the ground.
2. Using a safety stand, place a pointer (screwdriver, pen or pencil, etc.) to within ⅛ inch (3 mm) of the first step of the wheel (where the tire bead is seated).
3. Spin the wheel and watch the distance between the wheel and the pointer.
4. If wobble is a visible, remove that wheel, replace with a known good wheel, and repeat the check. Add the damaged bearings or wheels to the estimate.

DIMENSION MANUALS

When analyzing damage for making an estimate, you may need to use unibody/frame measuring equipment to determine the extent of the damage. See **Figure 28–9.**

After taking measurements on the vehicle, compare them to the body dimension manual. The manual will give illustrations of known good distances from specific body/frame points. By comparing your measurements to these known good measurements, you can determine the extent and direction of damage.

COLLISION ESTIMATING AND REFERENCE GUIDES

Collision estimating and reference guides help with filling out the estimate. Whether in manual or electronic form, estimating guides contain:

1. Illustrated parts breakdowns
2. Part names and numbers

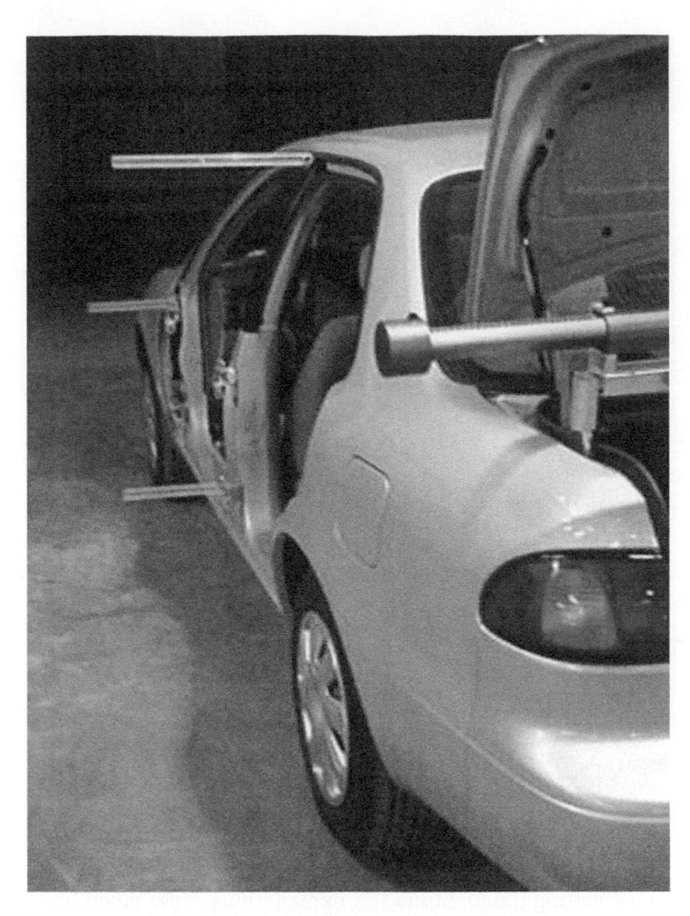

Figure 28–9. When in doubt about the extent of structural damage, use a measuring system. It will accurately show damage. (Courtesy of Lasermate)

3. Labor times
4. Refinish times
5. Part prices
6. Other miscellaneous information

Collision estimating guides can be used as a reference for pricing parts. However, never use them to determine the absolute price. Usually, these guides will list the name of the part, the year of the vehicle it will fit, its part number, the estimated time required to replace it, and the current price. The current prices are the factory-suggested list prices. Parts that have been discontinued are usually listed. The price that appears in the guide is the last available one at the time of printing.

Each collision estimating guide will have procedure ("P") pages. These procedure pages provide important information such as:

1. Arrangement of material
2. Explanation of symbols used
3. Definitions of terms used
4. How to read and use the parts illustrations
5. Procedure explanations for labor and refinishing, including which operations are included and which are NOT
6. How discontinued parts information is displayed
7. How interchangeable part information is displayed
8. Additions to labor times
9. Labor times for overlap items
10. How to identify structural operations
11. How to identify mechanical operations

DAMAGE REPORT TERMINOLOGY

Anyone working with collision estimating guides must be familiar with the terms and abbreviations used. See **Figure 28–10.** A few abbreviation examples are:

R & I—to remove and install.

R & R means to remove and replace.

Overhaul—to remove an assembly from the vehicle, disassemble, clean, inspect, replace parts as needed, reassemble, install, and adjust (except wheel and suspension alignment).

Included operations are those that can be performed individually but are also part of another operation.

Overlap occurs when replacement of one part duplicates some labor operation required to replace an adjacent part.

Refer to the procedure pages to identify all terms used.

PART COSTS

When should you repair or replace body parts? This question must be answered almost daily in collision repair shops. Actually, the decision often is a judgment call.

To help you decide whether to repair or replace panels, remember this statement.

If it is bent, repair it!
If it is kinked, replace it!

As explained in earlier chapters, a part is kinked if it is bent more than 90 degrees. A bend is damage of less than 90 degrees.

There are several other factors to consider: the type of surface, location of damage, and

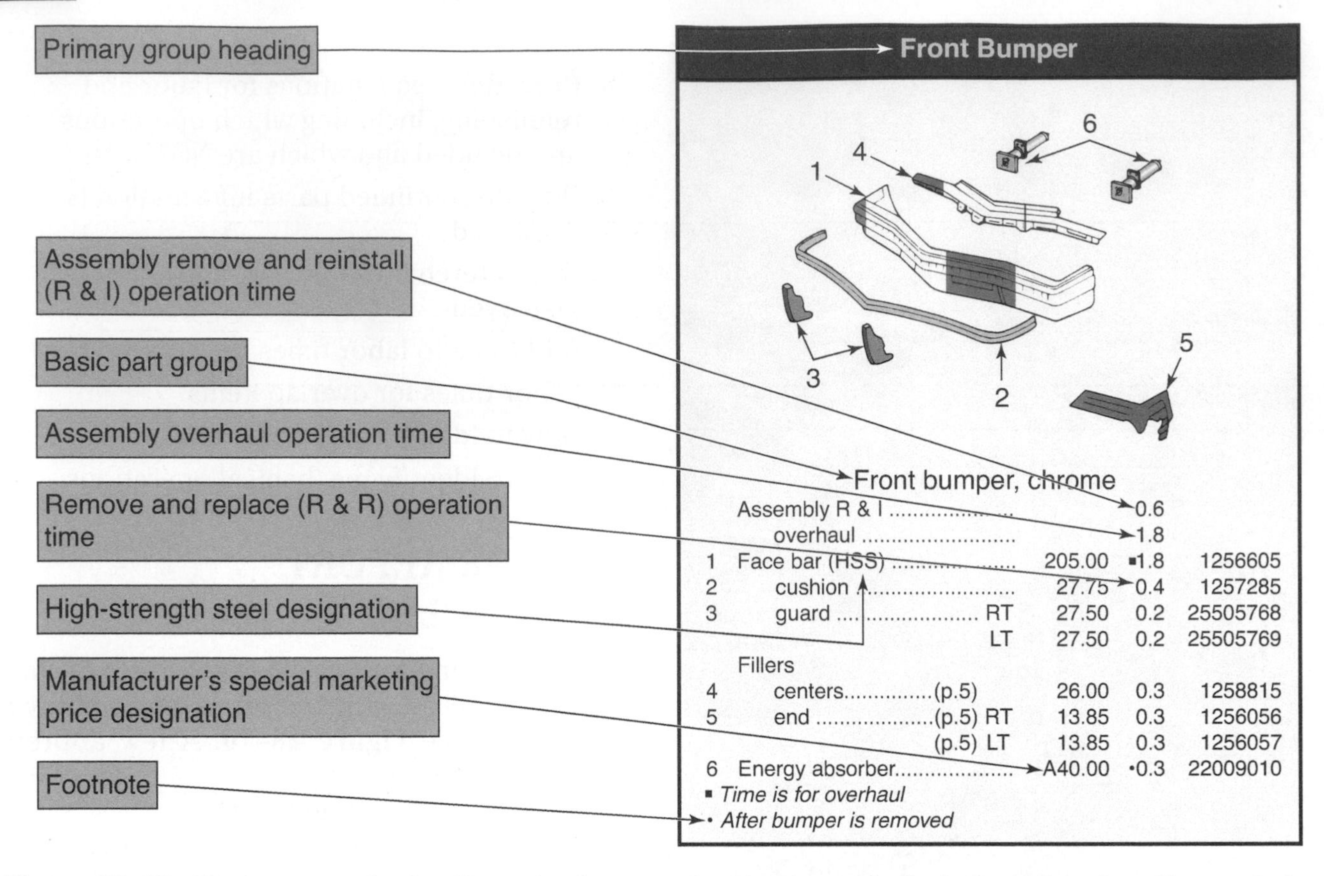

Figure 28–10. This is an example of an illustration from a crash estimating guide. Study the explanations. How much time would be charged to remove and install the energy absorber in the bumper?

extent of damage. The following are some useful guidelines:

1. If the damage is in a flat surface, it will straighten more easily than a sharp fold or buckle along a corner. Kinks along sharply formed edges almost always require replacement.
2. If the damage is located near the end of a rail, with the crush zone unaffected, replacement is NOT as critical as when the damage is in the crush zone or further into the rail. A kink in the crush zone calls for replacement.
3. If the damage is located near the engine or steering mounting areas, repeated stress loading can create fatigue failure. Kinks at these mounting points require replacement rather than repair.
4. Tightly folded metal that is "locked" due to severe work hardening requires replacement.

Part costs are also affected by whether the parts are new or recycled/salvaged. New parts might require more time to install than good recycled/salvaged parts. They will usually cost more too.

Recycled/salvaged parts will already have corrosion protection and sound deadening, whereas new parts might not. However, recycled/salvaged parts might have minor damage that must be repaired. All of this must be considered when writing the estimate. As can be seen, there are many variables that can affect the repair/replace decision.

WRITING ESTIMATES

An estimate or *damage report* must include basic information about the vehicle. A **manually written estimate** is done longhand by filling in information on a printed form, as shown in **Figure 28–11.** An **electronic/computer-written estimate** is done using a personal computer and printer. You should understand how both are done.

A damage report or estimate includes:

1. Customer information, including name, address, and phone number.

B & J
Collision Estimating Services

ESTIMATE OF REPAIRS
Nº 002128

SHEET NO. 1 OF 1 SHEETS

NAME	ADDRESS	PHONE	DATE
KAREN Miller	1143 RAILROAD ST. CRESSONA, PA. 17929	HOME 395-2719 BUS. 623 7347	12-17-07

YEAR	MAKE	MODEL	LICENSE NO.	MILEAGE	SERIAL/ V.I. NO.
2005	FORD	P.U.	MAE 917	14864	1FTDF15Y5GNA69994

INSURANCE COMPANY	TYPE OF INSURANCE	ADJUSTER	PHONE	CAR LOCATED AT
Amerisure	COL			

PARTS NECESSARY AND ESTIMATE OF LABOR REQUIRED	PAINT COST ESTIMATE	PARTS COST ESTIMATE	LABOR COST ESTIMATE
(1) FRONT FACE BAR Chrome NO gds OR PADS		205 82	.5
(1) " STONE deflector	1 0	40 50	.5
(1) Left Headlamp door (with argent grill)		52 32	2
(1) " " Shield		3 20	
(1) " FRONT fender	3 1	133 00	1 6
(1) " " " APRON		60 47	1 0
(2) wheels 15" 55.60 ea.		111 20	6
(2) stems and Balance		2 50	5
(2) HUB CAPS		43 46	—
Repair Radiator Support		—	2 0
Align FRONT End		—	1 5
(1) Left door trim Panel		73 40	
Stripe Left FRONT fender		15 00	.5
LABOR 25.0 HRS @ 23.00		575 00	
(note may be FRONT suspension damage)			
PAINT MAT.		89 10	
UNDERCOAT		15 00	
TOTALS		1,419 .97	

INSURED PAYS $______ INS. CO. PAYS $______ R. O. NO.______

INS. CHECK PAYABLE TO______

The above is an estimate, based on our inspection, and does not cover additional parts or labor which may be required after the work has been opened up. Occasionally, after work has started, worn, broken or damaged parts are discovered which are not evident on first inspection. Quotations on parts and labor are current and subject to change. Not responsible for any delays caused by unavailability of parts or delays in parts shipment by supplier or transporter.

ESTIMATOR______

AUTHORIZATION FOR REPAIRS. You are hereby authorized to make the above specified repairs to the car described herein.

SIGNED X DATE 19

GRAND TOTAL	1,419.97
TOWING & STORAGE	
TAX	85.20
TOTAL OF ESTIMATE	$ 1,505.17

Figure 28–11. Here is an example of a manually written estimate. Read it through carefully. Note how both the cost of parts and labor have been tabulated.

2. Vehicle information—year, make, model, body type, license number, odometer reading, VIN, paint code, and trim colors.
3. Options—remote mirrors, power windows, power door locks, antilock brake system (ABS), air conditioning, and so on.
4. Date the vehicle was received and promised completion date.
5. It may be helpful to make sketches of the damaged areas of the vehicle. Many damage report forms provide a place to do this. With computer estimating systems,

electronic photos or videos can also be helpful.

6. List whether new or recycled/salvaged parts will be used during the repair.
7. Summarize cost of parts and labor. See **Figure 28–12.**

At least three copies of the written estimate should be made. One is kept by the shop, one is given to the insurance company, and the other is given to the customer. An estimate is a **firm bid** for a given period of time—usually for 30 days. The reason for a given time period is obvious: part prices change and damaged parts can deteriorate.

The estimate is also considered the authorization to complete the repair work as listed, but ONLY when it is agreed upon and signed by the owner or by the owner and insurance company appraiser. The estimate explains the legal conditions under which the repair work is accepted by the collision repair shop. It protects the shop against the possibility of undetected damage that might be revealed later as repairs progress.

Many insurance policies contain a **deductible clause,** which means that the owner is responsible for the first given amount of the estimate (usually $100 to $500). The remaining cost is paid by the insurance company. In such cases, both the customer and insurance company should authorize the estimate.

Another important function of the estimate is that it serves as a basis for writing the work order or operational plan. The work order is usually prepared from the damage appraisal of the estimator (using the written estimate) and a visual inspection by the shop supervisor and/or a technician.

The **work order** outlines the procedures that should be taken to put the vehicle back in top condition. It is also a valuable tool to both the estimator and the shop foreman, since it lists the actual times necessary to do the job.

Following are additional factors to be considered when writing an estimate. Such added time is usually negotiated between the estimator and the insurance company or customer.

1. Time for the setup of the vehicle on frame straightening equipment and damage diagnosis
2. Time for pushing, pulling, cutting, and so on to remove collision damaged parts
3. Time to straighten or align related parts

Time/Dollar Conversion Table											
	Dollar per hour rates										
Time	.50	$1.00	$10.00	$15.00	$20.00	$25.00	$30.00	$35.00	$40.00	$45.00	$50.00
0.6	.30	.60	6.00	9.00	12.00	15.00	18.00	21.00	24.00	27.00	30.00
0.7	.35	.70	7.00	10.50	14.00	17.50	21.00	24.50	28.00	31.50	35.00
0.8	.40	.80	8.00	12.00	16.00	20.00	24.00	28.00	32.00	36.00	40.00
0.9	.45	.90	9.00	13.50	18.00	22.50	27.00	31.50	36.00	40.50	45.00
1.0	.50	1.00	10.00	15.00	20.00	25.00	30.00	35.00	40.00	45.00	50.00
1.1	.55	1.10	11.00	16.50	22.00	27.50	33.00	38.50	44.00	49.50	55.00
1.2	.60	1.20	12.00	18.00	24.00	30.00	36.00	42.00	48.00	54.00	60.00
1.3	.65	1.30	13.00	19.50	26.00	32.50	39.00	45.50	52.00	58.50	65.00
1.4	.70	1.40	14.00	21.00	28.00	35.00	42.00	49.00	56.00	63.00	70.00
1.5	.75	1.50	15.00	22.50	30.00	37.50	45.00	52.50	60.00	67.50	75.00
1.6	.80	1.60	16.00	24.00	32.00	40.00	48.00	56.00	64.00	72.00	80.00
1.7	.85	1.70	17.00	25.50	34.00	42.50	51.00	59.50	68.00	76.50	85.00
1.8	.90	1.80	18.00	27.00	36.00	45.00	54.00	63.00	72.00	81.00	90.00
1.9	.95	1.90	19.00	28.50	38.00	47.50	57.00	66.50	76.00	85.50	95.00
2.0	1.00	2.00	20.00	30.00	40.00	50.00	60.00	70.00	80.00	90.00	100.00
2.1	1.05	2.10	21.00	31.50	42.00	52.50	63.00	73.50	84.00	94.50	105.00
2.2	1.10	2.20	22.00	33.00	44.00	55.00	66.00	77.00	88.00	99.00	110.00
2.3	1.15	2.30	23.00	34.50	46.00	57.50	69.00	80.50	92.00	103.50	115.00
2.4	1.20	2.40	24.00	36.00	48.00	60.00	72.00	84.00	96.00	108.00	120.00
2.5	1.25	2.50	25.00	37.50	50.00	62.50	75.00	87.50	100.00	112.50	125.00

Figure 28–12. This chart can be used to convert time from an estimating guide into actual labor charges per hour. If the shop is charging $45 per hour and the labor time is 2.3 hours, how much labor in dollars will be charged?

4. Time to remove undercoating, tar, grease, and similar materials
5. Time to repair rust damage to adjacent parts
6. Time for the free-up of corroded or frozen parts
7. Time for drilling for ornamentation or mounting holes
8. Time to repair damaged replacement parts prior to installation
9. Time to check suspension and steering alignment/toe-in
10. Time for removal of shattered glass
11. Time to rebuild, recondition, and install after-market parts, NOT including refinishing time
12. Time for application of sound-deadening material, primecoating, caulking, and painting of the inner areas
13. Time to restore rust protection
14. Time to R & I main computer module when necessary in repair operations
15. Time to R & I wheel or hub cap locks
16. Time to replace accessories such as trailer hitches, sun roofs, and fender flares

ESTIMATING SEQUENCE

When estimating any type of damage, a logical sequence must be followed. Before making a written estimate, the estimator should visually inspect the entire vehicle, paying special attention to damaged subassemblies and parts that are mounted to (or part of) a damaged part.

The estimator must consider the same points as the technician does before making any decision on repair work. Most estimators start from the outside of the vehicle and work inward, listing everything on paper—by vehicle section—that is bent, broken, crushed, or missing.

For example, if the front grille and some of the related parts are damaged, list the needed repairs or replacements as follows:

1. Front Grille..Replace
2. Opening Panel............Straighten and replace
3. Deflector (or Valance Panel)..............Replace
4. Headlight Door ....Replace
5. Grille Opening Panel..........................Refinish

Notice that the parts are listed in a definite sequence according to factory disassembly operations or exploded views as provided in service manuals or collision estimating guides.

FLAT RATE OPERATIONS

The **flat rate** is a preset amount of time and money charged for a specific repair operation. As a rule of thumb, repair costs should never exceed replacement costs. If repairs and straightening will NOT produce a quality job, then the estimate should list the required new parts. Sheet metal parts usually offer the most opportunities for repair and straightening. As a result, sheet metal repair, replacement, and panel refinishing generally account for the largest number of estimate dollars.

To reduce part costs, many insurance appraisers and some customers might want to use recycled/salvaged parts. Recycled/salvaged parts are removed from damaged vehicles by *recyclers* (salvage yards). There is always a chance that such parts have been previously damaged and repaired. For this reason, it is important to carefully inspect all recycled/salvaged parts before they are installed to be sure that they are in usable condition.

Each damaged vehicle poses different problems that must be solved to arrive at a final decision concerning repair versus replacement. The most difficult questions arise when a vehicle is involved in a major collision.

LABOR COSTS

The procedure pages of crash estimating guides usually provide an explanation of what the labor time does and does NOT include. For example, replacing a panel or fender includes removing, installing, and aligning. It does NOT include the installation of molding or antennas, refinishing, pinstriping, or application of decals. Also NOT considered are corroded or inaccessible bolts, primecoating, and alignment or straightening of damaged adjacent parts.

The labor time reported in crash estimating guides is to be used as a guide only. The times are principally based on data reported by vehicle manufacturers or manual publishers who have arrived at them by repeated performance of each operation under normal shop conditions.

An explanation is listed in the guide of the established requirements for the average technician, working under average conditions and following the procedures outlined in the service manuals.

All labor times given in crash estimating guides include the time necessary to ensure proper fit of the new part. The times are based on new, undamaged parts installed as an individual operation. Additional time has NOT been added to compensate for collision damage to the vehicle. Removal and replacement of exchanged or used parts are also NOT considered. If additional aligning or repairs must be made, such factors should be considered when making an estimate.

When jobs overlap, reductions in the labor times must be considered. This occurs when replacement of one part duplicates some labor operations required to replace an adjacent part. For example, when replacing a quarter panel and rear body panel on the same vehicle, the area where the two parts join is considered overlap. Where a labor overlap condition exists, less time is required to replace adjoining parts collectively than is required when they are replaced individually.

Another labor cost reduction is noted as included operations. These are jobs that can be performed individually but are also part of another operation.

As an example, when replacing a door, the suggested time would include the replacement of all parts attached to the door, except for the ornamentation. It would be impossible to replace the door without transferring these parts. Consequently, the time involved in transferring them would be included operations and should be disregarded because the times for the individual items are already included in the door replacement time.

Flat rate manuals list a labor time plus a materials allowance; they do NOT, however, include the dollar value of the materials required.

REFINISHING TIME

Making a correct estimate of the amount of time required to refinish panels, doors, hoods, and so forth is a vital part of an estimator's job. Although the wide range of materials and conditions sometimes makes it difficult to arrive at a precise refinishing cost, there are a number of generally approved concepts that will help an estimator arrive at a fair judgment of the amount of materials that will be needed for the job.

Flat rate manuals list a labor time plus a materials allowance (in dollars) for many different refinishing operations. Independently published crash estimating guides list the labor times but NOT the dollar value of the materials required.

In most crash estimating guides on the market today, the time required for refinishing is shown in the parentheses adjacent to the part name. The refinishing time generally includes:

1. Cleaning/light sanding
2. Masking adjacent panels
3. Priming/scuff sanding
4. Final sanding/cleaning
5. Mixing paint/filling spray equipment
6. Applying colorcoat
7. Removing masking
8. Buffing or compounding (if required)
9. Cleaning equipment

Refinishing time generally does NOT include:

1. Cost of paints or materials
2. Matching and/or tinting
3. Grinding, filling, and smoothing welded seams
4. Blending into adjacent panels
5. Removal of protective coatings
6. Custom painting
7. Primecoating
8. Antirust materials
9. Sound-deadening materials
10. Refinishing the underside of hood or deck lids
11. Covering the entire vehicle prior to refinishing
12. Additional time to produce custom, non-OEM finishes

The refinishing times given in most estimates are for one color on new replacement parts—outer surfaces only. Additions to refinishing times are usually made for the following operations:

1. Refinishing the underside of the hood
2. Refinishing the underside of the trunk lid
3. Edging the new part

4. Two-tone operations
5. Stone chip (protective material)
6. Clearcoat (basecoat-clearcoat) after deduction for overlap

TOTAL LABOR COSTS

Once all the repairs and labor times have been entered on the estimate form, refer to the estimating guide's time/dollar conversion table. It is used to convert labor time into dollars to fit local labor or operating rates per hour.

When establishing labor rates, the shop overhead (including such items as rent, management and supervision, supplies, and depreciation on equipment) must be determined. Then the actual labor cost of all employees and the profit required to keep the business operating must be added to the shop overhead to obtain a dollar rate for repairs. This rate is usually figured on an hourly basis. Keep in mind that labor times shown in estimating guides are listed in tenths of an hour.

TOTALING THE ESTIMATE

Once all the columns of the estimating form—parts, labor, and refinishing cost—are filled out, they can be added together for a subtotal. To this figure, add any extra charges, such as wrecker and towing fees, storage fees, and state and local taxes. These figures, added to the subtotal, will give the grand total of the estimate.

While more and more large collision repair shops are doing repair jobs such as wheel alignment, rust protection, and tire placement, smaller operations still "farm-out" or "sublet" these jobs to specialty shops.

When the work is done, the specialty shop bills the collision repair shop for the work. Generally, this is done at a rate less than the normal retail labor cost. In this way, the collision repair shop can charge the normal retail cost and still make a small profit.

Shops that sublet work usually have a "sublet" column on the estimate where the retail labor cost is marked. This figure is added to the rest to obtain the grand total of the estimate.

If the customer wants extra work performed (damage that occurred prior to collision), this should be noted as *customer-requested,* or C/R, repairs. As a general rule, the insurance company will NOT pay for C/R repairs. Often a separate estimate must be made in such cases.

COMPUTERIZED ESTIMATING

Computerized estimating systems using a **PC** (personal computer) may provide more accurate and consistent damage reports. The use of computers makes dealing with thousands of parts on hundreds of vehicles more manageable. See **Figure 28–13.**

Computerized estimating systems store the collision estimating guide information in a computer. This eliminates a lot of time spent looking up parts and labor times and manually entering and totaling them on a form. The computer prepares a damage report, while still allowing the possibility of a manual override when necessary. See **Figure 28–14.**

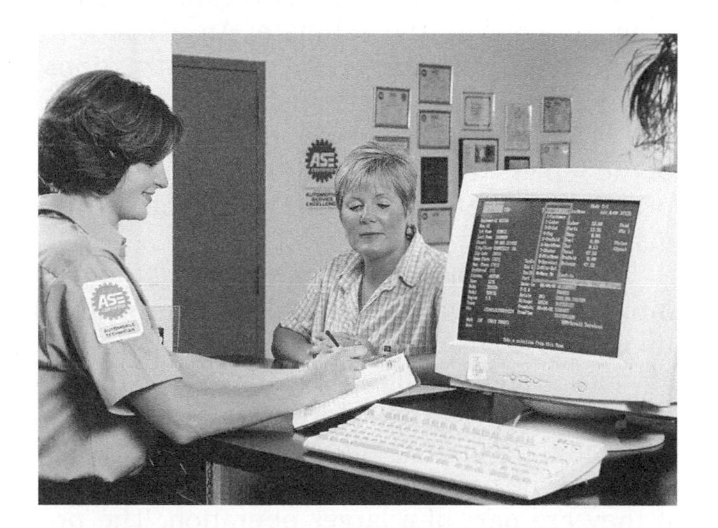

Figure 28–13. Computer estimating is much more efficient than trying to figure repair costs longhand. (Courtesy of ASE)

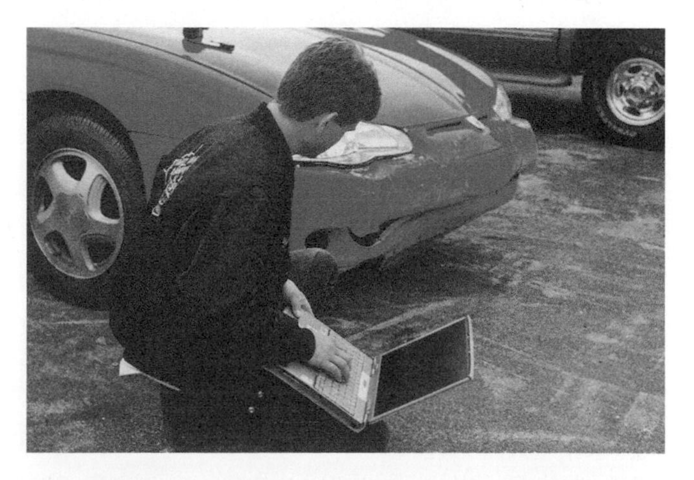

Figure 28–14. A laptop computer can be taken out to the vehicle during damage analysis. It can also be used in the office to finalize the damage report.

Computers have revolutionized the art of estimating by making enormous amounts of data readily accessible.

The **estimating system** has all of the data needed at the shop office, usually on CD-ROMs. Modern computer estimating systems store electronic databases containing up-to-date part prices and labor times that can be retrieved from the shop's computer system.

With the use of these sophisticated programs, estimators can now use the stored data to make virtually error-free estimates rapidly at a very low cost.

Computer Database

Once information has been gathered at the vehicle, the estimator will take these data into the office. The operator can then use the speed and convenience of a computer and estimating program to work up the estimate. An **estimating program** is software (computer instructions) that will automatically help find parts needed and labor rates and will calculate the total cost of the repairs. See **Figure 28–15.** The estimating program is often on a CD-ROM (optical data on disk).

To use the program, you must load the data into the PC's memory. This will then let you pull up images from an electronic dimension manual. Modern systems will retrieve exploded views of assemblies in electronic form. See **Figure 28–16.**

Many programs automatically deduct for overlap. The program notes operations as "Incl." if they are part of a larger operation. The program will also identify judgment times or user-entered information.

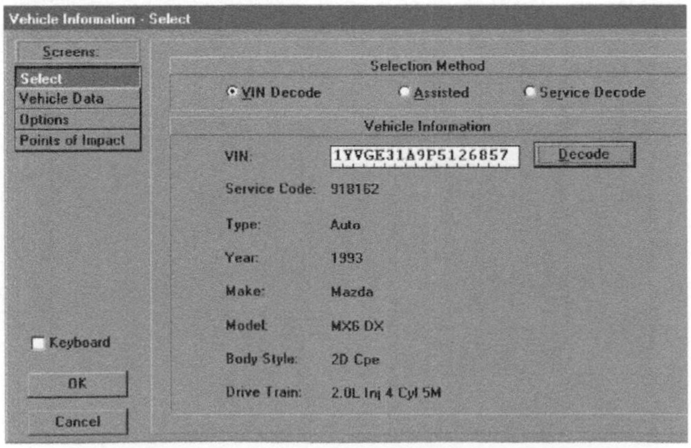

Figure 28–15. An estimating program is designed to help the estimator quickly and accurately identify vehicles and calculate repair costs. (Courtesy of Mitchell International, Inc.)

The estimating program can access a huge database (computer file) of information. The computer **database** includes part numbers, part illustrations, labor times, labor rates, and other data for filling out the estimate. Quick searches can be done to move through this database quickly and efficiently.

The most common and modern way of storing an estimating database is the CD-ROM. One or two **CD-ROMs** (compact discs) can hold all of the crash estimating guides and dimension manuals, as well as other information for every make and model vehicle. The compact disc database contains the same basic information that is in the collision estimating guide.

Labor time information for a given operation is taken from the same sources as in the collision estimating guides.

A CD-ROM allows access to a huge amount of data, which can be pulled into the PC's memory for manipulation.

Advanced computer estimating systems will even allow you to input photos of the damaged vehicle into the computer.

An **electronic or digital camera** can be used to take photos of the vehicle's damage and store them as electronic data. The camera can be connected to the computer to download these **digital images** (pictures stored as computer data) into memory or onto the computer's internal hard drive.

The estimator can look at these photos on the computer screen or monitor while finalizing the estimate. The electronic images can also be sent to the insurance adjuster for evaluating the vehicle's damage.

You can also select from either new or recycled/salvaged parts, and the program will help you enter the difference in costs and labor to install either type part. You can quickly compare the installation of like-kind and quality used parts with new parts. The difference in purchase price and labor times can be quickly analyzed.

If the headlights are damaged, for example, the program will remind you to include aiming headlights or will give an exploded view to make sure all damaged parts or part variations are noted.

When estimating painting/refinishing labor and materials, the program will let you select from solid color, base-clearcoat, tri-coat, two-tone paint, and other variables to accurately estimate painting costs. It will add costs for priming, tinting,

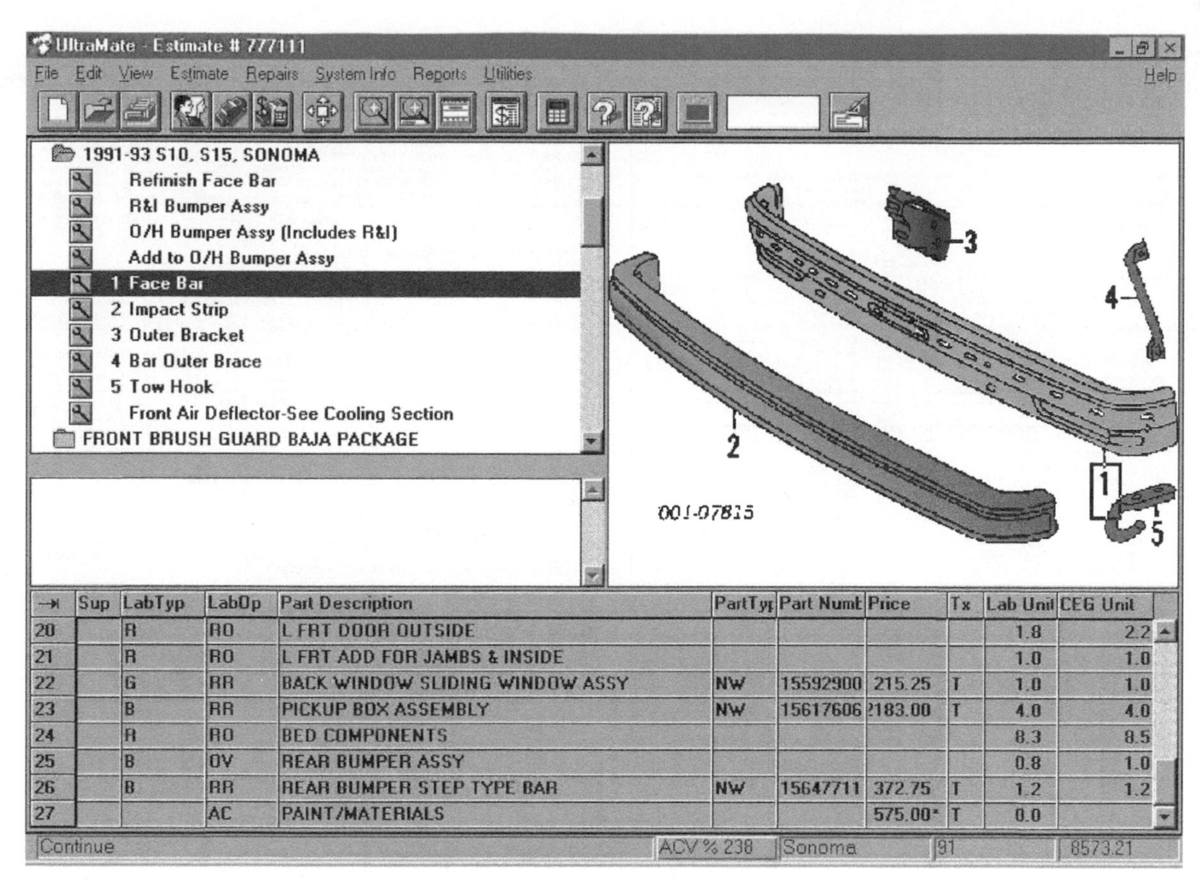

→	Sup	LabTyp	LabOp	Part Description	PartTyp	Part Numb	Price	Tx	Lab Unit	CEG Unit
20		R	RO	L FRT DOOR OUTSIDE					1.8	2.2
21		R	RO	L FRT ADD FOR JAMBS & INSIDE					1.0	1.0
22		G	RR	BACK WINDOW SLIDING WINDOW ASSY	NW	15592900	215.25	T	1.0	1.0
23		B	RR	PICKUP BOX ASSEMBLY	NW	15617606	2183.00	T	4.0	4.0
24		R	RO	BED COMPONENTS					8.3	8.5
25		B	OV	REAR BUMPER ASSY					0.8	1.0
26		B	RR	REAR BUMPER STEP TYPE BAR	NW	15647711	372.75	T	1.2	1.2
27			AC	PAINT/MATERIALS			575.00*	T	0.0	

Figure 28–16. Here is a computer display of an exploded view of a bumper assembly. The estimator can quickly see all the parts and select those that require replacement or repair. The lower section of the page also gives part costs and labor times for each part. (Courtesy of Mitchell International, Inc.)

blending, tape stripes, liquid mask, and other variables that will affect repair costs.

Mechanical repairs to the suspension, steering, or other parts can also be calculated. The estimating program will guide you through selecting parts and labor for correcting mechanical damage: wheel alignment, bleeding brakes, and similar tasks.

Most programs will also help you calculate frame/unibody repair time. You can select from a variety of straightening operations, which have general flat rate times.

Once all the information about the repair has been entered into the computer, the estimating program will automatically total all parts and labor, calculate taxes, and add other costs for a grand total.

The estimating program may also interface with other shop programs for payroll, maintenance, business reporting, document scanning, database storage, and shop management.

A **printer** can be used to make a hard copy (printed image on paper) for the customer, insurance adjusters, and shop personnel. You can quickly print vehicle dimension drawings, part views, or the estimate. Look at **Figure 28–17.**

FRONT CLIPS

In some situations, such as a severely damaged front end, an estimator might want to consider the purchase and installation of a recycled/salvaged front end assembly. In the body repair trade this is referred to as a **"front clip."** This assembly generally includes the front bumper and supports, grilles and baffles, radiator and its supporting members, the hood and its hinges (or hood torsion bars), the front fenders and skirts, all front lights, the wiring, and all other related parts. Often, this method of making collision repairs to the front end will decrease the total time the vehicle is in the shop.

TOTAL LOSS

A **total loss** occurs when the cost of the repairs would exceed the value of the vehicle. The insurance company or customer would normally

DAMAGE REPORT
02/17/98 at 11:34
JAMES
D.R. 34942-0003600
Est: R. GLEASON

RIVERDALE BODY SHOP
WHERE CUSTOMER SATISFACTION IS #1
7830 US 41
ST JOHN, IN 46373-
(219) 365-9600

Owner: DUFFY JAMES
Address: 123 W HILL
CROWN POINT IN 46307
Day Phone: (219) 555-1639-
Other Ph: ( ) - -
Deductible: $ 250.00

Insurance Co.:AMERICAN STATES INSURANCE Phone:
Claim No.:12651PD1.............2/98 Adj.:

90 GMC C15 4X2 WIDESIDE 2D SHORT BLACK 8-5.7L-FI
Vin: 1GTDC14K2LE535560 License: 52411S IN Prod Date: 2/90 Odometer: 64213

Automatic transmission	Power steering	Power brakes
Power windows	Power locks	Tinted glass
Body side moldings	Dual mirrors	Air conditioning
Tilt wheel	Cruise control	Fog lamps
Am radio	Fm radio	Stereo
Cassette	Cloth seats	Bucket seats
Recline/lounge seats	Aluminum wheels	Clear coat paint
Two tone paint	Rear step bumper	Sliding rear window

NO.	OP.	DESCRIPTION OF DAMAGE	QTY	PART COST	LABOR	PAINT	MISC
1		FRONT BUMPER					
2		O/H Front Bumper	1	0.00	1.6	0.0	
3**	Repl	A/M Fc br chrm w/o ar intk w/i	1	146.00	Incl	0.0	
4	Repl	Cntr fllr w/o grll vnt hls w/o	1	33.75	0.3	0.8	
5		Add for Clear Coat	1	0.00	0.0	0.2	
6	Repl	License bracket w/impact strip	1	19.66	0.3	0.0	
7							
8		FRONT LAMPS					
9*	Repl	LKQ RT Headlamp assy +20%	1	120.00	0.5	0.0	
10		Aim headlamps	1	0.00	0.5	0.0	
11							
12		HOOD					
13*	Repr	Hood	1	0.00	5.0	3.2	
14		Overlap Minor Panel	1	0.00	0.0	-0.2	
15		Add for Clear Coat	1	0.00	0.0	1.2	
16							
17		FENDER					
18**	Repl	A/M-CAPA RT Fender	1	87.00	2.8	2.6	
19		Overlap Major Adjacent Panel	1	0.00	0.0	-0.4	
20		Add for 2-Tone Refinish	1	0.00	0.0	0.9	
21		Add for Clear Coat	1	0.00	0.0	0.4	
22		Add for Edging	1	0.00	0.0	0.5	
23**	Repl	A/M RT Wheelhouse w/o 15000 GV	1	58.00	0.6	1.0	
24							
25		FRONT SUSPENSION					
26	Repl	RT Lower cntrl arm	1	291.00	1.4	0.0 M	
27							
28*		STRUCTURAL REPAIRS					
29*		FRAME SET UP ON RACK	1	0.00	1.0	0.0	
30*		PULL KNEE ASSY TO LENGTH	1	0.00	2.5	0.0 F	

DAMAGE REPORT
02/17/98 at 11:34
JAMES
D.R. 34942-0003600
Est: R. GLEASON

NO.	DESCRIPTION	QTY	PART COST	LABOR	PAINT	MISC
31	--					
32*	MISC. ITEMS					
33*	E-COAT PER PANEL	1	0.00	0.0	0.0	T 14.00
34*	TINT COLOR	1	0.00	0.0	0.5	
35*	BLEND ADJACENT PANELS	1	0.00	0.0	1.0	
36*	TAPE PIN STRIPES	1	0.00	0.0	0.0	X 30.00
37*	LIQUID MASK FOR OVERSPRAY	1	0.00	0.0	0.0	T 5.00
38*	HAZARDOUS WASTE DISPOSAL	1	0.00	0.0	0.0	X 2.50
	Towing Charges	1	0.00	0.0	0.0	X 50.00
	Subtotals ===>		755.41	16.5	11.7	101.50

NOTE HIDDEN DAMAGE: OPEN...RPG.

Parts		755.41
Body Labor	12.6 units @ $36.00	453.60
Paint Labor	11.7 units @ $36.00	421.20
Paint/Materials	11.7 units @ $18.00	210.60
Frame Labor	2.5 units @ $50.00	125.00
Mech. Labor	1.4 units @ $57.00	79.80
Sublet/Misc		101.50
SUBTOTAL		$ 2147.11
Tax on $ 985.01 at 5.0000%		49.25
GRAND TOTAL		$ 2196.36
ADJUSTMENTS: Deductible		-250.00
CUSTOMER PAYS		$ 250.00
INSURANCE PAYS		$ 1946.36

THIS ESTIMATE HAS BEEN PREPARED BASED ON THE USE OF ONE OR MORE REPLACEMENT PARTS SUPPLIED BY A SOURCE OTHER THAN THE MANUFACTURER OF YOUR MOTOR VEHICLE. WARRANTIES APPLICABLE TO THESE REPLACEMENT PARTS ARE PROVIDED BY THE MANUFACTURER OR DISTRIBUTOR OF THE REPLACEMENT PARTS RATHER THAN BY THE MANUFACTURER OF YOUR MOTOR VEHICLE.

Estimate based on MOTOR CRASH ESTIMATING GUIDE. Non-asterisk(*) items are derived from the Guide DR1GH88. Database Date 10/97
Double asterisk(**) items indicate part supplied by a supplier other than the original equipment manufacturer.
CAPA items have been certified for fit and finish by the Certified Auto Parts Association.
EZEst - A product of CCC Information Services Inc.

Figure 28–17. Once the computer estimate is done, it can be printed out on a laser printer. At least three copies should be generated. Read through this sample estimate.

NOT want the vehicle repaired in such a case. Instead, the insurance company will write a check to cover the cost of a replacement vehicle. An equivalent year, make, and model vehicle is then purchased by the customer.

The insurance company usually determines if a vehicle is a total loss. The company will evaluate the estimate and market prices for comparable vehicles when making this decision. Older vehicles are written up as a total loss more often than late model vehicles. This is because of their low replacement cost.

The totaled vehicle will usually be auctioned or sold to a salvage yard or recycler. The recycler will then disassemble the vehicle and sell its parts for a profit.

SUMMARY

- An estimate, also called a damage report or appraisal, calculates the cost of parts, materials, and labor for repairing a collision damaged vehicle.
- Direct damage occurs in the immediate area of the collision. Indirect damage is caused by the shock of collision forces traveling through the vehicle and by inertial forces acting on the rest of the unibody.
- Refer to literature such as dimension manuals and collision estimating guides to aid in the estimation process.
- Estimates may be manually written or electronically (computer) written. Computerized estimating uses a personal computer and printer.

TECHNICAL TERMS

damage analysis
direct damage
indirect damage
steering wheel center check
wheel run-out check
collision estimating and reference guides
R & I
R & R
overhaul
included operations

overlap
manually written estimate
electronic/computer-written estimate
firm bid
deductible clause
work order
flat rate
computerized estimating
PC
estimating system
estimating program
database
CD-ROMs
electronic or digital camera
digital images
printer
front clip
total loss

REVIEW QUESTIONS

1. How many copies of the written estimate should be made?
   a. One
   b. Two
   c. Three
   d. Four
2. An ______________, also called a ______________ ______________, or ______________, calculates the cost of parts, materials, and labor for fixing the collision damaged vehicle.
3. List six things you should do before starting damage analysis.
4. When inspecting damaged unibody vehicle, *Technician A* looks for damage only near the area of impact. *Technician B* looks for damage both in the area of impact and some distance away. Who is correct?
   a. Technician A
   b. Technician B
   c. Both Technicians A and B
   d. Neither A nor B
5. What is the smallest increment in which labor times are listed in crash estimating guides?
   a. Hours
   b. Half hours
   c. Quarter hours
   d. Tenths of an hour
6. Explain the difference between direct and indirect damage.
7. When you inspect the entire vehicle for damage, what 14 problems must you look for?
8. How do you analyze the center position of a steering wheel?
9. This check will find a bent wheel.
   a. Strut rotation check
   b. Strut position check
   c. Run-out check
   d. Overrun check
10. List five things included in collision estimating guides.
11. ______________ ______________ are those that can be performed individually but are also part of another operation.
12. ______________ occurs when replacement of one part duplicates some labor operation required to replace an adjacent part.
13. Give the statement or rule for determining whether to repair or replace a part.
14. A damage report or estimate includes these seven items.
15. The most common and modern way of storing an estimating database is the:
    a. CD-ROM
    b. Floppy disk
    c. Magnetic tape
    d. None of the above

ASE-STYLE REVIEW QUESTIONS

1. *Technician A* says that you should discuss the collision with the owner or driver of the vehicle to obtain information that may help during damage analysis. *Technician B* says that you should identify the vehicle completely, including VIN, year, make, model, engine, and optional equipment. Who is correct?
   a. Technician A
   b. Technician B
   c. Both Technicians A and B
   d. Neither Technician

2. *Technician A* says that when analyzing damage for an estimate, you may need to use unibody/frame measuring equipment. *Technician B* says that only a tape measure is needed during estimating. Who is correct?
   a. Technician A
   b. Technician B
   c. Both Technicians A and B
   d. Neither Technician

3. Estimating guides contain all of the following EXCEPT:
   a. Illustrated parts breakdowns
   b. Part names and numbers
   c. Labor times
   d. Paint mixing codes

4. Which of the following refers to tasks that can be performed individually but are also part of another operation?
   a. Included operations
   b. Estimated operations
   c. System operations
   d. Flat rate operations

5. *Technician A* says that if damage is located near the end of a rail, with the crush zone unaffected, replacement is always necessary. *Technician B* says that a kink in the crush zone can normally be repaired. Who is correct?
   a. Technician A
   b. Technician B
   c. Both Technicians A and B
   d. Neither Technician

6. *Technician A* says that new parts might require more time to install than good recycled parts. *Technician B* says that new parts usually cost more than recycled parts. Who is correct?
   a. Technician A
   b. Technician B
   c. Both Technicians A and B
   d. Neither Technician

7. If the labor time for a repair is 4.7 hours and the labor rate is $50 per hour, which of the following is the labor charge?
   a. $10
   b. $23.50
   c. $235
   d. $2,350

8. *Technician A* says that most estimating programs will NOT automatically deduct for overlap. *Technician B* says that estimating programs normally deduct for overlap. Who is correct?
   a. Technician A
   b. Technician B
   c. Both Technicians A and B
   d. Neither Technician

ACTIVITIES

1. Manually write an estimate for a vehicle with minor damage. Use manuals to find the cost of parts and labor. Calculate the total repair costs for the damage.
2. Visit a shop with a computerized estimating system. Ask the shop owner if you can observe the system in use.

CHAPTER

29 Entrepreneurship and Job Success

OBJECTIVES

After studying this chapter, you should be able to:

- Describe desirable traits of collision repair technicians.
- Summarize job responsibilities of industry personnel.
- Define the term "entrepreneur."
- Advance into other automotive-related professions.

INTRODUCTION

According to economic predictions, there will be a strong demand for collision repair technicians in the future.

Our nation is now, and always will be, a "nation on wheels." You have selected an excellent area of study—collision repair technology. With this knowledge base, you should be able to earn a good living for as long as there are vehicles on the road.

Job openings are common as people move up into other positions and retire. Always read newspapers to stay aware of job openings. Some may pay better or offer better **benefits** (insurance, vacation time, holiday pay, etc.) than your present job.

COLLISION REPAIR TECHNICIAN

A *collision repair technician* is a highly skilled professional capable of doing a wide variety of tasks. This person must have a working knowledge of mechanics, electronics, measurement, welding, cutting, straightening, painting, and so on.

Collision repair technicians earn good money and are in constant demand. After finishing your training and gaining practical experience, you should be proud of becoming a collision repair technician.

Specialized technicians concentrate their study in one area. Some shops have specialized paint technicians, sheet metal technicians, masking technicians, straightening technicians, and so on. This allows each person to be more efficient at their own skill area; more vehicles are repaired and greater profit is made.

RELATED PROFESSIONS

Related professions are jobs that require an understanding of auto body repair. See **Figure 29–1.** There are many related professions that you can advance into after gaining a working knowledge of collision repair. By understanding body repair and furthering your education, you may be able to get a job with:

1. Insurance company—adjuster, agent
2. Materials manufacturer—paint, filler, or other company

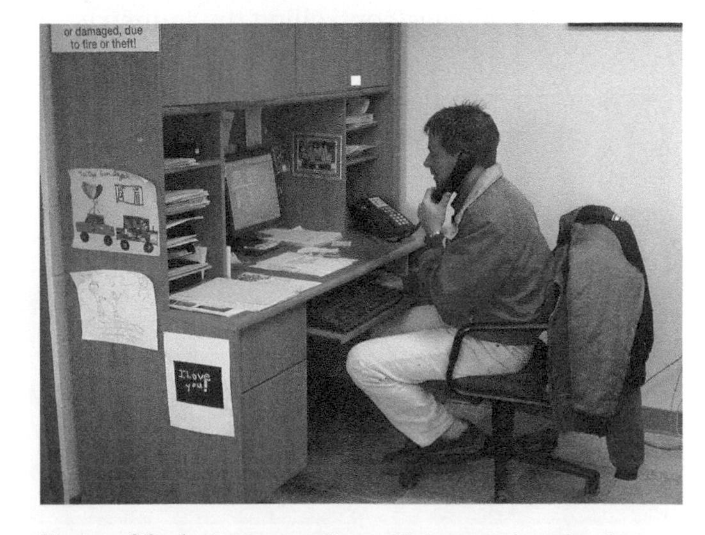

Figure 29–1. Understanding collision repair technology and terminology may help you get a job in a related profession, like this insurance adjuster position.

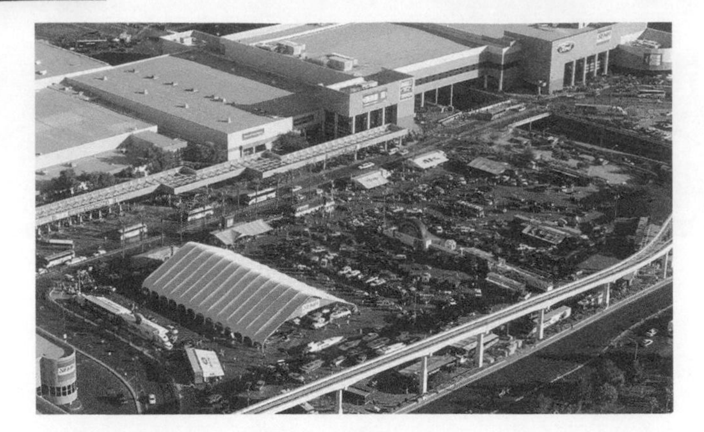

Figure 29–2. Proving yourself as a dependable collision repair technician will help you advance into other positions. This is an auto body equipment manufacturing show with numerous types of job offerings.

3. Parts suppliers—new, used, and remanufactured parts companies
4. Auto manufacturer—factory representative, designer, engineer (see **Figure 29–2**)
5. Instructor—teach collision repair classes

ENTREPRENEURSHIP

An **entrepreneur** is a person who starts his or her own business. See **Figure 29–3.** This business might be a repair shop, materials supply house, parts warehouse, or similar endeavor. You might want to consider being an entrepreneur someday.

If you start your own business, you would need to understand bookkeeping, payroll, and state and local laws controlling the industry.

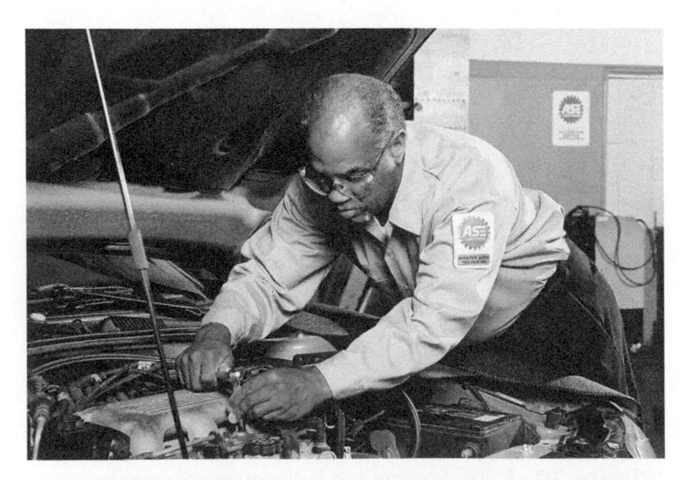

Figure 29–3. This certified technician worked hard and learned all aspects of running a business before starting his own collision repair shop. (Courtesy of ASE)

After mastering the knowledge needed to do collision repair work, you will become more marketable. Your skills as a collision repair technician can help when applying for other jobs or starting a business.

COOPERATIVE TRAINING PROGRAMS

Some schools offer **cooperative education programs** that allow you to have a job and get school credit at the same time. If such opportunities are available, you could be hired to work and train in a real collision repair shop. Some "co-op" programs pay a small wage while you learn.

During cooperative training, you might be a helper technician. You would work under and be further trained by an experienced professional. This is an excellent way of gaining practical, hands-on experience. And, remember, experience is the best teacher.

If you are still in school, check with your instructor and guidance counselor about cooperative education programs in your area.

KEEP LEARNING!

Try to learn something job related every day. Always learn from your mistakes. Read technical magazines and other publications. While working, try to think of more efficient ways of working. Consider new tools and techniques. This attitude will help you become more productive.

USE A SYSTEMATIC APPROACH

Develop a more **systematic approach** for doing your job. A systematic approach involves organizing and using a logical sequence of steps to accomplish a task or job. A systematic approach will result in your selecting more efficient ways of working.

Ask yourself these kinds of questions:

1. Did I take all needed tools to the vehicle?
2. Is there a better tool for a specific task?
3. Have I been reading the manufacturer's instructions (paints, body filler, equipment, and so on)?
4. Is my body in the right position to protect myself and feel comfortable?

WORK TRAITS

Work traits are those things, aside from skills, that make you a good or bad employee. Work traits often determine whether you keep a good job or get fired. The most important work traits are:

Reliability means being at work on time, being at work every day, and doing the job right. This is the most important job trait. Without it, you will have a difficult time keeping a job.

For example, if you often miss work, you will affect everyone in the shop. If the vehicle has been promised on Friday and you are not there, either someone else has to do your work, or the vehicle may not get done on time. Then the customer will be unhappy and will never return to your shop again. If this continues, the "word of mouth" will ruin the reputation of the shop and profits will decline.

Social skills are important so that other workers and customers like you. Many times you will need the help of another worker to complete a difficult, two-person task. If you are not liked by others, you will find many tasks almost impossible.

A good repair shop will have a "team of workers" who help each other succeed and prosper. They will exchange information, help each other with small tasks, and enjoy working together. You spend much of your life on the job; so why not enjoy it?

Productivity is a measure of how much work you get done. A highly productive technician will turn out a large amount of work. This will result in higher pay for the technician and more profits for the shop.

You want to balance productivity and quality. If you try to cut corners and get too much done too quickly, quality will often suffer. You must use proper work habits, common sense, and hard work to be productive.

Professionalism is a broad trait that includes everything from being able to follow orders to pride in workmanship. A professional does everything "by the book." He or she never cuts corners (for instance, leaving out the hard-to-reach bolt) trying to get the repair finished. Always think, dress, and act like a professional.

A professional:

1. Is customer oriented
2. Is up to date on vehicle developments
3. Keeps up with advancements in the repair industry
4. Pays attention to detail
5. Ensures that his or her work is up to specs
6. Participates in trade associations

SUMMARY

- A collision repair technician is a highly skilled professional capable of a wide variety of tasks. This person must have a working knowledge of mechanics, electronics, measurement, welding, cutting, straightening, painting, and so on.
- Specialized technicians concentrate their study in one area such as painting, sheet metal, or masking. This allows a person to be more efficient in a chosen skill; more vehicles are repaired and greater profit is made.
- An entrepreneur is a person who starts his or her own business. This business may be a collision repair shop, materials supply house, parts warehouse, or similar endeavor.

TECHNICAL TERMS

benefits
related professions
entrepreneur
cooperative education programs
systematic approach
work traits
reliability
social skills
productivity
professionalism

REVIEW QUESTIONS

1. According to economic predictions, there will be a strong demand for collision repair technicians in the future. True or false?
2. What are job benefits?
3. What are five areas of employment related to collision repair technology?
4. An ______________ is a person who starts his or her own business.
5. Some schools offer this type of program, which allows you to have a job and get school credit at the same time.
   a. Work release
   b. Work-Ed

c. Cooperative education
d. Continuing education

6. In your own words, describe the need for reliability, social skills, productivity, and professionalism when on the job.

ASE-STYLE REVIEW QUESTIONS

1. *Technician A* says that according to economic predictions, there will be a strong demand for collision repair technicians in the future. *Technician B* says that there will be no new job growth in the collision repair market. Who is correct?
   a. Technician A
   b. Technician B
   c. Both Technicians A and B
   d. Neither Technician

2. *Technician A* says that a collision repair technician needs little or no training and that the tasks could be done by anyone. *Technician B* says that a collision repair technician is a highly skilled professional capable of doing a wide variety of tasks. Who is correct?
   a. Technician A
   b. Technician B
   c. Both Technicians A and B
   d. Neither Technician

3. *Technician A* says that all collision technicians do all jobs in the shop. *Technician B* says that some technicians prefer to specialize and concentrate their studies in one area of collision repair. Who is correct?
   a. Technician A
   b. Technician B
   c. Both Technicians A and B
   d. Neither Technician

4. *Technician A* says that an entrepreneur is a person who specializes in frame repair. *Technician B* says that entrepreneurs are people who start their own businesses. Who is correct?
   a. Technician A
   b. Technician B
   c. Both Technicians A and B
   d. Neither Technician

5. *Technician A* says that learning new techniques is a lifelong process that requires continued training. *Technician B* says that when school is over the learning process stops. Who is correct?
   a. Technician A
   b. Technician B
   c. Both Technicians A and B
   d. Neither Technician

6. *Technician A* says that a collision worker who follows a systematic approach to repairs is more efficient. *Technician B* says that as long as all the work gets done no system is needed. Who is correct?
   a. Technician A
   b. Technician B
   c. Both Technicians A and B
   d. Neither Technician

7. Which of the following is NOT a work trait?
   a. Reliability
   b. Social skills
   c. Balance
   d. Productivity

8. *Technician A* says that "professionalism" is a broad trait that includes the ability to follow orders and pride in workmanship. *Technician B* says that "productivity" is a measure of how much work you get done. Who is correct?
   a. Technician A
   b. Technician B
   c. Both Technicians A and B
   d. Neither Technician

9. Which of the following is NOT part of being a professional?
   a. Being customer oriented
   b. Paying attention to detail
   c. Operating a computer
   d. Ensuring that work performed is up to specs

10. *Technician A* says cooperative training is two or more instructors cooperating with each other to provide instruction. *Technician B* says that cooperative education is a program in which a student has a job and gets school credit for it. Who is correct?

a. Technician A

b. Technician B

c. Both Technicians A and B

d. Neither Technician

ACTIVITIES

1. Visit a small collision repair–related business—parts house, parts supply store, repair shop, and so on. Ask the owner how he or she started the business. Write and give a class report.

2. Visit the library and obtain published materials on starting your own business. Create a wall display describing what it takes to start a business.

GLOSSARY

A

*__A-Pillars__—Either of the front pillars that support the windshield, the front of the roof, and the door hinges. Also called windshield pillar or A-post.

A/C High-Side—Section of the air conditioning system between the compressor and the orifice tube with smaller hoses and lines that carry high-pressure/high-temperature refrigerant, usually R-134a.

A/C Low Side—One side of the air-conditioning system. It contains low-pressure/low-temperature refrigerant.

Abrasive—Any material, such as sand, crushed steel grit, aluminum oxide, silicon carbide, or crushed slag, used for cleaning, sanding, smoothing, or material removal.

Abrasive Blasting—The process of using air pressure, a blasting gun, and an abrasive to remove old paint.

*__ABS__—Antilock brake system. A system that prevents wheel lock-up during braking.

AC Current—Alternating current voltage, the type of current that is found in your home wiring, inside an automotive alternator (generator), or a hybrid drive vehicle.

Accelerator—A fast evaporating thinner or reducer for speeding the drying time.

Accidents—Unplanned events that hurt people, break tools, damage vehicles, or have other adverse effects on the business and its employees.

Accumulators—Pressure storage tank between the evaporator and compressor that holds a desiccant bag to remove moisture from the air-conditioning system.

Acetylene Pressure—Pressure leaving acetylene pressure regulator of oxyacetylene welding outfit. Typically ranges from 1 to 12 psi (kPa).

Acid/Alkali Spotting—A discoloration of the paint surface caused by a chemical change of pigments from contact with acids or alkalies resulting from atmospheric contamination in the presence of moisture. This problem is found on older finishes that have been exposed to industrial pollution.

Acid Core Solder—Used for doing nonelectrical repairs, as on radiators.

Acid Rain Damage—Caustic, pitted paint damage caused by chemical etching from industrial fallout. *See* Minor Acid Rain Damage and Major Acid Rain Damage.

Acid Rain—Acidic materials released into the atmosphere from natural and industrial sources that cause paint surface damage.

Acorn Nuts—Nuts closed on one end for appearance and thread protection.

Actuators—Devices (solenoids or servo motors, for example) that move when responding to electrical signals from the vehicle's computer.

Active Gas—A type of shielding gas that combines with the weld to contribute to weld quality.

Active Restraint System—A restraint system that the occupants must make an effort to use, that is, fastening the seat belt.

Additives—Ingredients added to modify the performance and characteristics of the primer or paint product.

Adhesion Bonding—Uses oxyacetylene to melt a filler metal onto the workpiece for joining.

*__Adhesion Promoter__—A material applied to a surface, before the application of either adhesive or paint, to strengthen the bond.

*__Adhesives__—Any substance that is capable of bonding other substances together by surface attachment. In an auto glass replacement context, it is a high-strength polyurethane material unless otherwise specified.

Adhesive-Bonded Door Skin—A door skin that is bonded, not welded, to the door frame with structural adhesives.

Adhesive Bonded Parts—Metal or plastic parts that are held together by the use of a high-strength epoxy or special glue.

Adhesive Installation—Using an adhesive-sealer material to secure vehicle glass in place.

Adhesive Release Agent—A chemical that dissolves most types of adhesives, used to remove a glued or bonded part without damaging it.

Adhesive Remover—A chemical used to clean off the remaining vinyl glue after removal of a stripe or decal.

Adjustable Wrench—Also referred to as a crescent wrench, it has movable jaws to fit different head sizes.

Aftermarket Repair Manuals—Books published by publishing companies rather than the manufacturer. They are not as detailed but can give enough information needed for most repairs.

Air Bag—A strong nylon bag attached to the metal frame of the module. Vent holes in the bag allow for rapid

---

* Definitions of terms preceded by an asterisk (*) are supplied courtesy of 1-CAR.

deflation after deployment. When mounted on side of vehicle, long, elongated air bags can be called air curtains.

Air Bag Controller—This analyzes inputs from the sensor to determine if bag deployment is needed.

Air Bag Igniter—Produces a small spark that ignites propellant to deploy air bags and curtains when an electrical signal is sent from the control unit.

Air Bag Module—An assembly composed of the nylon bag and an igniter-inflator mechanism enclosed in a metal-plastic housing.

Air Bag System—Automatically deploys a large nylon bag(s) during a severe collision to help protect the driver and passengers from injury.

Air Blow Gun—Used to blow dust and dirt off a vehicle and its parts with a strong stream or blast of air.

Air Chisel—Similar to an air hammer, but it is smaller and is often equipped with a cold chisel type of cutter.

Air Compressor—Generates pressurized air for use by air tools and equipment.

Air-Conditioning Gauges—Used to measure operating pressures in a vehicle's air-conditioning system.

Air-Conditioning System—Used to cool and warm passenger compartment in different weather conditions.

Air Control Valve—It can be adjusted to control the volume of air flowing through air tools.

Air Couplings—These allow you to quickly install and remove air hoses and air tools.

Air Cutoff Tool—A tool that uses a small abrasive wheel to rapidly cut or grind metal.

Air Dams—A part that improves aerodynamics by restricting air passing under the vehicle body, thus reducing turbulence and resistance to airflow.

Air Drills—Uses shop air pressure to spin a drill bit.

Air Drying—Paint is allowed to dry in atmosphere.

Air File—A long, thin air sander for working large flat surfaces on panels.

Air Filter Drain Valve—Allows you to remove trapped water and oil from the filter.

Air Hammer—Uses back-and-forth hammer blows to drive a cutter or driver into the workpiece.

Air Hose Leak Test—A method used to find body leaks. Place a soapy water solution on possible leakage points and use low-pressure air on the inside of the vehicle. Bubbles will form wherever there is a leak.

Air Hoses—Reinforced, flexible rubber hoses that connect metal shop air lines to air tools and equipment. Connect the metal pipes to the air tools and equipment.

Air Hose Sizes—Given as inside diameters of passage through hose.

Air Leak Tape Test—Involves covering potential leaks with masking tape and driving the vehicle to test for air or wind noise. If covering an area stops the noise problem, you have found the air leak.

Air Leaks—Often result from improperly adjusted doors, window glass, or damaged weatherstripping.

Air Line Filter-Drier—Used in the air line to remove moisture and debris from the air flowing through the air lines. It is designed to trap and hold water and oil that passes out of the compressor air pump.

Air Nibbler—A tool used like tin snips to cut sheet metal. It has an air-powered snipping blade that moves up and down.

Air Polisher—Used to smooth and shine painted surfaces by spinning a soft buffing pad.

Air Pressure Regulator—Used to precisely control the amount of pressure fed to air tools and equipment.

Air Ratchet—A wrench, like the hand wrench, it has a special ability to work in hard-to-reach places.

Air Replacement System—Exhausts the air from spray booths continuously during the spraying process.

Air Sander—Uses an abrasive action to smooth and shape body surfaces and is one of the most commonly used air tools.

Air Saw—Air tool that uses a reciprocating (back-and-forth) action to move a hacksaw-type blade to quickly cut parts.

Air Spring Suspension—Uses air springs to support the vehicle load, replacing or supplementing the conventional spring suspension.

Air-Supplied Respirator—A half-mask, full face piece, hood, or helmet, to which clean, breathable air is supplied through a hose from a separate air source. It provides protection from isocyanate paint vapors and mists, as well as from hazardous solvent vapors.

Air Supply System—Provides clean, dry air pressure for numerous tools and equipment. It has an air compressor, metal lines, rubber hoses, quick disconnect fittings, a pressure regulator, filters, and other parts.

Air Tool Lubrication—A few drops of special air tool oil, lightweight motor oil, or a mixture of oil and automatic transmission fluid should be used on all air tools.

Air Tools—Tools that use air pressure for operation: including spray guns, impact guns, adhesive dispensers, and other tools in collision repair. They run cool and are very dependable.

Air Vent Hole—It allows atmospheric pressure to enter the cup of the spray gun.

Airless Plastic Welding—Uses an electric heating element to melt a 1/8 inch (3 mm) diameter rod with no external air supply. Airless welding with a smaller rod helps eliminate two troublesome problems: panel warpage and excess rod buildup.

Aligning Punch—A long and tapered tool used to align body panels and other parts.

Alignment Rack—Used to measure and adjust the steering and suspension of a vehicle after repairs. Also known as front end rack.

***Alkali**—Any caustic compound having a pH greater than 7.

Allen Wrench—A hex, hexagon, or six-sided wrench. It will install or remove set screws.

Allergens—Substances found in adhesives, hardeners, and nature that cause allergic reactions and physical illness.

All-Wheel Drive—A vehicle that uses two drive axle assemblies to power all four drive wheels.

***Ambient Temperature**—The temperature of the air in the work area.

***American Welding Society (AWS)**—An organization that sets standards for all types of welding.

Analog Multimeter (AVOM)—A multimeter with a pointer needle that moves across the face of a scale when making electrical measurements.
Anchor Chains—Attached from the floor anchors to the clamps attached to vehicle to hold the vehicle securely while straightening.
Anchor Clamps—A device bolted to specific points on the vehicle to allow the attachment of anchor chains. They distribute pulling force to prevent metal tearing.
Anchor Pots—Small steel cups imbedded in shop floor for anchoring vehicle when pulling out major damage.
Anchor Rails—Steel beams in floor for holding vehicle secure while straightening.
Anchoring Equipment—It holds the vehicle stationary while pulling and measuring.
Angle Measurements—Divide a circle into 360 or more parts called degrees.
Annealed—Metal that has been reheated and then cooled in a controlled manner to strengthen the metal and prevent it from becoming brittle.
Antichip Coating—A rubberized material used along a vehicle's lower panels; also called gravel guard, chip guard, and vinyl coating.
Anticorrosion Compounds—Wax- or petroleum-based coatings resistant to chipping and abrasion. Usually applied inside closed sections of structural members.
Anticorrosion Materials—A material used to prevent rusting and corrosion of metal parts. *See also* Undercoating.
Antifreeze—A liquid used to prevent freeze-up in cold weather and to lubricate moving parts. It also prevents engine overheating.
Antifreeze Tester—A hydrometer for measuring the strength of the cooling system solution (water-to-antifreeze concentration) and gives freezing temperature of antifreeze solution.
Anti-Lacerative Glass—Glass with one or more additional layers of plastic affixed to the inside of the glass. It gives added protection against shattering and cuts during impact.
Antispatter Compound—Spray that helps keep spatter from sticking to the nozzle during MIG welding.
Application Stroke—A side-to-side movement of the spray gun to distribute the paint mist properly on the vehicle.
Appraiser—Reviews the estimates and determines which one best reflects how, or if, the vehicle should be repaired or totaled.
Apprentice—Also known as a helper, learns new skills while assisting experienced personnel.
***Argon**—An inert gas used for shielding during welding.
Arm Sets—A resistance spot welding part that holds welding tips and conducts current to tips.
Arming Sensor—A sensor that ensures that the particular collision is severe enough to require that the air bag be deployed.
Asbestos Dust—Cancer causing particles once used in manufacture of older brake shoes/pads and clutch friction discs.
ASE Certification—A testing program to help prove that you are a knowledgeable collision repair or refinishing technician.
ASE Tests—Multiple-choice questions pertaining to the service and repair of a vehicle.
Asphyxiation—Refers to anything that prevents normal breathing.
Assembly—Several parts that fit together to make up a more complex unit.
Assembly Line Diagnostic Link (ALDL)—A connector provided for reading fault or trouble codes. It can be located in the passenger or engine compartment.
Asymmetrical—When the dimensions on the right side of the vehicle are NOT equal to those at the left.
Atomize—This term means to break the liquid into very tiny droplets or a fine mist.
Automatic Drain Valve—It periodically opens a solenoid-operated valve on the bottom of the air compressor to remove moisture from the storage tank.
Automatic Transmission—Transmission that shifts gear automatically using internal oil pressure and electronic control.
Automotive Recycler—"Salvage yard" that disassembles old or damaged vehicles to resell its parts collision and mechanical repair shops.
AWS—*See* American Welding Society.

B

***B-Pillars**—Either of the side pillars, near the middle of the vehicle, that support the roof. Also called B-posts.
Backing Patch—A patch bonded to the rear of repair area to restore the reinforced plastic's strength. The patch also forms a foundation for forming the exterior surface to match the original contour of the panel. The first part of a two-sided repair needed on damage that passes all the way through a panel.
Backing Strip—Also referred to as an insert, it is made of the same metal as the base metal and can be placed behind the weld. It helps proper fit-up and supports the weld.
***Backlite**—The glass installed in the rear window of a vehicle.
***Ball Joints**—A mechanical joint in which a ball moves freely within a socket. Used primarily to connect steering knuckles to the control arms. Also used to connect tie rods to the steering arms.
Ball Peen Hammer—A flat face hammer for general striking and a round peen end for shaping sheet metal, rivet heads, or other objects.
Banding Coat—The depositing of enough paint on edges or corners of surfaces.
Bare Metal Sanding—Sanding done to smooth rough metal surfaces.
Bare Metal Treatment—A process that prepares the metal for primer.
Base Gauges—First two body gauges hung near the center of the vehicle, usually at torque box area when measuring major damage.
Base Material—The material to be welded, usually metal or plastic.
Basecoat Patch—A small area on the vehicle's surface without clearcoat that enables the painter to check for color match with tri-coat colors.

Basecoat-Clearcoat—A vehicle refinishing system using sprayed-on colorcoats and transparent clearcoats of paint over primer materials, the most common paint system used today.

Battery—Stores electrical energy chemically. It provides current for the starting system and any hybrid drive system. It also provides current to all other electrical systems when the engine is not running.

Battery Charger—Converts 120 volts AC into 13 to 15 volts DC for recharging drained batteries.

Bay—A work area for one vehicle. Also termed a repair stall.

***Bead Height**—The height of a weld bead above the surrounding base metal.

***Bead Width**—The width of the weld bead, measured at its base.

Beam Splitters—Also referred to as laser guides, they are capable of reflecting the laser beam to additional targets.

Belt Retractor—Used to remove slack from the safety or seat belts so they fit snugly.

Bench Computer—A computer used to assist you in the straightening-measuring process.

Bench Grinder—A stationary, electric grinder mounted on a work bench or pedestal stand. It is used to sharpen chisels, punches, and to shape other tool tips.

Bench-Rack System—A frame-unibody straightening machine that allows quick loading like a rack but has the other features of a bench.

Bench Seat—A longer seat for several people.

Bench System—Generally a portable or stationary steel table for straightening severe vehicle damage.

Benefits—An employment term referring to insurance, vacation time, holiday pay, etc.

Bent—A term that describes a part where the change in the shape of the part between the damaged and undamaged areas is smooth and continuous, or straightening the part by pulling restores its shape to preaccident condition without areas of permanent deformation.

***Bevel**—The edge of a surface that has been tapered to remove a 90-degree angle. Also called a V-groove.

***Bezel**—A metal or plastic part, used as trim around lamps, knobs, or accessories.

Binder—Ingredient in a paint color that holds the pigment particles together.

Blasters—Air-powered tools for forcing sand, plastic beads, or another material onto surfaces for paint removal.

Bleed-Through—*See* Bleeding.

Bleeding—A problem in which colors in the primecoat or old paint chemically seep into the new paint, which can discolor new paint. Also called bleed-through.

Blistering—Small, swelled areas on finish, like a "water blister" on human skin, usually caused by rust under the surface, by spraying over oil or grease, by moisture in spray lines, trapped solvents, and prolonged or repeated exposure of the surface to high humidity.

Block—Foundation of the engine; all other engine parts are either housed in or attached to block.

Block Sanding—A simple back and forth scrubbing action with the sandpaper mounted on a rubber blocking tool.

Blown Fuse—A fuse that has been burned through by excess current. It will have infinite resistance.

Blushing—A problem that makes finish turn "milky," caused by fast solvents/reducers in high humidity or condensation on the vehicle surface while painting.

Body Center Marks—Locations stamped into the sheet metal in the unibody areas of a vehicle. They can save time when taking measurements to determine the extent and direction of major impact damage.

Body Clips—Specially shaped retainers for holding trim and other body pieces requiring little strength. The clip often fits into the back of the trim piece and through the body panel.

Body Files—Files that have very large, open teeth for cutting body filler. They often have a separate blade that fits into a handle.

***Body Filler**—Compounds used to build up and level low areas that cannot be brought back to their original contour by straightening.

Body Hammers—Designed to work with sheet metal. They often have a point or pick on one end and a flat, serrated, or rounded hammer head on the other.

Body ID Number—Gives information about how the vehicle is equipped, including paint codes or numbers for ordering the right type and color paint and trim. This number will be on the body ID plate. Also called service part number.

Body Jack—Also known as porta-powers, they can be used with frame/panel straighteners or by themselves. It produces a powerful pushing action.

Body Nuts—Special types of nuts used to hold specific parts onto the vehicle. Sometimes a washer is formed onto the nut. The flange on the nut helps distribute the clamping force of thin body panel or trim piece to prevent warping.

Body-Over-Frame (BOF)—This type of vehicle construction has separate body and chassis parts bolted to the frame.

***Body Repair Manual**—A model-specific repair manual published by the vehicle manufacturer.

Body Scanner—Part of a laser electronic measuring system, has two spinning lasers that strike and reflect off each target.

Body Shop Tools—Specialized tools designed for working with body parts.

Body Spoons—May be used like a hammer or as a dolly. Flat surfaces of a spoon distribute striking force over a wide area to prevent hammer dents.

Body Washers—Washers that have a very large outside diameter for the size hole in them. They provide better holding power on thin metal and plastic parts. Also called fender washers.

Bolt—A fastener with a shaft with a head on one end and threads on the other.

Bolt Diameter—Sometimes termed bolt size, it is measured around the outside of the threads.

Bolt Grade Markings—Lines or numbers on the top of the head to identify bolt hardness and strength.

Bolt Head—The part of a bolt that is used to torque or tighten the bolt.

Bolt Head Size—It is the distance measured across the flats of the bolt head.

Bolt Length—Measures the length of the bolt from the end of the threads to the bottom of the bolt head.
Bolt Size—*See* Bolt Diameter.
Bolt Strength—Indicates the amount of torque or tightening force that should be applied.
Bolt Strength Markings—These markings indicate bolt hardness and strength and are given as lines on the bolt head. The number of lines on the bolt head is related to its strength: as line number increases, so does strength.
Bolt Thread Pitch—A measurement of thread coarseness.
Bolt Torque—A measurement of the turning force applied when installing a fastener.
Bookkeeper—A person who performs the accounting duties, that is, invoices, checks, bills, banking, taxes.
Boots—They protect the rack in the rack-and-pinion steering unit from contamination by dirt, salt, and other road particles.
Box-End Wrench—A wrench with closed ends that surround the bolt or nut head.
Brake Lines—Carry fluid to wheel cylinders.
Brake Pads/Shoes—Use a friction lining pad or shoe for rubbing on the brake rotor or drum.
Brake Rotors/Drums—Provide round disc or drum friction surface lining or pads or shoes. They are bolted to each spindle of suspension system.
Brake System—It uses hydraulic pressure to slow or stop wheel rotation with brake pedal application.
Brake System Bleeding—A process that removes air from the brake fluid.
Brass Hammer—Also known as a lead hammer, it will make heavy blows without marring metal surfaces. The soft metal head will deform easily and protect the part from damage.
Brass Washers—Soft metal washers used to prevent fluid leakage, as on brake line fittings.
Brazing—Like soldering, but employs relatively low temperatures, around 800°F (427°C).
Breaker Bar—Also called a flex handle, it provides the most powerful way of turning bolts and nuts.
Bucket Seat—A single seat for one person.
Bump Cap—Protective head gear worn when working beneath the hood or under the vehicle.
Bumper Assembly—Bolts to the front or rear frame horns or rails to absorb minor impacts.
***Bumper Cover**—A flexible plastic cover that surrounds a bumper structure. Sometimes part of a fascia.
Bumper Shock Absorbers—A part used to absorb some of the impact of a collision and reduce damage.
Bumpers—A part designed to withstand minor impact without damage.
Bumping Hammers—Hammers used to bump out large dents.
Burnback—In MIG welding this occurs when the electrode wire melting rate is faster than the wire speed.
Burn Mark—A mark on the back of a weld that indicates a good weld penetration.
***Burn-Through**—A hole caused by excessive heat buildup which melts the base metal, allowing it to fall out of the weld joint.
Butt Welds—MIG welds formed by fitting two edges of adjacent panels together and welding along mating edges.

C

C-Clamp—A screw attached to a curved frame. It will hold objects on a work surface or drill press while working.
***C-Pillars**—Either of two pillars that support the rear door latch and the roof. Also called C-posts.
Cabinet Blaster—A stationary enclosure equipped with a sand or bead blast tool.
Cable Hood Release—A hood latch mechanism opened by means of a cable running into the passenger compartment.
Caliper—Holds the piston(s) and brake pads on disc brakes.
***Camber**—The inward or outward tilt of a tire at the top, measured in degrees from true vertical, when viewed from the front or rear of the vehicle. An outward tilt, away from the vehicle centerline, is positive camber, and an inward tilt is negative camber.
Camshaft—Controls valve operation. It can be located in the block or cylinder
***Canister Purge Valve**—A valve in an emission control system that allows hydrocarbons to flow from the charcoal canister to the engine intake manifold.
Cap—Protective head gear to keep hair safe and clean when sanding, grinding, and doing similar jobs.
Cap Screw—A term that describes a high-strength bolt.
Capillary Attraction—In brazing, it is the natural flow of the filler material into the joint.
Captive Spray Gun System—Individual guns that are set up and used for applying each different type of material.
Carbon Monoxide (CO)—An odorless, invisible gas that comes from vehicle exhaust.
Carburizing Flame—Also called a reducing flame, it is obtained by mixing slightly more acetylene than oxygen.
Carcinogens—Substances that can cause cancer.
Card Masking—Involves using a simple masking pattern to produce a custom paint effect.
Cartridge Filter Respirators—A rubber face piece that conforms to the face and forms an airtight seal. Used to protect against vapors and spray mists of nonactivated enamels, lacquers, and other nonisocyanate materials.
Cartridge Guns—Devices used to apply adhesive or sealer to body panels.
***Caster**—The angle of the steering axis, measured in degrees from true vertical, when viewed from the side of the vehicle. Caster is positive if the steering axis is tilted rearward, and negative if it is tilted forward.
Catalyst—An additive that causes a chemical reaction to cure paint, body filler, adhesives, etc.
***Catalytic Converter**—An emission control device in the exhaust system which uses a platinum-iridium catalyst to convert carbon monoxide gas and hydrocarbon particles to carbon dioxide gas and water.
Catalyzing—To add an ingredient to speed a chemical reaction in a collision repair product.
CD-ROMS—Compact discs that store information.
Center Link—It supports the tie-rods in position in parallelogram steering.
Center Orifice—Located at the spray gun fluid nozzle, it creates a vacuum for discharge of the paint, primer, clear, etc.

Center Pillars—Roof supports between the front and rear doors on four-door vehicles. Also called B-pillars.
Center Plane—An imaginary line that divides the vehicle into two equal halves: the passenger side and the driver side. Also called centerline.
Center Punch—A pointed tool used to start a drilled hole or mark parts. The indentation will keep a drill bit from wandering out of place.
Center Section—Also called midsection, it typically includes the body parts that form the passenger compartment.
Centerline—*See* Center Plane.
Certified Crash Tests—A test performed using a real vehicle and sensor-equipped dummies that show how much impact the people would suffer during a collision.
***cfh**—Cubic feet per hour. A unit for the flow rate of a gas.
Chain Wrench—A wrench used to grasp and turn round objects. It is used to remove stuck or damaged engine oil filters or to adjust exhaust systems.
***Channel**—A piece of U-shaped metal that is attached along the bottom edge of movable glass and connects the glass to the regulator.
Channellock® Pliers—Pliers that have several settings for grasping different size objects; also known as rib joint pliers.
Charging—A term used to describe filling the air-conditioning system with refrigerant.
Charging Station—A machine for automatically recharging an air-conditioning system with refrigerant.
Charging System—It recharges the battery and supplies electrical energy when the engine is running.
Charging System Voltage—Typically 13 to 15 volts.
Chassis—Mechanical systems that support and power the car. Include everything under the body—engine, transmission, suspension system, brake system, wheels and tires, steering system.
Chemical Burns—When a corrosive chemical such as paint remover injures your skin or eyes.
Chemical Stripping—Uses a chemical action to dissolve and remove paint down to bare metal.
Child Restraint Seat—A small removable appliance available from most automobile dealers or through various retail outlets. These restraint seats are available in either rearward-facing or forward-facing models, and in some cases may be used in either way. The seat should be tightly secured with the vehicle's shoulder or lap belt and held secure with a special locking clip supplied by the seat manufacturer.
Chisel—A tool used for some cutting operations such as shearing off rivet heads or separating sheet metal parts.
Chroma—Dimension of color that refers to the color's level of intensity, or the amount of gray (black and white) in a color. It is also called saturation, richness, intensity, or muddiness.
Chuck—Movable jaws that close down and hold the drill bit.
Circuit Breakers—Protect circuits by heating up and opening contact points when exposed to excess current draw.
Circular Sander—It spins its pad and sandpaper around and around in a circular motion.
Classroom—Venue for lectures, demonstrations, and meetings of school or shop personnel.
Clearance—Distance measured between two adjacent parts. Also called gap.
***Clips**—Devices which hold decorative chrome to the vehicle body, or hold moldings, etc.
Clock Spring—The electrical connection between the steering column and the air bag module.
Closed—A term that refers to an electrically connected electrical circuit.
Closed Coat Sandpaper—A type of grit on sandpaper and discs, the resin completely covers the grit. This bonds the grit to the paper or disc more securely.
***Closure Panel**—A movable, exterior body panel, such as a hood, door, deck lid, etc.
Cloth Polishing Pad—These are very tough pads and will cut paint smoothly and quickly. They are often used when heavy polishing is needed.
Clutch—A device used to couple and uncouple engine power to a manual transmission or transaxle.
***CO_2**—The chemical symbol for carbon dioxide. A gas used for shielding during welding.
Coarse File—In general, these work well to remove burrs and sharp edges on soft materials, such as brass, aluminum, and plastics.
Coarse Grit—A grit of 36 to 60, used for rough sanding and smoothing operations. This coarseness might be used to get the general shape of a large body filler area.
Coated Abrasives—*See* Sandpaper.
***Cold Solder Joint**—A solder joint that appears sound but is electrically defective.
Cold Weather Solvent—Designed to speed solvent evaporation, so the paint flows and dries in a reasonable amount of time.
Collapsible Steering Columns—They crush under force to absorb impact, thus reducing injuries.
Collision—An impact that causes damage to a vehicle body or chassis.
Collision Damage Manuals—Contain vehicle identification information, the price of new parts, time needed to install the parts, refinishing or painting data, and other information.
Collision Estimating and Reference Guides—Electronic or printed manuals containing illustrated part breakdown, part names and numbers, labor times, refinish times, part prices, and other miscellaneous information that help in filling out the estimate.
Collision Estimating Manuals—Guides or computer software programs that give information to help calculate the cost of repairs.
Collision Repair—Auto body repair, restoring a damaged vehicle back to its original condition, structurally and cosmetically.
Collision Repair Technician—A highly skilled professional who repairs damage from an accident.
Color—Caused by how objects reflect light at different frequencies into our eyes. The color seen depends on the kind and amount of light waves the surface reflects.
Color Blindness—A physical condition that makes it difficult for a person's eyes to see colors accurately.
Color Coded—Plastic welding rods are identified by color.
Color Corrected Lights—Used in the spray booth to make color show up properly.

Color Directory—A publication containing color chips and other paint-related information for most makes and models of vehicles.
Color Matching—The steps needed to make the new finish match the existing finish on the vehicle.
Color Matching Manuals—Guides that contain information needed for finishing panels, so that the repair has the same appearance as the old finish.
Color Spectrum—By passing light through a prism, light is broken down into its separate colors. White light contains all colors or the full spectrum.
Color Tree—A guide used to locate colors three dimensionally when matching colors.
Colorcoat—Layers of colored paint applied over primer or sealer followed by spray coats of clear paint.
Combination Pliers—Also known as slip-joint pliers, they will adjust to multiple sizes.
Combination Wrench—A wrench with an open end and a box end.
Combustibles—Substances capable of igniting and burning, such as paints, thinners, reducers, gasoline, dirty rags.
Combustion Chamber—A small enclosed area between the top of the piston and bottom of the cylinder head.
Compact Car—The smallest body classification, also known as economy car. It normally uses a small 4-cylinder engine, is very lightweight, and gets the highest gas mileage.
Complete Collision Services—May include wheel alignments, cooling system repairs, electrical system diagnosis and repair, suspension system work, and other collision and mechanical repairs.
Component—A part, refers to the smallest units on a vehicle.
Composites—Refers to a wide range of materials synthetically compounded from crude oil, coal, natural gas, glass strands, plastics, and other substances. *See also* Plastics.
Composite Force—The force of all pulls combined.
Composite Plastics—Also called "hybrids," they are blends of different plastics and other ingredients designed to achieve specific performance characteristics.
Composite Unibody—A unibody made of plastics and other materials, like carbon fiber, to form the vehicle structure.
***Compound Shape**—A structural shape where the opposite sides are not parallel over its length, or a surface that curves in two or more directions over its area.
Compounding—Also known as buffing, an air or electric buffing machine equipped with a pad is used to apply buffing compound to finish. The abrasive action cuts off a thin layer of topcoat to brighten color and shine paint.
Compressive Strength—Property of a material to resist being crushed.
Compressor Drain Valve—Located on the bottom of the compressor storage tank, it allows you to drain out water.
Compressor Oil Plugs—Provided for filling and changing air pump oil on a compressor.
Compressor Pressure Valve—It prevents too much pressure from entering the compressor tank.
Computer—A complex electronic circuit that produces a known electrical output after analyzing electrical inputs.
Computer Estimating—Preparing an estimate via computer. This streamlines the process by automating the written estimate.
Computer Self-Diagnostics—The computer can detect its own problems.
Computer System—Used to control/monitor fuel, ignition, charging, suspension and brake, climate control, and other systems in the vehicle.
Computerized Color Matching Systems—Software that uses data from the spectrophotometer to help in how to match the paint color.
Computerized Estimating—Uses a PC (personal computer) to provide more accurate cost of repairs.
Computerized Measuring Systems—A system that uses data from the measuring system for fast entry and checking of vehicle dimensions.
Computerized Mixing Scale—An electronic scale programmed to automatically indicate how much of each paint ingredient to use by weight.
Computerized Robotic Arm Measuring System—Uses a track-mounted robot arm to measure reference points on the damaged vehicle.
Computerized Service Information—Places service manuals, dimension manuals, estimating manuals, and other data on compact discs, allowing a personal computer to be used to more quickly to look up and print the desired information.
Conductor—It carries current to the parts of a circuit.
Cone Concept—Unibody vehicles are designed to absorb a collision impact. When hit, the body folds and collapses as it absorbs the impact. As the force penetrates the structure, it is absorbed by an ever increasing area of unibody. This characteristic spreads force until it is completely dissipated. Visualize the point of impact as the tip of the cone.
Connecting Rod—A link that attaches the piston to the crankshaft inside internal combustion engine.
Continuity—A continuous conductor path.
Continuous Weld—A single weld bead along a joint.
***Control Arms**—A suspension part, usually pivoted at each end, that keeps a wheel or axle in the proper position.
***Control Points**—Any of several identifiable points that are very accurately located during a vehicle's original assembly.
Conversion Charts—Show numbers or factors for changing from one measuring system to another or from one value to another mathematically.
***Conversion Coating**—The part of a treatment system that modifies the metal surface to improve rust protection and paint adhesion.
Convertible—Uses a retractable canvas roof with a steel tube framework. The top folds down into an area behind the seat. Some convertibles use a removable hardtop.
***Coolant**—A mixture of glycol and water, circulated through a cooling system to move heat from the engine to the radiator.
Cooling System—Maintains the correct engine operating temperature.

Cooling System Leak Test—Performed by installing a pressure tester on the radiator neck. Pump the tester handle until its gauge equals the cap pressure rating. A loss of pressure or coolant means there is a leak in the system.

Cooperative Education Programs—A curriculum offered by a school that allows you to have a job and get school credits at the same time.

Copper Washers—Washers used to prevent fluid leakage, as on brake line fittings.

***Corona**—The visible glow of the base metal at the weld site caused by the concentration of heat during GMA (MIG) welding.

***Corrosion**—The chemical reaction of air, moisture, or corrosive materials on a metal surface. Also called rust or oxidation.

Corrosion Converters—Anticorrosion materials that change ferrous (red) iron oxide to ferric (black/blue) iron oxide. Rust converters may also contain some type of latex emulsion that seals the surface after conversion is complete. These products offer an interesting alternative for areas that cannot be completely cleaned.

Corrosion Protection—Various methods used to protect body parts from rusting.

Corrosives—Acidic or alkaline substances that, when in contact with unprotected areas of the body, will cause injury.

Cosmetic Filler—Typically a two-part epoxy or polyester filler used to cover up minor imperfections on reinforced plastics.

***Cosmetic Surface**—A surface that is finished or decorated to improve its appearance. Includes paint, glass, upholstery, etc.

Cotter Pins—Pins that help prevent bolts and nuts from loosening; they fit through pins to hold parts together. They are also used as stops and holders on shafts and rods.

Cotton Polishing Pad—These are very tough pads and will cut paint smoothly and quickly. They are often used when heavy polishing is needed.

Covers—Protect the vehicle from damage.

Cowl—The body parts at the rear of the front section, right in front of the windshield.

Crankshaft—Changes the reciprocating (up and down) motion of the piston and rod into a more useful rotary (spinning) motion.

Crash Estimating Books—Contain vehicle identification information, the price of new parts, the time needed to install parts, refinishing or painting data, and other information.

Cream Hardeners—Used to cure body fillers.

Creeper—Allows you to lie and move around on the shop floor while working without getting dirty.

Crescent Wrench—Also referred to as an adjustable wrench, it has movable jaws to fit different head sizes.

CRI—Color Rendering Index, it is the index for measuring how close a lamp in indoor lighting is to actual daylight.

***Critical Temperature**—The maximum temperature allowed by a vehicle maker to prevent loss of strength in metal, when heating to relieve stress.

Crossflow Spray Booth—Moves air sideways over the car or truck. An air inlet in one wall pushes fresh air into the booth. A vent on the opposite wall removes the contaminated booth air.

***Crossmembers**—Any of the transverse structural or stiffening members of a vehicle frame or underbody structure.

Crush Zones—Areas of the frame or vehicle body engineered to collapse and absorb some of the energy of a collision.

Curb Height—Also called ride height, each of the front and rear wheels must carry the same amount of weight, thus allowing the vehicle to ride at a specific height.

***Cure**—The process of drying or hardening of a material.

***Cure Time**—The time required for a chemical or material to dry or set at a given temperature and humidity. Cure time varies with the type of material used and the thickness of the application.

Current—The movement of electricity (electrons) through a wire or circuit.

Custom Body Panels—Aftermarket parts that alter the appearance of the vehicle.

Custom Masks—Involves drawing a design on thin posterboard, then cutting it out, taping it onto the vehicle, and spray painting it for a custom pattern in the paint.

Custom-Mixed Colors—Paint colors that are mixed to order at the paint supply distributor.

Custom Painting—Using multiple colors, metal flake paints, multilayer masking, and special spraying techniques to produce a personalized look.

***Cutting Torch**—A common term for an oxyacetylene torch with a special tip used to cut metal. Can also be a plasma arc cutter.

CV-Axles—Constant velocity axles; they transfer torque from the transaxle to the wheel hubs.

***CV-Joint**—Constant velocity joint. A type of universal joint that allows the output shaft to rotate at the same instantaneous speed as the input shaft. Used in half shaft assemblies for driving wheels that are sprung independently of the differential.

Cyanoacrylates (CAs)—One-part, fast-curing adhesives used to help repair rigid and flexible plastics.

Cylinder—A round hole bored (machined) in the engine block that guides piston movement.

Cylinder Head—Covers and seals top of the engine cylinder. It contains valves, rocker arms, and sometimes the camshaft.

Cylinders—*See* Oxyacetylene Welding Outfit.

D

***D-Pillar**—Either of two pillars that support the roof and are located rearward of the C-pillars, as in station wagons and vans. Also called D-posts.

***D-Ring**—The seat-belt mounting point located on the B-pillar or the door surround panel.

Damage Analysis—Involves locating all damage, using a systematic series of inspections, measurements, and tests.

Damage Appraisal—*See* Estimate.

Dash Assembly—*See* Instrument Panel.

***Dash Lamp**—Any of the dash-mounted warning lamps that are used to display diagnostic trouble codes.

Dash Panel—*See* Firewall.

Database—A computer file. An estimating database would include part numbers, part illustrations, labor times, labor rates, and other data for filling out the estimate.

Datum Line—An imaginary flat surface parallel to the underbody of the vehicle at some fixed distance from the underbody. The plane from which all vertical or height dimensions are taken and that is used to measure the vehicle during repair. Also called a datum plane.

Datum Measurement—Refers to the distance between two points when measured from the datum plane/line.

Datum Plane—*See* Datum Line.

DC—Direct current flows through circuit in only one direction and voltage is relatively constant; type of electric current used in automobiles.

Dead Axle—A solid rear axle that holds two wheel and brake assemblies. Commonly used on front-drive vehicles, provides little, if any, independent movement of the rear wheels. Also known as trailing arm rear suspension.

Dead Blow Hammer—A hammer that has a metal face filled with lead shot (balls) to prevent rebounding. It will NOT bound back up after striking.

Dealership Body Shop—Is owned and managed under the guidance of a new car dealership, and often concentrates on repairs of the specific make of vehicles sold by the dealership.

Decimal Conversion Chart—It allows you to quickly change from fractions, to decimals, to millimeters.

Decimals—Measurements that divide an inch into tenths, hundredths, one-thousandths, ten-thousandths, and more divisions, used when high precision is important.

Deck Lid—Hinged panel over the rear storage compartment. Also called trunk lid.

Dedicated Bench and Fixture System—A measuring system that uses stationary jigs and fixtures to check body or frame alignment.

Deductible Clause— Statement on insurance policy giving amount of money owner must pay shop to cover costs of vehicle repairs.

Deep Sockets—Cylinder-shaped, box-end wrenches that are longer in length for reaching over stud bolts.

Defective (Bad) Hardener—Hardener that remains thin and watery, even after being kneaded thoroughly. It should not be used because it has broken down chemically.

Deformation—Refers to the new, undesired bent shape the metal takes after an impact or collision.

***Delamination**—The failure of the bond between layers, as when windshield glass separates from the inner layer of vinyl, or when paint peels from the substrate beneath it.

Dent Puller—A slide hammer with a threaded tip, a hood tip, or a suction cup.

Destructive Testing—A test that forces the weld apart to measure weld strength. Force is applied until the metal or weld breaks.

Detailing—A final cleanup and touch-up of vehicle.

Diagnosis Charts—Charts that give logical steps for finding the source of problems.

Diagnostic Tools—Meters, test lights, jumper wires, etc., used for locating an electrical fault in a vehicle's electrical system.

Diagonal Cutting Pliers—Pliers that have cutting jaws that will clip off wires flush with a surface; they are also known as side cut pliers.

Diagonal Line Measurement—Compares reading across an opening or between four reference points to determine damage.

Dial Indicator—Used to measure part movement and out-of-round in thousandths of an inch (hundredths of a millimeter).

Diamond Damage—A condition where one side of the vehicle has been moved to the rear or front, resulting in the frame being out of square. It is caused by a hard impact on a corner or off-center from the front or rear.

Die—A tool used for cutting threads on the outside of bolts or studs.

Diesel Injection System—Uses a high-pressure, mechanical pump to force fuel directly into the engine's combustion chambers (no spark plugs are needed).

Differential Assembly—A unit within the drive axle assembly. It uses gears to allow different amounts of torque to be applied to each drive while the vehicle is making a turn.

Digital Images—Pictures stored as computer data.

Digital Multimeter (DVOM)—A multimeter that gives a digital readout for the test value.

Dinging Hammer—A hammer used for final shaping.

Direct Damage—Damage that occurs in the area of immediate impact as a direct result of the vehicle striking an object.

Disarmed—All sources of electricity for air bag igniter are disconnected.

Disc Adhesive—A special nonhardening glue that comes in a tube. It can be placed on the pad to adhere the paper to the sander.

Disc Backing Plate—Plate mounted on the grinder spindle on thinner grinding discs for extra support.

Disc-Type Grinder—The most commonly used portable air grinder. It is operated like the single-action disc sander.

Discharging—The removal of refrigerant from the air-conditioning system.

Dividers—Have straight, sharp tips for taking measurements or marking parts for cutting. In collision repair work, dividers are sometimes used for layout or marking cut lines.

***Dogtracking**—A condition caused by excessive thrust angle where, as the vehicle's wheels move straight ahead, the body appears to be moving at an angle.

Dolly—Also referred to as a dolly block. Used like a small, portable anvil; generally used on the backside of a panel being struck with a hammer.

Door Alignment Tool—A tool used to slightly bend and adjust sprung doors and hatches.

Door Dust Cover—A paper or plastic cover that fits between the inner trim panel and door frame to keep out wind noise.

Door Frame—The main steel frame of the door.

Door Glass Channel—It serves as a guide for the glass to move up and down. It is a U-shaped channel lined with a low-friction material.

Door Hinge Spring Compressor—Used to remove and install the small spring used on some door hinges.
Door Hinges—Part of the door assembly, bolted between the pillars and door frame.
Door Intrusion Beam—A part that is welded or bolted to the metal support brackets on the door frame to increase door strength.
Door Latch—It engages the door striker on the vehicle body to hold the door closed.
Door Lock Assembly—It usually consists of the outside door handle, linkage rods, the door lock mechanism, and the door latch.
Door Regulator—A gear and arm mechanism for moving the glass.
Door Sills—*See* Rocker Panels.
Door Skin—The outer panel over the door frame. It can be made of steel, aluminum, fiberglass, or plastic.
Door Striker—It holds the door closed.
Door Striker Wrench—A special socket designed to fit over or inside door striker posts.
Door Trim Panel—An attractive cover over the inner door frame.
Door Weatherstripping—A rubber seal around the door or door opening to seal the door-to-body joint.
Double Masking—Using two layers of masking paper to prevent bleed-through or finish-dulling from solvents.
Dowel Pins—Small rods or pins that help hold or align parts.
Downdraft Spray Booth—Forces air from the ceiling down through exhaust vents in the floor.
Download—A computer term meaning to enter data.
***Drag Link**—A link found in some steering systems that connects the pitman arm to the steering arm. Also called center link.
***Dressing a Weld**—Grinding or sanding a weld bead or nugget to reduce the height or make it flush with the base metal.
Drift Punch—Also known as a starting punch, it has a fully tapered shank and will drive pins, shafts, and rods partially out of holes.
Drill Bits—Available in various sizes, these fit into the chuck on drills for making holes in parts.
Drills—Used to make accurately sized holes in metal and plastic parts. Both air and electric drills are available.
Drive Shaft—A long tube that transfers power from the transmission to rear axle assembly.
Driver's-Side Air Bag—Mounted inside the steering wheel center pad, it is activated during a frontal collision but may not deploy from side collisions.
Dry Application of Paint—Spraying with spray gun tip slightly further from the surface or by moving the gun more quickly to apply less paint to the surface; commonly used with colorcoats prior to applying the clearcoats with wet application.
Dry Metallic Paint Spray—Aluminum flakes are trapped at various angles near the surface of the paint film making the paint appear lighter and more silver.
Dry Sanding—A term describing sanding done with coarser nonwaterproof sandpaper, without using water.
Dry Sandpaper—Designed to be used without water.
***Dry-Set**—To trial fit a glass assembly before applying adhesive.
***Dry Spray Appearance**—A paint defect where the paint droplets flash before they flow together, resulting in a dull, overspray appearance.
Drying—Use of different methods to cure fresh paint.
Dual Action Sander—An orbital sander that moves in two directions at the same time. It produces a much smoother surface finish.
Duct Tape—A thick tape with a plastic body. It is sometimes used to protect parts from damage when grinding, sanding, or blasting.
Dust Coat—A light, dry coating that is similar to a mist coat.
Dust Respirator—A filter that fits over your nose and mouth to block small airborne particles while sanding or grinding.
Dustless Sanding System—A system designed to draw airborne dust into a storage container, much like a vacuum cleaner, by using a blower or air pump.
Duty Cycle—The number of times the welder can safely operate at a given amperage level continuously over 10 minutes.
***DVOM**—Digital volt-ohmmeter. A high-impedance instrument used to test electrical systems.

E

***E-Coat**—Electro-deposition primer applied to metal parts during vehicle assembly and replacement part manufacture to prevent rust.
Earmuffs—Safety gear that protects your eardrums from damaging noise levels.
Earplugs—Provides protection to your eardrums from damaging noise levels in the metalworking areas.
Edge Masking—Taping over panel edges and body lines prior to machine buffing or polishing to protect the paint from burn-through.
EGR—Exhaust gas recirculation. A valve that opens to allow engine vacuum to siphon exhaust into the intake manifold.
Elastic Deformation—The ability of metal to stretch and return to its original shape.
Elastomer—*See* Flex Agent.
Electric Adhesive Cutters—Devices that plug into 120 volts to produce a vibrating action to assist in cutting the adhesive around glass.
Electric Circuit—Made up of a power source, conductors, and a load.
Electrical Fires—Fires that result when excess current causes wiring to overheat, melt, and burn.
Electrical Repairs—Include tasks like repairing severed wiring, replacing engine sensors, and scanning for computer or wiring problems.
Electrical Symbols—Graphic representations of electrical-electronic components.
Electrical Systems—Anything powered by the battery, that is, ignition, lights, radio, heat, air conditioning.
Electrical Tape—Made of flexible, thin plastic, it can be used around wire splices when the connection will NOT be exposed to moisture.
Electrocution—Results when excessive electricity passes through your body, causing severe burns, injury, or death.
Electrode Tips—A resistance spot welding part that allows current flow through spot weld.

Electrolyte—A mixture of water and sulfuric acid or another caustic agent in the battery.

Electromagnet—A set of windings.

Electronic Leak Detector—A device that uses a signal generator tool and signal detector to find body leaks.

Electronic Measuring Systems—Measuring systems that use a computer to control the measuring system operation, using laser scanners, ultrasound probes, or robotic measuring arms.

***Electronic Memory**—The storage capability of a programmable electronic device, such as a security system, memory seat, mirror, or radio.

Electronic Mil Gauge—Measures paint/refinishing materials and displays resulting mil thickness with a digital readout.

Electronic Mixing Scales—Computerized scale that helps automate paint mixing. After the technician programs in the amount of paint needed for the area to be refinished, a computerized scale will state how much of each material (pigment, tint, flake, and binder), by weight, to pour into the mixing cup. As you pour each ingredient into the cup on the scale, the scale will go to zero. Once zeroed, you have added the correct amount of that ingredient. The scale will then prompt you to add a specific amount of the next ingredient. This allows you to quickly produce the correct ingredient mix for a specific color paint.

Electronic or Digital Camera—A camera used to take photos of the vehicle's damage and store them as digital data.

Electronic/Computer Written Estimate—A damage report that is completed by using a personal computer and printer.

Electrostatic Spray Guns—Electrically charge the paint particles at the gun to attract them to the vehicle body.

Emblem Adhesive—Designed to hold hard plastic and metal parts. It is also referred to as plastic adhesive.

Emergency Telephone Numbers—This list should include a doctor, hospital, and fire and police departments and should be clearly posted next to the shop's telephone.

Emission Control Systems—Used to prevent potentially toxic chemicals from entering the atmosphere.

Enamel—Sprayed-on synthetic primer or paint coating that normally uses a hardener or catalyst additive to speed curing or drying time.

Encapsulated Glass—*See* Modular Glass.

Energy Reserve Module—It allows the air bag to deploy in the event of a power failure.

Engine—A machine that provides energy to move the vehicle and power all accessories.

***Engine Cradle**—A sub-frame bolted to the vehicle frame or underbody that supports the engine. The engine cradle may also support the transmission and the suspension system. Sometimes called the powertrain cradle.

Engine Crane—A device that can be formed on most racks or benches to raise and remove an engine.

Engine Holder—A device used to support the engine-transmission assembly when the cradle must be unbolted or removed.

Engine Stand—Used to hold a power plant after removal from the vehicle. It will hold the engine on a small roll-around framework for convenience.

English Measuring System—Fractions and decimals are used for giving number values.

English-Metric Conversion Chart—It allows you to convert from English to metric or from metric to English values.

Entrepreneur—A person who starts and successfully runs his or her own business.

EPA (Environmental Protection Agency)—A government agency responsible for environmental protection.

Epoxy—A two-part bonding agent that dries harder than adhesive. It comes in two separate containers, usually tubes; one contains epoxy resin and the other contains a hardener.

***Epoxy Primer**—A primer that uses a thermoset resin to increase corrosion protection and adhesion, with minimal shrinkage.

Eraser Wheel— A rubber wheel and arbor designed to remove vinyl tape stripes without damaging paint.

Estimate—Also called a damage report or appraisal, it calculates the cost of parts, materials, and labor for repairing a collision damaged vehicle.

Estimating—Involves analyzing damage and calculating how much it will cost to repair the vehicle.

Estimating Program—Software that will automatically help find parts needed, labor rates, and calculate total for the repairs.

Estimating System—Electronic databases containing the part and labor information needed for computerized estimating; usually the software comes on CD-ROMs.

Estimator—Makes an appraisal of vehicle damage and determines the parts, materials, and labor needed to repair the vehicle.

***Etch**—The process of chemically roughing a metal surface.

Evacuating—An A/C system must be evacuated anytime air has entered the system. Evacuating is done by vacuum lowering the boiling point of the moisture, converting it to vapor, and removing it.

***Evaporator**—The part of an air-conditioning system where the refrigerant changes from a low-pressure liquid to a low-pressure gas by absorbing heat from the air in the vehicle's passenger compartment.

Exhaust System—It collects and discharges exhaust gases caused by the combustion of the air-fuel mixture within the engine.

Explosions—Air pressure waves that result from extremely rapid burning.

Extensions—Fit between the socket and its drive handle and allow you to reach in and install the socket when it is surrounded by obstructions.

F

Factory Packaged Colors—Ready-mixed paint supplied by refinish suppliers.

***Factory Seams**—The edges and seams where panels were joined during vehicle assembly. Also called factory joints.

Fastened Parts—Parts held together with various fasteners (bolts, nuts, clips, etc.); fenders, hood, and grille.

Fault Code—A code representing a specific circuit or part with a problem.

Featheredged—A tapered edge of a repair area, or the process of making a taper by sanding.

Feeler Gauges—Small blades that measure small clearances inside parts. Blade thickness is given on each blade in thousandths of an inch (0.001, 0.010, 0.020) or in hundredths of a millimeter (0.01, 0.07, 0.10). *See also* Flat Feeler Gauges and Wire Feeler Gauges.

Fender Cover—Material placed over the vehicle body to protect the paint from chips and scratches while working.

Fender Shimming—An adjustment method that uses spacers under the bolts that attach the fender to the cowl or inner fender panel. By changing shim thicknesses, you can move the fender position for proper alignment.

Fender Washers—*See* Body Washers.

Fiber-Reinforced Plastics (FPR)—Plastic panels reinforced with fiber.

Fiber Washers—Washers that prevent vibration or leakage but cannot be tightened to a great extent.

Fiberglass Body Filler—A plastic filler with fiberglass material added. It is used for rust repair or where strength is important.

Fiberglass Cloth—Made by weaving the fiberglass strands into a stitched pattern.

Fiberglass Mat—A series of long fiberglass strands irregularly distributed to form a patch. It is used to strengthen and form a shape for the resin liquid.

Fiberglass Resin—Another form of plastic body repair material. It is a thick resin liquid.

Files—Hand tools used to remove burrs, sharp edges, and to do other smoothing tasks.

Filler—Any material used to fill (level) a damaged area.

Filler Filing—Using a coarse "cheese grater" or body file to rough shape the semihard filler. You will knock off the high spots and rough edges.

Filler Material—Material from a wire or rod that is added to the weld joint.

Filler Mixing Board—A clean, nonporous surface for mixing filler and hardener.

Filler Over-Catalyzation—A condition caused by using too much hardener for the amount of filler.

Filler Oversanding—A condition that results when the filled-in area is below the desired level, which makes it necessary to apply more filler.

***Filler Rod**—A plastic rod used in a plastic weld to form a bond and fill a damaged area. Also, a metal rod when welding metal.

***Filler Strip**—A strip inserted into a rubber gasket after the glass is installed, forcing the gasket against the glass to form a seal and improve the grip. Sometimes called locking bead or spline.

Filler Undersanding—A condition that results when the filled area is higher or thicker than the surrounding panel.

***Filler Wire**—The wire used to add metal to a weld puddle, to create a bead or nugget.

***Fillet Weld**—A weld where the bead fills the junction between two pieces of base metal joined at an angle, as in a tee or lap joint.

Final Detailing—Term used to describe the location and correction of any defect that may cause customer complaints. The steps are sanding and filing; compounding; machine glazing; and hand glazing.

Fine File—Normally used to smooth steel, it will give a smoother surface on harder materials.

Fine Grit—A grit of 150 to 180, used to sand bare metal and for smoothing existing paint.

Fine-Line Masking Tape—A very thin, smooth surface plastic masking tape. Also termed flush masking tape.

Finesse Sanding—Using ultra fine grit sandpapers to repair minor paint flaws.

Finishing Area—Area in shop where the vehicle surface is prepared for painting before going into the paint booth, which has a large metal enclosure to keep out dirt and circulate clean, fresh air.

Finishing Hammers—Hammers used to achieve the final sheet metal contour.

Finishing Washers—Washers that have a curved shape for a pleasing appearance. They are used on interior pieces.

Fire—A rapid oxidation of a flammable material, producing high temperatures.

Fire Extinguisher—An instrument designed to quickly smother a fire. There are several types available for putting out different kinds of fires.

Fire Wall—The panel dividing the front section and center, passenger compartment section. Sometimes termed dash panel or front bulkhead.

Firm Bid—A written estimate that is good for a given period of time, usually 30 days.

First Aid Kit—This includes many medical items such as sterile gauze, bandages, scissors, bandaids, and antiseptics that are needed to treat minor shop injuries.

Fisheye Eliminator—A paint additive that helps smooth the paint when small craters or holes in the paint film are a problem.

Fisheyes—A paint problem involving the separation of wet paint film. Small indentations will form in the fresh paint. Sometimes, the previous finish under the new material can be seen in these spots or indentations in the paint film.

Fit Test—A test performed prior to using a respirator. It checks for respirator air leaks, making both negative and positive pressure checks.

Fixtures—Thick metal parts that bolt between the vehicle and bench to check alignment.

***Flame Treatment**—The light scorching of a plastic repair area with a torch, to strengthen the bond of the adhesive to be applied.

***Flange**—A bend or offset formed along the edge of a panel, or around a hole in a panel.

***Flare**—A tapered expansion of an opening. A flare is often used when connecting joints in tubing.

Flare Nut Wrench—Also referred to as tubing or line wrench, it has a small split in its jaw to fit over lines and tubing.

***Flash Time**—The first stage of drying where some of the solvents evaporate. The surface dulls from a high gloss to a normal gloss.

Flat Feeler Gauges—Feeler gauges used for measuring between parallel surfaces.

Flat Rate—A preset amount of time and money charged for a specific repair operation.

Flat Washers—Washers used to increase clamping surface area. They prevent the smaller bolt head from pulling through sheet metal or plastic.

Flat Welding—Welding position in which the pieces are parallel to the bench or shop floor.
Flattener—An agent added to paint to lower gloss or shine.
***Flex Agent**—An additive that increases the flexibility of paint for use on plastic parts.
Flex Handle—Also called a breaker bar, it provides the most powerful way to turn bolts and nuts.
***Flexible Filler**—A material used to fill and level repair areas on plastic parts.
Floating Test—A test that can be used to help determine the type of plastic. A plastic that floats in water is thermoplastic. A plastic that sinks in water is thermoset plastic.
Floor Pan—Main structural section in the bottom of the passenger compartment.
Flop—Also termed flip-flop, it refers to a change in color hue when viewing from head-on and then from the side.
Flow Meter—A device that measures the movement of air, gas, or a liquid past a given point.
Fluid Control Knob—A part of the spray gun; it changes the distance the fluid needle moves away from its seat in the nozzle when the trigger is pulled. This controls paint flow.
Fluid Control Valve—On a spray gun, it can be turned to adjust the amount of paint or other material emitted.
Fluid Needle Valve—It seats in the fluid tip on a spray gun to prevent flow or can be pulled back to allow flow.
Fluid Needle—A part of the spray gun; it open or shuts off the flow of paint.
Fluid Nozzle—A part of the spray gun; it forms an internal seat for the fluid needle.
Fluorescent Light—Artificial light that has more violets and reds than daylight.
Fluorine Clearcoat—Used to improve resistance to UV radiation; protect from weathering, chalking, oxidation, and industrial fallout; improve luster of the finish; and reduce required maintenance, such as waxing and polishing.
Flux—Cleaning material used when heat soldering electrical wires.
***Flux-Cored Wire**—A type of welding wire having a central core of flux that creates a shielding gas when heated.
Flywheel—A heavy metal disc that helps keep the crankshaft turning smoothly and connects engine power to the transmission.
Flywheel Ring Gear—Meshes with the starter-mounted gear while cranking.
***Foam Fillers**—Plastic foam used in body cavities, primarily to stop the transmission of sound.
Foam Rubber Polishing Pad—Commonly used for final polishing to remove swirl marks and is very soft and will produce a higher luster than a cloth or cotton pad.
Forced Drying—Curing fresh paint by using special heat lamps or other equipment to speed the process.
Forked Trim Tool—Tool designed to remove body clips in trim parts.
Four-Wheel Drive—Vehicles that use a transfer case to send power to both axle assemblies and all four wheels. The transfer case can be engaged and disengaged to select two- or four-wheel drive as desired.
Fractions—They divide an inch into thirty-seconds, sixteenths, and larger parts of an inch.
Frame—An independent, separate part not welded to any major units of the body shell.
Frame Horn—The very front of the frame rails where the bumper attaches.
Frame Rack—Frame straightening equipment that uses a large steel framework (bench or rack), pulling chains, and hydraulic power to push out the vehicle frame or unibody damage.
Frame Rack Accessories—The many chains, special tools, and other parts needed to perform the many different frame straightening operations.
***Frame Rails**—The fore-and-aft members of a frame or underbody structure.
Frame Straightening Accessories—The many chains, special tools, and other parts needed to perform the many different frame straightening operations.
Framed Doors—A type of door design, it surrounds the sides and top of the door glass with a metal frame, helping keep the window glass aligned.
Franchise Facility—Is tied to a main headquarters that regulates and aids the business operation.
Front Bulkhead—*See* Firewall.
"Front Clip"—The purchase and installation of a recycled/salvaged vehicle front end assembly.
Front End Rack—Used to measure and adjust the steering and suspension of a vehicle after repairs. Also known as an alignment rack.
Front-Engine, Rear-Wheel Drive (RWD)—A vehicle that has the engine in the front and the drive axle in the rear.
Front Fender Aprons—The inner panels that surround the wheels and tires to keep out road debris.
Front Fenders—Part that extends from the front doors to the front bumper. They cover the front suspension and inner aprons.
Front Pillars—Pillars that extend up next to windshield edges, also called A-pillars.
Front Section—Also called nose section, it includes everything between the front bumper and the fire wall.
Front-Wheel Drive—Vehicles that use a transaxle to transfer engine torque to front drive wheels.
Fuel Evaporative System—It pulls fumes from the gas tank and other fuel system parts into a charcoal canister.
Fuel Filter—Used for straining out debris in gasoline or diesel fuel.
Fuel Injectors—Electrically operated fuel valves located in the engine intake manifold or combustion chambers.
Fuel Pressure Regulator—A spring-loaded device that controls the amount of fuel pressure that is fed into the fuel rail and fuel injectors.
Fuel Pump—A mechanical or electric part for forcing fuel to engine.
Fuel Rail—Large fuel log or line that feeds gasoline to fuel injectors on the engine.
Fuel System—Feeds the correct amount of fuel into the engine.
Full Body Sectioning—Replacing the entire rear section of a collision damaged vehicle with the rear section of a salvage vehicle.

Full Cutout Method—A method of windshield replacement used when the original adhesive is defective or requires complete removal.
Full-Face Shield—Safety gear worn when there is more danger from flying particles, as when grinding.
Full-Size Car—Large, heavy, high fuel consumption automobile that can have either unibody or body-over-frame construction.
Full Wet Coat—A heavy, glossy coat applied over the tack coat. It makes the paint lay down smooth and shiny.
Funnels—Instruments used when pouring fluid from a container into a small opening.
Fuse Box—This holds the various circuit fuses, breakers, and flasher units.
Fuse Ratings—The current at which the fuse will blow.
Fuses—Circuit protection devices.
***Fusible Link**—A short length of wire, smaller in diameter (lower current capacity) than the rest of the circuit, spliced into a primary circuit to act as a time-delay fuse.
***Fusion**—The melting and flowing together of two pieces of metal during welding.
Fusion Welding—Joining different pieces of metal together by melting and fusing them into each other.

G

***Galvanic Corrosion**—Rust caused by contact between dissimilar metals when moisture is present.
***Galvanizing**—A protective zinc coating applied during the production of steel.
Gap—Distance measured between two adjacent parts, also called clearance.
Gas Flow Rate—A measurement of how fast gas flows over the weld puddle in MIG welding.
***Gas Metal Arc Welding (GMAW)**—A welding process in which the electrode filler wire is fed continuously into the weld puddle while the puddle is protected by the shielding gas. Also called metal inert gas (MIG) welding.
Gaskets—Used to prevent air and water leakage between body parts.
Gasoline—A highly flammable petroleum- or crude oil–based liquid that vaporizes and burns rapidly.
Gasoline Injection System—Uses sensors and a computer to control electrically operated fuel valves, called fuel injectors, located in the intake manifold.
Gauge Measuring Systems—A method that uses sliding metal rods or bars and adjustable pointers with rules scaled to measure body dimensions.
General Bolt Torque Chart—Gives a general torque value for the size and grade of bolt.
Get Ready—A thorough clean-up before returning the vehicle to the customer.
Glazing Putty—A material made for filling small holes or sand scratches.
Goggles—Eye protection suitable when handling chemicals.
Good Spray Pattern—Deposits an even, oval-shaped mist of paint on the surface being painted, resulting from proper mixture of air and paint droplets and dependent on proper spray gun operation and adjustment.
Gouge—A sharp dent or crease into a panel caused by a focused impact.
Graduated Mixing Cup—A clear plastic cup with paint ratio markings for mixing spray materials.
Graduated Pail—Used to measure liquid materials when mixing.
Grain Structure—In a piece of steel, it determines how much it can be bent or shaped.
Gravity Feed Spray Gun—The cup is mounted on top of the spray gun head so the material flows down without external air pressure.
Grease Gun—A device used to lubricate high-friction points on a vehicle's steering and suspension systems.
Grinders—Used for fast removal of material. They are often used to smooth metal joints after welding and to remove paint and primer.
Grinding Discs—Round, very coarse abrasives used for initial removal of paint, plastic, and metal (weld joints).
***Grit**—A numerical system that rates sandpaper and sanding disc coarseness, a smaller number (36 for example) denotes coarser sandpaper and vice versa (1200 would be very fine). *See also* Very Coarse Grit, Coarse Grit, Medium Grit, Fine Grit, and Very Fine Grit.
Grit Numbering System—Denotes how coarse or fine the abrasive is.
Grit Sizes—A term that refers to the coarseness of sandpaper.
Ground—Electrical path back to the battery negative cable through wires, cables, or body structure.
Grounded Circuit—When negative side of an electric circuit is connected to the battery negative terminal or metal unibody or frame. A grounded circuit problem occurs when the insulation on a wire is worn and the metal conductor accidentally touches the metal body or frame of the vehicle.
Guide Coat—A thin layer of a different color primer or a special powder applied to the repair area often used to check for high and low spots on your repair area. By watching what happens to the guide coat with light sanding, you can find low and high spots.
Gun Angle—Consists of two different angles: the angle of the gun to the workplace and the angle of direction of travel.
Gun Arching—Uneven film thickness, paint runs, excessive overspray, dry spray, and orange peel caused by not moving the spray gun parallel with the surface.
Gun Body—The part of the spray gun that holds the parts that meter air and liquid. It also holds the spray pattern adjustment valve, fluid control valve, air cap, fluid tip, trigger, and related parts.
Gun Heeling—Uneven film thickness, excessive overspray, dry spray, and orange peel caused by allowing the spray gun to tilt.
Gun-Mounted Pressure Gauge—A gauge or regulator installed between the hose coupler and the gun that lets you set actual pressure at the gun. It is the best method to measure and adjust spray gun air pressure. Also called gun-mounted gauge-regulator

H

Hacksaw—A tool sometimes used to cut metal parts.
1/2 Inch Impact—An impact wrench with a 1/2-inch size drive head. It is shaped like a pistol with a hand grip

hanging down. It is frequently used to service wheel lug nuts.
***Half Shaft**—A rotating shaft assembly using two CV-joints to transmit power from a differential to a wheel that is sprung independently of the differential. Commonly used in front-wheel-drive vehicles and some rear-wheel-drive vehicles.
Halo Effect—An unwanted shiny ring or halo that appears around a pearl or mica paint repair. It is caused by the paint being wetter in the middle and drier near the outer edges of the repair.
Hammer-Off-Dolly—A method used to straighten metal just before the final stage of straightening.
Hammer-On-Dolly—A method used to stretch metal and to smooth small, shallow dents and bulges.
Hammers—Used for striking and exerting an impact on a part.
Hand Blaster—A small, portable tool for blasting parts and panels on the vehicle.
Hand Cleaner—Always use proper hand cleaners, as many chemicals, like thinner, can be absorbed into the skin, eventually causing long-term illnesses.
Hand Compound—An oil-based rubbing compound that provides lubrication; best on small or blended areas.
Hand Glazes—Used for final smoothing and shining of the paint.
Hand Scrapers—Used on flat surfaces, they will easily remove gaskets and softened paint (when paint stripping chemicals are used).
Hand Tools—Generally include tools such as wrenches, screwdrivers, and pliers, which are commonly used to remove parts, fenders, doors, and similar assemblies.
Hard Brazing—Brazing with materials that melt at temperatures above 900°F (486°C).
***Hardener**—An additive that causes a chemical reaction to cure paint, body filler, adhesives, etc.
Hardtop—A body design that does not have a center pillar to support the roof but must be reinforced to provide extra strength. It is available in 2- and 4-door versions.
Hardtop Doors—A type of door design, it has the glass extending up out of the door without a frame around it.
Hard Water Spotting Damage—Damage that forms when rain or tap water dries on the paint surface and evaporates, leaving hard minerals on the paint surface. Hard water spotting leaves a round white ring on the paint surface.
Hardware—Computer, printers, hard drives, and CD-ROM drives used to speed up the estimating process.
Hatchback—A body design that has a large third door at the back. This design is commonly found on small compact cars, allowing for more rear storage space.
Hazardous Material—Any substance that can harm people or the environment.
Head-On View—Compares the test panel to the vehicle straight on or perpendicular.
Header Pipe—Steel tubing that carries exhaust gases from the engine's exhaust ports to the catalytic converters, mufflers, and rest of exhaust system.
Headlight Aimers—Equipment used to adjust the direction of the vehicle headlights.
Headlight Aiming Screws—Screws with a special plastic adapter mounted on them. The adapter fits into the headlight assembly.
Headliner—A cloth or vinyl cover over the inside of the passenger compartment roof.
Headrest—The padded frame that fits into the top of the seat back.
Headrest Guide—Sleeve that accepts the headrest post and mounts in the seat back.
***Heat-Affected Zone**—A metal area that has been heated beyond its critical temperature, causing it to lose strength.
Heat Crayons—Used to determine the temperature of the aluminum or other metal being heated. They will melt at a specific temperature and warn you to prevent overheating.
Heat Setting—Determines the length of the arc when MIG welding. Also called voltage.
***Heat Sink**—A piece of metal that protects wiring, or other sensitive parts, by absorbing excessive heat. Clamp-on heat sinks are often used during repair operations such as soldering.
Heat Sink Compound—A paste that can be applied to parts during welding to absorb heat and prevent warpage.
***Heat-Treatable Alloy**—Any substance whose strength will not be affected by the application of a controlled amount of heat. Usually refers to metals, such as alloys of aluminum or iron (steel).
Heater System—Uses coolant heat and a heater core (small radiator under the dash) to warm the passenger compartment.
Helicoil®—A tool used to repair badly damaged internal threads. Also called a Thread Insert.
Helper—Also known as an apprentice, learns new jobs while assisting experienced personnel.
***HEPA Filter**—A high-efficiency particulate air filter. A type of air filter that traps at least 99.97% of all particles that are 0.3 micron or larger in size.
***Hg**—The chemical symbol for mercury. The height of a column of mercury, expressed in inches, is a measure of pressure or vacuum. One inch Hg equals 0.491 psi.
High-Efficiency Spray Guns—Designed to reduce VOC emissions by only using 10 psi air pressure at the gun head. Also called HVLP for high volume, low pressure or LVLP for low volume, low pressure.
High-Solids Materials—The nonliquid contents of paint needed to reduce air pollution or emissions when painting.
High Spot—Also called a bump, it is an area that sticks up higher than the surrounding surface.
High-Strength Steel (HSS)—Sheet metal that is stronger than low-carbon or mild steel because of heat treatment.
High Transfer Efficiency—Means that more of the paint applied by a spray gun will remain on the surface.
Hinged Parts—Parts that swing up and open, such as doors, hoods, and decklids.
Hog Rings—A device that stretches and holds the seat cover over the seat frame and padding.
Hole Saws—Special cutters that fit into a drill like a drill bit to make large holes in body panels.
Hood—The hinged panel for accessing the engine compartment (front-engine vehicle) or trunk area (rear-engine vehicle).
Hood Adjustments—Adjustments made at the hinges, at the adjustable stops, and at the hood latch.

Hood Hinge Spacers—A part that helps adjust the hood.

Hood Hinge Spring Tool—Used to stretch hood springs off and on. It is a hooked tool that will easily pry the end of the spring off of and onto its mount.

Hood Hinges—A part that allows the hood to open and close while staying in alignment.

Hood Latch—Part of the cable hood release, it has metal arms that grasp and hold the hood striker.

Hood Latch Adjustment—This controls how well the hood striker engages the latch mechanism.

Hood Latch Mechanism—Keeps the hood closed and releases the hood when activated.

Hood Release Cable—Part of the cable hood release, it is a steel cable that slides inside a plastic housing. One end fastens to the release handle and the other to the hood latch.

Hood Stop Adjustment—A device that controls the height of the front of the hood.

Hood Striker—Part of the cable hood release, it bolts to the hood and engages the hood latch when closed.

Hood/Trunk Tool—A telescoping rod that can be used to prop open the hood or trunk lid.

***Horizontal Datum Plane**—A horizontal plane, located at or below a vehicle's underbody, that serves as a reference for height measurements.

Horizontal Welding—The pieces are turned sideways. Gravity tends to pull the puddle into the bottom piece.

Hose Clamps—Used to hold radiator hoses, heater hoses, and other hoses onto their fittings.

Hoses—*See* Oxyacetylene Welding Outfit.

Hot Air Plastic Welding—Uses a tool with an electric heating element to produce hot air that blows through a nozzle and onto the plastic.

Hot Weather Solvent—A reducer or thinner. It is designed to slow solvent evaporation to prevent problems.

"Hot Wires"—Wires that connect the battery positive to the components of each circuit.

Hue—Dimension of color that describes what we normally think of as color, the color that is seen. Also called color, cast, or tint.

HVLP—*See* High-Efficiency Spray Gun.

Hybrid Bonding—Refers to using more than one method to join structural body parts on a vehicle. It is now being used during the manufacture of today's steel and aluminum unibody structures.

Hydraulic—Equipment operated by oil under pressure.

Hydraulic Equipment—Uses a confined fluid or oil to develop the pressure necessary for operation.

Hydraulic Jacks—A device used to raise the vehicle.

Hydraulic Rams—Use oil under pressure from a pump to produce a powerful linear motion.

Hydrometers—Used to measure the specific gravity or density of a liquid such as antifreeze, battery acid, etc.

I

Idler Arm—An arm that duplicates the motion of the pitman arm on the opposite side of the vehicle in order to maintain steering geometry.

Ignition Coil—A step-up transformer that produces high voltage (30,000 volts or more) needed to make current jump the spark plug gap.

Ignition Switch—Switch in the steering column is used to connect battery voltage to a starter solenoid or relay.

Ignition System—This produces an electric arc in a gasoline engine to cause the fuel to burn. It must fire the spark plugs at the right time. The resulting combustion pressure forces the pistons down to spin the crankshaft.

Impact Adapters—It is important that when using an air impact wrench these (usually black) adapters are used, rather than other types of adapters (chrome plated), which might shatter and fly off, endangering everyone in the immediate area.

Impact Driver—A screwdriver that is hit with a hammer to rotate tight or stuck screws. The body of the driver can be rotated to change directions for installing or removing.

Impact Sensor—The first sensor to detect a collision; it is mounted at the front of the vehicle.

Impact Sockets—These cylinder-shaped, box-end wrenches are thicker and case hardened for use with an air-powered impact wrench.

Impact Wrench—This portable, hand-held, reversible air tool is shaped like a pistol with a handgrip hanging down and is frequently used to service wheel lug nuts. It is available with different size drive heads.

Improper Coverage—A term that means the paint film thickness is not uniform or too thin. It is caused by not triggering exactly over the edge of the panel or from improper spray overlap.

Improper Spray Overlap—A term that means you are not covering half of the previous pass with the next pass.

In-Line Oiler—An attachment that will automatically meter oil into air lines for air tools.

In-Shop Estimating System—A system that has all of the data needed at the shop office, usually on CD-ROMs.

Incandescent Light—Artificial light that has more yellows, oranges, and reds than daylight.

Included Operations—A repair that can be performed individually but is also part of another repair.

Incorrect Gun Stroke Speed—A term that means you are moving the gun too slowly or quickly.

Independent Body Shop—Is owned and operated by a private individual and is not associated with other shops or companies.

Indirect Damage—Damage caused by the shock of collision forces traveling through the body and inertial forces acting upon the rest of the unibody.

Inductive Pickup—A device that slips over the wire or cable to measure current.

Industrial Fallout—Occurs when metallic particles are released into the atmosphere from steel mills, foundries, and railroad operations. A source of paint damage.

Inert Gas—A type of shielding gas that protects the weld, but does not combine with the weld.

Inertia Sensors—Part of the air bag system, they detect a rapid deceleration to produce an electrical signal.

***Inertia Switch**—A switch that shuts off the electrical power to the fuel pump and other circuits during a collision.

Infinite Reading—Indicates maximum resistance in a circuit, showing an open within the circuit.

Infrared Drying Equipment—Uses special bulbs to generate infrared light for fast drying of paint materials.

Initial Washing—Complete cleaning of the vehicle to remove mud, dirt, and other foreign matter before bringing the vehicle into the shop, preventing road debris from entering shop area.

Inner Wheel Housings—Housings that surround the rear wheels.

Inserts—Metal backing sometimes installed in weld repairs of closed sections, such as rocker panels, R- and B-pillars, and rails.

Inside Calipers—A tool designed for measuring inside parts. They are accurate to about 1/64 in.

Instrument Cluster—Contains the speedometer, gauges, indicating lights, and similar parts.

Instrument Panel—The assembly that includes the soft dash pad, instrument cluster, radio, heater and AC controls, vents, and similar parts. Also known as dash assembly.

Insulation—It stops current flow and keeps the current in the metal wire conductor.

Insurance Adjuster—Reviews estimates and determines which one best reflects how the vehicle should be repaired.

Integral—Unit is built as one piece instead of two or more.

Intermediate Car—Medium-size body classification, uses a 4-, 6-, or 8-cylinder engine and has average weight and physical dimensions. It usually has unibody construction, but a few vehicles have body-over-frame construction.

Intermix System—A full set of paint pigments and solvents that can be mixed at the body shop.

International Symbols—A way of identifying an unknown plastic. The code is molded into the plastic part.

Intrusion Beam—A beam, welded inside the door frame, that protects the occupants during a side impact.

Irritants—Hazardous materials that can affect your lungs, skin, and eyes.

ISO Codes—"International symbols" is a way of identifying an unknown plastic. The code is molded into the plastic part.

***Isocyanates**—Toxic additives used in some refinish materials to force curing by molecular cross-linking.

***Isolator**—A friction type of energy absorber.

J

Jack Stands—Strong steel pieces of equipment designed to support a vehicle when someone works underneath it. They have four legs to hold them steady and an extendible shoe on which the vehicle rests. Also known as safety stands.

Jam Nuts—Thin nuts used to help hold larger, conventional nuts in place.

Jigs—Used to help locate and guide the cut when sectioning and to check the vehicle body/frame alignment.

Joint Fit-Up—Refers to holding workpieces tightly together, in alignment, to prepare for welding. It is critical to the replacement of body parts.

Jounce—Motion caused by a wheel going over a bump and compressing the spring.

Jounce/Rebound Check—A test that involves pushing down on the front or rear of the vehicle to load the suspension, and then allowing the vehicle to bounce back up. It is used to identify damage to the steering gear, column, or tie-rods.

Jumper Cables—Cables used to connect two batteries together when one is discharged.

Jumper Wires—A device used to temporarily bypass circuits or components for testing.

Jumpsuit—The proper clothing to wear in the paint spraying area.

K

Keys—Devices used by equipment manufacturers to retain parts in alignment or used to tighten the chuck on the drill.

Kick Panels—The small panels between the front pillars and rocker panels.

***Kingpin**—The shaft that a steering knuckle pivots around.

Kinked—A term that describes a part that has a sharp bend or a small radius, usually more than 90 degrees, or a part where after straightening, there is a visible crack or tear in the metal or a permanent deformation that cannot be straightened to its preaccident shape without the use of excessive heat.

Kneading Hardener—Squeezing the tube of hardener back and forth with your fingers to mix the material.

Knee Bolster—Located underneath the steering column and behind the steering column trim, it cushions the driver's knees from impact and helps prevent the driver from sliding under the air bag during a collision.

***kPa, Kilopascal**—A metric unit for measuring pressure. One kPa equals 0.145 psi.

L

Lace Painting—Involves spraying through lace fabric to produce a custom pattern in the paint.

Ladder Frame—A frame that has long frame rails with a series of straight crossmembers formed in several locations. It is a seldom-used modification of the perimeter frame.

Laminated Plate Glass—Two thin sheets of glass with a layer of clear plastic between them. It is used for windshields.

Lap Belts—Seat belts that extend across a person's lap.

***Lap Joints**—A type of weld joint made by overlapping two pieces of metal and joining them with a bead along one or both edges.

Laser—An acronym for "light amplification by stimulated emission of radiation." Lasers are used in electronic measuring systems.

Laser Guides—Also referred to as beam splitters or targets, they are capable of reflecting the laser beam so alignment equipment can measure extent and direction of structural damage.

***Lateral Acceleration**—A sensor that provides an electrical acceleration signal to a control module.

Lateral Dimensions—Vehicle measurements involving width.

Lead Hammer—Also know as a soft hammer, it will make heavy blows without marring the metal surface. The soft metal head will dent and protect the part.

Leak Detector—A tool for finding refrigerant leaks in lines, hoses, and other parts of an air-conditioning system.

Leather Shoes—Thick leather shoes with nonskid soles that help prevent falls and foot injuries from falling parts and tools.

Left-Hand Threads—Nuts and bolts that must be turned counterclockwise to tighten.

***Let-Down Panel**—A test panel used to determine the color match and the number of coats required to match a multistage finish.

Lid Shock Absorbers—Usually a spring-loaded, gas-filled unit that holds the lid open and causes it to close more slowly.

Lid Torsion Rods—Spring steel rods used to help lift the lid weight. They extend horizontally across the body and engage a stationary bracket.

Lifetime Tool Guarantee—This type of guarantee will cover the replacement or repair of a tool if it ever fails or breaks.

Lift Safety Catch—A device on a hydraulic jack. When engaged, it ensures that the lift cannot lower while working underneath the vehicle.

Lifter—A cylindrical part that rides on the camshaft lobes and transfers motion to the pushrods.

Light Body Filler—A filler formulated for easy sanding and fast repairs. It is used as a very thin top coat of filler for final leveling.

Light Temperature—A rating of lighting in "Kelvin." For painting, a lamp rating or temperature of 6,000–7,000 Kelvin is recommended.

Line Wrench—Also referred to as tubing or flare nut, it has a small split in its jaw to fit over lines and tubing.

Linear Measurements—Straight line measurements of distance. Commonly used when evaluating major structural damage after a collision.

Lint-Free Coveralls—Proper clothing to wear in a paint spraying area.

Liquid Electrical Tape—Liquid plastic material applied with a brush to a soldered joint to help make the electrical connection waterproof.

Liquid Masking Material—A masking system that seals off the entire vehicle to protect undamaged panels and parts from paint overspray.

Load—Circuit part that converts electrical energy into another form of energy (light, movement, heat, etc.).

Lock Cylinders—A tumbler mechanism that engages the key so that you can turn the key and disengage the latch.

Locking Pliers—Also known as Vise-Grips, these have adjustable-width jaws that lock into position on parts.

Locksmith Tool—Also termed "slim jim," it is used to open locked doors on cars and trucks.

Long-Hair Fiberglass Filler—A fiberglass filler with long strands of fiberglass for even more strength.

Long Spray Distance—A spray gun distance that causes a greater percentage of the thinner to evaporate, resulting in orange peel or dry spray.

Longitudinal Engine—An engine-mounting configuration that has the crankshaft centerline front-to-rear when viewed from the top of the vehicle. Used in front-engine, RWD vehicles.

Low Impedance—Refers to low resistance in meters used to test modern electronic circuits.

Low Spot—Also called a dent, it is an area that is recessed below the surrounding surface.

Lower Cabinet—Often, heavier tools are stored in the toolbox lower cabinet.

Lower Rear Panel—Panel that fits between the trunk compartment and rear bumper between the quarter panels.

Lowering—To work a high spot or bump down or into the body panel so it is level with undamaged area.

***LPG**—Liquefied petroleum gas.

Lubrication System—Keeps the moving parts from quickly wearing and failing by forcing oil to friction points in the engine.

Lumen Rating—The measurement of a lamp's brightness.

LVLP—See High-Efficiency Spray Guns.

M

Machine Compound—A compound formulated to be applied with an electric or air polisher.

Machine Grinding—A process used to remove old finish from small flat areas and gently curved areas.

Machine Screws—Screws that are threaded their full length and are relatively weak.

MAG—Metal active gas. Describes the welding process when the primary gas of the shielding gas is active.

***Magnaflux**—A method of detecting cracks in steel parts, using an electric current to activate a magnetic dye.

Magnetic Field—Also known as flux, it is an invisible energy present around permanent magnets and current carrying wires.

Magnetic Guide Strip—Used to help guide the pin striping tool for making straight or slightly curved pin stripes.

Magnetism—Involves the study of how electric fields act upon ferrous (iron-containing) objects.

Major Acid Rain Damage—Severe chemical etching that has eaten completely through the paint.

Major Repairs—Refers to the replacement of large body sections and frame straightening.

Manometer—An instrument that indicates when the intake filters in a spray booth are overloaded.

Manual Estimating—Preparing a written estimate using crash estimating books and collision damage manuals.

Manual Mixing Scales—Weigh each paint ingredient as it is poured into the mixing cup on the scale.

Manual Transmission—A transmission that must be hand shifted through each forward gear.

Manually Written Estimate—A damage report that is completed in longhand by filling in information on a printed form.

Manufacturer's Instructions—Very detailed procedures for the specific product.

Manufacturer's Specifications—Measurements given by a manufacturer for proper repair of their vehicles.

Manufacturer's Warnings—Procedures given by the manufacturer for the safe use of their product.

Marble Effect—A custom paint job made by forcing crumpled plastic against a freshly painted stripe or area.

Mash Damage—Has occurred when any section or member of the vehicle is shorter than factory specifications. Mash is usually limited to forward of the cowl or rearward of the rear window.

Masking—A special tape, paper, or plastic used to cover vehicle surfaces and parts to protect it from paint overspray.

Masking Area—This area is usually equipped with masking paper and tape dispensers, tire covers, and other needed materials.

Masking Coating—Also called masking liquid, it is usually a water-based sprayable material for keeping overspray off body parts.

Masking Covers—Specially shaped cloth or plastic covers for masking specific parts.

Masking Foam—A self-stick foam rubber cord designed for quickly and easily masking behind doors, hoods, gas cap lids, and other panels to block overspray. Also called Masking Rope.

Masking Machine—A machine designed to feed out masking paper while applying masking tape to one edge of the paper.

Masking Paper—A special paper designed to be used to cover body parts not to be painted.

Masking Paper Dispenser—A device that automatically applies tape to one edge of the masking paper as the paper is pulled out.

Masking Plastic—Used just like masking paper to cover and protect parts from overspray.

Masking Rope—*See* Making Foam.

Masking Tape—An adhesive used to hold masking paper or plastic into position. It is a high tack, easy-to-tear tape.

Master Cylinder—It develops hydraulic pressure for the brake system.

Material Safety Data Sheets (MSDS)—Documents that provide safety, handling, storage, and clean-up information for hazardous materials.

Measurement Gauges—Special tools used to check specific frame and body points. They allow you to quickly measure the direction and extent of vehicle damage.

Measurements—Number values that help control processes in collision repair.

Measuring System—A special machine used to gauge and check the amount of frame and body damage. It compares known good measurements with those on the vehicle being repaired.

Mechanical Repairs—Repairing mechanical components such as water pump, radiator, etc.

Mechanical Systems—Chassis parts of an automobile such as steering, braking, and suspension systems.

***Media**—The material that is used, under air pressure, to remove paint from a surface in a process called media blasting. Types of media are ground-up plastic, sand, or other material.

Medium Grit—A grit of 80 to 120, used for sanding body filler high spots and for sanding paint.

Melt-Flow Plastic Welding—Most commonly used airless welding method.

***Metal Conditioner**—An acid-based material that is part of a metal treatment system. This material etches the metal surface to improve paint adhesion.

Metal Dust Damage—A problem that occurs when metallic particles from industrial fallout settle onto the paint. The particles soon begin to corrode, eating into the finish. Also known as "rail dust."

Metal Inert Gas (MIG) Welding—One of two general types of gas metal arc welding methods; it is a wire-feed fusion welding process commonly used in collision repair. It is the accepted industry name for gas metal arc welding (GMAW).

Metallic Color—Paint with large reflective pigment flakes added.

Metalworking Area—An area where parts are removed, repaired, and installed.

Metamerism—How different light sources affect the appearance of paint pigments and metallics.

Meter Stick—*See* Metric Rule.

Metric Bolt Strength Markings—These markings, which apply to both bolts and nuts, indicate metric bolt hardness and strength and are given as numbers, the higher the number, the stronger the bolt.

Metric Measuring System—Uses a power of ten as its base. It is a simpler system than our conventional system, because multiples of metric units are related to each other by the factor *ten*. Every metric unit can be multiplied or divided by a factor of ten to get larger units (multiples) or smaller units (submultiples). Also called the scientific international (SI) system.

Metric Rule—Measuring scale marked in millimeters and centimeters. The numbered lines usually equal 10 millimeters (1 centimeter). Also called a meter stick.

Micrometers—Devices that are used to measure mechanical parts when high precision is important.

Mid-Engine, Rear-Wheel Drive (MRD)—A vehicle that has the engine located right behind the front seat, or centrally located.

MIG Contact Tip—It transfers current to the welding wire as the wire travels through the hole in the tip.

MIG-MAG—The welding process, when nearly equal active and inert combinations of shielding gases are used.

MIG Nozzle—It protects the contact tip and directs the shielding gas flow.

MIG Welding Gun—Also called a torch, it delivers wire, current, and shielding gas to the weld site.

Mil Gauge—Used to measure the thickness of the paint on the vehicle.

***Mild Steel (MS)**—Steel that can withstand stress up to 30,000 psi. Also called low-carbon steel, it is a sheet metal that has a low level of carbon and is relatively soft and easy to work.

Mils—A measurement of paint thickness represented in thousandths of an inch (hundredths of a millimeter).

Minivan—A van that is smaller and often uses front-engine, FWD with unibody construction.

Minor Acid Rain Damage—A form of paint damage that produces shallow craters, dulling, fading, and chalking, damage which does not eat fully through the paint.

Minor Repairs—Repairs requiring minimum time and effort, for example, small dents, scratches.

Mixing Board—The surface used for mixing the filler and its hardener.

Mixing By Parts—For a specific volume of paint or other material, a specific amount of another material must be added.

Mixing Chart—A guide that converts a percentage into how many parts of each material must be mixed.

Mixing Instructions—Instructions normally given on the material's label, usually as a percentage or parts of one ingredient compared to the other(s).

Mixing Scales—Used by paint suppliers and technicians to weigh the various ingredients when mixing paint materials.

Mixing Sticks—Have graduated scale markings that allow you to easily mix paint, primer, clear, solvent, and additives in the correct proportions.

Modular Glass—Also known as encapsulated glass, it has a plastic trim molding attached to its edge to fit the contours of the vehicle more closely.

Molding Removal Tool—A tool used to separate adhesive-held molding or trim.

***Motorized Seat Belt**—An automatic seat belt that is applied to an occupant and pretensioned by a motor-driven mechanism.

Motors—A machine that uses permanent and electromagnets to convert electrical energy into a rotation motion for doing work.

Mottling—Streaking of the color, usually with metallic finishes. It is caused by excessive wetting or a heavier film thickness in some areas.

***MSDS**—Material Safety Data Sheet. A document that provides safety, handling, storage, and clean-up information for hazardous materials.

Muffler—A metal chamber for dampening pressure pulsations to reduce exhaust noise.

Multimeter—A voltmeter, ohmmeter, and ammeter combined into one case. Also called a volt-ohm-milliammeter (VOM), it can be used to measure actual electrical values for comparison to known good values.

Multiple Part Rocker—An assembly of several pieces of sheet metal with internal reinforcements.

Multiple Pull Method—A method used on major damage, it involves several pulling directions, and steps are needed.

Multistage Finishes—A type of glamor finish.

N

National Institute for Automotive Service Excellence (ASE)—Offers a voluntary certification program that is recommended by the major vehicle manufacturers in the United States.

Needlenose Pliers—Pliers that have long, thin jaws for reaching in and grasping small parts.

Negative Camber—Top of the wheel is tilted inward when viewed from the front.

Negative Caster—Tilts the tops of the steering knuckles toward the front of the vehicle.

Negative Pressure Test—Part of the fit test. Performed by placing the palms of both hands over the cartridges and inhaling. A good fit is evident if the face piece collapses onto your face.

***Neoprene**—A synthetic rubber material that is resistant to acid and fuels.

***Neutral Flame**—A flame created by balancing the amounts of oxygen and fuel gas so that the inner and outer cones are at equal heights.

***Neutralize**—To cause a substance or surface to be neither acidic nor alkaline.

New Part Primer Coat—Replacement panels that are primed by the manufacturer or part supplier to protect the metal against rust.

***NGA**—National Glass Association. A national trade association that represents companies involved in both auto glass installations and architectural glass work.

***NIOSH**—National Institute for Occupational Safety and Health. A U.S. research group that develops methods for controlling worker exposure to chemical and physical hazards.

***Nitrile Rubber**—A type of fuel-resistant rubber used for the manufacture of protective gloves.

Nonbleeder Spray Gun—A type of spray gun that releases air only when the trigger is pulled back. It has an air control valve. The trigger controls both fluid needle movements and the air control valve.

Nonthreaded Fasteners—Fasteners that, as implied, do not use threads. They include keys, snaprings, pins, clips, adhesives, etc.

***Nugget**—The fused area of a plug weld or spot weld.

Nut—A fastener that uses internal (inside) threads and an odd shaped head that often fits a wrench. When tightened onto a bolt, a strong clamping force holds the parts together.

O

***OEM**—Original equipment manufacturer. The original maker of a vehicle or equipment.

OEM Finishes—Factory paint jobs.

Office Manager—This employee's duties include various aspects of the business such as handling letters, estimates, and receipts. In many small shops, the office manager also acts as the parts manager and bookkeeper.

Offset Butt Joint—A basic joint without an insert. It is also known as a staggered butt joint.

Offset Screwdrivers—Have a shank at a 90-degree angle to the tip and are used in restricted areas like inside glove boxes.

Ohm's Law—A math formula for calculating an unknown electrical value (amps, volts, or ohms) when two values are known.

Oil Can—A can with a long spout for applying oil to hard-to-reach areas. Often is used to lubricate parts and air tools.

Oil Dipstick—A device used to check the oil level.

Oil Drain Plug—It is located in the oil pan for draining and changing the engine oil.

Oil Filter—It traps debris and prevents it from circulating through the engine oil galleries.

Oil Pan—It holds an extra supply of motor oil. Also known as the sump, it bolts to the bottom of the engine block.

One-Part Putty—Spot putty applied directly out of tube or container. It takes longer to harden than two-part and can shrink more easily.

Open Circuit—An unwanted break in an electrical circuit.

Open Coat Sandpaper—A type of grit on sandpaper and discs; the resin that bonds the grit to the paper only touches the bottom of the grit.

Open-End Wrench—A wrench with three-sided jaws on both ends.
Open Time—*See* Work Life.
Opened—A circuit that is disconnected.
Operating Manual—Publications provided to give detailed information on using the exact type of tool or equipment properly.
Orange Peel—A paint roughness problem that looks like tiny dents in the paint surface, caused when droplets formed in the spray pattern hit the surface and dry before they have time to flow out. This paint problem resembles the skin of an orange.
Orbital Action Polisher—Power tool that moves polishing compound in a random manner to prevent swirl marks left from machine compounding.
Orbital Sander—A dual action sander that moves in two directions at the same time. It produces a much smoother surface finish.
Orifice—A hole in the bottom of the viscosity cup.
Oscillating Sander—This sander spins a sanding pad that is mounted to a concentric shaft that also has a counterweight on it. It sands more smoothly and faster than some other sanders.
OSHA-Approved Blow Gun—Approved by the Occupational Safety and Health Administration, this blow gun has pressure-relief holes in the nozzle tip that help prevent injury if the blow gun is accidentally pressed against your body.
Overhaul—To remove an assembly from the vehicle, disassemble, clean, inspect, replace parts as needed, reassemble, install, and adjust (except wheel and suspension alignment).
Overhead Welding—Welding position in which the piece is turned upside down.
Overlap—Occurs when replacement of one part duplicates some labor operation required to replace an adjacent part.
Overlap Strokes—The process of making each spray gun coat cover about half of the previous coat of paint.
Overlay—A large, self-adhesive vinyl material applied to the finish that provides an easy way to customize the looks of a vehicle.
Overlay Dry Method—A method of installing stripes or decals that does not involve the use of soapy water. All surfaces are clean and dry.
Overlay Wet Method—A method of installing stripes or decals that involves using soapy water to help simplify the application of larger decals and striping.
Overmasked—A term that means the painter must touch up the part of the vehicle that should have been painted.
Overpulling—Pulling the damage slightly beyond its original dimension in a controlled way so that the metal will flex back slightly when tension is released and line up properly.
Overpulling Damage—Results from failing to measure accurately and often when pulling on unibody vehicles.
***Overspray**—Sprayed material that falls outside the intended spray area.
Overspray Leak—The term that describes the results of not sealing the masking paper or plastic and getting overspray on unwanted surfaces.
***Oxidation**—The residue that forms on metal, or the dull layer which forms on the surface of paint. Oxidation occurs when the base material combines with oxygen.
Oxidizing Flame—It is obtained by mixing slightly more oxygen than acetylene.
Oxyacetylene Welding—A form of fusion welding in which oxygen and acetylene are used in combination.
Oxyacetylene Welding Outfit—Parts of an oxyacetylene welder: These include a tank, called a cylinder, that holds acetylene and the other oxygen; special valves, called regulators, that control the amount of gas pressure going to the welding torch; hoses that run from the regulators to the torch; and the torch itself, which mixes oxygen and acetylene in the proper proportions and produces a flame capable of melting steel.
Oxygen Pressure—Pressure leaving oxygen pressure regulator of oxyacetylene welding outfit. Typically ranges from 5 to 100 psi (kPa).

P

Package Tray—*See* Rear Shelf.
Pad Cleaning Tool—A metal star wheel and handle that will clean dried polishing compound out of the pad.
Paint—A term that generally refers to the visible paint.
Paint Adhesion Check—A test to see if the old paint is adhering properly.
Paint Binder—The ingredient in a paint that holds the pigment particles together.
Paint Blending—Tapering the new paint gradually into the old paint.
Paint Booth Area—An area where the body is painted. Also known as the finishing area.
Paint Drying Room—A dust-free room that speeds up drying, produces a cleaner job, and increases the volume of refinishing work.
Paint Film Breakdown—A term for checking, cracking, or blistering of paint.
Paint Formula—The percentage of each ingredient that is needed to match an OEM color.
Paint Gloss—Surface shine of paint.
Paint Mixing—Blending the paint and thinner or reducer to the correct thickness or viscosity.
Paint Mixing Instructions—Directions on how to mix the paint; usually given on the paint can label.
Paint Mixing Room—A safe, clean, well-lit area for a painter to store, mix, and reduce paint materials.
Paint Mixing Sticks—Used to help mix paints, solvents, catalysts, and other additives right before spraying.
Paint Overlap—The area where one vertical painted area overlaps the new area being painted.
Paint Overspray—An unwanted paint mist that spreads away from the surface being painted.
Paint Part Edge—Edge where old paint and new paint meet.
Paint Prep Area—An area where the vehicle is readied for painting or refinishing.
Paint Preparation—Preparing the vehicle for spraying or refinishing.

Paint Reference Charts—Found in service manuals, they give comparable paints manufactured by different companies.
Paint Runs—Excess paint thickness flows down when spraying.
Paint Sanding—Needed before painting or when the finish is rough or in poor shape and to level and smooth primed areas.
Paint Scuffing—A term used to describe roughing the paint for better paint adhesion.
Paint Sealer—An innercoat between the paint and the primer or old finish to prevent bleeding.
Paint Selection—Determining the right paint for the job, so that the new paint matches the old and to ensure long life.
Paint Settling—A term that describes when the paint sits idle and pigments, metallic flakes, or mica particles settle to the bottom.
Paint Shop Area—Area in facility where the vehicle is refinished.
Paint Solvent—The liquid solution that carries the pigment and binder so it can be sprayed.
Paint Stirring Sticks—Wooden sticks for mixing the contents after they are poured into the spray gun cup or container.
Paint Strainer—A paper funnel-mesh strainer that keeps debris out of the spray gun.
Paint Stripper—A powerful chemical that dissolves paint for fast removal of an old finish.
Paint Surface Chips—A result of mechanical impact damage to the paint film: door dings, damage from road debris, etc.
Paint Surface Protrusion—A particle of paint or other debris sticking out of the paint film after refinishing.
Paint System—All materials (primers, catalysts, paints) are compatible and manufactured by the same company.
Paint Thickness—Measurement of distance between surface of paint and body of vehicle. Viscosity of paint; affected by reduction or thinning.
Paint Viscosity—A term that refers to the paint's thickness or ability to resist flow.
Painted Flames—A custom painting technique often used on "hot rods" or older street rods.
Painter Prep Area—A shop area that provides a clean area for a painter to dress, a clean storage for painting suits, and a place to clean and store personal safety equipment.
Painter's Stretch Hood—Protective head gear for the paint booth.
Painting—This involves spraying primer and paint over the properly prepared vehicle body surface.
Painting Environment—The suitable conditions for painting, that is, cleanliness, temperature/humidity, light, and compressed air/pressure.
Paintless Dent Removal—A method of using picks to remove small dents without having to repaint the panel.
Pan—A floor-related component, for example, front floor pan.
Panel—A general term that refers to a large removable body part.
Panel Alignment Marks—Marks that can be provided on new parts to help position them for welding.
Panel Cutters—A tool that will precisely cut sheet metal, leaving a clean, straight edge that can be easily welded.
Panel Repairs—Repairs that involve painting/refinishing a complete body part separated by a definite boundary, such as a door or fender.
Panel Replacement—Removing and installing a new panel or body part.
Panel Straightening—Bending or shaping the panel back to its original position, using hand tools and equipment.
Parallax Error—Results when you read a rule or scale from an angle, instead of looking straight down. Viewing at an angle causes you to read the wrong line on the scale.
Parallel Circuit—A circuit that has two or more legs or paths for current. Current can flow through either leg independently.
Parallelogram Steering—Uses two tie-rod assemblies connected to the steering arms to support a long center link.
Part Gap—Also known as clearance, it is the distance measured between two adjacent parts, hood-to-fender gap, for example.
Part Location Diagram—Diagram included in some service manuals for finding electrical parts (harnesses, sensors, switches, computers, etc.).
Partial Cutout Method—Method of windshield replacement that uses some of the original adhesive, which serves as a base for the new adhesive.
Partial Frame—A frame that is a cross between a solid frame and a unibody.
Particle Respirator—*See* Dust Respirator.
Parts Manager—A person in charge of ordering, receiving, and distributing parts.
Passenger-Side Air Bag—Mounted behind a small door in the side of the instrument panel, deploys during frontal impacts.
***Passive Restraint System**—Any restraint system that does not require activation by the occupant to be effective, such as an automatic seat belt or supplemental air bag system.
***Pathogen**—A disease-causing agent, usually in a medium such as blood.
Pattern Control Knob—A part of the spray gun; when closed, the spray pattern is round. As the knob is opened, the spray becomes more oblong in shape.
PC—*See* Personal Computer.
PCV—Positive crankcase ventilation system. It channels engine crankcase blowby gases into the engine intake manifold.
Pearl Paint—Paint with medium size reflective pigment particles, such as mica, that give it luster or shine that tends to change color with the viewing angle.
Peeling—A paint problem that shows up as a separation of the surface film from the subsurface, caused by improper surface preparation or incompatibility of one coat to another.
Pencil Mil Gauge—Measures paint/refinishing materials with a calibrated magnet and spring setup.
Percentage Reduction—Materials must be added in certain proportions or parts.
Perimeter Frame—A frame that has the frame rail near the outside or perimeter of the vehicle.

Personal Computer—Also referred to as a PC, it is used to keep track of business transactions, complete damage reports, and perform electrical tests on vehicles.

Phillips Screwdriver—A hand tool that has two crossing blades for a star-shaped screw head.

Physical Injury—A general category that includes cuts, broken bones, strained backs, and similar injuries.

Piano Wire—Fine steel wire that can be used to cut the adhesive around glass.

Picking Hammers—Hammers with a pointed end used to raise small dents from the inside, and a flat end for hammer-and-dolly work to remove high spots and ripples.

Picks—Tools used to reach into confined spaces for removing tiny dents or dings.

Pickup Truck—A body style that has a separate cab and bed, typically with a front-engine, RWD.

Pigments—Fine powders that impart color, opacity, durability, and other characteristics to the primer or paint.

Pillars—Vertical body members that hold the roof panel in place and protect in case of a rollover accident.

Pin Holes—Small holes or blistering over plastic filler caused by air bubbles raising the surface film.

Pin Punch—It has a straight shank for use after a starting punch. It will push a shaft completely out of a hole.

Pin Striping Brushes—Brushes with very long soft horse hairs that are used to apply paint in a small, controlled area.

Pin Striping Tool—A serrated roller to deposit a painted pin stripe.

Pinchweld Clamps—Attached to the body at the front and rear of the rocker panel pinchwelds; four are normally used.

***Pinchweld**—A flange extending from the body of a vehicle into the opening for glass parts, usually extending from the side pillars and roof.

Pins—Devices used by equipment manufacturers to retain parts in alignment.

Pinstripe Brushes—Used to apply paint in small, controlled areas and can also be used to touch up chips along the lower body panel that were not painted.

Pipe Wrench—A type of adjustable wrench for holding and turning round objects. It has sharp jaw teeth that dig into and grasp the part.

Piston—Part of the engine that transfers the energy of combustion (burning of an air-fuel mixture) to the connecting rod.

Pitch—Spacing between resistance spot welds.

***Pitman Arm**—The arm that converts the rotary motion of the steering gear sector shaft to the side-to-side movement of the center link in a parallelogram steering system.

Pitting—A problem where small holes form in the paint film. Similar to blistering. Also called cratering.

Plasma Arc Cutting—Method of cutting metal that creates an intensely hot air stream over a very small area that melts and removes metal, making extremely clean cuts possible. Because of the tight focus of the heat, there is no warpage, even when cutting thin sheet metal.

***Plastic Adhesion Promoter**—A special primer containing adhesion promoters for refinishing plastics.

Plastic Adhesive Repair System—A high-strength glue or epoxy used to repair damage to plastic parts.

Plastic Bleed-Through—A discoloration, often a yellowing, of the color due to chemicals from the body filler. Although it is very rare today, it may be caused by too much hardener or by applying the paint before the body filler is fully cured.

***Plastic Cleaner**—A cleaner used to remove contaminants from a plastic repair area before starting a repair, and again before applying primers or paint.

Plastic Deformation—Ability of metal to be bent or formed into different shapes.

Plastic Flame Treating—A torch flame is used to oxidize and chemically prepare the plastic for adhesion.

Plastic Gloves—Used to protect hands from the harmful effects of corrosive liquids, undercoats, and finishes.

Plastic Hammer—A hammer used for making light blows where parts can be easily damaged.

Plastic Memory—A term that refers to plastic that wants to keep or return to its original molded shape.

Plastic Speed Welding—A type of welding that uses a specially designed tip to produce a more uniform weld and at a high rate of speed.

Plastic Stitch-Tamp Welding—A type of welding used primarily on hard plastics, like ABS and nylon, to ensure a good base/rod mix.

Plastic Welder—A tool used to heat and melt plastic for repairing or joining plastic parts.

Plastic Welding—Uses heat and sometimes a plastic filler rod to join or repair plastic parts.

Plastics—Refers to a wide range of materials synthetically compounded from crude oil, coal, natural gas, and other substances. *See also* Composites.

Pliers—A hand tool used for working with wires, clips, and pins. They will grasp and hold parts, like your fingers.

***Plug Weld**—A weld where two or more pieces of metal are joined by filling a hole in the outer pieces while penetrating into the underlying pieces.

Pneumatic—Equipment operated by air under pressure.

Pneumatic Windshield Cutters—Devices that use shop air pressure and a vibrating action to help cut the adhesive around glass.

Pocket Scale—Very small measurement tool (typically 6 in. or 152 mm long). It will clip into your shirt pocket and can be handy for numerous small measurements. Also called a pocket rule.

Point-to-Point Measurement—A term that refers to the shortest distance between two points.

Polishing—Using very fine compound to bring the paint surface up to full gloss.

Polishing Compound—Also called machine glaze, it is a fine grit compound designed for machine applications.

Polishing Pad—A cotton or synthetic cloth cover that fits over the polisher's backing plate.

***Polyester Putty**—A material used to fill and level minor surface imperfections and low areas.

***Polypropylene Primer**—A special primer containing adhesion promoters for refinishing polyolefin plastics.

Pop Rivets—A fastener used to hold two pieces of sheet metal together.

***Porosity**—The presence of holes or voids within a weld bead or nugget.

Portable Hydraulic Rams—Small oil-filled piston and cylinder assemblies for removing minor damage.

Portable Power Units—Small hydraulic piston and cylinder assemblies for removing minor damage.

Portable Puller—A hydraulic ram and post mounted on caster wheels.

Portable Pulling/Pushing Arm—Hydraulic operated metal beam that pulls on the chain to remove major structural damage to the vehicle.

Positive Camber—Top of the wheel is tilted out, when viewed from the front.

Positive Caster—Tilts the tops of the steering knuckles toward the rear of the vehicle.

Positive Pressure Test—Part of the fit test. Performed by covering up the exhalation valve and exhaling. A proper fit is evident if the face piece billows out without air escaping from the mask.

Postpainting Operations—Things done after painting, such as removing masking tape, reinstalling parts, and cleaning the vehicle.

Power Brakes—A standard hydraulic brake system with the addition of a vacuum, hydraulic, or electric assist. A booster unit is added to help apply the master cylinder and brakes.

Power Grinding—Using an air grinder to quickly remove large amounts of paint and other materials.

Power Sanding—Using an air sander to begin smoothing operations, often to level surface imperfections.

Power Steering Hoses—Carry the oil to and from the power steering pump.

Power Steering Pump—Forces pressurized oil through the steering system.

Power Tools—Use air pressure or electrical energy to aid repairs. These include air wrenches, air and electric drills, sanders, and similar tools.

Power Winch—Uses an electric motor and steel cable to provide a means of pulling the damaged vehicle onto the rack or tow truck.

Powertrain/Drivetrain—Includes all of the parts that produce and transfer power to the drive wheels, including the engine, transmission or transaxle, drive axle(s), and other related parts.

Preexisting Damage—Damage that includes paint cracking, scratches in paint, and acid rain damage that is unrelated to current repairs and may have to be repaired before the new finish can be applied.

Premixed—Material that is ready to spray.

Prep Solvent—A fast-drying solvent often used to clean a vehicle. It removes wax, oil, grease, and other debris that could contaminate and ruin the paint job.

Pressure-Feed Spray Guns—Air tools that force primer or paint into the air stream to atomize liquid material into a fine mist that adheres to and thinly coats the surface of vehicle.

Pressure Gauge—A device that reads in pounds per square inch or kilograms per square centimeter.

Pressurized Pot—Also referred to as a pressure cup spray gun, it uses air pressure inside the paint cup or tank to force the material out of the gun.

***Primary Damage**—Damage, at or near the point of impact, caused by the collision. Also called direct damage.

Primecoat Show-Through—A problem in which the color of the primecoat is seen through the paint, caused by insufficient colorcoats or repeated compounding, as well as not having uniform color under the paint.

***Primer**—An undercoat or chemical applied to a surface to improve the adhesion, durability, and appearance of a paint or the bond of an adhesive.

Primer-Filler—A very thick form of primer-surfacer. It is sometimes used when a very pitted or rough surface must be a filled and smoothed quickly.

***Primer-Sealer**—An undercoat used to protect the primer from the solvents in the paint.

***Primer-Surfacer**—A high-solid type of primer used to level and fill small imperfections in a surface.

Priming—Primarily is done to help smooth the body surface and help topcoats of paint adhere or stick to the body. It is done before painting.

Printer—Used to make hard copies (printed images on paper) of electronic estimates for the customer and repair information for technicians.

Productivity—A measure of how much work you get done.

Professionalism—A broad trait that includes everything from being able to follow orders, to pride in workmanship. A professional does everything "by the book." He or she never cuts corners (for instance, leaving out a hard-to-reach bolt) trying to get a repair finished.

Progression Shop—An assembly line type of organization with specialists in each area of repair.

Propellant Charge—Part of the air bag assembly, converts sodium azide to nitrogen gas as it burns, filling the air bag in a fraction of a second. As the air bag inflates, the steering wheel cover or dash is forced to split open allowing full inflation.

Proportional Numbers—Denote the amount of each material needed. The first number is usually the parts of paint needed. The second number is usually the solvent (or reducer). A third number might be used to denote the amount of hardener or other additives required.

***psi**—Pounds per square inch. A unit of pressure or stress activation by the occupant to be effective, such as an automatic seat belt or supplemental airbag system.

Pull Rods—These have a handle and curved end for light pulling of dents.

Pull Welding—You aim or angle the gun back toward the weld puddle.

Pulling Adaptors—Special straightening equipment accessories that allow you to pull in difficult situations.

Pulling Clamps—They bolt around or onto the vehicle, so a pulling chain can be attached to the vehicle.

Pulling Equipment—It uses hydraulic power to force the body structure or frame back into position.

Pulling Posts—Also known as towers, they are strong steel members used to hold the pulling chains and hydraulic rams.

Punches—Tools used for driving and aligning operations.

Purging—Uses refrigerant to push air and dirt out of the hoses to prevent air and other contaminants from being pushed into the vehicle's A/C system.

Push-In Clips—Usually made of plastic, they are used to hold body panels.

Push Welding—You aim or angle the gun ahead of the weld puddle.
Pushrods—Hollow tubes that transfer motion from the lifters to rocker arms in engine.

Q

Quarter Panels—Large, side body sections that extend from the side doors back to the rear bumper, usually welded in place and form a vital part of the rear body structure.

R

R & I—To remove and install.
R & R—To remove and replace.
***R-12 Refrigerant**—A type of refrigerant containing chlorofluorocarbon (CFC).
***R-134a Refrigerant**—A type of refrigerant containing hydrochlorofluorocarbon (HFC).
***Race**—The inner or outer bearing surface of a ball- or roller-bearing assembly. The balls or rollers support the load by rolling between the surfaces of the races.
Rack—A toothed shaft (a bar with a row of teeth cut into one edge) that meshes with a pinion gear in rack-and-pinion steering systems.
***Rack-and-Pinion Assembly**—A steering gear system in which the rotary motion of a pinion gear is converted to a side-to-side movement of a rack, the ends of which are attached to the steering arms by tie rods.
Rack-and-Pinion Steering—Uses a simplified steering system that weighs less and takes up less space than parallelogram steering. Now used on most passenger vehicles.
Rack Straightening System—Generally a drive-on system with a built-in anchoring and pulling mechanism.
Radiator—Transfers coolant heat to the outside air.
Radiator Cap Pressure Rating—Stamped on the cap, it is the amount of pressure the cap is designed to maintain.
Radiator Cap Pressure Test—A test done using a cooling system pressure tester. The tester gauge should stop increasing its pressure reading when the cap rating is reached.
Radiator Core Support—The framework around the front of the body structure for holding the cooling system radiator and related parts.
Radiator Fan—Draws outside air through the radiator to remove heat.
Radiator Pressure Cap—Prevents the coolant from boiling.
Raising—To work a dent outward or away from the body.
Ratchet—A common type of socket drive handle with a small lever that can be moved for either loosening or tightening bolts and nuts.
Reading Tires—Involves inspecting tire tread wear and diagnosing the cause.
Rear Axle Assembly—Housing that contains the ring gear, pinion gear, differential assembly, and axles.
Rear Bulkhead Panel—A panel that separates the passenger compartment from the rear trunk area.
Rear-Engine, Rear-Wheel Drive (RRD)—A vehicle that has the engine in the back and a transaxle transfers power to the rear drive wheels.
Rear Hatch—A large panel and glass assembly hinged for more access to the rear of the vehicle.
Rear Pillars—Pillars that extend up from the quarter panels to hold the rear of the roof and rear window glass. Also called C-pillars.
Rear Seat Air Bags—Fit into the rear cushion of the front seats. They inflate to protect the passengers in the rear seat from injury in a frontal collision. They are not very common but can be found in a few expensive luxury vehicles.
Rear Section—Also known as tail section or rear clip, it consists of the rear quarter panels, trunk or rear floor pan, rear frame rails, trunk or deck lid, rear bumper, and related parts.
Rear Shelf—A thin panel behind the rear seat and in front of the back glass. It often has openings for rear stereo speakers. Also known as package tray.
Rear Shock Towers—Parts that hold the top of the rear suspension.
Rear Spoiler—A part that mounts in the trunk lid to alter the airstream at the rear of the body to increase body down force. This helps rear wheel traction at highway speeds.
Rear-Wheel Drive—Vehicles that use a conventional transmission, drive shaft, and rear axle assembly to transfer power to the rear drive wheels.
Rebound—Motion caused by a wheel going into a dip or returning from a jounce and extending the spring.
Receiver-Driers—Part in the air-conditioning system that removes moisture and acids, located between the condenser and expansion device.
Recovery Station—A machine used to capture the old, used refrigerant so that it does not enter and pollute the atmosphere.
Recovery System—Service equipment that captures the old used refrigerant from the vehicle and keeps it from entering and contaminating the earth's atmosphere. It can clean and process used refrigerant for reuse or recycling in another vehicle.
Recycled Assemblies—Undamaged parts from another damaged vehicle that are used for repairs.
Recycling—Process of capturing and filtering used materials (like paint solvent or refrigerant) so that they can be reused again.
***Reference Points**—Identifiable points on a vehicle that may be used for measurement when a control point is not available.
Refinishing—This involves applying primer, sealer, and paint over the properly prepared vehicle body.
Refinishing Materials—A general term referring to the products used to repaint the vehicle.
Refinishing System—Indicates that all materials used in refinishing (primers, catalysts, reducers, colors, and clears) are compatible and manufactured by the same company.
***Refractometer**—An instrument used to measure the specific gravity of a liquid.
***Regulator**—The mechanism that moves the glass when activated by a switch or crank.
Reinforced Reaction Injection Molded (RRIM) Polyurethane—A two-part polyurethane composite plastic. Part A is the isocyanate. Part B contains the

reinforced fibers, resins, and a catalyst. The parts are mixed and injected into a mold.

Related Professions—Jobs that require an understanding of auto body repair, such as an insurance agent or adjuster or paint manufacturer sales representative.

***Relative Humidity**—The amount of water vapor in the air, expressed as a percentage of the maximum amount the air can hold under current conditions of temperature and pressure. Rain or fog forms when the relative humidity reaches 100%.

Relay—A remote control switch, used in electrical components.

***Release Agent**—A solvent used to soften adhesives or sealants.

Reliability—Being at work on time, being at work every day, and doing the job right.

Repair Charts—Give diagrams that guide you through logical steps for making repairs. They can vary in content and design. Most use arrows and icons (graphic symbols) that represent repair steps.

Repair Stall—A work area for one vehicle. Also termed a bay.

Resistance—A restriction or obstacle to current flow.

Respirators—Safety gear worn over the nose and mouth to keep airborne materials from being inhaled.

Restraint System—Designed to help hold people in their seats and prevent them from being injured during a collision.

Retarder—A slow-evaporating thinner or reducer used to retard or slow drying.

***Retrofit**—A postproduction change to improve the performance, or change the function, of a part or system using parts and procedures that have been tested.

Reveal Molding—Used to cover the adhesive, it is held in place by adhesive grooves in the body or by clips.

Reverse Masking—A masking method that requires you to fold the masking paper back and over the masking tape.

Reverse Polarity—Also called "DC reverse," it is when the electrode is positive and the workpiece is negative.

Rib Joint Pliers—Pliers that have several settings for grasping different size objects; also known as Channellock pliers.

Ribbon Sealers—Sealers that come in strip form and are applied by hand.

***Ride Height**—The height measurement, from the surface supporting tires to designated points on the vehicle structure, under conditions specified by the vehicle maker.

Right-Hand Threads—Nuts and bolts that must be turned clockwise to tighten.

Right-to-Know Laws—These regulations require that companies provide essential information and stipulations for safely working with hazardous materials.

Rivet Bonding—Uses adhesive and self-piercing metal rivets to join body panels on some aluminum unibody vehicles.

Rocker Arms—Levers that transfer camshaft action from the pushrods to the valves.

***Rocker Panels**—Either of two structural members, located below the doors, that support the door pillars and the floor pan. Also called door sills.

Rod Color Coding—A coding system for plastic rods indicating compatibility with various base materials.

Roof Panel—A large multipiece panel that fits over the passenger compartment.

Rosin-Core Solder—A type of solder designed for doing electrical repairs.

RRIM—Reinforced reaction injection molded, a two-part polyurethane composite plastic. Part A is the isocyanate. Part B contains the reinforced fibers, resins, and a catalyst. The parts are mixed and injected into a mold.

Rubber Body Insulators—Used between the frame and body to reduce noise and vibration.

Rubber Gloves—Used to protect hands from the harmful effects of corrosive liquids, undercoats, and finishes.

Rubber Mallet—A solid rubber head that is fairly heavy. It is often used to gently bump sheet metal without damaging the painted finish.

Rubber Seals—Used to prevent air and water leakage between body parts.

Rubberized Undercoat—A synthetic-based rubber material applied as a corrosion or rust preventive layer.

Rubbing Compound—Coarsest type of hand applied abrasive paste or compound. It will rapidly remove paint or clear but will leave tiny but visible scratch marks.

Ruler—Most basic tool for linear measurement. It has an accuracy of approximately 1/64 in. or 0.5 mm. Also called a scale.

***Runout**—Any radial or lateral variation in the dimensions of a part such as a wheel, brake rotor, or brake drum, measured as the part is rotated on its side.

***Runs and Sags**—A paint defect caused by excessive paint flowing unevenly down a surface, causing ridges and lines to form.

Rust Under Finish—Metal corrosion causes finish to peel or blister, or causes raised spots on the surface of paint film. Broken film has allowed moisture to creep under the surrounding finish. Usually caused by improper metal preparation, stone chips, or other problems.

S

***SAE**—Society of Automotive Engineers.

SAE-Metric Conversion Chart—Gives multipliers that can be used to convert from SAE to metric or from metric to SAE values.

SAE Rule—Measuring tool that has markings in fractions of an inch (1/2, 1/4, 1/8, 1/16) or in decimal parts of an inch (0.10, 0.20, 0.30, 0.40).

Safety—Involves working intelligently to prevent personal injury and property damage.

Safety Glasses—Eye protection suitable for minor danger.

Safety Program—A written shop policy designed to protect the health and welfare of personnel and customers.

Safety Signs—Provided to give information that helps to improve shop safety, such as fire exits, fire extinguisher locations, dangerous or flammable chemicals, and other information.

Safety Stands—Strong steel equipment designed to support a vehicle when someone works underneath it.

They have four legs to hold them steady and an extendible shoe on which the vehicle rests; also known as jack stands.

Safety Trigger—Safety catch on tool trigger that prevents a power tool from being turned on by accident.

Sag—*See* Runs and Sags.

Sag Damage—A condition where a section of the frame is lower than normal, generally is caused by a direct impact from the front or rear. It can occur on one side of the vehicle or on both sides.

***Salvage Part**—A part, removed from a vehicle being scrapped, that is intended to be used as a replacement part.

Sand Scratches—A result of final sanding with too coarse a sandpaper, or not allowing materials (usually primer-surfacer or spot putty) to dry fully before painting.

Sander Pad—A soft mounting surface for the sand paper.

Sanding—A method where an abrasive coated paper is used to level and smooth a body surface being repaired.

Sanding Blocks—Plastic or synthetic rubber support tool for sandpaper that comes in various shapes and sizes to match the shape of the body part being repaired.

Sanding Discs—Round sandpaper normally used on an air-powered orbital sander.

Sanding Sheets—Sandpaper in square sheets that can be cut to fit sanding blocks.

Sandpaper—A heavy paper coated with an abrasive grit. It is the most commonly used abrasive in auto body repair.

***Sandscratch Swelling**—A paint defect caused by solvents being absorbed into sandscratches.

Scale—Most basic tool for linear measurement. It has an accuracy of approximately 1/64 in. or 0.5 mm. Also called a ruler.

Scan Tool—A device used to read and convert computer fault codes.

Scanner Cartridge—Installed into the scanner for the specific make and model car or truck being tested. It holds the information needed for that vehicle.

Scanners—Devices used to diagnose or troubleshoot vehicle computer systems and wiring problems.

Scientific International (SI) System—*See* Metric Measuring System.

Screw-On Slide Hammer—Removes deeper dents and creases.

Screwdrivers—Hand tools used to rotate screws for installation or removal.

Screws—Threaded fasteners often used to hold nonstructural parts on a vehicle; trim pieces, interior panels, and so forth are often secured by screws.

Scuff Padding—The process of roughing a surface by light sanding or rubbing with a nylon scuff pad.

Scuff Pads—Tough synthetic pads used to clean and lightly scratch the surface of paints so the new paint will stick.

***Sealant**—Any of various liquids which, when applied to a joint, dry to form an airtight seal.

Sealer—Used to prevent water and air leaks between parts. It is flexible, which prevents cracking.

***Seam Sealer**—A material designed to keep moisture and fumes out of the passenger compartment and protect seams and joints from corrosion.

Seat Back—Rear seat assembly that includes the cover, padding, and metal frame.

Seat Belt Anchors—Devices that allow one end of the seat belt to be bolted to the body structure.

Seat Belt Buckle Mechanism—Allows you to put the seat belt on and take it off.

Seat Belts—Strong nylon straps with special ends attached for securing people in their seats.

Seat Covers—These protective covers help prevent vehicle seats from being stained.

Seat Cushion—Bottom section of the seat, which includes cover, padding, and frame.

Seat Cushion Sensors—Detect the weight of a person sitting in the passenger seat so that if no one is sitting in the passenger seat, the air bag system may not deploy the passenger air bag.

Seat Track—The mechanical slide mechanism that allows the seat to be adjusted forward or rearward.

***Secondary Damage**—Damage, beyond the point of impact, that resulted from the force of the collision. Also called indirect damage.

***Sectioning**—A repair made by cutting and removing the damaged portion of a panel and replacing it with an undamaged part, as opposed to replacing the damaged panel at factory seams.

Sedan—A body design with a center pillar that supports the roof. Sedans come in both 2- and 4-door versions.

Self-Centering Gauges—Gauges that show alignment or misalignment by projecting points on the vehicle's structure into the technician's line of sight.

Self-Darkening Filter Lenses—A welding filter lens that instantly turns dark when the arc is struck.

Self-Defrosting Glass—Windshield/window glass that has a conducting grid or invisible layer that carries electric current to heat the glass.

***Self-Etching Primer**—A primer which contains an etching agent, used in place of metal treatment before priming, to provide rust protection.

Self-Locking Nuts—Nuts that produce a friction or force fit when threaded onto a bolt or stud.

Self-Stick Sandpaper—Sandpaper with adhesive applied to it during manufacturing.

Self-Tapping Screws—Screws that have pointed tips to help cut new threads in parts.

Sensors—Devices that convert a condition (temperature, pressure, part movement, etc.) into an electrical signal. They send electrical input signals back to the computer, providing feedback for computer-assisted vehicle systems, such as with a computer-assisted steering system.

Series Circuit—A circuit with only one conductor path or leg for current through the circuit. Current must flow through the wires and components one after the other.

Series-Parallel Circuit—A circuit that has both series and parallel branches in it. It has characteristics of both circuit types.

Service Manual Abbreviations—Represent technical terms or words and saves space in the service manual.

Service Manuals—Yearly manuals published by the automotive manufacturers that describe the construction and repair of their vehicle makes and models.

Service Part—*See* Body ID Number.

Service Ports—Small test fittings in the air-conditioning system to which the air-conditioning gauges are connected.

Set-Back—When one wheel is moved back, creating an unequal wheelbase between the left and right sides of a vehicle.

Set Screws—Screws that frequently have an internal drive head for an Allen wrench. They are used to hold parts onto shafts.

Shading Coats—A progressive application of paint on the boundary of spot repair areas so that a color difference is not noticeable. Also referred to as blend coats.

Shakeproof Washers—Washers that have teeth or bent lugs that grip both the work and the nut. Several designs, shapes, and sizes are available. An external type has teeth on the outside and an internal type has teeth around the inside. Also called teeth lock washers.

Shear Strength—A measure of how well a material can withstand forces acting to cut or slice it apart.

Sheet Metal Gauge—Instrument used to measure body or repair panel thickness or gauge size (a number system that denotes the thickness of sheet metal).

Sheet Metal Screws—Screws that have pointed or tapered tips. They thread into sheet metal for light holding tasks.

Sheet Molded Compound (SMC)—Fiber-reinforced composite plastic panel.

***Shielding Gas**—A gas or mixture of gases used to protect a weld site from atmospheric contamination.

Shock Absorbers—Dampening devices that absorb spring oscillations (bouncing) to smooth the vehicle's ride quality. It is a part of the suspension system.

Shop Air Lines—Thick steel pipes that feed out from the air compressor tank to work stalls in the shop. Flexible air hoses connect to stationary air lines.

Shop Layout—General organization or arrangement of work areas in the repair facility, including fire exit routes, fire extinguisher locations, storage areas, frame racks, paint booth, etc.

Shop Office—Financial hub of the shop. Office workers handle paperwork, ensure estimates are accurate, pay bills, order parts, and distribute payroll checks.

Shop Owner—Maintains knowledge of all phases of the work done in the shop as well as its business operations.

Shop Supervisor—Handles the everyday operation of the shop and communication with all personnel.

Short Circuit—An unwanted wire-to-wire or wire-to-ground connection in an electrical circuit.

Short-Hair Fiberglass Filler A fiberglass filler with tiny particles of fiberglass in it. It works and sands almost like a conventional filler but is much stronger.

Short Spray Distance—A spray gun distance that causes the high-velocity mist to ripple the wet film.

Shoulder Belts—Seat belts that extend over a person's chest and shoulder.

Show-Through—When the old finish can be seen, to varying degrees, through the newly applied paint.

Shrinking Hammers—Finishing hammers with a serrated or cross-grooved face. They are used to shrink spots that have been stretched by excessive hammering.

Shrinking Metal—Removes strain or tension on damaged, stretched sheet metal.

Side Cut Pliers—Pliers that have cutting jaws that will clip off wires flush with a surface; they are also known as diagonal cutting pliers.

Side Draft Spray Booth—Moves air sideways over the car or truck. An air inlet in one wall pushes fresh air into the booth. A vent on the opposite wall removes the booth air.

Side Impact Air Bags—Deploy from the door panels, headliner, or from the side of the front seats.

Side Impact Beams—Strong metal bars or beams that bolt or weld inside the doorframe to protect the passengers from side impact damage during collision.

Side Orifices—Located on the spray gun air cap, they determine the spray pattern by means of air pressure.

Side Sway Damage—Damage that results from collision impacts that occur from the side.

Side-Tone View—Compares the test panel to the vehicle on a 45–60-degree angle.

Single Pull Method—A method that uses only one pulling chain; it works well with minor damage on one part.

Single-Sided Damage—Surface damage that does NOT penetrate or fracture the rear of the panel.

Single-Sided Plastic Welds—Plastic welding method used when the part cannot be removed from the vehicle.

Siphon Spray Guns—These use airflow through the gun head to form a suction that pulls paint into the air stream.

***Skim Coat**—A thin layer of material applied to a surface to cover imperfections.

Skin Hem—Folded door edge.

Skip Welding—It produces a continuous weld by making short welds at different locations to prevent overheating.

Slide Hammer—A type of puller that uses a hammering action to remove parts or straighten minor dents in the panels.

***Slip Yoke**—The yoke in a universal joint that is splined, transmitting torque to or from the driveshaft while allowing the effective length of the driveshaft to vary as the driven wheels move through the range of the suspension system.

Slip-Joint Pliers—Also known as combination pliers, they will adjust for two sizes.

Slotted Nuts—Also known as castellated nuts, they are grooved on top, so that a safety wire or cotter pin can be installed into a hole in the bolt.

Smoke Gun—A device used to find air leaks around doors and windows.

Snap-Fit Parts—Parts that use clips or interference fit to hold together.

Snap Ring Pliers—Pliers that have tiny tips for fitting into clips or snaprings. Both external and internal types are available.

Snap Rings—Nonthreaded fasteners that install into a groove machined into a part. They are used to hold parts on shafts.

Social Skills—Interpersonal skills that allow you to work as part of a team. Important so that other workers and customers like you.

Society of Automotive Engineers (SAE)—Developed a system of measurements that use fractions and decimals for giving number values. This system is primarily used in the U.S., not other countries.

Society of Automotive Engineers (SAE) Measuring System—First developed using human body parts as the basis for measurements. The length of the human arm was used to standardize the yard and the human foot devised the foot. Also called the English, U.S., customary, or conventional system. It is primarily used in the United States, but NOT in other countries.

Socket Drive Size—The size of the square opening for the drive handle.

Sockets—Cylinder-shaped, box-end wrenches for rapid turning of bolts and nuts.

***Sodium Hydroxide**—A caustic chemical (lye) found in small amounts with the talc residue, following an air bag deployment.

Soft Brazing—Brazing with materials that melt at temperatures below 900°F (468°C).

Softer Bristle Brushes—Brushes often used with cleaning solvent to remove oil and grease from parts.

Software—Computer programs and CDs used to speed up the estimating process.

Soldering—A process using moderate heat and solder to join wires or other parts.

Soldering Gun—A tool used to heat and melt solder for making electrical repairs.

***Solenoid**—A remotely operated device that converts an electrical input into a mechanical output for the purpose of actuating a latch, valve, switch, etc.

***Solid Axle**—A part of a suspension system in which the wheels are mounted at each end of a rigid beam or axle housing.

Solids—Nonliquid contents of the paint or primer.

***Solvent Reducer**—Any volatile liquid in which a substance can be dissolved, such as cleaning fluids, thinners, and fuels.

Sound-Deadening Materials—Insulation materials that prevent engine and road noise from entering the passenger compartment.

Sound-Deadening Pads—Plastic or asphalt-based material bonded to the inside surface of trunk cavities and doors to reduce noise, vibration, and harshness.

Space Frame—Similar to a unibody vehicle, a space frame vehicle has a metal body structure covered with an outer skin of plastic or composite panels.

Spacer Washers—Washers that come in specific thicknesses to allow for adjustment of parts or panels.

Spark Lighter—A device that produces a spark and ignites an oxyacetylene torch.

Spark Plug Wires—High-tension conductors with thick insulation that carry high coil voltage to each spark plug.

Spark Plugs—Use ignition coil high voltage to ignite the fuel mixture in the engine's combustion chambers.

Spatulas—Tools used to apply filler to low spots in body panels.

Specialty Shop—Repair facility that only works on one part or system of a vehicle.

Specific Gravity—Density of a liquid.

Specifications—Measurements for numerous body dimensions and mechanical parts.

Speed Handle—A tool that can be rotated to quickly remove or install loose bolts and nuts.

***Speed Sensor**—A sensor that provides an electrical speed signal to a control module.

Speed Welding Rate—Plastic speed welding rate, determined by the angle between the torch and the base material.

Spider Webbing—A technique accomplished by forcing paint through the air brush in a very thin, fibrous-type spray.

***Spindle**—The shaft-like portion of a suspension system that supports the wheel and bearings of an undriven wheel. May also refer to the hub of a driven wheel.

Split Lock Washers—Washers used under nuts to prevent loosening by vibration. The ends of these spring-hardened washers dig into both the nut and the work to prevent rotation.

Spontaneous Combustion—Occurs when a fire starts by itself.

Spoons—An instrument used to pry out damage, struck with a hammer to drive out damage, and as a dolly in hard-to-reach areas.

Spot Putty—Also called glazing putty, is used to fill minor surface imperfections in primer and paint.

Spot Repair—Involves minor body repair and painting an area smaller than the panel. The paint must be blended out to match the existing finish.

***Spot Weld**—A type of weld where two pieces of metal are fused together at a spot, using pressure and electric current, with no filler material.

Spot Weld Drill—A specially designed drill for removing spot-welded body panels.

Spouts—Insert these into a can for handy pouring.

Spray Booth—Designed to provide a clean, safe, well-lit enclosure for painting.

Spray Gun Air Cap—Works with the air valve to control the spray pattern of the paint. It screws over the front of the gun head.

Spray Gun Angle—A term that refers to whether the gun is tilted up or down or sideways.

Spray Gun Cap—It often fits onto the bottom of the spray gun body to hold the material to be sprayed.

Spray Gun Cup—A cup that fits onto the body of the spray gun and holds the material to be sprayed.

Spray Gun Distance—The distance from the gun tip to the surface being painted.

Spray Gun Lubrication—Placing a small amount of oil on packing and high friction points.

Spray Gun Speed—A term that refers to how fast the gun is moved sideways while painting.

Spray Gun Triggering—Involves stopping the paint spray before you stop moving the gun sideways.

Spray Gun Washer—Enclosed equipment that automatically cleans a spray gun.

Spray Guns—They atomize sealer, primer, paint, and other liquid so that it applies to vehicle surfaces smoothly and evenly.

Spray-Out Panel—A test panel that checks the paint color and also shows the effects of the painter's technique.

***Spray Pattern**—The pattern made by material sprayed from a stationary spray gun as it strikes a flat surface.

Spray Pattern Test—A process to check the operation of the spray gun on a piece of paper.

Spraying—The physical application of paint using a spray gun.

Spreaders—Tools used to apply filler to low spots in body panels.

Spring-Back—The tendency for metal to return to its original shape deformation.
Spring Hammering—A method of bumping damage with a hammer and a dinging spoon.
Spring Hangers—Chassis parts sometimes formed on the frame to hold the suspension system springs.
Spring Scale—A device that measures pulling force.
Square Keys—A type of nonthreaded fastener used to prevent hand wheels, gears, cams, and pulleys from turning on their shafts. These keys are strong enough to carry heavy loads if they are fitted and seated properly.
Squeeze-Type Resistance Spot Welding—A type of welding that uses electric current through the base metal to form a small, round weld between the base metals.
***Stabilizer Bar**—A transverse torsion bar, attached to the suspension system on the underside of the vehicle, to reduce roll. Also called antiroll bar.
Standard Screwdriver—A screwdriver with a single flat blade tip that fits into screws with slotted heads.
Starter Solenoid—When energized electrically, it connects the battery to the starting motor and sometimes pushes starter pinion gear into engagement with the flywheel ring gear on engine.
Starting Motor—A large DC motor for rotating the engine flywheel.
Starting Punch—Also known as a drift punch, it has a fully tapered shank and will drive pins, shafts, and rods partially out of holes.
Starting System—A large electric motor that turns the engine flywheel. This spins or "cranks" the crankshaft until the engine starts and runs on its own power.
Station Wagon—A roof/body style that extends the roof straight back to the rear of the body.
Stationary Parts—Parts that are permanently welded or adhesive-bonded into place, like the floor, roof, and quarter panels.
Steel Brushes—These metal brushes can be used to remove rust and dirt from parts.
Steering Axis Inclination (SAI)—Angle between true vertical and a line through the upper and lower pivot points, as viewed from the front.
Steering Column—Part of the steering system that transfers steering wheel rotation through firewall and to steering rack or pitman arm.
Steering Gearbox—Changes the wheel rotation into side movement for turning the front wheels of the vehicle.
***Steering Knuckles**—That part of the steering system that supports the wheel spindle or hub and pivots about the steering axis.
Steering System—It transfers steering wheel motion through gears and linkage rods to swivel the front wheels.
Steering Wheel Center Check—A test that involves making sure the steering wheel has not been moved off center to do part damage.
Stick Arc Welding—Also known as shielded arc welding, it uses a welding rod coated with a flux for fusion welding.
Stitch Welding—A continuous weld in one location, but with short pauses to prevent overheating.
Stool Creeper—A small seat with caster wheels that allows you to sit and move around on the shop floor while working; provides a handy place to lay tools.
Straight Polarity—Also called "DC straight," it is when the electrode is negative.
Straightening—Refers to using alignment equipment to pull or push damaged metal back out to its original shape.
Straightening Equipment—Anchoring equipment, pulling equipment, and other accessories used to apply tremendous force to move the frame or body structure back into alignment.
Straightening System Accessories—Various pulling chains, clamps, hooks, adapters, straps, and stands needed to mount, pull, and repair all makes and models of vehicles.
Stress Concentrators—Designed into unibody vehicles to control and absorb collision forces, minimize structural damage, and increase occupant protection.
Stress Relieve—A process using heat and or hammering to relax work-hardened metal while pulling.
Stressed Hull Structure—Engineering concept behind unibody design, in which a sheet metal is welded to form a box- or egg-like configuration so that strength is achieved through shape and design of the individual parts instead of their mass and weight and the entire inner structure works together for structural integrity.
Stretched Metal—Metal that has been forced thinner in thickness and larger in surface area by impact.
Stripping—Applying a chemical remover or air-powered blasting equipment to soften and lift off paint.
Structural Adhesive—An adhesive used to bond parts together; used in place of welds.
Structural Filler—Used to fill the larger gaps in the panel structure while maintaining strength. It adds to the structural rigidity of the part.
Structural Parts—Those parts of a vehicle that support the weight of the vehicle, absorb collision energy, and absorb road shock.
Strut Position Check—A test to check the position of the struts, thus determining if there is any damage.
Strut Pulling Plates—A device designed to bolt onto the top of shock towers for pulling.
Strut Rotation Check—A test to see if the strut is damaged.
Strut Tower Gauge—Allows visual alignment of the upper body area. It shows misalignment of the strut tower/upper body parts in relation to the vehicle's centerline plane and datum plane.
Strut Towers—Reinforced body areas for holding the upper parts of the suspension system. Also called shock towers.
Stubby Screwdrivers—These drivers have very short shanks to fit into tight or restricted areas.
Stud Spot Welder—It joins pull rods on the surface of a panel so that you do not have to drill holes. It is the best way to pull dents.
Sub-Frame Assemblies—Part of a partial frame, used at the front and rear while the unibody supports the middle area of the vehicle. The sub-frame is used to support the suspension and drivetrain.
Substrate—Steel, aluminum, plastic, and composite materials used in the vehicle's construction.
Suction Cup Tools—Large synthetic rubber cups for sticking onto parts. They are often used to hold

window glass when holding or moving the glass, and also to pop out large surface area dents in panels.

Suction Gun—Removes or extracts liquid. Pull on the handle and a fluid is sucked into the tool.

Sunlight—The standard by which other light sources are measured. It contains the entire visible spectrum of light.

Support Members—Used in high-stress areas and often bolted to the bottom of the unibody to hold the engine, transmission, and suspension in alignment, and to reduce body flex.

Surface Evaluation—A close inspection of the old paint to determine its condition.

Surface High Spot—An area that shows up when sanding quickly cuts through the guide coat.

Surface Inspection—Examining the old body surface condition before preparing it for new paint.

Surface Low Spot—An area that shows up when sanding will not remove the guide coat.

Surface Paint Chips—Paint damage resulting from mechanical impact to the finish: door dings, damage from road debris, etc.

Surface Preparation—Careful cleaning and sanding of surfaces to be painted ensures that the repairs and new paint will hold up over time.

Surface Protrusion—A particle of dirt, paint, or other debris sticking out of the film after refinishing, caused by a lack of cleanliness.

Surface Roughness—A measurement of paint film or other surface smoothness in a limited area.

Surface Temperature Thermometer—When using a paint drying room, it measures panel temperatures to prevent overheating damage.

Surface Waviness—A measurement of an area's general levelness or trueness.

Suspension System—It allows the tires and wheels to move up and down with road surface irregularities.

Swirl Marks—Round or curved lines in the paint caused by buffing.

Swivel Sockets—Cylinder-shaped, box-end wrenches that have a universal joint between the drive end and socket body.

Symmetrical—When the dimensions on the right side of the vehicle are equal to the dimensions on the left side of the vehicle.

Systemic Approach—An organized and logical sequence of steps to accomplish a task or job.

T

T-Handles—Two-part tools that fit over the tap, die or socket wrench for turning.

Tabulation Chart—A chart used to log reference point measurements during a repair.

***Tack**—To wipe very small particles from a surface using a special cloth, called a tack cloth.

Tack Cloth—A rag with coating that holds dust and debris.

Tack Coat—Also known as mist coat, it is a very light mist coat applied to the surface first. It allows the application of heavier wet coats without sagging or runs.

Tack Rag—A cloth used to remove any loose dust and other debris on vehicle surfaces.

***Tack Weld**—A small, temporary weld placed at intervals along a joint to hold the pieces in alignment.

Tailgate—A door that allows access to the rear of a station wagon.

Tap—A tool for cutting inside threads in holes, used to repair damaged threaded holes.

Tape Rule—Also known as a tape measure, it will extend out for making very long measurements.

Taper Pins—Pins with a larger diameter on one end than on the other. They are used to locate and position matching parts or to secure small pulleys and gears to shafts.

Teeth Lock Washers—*See* Shakeproof Washers.

***Tempered Glass**—A strong, break-resistant type of safety glass that, if broken, shatters into small granular pieces.

***Tensile Strength**—The maximum force per unit area that a material can withstand in tension before failure occurs. Commonly expressed in kilopascals (pounds per square inch).

Tension—Measures both yield stress and ultimate strength of a material.

***Tensioner**—A device in a seat belt system which automatically tightens the belt around an occupant when there is sudden deceleration of the vehicle.

Test Light—An instrument used to determine if there is current flowing through the circuit.

Thermal Melt Stick—*See* Heat Crayon.

Thermal Paint—Used to determine the temperature of the aluminum or other metal being heated. It melts at a specific temperature and warns you of high heat to prevent overheating damage.

Thermometers—Devices used to measure temperature.

Thermoplastics—Plastics that can be repeatedly softened and reshaped by heating, with no change in their chemical makeup. They soften or melt when heated and harden when cooled.

***Thermosetting Plastics**—Plastics that are heated during manufacture and molded into a fixed shape. After manufacture, the shape cannot be altered by heat.

Thermostat—Regulates coolant flow and system operating temperature.

Thread Pitch—A measurement of bolt and nut thread coarseness. Bolts and nuts can have coarse, fine, and metric threads.

Thread Pitch Gauge—A device that measures bolt thread pitch.

Three Body Sections—For simplicity and to help communication in the auto body repair, a vehicle is divided into front, center, and rear sections.

***Three-Dimensional Measuring System**—A measuring system that can locate points with the dimensions of length, width, and height relative to three defined reference planes.

***Thrust Angle**—The angle between the centerline of the vehicle and an imaginary line that is parallel to the track of the rear wheels. Ideally, the thrust angle should be zero.

Tie-Rod Ends—There are two that thread onto the end of the rack and are covered by rubber bellows boots in the rack-and-pinion steering unit.

Tin Snips—This common metal cutting tool can be used to cut straight or curved shapes in sheet metal or to trim panels to size.

Tinted Glass—Window/windshield glass that contains a shaded vinyl material to filter out most of the sun's glare, helpful in reducing eye strain and prevents fading of the interior.

Tinting—Altering the paint color slightly to better match the new finish with the old finish.

Tire Pressure Gauge—Tool that accurately measures tire air pressure in pounds per square inch (psi) or kilopascals when pressed over the tire valve stem.

***Toe**—The angle that the tires point inward or outward relative to straight ahead when viewed from above the vehicle.

Toe-In—Results when the front of the wheels are set closer than the rear. The wheels point in at the front.

Toe-Out—Results when the front of the wheels are farther apart than at the rear. The wheels point out at the front.

***Tolerance**—The allowable plus-or-minus variation from a specified value.

Tool and Equipment Storage Room—An area for safely keeping specialized tools and equipment.

Tool Box—Stores and protects your tools. Most are comprised of a large, bottom roll-around cabinet and an upper tool chest.

Tool Holders—Clip racks, pouches, or trays that help you organize small tools.

Torch—*See* Oxyacetylene Welding Outfit.

Torch Shrinking—Uses the heat of an oxyacetylene torch to release tension in the panel.

Torque—This measurement of twisting force is given in both inch-pounds and foot-pounds, or in metric measurements of Newton-meters.

Torque Boxes—The structural parts of the frame designed to allow some twisting to absorb road shock and collision impact.

Torque Converter—Fluid coupling used in place of a clutch in automatic transmissions.

Torque Pattern—A tightening sequence that ensures that parts are clamped down evenly by several bolts or nuts.

Torque Specifications—Tightening values for the specific bolt or nut.

Torque Wrench—A tool used to measure tightening or twisting force.

***Torsion Bar**—A steel rod that, when twisted, functions as a spring in a suspension system.

***Torsion Rod**—A type of rod that, when twisted, acts as a spring. Also called torsion spring.

Torsional Strength—The property of a material that withstands a twisting force.

Torx® Screwdrivers—These specialty drivers have uniquely shaped tips.

Total Loss—When the cost of repairs would exceed the cost of buying another vehicle.

Touch-Up Spray Guns—Very small guns, ideal for painting small repair areas.

Toxins—Poisonous substances found in many hazardous materials.

Tracking—Parallel alignment of the rear wheels, the vehicle centerline, and the front wheels.

Tram Gauge—A special body dimension measuring tool usually having a lightweight frame with pointers. The pointers can be aligned with body dimension reference points to determine the direction and amount of body misalignment damage.

Transaxle—A transmission and differential combined into a single housing or case. Both automatic and manual transaxles are available.

Transfer Efficiency—The percentage of paint a spray gun is capable of depositing on the surface.

Transmission—An assembly with a series of gears for increasing torque to the drive wheels so the car can accelerate properly.

Transverse Engine—An engine mounting configuration that locates the engine sideways in the engine compartment. The engine crankshaft centerline extends toward the right and left of the body. Both front-engine and rear-engine vehicles sometimes use this configuration.

Travel Speed—When welding, it is the speed you move the gun across the joint.

Tread Depth Gauge—An instrument that will quickly measure tire wear.

Trim Adhesive—Glue used to install various trim pieces (letters, molding, emblems) onto a body surface.

Trim Pad Tools—Tools designed to reach behind interior panels to pop out and remove clips.

Trim Screws—Screws that have washers attached to them. They improve the appearance and help keep the trim from shifting.

Troubleshooting Charts—Give logical steps for finding the source of problems. Mechanical, body, electrical, and other types of troubleshooting charts are provided in service manuals or computerized service information. Also called diagnostic charts.

Trunk Floor Panel—A stamped steel part that forms the bottom of the rear storage compartment.

Trunk Lid—*See* Deck Lid.

Tube Sealers—Seam sealers applied directly from the tube or by using a caulking gun.

Tubing Wrench—Also referred to as a flare nut or line wrench, it has a small split in its jaw to fit over lines and tubing.

Tunnel—Space formed in the floor pan for the transmission and drive shaft.

Turning Radius—Different amount each wheel moves during a turn.

Twist Damage—A condition where one corner of the vehicle is higher than normal; the opposite corner might be lower than normal.

Two-Part Adhesive Systems—An adhesive that consists of a base resin and a hardener (catalyst). When mixed together they form an acceptable alternative to welding for many plastic repairs.

Two-Part Putty—Spot putty that comes with its own hardener for rapid curing.

Two-Sided Plastic Weld—The strongest type of weld because you weld both sides of the part.

Two-Stage Paints—Consists of two distinct layers of paint: basecoat and clearcoat.

U

***U-Joint**—Universal joint. A device that couples rotary motion between shafts that meet at an angle.

***UHSS**—Ultra-high-strength steel. A type of steel that is stronger than high-strength steel and is able to withstand stresses of up to 110,000 psi.

Ultimate Strength—Measure of the load that breaks a specimen.

Ultrasonic Receiver Beam—Part of an ultrasound measuring system, mounts under the vehicle center section.

Ultrasound Measuring Systems—Employs many of the same principles as electronic laser systems, but uses sound waves, not light beams, to measure vehicle reference point locations.

Ultrasound Probes—Part of an ultrasound measuring system, mounted on vehicle reference points and generates high-frequency sound waves.

Undercoating—An anticorrosion material, often a thick tar or synthetic rubber-based material, sprayed onto the underbody of the vehicle to prevent rusting.

Undermasked—A term describing an area that must be cleaned with solvent or polishing compound to remove overspray.

Underwriters Laboratories (UL)—Nonprofit organization that operates laboratories to investigate materials, devices, products, equipment, and construction methods to define any hazards that may affect life and property.

Unibody—A type of construction where body parts are welded and bolted together to form an integral frame. Lighter, thinner, high-strength steel alloys or aluminum alloy are used.

Universal Joint—*See* U-Joint.

Universal Measuring Systems—Systems that have the ability to measure several reference points at the same time, making the job much easier and more accurate.

Upper Chest—Top chest of a toolbox; usually holds commonly used tools at eye level.

***Urethane Adhesive**—Any of several strong polymer adhesives that are used to install auto glass. Urethane adhesives are necessary to meet government standards for windshield retention in most late-model passenger vehicles.

Utility Knife—A hand tool with a retractable blade used for cutting or trimming.

UV Radiation Damage—Discoloration, cracking, checking, dulling, or yellowing resulting from excessive exposure of the paint film to the sun's radiation.

V

Vacuum Gauge—A device that reads vacuum, negative pressure or "suction." It reads in inches of mercury or kilograms per square centimeter.

Vacuum Suction Cup—A tool that uses a remote power source (separate vacuum pump or air compressor airflow) to produce negative pressure (vacuum) in the cup. It is used to pull out larger, deeper dents than a suction cup.

***Valance**—A decorative exterior panel used to fill a gap or hide other parts.

Value—Dimension of color that refers to the degree of lightness or darkness of the color.

Valves—Flow control devices that open to allow air-fuel mixture into and exhaust out of the combustion chamber.

Variance Chips—Several samples of color used to help match paint color variations.

Vehicle Classification—Relates to the terms used to characterize the construction, size, shape, number of doors, type of roof, and other criteria of a motor vehicle.

Vehicle Dimension Manual—A guide that gives body and frame measurements from undamaged vehicles.

Vehicle Doors—Structural units that allow entry into and exit from the passenger compartment.

***Vehicle Identification Number (VIN) Plate**—A permanently installed plate displaying the vehicle identification number, which is viewable through the windshield from outside the vehicle.

Vehicle Left Side—The steering wheel side on vehicles built for American roads.

Vehicle Measurement—Using specialized tools and equipment to measure the location of reference points on the vehicle so that these measurements can then be compared to published dimensions from an undamaged vehicle. By comparing known good and actual measurements, you can determine the extent of damage.

Vehicle Preparation—The final steps prior to painting, including cleaning, sanding, stripping, masking, priming, and other related tasks.

Vehicle Right Side—Passenger side or side opposite the steering wheel.

Ventilated—Has a good supply of fresh air flowing through it.

Vertical Welding—The pieces are turned upright. Gravity tends to pull the puddle down the joint.

Very Coarse Grit—A grit of 16 to 60, generally used for fast material removal. It will quickly remove paint and take it down to bare metal.

Very Fine Grit—Grit ranges from 220 to about 2000, used for numerous final smoothing operations. Larger grits of 220 to 320 are for sanding primer-surfacers and paint. Finer grits of 400 to 2000 are for colorcoat sanding and sanding before polishing or buffing. Very fine grits are usually wet sandpapers to keep the paper from becoming clogged or filled with paint.

Vinyl—A soft, flexible, thin plastic material often applied over a foam filler.

Vinyl Adhesive—An adhesive designed to bond a vinyl top to the vehicle body.

Vinyl Decals—A more complex and decorative pressure-sensitive material than tape stripes.

Vinyl Overlay Remover—A chemical that dissolves plastic vinyl to aid its removal.

Vinyl Prep—A chemical solution that opens the pores of the vinyl material, preparing it for color and/or clearcoating.

Vinyl Tape—A tough, durable, decorative striping material adhered to the vehicle's finish. It has a pressure-sensitive backing that bonds securely to the finish

***Viscosity**—The thickness of a liquid that affects its ability to flow.

Viscosity Cup—A device used to measure the thickness or fluidity of the mixed materials, usually paint. It is a small stainless steel cup attached to a handle.

Viscosity Cup Seconds—Number of seconds that paint should take to flow out of viscosity cup if thinned or reduced properly.

Vise—A device used to secure or hold parts during hammering, cutting, drilling, and pressing operations. It normally bolts onto a work bench.

Vise Caps—Soft lead, wood, or plastic vise jaw covers that will protect a part from marring.

Vise-Grip® Pliers—Also known as locking pliers, these have adjustable-width jaws that lock into position on parts.

Visual Weld Inspection—The most practical method of inspection on a repaired vehicle because the weld is not taken apart. It involves looking at the weld for flaws, proper size and proper shape.

VOC Tracking Systems—A computerized system that helps monitor and record materials used in order to abide by environmental regulations.

***Volatile Organic Compounds (VOCs)**—A solvent that, when released into the atmosphere, forms ozone.

Voltage—The pressure that pushes the electricity through the wire or circuit.

Voltage Regulator—Usually mounted in the alternator, controls alternator output.

Voltage Spikes—Voltage surges that can destroy many microcircuits in today's electronic systems.

VOM—*See* Multimeter.

W

***Warning Lamp**—Any of several dash-mounted lamps that alert the driver of a problem or dangerous condition, such as check engine, low fuel, door ajar, brakes, etc.

Washers—Used under bolts, nuts, and other parts to prevent damage to the surfaces of parts and provide better holding power.

Washup—A thorough cleaning of the vehicle before repairs begin.

Water-Base/Waterborne Paints—Paints that use water to carry the pigment.

Water Hose Test—A method used to find body leaks. Water is sprayed onto the possible leakage areas while someone watches for leaks inside the vehicle.

Water Leaks—Result from poor seal around the windshield, window glass, sunroof, doors, or lids.

Water Pump—It circulates coolant through the inside of the engine, hoses, and radiator.

Water Spotting—Dulling of gloss on areas of the finish. It can occur as a mass of spots that appear as a large distortion of the film. It is due to spots of water drying on a finish that is not thoroughly dry.

***Wax and Grease Remover**—A cleaner used to remove contaminants from a repair area before starting a repair, and again before applying primers or paint.

Weatherstrip Adhesive—An adhesive designed to hold rubber seals and similar parts in place.

Weatherstripping—A rubber seal that prevents leakage at the joint between a movable part (lid, hatch, door) and the body.

Weld—Formed when separate pieces of material are fused together using heat.

***Weld-Bond Adhesive**—An adhesive used between the weld surfaces of a joint to seal and strengthen the joint.

Weld Bonding—Uses adhesive and resistance spot welds to join steel or aluminum body panels together during vehicle manufacture.

Weld Distortion—Uneven weld bead.

Weld Face—The exposed surface of the weld on the side where you welded.

Weld Legs—The width and height of the weld bead.

Weld Overlap—Excess weld metal mounted on top and either side of weld bead.

Weld Penetration—Indicated by the height of the exposed surface of the weld on the back side. It is needed to assure maximum weld strength.

Weld Porosity—Holes in the weld.

Weld Root—Part of the joint where the wire electrode is directed.

Weld Spatter—Drops of electrode on and around weld bead.

Weld Throat—This refers to the depth of the triangular cross section of the weld.

***Weld-Through Primer**—A rust-resistant primer applied before welding to mating surfaces that are uncoated, or where a zinc coating has been removed.

Weld Undercut—A groove melted along either side of the weld and left unfilled.

Welded Door Skin—Spot welds hold the skin onto its frame.

Welded Parts—Metal or plastic parts that are permanently joined by melting the material so that it flows together and bonds when cooled.

Welded Pull-Tab—A small piece of steel plate welded onto the unibody. It is used if you need to pull where there is no place to attach a clamp.

Welder Amperage Rating—It gives the maximum current flow through the weld joint. The thickness of the metal being welded determines the amperage needed.

Welding Filter Lens—Sometimes called filter plate, it is a shaded glass welding helmet insert for protecting your eyes from ultraviolet burns.

Welding Torch—One of two types of welding torches, has two valves for adjusting gas flow.

Weldroot—The part of the joint where the wire electrode is directed.

Wet Application—Spray gun is used to apply thicker coat of primer, sealer, or paint so that film is smooth and glossy.

Wet Edge—The area just painted that is still wet when starting to paint a new adjoining area.

Wet Metallic Paint Spray—The aluminum flakes have sufficient time to settle in the wet paint, making the color appear darker and less silver.

Wet Sanding—Involves using a water-resistant, ultrafine sandpaper and water to level and smooth the paint.

Wet Sandpaper—Sandpaper that can be used with water for flushing away sanding debris that would otherwise clog fine grits.

Wet Spots—A finish problem seen as off-colored and/or slow drying spots of various sizes, usually due to improper cleaning, heavy primecoats not properly dried, or contamination with gasoline or other incompatible solvents.

Wheel Alignment—Involves positioning the vehicle's tires so that they roll properly over the road surface.

Wheel Alignment Machine—A machine used to measure wheel alignment angles so they can be adjusted.

Wheel Clamps—Wheel clamps are used to load and hold suspension with wheels and tires removed with vehicle on the rack or bench.

Wheel Cylinders—Use hydraulic pressure to push the brake pads or shoes outward.
Wheel Pullers—Devices used to remove steering wheels, engine pulleys, and similar pressed-on parts.
Wheel Run-Out Check—A test that will show if there is damage to a rotating part of a wheel assembly.
Wheelbase—Measurement between the center of the front and rear wheel hubs.
White Light—A mixture of various colors of light.
Windings—Wires wrapped around an iron core that make up an electromagnet.
Window Antenna Wire—A wire for radio reception, placed either between the layers of laminated glass (windshield) or printed on the surface of the glass (rear window).
Window Regulator—A gear mechanism that allows you to raise and lower the door glass.
Windshield Gasket—A rubber molding shaped to fit the windshield, body, and trim.
Windshield Knife—A hand tool designed to cut through the sealant used on some windshields. It has a sharp cutter blade and two handles.
Wing Nuts—Nuts that have two extended arms for turning the nut by hand. They are used when a part must be removed frequently for service or maintenance.
Wire Color Coding—The wire insulation is colored for easy identification.
Wire Feeler Gauges—Round feeler gauges used for measuring distances between nonparallel or curved surfaces.
Wire Speed—In welding, it is how fast the rollers feed the wire into the weld puddle.
Wire Stick-Out—The distance between the end of the gun's contact tip and the metal being welded.
Wiring Diagram—A drawing of an electrical circuit used to determine and isolate problems.
Wiring Harness—Several wires are enclosed in a protective covering.
Woodruff Keys—Keys used to prevent hand wheels, gears, cams, and pulleys from turning on their shaft.
Work Hardening—The limit of plastic deformation that causes the metal to become hard where it has been bent.
Work Life—Time when it is still possible to disturb the adhesive and still have the adhesive set up for a good bond. Also called open time.
Work Order—Outlines the procedures that should be taken to put the vehicle back in top condition.
Work Traits—Those things, aside from skills, that make you a good or bad employee, such as reliability and professionalism.
Worm Hose Clamp—A clamp that uses a screw that engages a slotted band. Turning the screw reduces or enlarges clamp diameter.
Wrench Size—The distance across the wrench jaws.
Wrenches—Tools used to loosen or tighten nuts and bolts.
Wrinkling—Severe puckering of the film that appears like the skin of a prune (fruit), caused by under reduction, insufficient air pressure causing excessive film thickness, excessive coats, overloading caused by fast reducers, solvents trapped by surface drying, or fresh film being exposed to heat too soon.

X

X-Frame—A frame that has two long members crossing over in the middle of the frame rails. Also called a backbone frame.

Y

Yardstick—Long rule or scale (3 feet in length) used for some larger linear measurements.
Yield Point—The amount of force that a piece of metal can resist without tearing or breaking.
Yield Stress—The amount of strain needed to permanently deform a test specimen of sheet metal.

Z

Zahn Cup—Least expensive type of paint viscosity measuring tool; it is a small cylinder with a hole or orifice in the bottom. The amount of time needed for the liquid to pour out of the hole can be used to determine the thickness or fluidity of the liquid material.
***Zinc Coating**—A coating of zinc applied to metal during manufacture to improve rust resistance. Also called galvanizing.
Zone Concept—It divides the horizontal surfaces of the vehicle into zones defined by character lines and moldings. It requires refinishing of an entire zone or zones with basecoat, mica intermediate coats, and clearcoats.

APPENDIX A

ABBREVIATIONS USED BY COLLISION REPAIR TECHNICIANS AND ESTIMATORS

The estimator and collision repair technician must be able to communicate verbally as well as in writing. Both in estimates and work procedure reports, most estimators use abbreviations. Generally, these abbreviations are the same as those used in crash estimating guides. Some abbreviations are even used verbally. For example, three of the most commonly used abbreviations in a body shop are:

- **R&I: Remove and Reinstall**—The item is removed as an assembly, set aside, and later reinstalled and aligned for a proper fit. This is generally done to gain access to another part. For example, "R&I bumper" would mean that the bumper assembly would have to be removed to install a new fender or quarter panel.
- **R&R: Remove and Replace**—Remove the old parts, transfer necessary items to new part, replace, and align.
- **O/H: Overhaul**—Remove an assembly from the vehicle, disassemble, clean, inspect, replace parts as needed, then reassemble, install, and adjust (except wheel and suspension alignment).

In addition to these abbreviations, the following terms are those accepted by most estimating guides, shop manuals, and estimators. They are the ones used in most written forms.

A	Manufacturer has no list price for the part.
ABS	antilock brake system
A/C	air conditioner
ACRS	air cushion restraint system
adj	adjuster or adjustable
A/F	air-fuel ratio
AIR	air injector reactor
alt	alternator
alum	aluminum
amp	ampere
approx.	approximately
assy	assembly
A/T	automatic transaxle
AT	automatic transmission
auth	authority
auto	automatic
aux	auxiliary
B+	battery voltage
bat.	battery
bbl	barrel
bk	back
blwr	blower
bmpr	bumper
brg	bearing
brk	brake
brkt	bracket
Bro	Brougham
btry	battery

btwn	between
B-U	back-up
bush	bushing
Calif	California
chnl	channel
c/mbr	crossmember
cntr	center
col	column
comp	compressor
compt	compartment
conn.	connector
cond	conditioning or conditioner
cont	control
conv	converter or convertible
cor	corner
cov	cover
Cpe	coupe
C/R	customer requested
crossmbr	crossmember
c/shaft	crankshaft
ctl	control
Ctry	country
Cust	custom
CV	constant velocity
cyl	cylinder
D	discontinued part
d	drilling operational time
da	dash
dbl	double
def	deflector
dehyd	dehydrator
desc	description
dia	diameter
diag	diagonal
dist	distributor
div	division
Dixe	deluxe
DP	dash pot
dr	door
ea	each
ECU	electronic control unit
EFI	electronic fuel injection
EGR	exhaust gas recirculation
elec	electric
emiss	emission
eng	engine
EP	exhaust purging
equip	equipment
evap	evaporator
exc	except
exh	exhaust
extn	extension
FED	federal (All States Except Calif.)
flr	floor
Fndr	fender
Fr & Rr	front and rear
frm	from
fr or rr	front or rear
ft	foot
ft-lb	foot-pounds
FWD	front wheel drive
gal	gallon
gen	generator
GND	ground
grds	guards
grv	groove
harn	harness
H'back	hatchback
hd	heavy duty
HDC	heavy duty cooling
hdr	header
HEI	high energy ignition
Hi Per	high performance
horiz	horizontal
H.P.	high performance
hp	horsepower
hsg	housing
HSLA	high strength alloy steel
HSS	high strength steel
HT	hard top
H'Top	hard top
hyd	hydraulic
Hydra	hydramatic
ID	inside diameter
ign	ignition

in	inch
incl	includes
INJ	Injection
in.-lb	inch-pounds
inr	inner
inst	instrument
inter	intermediate
IP	instrument control panels
L	left
LED	light-emitting diode
LF	left front
LH	lefthand
lic	license
lp	lamp
LR	left rear
LS	left side
lwr	lower
max	maximum
mdl	model
mldg	molding
MT	manual transmission
mtd	mounted
mtg	mounting
muff	muffler
NAGS	National Auto Glass Specification
neg	negative
OD	outside diameter
OD, O/D	overdrive
OEM	original equipment manufacturer
opng	opening
orna	ornament
O/S	oversize
otr	outer
p	paint operational time
pass	passenger
PCV	positive crankcase ventilation
pkg	package
plr	pillar
pnl	panel
pos	positive
PS	power steering
psi	pounds per square inch
pt	pint
Pwr	power
qtr	quarter
R	right
rad	radiator
R-L	right or left
rec	receiver
refl	reflector
reg	regulator
reinf	reinforcement
reson	resonator
RH	right-hand
Sed	sedan
ser	serial or series
shid	shield
sidembr	side member
sig	single
SIR	supplemental inflatable restraint
spd	speed
spec	special
SRS	supplemental restraint system
Sta	station
stab	stabilizer
stat	stationary
Std	Standard
stl	steel
strg	steering
Sub	suburban
sup	super
supt	support
surr	surround
susp	suspension
SW	station wagon
tach	tachometer
t & t	tilt and telescope or tilt and travel
TE	thermactor emission
tel	telescope
trans	transmission
TWC	three-way catalyst
U/D	underdrive
upr	upper
U/S	undersize

vent ventilator
vert vertical
vib vibration
VIR valve-in-receiver

w/ with
w/b wheel base
WB wheelbase
WD wheel drive
Wgn wagon
w'house wheelhouse
whl wheel
whise wheelhouse
wndo window
w/o without
wo/ without
wshd windshield
w'strip weatherstrip

APPENDIX B

MEASUREMENT EQUIVALENTS

Conversion Factors		
Multiply	**By**	**To obtain**
Length		
Millimeters (mm)	0.03937	Inches
	0.1	Centimeters (cm)
Kilometers (km)	0.6214	Miles
	3281	Feet
Inches	25.4	Millimeters (mm)
Miles	1.6093	Kilometers (km)
Area		
Inches^2	645.16	Millimeters^2 (mm^2)
	6.452	Centimeters^2 (mm^2)
Feet^2	0.0929	Meters^2 (m^2)
	144	Inches^2
Volume		
Centimeters^3 (cc)	0.06102	Inches^3
	0.001	Liters (L)
Liters (L)	61.024	Inches^3
	0.2642	Gallons
	1.0567	Quarts
Inches^3	16.387	Centimeters^3 (cc)
Feet^3	1728	Inches^3
	7.48	Gallons
	28.32	Liters (L)
Fluid ounces (oz)	29.57	Milliliters (mL)
Mass		
Gram (g)	0.03527	Ounce
Kilograms (kg)	2.2046	Pounds
	35.274	Ounces

(*Continued*)

Conversion Factors

Multiply	By	To obtain
Length		
Force		
Ounce	0.278	Newton (N)
Pound	4.448	Newton (N)
Kilogram	9.807	Newton (N)
Torque		
Foot-pounds	1.3558	Newton-meters (Nm)
	0.1383	Kilogram/meter (kg/m)
Inch-pounds	0.11298	Newton-meters (Nm)
	0.0833	Foot-pounds
Kilogram-meters (Kg/m)	7.23	Foot-pounds
	9.80665	Newton-meters (Nm)
Pressure		
Atmospheres	14.7	Pounds/square inch (psi)
	29.92	Inches of mercury (In. Hg)
Inches of mercury (In. Hg)	0.49116	Pounds/square inch (psi)
	13.1	Inches of water
	3.377	Kilopascals (kPa)
Bars	100	Kilopascals (kPa)
	14.5	Pounds/square inch (psi)
Kilogram/cu^2 (Kg/cm^2)	14.22	Pounds/square inch (psi)
	98.07	Kilopascals (kPa)
Kilopascals (kPa)	0.145	Pounds/square inch (psi)
	0.2961	Inches of mercury (In. Hg)
Pascal	1	Newton/square meter (N/m^2)
Fuel Performance		
Miles/gallon	0.4251	Kilometers/liter (km/L)
Velocity		
Miles/hours	1.467	Feet/second
	88	Feet/minute
	1.6093	Kilometers/hour (km/h)
Kilometers/hour	0.27778	Meters/second (m/s)

Torque Conversions (Foot-Pounds, Newton-Meters, Meter-Kilograms)

ft/lb	0	1	2	3	4	5	6	7	8	9
0	0	1.35	2.70	4.05	5.40	6.75	8.10	9.45	10.8	12.1
10	13.5	14.9	16.2	17.6	18.9	20.3	21.6	22.9	24.3	25.6
20	27.0	28.3	29.7	31.0	32.5	33.7	35.1	36.4	37.8	39.1
30	40.5	41.8	43.2	44.5	45.9	47.2	48.6	49.9	51.3	52.6
40	54.0	55.3	56.7	58.0	59.4	60.7	62.1	63.4	64.8	66.1
50	67.5	68.8	70.2	71.5	72.9	74.2	75.6	76.9	78.3	79.6
60	81.0	82.3	83.7	85.0	86.4	87.7	89.1	90.4	91.8	93.1
70	94.5	95.8	97.2	98.5	99.9	101	102	103	105	106
80	108	109	110	112	113	114	116	117	118	120
90	121	122	124	125	126	128	129	130	132	133
100	135	136	137	139	140	141	143	144	145	147
110	148	149	151	152	153	155	156	157	159	160
120	162	163	164	166	167	168	170	171	172	174
130	175	176	178	179	180	182	183	184	186	187

Note: The following formulas can be used:

ft-lb × 1.35 = Nm

ft-lb + 7.23 = mkg

For meter-kilograms within 5%, divide Newton-meters by 10 (move the decimal point one place left).

For greater accuracy, divide by 9.81.

APPENDIX C

TAP AND DRILL BIT DATA

Decimal Equivalents and Tap Drill Sizes			Decimal Equivalents and Tap Drill Sizes		
Drill Size	Decimal	Tap Size	Drill Size	Decimal	Tap Size
1/64	.0156		39	.0995	
1/32	.0312		38	.1015	5–40
60	.0400		37	.1040	5–44
59	.0410		36	.1065	6–32
58	.0420		7/64	.1093	
57	.0430		35	.1100	
56	.0465		34	.1110	6–36
3/64	.0469	0–80	33	.1130	6–40
55	.0520		32	.1160	
54	.0550	1–56	31	.1200	
53	.0595	1–64, 72	1/8	.1250	
1/16	.0625		30	.1285	
52	.0635		29	.1360	8–32, 36
51	.0670		28	.1405	8–40
50	.0700	2–56, 64	9/64	.1406	
49	.0730		27	.1440	
48	.0760		26	.1470	
5/64	.0781		25	.1495	10–24
47	.0785	3–48	24	.1520	
46	.0810		23	.1540	
45	.0820	3–56, 4–32	5/32	.1562	
44	.0860	4–36	22	.1570	10–30
43	.0890	4–40	21	.1590	10–32
42	.0935	4–48	20	.1610	
3/32	.0937		19	.1660	
41	.0960		18	.1695	
40	.0980				

(*Continued*)

Decimal Equivalents and Tap Drill Sizes			Decimal Equivalents and Tap Drill Sizes		
Drill Size	Decimal	Tap Size	Drill Size	Decimal	Tap Size
11/64	.1719		O	.3160	
17	.1730		P	.3230	
16	.1770	12–24	21/64	.3281	
15	.1800		Q	.3320	3/8–24
14	.1820	12–28	R	.3390	
13	.1850	12–32	11/32	.3437	
3/16	.1875		S	.3480	
12	.1890		T	.3580	
11	.1910		23/64	.3594	
10	.1935		U	.3680	7/16–14
9	.1960		3/8	.3750	
8	.1990		V	.3770	
7	.2010	1/4–20	W	.3860	
13/64	.2031		25/64	.3906	7/16–20
6	.2040		X	.3970	
5	.2055		Y	.4040	
4	.2090		13/32	.4062	
3	.2130	1/4–28	Z	.4130	
7/32	.2187		27/64	.4219	1/2–13
2	.2210		7/16	.4375	
1	.2280		29/64	.4531	1/2–20
A	.2340		15/32	.4687	
15/64	.2344		31/64	.4844	9/16–12
B	.2380		1/2	.5000	
C	.2420		33/64	.5156	9/16–18
D	.2460		17/32	.5312	5/8–11
E, 1/4	.2500		35/64	.5469	
F	.2570	5/16–18	9/16	.5625	
G	.2610		37/64	.5781	5/8–18
17/64	.2656		19/32	.5937	11/16–11
H	.2660		39/64	.6094	
I	.2720	5/16–24	5/8	.6250	11/16–16
J	.2770		41/64	.6406	
K	.2810		21/32	.6562	3/4–10
9/32	.2812		43/64	.6719	
L	.2900		11/16	.6875	3/4–16
M	.2950		45/64	.7031	
19/64	.2968		23/32	.7187	
N	.3020		47/64	.7344	
5/16	.3125	3/8–16			

(*Continued*)

Decimal Equivalents and Tap Drill Sizes			Decimal Equivalents and Tap Drill Sizes		
Drill Size	Decimal	Tap Size	Drill Size	Decimal	Tap Size
3/4	.7500		57/64	.8906	
49/64	.7656	7/8–9	29/32	.9062	
25/32	.7812		59/64	.9219	
51/64	.7969		15/16	.9375	1–12, 14
13/16	.8125	7/8–14	61–64	.9531	
53–64	.8281		31/32	.9687	
27/32	.8437		63/64	.9844	
55/54	.8594		1	1.000	
7/8	.8750	1–8			

Decimal Equivalents of Number Size Drills							
No.	Size of Drill (Inches)	No.	Size of Drill (Inches)	No.	Size of Drill (Inches)	No.	Size of Drill (Inches)
1	.2280	21	.1590	41	.0960	61	.0390
2	.2210	22	.1570	42	.0935	62	.0380
3	.2130	23	.1540	43	.0890	63	.0370
4	.2090	24	.1520	44	.0860	64	.0360
5	.2055	25	.1495	45	.0820	65	.0350
6	.2040	26	.1470	46	.0810	66	.0330
7	.2010	27	.1440	47	.0785	67	.0320
8	.1990	28	.1405	48	.0760	68	.0310
9	.1960	29	.1360	49	.0730	69	.0292
10	.1935	30	.1285	50	.0700	70	.0280
11	.1910	31	.1200	51	.0670	71	.0260
12	.1890	32	.1160	52	.0635	72	.0250
13	.1850	33	.1130	53	.0595	73	.0240
14	.1820	34	.1110	54	.0550	74	.0225
15	.1800	35	.1100	55	.0520	75	.0210
16	.1770	36	.1065	56	.0465	76	.0200
17	.1730	37	.1040	57	.0430	77	.0180
18	.1695	38	.1015	58	.0420	78	.0160
19	.1660	39	.0995	59	.0410	79	.0145
20	.1610	40	.0980	60	.0400	80	.0135

APPENDIX D

REFERENCE TABLES

Dry Torque Recommendations

Diameter	Grade 5 Coarse	Grade 5 Fine	Grade 6 Coarse	Grade 6 Fine	Grade 8 Coarse	Grade 8 Fine
1/4	108[a]	120[a]	132[a]	156[a]	17	19
5/16	17	20	23	25	34	37
3/8	31	35	40	45	60	68
7/16	50	55	64	72	96	108
1/2	75	85	98	110	145	165
9/16	110	120	140	160	210	235
5/8	150	170	195	220	290	330

[a]Any torque less than 15 lb is given in in.-lb

Lubricated Torque Recommendations (Reduced 33 Percent)

Diameter	Grade 5 Coarse	Grade 5 Fine	Grade 6 Coarse	Grade 6 Fine	Grade 8 Coarse	Grade 8 Fine
1/4	72[a]	80[a]	88[a]	104[a]	136[a]	152[a]
5/16	135[a]	160[a]	15	17	22	25
3/8	21	23	26	30	40	45
7/16	33	37	43	48	64	72
1/2	50	57	65	73	96	110
9/16	73	80	93	107	140	157
5/8	100	113	130	147	193	220

[a]Any torque less than 15 lb is given in in.-lb

Metric Dry Torque Recommendations

Diameter (mm)	Pitch	Grade 8.8	Grade 12.9
6	1.00	84[a]	132[a]
7	1.00	132[a]	20
8	1.25	18	29
8	1.00	20	32
10	1.50	33	58
10	1.25	35	61
10	1.00	38	64
12	1.75	59	100
12	1.50	65	110

[a]Any torque less than 15 ft lb is given in in.-lb

Metric Lubricated Torque Recommendations (Reduced 33 percent)

Diameter (mm)	Pitch	Grade 8.8	Grade 12.9
6	1.00	56[a]	88[a]
7	1.00	88[a]	160[a]
8	1.25	144[a]	19
8	1.00	160[a]	21
10	1.50	22	39
10	1.25	23	41
10	1.00	25	43
12	1.75	39	67
12	1.50	43	73

[a]Any torque less than 15 ft lb is given in in.-lb

INDEX

A

D

E

F

G

J

K

L

M

T

U

V

W

Y

Z